Sport Nutrition

Third Edition

Asker Jeukendrup, MSc, PhD
Loughborough University, Mysportscience

Michael Gleeson, BSc, PhD
Loughborough University

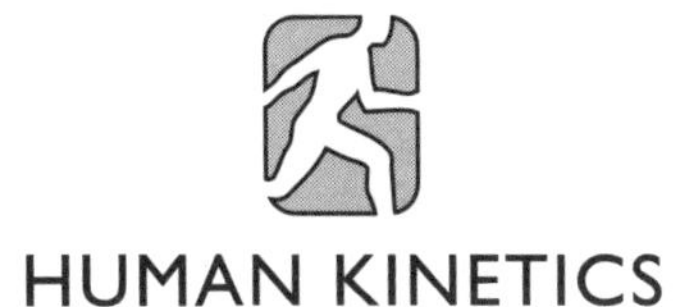

HUMAN KINETICS

Library of Congress Cataloging-in-Publication Data

Names: Jeukendrup, Asker E., 1969- author. | Gleeson, Michael, 1956- author.
Title: Sport nutrition / Asker Jeukendrup, Michael Gleeson.
Description: Third edition. | Champaign, IL : Human Kinetics, [2019] |
Includes bibliographical references and index.
Identifiers: LCCN 2017049720 (print) | LCCN 2017050304 (ebook) | ISBN
9781492567288 (e-book) | ISBN 9781492529033 (print)
Subjects: | MESH: Sports Nutritional Physiological Phenomena | Athletes |
Food | Exercise--physiology | Physical Fitness--physiology
Classification: LCC TX361.A8 (ebook) | LCC TX361.A8 (print) | NLM QT 263 |
DDC 613.2/024796--dc23
LC record available at https://lccn.loc.gov/2017049720

ISBN: 978-1-4925-2903-3 (print)

The web addresses cited in this text were current as of June 2018, unless otherwise noted.

Senior Acquisitions Editor: Amy N. Tocco
Developmental Editors: Kevin Matz and Carly S. O'Connor
Managing Editor: Carly S. O'Connor and Kirsten E. Keller
Proofreader: Rodelinde Albrecht
Indexer: Nancy Ball
Permissions Manager: Dalene Reeder
Graphic Designer: Julie L. Denzer
Cover Designer: Keri Evans
Cover Design Associate: Susan Rothermel Allen
Photograph (cover): vm/E+/Getty Images
Photo Production Manager: Jason Allen
Senior Art Manager: Kelly Hendren
Illustrations: © Human Kinetics, unless otherwise noted
Printer: Walsworth

Printed in the United States of America 10 9 8 7 6 5 4 3

The paper in this book was manufactured using responsible forestry methods.

Human Kinetics
1607 N. Market Street
Champaign, IL 61820
USA

United States and International
Website: **US.HumanKinetics.com**
Email: info@hkusa.com
Phone: 1-800-747-4457

Canada
Website: **Canada.HumanKinetics.com**
Email: info@hkcanada.com

E6770

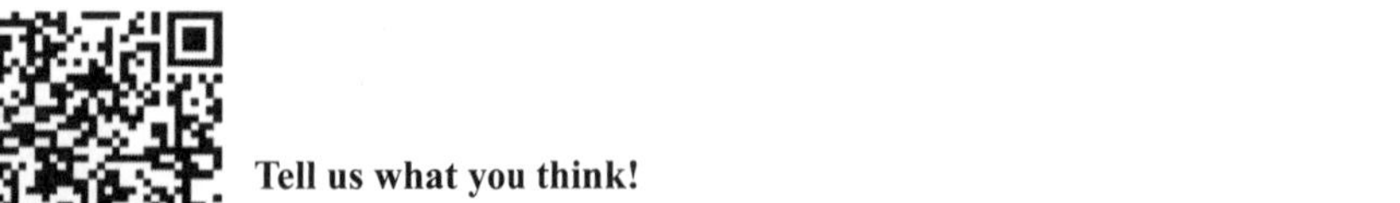

I would like to dedicate this book to my two wonderful daughters, Natasha and Sienna.
And to Zita, my fiancée, who must be one of the most patient people in the world.
And to my parents, Jos and Loes, who encouraged me and supported me.
And to Bengt Saltin, who inspired me as a mentor and was one of the pioneers
in our field. Bengt passed away on September 12, 2014 but will never be forgotten.

—AJ

For Laura, my wife, sweetheart, and soulmate.

—MG

Contents

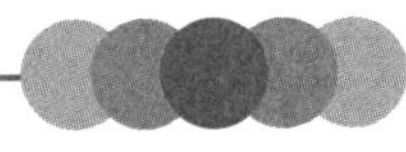

Preface

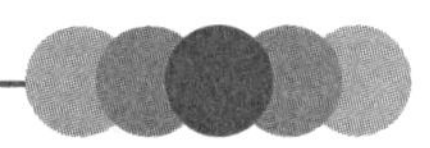

Nutrition plays an essential role in exercise and sport because it is important for health, adaptations to physical activity and exercise, weight maintenance, and exercise performance. Nutrition influences nearly every process in the body involved in energy production and recovery from exercise. To apply the principles of sport nutrition, you should have a basic understanding of nutrition and knowledge of the biochemical and physiological processes that occur in cells and tissues and the way those processes are integrated throughout the body.

We wrote this book primarily for students of sports science, exercise physiology, and other sport-related or exercise-related degree programs. Many degree courses in sports-related subjects now include some coverage of nutrition, and the aim of this book is to introduce students, as well as athletes and coaches, to the underlying principles of sport nutrition and to show how these relate to sports performance. Because this background information is often missing from current texts, it can be difficult to understand the reasoning behind specific nutritional guidelines. The wide range of sport nutrition products on the market—and manufacturers' claims about them (which are often based on selective evidence or pseudoscience)—can be confusing. In contrast, with a few notable exceptions, little confusion exists among scientists in most areas of sport nutrition, which emphasizes the importance of providing accurate and adequate information. Therefore, this book provides the scientific underpinnings of sport nutrition guidelines and advice at a level that is appropriate for students. We attempt to provide a scientific basis for sport nutrition that covers the principles, background, and rationale for current nutrition guidelines for athletes.

Readers of this book do not need a deep understanding of biochemistry, biology, chemistry, or physiology, but they should be familiar with some of the main concepts, because the physical, chemical, and biochemical properties of cells and tissues determine the physiological responses to exercise and the effects that nutrition has on these responses. This book aims to develop the knowledge of these disciplines from a basic level to a relatively advanced level. Readers who are unfamiliar with or are a bit rusty on fundamental concepts are advised to study appendix A before reading the chapters. Appendix A contains a brief explanation of the basic physical, chemical, and biological processes and the structures of molecules, membranes, cells, and organelles they contain. Any confusion about terms used in this book can be overcome by referring to the extensive glossary, which defines many of the terms and common abbreviations related to nutrition, physiology, and metabolism.

After reading this book, you should have a comprehensive understanding of the basics of nutrition as it relates to sport. You should also have an excellent grasp of how nutrition can influence exercise performance, training, and recovery from exercise. As a result, you should be able to explain the basis for sport nutrition advice given to athletes or coaches. The book should also encourage you to be critical toward information that is published in magazines, on the Internet, or even in scientific publications. Rather than accepting claims that are made, you should think about underlying mechanisms and the strength of the evidence that supports the claims. Every sport has specific nutritional requirements, and these requirements may be influenced by environmental factors and differences among individuals (e.g., gender, body mass). For example, after reading this book, you will understand why endurance athletes benefit from carbohydrate feedings during competition but weightlifters do not; be able to explain why creatine supplements benefit game players and athletes in strength sports but have no effect on performance in endurance sports; and be able to appreciate why fluid intake can influence performance in prolonged exercise but is unlikely to affect performance in events that last fewer than 30 minutes.

How This Book Is Organized

In each chapter, we have tried to explain the specific role of nutrition in enhancing exercise performance and to provide the reader with up-to-date findings from the most current research. Topics discussed in this book include the following:

- General principles of nutrition and nutrient requirements
- Guidelines for a healthy diet
- Fuel sources for muscle and exercise metabolism

- Energy requirements of different sports
- Digestion and absorption of food
- Macronutrients: carbohydrate, fat, and protein
- Water requirements and fluid balance
- Micronutrients: vitamins and minerals
- Nutrition supplements
- Effects of nutrition on training adaptations
- Nutrition and immune function in athletes
- Body composition
- Weight management
- Eating disorders in athletes
- Personalized nutrition

In chapter 1, we explain some of the important principles of nutrition and describe appropriate dietary intake guidelines such as the dietary reference value (DRV) and the recommended dietary allowance (RDA). Chapter 2, which is new to this edition, addresses guidelines for a healthy diet and the potential health problems associated with consuming too much or too little of certain nutrients, foods, or beverages. We cover the biochemistry of exercise in chapter 3, and we discuss the metabolic pathways that provide muscles with energy to perform physical work. Chapter 4 considers how the energy content of foods and the energy needs of athletes in different sports can be estimated. Chapter 5 explains how food is digested and absorbed in the gastrointestinal tract and how exercise can influence these processes. In chapters 6 through 9, the roles of each of the major macronutrients—carbohydrate, fat, and protein—and the importance of adequate fluid intake in relation to exercise performance are discussed. Chapter 10 explains the role of micronutrients (vitamins and minerals) and contains new information about the role of vitamin D, including an explanation of why many people can become deficient in this vitamin. Chapter 11 provides guidance on distinguishing fact from fallacy with regard to nutrition supplements and discusses the claims and the scientific evidence that support or refute the claims of specific supplements. The remaining chapters delve into other nutrition-related issues that are important for athletes: the influence of nutrition on adaptation to training (chapter 12), the effects of nutrition and exercise on immune function (chapter 13), methods available to assess body composition (chapter 14), suitable ways for athletes to lose or gain weight (chapter 15), and the risks, consequences, and characteristics of eating disorders (chapter 16). Finally, a new chapter to this edition (chapter 17), discusses the recently introduced topic of personalized nutrition. This is also the most practical of all the chapters. In it we discuss some of the practical issues a practitioner faces, and in a few examples we bring advice with regards to fluid, carbohydrates, protein, and other nutrients together in a number of sports.

Special Chapter Elements

Each chapter begins with objectives that explain what students should learn from the chapter. These can be used to preview the chapter and check your comprehension after reading the material. Key terms are bolded in the text and definitions for each, together with some other terms that may be unfamiliar to readers, are provided in the glossary. The figures and tables used in each chapter promote in-depth understanding of concepts and ideas, and the sidebars provide more detailed coverage of selected topics. At the end of each chapter, there is a list of key points that reemphasizes the most important facts discussed. Appendix B provides useful explanations of units of measurement and tables you can use to convert units. Appendixes C, D, and E provide at-a-glance information on recommended daily allowances, reference nutrient intakes, and recommended dietary intakes for North America, the United Kingdom, and Australia and New Zealand, respectively.

New to This Edition

The third edition contains a complete update of the nutrition guidelines, which have changed considerably since the last edition. We have also included a new chapter on healthy eating. Some areas have developed significantly in the last few years; for example, developments in the field of carbohydrate metabolism have altered the recommendations given to athletes. The role of protein has been studied more extensively, and our understanding has improved significantly; therefore, guidelines can now be given on the type, amount, and timing of protein intake to maximize training adaptation. An important new area of study examines adaptations to training and how they can be altered by nutrition. Major advances in this area have occurred, mostly because of developments within molecular biology. To understand the role of nutrition on adaptations to exercise training, it is essential to understand the underlying molecular changes. For example, how is it possible that resistance exercise results in more muscle, but endurance training does not change muscle mass but may improve the quality of the muscle (e.g., its capacity to oxidize fat)? Molecular processes underlie these distinctly different adaptations to exercise. We have incorporated more basic knowledge of the regulation of protein synthesis and gene expression in appendix A. We discuss the molecular and cellular changes to exercise training in chapter 12. Another rapidly developing field is immunonutrition, and chapter 13, which is devoted to that topic, has been updated and expanded and covers information that is based on the latest expert consensus reviews.

In this edition, all chapters have been updated with information that has become available since the previous edition was published. The following are among the topics addressed by new additions to the text:

- Updated dietary guidelines for healthy eating
- Nutrients and supplements and their influence on exercise metabolism and, consequently, sport performance
- The role of the gut microbiota
- Carbohydrate mouth rinses
- Low-carbohydrate diets, ketogenic diets, and intermittent fasting diets for weight loss
- Recommendations on the type, amount, and timing of protein intake to maximize adaptation
- The role of leucine in stimulating protein synthesis
- New thoughts on fluid requirements for exercise
- The latest ergogenic supplements, including nitrates, ß-alanine, and polyphenols, and combinations of ergogenic supplements
- The latest on antioxidants and training adaptation, nutrition and sleep, and nutrition and recovery from injury
- Nutritional strategies to reduce infection risk (e.g., vitamin D, probiotics, colostrum, polyphenols)

Perhaps most important, chapter 17 is entirely new and is devoted to personalized nutrition. This chapter covers nutrigenomics, periodized nutrition, sex differences, nutrition requirements for young and older athletes, nutrition challenges for athletes with type 1 diabetes, and nutrition recommendations for specific sports and situations. This chapter should help you apply the theoretical knowledge from the previous chapters in a practical way.

Notes for Instructors

The accompanying ancillaries should make it easy to teach a quality sport nutrition course when adopting this book. Each chapter of the instructor guide includes a recommended class format, chapter objectives, a detailed outline of each chapter (which could form the structure of a lecture), and sample student assignments. In addition, suggestions for practical lab classes are offered for some of the chapters. The presentation package contains over 700 PowerPoint slides that can be used to put together one or more lectures for each chapter; they include the most important text, figures, and tables from each chapter. The image bank includes most of the figures and tables from the text, and instructors can use these images to create handouts, illustrate a PowerPoint presentation, or create other learning aids for their students. Finally, the test package contains over 670 multiple-choice, fill-in-the-blank, short answer, and true–false questions (with answers) that can be used for exams.

All chapters have been updated, and students will learn about the basics and about rapidly developing areas in which cutting-edge research is performed. With the extensive updates and provided ancillaries, course instructors should be able to put together an informative and successful course from which students will gain knowledge and enjoyment. In the many years we have been teaching this subject (with similar materials), we have learned that this course is one that students most enjoy and appreciate.

Our approach in writing this book comes from years of experience in teaching sport nutrition at the university level. Thus, we are conscious of the needs of course instructors. Above all, we wanted to create a book that is a useful resource to students and instructors alike. Therefore, the chapters of the book are constructed based on the way we would deliver a lecture on the topic. The figures, tables, and photos that we present in the book are similar to the ones we use in our own lectures and tutorials to illustrate important concepts, methods, and research findings. The book can be used in support of teaching for one- or two-semester courses.

The book provides broad coverage of nutrition as it relates to sport and includes some unique topics, such as immunonutrition and the newly introduced issue of personalized nutrition. We describe the main findings of influential research studies without going into too much detail (except where absolutely necessary) about experimental protocols, and we critique the limitations of some of these studies. Although most of the text is based on appropriate scientific studies, not every statement is referenced by a bibliographic source, because too many citations tend to interrupt the flow of the text. We have used references selectively so students can look at appropriate primary sources of information to find more details for themselves without being overwhelmed by extensive reference lists. The recommended readings at the end of each chapter mostly include key papers, suitable books or book chapters, and up-to-date reviews that provide evidence-based information by experts and active researchers in the field of the chapter topic. We hope that the unique features of our book will help instructors deliver a better course and expend less time preparing lectures and tutorials.

We hope this book inspires instructors as well as students, coaches, and athletes to achieve their potential in many ways. Most of all, we hope you enjoy reading our book on this fascinating subject.

Acknowledgments

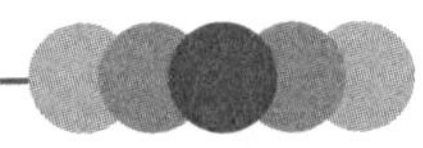

For many years we have worked with students, athletes, coaches, sport science and nutrition support staff, industrial partners, governing bodies, and scientists. These interactions have not only shaped this book but also inspired us in our careers and our own participation in and enjoyment of sport.

We acknowledge the discussions with many of our colleagues who have inspired us to write this book and with whom we had the pleasure to interact both socially and academically: Keith Baar, Stéphane Bermon, Nicolette Bishop, Louise Burke, Philip Calder, George Chiampas, Graeme Close, Kevin Currell, William Fraser, Martin Gibala, Bret Goodpaster, Mark Hargreaves, John Hawley, Jorn Helge, Peter Hespel, Hans Hoppeler, Andrew Jones, David Jones, Luc van Loon, David Martin, Ronald Maughan, Romain Meeusen, Sam Mettler, David Nieman, Timothy Noakes, Jeni Pearce, Stuart Phillips, Scott Powers, David Pyne, Matthew Reeves, David Rowlands, Bengt Saltin, Susan Shirreffs, Lawrence Spriet, Trent Stellingwerff, Mark Tarnopolsky, Kevin Tipton, Anton Wagenmakers, Gareth Wallis, Neil Walsh, and Clyde Williams. We are very grateful to others who have assisted us in writing this book.

We also thank the dedicated team at Human Kinetics, particularly Amy Tocco and Carly O'Connor, who have been very professional, patient, and helpful throughout the editorial process. Finally, we thank our partners, Zita and Laura, for their love, continuing support, and patience during the many hours we spent writing this book.

1

Nutrients and Recommended Intakes

Objectives

After studying this chapter, you should be able to do the following:

- Describe the main classes of nutrients
- Describe the different types of carbohydrates (monosaccharides, disaccharides, polysaccharides, and dietary fiber)
- Describe the main composition of the average Western diet
- Describe the chemical properties of various lipids (fats), including the differences between saturated and unsaturated fatty acids and between *cis* and *trans* fatty acids, and the functions of dietary lipids
- Describe the chemical properties of amino acids and proteins and the functions of protein in the body
- Describe the general role of water in the human body
- Describe the different classes of and the general role of micronutrients in the body
- Discuss the differences between essential and nonessential nutrients
- Discuss the basis of recommended daily intakes of nutrients
- Discuss the differences in the various methods to assess food intake and diet composition

Nutrition is often defined as the total of the processes of ingestion, digestion, absorption, and metabolism of food and the subsequent assimilation of nutrient materials into the tissues. A **nutrient** is a substance found in food that performs one or more specific functions in the body. We eat foods, but we do not eat nutrition or nutrients. The food we eat is part of our nutrition and contains nutrients.

This chapter discusses the properties and functions of various components of the diet and the recommended intake amounts for various nutrients. Subsequent chapters discuss the specific nutritional needs of athletes and other physically active people. These needs are often higher than those for relatively sedentary individuals, and, in preparation for and during competition, different nutrition guidelines apply to athletes compared with the general public. In principle, however, the guidelines for healthy nutrition apply to everyone. In a few cases or situations, guidelines for athletes will be different, but during periods of training, guidelines will be similar after taking into account the higher dietary energy requirements of most athletes. To optimize athletic performance, however, sport nutrition recommendations may deviate from general recommendations. For example, a high fiber intake is often recommended because it protects against cardiovascular disease and possibly against some forms of cancer. But the consumption of dietary fiber before or during prolonged endurance exercise may reduce gastric emptying, increase the risk of gastrointestinal problems, and impair athletic performance. Therefore, fiber should be consumed on training days, when performance is usually less critical, and should probably be avoided by some athletes before and during a race. Another example of different recommendations for the public and for athletes involves sodium intake. A low-sodium diet is usually recommended to the public (see chapter 2), but, as will be discussed in chapter 9, endurance athletes competing in hot conditions may experience sodium losses. For these athletes, relatively high intakes of sodium are no problem and are even recommended. Similarly, although the general population likely consumes too much sugar, athletes can benefit from the ingestion of sugars during exercise or during recovery from exercise.

Function of Nutrients

Food provides nutrients that have one or more physiological or biochemical functions in the body. Nutrients are usually divided into six different categories: **carbohydrate**, **fat**, **protein**, **water**, **vitamins**, and **minerals**. The functions of nutrients are often divided into three main categories:

1. *Promotion of growth and development.* This function is mainly performed by protein. Muscle, soft tissues, and organs consist largely of proteins, and proteins are required for any tissue growth or repair. In addition, calcium and phosphorus are important building blocks for the skeleton.
2. *Provision of energy.* This function is predominantly performed by carbohydrate and fat. Although protein can also function as a fuel, its contribution to energy expenditure is usually limited, and energy provision is not a primary function of protein.
3. *Regulation of metabolism.* Nutrients used in this function are vitamins, minerals, and protein. Enzymes are proteins that play an important role as catalysts that allow metabolic reactions to proceed at far higher rates than they would spontaneously. An example of an enzyme is **phosphorylase**, which breaks down carbohydrate stores in the liver and muscles. Another important protein is **hemoglobin**, which is found in **erythrocytes** (red blood cells). Erythrocytes are essential for the transport of oxygen from the lungs to the tissues, and the hemoglobin molecule acts as an oxygen carrier. The hemoglobin molecule is a complex of protein (**polypeptide** chains) and nonprotein groups (porphyrin rings) that hold iron (to which oxygen molecules can be bound). For the synthesis of this complex, other enzymes, minerals, and vitamins are required. Thus, the interaction between vitamins, minerals, and proteins in the regulation of metabolism can be complex.

CATEGORIES OF NUTRIENTS

Macronutrients are present in relatively large amounts in the human diet, whereas micronutrients are present in minuscule amounts.

Macronutrients
Carbohydrate
Fat
Protein
Water

Micronutrients
Vitamins
Minerals
Trace elements

The body requires substantial amounts of certain nutrients every day, whereas other nutrients may be ingested in small amounts. Nutrients for which the daily intake is more than a few grams are usually referred to as **macronutrients**. Macronutrients are carbohydrate, fat, protein, and water. Nutrients that are needed in only small amounts (less than 1 g/day) are referred to as **micronutrients**. Most nutrients are micronutrients, and they consist of vitamins, minerals, and trace elements.

Carbohydrate

Carbohydrates are molecules built of carbon (*carbo*), hydrogen, and water (*hydrate*). The general formula of a carbohydrate is CH_2O. In other words, the molar ratio of carbon, hydrogen, and oxygen is 1:2:1 in all carbohydrates. A carbohydrate can be one or a combination of many of these CH_2O units, and this is often written as $(CH_2O)n$, where n is the number of CH_2O units. For example, in glucose, $n = 6$; thus, a molecule of glucose contains 6 carbon atoms, 12 hydrogen atoms, and 6 oxygen atoms ($C_6H_{12}O_6$). The chemical structure of glucose is depicted in figure 1.1. Glucose is formed during

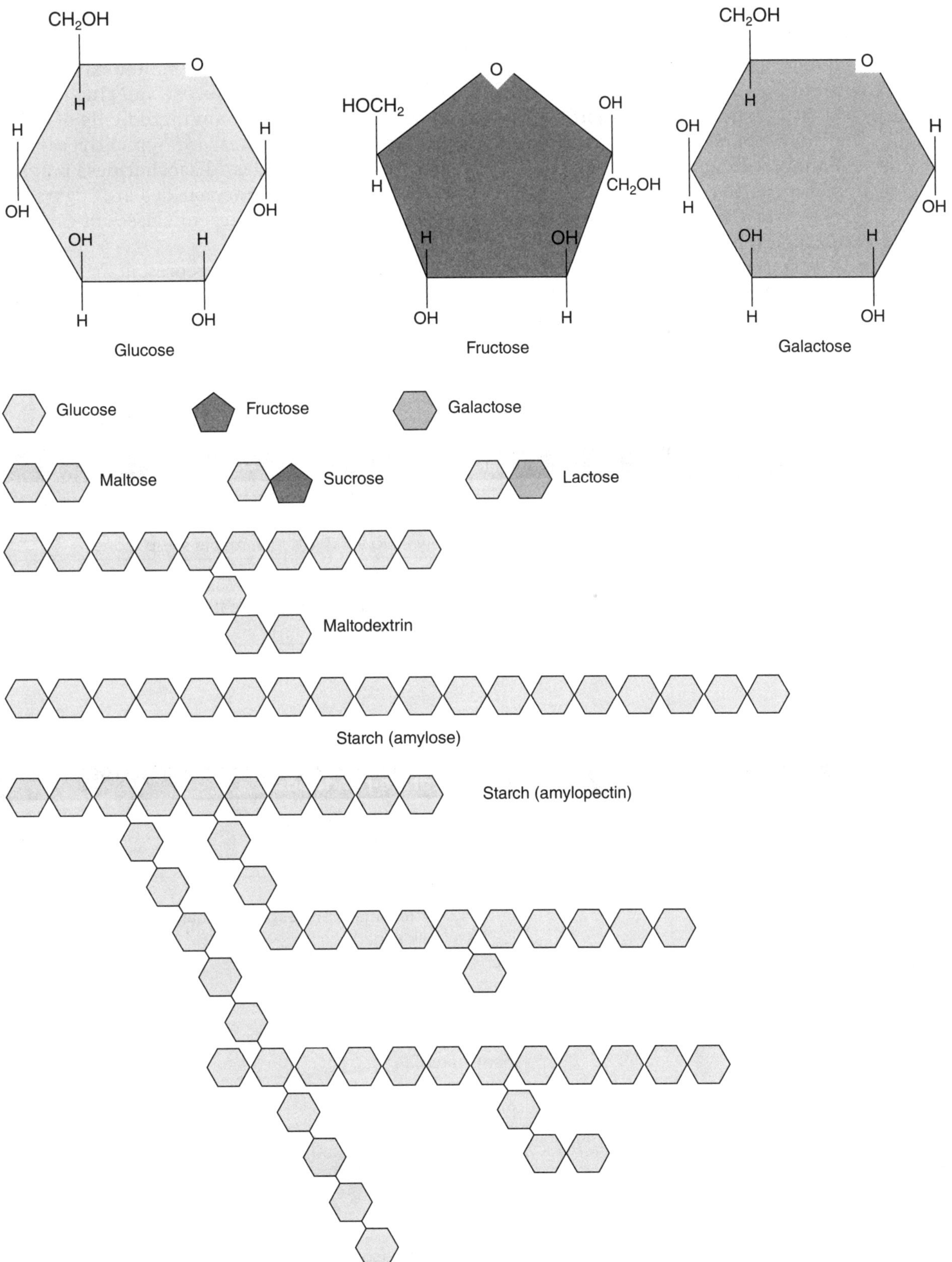

Figure 1.1 Carbohydrates and their structures. Human nutrition requires three monosaccharides (glucose, fructose, and galactose) and three disaccharides (maltose, sucrose, and lactose). Glucose polymers (**maltodextrins**) and starch are series of coupled glucose molecules.

From Jeukendrup and Jentjens (2000)

photosynthesis, and we obtain almost all our carbohydrate from plants. Carbohydrates can be found in all living cells.

Carbohydrate is an important fuel during exercise and is a crucial component of the athlete's diet. In preparation for competition it becomes even more important (as discussed in chapter 6), and it is also crucial in the recovery phase postexercise. Carbohydrate-rich foods include grains, potatoes, pasta, and rice, which contain mostly starches and fiber, but a large percentage of carbohydrate in the Western world is obtained from sugar (for examples of carbohydrate sources, see table 1.1). The most important carbohydrates in our diet are glucose, fructose, sucrose, glucose polymers (maltodextrins), and starch (amylopectin). Glucose and glucose polymers are usually the main ingredients of sports drinks. Carbohydrates are typically divided into monosaccharides, disaccharides, polysaccharides, and fiber. Saccharides are sugars. For an overview of the different classes of carbohydrate, see table 1.2.

The **monosaccharides** represent the basic unit of a carbohydrate, and three monosaccharides—glucose, fructose, and galactose—are present in

TABLE 1.1 Types of Carbohydrate and Their Food Sources

Carbohydrate	Carbohydrate-rich foods
Sugars (simple carbohydrate)	Fruit juices, fruits, sweetened cereals and baked goods, jam, candy, chocolate, toffee, most sports drinks, beet and cane sugar, brown sugar, table sugar, maple syrup, honey
Starches	Cereal, potatoes, pasta, rice, bread
Fiber	Whole-grain cereals and breads, oats, dried beans and peas, fruits and vegetables

TABLE 1.2 Classes of Carbohydrate

Carbohydrate	Carbohydrate-rich foods
Monosaccharides	Glucose or dextrose (grape sugar) Fructose or levulose (fruit sugar) Galactose
Disaccharides	Maltose (malt sugar) Sucrose (table sugar, cane sugar, saccharose, or beet sugar) Lactose (milk sugar) Trehalose or mycose Isomaltulose
Polysaccharides	Maltodextrin Starch Plant starch Amylose Amylopectin Resistant starch Glycogen
Fiber	Dietary fiber Functional fiber Hemicellulose Resistant starch (some forms) Dietary and functional fiber Cellulose ß-glucans Gums Pectins

our diet. Glucose is often called dextrose or grape sugar, and fructose is often referred to as fruit sugar. Galactose is usually present in only small amounts in our diet, but relatively large amounts are released after the digestion of the disaccharide milk sugar (lactose). The monosaccharides glucose, fructose, and galactose have similar structures and identical numbers of carbon, hydrogen, and oxygen atoms, but they have slightly different carbon-hydrogen-oxygen linkages that give them different biochemical characteristics (see figure 1.1). Glucose is the only carbohydrate that can be oxidized in muscle. Fructose and galactose must be converted into glucose (or lactate) before they can be oxidized. The conversion of fructose and galactose into glucose occurs in the liver at relatively slow rates.

Disaccharides are combinations of two monosaccharides. Disaccharides and monosaccharides are collectively called sugars, simple sugars, or simple carbohydrates. The most important disaccharides are **sucrose**, **lactose**, and **maltose**. Sucrose, which is by far the most abundant dietary disaccharide, provides about 20% to 25% of the daily energy intake in the Western world. Sucrose is composed of a glucose molecule and a fructose molecule. Foods that contain sucrose include beet and cane sugar, brown sugar, table sugar, maple syrup, and honey. Lactose, or milk sugar, is found in milk and consists of glucose and galactose. Maltose, or malt sugar, is present in beer, cereals, and germinating seeds and consists of two glucose molecules; it is present in small amounts in our diet.

Oligosaccharides are three to nine monosaccharides combined and can be found in most vegetables. **Polysaccharides** contain 10 or more monosaccharides in one molecule. Polysaccharides can contain 10 to 20 monosaccharides (often referred to as glucose polymers or maltodextrins) or up to thousands of monosaccharides (starch, glycogen, or fiber). Starch, glycogen, and fiber are the predominant forms of polysaccharides. Essentially, these polysaccharides are the storage forms of carbohydrate.

- **Starch**, or **complex carbohydrate**, is present in seeds, rice, corn, and various grains that make bread, cereal, pasta, and pastries. Starch is the storage form of carbohydrate in plants. The two apparently different forms of starch are **amylopectin** and **amylose**. Amylopectin is a highly branched molecule that consists of many glucose molecules (2,000-200,000), whereas amylose is a long chain of glucose molecules (200-4,000) twisted into a helical coil. Starches with relatively large amounts of amylopectin are rapidly digested and absorbed, whereas those with high amylose contents are digested more slowly. Most starches contain both amylase and amylopectin, and the relative contribution determines the properties of the food. For example, the quantity of amylose in rice kernels has a big effect on the properties of the cooked rice; rice with little amylose will be sticky and soft, whereas rice with a large amount of amylose will be firmer and not sticky. Approximately 50% of our total daily carbohydrate intake is in the form of starch.
- **Glycogen** is the storage form of carbohydrate in animals, including humans. It is stored in the liver (80-100 g) and in skeletal muscles (300-900 g), and its structure is comparable to amylopectin (see chapters 3 and 6 for detailed discussions).
- Dietary fiber used to be known as roughage. It comprises the edible parts of plants that are not broken down and absorbed in the human gastrointestinal tract. **Fiber** consists of structural plant polysaccharides such as **cellulose**. The human small intestine has no enzymes to break down these polysaccharides (and thus they cannot be digested). Although cellulose may be the most common type of fiber, there are many other types of fiber, including gums, hemicellulose, ß-glucans, and pectin.

The National Academy of Sciences in the United States assembled a panel that came up with the following definitions that were published (Food and Nutrition Board 2005) in a report on dietary reference intakes:

- Dietary fiber consists of nondigestible carbohydrate and lignin that are intrinsic and intact in plants.
- Functional fiber consists of isolated, nondigestible carbohydrate that has beneficial physiological effects in humans.
- Total fiber is the sum of dietary fiber and functional fiber, and it is the intake of total fiber that matters most.

Dietary fiber is also often divided into soluble and insoluble fiber. **Soluble fiber** dissolves well in water, whereas insoluble fiber does not. Both types of fiber are present in plant foods. Some plants contain more soluble fiber, and others have more insoluble fiber. **Insoluble fiber** possesses water-attracting properties that help increase bulk, soften stool, and shorten transit time through the intestinal tract. Soluble fiber undergoes metabolic processing through fermentation and yields end products that have broad, significant health effects. For example, plums have a thick skin covering a juicy pulp. The skin is an example of an insoluble fiber source, whereas the pulp contains soluble fiber sources. Good sources of fiber are listed in table 1.3.

Dietitians and nutritionists commonly classify carbohydrate as simple (sugars) or complex (starches). The term *complex carbohydrate* was first used in the Senate Select Committee on Nutrition and Human Needs publication *Dietary Goals for the United States* (1977), where it denoted "fruit, vegetables and whole grains." Dietary guidelines generally recommend that complex carbohydrate and nutrient-rich simple carbohydrate, which are in fruit and dairy products, make up the bulk of carbohydrate consumption (see chapter 2). Since its introduction, complex carbohydrate has been used to describe either starch alone or the combination of all polysaccharides and sometimes includes dietary fiber. Originally, the term complex carbohydrate was used to encourage consumption of what were considered healthy foods, such as whole-grain cereals. But the term becomes meaningless when it is used to describe fruit and vegetables, which are low in starch and contain mostly simple sugars. In addition, we now realize that different starches can have different metabolic effects. Some forms can be rapidly absorbed and have a high glycemic index, whereas others are resistant to digestion. As a substitute term for starch, the term complex carbohydrate seems to have little merit, and it is better to discuss carbohydrate components using their common chemical names. The U.S. Department of Agriculture's *Dietary Guidelines for Americans* (2005) dismissed the simple–complex carbohydrate distinction and instead recommended fiber-rich foods and whole grains.

The glycemic index (GI) and glycemic load systems are popular alternative classification methods that rank carbohydrate-rich foods based on their effects on blood glucose levels. The insulin index is a similar, more recent classification method that ranks foods based on their effects on blood insulin levels. The glycemic index and glycemic load are further discussed in chapter 6.

Functions of Carbohydrate

Carbohydrate has an important role in energy provision and exercise performance. It is the predominant fuel during high-intensity exercise (see chapter 3). Muscle glycogen and blood-borne glucose can provide more than 130 kJ/min (32 kcal/min) during very high-intensity exercise. Carbohydrate is stored in relatively small amounts in muscle and the liver and can become completely depleted after prolonged strenuous exercise. Ingestion of carbohydrate will rapidly replenish carbohydrate stores, and excess carbohydrate is converted into fat and stored in adipose tissue.

TABLE 1.3 Dietary Fiber and Food Sources

Type of fiber	Food sources
Soluble fiber	Legumes (peas, soybeans, and other beans) Oats, rye, barley Some fruits and fruit juices (particularly prune juice, plums, and berries) Vegetables such as broccoli and carrots Root vegetables such as potatoes, sweet potatoes, and onions (skins of these vegetables are sources of insoluble fiber) Psyllium seed husk
Insoluble fiber	Whole-grain foods Bran Nuts and seeds Vegetables such as green beans, cauliflower, zucchini (courgette), and celery Skins of some fruits, including tomatoes

In normal conditions, blood glucose is the only fuel used by the cells of the central nervous system. After prolonged fasting (about 3 days), **ketone bodies** are produced by the liver (from **fatty acids**), and these can serve as an alternative fuel for the central nervous system (especially after prolonged starvation). The central nervous system functions optimally when the blood glucose concentration is maintained above 4 mmol/L. Normal blood glucose concentration is about 5.5 mmol/L. At concentrations below 3 mmol/L, symptoms of hypoglycemia (low blood sugar) may develop, including weakness, hunger, dizziness, and shivering. Prolonged and severe hypoglycemia can result in unconsciousness and irreversible brain damage. Therefore, tight control of blood glucose concentration is crucial. Blood glucose also provides fuel for the red and white blood cells. New dietary guidelines for children and adults state that an intake of at least 130 g of carbohydrate each day should be achieved. This recommendation is based on the minimum amount of carbohydrate needed to produce sufficient glucose for the brain to function. Most people, however, consume far more than 130 g/day.

Functions of Fiber

The functions of a specific type of fiber are determined by whether the fiber is classified as soluble or insoluble. Insoluble fiber has its effects mainly in the colon, where it adds bulk and helps retain water, which results in a softer and larger stool. Fiber decreases the transit time of fecal matter through the intestines. So, a diet high in insoluble fiber is most often used in treatment of constipation resulting from poor dietary habits and is known to promote bowel regularity. Soluble fiber lowers blood cholesterol concentrations and normalizes blood glucose.

In addition, most soluble fiber is highly fermentable, and fermentable fibers help maintain healthy populations of friendly bacteria. Besides producing necessary short-chain fatty acids, these bacteria play an important role in the immune system by preventing pathogenic (disease-causing) bacteria from surviving in the intestinal tract. Fiber also has several effects on nutrient digestion and absorption. It reduces the rate of gastric emptying and can influence the absorption of various micronutrients. Fiber increases food bulk, which increases satiety, and it can reduce energy intake by 400 to 600 kJ/day (96-143 kcal/day). Fiber is associated with various health effects that will be discussed in more detail later.

Fat

Fats or **lipids** are compounds that are soluble in organic solvents such as acetone, ether, and chloroform. The term *lipid,* derived from the Greek word *lipos* (fat), is a general name for oils, fats, waxes, and related compounds. Oils are liquid at room temperature, whereas fats are solid. Lipid molecules contain the same structural elements as carbohydrates: carbon, hydrogen, and oxygen. Lipids, however, have little oxygen relative to carbon and hydrogen. A typical structure of a fatty acid is $CH_3(CH_2)_{14}COOH$ (palmitic acid or palmitate): 16 carbons, 32 hydrogens, and 2 oxygens.

Fatty acids have a carboxylic acid (COOH) at one end of the molecule and a methyl group at the other end that are separated by a hydrocarbon chain that can vary in length (see figure 1.2). The carboxylic acid group can bind to glycerol to form a mono-, di-, or triacylglycerol.

Although the solubility of the different lipids varies considerably, they generally dissolve poorly in water. The three classes of lipids most commonly recognized are simple lipids, compound lipids, and derived lipids (see table 1.4). An overview of various lipids and their structures is provided in figure 1.2. **Triacylglycerols**, or triglycerides, are the most abundant dietary lipids consumed by humans. They are composed of a three-carbon glycerol backbone esterified with three fatty acids. Triacylglycerols differ in their fatty acid composition.

In humans, the chain length of fatty acids typically varies from C14 to C24, although shorter or longer chains may occur (see table 1.5). Fatty acids with a chain length of C8 or C10 are **medium-chain fatty acids (MCFAs)**, and those with a chain length of C6 or fewer are **short-chain fatty acids (SCFAs)**. The most abundant fatty acids are the **long-chain fatty acids (LCFAs)**, which have a chain length of C12 or more. Of the long-chain fatty acids, palmitic acid (C16) and oleic acid (C18, one double bond) are the most abundant. Fatty acids with no double bonds in their hydrocarbon chains are called saturated fatty acids (SFAs). Those with one or more double bonds are **unsaturated fatty acids (UFAs)**. Fatty acids are usually described with numbers that indicate the length of the fatty acid (the number of carbons), the number of double bonds in the molecule, and the location of the first double bond. For example, C18:3 (*n*-3) is an 18-carbon fatty acid with three double bonds. The first double bond starts at the third carbon counting from the terminal methyl (CH_3) group (see figure 1.2). Another way of indicating the fatty acid and

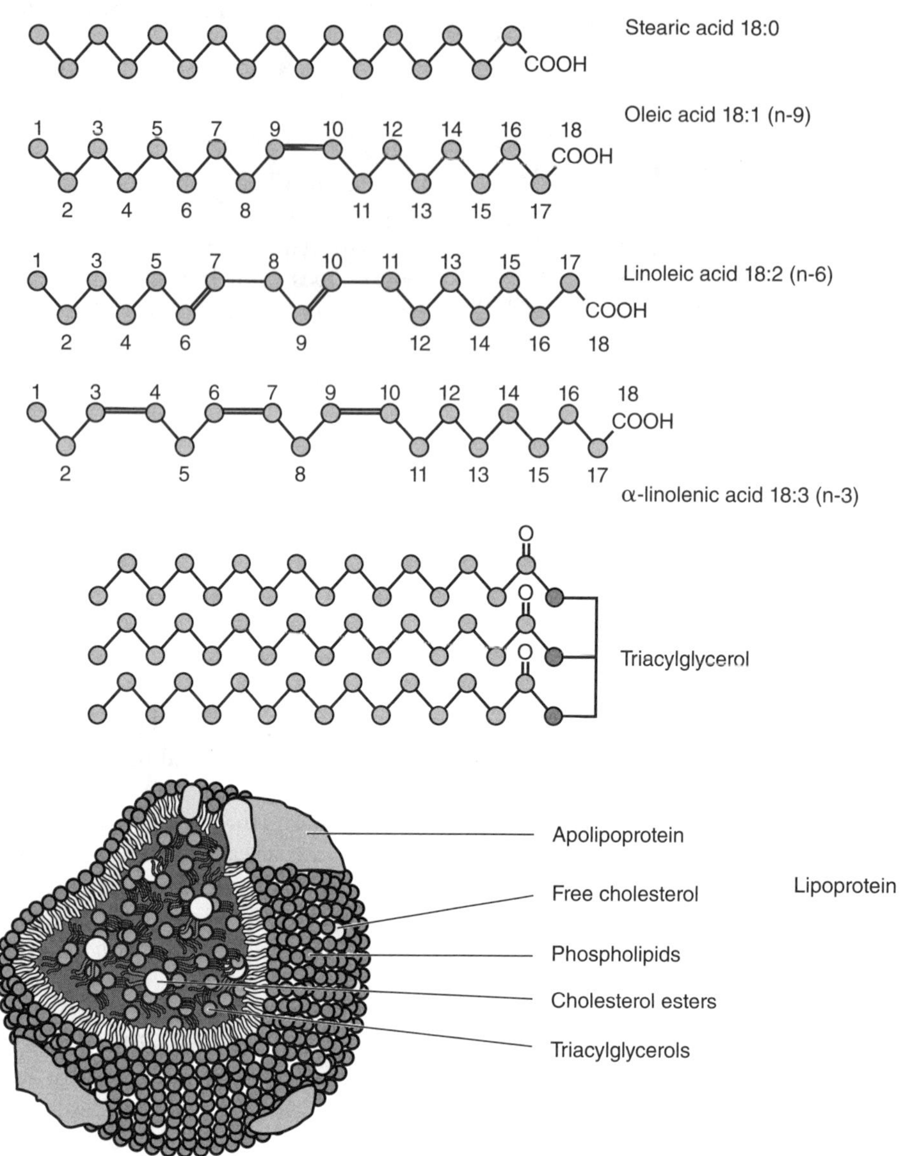

Figure 1.2 Lipids in the human body include fatty acids, triacylglycerols, lipoproteins, and phospholipids. Fatty acids differ in their chain length (number of carbons) and the number and location of double bonds.

TABLE 1.4 Three Classes of Lipids

Lipid class	Lipid type	Examples
Simple lipids	Neutral fats Waxes	Triacylglycerol (triglyceride) Beeswax
Compound lipids	Phospholipids Glycolipids Lipoproteins	Lecithins, cephalins, lipositols Cerebrosides, gangliosides Chylomicrons, very low-density Lipoproteins (VLDL), low-density Lipoproteins (LDL), high-density Lipoproteins (HDL)
Derived lipids	Fatty acids Steroids Hydrocarbons	Palmitic acid, oleic acid, stearic acid, linoleic acid Cholesterol, ergosterol, cortisol, bile acids, vitamin D, estrogens, progesterone, androgens Terpenes

TABLE 1.5 Overview of Different Fatty Acids and Their Nomenclature

Fatty acids	Double bonds	Common name	Chemical formula
2:0	—	Acetic	CH_3COO^-
4:0	—	Butyric	$CH_3(CH_2)_2COO^-$
6:0	—	Capronic	$CH_3(CH_2)_4COO^-$
8:0	—	Caprylic	$CH_3(CH_2)_6COO^-$
10:0	—	Caprynic	$CH_3(CH_2)_8COO^-$
12:0	—	Lauric	$CH_3(CH_2)_{10}COO^-$
14:0	—	Myristic	$CH_3(CH_2)_{12}COO^-$
16:0	—	Palmitic	$CH_3(CH_2)_{14}COO^-$
16:1	*n*-6	Palmitoleic	$CH_3(CH_2)_5CH{=}CH(CH_2)_7COO^-$
18:0	—	Stearic	$CH_3(CH_2)_{16}COO^-$
18:1	*n*-9	Oleic	$CH_3(CH_2)_7CH{=}CH(CH_2)_7COO^-$
18:2	*n*-6	Linoleic	$CH_3(CH_2)_4(CH{=}CHCH_2)_2(CH_2)_6COO^-$
18:3	*n*-6	γ-linolenic	$CH_3(CH_2)_4(CH{=}CHCH_2)_3(CH_2)_3COO^-$
18:3	*n*-3	α-linolenic	$CH_3(CH_2)(CH{=}CHCH_2)_3(CH_2)_6COO^-$
20:0	—	Arachidonic	$CH_3(CH_2)_{18}COO^-$
20:2	*n*-6	Eicosadinoic	$CH_3(CH_2)_4(CH{=}CHCH_2)_2(CH_2)_8COO^-$
20:3	*n*-6	Eicosatrinoic	$CH_3(CH_2)_4(CH{=}CHCH_2)_3(CH_2)_5COO^-$
20:4	*n*-6	Arachidonic	$CH_3(CH_2)_4(CH{=}CHCH_2)_4(CH_2)_2COO^-$
20:5	*n*-3	Eicosapentaenoic (EPA)	$CH_3(CH_2)(CH{=}CHCH_2)_5(CH_2)_2COO^-$
22:0	—	Behenic	$CH_3(CH_2)_{20}COO^-$
22:5	*n*-3	Docosapentaenoic	$CH_3(CH_2)(CH{=}CHCH_2)_5(CH_2)_4COO^-$
22:6	*n*-3	Docosahexaenoic (DHA)	$CH_3(CH_2)(CH{=}CHCH_2)_6(CH_2)COO^-$
24:0	—	Lignoceratic	$CH_3(CH_2)_{22}COO^-$

the position of the double bond is C20:4 ω3. The latter is called an **omega-3 fatty acid**.

Monounsaturated fatty acids (MUFAs) have one double bond, and the hydrogen atoms are present on the same side of the double bond. Typically, plant sources rich in monounsaturated fatty acids (e.g., canola oil, olive oil, and safflower and sunflower oils) are liquid at room temperature. Monounsaturated fatty acids are present in foods with a double bond located at 7 (*n*-7) or 9 (*n*-9) carbon atoms from the methyl end. Monounsaturated fatty acids that are present in the diet include oleic acid (18:1*n*-9), palmitoleic acid (16:1*n*-7), eicosenoic acid (20:1*n*-9), and erucic acid (22:1*n*-9). Oleic acid accounts for more than 90% of dietary monounsaturated fatty acids. Monounsaturated fatty acids, including oleic acid and nervonic acid (24:1*n*-9), are important in membrane structural lipids, particularly nervous tissue myelin. Other monounsaturated fatty acids, such as palmitoleic acid, are present in minor amounts in the diet.

The **polyunsaturated fatty acids (PUFAs)** have two or more double bonds and can be roughly divided into two categories: *n*-6 and *n*-3 fatty acids. The most important *n*-6 polyunsaturated fatty acids are linoleic acid (18:2), γ-linolenic acid (18:3), dihomo-γ-linolenic acid (20:3), arachidonic acid (20:4), adrenic acid (22:4), and docosapentaenoic acid (22:5).

Humans cannot synthesize **linoleic acid**, and a lack of it results in adverse clinical symptoms, including a scaly rash and reduced growth. Linoleic acid is also the precursor to arachidonic acid, which is the substrate for eicosanoid production in tissues, is a component of membrane structural lipids, and is important in cell signaling pathways. The *n*-6 polyunsaturated fatty acids also play critical roles in normal epithelial cell function. The *n*-3 polyunsaturated fatty acids tend to be highly unsaturated, and one of the double bonds is located three carbon atoms from the methyl end. The *n*-3 polyunsaturated fatty acids include α-linolenic acid (18:3), eicosapentaenoic acid (20:5), docosapentaenoic acid (22:5), and docosahexaenoic acid (22:6). Humans do not synthesize **α-linolenic acid** (18:3), and a lack of it results in adverse clinical symptoms, including neurological abnormalities and poor growth. It is also the precursor for synthesis of eicosapentaenoic acid (EPA) and docosahexaenoic acid (DHA). EPA is the precursor of *n*-3 eicosanoids, which have been shown to have beneficial effects in preventing coronary heart disease, arrhythmias, and thrombosis. All the fatty acids listed have a *cis* configuration, which refers to the arrangement of the double bond (see figure 1.3). Fatty acids that have a *trans* configuration are called the ***trans* fatty acids**.

Trans fatty acids are unsaturated fatty acids that contain at least one double bond in the *trans* configuration. The *trans* double-bond configuration results in a larger bond angle than the *cis* configuration, which in turn results in a more extended fatty acid carbon chain that is more like that of saturated fatty acids than that of *cis* unsaturated, double-bond-containing fatty acids. The conformation of the double bond affects the physical properties of the fatty acid. Fatty acids containing a *trans* double bond have the potential for closer packing or aligning of acyl chains, which results in decreased mobility; hence, fluidity is reduced when compared with fatty acids that contain a *cis* double bond. Partial hydrogenation of polyunsaturated oils causes isomerization of some of the remaining double bonds and migration of others, which results in an increase in *trans* fatty acid content and hardening of fat. Hydrogenation of oils, such as corn oil, can result in both *cis* and *trans* double bonds anywhere between carbon 4 and carbon 16. A major *trans* fatty acid is elaidic acid (9-*trans* 18:1) (figure 1.3). Production of hydrogenated fats increased steadily until the 1960s as processed vegetable fats replaced animal fats in the United States and other Western countries. These more saturated fats have a higher melting point, which makes them attractive for baking and extends their shelf life. Unlike other dietary fats, *trans* fats are neither essential nor salubrious, and, in fact, the consumption of *trans* fats increases the risk of coronary heart disease by raising levels of "bad" LDL cholesterol and lowering levels of "good" HDL cholesterol (see chapter 2).

During hydrogenation of polyunsaturated fatty acids, small amounts of several other *trans* fatty acids (9-*trans,*12-*cis* 18:2; 9-*cis,*12-*trans* 18:2) are produced. In addition to these isomers, dairy fat and meats contain 9-*trans* 16:1 and conjugated dienes (9-*cis,*11-*trans* 18:2). The *trans* fatty acid content in foods tends to be higher in foods containing hydrogenated oils.

Cholesterol is a lipid found in the cell membranes of all animal tissues, and it is transported

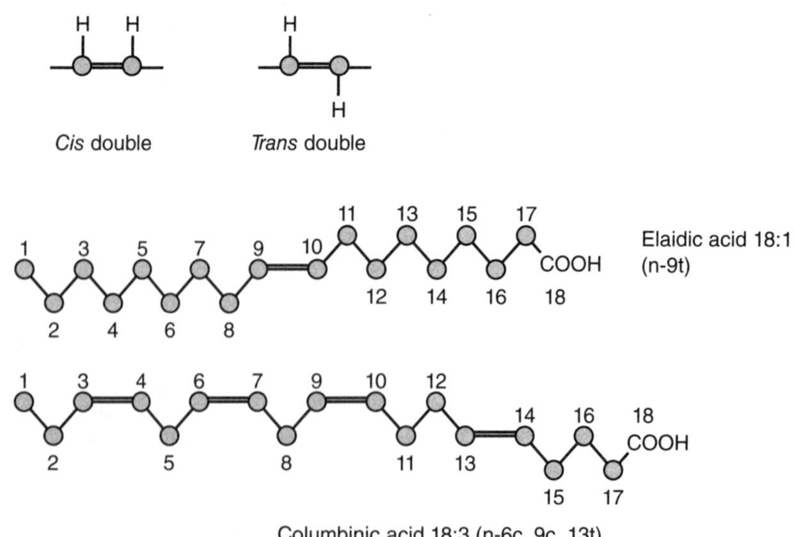

Figure 1.3 *Trans* fatty acids have a slightly different chemical configuration than *cis* fatty acids and are recognized as a cardiovascular risk factor.

in the blood plasma. Cholesterol, which is also considered a sterol (a combination steroid and alcohol), is required to build and maintain cell membranes; it regulates membrane fluidity over a wide range of temperatures. Cholesterol aids in the manufacture of bile (which is stored in the gallbladder and helps digest fats), is important for the metabolism of fat soluble vitamins, and is the major precursor for the synthesis of vitamin D and various steroid hormones.

Triacylglycerols (and cholesterol esters) found in plasma are usually incorporated into the core of a lipoprotein with **phospholipids**, free cholesterol, and apolipoproteins surrounding it. Apoprotein is a general name given to a protein that combines with another type of molecule to form a complex conjugated protein. Apolipoproteins are proteins that combine with lipids to form a complex as in the various lipoprotein particles. Various lipoproteins differ in their density, triacylglycerol content, and cholesterol content, but they also fulfill different functions. Examples of such lipoproteins are chylomicrons, **very low-density lipoproteins (VLDLs)**, **low-density lipoproteins (LDLs)**, intermediate-density lipoproteins (IDLs), and **high-density lipoproteins (HDLs)** (see figure 1.4).

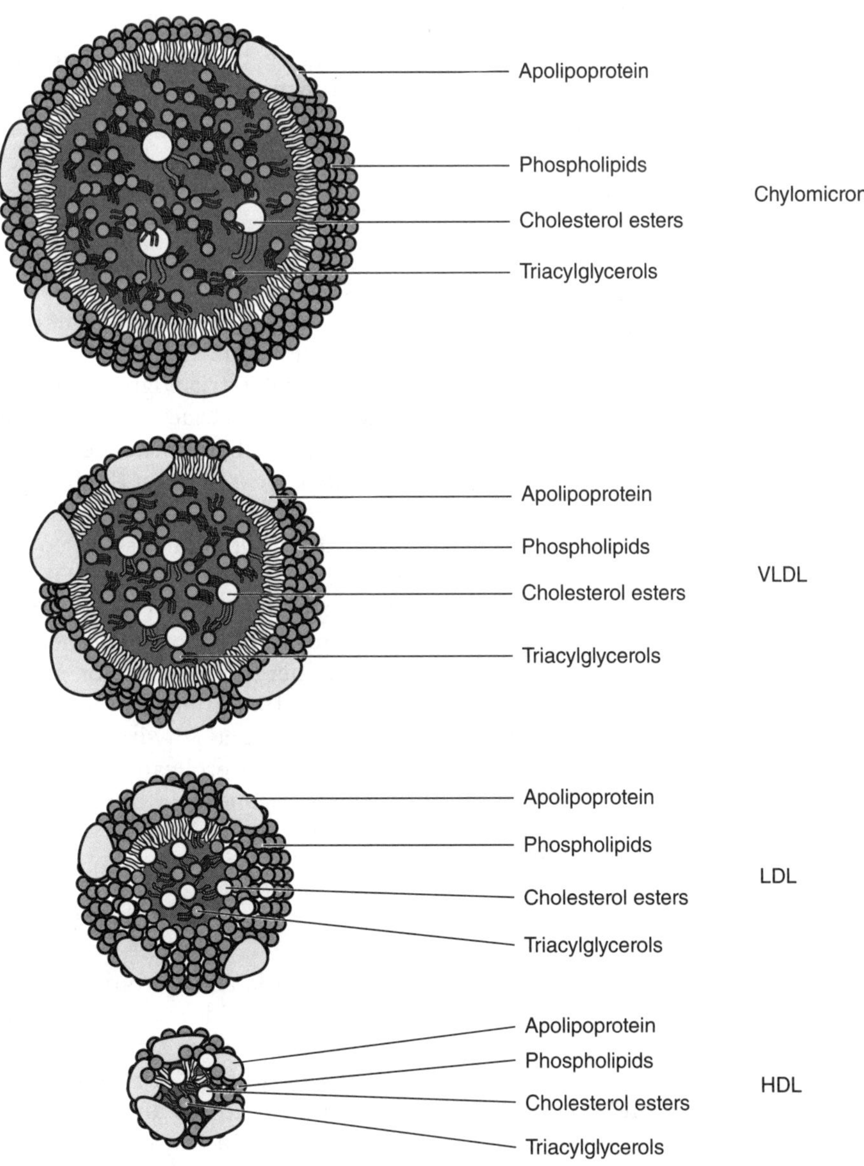

Figure 1.4 Various lipoproteins. The various shades of blue represent different types of apolipoproteins.

NOMENCLATURE OF FATTY ACIDS

In the literature, various nomenclature is used with regard to fatty acids. To avoid misunderstandings or misinterpretations, the nomenclature in this book will be explained. Distinction must be made between fatty acids that are incorporated into triacylglycerols or other particles and fatty acids that are not incorporated into triacylglycerols. The fatty acids that are not esterified to form a monoacylglycerol, diacylglycerol, or triacylglycerol are **nonesterified fatty acids (NEFAs)** or **free fatty acids (FFAs)**. The term *free fatty acid* might be somewhat ambiguous because, for example, in plasma, these fatty acids are bound to albumin and are not free. Only a minuscule fraction of fatty acids (less than 0.01% of the plasma fatty acid pool) are not bound to any other compound (non-protein-bound fatty acids). In this book, the term *fatty acid* (not free fatty acid) is used to designate fatty acids that are not esterified to monoacylglycerols, diacylglycerols, or triacylglycerols but might be bound to albumin or **fatty acid–binding proteins (FABPs)**.

Functions of Lipids

Lipids are an important energy source, especially during prolonged exercise. Large amounts of fat can be stored in the body. Fat is stored mainly in subcutaneous adipose tissue from which it is mobilized and transported to the organ that uses it. Skeletal muscle contains a directly accessible store of fat (intramuscular triacylglycerol). Lipids have many other important functions, including the following:

- Lipids fuel most cells and are important fuels for the contracting muscle.
- Fat protects vital organs such as the heart, liver, spleen, kidneys, brain, and spinal cord. A layer of adipose tissue covers these organs to protect them against trauma. About 2% to 4% of total body fat is stored around vital organs.
- The intake of fat-soluble vitamins A, D, E, and K and carotenoids depends on daily fat intake, and fats provide the transport medium in the body.
- Phospholipids and cholesterol are important constituents of cell membranes.
- Cholesterol is also an important precursor in the formation of bile and is itself an important component of bile.
- Cholesterol is a precursor for important hormones (particularly steroids such as testosterone).
- Linoleic acid plays an important role in the formation of eicosanoids, which are hormone-like substances formed in cells with a regulatory function. Eicosanoids play a role in the maintenance of blood pressure, platelet aggregation, intestinal motility, and immune function.
- Fat often makes food more tasty and attractive. It carries many aromatic substances and makes food creamier and more appetizing.

Lipids as Fuel

Only some of the lipid forms can be used as a fuel. Oxidizable lipid fuels include fatty acids, intramuscular triacylglycerols (IMTGs), and circulating plasma triacylglycerols (chylomicrons and VLDLs). VLDL, for instance, is the main transport of triacylglycerols from the liver to adipose tissue and muscle, whereas HDL transports cholesterol from the peripheral tissues to the liver. Therefore, chylomicrons and VLDL may play a role in energy metabolism during exercise, but LDL, IDL, and HDL probably do not play a significant role in energy provision for muscle. In addition, fat-derived compounds, such as ketone bodies (acetoacetate and ß-hydroxybutyrate), can serve as a fuel, and glycerol can be converted into glucose in gluconeogenesis in the liver and subsequently oxidized.

Protein

Amino acids are the building blocks of all proteins. Amino acids are bound by **peptide bonds**, and once the amino acids are connected they are called a **peptide**. Most proteins are polypeptides combining up to 300 amino acids. Some examples of proteins are actin, tropomyosin, troponin, and myosin, which together make up the contractile apparatus in the muscle (see chapter 3 for a detailed discussion). Because muscle is mostly protein, meat is a good source of protein. Twenty different amino acids are commonly found in proteins. Each amino acid consists of a carbon atom bound to four chemical groups: a hydrogen atom; an amino group, which contains nitrogen; a carboxylic acid group; and a side chain, which varies in length and structure (see figure 1.5). Different side chains give different properties to the amino acid.

Of the 20 amino acids normally found in dietary protein, humans can synthesize 11. The human body cannot manufacture the other nine amino acids. Those that can be synthesized are called **nonessential amino acids**. Those that cannot be synthesized and must be derived from the diet are called the **essential amino acids** (see the sidebar). Figure 1.5 lists the various amino acids and their structures.

Amino acids have central roles in the metabolism of many organs and tissues. Amino acids are not only precursors for the synthesis of body proteins but also precursors and regulators of the synthesis of important metabolic mediators and compounds with a regulatory biological activity (e.g., **neurotransmitters**, hormones, **DNA**, and **RNA**).

Proteins provide structure to all cells in the human body. They are an integral part of the cell membrane, the cytoplasm, and the organelles. Muscle, skin, and hair are composed largely of proteins. Bones and teeth are composed of minerals embedded in a protein framework. When a diet is deficient in protein, these structures break down, resulting in reduced muscle mass, loss of skin elasticity, and thinning hair. Many proteins are enzymes that increase the rate of metabolic reactions.

Unlike fat and carbohydrate, protein is not usually linked with diseases such as cancer, tooth caries, or arteriosclerosis. For this reason, protein is often associated with health, and many companies use this association in their marketing strategies (e.g., protein shampoo). Indeed, in the developed world, where protein deficiency is uncommon, dietary protein intake is less critical and is not related to disease. Prolonged deficiencies of dietary protein, however, have devastating consequences for health that result in immunodeficiency, edema, and muscle wasting; ultimately, organ failure will result in death. Excess intake of protein is relatively rare and is not considered to be a health issue except for people with impaired kidney function.

Recommended intakes are generally based on data from nitrogen balance studies (see chapter 8). Recommended protein intake varies worldwide from 0.8 to 1.2 g/kg of body weight. Protein intake in the Western world usually well exceeds the recommendations and averages at about 80 to 100 g/day. Because meat and fish are the most common sources of protein, vegetarians could be at risk for marginal protein intake. Vegetarians often compensate by eating more grains and legumes, which both are excellent protein sources. But grains and legumes do not contain all essential amino acids. Grains lack the essential amino acid lysine, and legumes lack methionine. An exception may be well-processed soybean protein, which is a high-quality protein comparable to protein from animal sources. Although some cultures have a much higher protein intake, most Western countries have protein intakes between 10% and 15% of the total daily energy intake. The Centers for Disease Control and Prevention (CDC) reported an average protein intake of 16.1% of energy intake for men and 15.6% for women in the United States for the period 2011-2014.

The data on which recommendations are based are typically obtained from studies in sedentary people. Are protein requirements greater for athletes involved in strenuous training programs? Although many national committees recognize the possibility that strenuous daily activity may increase protein needs, most experts do not suggest increased protein intake for active people. It has also been observed that after a period of training,

NONESSENTIAL AND ESSENTIAL AMINO ACIDS

Dispensable (Nonessential) Amino Acids

- Alanine
- Arginine
- Asparagine
- Aspartate
- Cysteine
- Glutamate
- Glutamine
- Glycine
- Proline
- Serine
- Tyrosine

Indispensable (Essential) Amino Acids

- Histidine
- Isoleucine
- Leucine
- Lysine
- Methionine
- Phenylalanine
- Threonine
- Tryptophan
- Valine

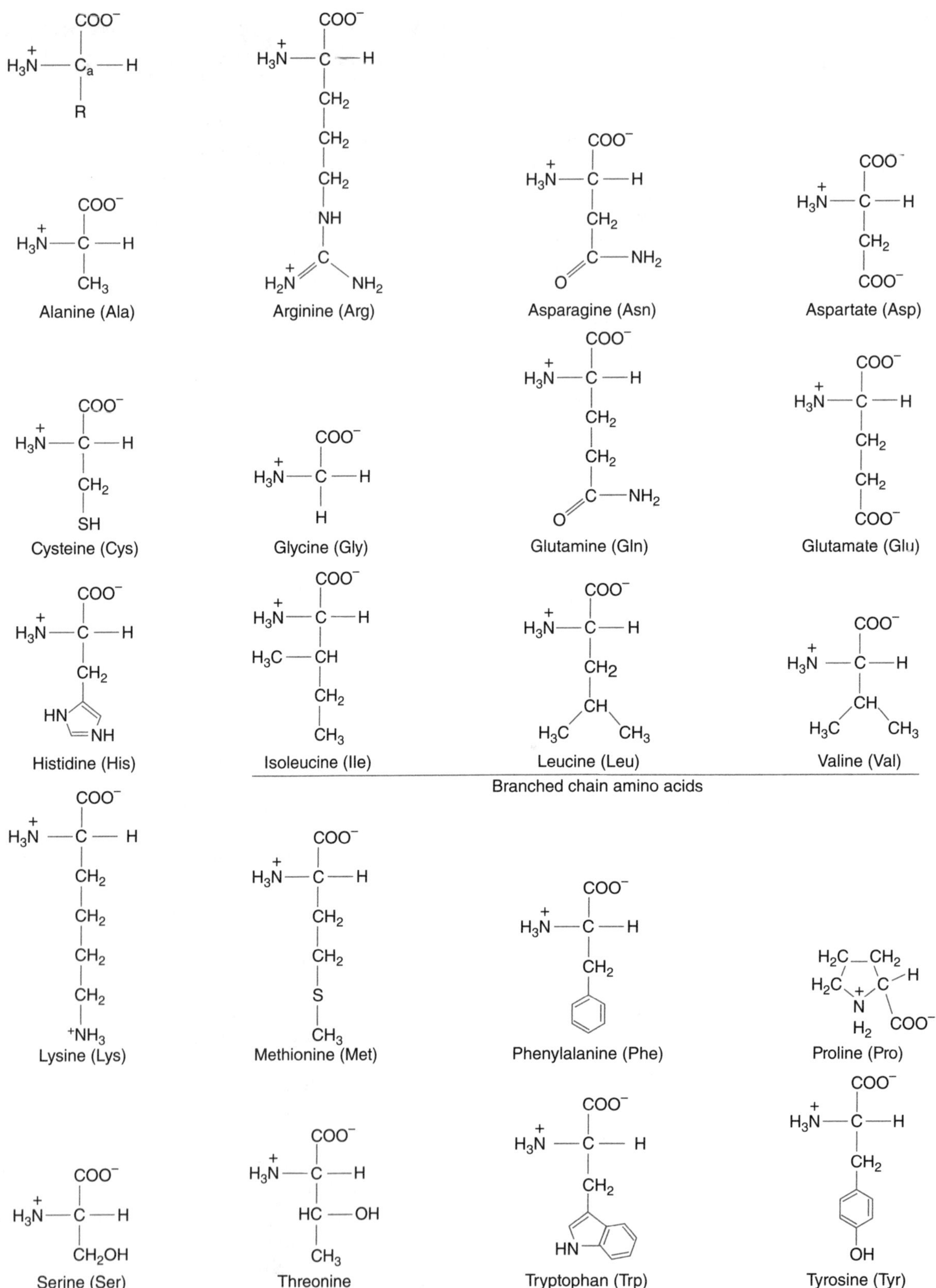

Figure 1.5 Chemical structures and abbreviations of amino acids.

QUALITY OF PROTEIN

The quality of a protein relates to the degree to which that protein contributes to daily requirements. Various methods have been proposed to measure the protein quality of a food. The most recent method is the protein digestibility corrected amino acid score (PDCAAS). PDCAAS is a method of evaluating protein quality based on the amino acid requirements of humans. Using the PDCAAS, protein-quality rankings are determined by comparing the amino acid profile of a specific food protein against a standard amino acid profile. The maximum score of 1.0 means that after digestion of the protein, it provides, per unit of protein, 100% or more of the indispensable amino acids required. Although this classification was adopted by the U.S. Food and Drug Administration (FDA), the Food and Agricultural Organization of the United Nations, and the World Health Organization in 1993 as "the preferred best" method to determine protein quality, it has received much criticism. People rarely eat a single source of protein; therefore, having the information for individual sources of protein does not give information about the protein quality of the overall diet unless all protein-containing food sources are considered to calculate an average score. In addition, the fact that common protein sources, which have different amino acid profiles, receive identical scores of 1.0 limits its usefulness as a comparative tool. But in the absence of a better method, the PDCAAS is frequently used.

A PDCAAS value of 1.0 is the highest and 0.0 is the lowest. The following are the ratings of some common foods:

Whey (milk protein)	1.0
Egg white	1.0
Casein (milk protein)	1.0
Milk	1.0
Soy protein isolate	1.0
Beef	0.92
Soybean	0.91
Kidney bean	0.68
Rye	0.68
Whole wheat	0.54

the efficiency of protein use increases. Therefore, protein requirements to maintain muscle mass may not increase. The requirements are discussed in more detail in chapter 8. Note, however, that the diets of endurance-trained people often contain twice the recommended amounts of protein, mainly because the increased energy intake also increases the protein intake.

As mentioned earlier, the amount and the quality of protein are important. Protein that contains all the essential amino acids is called complete protein or high-quality protein. Protein that is deficient in one or more amino acids is called incomplete protein or low-quality protein. Incomplete protein is unable to support human life and growth. Animal protein is generally of higher quality than plant protein because all essential amino acids are present, and they are present in larger quantities and in proper proportions. The individual amino acids in animal protein and plant protein are identical and of equal quality. The quality of the protein depends purely on the kinds of amino acids present in the protein.

Because the metabolism of all amino acid is integrated, all essential amino acids must be obtained by dietary intake. A short supply of any essential amino acid can interfere with normal protein synthesis. An appropriate selection of plant protein sources can provide an adequate supply of amino acids, but consumption of animal protein is more likely to ensure a balanced intake. By combining plant foods such as rice and beans, it is possible to obtain a balanced intake of amino acids. Essential amino acids that are deficient in one food can be obtained from another. Protein from different sources that balances the amino acid intake is called complementary protein.

Water

Water, the most abundant molecule on the surface of the Earth, is essential for the survival of all known forms of life. One molecule of water has two hydrogen atoms covalently bonded to a single oxygen atom. Oxygen attracts electrons much more strongly than hydrogen does, resulting in a net positive charge on the hydrogen atoms and a net negative charge on the oxygen atom. The presence of a charge on each of these atoms gives each water molecule a net dipole moment and explains many of the properties of water.

The adult body is about 60% water by weight; therefore, a person who weighs 70 kg (154 lb) consists of approximately 40 kg (88 lb) of water. The percentage of water is highest in infants and generally decreases with age. Water content varies among different tissues of the body. Blood is about 90% water, muscle is about 75%, bone is about 25%, and adipose tissue is about 5%. The proportion of water in various body compartments also varies. About two-thirds of body water is found inside cells as intracellular fluid. The remaining one-third is found outside cells as **extracellular fluid**. Extracellular fluid includes water in the blood, lymph, and cerebrospinal fluid as well as in the fluid found between cells, which is called **interstitial** fluid (see appendix A for detailed explanations).

Water transports nutrients, provides protection, helps regulate body temperature, participates in biochemical reactions, and provides the medium in which these reactions take place (blood transports nutrients and oxygen to the tissues and transports carbon dioxide and waste products away from the tissues). Water in urine transports waste products such as urea, excess salt, and ketones out of the body.

The protective functions of water are lubrication, cleansing, and cushioning. Tears lubricate the eyes and wash away dirt. Synovial fluid lubricates the joints. Saliva lubricates the mouth, making chewing and swallowing food possible. Water inside the eyeballs and spinal cord acts as a cushion against shock. During pregnancy, water in the amniotic fluid provides a protective cushion for the fetus.

An important role of water during exercise is regulating body temperature (see chapter 9). When body temperature starts to rise above the normal temperature of around 37 °C (98.6 °F), the blood vessels in the skin dilate, causing blood to flow close to the surface of the body and release some of the heat. This release occurs with fever, with an increase in the environmental temperature, and with exercise. In a cold environment, blood vessels in the skin constrict, restricting blood flow near the surface and conserving body heat. The most obvious way that water helps regulate body temperature is through sweat. When body temperature increases, the sweat glands in the skin secrete sweat. As the sweat evaporates, heat is removed from the body surface.

In the body, water also acts as a **solvent**, which is a fluid in which solutes dissolve to form a solution. Water is an ideal solvent for some substances because it is polar, which means that the two sides, or poles, of the water molecule have different electrical charges. The oxygen side of a water molecule has a slightly negative charge, and the hydrogen side has a slightly positive charge. This polarity allows water to surround other charged molecules and disperse them. Table salt (sodium chloride), which dissolves well in water, consists of a positively charged sodium ion bound to a negatively charged chloride ion. In water, the sodium and chloride ions dissociate because the positively charged sodium ion is attracted to the negative pole of the water molecule and the negatively charged chloride ion is attracted to the positive pole. Substances such as sodium chloride, which dissociate in water to form positively and negatively charged ions, are known as **electrolytes** because they can conduct an electrical current when dissolved in water.

As with all other nutrients, regular and sufficient water intake is required to maintain health and good physical performance. The hydration status of the body is determined by the balance between water intake and water loss. Loss of water (through diarrhea or sweating) may result in dehydration, and failure to drink fluid for more than a few days can result in death. With a water loss of 3% of total body weight, blood volume decreases and exercise performance deteriorates. A 5% loss can result in confusion and disorientation, and a loss greater than 10% can be life threatening. Dehydration frequently occurs in many sports but can be prevented through adequate water intake (see chapter 9 for a detailed discussion).

Water intake of an adult is typically 2 to 2.8 L/day (68-95 fl oz/day). Because water requirements are highly dependent on sweat rates and sweat rates are dependent on energy expenditure, as a rule of thumb, fluid requirements are 1 ml (0.03 fl oz) for every 4 kJ (1 kcal) of energy expended. Of the daily 2 to 2.8 L consumed, 1 to 1.5 L (34-51 fl oz) is usually in the form of fluids, and the remainder is obtained from foods. Athletes who train and compete in hot conditions may have fluid requirements greater than 15 L/day (4 gal/day).

Alcohol

Alcohol (ethanol) is consumed as a beverage. Alcohol is a nutrient that provides 28 kJ (7 kcal) of energy per gram, but it is not essential in the diet. Most of it gets converted to fat. Although alcohol may have health benefits when ingested in moderation, excessive consumption impairs brain function and has other detrimental effects on health (see chapter 2 for further details).

Vitamins, Minerals, and Trace Elements

Vitamins are organic compounds, and minerals and trace elements are inorganic compounds. Collectively known as micronutrients, these essential compounds have many biological functions. They serve as regulators and links in the processes of energy release from food. They are important cofactors in various chemical reactions and, as such, are important in maintaining homeostasis (relatively constant internal conditions). People often consider vitamin intake to be synonymous with good health (e.g., folic acid prevents birth defects, vitamin E protects the heart, vitamin A prevents cancer), and some minerals are reputed to have strong relations to health (e.g., calcium helps to prevent osteoporosis).

All the 13 known vitamins have important functions in most metabolic processes in the body. Vitamins must be obtained from the diet except vitamin D, which can be synthesized from sunlight, and vitamin K, which is synthesized by bacteria in the intestine. When a vitamin becomes unavailable in the diet, a deficiency may develop within 3 to 4 weeks. Vitamins are either water soluble or fat soluble (see the sidebar). Water-soluble vitamins dissolve in water; fat-soluble vitamins dissolve in organic solvents and are usually ingested with fats. Minerals can be divided into macrominerals, which have a required daily intake of more than 100 mg or presence in the body in amounts greater than 0.01% of the body weight, and microminerals (trace elements), which have a required daily intake of less than 100 mg or presence in the body in amounts less than 0.01% of body weight (see chapter 10 for a detailed discussion).

Sodium, which is often ingested as sodium chloride, has various functions in the body, including some related to muscle contraction (see chapter 10), nerve function, and maintenance of normal blood pressure. Muscles and nerves require electrical currents to function properly. Muscle and nerve cells generate these electrical currents by controlling the flow of electrically charged ions, including sodium. For muscle cells, these electrical currents stimulate contraction of the muscle. Nerves, on the other hand, need electrical activity to communicate with other nerves. Cells use molecular pumps to keep sodium levels outside the cell high. When an electrical current is needed, cells can allow the positively charged sodium ions into the cell, which generates a positive electrical current. This concentration difference for sodium

FAT-SOLUBLE VITAMINS (A, D, E, AND K) AND WATER-SOLUBLE VITAMINS

- Biotin
- Choline*
- Folic acid
- Pantothenic acid
- Vitamin A
- Vitamin B_1 (thiamin)
- Vitamin B_2 (riboflavin)
- Vitamin B_3 (niacin)
- Vitamin B_6 (pyridoxine)
- Vitamin B_{12}
- Vitamin C (ascorbic acid)
- Vitamin D
- Vitamin E (α-tocopherol)
- Vitamin K

*Choline is not classed as a vitamin but it is considered to be an essential vitamin-like nutrient.

between the outside and inside of cells can also be used to drive the cotransport of other substances (e.g., glucose) into cells. Sodium is dissolved in the body fluids and it attracts and holds water, so sodium in the blood helps maintain the volume of the liquid portion of the blood (plasma), which in turn helps maintain normal blood pressure (normotension) of around 120 mmHg (**systolic**, when the heart contracts) and 80 mmHg (**diastolic**, when the heart is relaxed). If you consume too much sodium, however, your body may hold onto extra water, which increases the volume of your blood. Since your blood vessels cannot expand to accommodate this increased blood volume, your blood pressure will rise. High blood pressure is a risk factor for many diseases, heart problems, and stroke (see chapter 2 for further details of the health effects of sodium).

Phytonutrients

Phytonutrients are certain organic components of plants (*phyto* is Greek for plant) that are thought to promote human health. They differ from vitamins because they are not considered essential nutrients, which means that people will not develop nutritional deficiencies without them.

The many types of phytonutrients can be divided into different classes (see the sidebar). The most well known and most researched of these are probably the carotenoids, which are found in carrots, broccoli, yellow and leafy green vegetables, and other vegetables, and polyphenols, which are found in various berries, fruits, tea, beer, and wine.

Of all the phytonutrients, carotenoids are the ones that receive the most attention and are the most researched. Carotenoids are the red, orange, and yellow pigments in fruits and vegetables. The carotenoids most commonly found in vegetables are listed in table 1.6 along with common sources of these compounds. Fruits and vegetables that are high in carotenoids appear to protect humans against certain cancers, heart disease, and age-related macular degeneration.

Polyphenolic compounds are natural components of a wide variety of plants. Food sources rich in polyphenols include onions, apples, tea, red wine, red grapes, grape juice, strawberries, raspberries, blueberries, cranberries, and certain nuts (table 1.7). The average polyphenol intake in most countries has not been precisely determined largely because no food database currently exists for these compounds. It has been estimated that in the Dutch diet, a subset of flavonoids (flavonols and flavones) provides 23 mg/day. These small amounts, however, may have significant effects.

Polyphenols can be classified as nonflavonoids and flavonoids. The flavonoids quercetin and catechins are the most extensively studied polyphenols relative to absorption and metabolism. Green tea is a good source of catechins.

COMMON CLASSES OF PHYTONUTRIENTS

Carotenoids

Flavonoids (polyphenols) including isoflavones (phytoestrogens)

Inositol phosphates (phytates)

Isothiocyanates and indoles

Lignans (phytoestrogens)

Phenols and cyclic compounds

Saponins

Sulfides and thiols

Terpenes

TABLE 1.6 Carotenoids and Their Food Sources

Carotenoid	Common food sources
α-carotene	Carrots
ß-carotene	Orange and yellow vegetables (e.g., sweet potato, pumpkin, carrots, squash) and leafy green vegetables (e.g., spinach, kale)
ß-cryptoxanthin	Citrus, peaches, apricots
Lutein	Leafy greens (e.g., kale, spinach, turnip greens)
Lycopene	Tomatoes, pink grapefruit, watermelon, guava
Zeaxanthin	Green vegetables, eggs, citrus

TABLE 1.7 Polyphenols and Their Food Sources

Nonflavonoids	Sources
Ellagic acid	Strawberries, blueberries, raspberries
Coumarins	Bell peppers, bok choy, cereal grains, broccoli
Flavonoids	**Sources**
Anthocyanins	Red fruits
Catechins	Tea, wine
Flavanones	Citrus
Flavones	Fruits and vegetables
Flavonols	Fruits, vegetables, tea, wine
Isoflavones	Soybeans

Recommended Intakes of Nutrients

We previously described the various nutrients and their functions. In the next chapter, we discuss appropriate food and beverage choices that will provide the required amounts of nutrients and guidelines for healthy eating. In subsequent chapters, we examine the energy requirements of exercise and the specific needs for macronutrients and micronutrients in the athletic population. We now explain the basis for consumption recommendations of nutrients. We discuss how recommendations for certain nutrients are established and how these are translated into practical advice for the public. Finally, we discuss how to assess whether a person or group is achieving the recommendations.

As mentioned earlier, nonessential nutrients can be synthesized in the body and essential nutrients cannot. This terminology is sometimes confusing because a nutrient that is essential for the body can be classified as nonessential because it can be synthesized within the body. To avoid confusion, nutritionists often prefer the terms *indispensable* (essential) and *dispensable* (nonessential). In this book, we use the terms *essential* and *nonessential*.

Although Hippocrates practiced a form of dietetic medicine in 400 BC, this area has evolved exponentially over the past 200 to 250 years. In ancient times, people were already aware that certain food components could prevent disease or be used to treat diseases. But only during the past two centuries have some nutrients been recognized as essential for human life. Scurvy was a disease common among sailors, pirates, and others aboard ships at sea longer than perishable fruits and vegetables could be stored. In 1740, British naval surgeon James Lind discovered that the consumption of citrus fruits by sailors could prevent and cure scurvy. Other shipboard foods and medicine did not have this effect. Although scurvy was not attributed to a deficiency in vitamin C at that time, the essentiality of certain nutrients for the maintenance of health was later established.

Tragic studies with prisoners in Nazi death camps have revealed the importance of various vitamins and minerals. Prisoners received a diet deficient in a certain vitamin or mineral, and their health status was recorded. With diets deficient in certain nutrients, specific diseases developed and ultimately resulted in death. In early studies with rats, diets deficient in one or more nutrients retarded growth, and the animals experienced specific disease symptoms. But when the animals were subsequently fed with the missing nutrient, they recovered completely and growth was promoted. The nutrients that exhibited these health effects were classified as essential. According to more recent definitions (Harper 1999), a nutrient is considered essential if it meets the following criteria:

- The substance is required in the diet for growth, health, and survival.
- Absence of the substance from the diet or inadequate intake results in characteristic signs of a deficiency, disease, and ultimately death.
- Growth failure and characteristic signs of deficiency are prevented only by the nutrient or a specific precursor of it and not by other substances.
- Below some critical level of intake of the nutrient, growth response and severity of signs of deficiency are proportional to the amount consumed.

- The substance is not synthesized in the body and is therefore required for some critical function throughout life.

Some nutrients are classified as conditionally essential (or conditionally indispensable). This term was introduced in 1984 because some nutrients that were normally not essential seemed to become essential under certain conditions. Conditionally essential nutrients must be supplied exogenously to people that do not synthesize them in adequate amounts. Deficiencies can be the result of defects in the synthesis of certain nutrients or a temporary increased need for certain nutrients. An example of defective synthesis is a genetic defect in the synthesis of carnitine. Without carnitine supplementation, people with this condition experience muscle-wasting disease (myopathy). When carnitine is supplemented, however, the condition is corrected. An example of increased need can been seen in surgical patients in an intensive care unit who usually have lower than normal plasma and muscle glutamine concentrations. These deficits are associated with negative nitrogen balance,

ESSENTIAL (INDISPENSABLE) NUTRIENTS

Amino acids

- Histidine
- Isoleucine
- Leucine
- Lysine
- Methionine
- Phenylalanine
- Threonine
- Tryptophan
- Valine

Fatty acids

- α-Linolenic
- Linoleic

Minerals

- Calcium
- Chloride
- Magnesium
- Phosphorus
- Potassium
- Sodium

Trace minerals

- Chromium
- Copper
- Iodine
- Iron
- Manganese
- Molybdenum
- Selenium
- Zinc

Ultratrace elements

- Arsenic
- Boron
- Cobalt
- Nickel
- Silicon
- Vanadium

Vitamins and choline (which is an essential vitamin-like nutrient)

- Biotin
- Choline
- Folic acid
- Niacin
- Pantothenic acid
- Riboflavin
- Thiamin
- Vitamin A
- Vitamin B_6 (pyridoxine)
- Vitamin B_{12} (cobalamin)
- Vitamin C (ascorbic acid)
- Vitamin D
- Vitamin E
- Vitamin K

Water

decreased protein synthesis, and increased protein breakdown, which result in muscle wasting. The patients improve when glutamine is supplemented. In these examples, carnitine and glutamine are classified as conditionally essential nutrients.

Development of Recommended Intakes

The list of nutrients classified as essential or indispensable is quite extensive (see the sidebar). For many centuries, people have tried to define the minimum and optimum intakes of various nutrients. In 1941, the first Food and Nutrition Board was formed in the United States. In 1943, dietary standards for evaluating nutritional intakes of large populations and for planning agricultural production were published. Since then, the guidelines have been revised several times. Initially, reference values for 10 nutrients were established. Current guidelines in the United States and Canada, which were established between 1997 and 2004, cover 46 nutrients.

When the first set of **recommended dietary allowances (RDAs)** was created in 1941, the primary goal was to prevent diseases caused by nutrient deficiencies. The RDAs were originally intended to evaluate and plan for nutritional adequacies in groups such as the armed forces and children in school lunch programs rather than to determine individuals' nutrient needs. But, because the RDAs were essentially the only nutrient values available, they began to be used in other ways. Health professionals often used RDAs to size up the diets of patients or clients. Statistically speaking, RDAs would prevent deficiency diseases in 97% of a population, but there was no scientific basis that RDAs would meet the needs of a single person.

It was evident that the RDAs were not addressing individual needs and new science needed to be included. Therefore, the Food and Nutrition Board sought to redefine nutrient requirements and develop specific nutrient recommendations for individuals and groups. Along with these changes, concepts such as tolerable upper intakes and adequate intakes emerged to meet individuals' needs. A more recent development was the recommended range of macronutrient intakes associated with reduced risk of chronic metabolic and cardiovascular disease while providing sufficient essential nutrients.

RDAs and various national dietary guidelines are no longer focused only on preventing deficiency diseases such as scurvy or beriberi; they are also aimed at reducing the risk of diet-related chronic conditions such as **coronary heart disease (CHD)**, diabetes, hypertension, and **osteoporosis**. The guidelines have also become more specific and have been developed for various sex and age groups and for pregnant and lactating women; different groups have different reference values.

Current Recommended Intakes

The framework for a set of new recommendations is the **dietary reference intake (DRI)**. The DRI has been released in stages over the past decade. Under the umbrella of the DRI, five standards have been developed: the estimated average requirement (EAR), the acceptable macronutrient distribution range (AMDR), the recommended dietary allowance (RDA), the adequate intake (AI), and the tolerable upper intake level (UL). Establishment of these reference values requires that a criterion of nutritional adequacy be carefully chosen for each nutrient and that the population for whom these values apply be carefully defined.

The **estimated average requirement (EAR)** represents the amount of a nutrient that is deemed sufficient to meet the needs of the average individual in a certain age and gender group (see figure 1.6). At an intake level equal to the EAR, half of a specified group would not have their nutritional needs met. This is equivalent to saying that randomly chosen individuals from the population would have a 50% chance of having their requirements met at this intake level.

The RDA is an estimate of the minimum daily average dietary intake level that meets the nutrient requirements of nearly all (97%-98%) healthy people in a particular life stage and gender group. The RDA is intended to be used as a goal for daily intake by individuals because this value estimates an intake level that has a high probability of meeting the requirement of a randomly chosen individual (about 97.5%). The process for setting the RDA depends on being able to set an EAR and estimating the variance of the requirement itself. Note that if an EAR cannot be set due to limitations of the data available, no RDA can be set.

The RDA is a safe excess of nutrients that prevents nutritional deficiencies in most of the population. When the distribution of a requirement among individuals in a group can be assumed to be approximately normal (or symmetrical) and a standard deviation (SD) of requirement ($SD_{requirement}$)

DEFINITIONS

Dietary Reference Intake (DRI)

The new standards for nutrient recommendations that can be used to plan and assess diets for healthy people. Think of DRI as the umbrella term that includes the following values.

Acceptable Macronutrient Distribution Range (AMDR)

The AMDR is the range of intake for a specific energy source (i.e., carbohydrate, fat, or protein) that is associated with reduced risk of chronic disease and provides essential nutrients. If a person's intake is outside of the AMDR, there is a potential for increased risk of chronic diseases and insufficient intake of essential nutrients.

Estimated Average Requirement (EAR)

An EAR is a nutrient intake value that is estimated to meet the requirement of half of the healthy individuals in a group. It is used to assess nutritional adequacy of intakes of population groups. In addition, EARs are used to calculate RDAs.

Recommended Dietary Allowance (RDA)

The RDA is the daily dietary intake level that is sufficient to meet the nutrient requirement of 97% to 98% of all healthy people in a group. This value is a goal for individuals and is based on the EAR. If an EAR cannot be set, no RDA value can be proposed.

Adequate Intake (AI)

This value is used when an RDA cannot be determined. It is a recommended daily intake level based on an observed or experimentally determined approximation of nutrient intake for a group (or groups) of healthy people.

Tolerable Upper Intake Level (UL)

The UL is the highest level of daily nutrient intake that is likely to pose no risks of adverse health effects to almost all individuals in the general population. As intake increases above the UL, the risk of adverse effects increases.

can be determined, the EAR can be used to set the RDA as follows:

$$\text{RDA} = \text{EAR} + 2 \times 3\ \text{SD}_{\text{requirement}}$$

The RDA is intended to be used as a goal for daily intake by individuals and will vary depending on age and gender (and, for women, whether they are pregnant or lactating); they do not apply to other populations or to conditions that may have specific requirements. The RDA is based on the median heights and weights of a population; therefore, groups of adults who weigh more or less than this median may have slightly higher or lower requirements, respectively. In addition, stress, disease, injury, and total energy expenditure can influence the need for certain nutrients. RDAs are currently available for energy intake, protein, 11 vitamins, and seven minerals (see appendixes C, D, and E).

When available scientific evidence to estimate an EAR is insufficient, an AI will be set. People should use the AI as a goal for intake when no RDA exists. The AI is derived through experimental or observational data that show a mean intake that appears to sustain a desired indicator of health, such as calcium retention in bone for most members of a population. AIs have been set for two B vitamins, the vitamin-like choline, vitamin D, and some minerals such as calcium and fluoride (see appendix C).

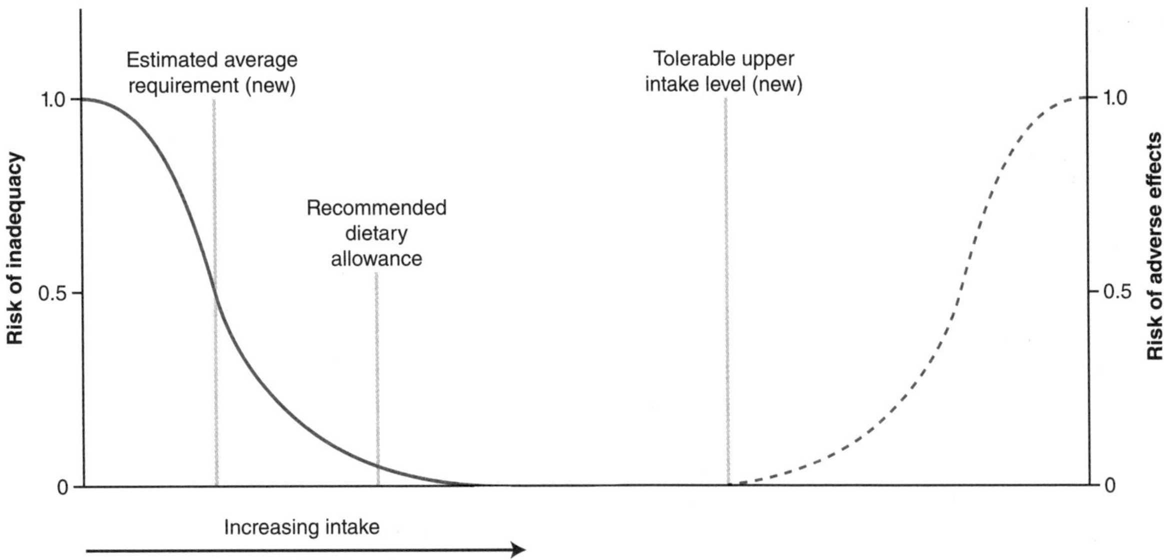

Figure 1.6 Risk of inadequacy and risk of adverse effects at increasing levels of intake.

The **upper limit (UL)** is the maximum level of daily nutrient intake that is unlikely to pose health risks to the greatest number of individuals in the group for whom it is designed (see figure 1.6). The UL is not intended to be a recommended level of intake; no benefit has been established for individuals to consume nutrients at levels above the RDA or AI. For most nutrients, the UL refers to total intakes from food, fortified food, and nutrient supplements. The need for setting the UL grew out of the increased practice of fortifying foods with nutrients and the popularity of dietary supplements that resulted in high intakes of some nutrients. In excess, some nutrients can be toxic.

The **acceptable macronutrient distribution range (AMDR)** is the range of intake for a dietary energy source (i.e., carbohydrate, fat, or protein) that at the lower end of the range will provide adequate intake of essential nutrients (such as essential fatty acids or essential amino acids) but below the upper end of the range will be associated with reduced risk of chronic disease. If an individual's intake is outside of the AMDR, for example, eating too much fat or too little protein, there is a potential of increasing the risk of chronic metabolic or cardiovascular diseases or getting insufficient intakes of the essential amino acids, respectively.

DRIs are mainly intended for diet planning. Specifically, a diet should aim to meet any RDA (or AI) set and not exceed the UL. DRIs are based on averages of large populations and thus are not designed to detect nutrient deficiencies in individuals. A person whose intake of a particular nutrient is below the recommendations may not be deficient in that nutrient. Only a clinical and biochemical examination can determine whether a person has a nutritional deficiency. Comparison of a person's intake to the RDA, however, can help determine whether the person is at risk for a deficiency. To determine whether a person's nutrient intake meets the RDA, it should be calculated over a period of 5 to 8 days. A person whose diet does not contain the full RDA on one day is not necessarily at risk for deficiencies because the inadequacy can be compensated the next day. Note that the RDA does not reflect the minimum requirements but rather a safe excess intake. Of course, people who do not consistently take in the RDA for a number of nutrients have a chance of becoming deficient over time. In the case of vitamin D, requirements have been determined based on bone health, but it is now recognized that the requirement may be higher for optimal immune function (see chapter 13 for further details). Another issue with vitamin D is that, unlike all the other fat- and water-soluble vitamins, it (specifically vitamin D_3 or cholecalciferol) can be synthesized in the skin, from cholesterol, when exposure from sunlight ultraviolet B radiation is adequate. Evidence indicates the synthesis of vitamin D from sunlight exposure is regulated by a negative feedback loop that prevents toxicity, but because of uncertainty about the cancer risk from overexposure to sunlight, no recommendations have been issued by national bodies regarding the amount of sunlight exposure required to meet vitamin D requirements. Accordingly, the RDA of vitamin D for adults (5 µg or 200 IU in the European Union, 10 µg or 400 IU in the United Kingdom, and 15 µg or 600 IU in the United States) assumes that no synthesis occurs and all vitamin D is from food intake, although that will rarely occur in practice. Studies indicate that in the winter months, many people (including athletes) can become deficient in vitamin D, and this may be partly responsible for the higher incidences of colds and flus during the winter months (He et al. 2016). Some countries, including the United Kingdom, now advise a daily vitamin D intake of up to 25 µg or 1,000 IU during wintertime, and there are ongoing debates about the need for fortification of foods with vitamin D. Some countries, including several in Europe and the United States, encourage fortification of selected foods (usually milk, margarine, and cereal products).

RDAs do not account for unusual requirements caused by disease or environmental stress. In addition, the data used to determine the RDAs often did not include athletes, or the activity levels of the subjects were not reported. Therefore, the RDAs may not be an accurate means of evaluating the nutritional needs of people engaged in regular strenuous exercise.

Simplifying Nutrient Reference Values for Food Label Recommendations

The reference values used to determine RDAs are age and gender specific, but for food-labeling purposes, an additional set of reference values had to be produced. Packages must be the same for men and women and for children and adults, so the RDA values had to be condensed into acceptable recommendations for all groups (except for children under 4 years of age and pregnant or lactating women, for whom the RDAs are still the standard). Originally, product labels contained U.S. RDAs, but these have been replaced by **daily values (DVs)**.

The U.S. RDAs, which were based on RDAs, were developed by the FDA in 1973 for use in food labeling. The U.S. RDAs did not vary by age and gender. The FDA usually picked the highest RDA levels across all age and gender groups to determine the U.S. RDAs. These values were adopted not only for simplicity in food packaging but also to reflect advances in scientific knowledge with respect to essential nutrient requirements.

The DVs used today are based on two sets of references: (1) the reference daily intakes (RDIs; a new name for the U.S. RDAs), which make up most of the DVs and provide dietary references for essential vitamins and minerals, and (2) the **daily reference values (DRVs)**, which are standards for proteins and various dietary components that have no RDAs or other established nutrient standards (e.g., cholesterol, total fat, carbohydrate, dietary fiber, sodium, and potassium) (see table 1.8). On food labels (known as nutrition facts labels), all reference values are listed as DVs, but they can be either DRVs or RDIs. On current food labeling, the percentage of daily value is the percentage of RDI or DRV available in a single serving. For further details of nutrition facts labels and how they should be used see chapter 2.

Differences Between Countries and Organizations

The United Nations and the European Union, as well as many individual countries, have formulated recommendations with respect to the amount of each nutrient that should be consumed. Therefore,

TABLE 1.8 Daily Reference Values

Food component	DRV
Total fat	Less than 65 g (30% of energy intake)
Saturated fat	Less than 20 g (10% of energy intake)
Cholesterol	Less than 300 mg
Total carbohydrate Sugars	300 g (60% of energy intake) Less than 10% of energy intake
Dietary fiber	25 g
Sodium	Less than 2,400 mg
Potassium	3,500 mg
Protein	50 g (10% of energy intake)

DRV based on 8.4 MJ (2,000 kcal) guideline.

definitions of RDA differ slightly in different countries (see appendixes C, D, and E). In the United Kingdom (appendix D) and Germany, the RDA is called the **reference nutrient intake (RNI)**, and in Australia it called the RDI (appendix E). Canada now uses the same system as the United States, and Canada's RNI has been replaced by the DRI.

United Kingdom

In the United Kingdom, the RNI, which is similar to the original RDA, is the level of intake required to meet the known nutritional needs of more than 97.5% of healthy persons. The EAR in the United Kingdom is similar to the EAR in the United States, but unlike the United States, the United Kingdom also has a lower reference nutrient intake (LRNI) value. The LRNI is the amount of a nutrient that is virtually certain to be inadequate (it is defined as the amount of a nutrient that is enough for the 2.5% of people who have low requirements). (Notably, the average intake of the trace element selenium falls well below the LRNI.) In the United Kingdom, estimated requirements for certain groups of the population are based on advice that was given by the Committee on Medical Aspects of Food and Nutrition Policy (COMA) back in the early 1990s. COMA examined the available scientific evidence and estimated nutritional requirements of various groups within the UK population. These were published in the 1991 report Dietary Reference Values for Food Energy and Nutrients for the United Kingdom. Since this time, COMA has been superseded by the Scientific Advisory Committee on Nutrition (SACN). SACN will likely review the UK nutritional requirements soon because they are now more than 105 years old. In recent years, SACN has been focusing on nutrients about which there is cause for concern (e.g., iron, folate, selenium, calcium, and vitamin D as well as energy and carbohydrate).

Australia

Australia followed guidelines that were referred to as the RDIs for use in Australia. The last version of the RDIs was published in 1991 by the National Health and Medical Research Council in Australia. These RDIs were later adopted in New Zealand as well. In July 1997, a workshop of invited experts, including representatives from New Zealand, was held in Sydney to discuss the need for a revision of the 1991 RDIs. This was the beginning of the development of a new set of reference values for each nutrient; these are now referred to as nutrient reference values (NRVs), an umbrella term that includes the EAR, RDI, AI, and UL. The NRVs were further updated in 2005.

In contrast to the U.S. and Canadian approach, the method used by Australia and New Zealand retained the traditional concept of adequate physiological or metabolic function or avoidance of deficiency states as the prime reference point for establishing the EARs and RDIs and dealt separately with the issue of chronic disease prevention.

World Health Organization

The World Health Organization (WHO), the Food and Agriculture Organization of the United Nations (FAO), and the International Atomic Energy Agency (IAEA), in their publication *Trace Elements in Human Nutrition and Health* (WHO 1996), use the term *basal requirement* to indicate the level of intake needed to prevent pathologically relevant and clinically detectable signs of a dietary inadequacy.

Although recommendations can provide guidance on nutrient requirements, they are not a practical way of informing people about appropriate food choices. For example, how do people know whether they are consuming 0.8 g/kg of body weight of protein per day or meeting the RDIs for calcium, vitamin A, and other essential minerals and vitamins? Achieving a healthy, balanced diet is discussed in chapter 2.

Analyzing Dietary Intakes

People must analyze their diets to determine whether their nutrient intakes align with the previously discussed guidelines. Analyzing dietary intakes can be useful for several reasons. For example, the average intake in a group of athletes can be studied, and the data can be used in conjunction with biochemical or anthropometric data to determine whether their diets are adequate. Dietary intake data can also be used in conjunction with a medical report or to explain the incidence or prevalence of health problems. Such measurements can also be used for educational purposes, and the efficacy of nutritional advice or intervention programs can be investigated. Several methods have been developed to measure dietary intake (see table 1.9), and each method has advantages and disadvantages.

After the nutrient intake information is obtained, it can be compared with the recommendations. A simple but not especially accurate comparison can be made with a guide such as the food guide pyramid (see chapter 2). When a 3- to 7-day dietary survey is completed, however, the intake can be analyzed in detail. To calculate the intake of specific nutrients, food labels or one of many food composition databases can be used. In the United States, the major source of information

TABLE 1.9 Methods to Estimate Nutrient Intake

Method	Short description	Advantages	Disadvantages
Prospective methods			
3-day dietary survey	Recording all foods consumed for 3 days	• Fairly accurate • Inexpensive • Provides detailed information • Provides information about eating habits	• May not represent normal diet • Tends to underestimate energy intake
3-day weighed food record	Weighing and recording all foods consumed for 3 days	• Accurate • Inexpensive • Provides detailed information • Provides information about eating habits	• Demanding for respondent • Potential compliance problems • May not represent normal diet • Tends to underestimate energy intake
7-day dietary survey	Recording all foods consumed for 7 days	• Fairly accurate • Inexpensive • Provides detailed information • Provides information about eating habits	• Demanding for respondent • Compliance may diminish after 4 days • May not represent normal diet • Tends to underestimate energy intake
7-day weighed food record	Weighing and recording all foods consumed for 7 days	• Accurate • Inexpensive • Provides detailed information • Provides information about eating habits	• Highly demanding for respondent • Compliance may diminish after 4 days • May not represent normal diet • Tends to underestimate energy intake
Duplicate food collections	Saving a duplicate of each food for chemical analysis	• Probably the most accurate method • Provides detailed information	• Expensive (analysis) • Time consuming • May affect food choice • Demanding for respondent • Likely to underestimate food intake
Retrospective methods			
24-hour recall	Questionnaire or interview to assess dietary intake in the previous 24 hours	• Good response rate • Relatively easy • Inexpensive • Can be used to rank nutrient intakes in groups of people	• May not represent usual food intake • Memory bias • Underestimates total energy intake • Does not provide quantitative data
Food frequency	Questionnaire or interview with questions about the frequency of intake of certain foods	• Good response rate • Relatively easy • Inexpensive • Can be used to rank nutrient intakes in groups of people in qualitative terms	• Memory bias • Underestimates total energy intake • Does not provide quantitative data • Overestimates actual energy intake at low energy intakes and underestimates actual energy intake at high energy intakes • May not represent normal food intake
Diet history	Combination of 24-hour recall and food frequency questionnaire	• Can be used to rank nutrient intakes in groups of people	• Requires trained interviewer • Takes longer to complete than 24-hour recall or food frequency questionnaire

is the U.S. Department of Agriculture (USDA) Nutrient Database, which is available online (U.S. Department of Agriculture 2003). Various software packages and some online programs use this database or other databases to calculate food intake. In all cases, the exact amount and kind of food must be recorded. If a food is not included in the database, an appropriate substitute should be chosen. Most programs allow the user to add new products to the database, which can be done using information on the food label. The software will usually produce an average intake over 24 hours for all macronutrients and micronutrients. These values can then be compared with the recommended amounts.

Three-Day Food Record

The 3-day dietary survey is a relatively simple and reasonably accurate way to determine the total daily energy intake and the quality of food. The 3-day log should represent a normal eating pattern. Inclusion of two weekdays and one weekend day is recommended. Calculations of energy intake from records of daily food consumption are usually within 10% of the actual energy intake. This method provides reliable results for the intake of some nutrients, such as carbohydrate and water, but longer periods may be required to get a more reliable classification of individual intake for nutrients such as cholesterol and fat and some of the micronutrients.

To obtain an accurate measure of food, people can use common measuring tools such as a ruler to measure the length, width, and height of food; standard measuring cups and measuring spoons to determine volume; and a scale to determine weight to the nearest gram. Weighed food records are accurate, but people must be motivated to log food by weight. Poor compliance has been reported with weighed food records, and the use of household measuring devices is often the preferred method. Weighed food records, however, may be the method of choice for highly motivated athletes.

All foods consumed, including beverages, should be recorded using a blank 3-day food log (a sample entry is shown in figure 1.7). When completing a diet record, people should always keep the sheets nearby and record the food while consuming it. When the food log is completed, the energy and nutrient intakes can be calculated using a software package or a food table. People should use a software package or food table for the country in which they live, because many products are specific to particular countries.

Most people are only vaguely aware of what they eat. Without instruction, food records lack sufficient detail to be useful for most research purposes. Errors occur mainly because of memory failures. In general, common foods are recorded accurately, but uncommon foods are sometimes poorly recorded. Most errors are made in reporting the frequency of consumption. Errors in estimating portion size are common as well. If food is not weighed, the mass of various foods may be considerably under- or overestimated. Errors are sometimes as large as 50% for foods and 20% for nutrients (Burke and Deakin 2000; Shils, Olson, Shike, and Ross 1999). Training and instructing the people who are recording food intake can reduce errors, but the instructions should be repeated several times. On an individual level, the 3-day food survey is generally accepted as one of the best methods to assess nutritional intake. But this method also has disadvantages. Overweight people tend to underestimate their portion sizes, whereas underweight people tend to overestimate portions (Johansson et al. 1998). People may not report their food intakes accurately, which makes coding the specific food type difficult. For example, writing "four potatoes" is not sufficiently informative. Were the potatoes large or small? Were they boiled, baked, fried, or raw? Were the skins removed? Some food records may be illegible, which introduces more coding errors. Therefore, people must be carefully instructed and asked to provide as much detail as possible.

Seven-Day Food Record

The 7-day dietary survey is the same as the 3-day survey, but the recording period is longer. The

Time	Place	Food or beverage	Preparation method	Amount
7:00 a.m.	Home	Corn Flakes, Kellogg's		1 small bowl (35 g cereal)
		Whole milk		200 ml (7 fl oz)
9:00 a.m.	Office	Coffee	Filter	240 ml (8 fl oz)
		Sugar		1 teaspoon

Figure 1.7 Sample of an accurate food diary.

extended recording time may allow for a more reliable classification of a person's normal diet and nutrient intake. The 7-day survey includes all weekdays and weekend days. The disadvantage of this method is that people may become tired of recording and forget to write down foods consumed, which results in a less accurate nutritional assessment. Often, lack of compliance is reported after about 4 days. Besides the 3-day and 7-day options, dietary surveys of other lengths (e.g., 5 days, 1 month, 12 months) have been used.

Duplicate Food Collections

The duplicate food collections method, which involves preparing two portions of food and saving a duplicate of everything that is eaten, is a highly accurate recording method. The duplicate portions are collected and put in a blender for chemical analysis of the nutrient content. This method, which is used mainly for research purposes, is extremely expensive because of the costs of the chemical analyses, especially when many nutrients are investigated. The method also places a burden on the individual and is likely to affect food choices. This method may result in underreporting of food intake.

Twenty-Four-Hour Recall

The most common technique of assessing food intake is the 24-hour recall. A trained interviewer asks participants on one or more occasions to describe the food, drinks, and dietary supplements they consumed during the previous 24 hours. The data obtained may include information about the time of food intake, preparation of the food, and the eating environment.

The advantages of the 24-hour recall technique are that it is easy to administer, time efficient, and inexpensive. Disadvantages include the likelihood of underreporting, even when participants are interviewed by a skilled dietitian; the underestimation of energy and nutrient intake, sometimes by as much as 20%; and the tendency of overweight people to underestimate their portions (underweight persons tend to overestimate portions) (Johansson et al. 1998). In addition, this technique relies heavily on memory, which makes it unsuitable for certain groups, such as the elderly.

The data obtained from 24-hour recalls are more accurate when they are repeated several times at random. This approach also corrects somewhat for day-to-day variations in food intake. Obtaining more than one 24-hour recall within a week and including at least one weekend day is the preferred method. One recall per week is unlikely to represent usual intake. The 24-hour recall method is a reasonably good way to estimate nutrient intake in a group of people, but it is less valuable for individual use. It can, however, provide a foundation for pursuing a more detailed recording method.

Food Frequency Questionnaire

A food frequency questionnaire (see figure 1.8) is often used to get a general picture of someone's patterns of food intake. A person responds to a series of questions about the frequency of food intake: How often do you eat red meat? How often do you eat fruit? How often do you drink milk? Questions about portion size, food preparation, and supplement use can be included, but their use is not a standard procedure. A problem with this method is that the products mentioned in the questionnaire may not represent the respondent's actual food intake.

The food frequency questionnaire is a relatively easy and quick method, but it does not itemize intake on a specific day. The information obtained is qualitative rather than quantitative. The food frequency questionnaire is regularly used in clinical or research settings. If investigators are interested in only one food item or food group, the food frequency questionnaire can be extremely useful. Food frequency questionnaires have been developed for specific populations to address intakes in various cultures and in populations of differing ages (e.g., children).

Diet History

A diet history provides general information about dietary habits and patterns. This technique was originally described by Burke in 1947 and combines the 24-hour recall with a food frequency questionnaire. Combining these different methods usually gives a better view of a person's dietary habits by asking questions such as the following: Do you always have breakfast? Do you skip lunch? Did you drink milk as an adolescent? A diet history can provide information about changes in dietary habits, including seasonal changes. A diet history takes about 20 minutes to complete. This method requires an interviewer who is a well-trained dietitian.

	Once a day	Twice or more a day	Once a week	Twice or more a week	Once a month	Twice or more a month
Milk						
• Whole		✓				
• Reduced fat			✓			
• Nonfat						
Yogurt						
• Whole					✓	
• Reduced fat						
• Nonfat						
Cheese						
• Hard		✓				
• Soft				✓		
• Reduced fat						
Ice cream						
• Regular					✓	
• Reduced fat						

Figure 1.8 Food frequency questionnaire.

Key Points

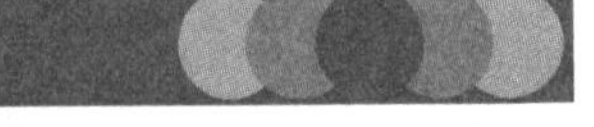

- Food provides nutrients that have physiological or biochemical functions in the body.
- Nutrients are usually divided into six different categories: carbohydrate, fat, protein, vitamins, minerals, and water.
- Functions of nutrients include promotion of growth and development, provision of energy, and regulation of metabolism.
- Among the several different classes of carbohydrate are sugars, starches, and fiber.
- Fiber, although it is not absorbed, has several important functions, including maintaining normal gut function. For most people, the recommended intake would be 20 to 35 g/day, but the typical fiber intake in Western countries is only 14 to 15 g/day.
- There are several classes of fats, including fatty acids, triacylglycerols, and lipoproteins. Triacylglycerol is the main storage form.
- Amino acids are the building blocks of proteins. Of the 20 amino acids normally found in dietary protein, humans can synthesize 11. Those that can be synthesized are called nonessential amino acids. Those that cannot be synthesized and must be derived from the diet are called essential amino acids.
- Proteins that contain all the essential amino acids are called complete proteins or high-quality proteins. Proteins that are deficient in one or more amino acids are called incomplete proteins, and they are commonly referred to as low-quality proteins.
- Water is an extremely important nutrient. The adult body is about 60% water by weight. Two-thirds of the water is intracellular fluid, and the remaining one-third is extracellular fluid.

- Vitamins, minerals, and trace elements are micronutrients. Vitamins are organic compounds, and minerals and trace elements are inorganic compounds.
- Phytonutrients are certain organic components of plants that are thought to promote human health but are nonnutrients. They differ from vitamins because they are not considered essential nutrients, meaning that people who lack them will not develop nutritional deficiencies.
- Essential nutrients cannot be synthesized in the body, but they are required for growth, health, and survival. Inadequate intake of essential nutrients results in characteristic signs of a deficiency, disease, and ultimately death.
- Humans have essential requirements for more than 40 nutrients. Nonessential nutrients can be synthesized in the body from their precursors.
- Several methods are used to assess food intake and diet composition. These methods include diet histories, 24-hour recalls, food frequency questionnaires, self-reported food records, and weighed food records. The methods differ substantially in their accuracy and practicality.

Recommended Readings

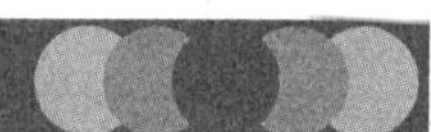

Bender, D.A., and A.E. Bender. 1997. *Nutrition. A reference handbook.* Oxford: Oxford University Press.

Food and Nutrition Board. 2005. *Dietary reference intakes for energy, carbohydrate, fiber, fat, fatty acids, cholesterol, protein, and amino acids (macronutrients).* Washington, DC: National Academies Press.

Gibney, M.J., I. Macdonald, and H. Roche, eds. 2008. *Nutrition and metabolism (the Nutrition Society textbook).* Oxford: Blackwell Science.

Mann, J., and A.S. Truswell. 2002. *Essentials of human nutrition.* Oxford: Oxford University Press.

Shils, M.E., J.A. Olson, M. Shike, A.C. Ross, B. Caballero, and R.J. Cousins, eds. 2005. *Modern nutrition in health and disease.* Baltimore: Williams and Wilkins.

UK Government. 2016. *Government dietary recommendations: The eatwell guide.* www.gov.uk/government/publications/the-eatwell-guide

U.S. Department of Agriculture. 2005. *Dietary guidelines for Americans, 2005.* Chapter 7, Carbohydrate. https://health.gov/dietaryguidelines/dga2005/document/default.htm

U.S. Department of Agriculture. 2015. *2015-2020 dietary guidelines for Americans.* https://health.gov/dietaryguidelines/2015/guidelines/

2

Healthy Eating

Objectives

After studying this chapter, you should be able to do the following:

- Discuss the basis of the guidelines for establishing a balanced, healthy diet
- Understand that for some sports, the dietary guidelines are not different from those given to the general population
- Understand why excessive intakes of some nutrients or certain nutrient subgroups and nonessential nutrients can have harmful effects on health
- Understand why diets that are deficient in some nonessential nutrients will not deliver what is needed for optimal function and health
- Understand the current guidelines for a healthy diet
- Appreciate the differences in the dietary guidelines from different countries
- Understand the regulations for food labeling and health claims
- Understand the effects of food processing

In the previous chapter, we described the various nutrients and their functions. When most people sit down for meals, they do not think about the nutrients; instead, they are concerned about the taste, texture, and smell of the food. Although many people recognize the importance of the nutritional value of food and may be aware of some of the health implications of what they eat and drink, food choices are based on many factors, including personal preferences, availability, cost, and convenience. Advice is offered by numerous government departments (e.g., health, agriculture) and other agencies (e.g., World Health Organization) about foods or combinations of foods that will deliver certain amounts of nutrients. This chapter explores the dietary recommendations in various countries. We discuss how recommendations for certain nutrients and foods are established and how these are translated into practical advice for the public. Although the focus of this book is sport nutrition and the dietary and supplement requirements of athletes engaged in sports that require endurance, strength, power, and speed, not all sports involve these characteristics (e.g., lawn bowls, bowling, curling, darts, golf, snooker, target shooting). The dietary requirements of competitors in such sports are the same as those for the general population, so it is important to know the general requirements and how they can be attained through appropriate food and beverage choices. In addition, when athletes retire from competition, their dietary needs will change. In this chapter, we will examine how a healthy diet relates to long-term health, avoiding weight gain, and reducing the risk of chronic cardiovascular and metabolic diseases. This includes a discussion about nutrition in the general population, which assumes relatively low physical activity levels, and how people can achieve a healthy diet through appropriate food choices and eating to maintain energy balance. In subsequent chapters, we will discuss the energy requirements of exercise and the specific needs for macronutrients and micronutrients in those who are more athletic. Food choices and supplements that help maintain robust immunity and reduce infection risk are discussed in chapter 13.

Health Effects of Consuming Excess Nutrients

Consuming adequate amounts of essential nutrients does not negate the potentially harmful health effects of the foods that we consume. Excessive intake of some nutrients (e.g., carbohydrate, fat) or certain nutrient subgroups (e.g., simple **sugars**, corn syrup, saturated fats, *trans* fatty acids) and other nonessential nutrients (e.g., alcohol, **salt**) can have harmful effects on health, particularly in the long term, and increase the risk of developing chronic metabolic and cardiovascular diseases and cancer. Even the excessive consumption of vitamin or mineral supplements will have negative health effects, and this issue is covered in chapter 10. Conversely, diets that are deficient in some of the nonessential nutrients (e.g., fiber, phytonutrients) will not deliver what is needed for optimal function and health. Here we will examine these important health issues and summarize the current conclusions and recommendations.

Carbohydrate Intake and Health Effects

Carbohydrate intake varies enormously in different parts of the world. In many parts of Africa, for instance, a typical diet consists of 80% carbohydrate (as a percentage of total daily energy intake), but in the Western world, carbohydrate intake is often 40% to 50%. In Caribbean countries, carbohydrate intake averages 65%, which is closer to the recommended daily intake. A carbohydrate intake of 40% to 50% is about 300 g of carbohydrate per day in a relatively sedentary person. An athlete in a strenuous training program may consume as much as 1,000 g of carbohydrate per day. Athletes are usually encouraged to consume more than 60% of their total energy intake as carbohydrate; however, the carbohydrate needs of athletes are usually best expressed in relation to their body mass (grams of carbohydrate per kilogram of body weight) to address their needs for training and competition (see chapter 6).

There is compelling evidence that carbohydrate quality has important influences on obesity, cardiovascular disease, metabolic syndrome, and type 2 diabetes (Slyper 2013). Numerous studies indicate that dietary fiber has an important influence on satiety and that relatively high intakes of dietary fiber can reduce weight gain and protect against cardiovascular disease. Other studies have shown that vegetables and fruits protect against coronary heart disease (CHD) and whole grains protect against cardiovascular disease, type 2 diabetes, and weight gain. Sugar consumption is a proven cause of weight gain, and obesity is strongly associated with increased risk of cardiovascular and metabolic diseases. In the Western diet, about 50% of the carbohydrate intake is in the form of sugars, especially sucrose and high-fructose corn syrup. It has been suggested that the consumption of a diet high in total carbohydrate adversely affects insulin sensitivity compared with consumption of a high-fat diet. Animal studies suggest that simple sugars, particularly fructose in large amounts, can have adverse effects on insulin action, and some studies in humans seem to confirm this. Note, however, that these findings apply to a population with extremely low levels of physical activity, so these observations may not relate to the carbohydrate intake per se. Endurance athletes, who generally consume high-carbohydrate diets, display high insulin sensitivity. Furthermore, increased intake of dietary fiber appears to improve insulin action and may offer protection against type 2 diabetes.

Fiber Intake and Health Effects

In the United States and Canada, a fiber intake of 10 to 13 g per 4,200 kJ (1,000 kcal) of dietary energy intake is recommended. For most people, this intake would equal 20 to 35 g of fiber per day. The typical fiber intake in Western countries, however, is about 15 g/day for women and 18 g/day for men (Hoy and Goldman 2014). In African countries, the intake of fiber is about 40 to 150 g/day. Although earlier studies may have been confounded by the fact that populations with a high fiber intake generally were also poorer and had different nutritional habits (e.g., less meat intake), the findings of reduced cardiovascular disease incidence with high fiber intake seem to be confirmed by more recent studies that suggest that low fiber intake is associated with increased risk of cardiovascular disease (Slyper 2013). A recent meta-analysis that included 22 cohort study publications that reported total dietary fiber intake, fiber subtypes, and fiber from food sources and primary events of cardiovascular disease or CHD found that total dietary fiber intake was inversely associated with the risk of cardiovascular disease (risk ratio of 0.91 per 7g/day [95% confidence intervals (CI) 0.88 to 0.94]) and CHD (0.91 [0.87-0.94]) (Threapleton et al. 2013). Insoluble fiber and fiber from cereal and vegetable sources were inversely associated with the risk of CHD and cardiovascular disease. Fruit fiber intake was inversely associated with the risk of cardiovascular disease. Fruits, vegetables, and plant fiber have long been thought to protect against cancer. Indeed, high intake of fruits and vegetables is associated with reduced incidence of some cancers; however, this may be related not only to fiber intake but also to intake of folic acid (Willett 2000) and other phytonutrients (discussed later in this chapter). The European Prospective Investigation into Cancer and Nutrition is a prospective cohort study that includes more than 500,000 participants from 10 European countries that has examined associations between fruit, vegetable, and fiber consumption and the risk of cancer at 14 different sites (Bradbury, Appleby, and Key 2014). This large-scale study reported that the risk of cancers of the upper gastrointestinal tract was inversely associated with fruit intake but was not associated with vegetable intake. The risk of colorectal cancer was inversely associated with total fruit and vegetable and total fiber intakes, and the risk of liver cancer was also inversely associated with the total fiber intake. The risk of lung cancer among smokers was inversely associated with fruit intake but was not associated with vegetable intake. There was a borderline inverse association of fiber intake with breast cancer risk. For the other nine cancer sites studied (stomach, biliary tract, pancreas, cervix, endometrium, prostate, kidney, bladder, and lymphoma) there were no reported significant associations of risk with total fruit, vegetable, or fiber intakes.

One potential mechanism for reduced cancer risk is the reduced transit time of food (the time that food spends in the gut) due to fiber intake, which could reduce the uptake of carcinogenic substances. Another possible mechanism is that the fiber absorbs some of these carcinogenic substances. In addition, a change in fiber intake may be the result of altered nutritional habits that reduce the presence of carcinogenic substances (i.e., increased fiber intake is often accompanied by decreased fat intake). Higher fiber intake has also been associated with better weight maintenance. Increasing dietary fiber intake is often recommended because of its apparent protective effects against cancers, cardiovascular diseases, and type 2 diabetes.

Sugar Intake and Health Effects

Over the past century, the yearly intake of simple sugars has increased dramatically to approximately 50 kg (110 lb) per person, which is 25 times more than 100 years ago. This change is largely due to increased consumption of soft drinks, but consumption of candy and baked goods also contributes (figure 2.1).

Accumulating evidence indicates that the intake of large amounts of simple sugars is linked to increased risk of obesity and cardiovascular disease, but considerable debate exists about this topic (Gibson 1996; Rippe and Angelopoulos 2016; Slyper 2013). Although sugar consumption is often plotted against obesity rates and a linear correlation is shown, in the last 10 years, sugar consumption has decreased but the development of obesity has not slowed down. Also, the results of studies are not conclusive. Often, epidemiological studies are quoted to support the role of carbohydrate, specifically sugar, in increasing the prevalence of obesity and related diseases. However, a higher sugar intake is often accompanied by higher saturated fat intake and higher energy intake. Therefore, sugar could simply be an indicator of a higher energy intake. A recent analysis of food availability data in the United States confirmed that this is the case. A report by the U.S. Department of Agriculture presented data about the amount of food available for consumption between 1970 and 2014 and estimated what American food consumption was by subtracting food waste. It was found that between 1970 and 2014, food intakes from all major **food groups** increased (Bentley et al. 2017). In fact, the average total energy intake increased by 474 calories per person; however, most of this increase in energy intake (about 94%) was attributed to an increased consumption of flour, cereal products, and added fats rather than added sugars.

Given that Americans have been eating more and many have sedentary lifestyles (e.g., driving rather than walking or cycling, watching TV, playing video games), it is easy to understand how the obesity epidemic has developed. Carbohydrate and sugar intakes might not be solely to blame, but they are contributing factors.

Generally, diets low in fiber and high in simple sugars are associated with increased risk of non-insulin-dependent **diabetes mellitus** (NIDDM), or **type 2 diabetes**. This disease is characterized by resistance of different tissues to insulin, which results in various metabolic and related complications. For example, in people with type 2 diabetes, insulin-stimulated glucose uptake into tissues is impaired, and fasting blood glucose concentrations are often extremely high. Fat mobilization is normally inhibited by insulin, and reduced insulin action will therefore result in increased fatty acid

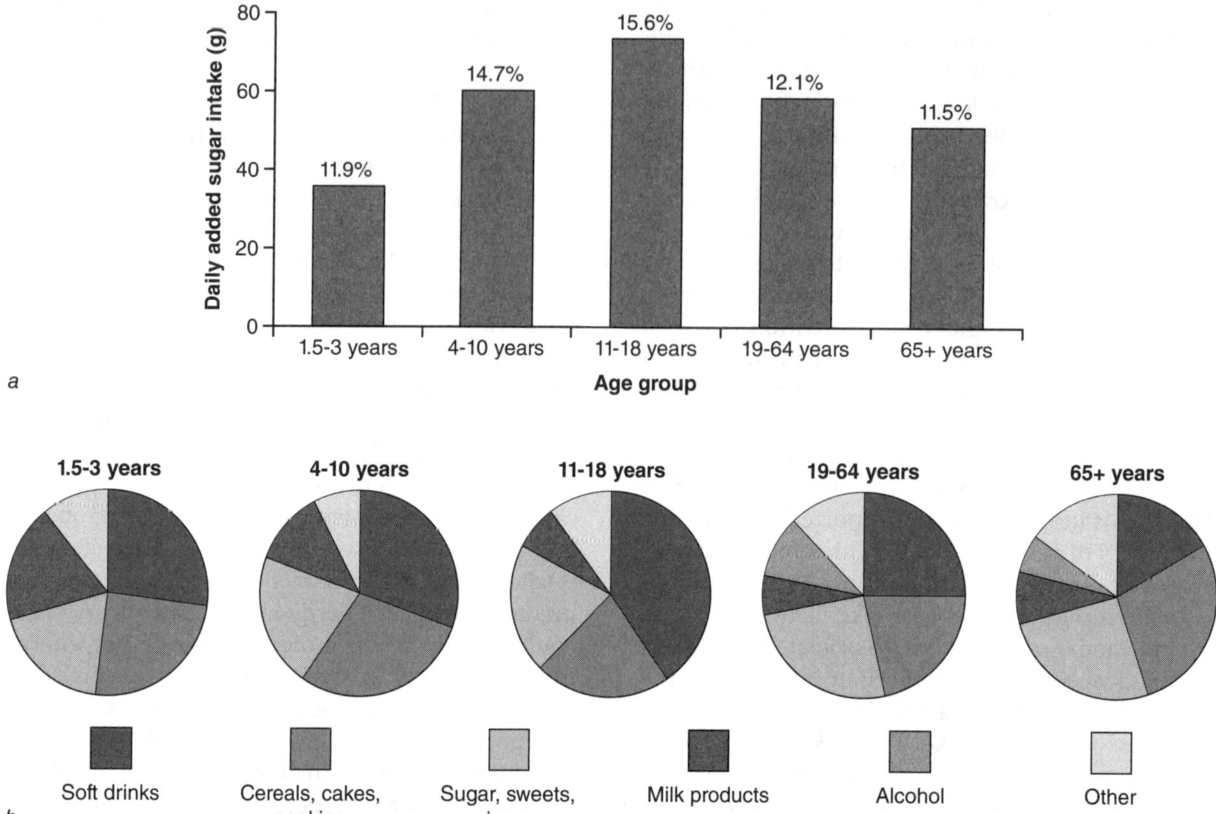

Figure 2.1 Sources of sugar intake in the Western diet: *(a)* daily added sugar intake by age group and *(b)* where different age groups get their added sugar.

Data from UK National Diet and Nutrition Survey Rolling Programme (2008/2009 – 2011/12), published 2014. Available: www.gov.uk/government/collections/national-diet-and-nutrition-survey

concentrations in the blood. This reduced insulin sensitivity (or increased insulin resistance) has far-reaching consequences and may result in many serious clinical complications. A high intake of fiber-rich foods seems to protect against this disease (American Dietetic Association 1997; Slyper 2013).

Although a dose–response relationship between sugar consumption and obesity has not been definitively determined, sufficient evidence prompted the WHO to launch guidelines for sugar intake in adults and children (WHO 2015a). These guidelines recommend that adults and children reduce their daily intake of free sugars to less than 10% of total energy intake, and they suggest that a further reduction to below 5%, or roughly 25 g/day (6 teaspoons), would provide additional health benefits.

Another adverse effect of certain carbohydrates (primarily glucose, fructose, and sucrose but also starches) is dental caries (bacterial tooth decay). These carbohydrates provide a substrate for bacterial fermentation. The bacteria in dental plaque metabolize dietary sugars to acids that then dissolve dental enamel and dentine. In many countries, the severity of dental caries increased in parallel with importation of sugar and reached its peak in the 1950s and 1960s. Since then, severity has declined in many countries due to the wide use of fluoride, especially in toothpaste, but dental caries is still a relevant concern. The evidence that dietary sugars are the main cause of dental caries is extensive; without sugar, caries would be negligible (Rugg-Gunn 2013). Sucrose, in particular, increases the prevalence and progression of dental caries (Depaola, Faine, and Pamer 1999). Sugars are most detrimental if they are consumed between meals and in forms that are retained in the mouth for a long time. For example, candy often contains sucrose and has a relatively long contact time with teeth (Kandelman 1997). If sugar is consumed in beverages with low pH (such as soft drinks or sports drinks), the risks of dental caries and tooth erosion are further increased. Risks can be decreased by drinking fluoridated water, brushing or flossing teeth (removing plaque), and reducing frequency and duration of contact with sugar by reducing sugar consumption.

Health Effects of Sugar-Sweetened Beverage Intake

Consumption of soft drinks in the United States increased 130% (from 144 to 332 ml) between 1977 and 1996 (Tippett and Cleveland 1999). However, a decrease in sugar-sweetened beverage (SSB) consumption among youth and adults in the United States was observed between 1999 and 2010 (Kit et al. 2013). In 2009-2010, U.S. youth consumed a daily mean of 650 kJ (155 kcal) from SSBs, and adults consumed a mean of 632 kJ (151 kcal) per day from SSBs, a decrease from 1999 to 2010 of 285 kJ/day (68 kcal/day) and 188 kJ/day (45 kcal/day), respectively. In 2009-2010, 64% of youth and 51% of adults drank SSBs on a given day and SSBs contributed 8.0% and 6.9% of daily energy intake among youth and adults, respectively (Kit et al. 2013). Although the reduction in SSB consumption may be a promising and continuing trend, SSB intake is still higher in the United States than in any other country, and it is much higher than is recommended. In the United States between 2011 and 2014, the percentage of total daily calories obtained from SSBs was 7.3% for boys and 7.2% for girls and 6.9% for men and 6.1% for women (Quickstats 2017). This is still higher than desirable for health, and, as a result, some U.S. states and some countries have imposed a sugar tax on SSBs to discourage sales.

Experimental studies have shown that children who regularly consume SSBs show larger weight gain compared to children who consume SSBs less often. This may relate to the lack of satiation provided by these drinks, meaning that just as much food is eaten and there is no compensatory reduction in calorie intake despite the extra calories ingested in the SSBs. Substituting SSBs with noncaloric beverages has been found to reduce weight gain in children (de Ruyter et al. 2012). Several meta-analyses (large-scale statistical analyses based on study data) have suggested that SSBs are associated with weight gain and obesity in children and adults (Malik, Schulze, and Hu 2006; Olsen and Heitmann 2009). There have been three recent systematic reviews and meta-analyses of randomized control trials on sugar or SSB consumption and body weight (Kaiser et al. 2013; Malik et al. 2013; Te Morenga, Mallard, and Mann 2013). These trials suggested that increasing energy consumption through sugar intake may lead to modest weight gain in adults, but the weight gain appears to be due to the increased energy consumption rather than any unique aspect of sugar. One systematic review and meta-analysis that included 30 randomized controlled trials (19 of which were ad libitum and 11 of which were isoenergetic) and 38 prospective cohort studies found that the ad libitum randomized controlled trials and cohort studies agreed with each other; when individuals reduced or increased sugar consumption, there was a "small but significant" effect on body weight (Te Morenga, Mallard, and Mann 2013). On average, individuals in the ad libitum trials and cohort studies lost an average of 0.8 kg (1.8 lb) when they reduced their sugar intake and gained an average of 0.75 kg (1.7 lb) when they increased their sugar consumption. The 11 isocaloric trials (in which the dietary sugars were replaced by the same number of calories from other macronutrients), however, showed no association between body weight change and sugar intake, which led to the conclusion that increased sugar intake promoted weight gain by increasing energy intake in excess of energy expenditure.

Three prospective cohort studies examined the association between SSB consumption and incidence of CHD in populations with predominantly sedentary lifestyles. Data from a large prospective cohort study found no association between SSB consumption and myocardial infarction (Eshak et al. 2012). Data from the Male Health Professional Follow-Up Study found a significant association between CHD events and the highest quintile of SSB consumption compared to the lowest (de Koning et al. 2012). Data from the Nurses' Health Study showed significantly elevated CHD risks for people who consumed two or more servings of SSBs per day compared with those who consumed less than one serving per month (Fung et al. 2009). The studies that found a correlation show that high SSB consumption may increase the risk of CHD in those with sedentary lifestyles when SSB intake contributes to a positive energy balance (i.e., daily energy intake that exceeds daily energy expenditure).

Health Effects of High Fructose Intake

Some of the debate about the health effects of excess carbohydrate intake has specifically targeted the monosaccharide fructose and high-fructose corn syrup (HFCS). Fructose was virtually absent from the diet a few hundred years ago, but it is now a major component of the diet. The main dietary sources of fructose are disaccharide sucrose from beet or cane, HFCS, fruit, fruit juices, and honey. Fructose has the chemical formula $C_6H_{12}O_6$, the same as glucose, but its metabolism differs markedly from that of glucose due to its almost complete uptake by the liver, where it is converted into glucose, glycogen, lactate, and fat. Fructose was initially thought to be a good sugar choice for diabetic patients due to its low glycemic index. Chronic consumption of large amounts of fructose in rodents, however, led to insulin resistance, obesity, type 2 diabetes, and high blood pressure. The evidence is less compelling in humans, but high fructose intake has been shown to increase blood cholesterol and impair liver insulin sensitivity. In large amounts, dietary fructose leads to greater adverse metabolic changes than equivalent amounts of glucose, although the extent to which fructose per se (rather than the calories it provides) contributes to many of the metabolic changes found in the obese is still a matter of debate (Slyper 2013). Excess fat production in the liver, lipotoxicity, oxidative stress, and elevated blood levels of uric acid have all been proposed as mechanisms responsible for the adverse metabolic effects of fructose. Although there is compelling evidence that very high fructose intake can have deleterious metabolic effects in humans, the role of fructose in the development of the current epidemic of metabolic disorders remains controversial (Tappy and Lê 2015). Epidemiological studies show growing evidence that consumption of sweetened beverages (containing either sucrose or a mixture of glucose and fructose) is associated with a high energy intake, increased body weight, and the occurrence of metabolic and cardiovascular disorders. There is, however, no unequivocal evidence that fructose intake at moderate doses is directly related with adverse metabolic effects. There has also been much concern that consumption of free fructose, as provided in HFCS, may cause more adverse effects than consumption of fructose consumed as the disaccharide sucrose, but there is no direct evidence for more serious metabolic consequences of HFCS versus sucrose consumption (Tappy and Lê 2010). Indeed, multiple studies have not demonstrated any unique properties of HFCS compared to sucrose with regard to energy-regulating hormones, appetite, or weight gain in normal weight and obese individuals (Rippe and Angelopoulos 2016). Thus, the current evidence indicates that there are no differences between HFCS and sucrose regarding the likelihood of causing obesity. The extent to which fructose itself, rather than the calories it provides, contributes to the metabolic changes associated with obesity is still a matter of debate.

Health Effects of Fat Intake

According to a large nutrition survey in the United States called the National Health and Nutrition Examination Survey (NHANES), fat intake declined from 36.9% to 33.5% for men and from 36.1% to 33.9% for women from 1971 to 2004. Although the percentage of fat in the diet decreased, the actual fat intake (in grams) increased slightly because of an increase in total daily energy intake. From 2004 to 2010, there was a slight reduction in total energy and fat intake. Few people in Western countries have fat intakes below 20%. More than 95% of the daily fat intake is in the form of triacylglycerols; phospholipids, fatty acids, cholesterol, and plant sterols make up the remainder. The daily triacylglycerol intake in the North American diet is about 100 to 150 g/day. The average person in the United States consumes about one-third of their fat from plants (vegetables) and two-thirds from animal sources. Saturated fatty acids typically represent 11% of the total energy intake (NHANES 2007-2010).

Health Effects of Saturated Fat Intake

High levels of blood cholesterol are associated with high intake of saturated fats. More than half of the cholesterol in the body is synthesized by the body; the liver and intestines each produce about 10% to 15% of total daily amounts. Only about 20% of cholesterol is directly obtained from the diet. Normal adults typically synthesize about 1 g of cholesterol per day, and the total body content is about 35 g. In the United States and other Western countries, typical daily dietary intake of cholesterol is about 200 to 300 mg. The body compensates for cholesterol intake by reducing the amount that is synthesized. Cholesterol is found in eggs, red meat, organ meat (e.g., heart, liver, kidney), shellfish, and dairy products such as whole milk, butter, cheese, and cream. Foods of plant origin contain no cholesterol.

Cholesterol is synthesized from acetyl coenzyme A (acetyl-CoA), which is the end product of fat and carbohydrate metabolism (see chapter 3 for further details). In the bloodstream, cholesterol is mostly transported within lipoprotein particles. Epidemiological research has shown that people who consume diets that are high in saturated fats have relatively high levels of blood cholesterol and suffer a high prevalence of CHD. LDL cholesterol promotes the development of **arteriosclerosis** and predisposes people to cardiovascular disease. HDL cholesterol, on the other hand, seems to protect against cardiovascular disease. Reducing blood LDL cholesterol decreases the risk for CHD.

Various ways of lowering LDL cholesterol, such as reducing the intake of saturated fat (Hooper et al. 2015), increasing physical activity, and consuming cholesterol-lowering drugs such as statins, which inhibit cholesterol synthesis, are effective in reducing the risk of cardiovascular disease. A reduction in cardiovascular events was seen in studies that primarily replaced saturated fat calories with polyunsaturated fat, but no effects were seen in studies that replaced saturated fat with carbohydrate or protein (Hooper et al. 2015).

The Seven Countries Study compared CHD mortality in 12,000 men aged 40 to 59 years in seven countries and found positive correlations between CHD mortality and total fat intake in 1970 and between CHD mortality and saturated fat intake in 1986 (Keys et al. 1986; Thorogood 1996). Migrant studies of Japanese men living in different cultures confirmed that men in California had the diets richest in saturated fat and cholesterol and the highest CHD rates, those in Hawaii had intermediate saturated fat intakes and CHD rates, and those in Japan had the lowest in saturated fat and cholesterol intakes and the lowest CHD rates (Kagan et al. 1974; Robertson et al. 1977). However, systematic reviews of the observational data have not confirmed these studies. A study by Skeaff and Miller (2009) included 28 U.S. and European cohorts (including 6,600 CHD deaths among 280,000 participants) that investigated the effects of total, saturated, monounsaturated, *trans*, and omega-3 fats on CHD deaths and events. They found no clear relationship between total, saturated, or monounsaturated fat intakes and CHD events or deaths. There was evidence that *trans* fats increased CHD events and deaths and that total polyunsaturated fats and omega-3 fats decreased them. More large-scale intervention studies are needed to clarify cause and effect to ensure that confounding is not hiding true relationships or suggesting relationships where they do not exist.

Some studies have suggested a correlation between high dietary fat intake and obesity, but other studies seem to raise questions about the effects of the dietary fat intake on body weight. The evidence that high fat intake contributes to obesity is insufficient to make definitive recommendations for a very low-fat diet. Therefore, the Dietary Guidelines for Americans (U.S. Department of Agriculture 2005, 2015) state that fat intake should be moderate (rather than low). In fact, a very low fat and high carbohydrate intake may have adverse health effects. Reducing dietary fat to below 20% of energy intake and replacing the calories with those from high-glycemic carbohydrate results in elevated plasma triacylglycerols, increased LDL cholesterol, and decreased HDL cholesterol. These metabolic changes increase the risk of cardiovascular disease and predisposition to CHD (Slyper 2013).

High fat intake (along with low fiber intake) has been linked with increased incidence of colon and prostate cancer and with increased body weight. Epidemiological studies suggest that, as with cardiovascular diseases, the type of fat is important to cancer risk. The associations between high fat intake and cancer may be due to the intake of animal fat (saturated fat) rather than vegetable fat (unsaturated fat), which raises the possibility that fat itself is not the most important factor (Willett 2000). Omega-3 (*n*-3) fatty acids, which are found in fish, seem to protect against cancer. For example, Alaskan natives and Japanese, whose diets rely heavily on fish and thus have a relatively high intake of fish oil, also seem to have lower incidences of cancer.

Health Effects of *Trans* Fatty Acid Intake

Trans fatty acids are unsaturated fatty acids that contain at least one double bond in the *trans* configuration. Unlike other dietary fats, *trans* fats are neither essential nor desirable, and there is evidence that indicates *trans* fatty acid intake raises blood LDL cholesterol levels and lowers HDL cholesterol levels (Brouwer et al. 2010; Lichtenstein et al. 1999; Mensink and Katan 1990), which increases the risk of cardiovascular disease (Lichtenstein 2014). There are two main sources of dietary *trans* fatty acids: meat and dairy fats and partially hydrogenated fats. Due to changes in federal labeling requirements for packaged foods and some bans on the use of partially hydrogenated fats, *trans* fat intake has declined in recent years. Similar to saturated fatty acids, *trans* fatty acids increase plasma LDL cholesterol concentrations. In contrast to saturated fatty acids, *trans* fatty acids do not increase HDL cholesterol concentrations. These differences have been attributed to an alteration in lipoprotein catabolic rate rather than production rate. Although some issues remain unresolved regarding *trans* fatty acids and cardiovascular disease risk factors other than plasma lipoprotein concentrations, this should not affect the dietary recommendation to limit *trans* fat intake.

Results from the U.K. National Diet and Nutrition Survey (NDNS) rolling program for 2012/2013 to 2013/2014 (2016) show that children and adults, including older adults, are eating 0.5% to 0.6% of food energy as *trans* fats. The UK Scientific Advisory Committee on Nutrition recommends that average intakes of *trans* fatty acids should not

THE BUTTER VERSUS MARGARINE DEBATE

For the last few decades, there has been controversy over the health risks associated with regular consumption of butter and margarine. Although butter and margarine cannot be distinguished by their energy density or fat content, they can be distinguished by the composition of their fatty acids. Margarine is manufactured from plant-derived unsaturated fatty acids that are hydrogenated to convert the lipids into a hardened form (although not as hard as butter). Until the 1980s, about 20% of the fatty acids in margarine were *trans* fatty acids compared with 7% in butter. Health concerns about these fats led to the reformulation of many margarines and spreads to make the *trans* fat content much lower. Margarine does not contain cholesterol because it is manufactured from vegetable oil, but each gram of butter contains 10 to 15 mg of cholesterol and much more saturated fat than margarine. Currently, margarine is probably healthier than butter. Butter should be used sparingly because it is high in saturated fat, which aggressively increases levels of LDL.

exceed 2% of food energy; therefore, on average, the UK is well within the recommended maximum levels. That doesn't mean UK consumers should be complacent about *trans* fats in foods.

Health Effects of Protein Intake

In developing countries, protein deficiency is common and can result in kwashiorkor (a pure protein deficiency that is characterized by a bloated belly, which is caused by edema, and impaired immunity with increased susceptibility to infections) or marasmus (a protein deficiency that results from a total dietary energy deficiency and is characterized by extreme muscle wasting). In the developed world, dietary protein intake is less critical and is not related to disease.

It has been suggested that long-term consumption of a high-protein diet may result in impaired kidney function, but evidence for this is nonexistent. Circumstances may differ in cases of preexisting kidney problems.

Health Effects of Sodium Intake

Sodium is found in many foods. It is the major electrolyte in the extracellular fluids of animals, and it is added to foods to enhance flavor and act as a preservative. Sodium deficiency results in a loss of water on the outside of cells, which decreases blood volume. Low blood volume may lead to low blood pressure, which is a serious health condition that can present symptoms such as fatigue and lethargy. A low level of sodium in the blood (hyponatremia) can be caused by drinking too much water. This has been observed in people who take part in long-duration events such as marathons. Symptoms are not usually very specific and can include changes in mental state, headache, nausea and vomiting, tiredness, muscle spasms, and seizures. Severe hyponatremia can lead to coma and can be fatal.

Excess sodium intake is related to the development of high blood pressure (hypertension). Normal blood pressure (normotension) is less than 120 mmHg (systolic) and 80 mmHg (diastolic). Blood pressure is largely regulated by the degree of blood vessel constriction and by sodium and water retention in the kidneys. When blood volume increases or blood vessels are narrowed, blood pressure rises. If blood pressure is chronically above 140/90 mmHg, risk of arteriosclerosis, heart attack, stroke, kidney disease, and early death increases. Blood pressure between 120/80 and 139/89 mmHg is referred to as prehypertension and may indicate increased risk for the diseases mentioned.

Epidemiological, migration, intervention, and genetic studies in humans and animals provide very strong evidence of a causal link between high dietary salt intake and high blood pressure. The mechanisms by which dietary salt increases arterial pressure are not fully understood, but they seem related to the inability of the kidneys to excrete large amounts of salt. From an evolutionary viewpoint, humans are adapted to ingest and excrete less than 1 g of salt per day. This is about eight times less than the average salt intakes currently observed in many industrialized and urbanized countries. Independent of the rise in blood pressure, excess dietary salt also increases cardiac left ventricular mass, arterial thickness and stiffness, the incidence of stroke, and the severity of cardiac failure (Meneton et al. 2005). Thus, a high-salt diet appears to be a major factor in the frequent occurrence of hypertension and cardiovascular diseases.

The Dietary Guidelines for Americans (U.S. Department of Agriculture 2015) recommend a low-sodium diet with an intake of no more than 2.3 g of sodium (equivalent to 5.8 g of salt) per day, but this recommendation is controversial. Salt reduction in normotensive individuals has little or no effect on blood pressure, and high sodium intake does not affect blood pressure in all people (Graudal, Galloe, and Garred 1998). About 50% of people may be "salt sensitive," and others may be considerably less affected by increased sodium intake. Because targeting only those who are salt sensitive would be difficult, and because moderate salt intake has no reported negative effects (Kumanyika and Cutler 1997), dietary guidelines in most other countries recommend that people choose and prepare foods with less salt and limit their salt intake to no more than 6 g per day.

Health Effects of Phytonutrient Intake

Phytonutrients are certain organic components of plants that are thought to promote human health but are non-nutrients. They differ from vitamins because without them people will not develop nutritional deficiencies. Phytonutrients, such as carotenoids and polyphenols, may protect human health by

- serving as antioxidants,
- enhancing immune response,
- enhancing cell-to-cell communication,
- altering estrogen metabolism,
- converting to vitamin A (by metabolizing beta-carotene),
- causing cancer cells to die (apoptosis), and
- repairing DNA damage caused by smoking and other toxic exposures.

Evidence that fruit and vegetable consumption protects human health is accumulating from large-population (epidemiological) studies, human feeding studies, and cell culture studies. For example, fruit and vegetable consumption has been linked to decreased risk of stroke. In one study, each additional daily serving of fruits and vegetables equated to a 22% decrease in risk of stroke, including transient ischemic attack. A recent meta-analysis of 20 prospective cohort studies involving 16,981 stroke events among 760,629 participants (Hu et al. 2014) found that the relative risk (95% CI) of stroke for people with the highest versus the lowest total fruit and vegetable consumption was 0.79 (CI: 0.75-0.84). The effect was 0.77 (CI: 0.71-0.84) for fruit consumption and 0.86 (CI: 0.79-0.93) for vegetable consumption, and the risk of stroke decreased by 32% (0.68 [CI: 0.56-0.82]) and 11% (0.89 [CI: 0.81-0.98]) for every 200 g of fruit and vegetable consumption per day, respectively.

In another study, older men who had the highest intakes of dark green and deep yellow vegetables had about a 46% decrease in risk of heart disease relative to men with the lowest intakes. Men with the highest intakes had about a 70% lower risk of cancer than did their counterparts with the lowest intakes. The differences in vegetable consumption between high and low intake rankings were not striking. Men with the highest intakes consumed between 2.05 and 2.2 servings of dark green or deep yellow vegetables per day, and those with the lowest intakes consumed between 0.7 and 0.8 servings. This evidence suggests that small, consistent changes in vegetable consumption can make important changes in health outcomes.

In a meta-analysis that examined 95 prospective studies of combined fruit and vegetable intake and risk of cardiovascular disease, total cancer, and all-cause mortality (Aune et al. 2017), the relative risk per 200 g of fruit and vegetables per day was 0.92 (CI: 0.90-0.94, n = 15) for CHD, 0.84 (CI: 0.76-0.92, n = 10) for stroke, 0.92 (CI: 0.90-0.95, n = 13) for cardiovascular disease, 0.97 (CI: 0.95-0.99, n = 12) for total cancer, and 0.90 (CI: 0.87-0.93, n = 15) for all-cause mortality. Similar associations were observed for fruits and vegetables separately. Reductions in risk were observed in a dose-response manner when participants ate up to 800 g of fruit and vegetables per day for all outcomes except cancer (600 g/day). Inverse associations were observed between the intake of apples and pears, citrus fruits, green leafy vegetables, cruciferous vegetables (e.g., cauliflower, cabbage, garden cress, bok choy, broccoli, Brussels sprouts), and salads and cardiovascular disease and all-cause mortality and between the intake of green and yellow vegetables and cruciferous vegetables and total cancer risk. In summary, it is reasonable to conclude that fruit and vegetable intake is associated with reduced risk of cardiovascular disease, cancer, and all-cause mortality.

On average, Americans consume 3.3 servings of vegetables per day (NHANES), but dark green vegetables and deep yellow or orange vegetables each represent only 0.2 daily servings. On any given day, about half the U.S. population does not consume the recommended minimum three servings of vegetables About 10% of the population consumes less than one serving of vegetables per day. On any given day, about 71% of the population does not consume the recommended minimum two servings of fruit. About half the population consumes less than one serving of fruit per day. This seems to be a worldwide trend; one study showed that 77.6% of men and 78.4% of women from 52 mainly low- and middle-income countries consumed fewer than the minimum recommended five daily servings of fruits and vegetables (Hall et al. 2009).

For one class of phytonutrients, flavonoids, consumption has been linked to a lower risk of heart disease in some studies. Older Dutch men with the highest flavonoid intakes had a 58% lower risk of heart disease than their counterparts with the lowest intakes (Geleijnse et al. 2002). Similarly, Finnish men with the highest flavonoid intakes had a 40% lower risk of mortality from heart disease than men with the lowest intakes (Mursu et al. 2008). Other studies, however, could not confirm the protective effect of flavonoids. In one study, flavanol intake did not predict a lower rate of ischemic heart disease and was weakly and positively associated with ischemic heart disease mortality (Rimm et al. 1996). In another study in U.S. women, data did not support a strong link between flavonoid intake and CHD (Lin et al. 2007). In a meta-analysis of 10 epidemiological studies (Liu et al. 2017), the relative risk of all-cause mortality for the highest versus lowest categories of total flavonoid intake was 0.82 (95% CI: 0.72-0.92). Dose-response analysis showed that people who consumed 200 mg/day of total flavonoids had the lowest risk of all-cause mortality. Furthermore, a marginally significant association was found between total dietary flavonoid consumption and relative risk (RR) of death from cardiovascular disease (summary RR: 0.85; 95% CI: 0.70-1.03) and CHD (summary RR: 0.74; 95% CI: 0.54-1.02), respectively. This provides strong evidence for the recommendation that adults consume flavonoids-rich foods (see chapter 1) as part of a healthy diet to reduce the risk of all-cause mortality.

Although large studies have linked fruit and vegetable consumption with lowered risk of chronic diseases such as specific cancers and heart disease, claims made in the media about phytonutrients and functional foods (i.e., those containing health-promoting compounds) seem far ahead of established proof that documents the health benefits of these foods or food components. Our knowledge of phytonutrients and their effects is improving, and more specific information on phytonutrient consumption and human health will be forthcoming.

Practical Guidelines for a Balanced, Healthy Diet

Although recommendations such as the DRI may provide guidance on nutrient requirements, they are not a practical way of informing people about appropriate food choices. For example, how do we know whether we are consuming about 0.8 g of protein per kilogram of body weight per day or meeting the RDI for calcium, vitamin A, and other essential minerals and vitamins? A healthy diet is often referred to as a balanced diet that stresses variety and moderation. But how do we achieve a balanced diet? Nutritionists addressed this question early in the 20th century and developed several simple and comprehensive food guides, the most important of which is the Food Guide Pyramid (see table 2.1).

In 2005, a food guide called **MyPyramid** was developed (see figure 2.2) based on the Food Guide Pyramid, and it contained the same six food categories. The latest U.S. food guide is called **MyPlate** (figure 2.3) (www.ChooseMyPlate.gov), and it is based on the 2015-2020 Dietary Guidelines for Americans (www.health.gov/dietaryguidelines).

TABLE 2.1 Categories of the Food Guide Pyramid and the Most Important Nutrients They Provide

Food categories	Essential nutrients
Breads, cereals, rice, pasta	Thiamin, niacin, riboflavin, iron
Milk, yogurt, cheese	Calcium, protein, riboflavin, vitamin A
Meat, poultry, fish, eggs, dry beans, nuts	Protein, thiamin, niacin, iron
Vegetables	Vitamin A, vitamin C
Fruit	Vitamin A, vitamin C
Fats, oils, sweets*	Vitamin A, vitamin D, vitamin E

*A component that mainly adds to energy intake and does not provide micronutrients.

ALCOHOL: GOOD OR BAD?

Alcohol, or ethanol, is a nonessential nutrient that provides 28 kJ (7 kcal) of energy per gram. Average alcohol intake in the United States is about 2% to 3% of daily energy intake. Alcohol is the most widely abused addictive drug and causes intoxication (impaired mental function), liver damage, and other organ damage. It is responsible for approximately 6% of deaths worldwide. In the United States between 2006 and 2010, an estimated 88,000 people (approximately 62,000 men and 26,000 women) died from alcohol-related causes annually. This does not include alcohol-related homicides and alcohol-impaired driving fatalities, which accounted for about 10,000 deaths annually (Centers for Disease Control and Prevention 2013). In moderation, however, alcohol may have health benefits. Moderate alcohol consumption (no more than 3-4 standard drinks per drinking episode, no more than 9 drinks per week for women and 12-14 for men) reduces stress and raises levels of HDL cholesterol, which has a protective effect against cardiovascular diseases. Protection may also be provided by phenols in red wine, which are antioxidant compounds that reduce lipoprotein oxidation and thereby prevent or reduce the formation of atherosclerotic plaques. Heavy alcohol consumption (8 or more drinks a week for women, 15 or more for men), however, increases blood pressure, and this risk outweighs the positive effects of alcohol consumption. Consumption of alcohol in any amount has been shown to increase the risk of oropharyngeal, esophageal, and breast cancers. The energy content of alcohol can also be a significant contributor to obesity. A 750 mL (26.4 fl oz) bottle of red wine contains about 2,500 kJ (597 kcal), which is the equivalent to two hamburgers. Therefore, in the interest of health, alcohol should only be consumed in moderation and at appropriate times (i.e., not before driving or participating in sport or work). Furthermore, alcohol should be avoided during pregnancy. Note that one drink is defined as 360 ml (12 fl oz) of beer with 5% alcohol content, 150 ml (5 fl oz) of wine with 12% alcohol content, or 45 ml (1.5 fl oz) of spirits with 40% alcohol content. In the United Kingdom, alcohol intake is measured in units. One unit is 10 ml (0.3 fl oz) of pure alcohol, regardless of the type of alcohol being consumed. Intake recommendations are two to three units of alcohol per day for women and three to four units for men. Units are often defined as one small glass of wine, a half pint of beer, or one pub measure of spirits. The alcohol content of different products varies; some stronger beers and lagers may contain as many as five units of alcohol per 500 ml (17 fl oz).

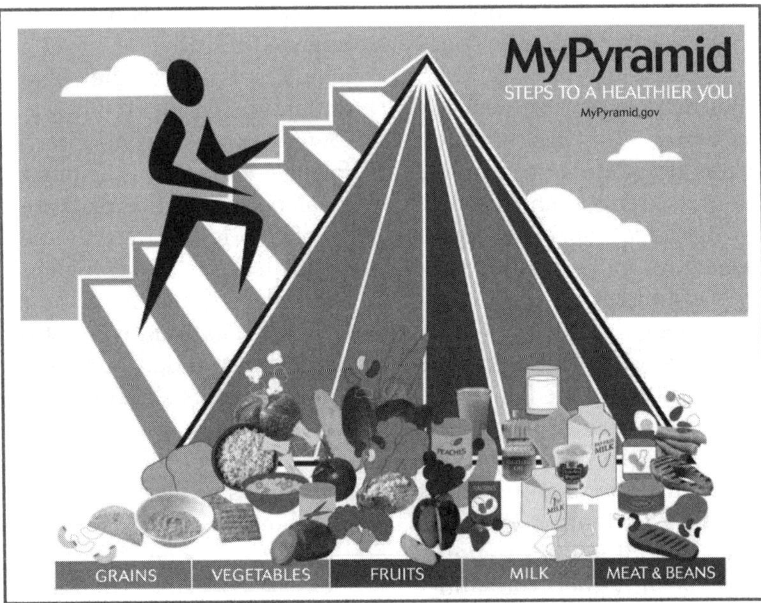

Figure 2.2 MyPyramid.

U.S. Department of Agriculture and the U.S. Department of Health and Human Services.

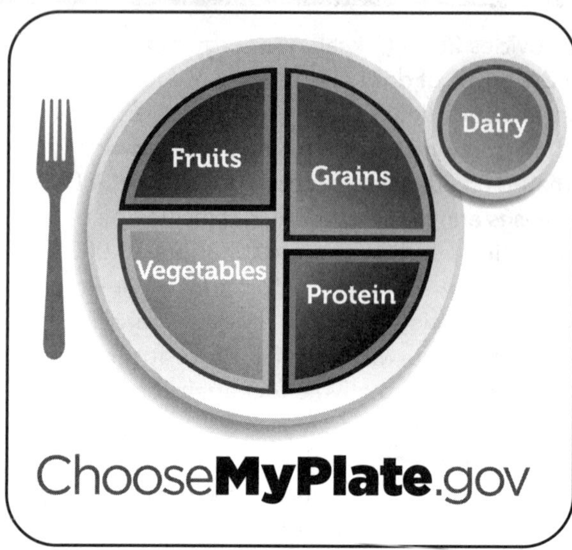

Figure 2.3 MyPlate.
USDA's Center for Nutrition Policy and Promotion.

The foods in each category make similar nutrient contributions. In previous versions of the dietary guidelines, the only macronutrient with an RDA was protein. The latest version of the dietary guidelines, however, includes recommendations for carbohydrate and fat to minimize the risk of chronic diseases. The recommendation for adults is that 45% to 65% of energy intake should be from carbohydrate, 20% to 35% should be from fat, and 10% to 35% should be from protein. Carbohydrate can be found in bread, cereal, rice, pasta, vegetables, fruits, beans, and sweets. Protein is found mostly in meat, poultry, fish, eggs, dry beans, and nuts. Fat is found in meat, poultry, fish, eggs, nuts, oils, and sweets.

The Dietary Guidelines for Americans are considered an essential resource for health professionals and policymakers who design and implement food and nutrition programs such as school lunches. In addition, they provide information to help people make healthy food and beverage choices. The guidelines are based on the recommendations of the 2015 Dietary Guidelines Advisory Committee, which was composed of experts in the fields of nutrition, health, and medicine who analyzed the current body of scientific evidence. They produced a report that provided advice and recommendations to the federal government based on the current state of scientific evidence on nutrition and health. In addition to providing guidance for choosing a healthy diet, the guidelines focus on preventing (rather than treating) the diet-related chronic diseases that continue to affect the U.S. population. The latest edition of the guidelines also includes data that describe the significant differences between Americans' current consumption habits and the recommendations. It recommends the areas in which shifts to healthier food and beverage choices are encouraged to help people achieve more healthy eating patterns. The emphasis is on helping people improve and maintain overall health and reduce their risk of developing chronic diseases. The body of scientific literature on healthy eating patterns and their effects on disease prevention is more robust now than ever before. Chronic diet-related diseases continue to rise, and levels of physical activity in the general U.S. population remain low. Progress in reversing these trends will require comprehensive and coordinated strategies, and the dietary guidelines are an important part of a complex and multifaceted solution to promote health and help reduce the risk of chronic disease (U.S. Department of Agriculture 2015).

Many countries have developed their own guidelines. The UK food guide was also depicted as a plate until 2016, when the Eatwell Guide (www.gov.uk/government/publications/the-eatwell-guide) was introduced (see figure 2.4). The change from the plate depiction was a result of consumer-research findings that the approach no longer resonated with the public. Food group segments are still used, but they have been updated to emphasize certain food products that are less expensive and more environmentally sustainable. For example, the main protein segment is titled "beans, pulses, fish, eggs, meat and other proteins" to highlight the contribution of nonmeat sources to protein intake. The segment sizes of the food groups have been adjusted to reflect current government advice on a healthy balanced diet. The Eatwell Guide differentiates unsaturated oils (e.g., vegetable, olive) and low-fat spreads from other foods that are high in fat, salt, and sugar. The oils and spreads segment is small because these foods are high fat and contain a lot of calories, so they should only be consumed in small amounts. Foods high in fat or sugar have now been placed outside of the main image. Research indicated that removal of these products from the main image aided consumer understanding that these products should be consumed infrequently and only in small quantities. Having these food products outside of the main image also helped consumers understand the need to shift toward a healthier lifestyle.

The Eatwell Guide also introduced a hydration message, because staying hydrated is part of a healthy diet. The Eatwell Guide reinforces fluid recommendations and the best drinks to choose: water, low-fat milk, and sugar-free drinks such

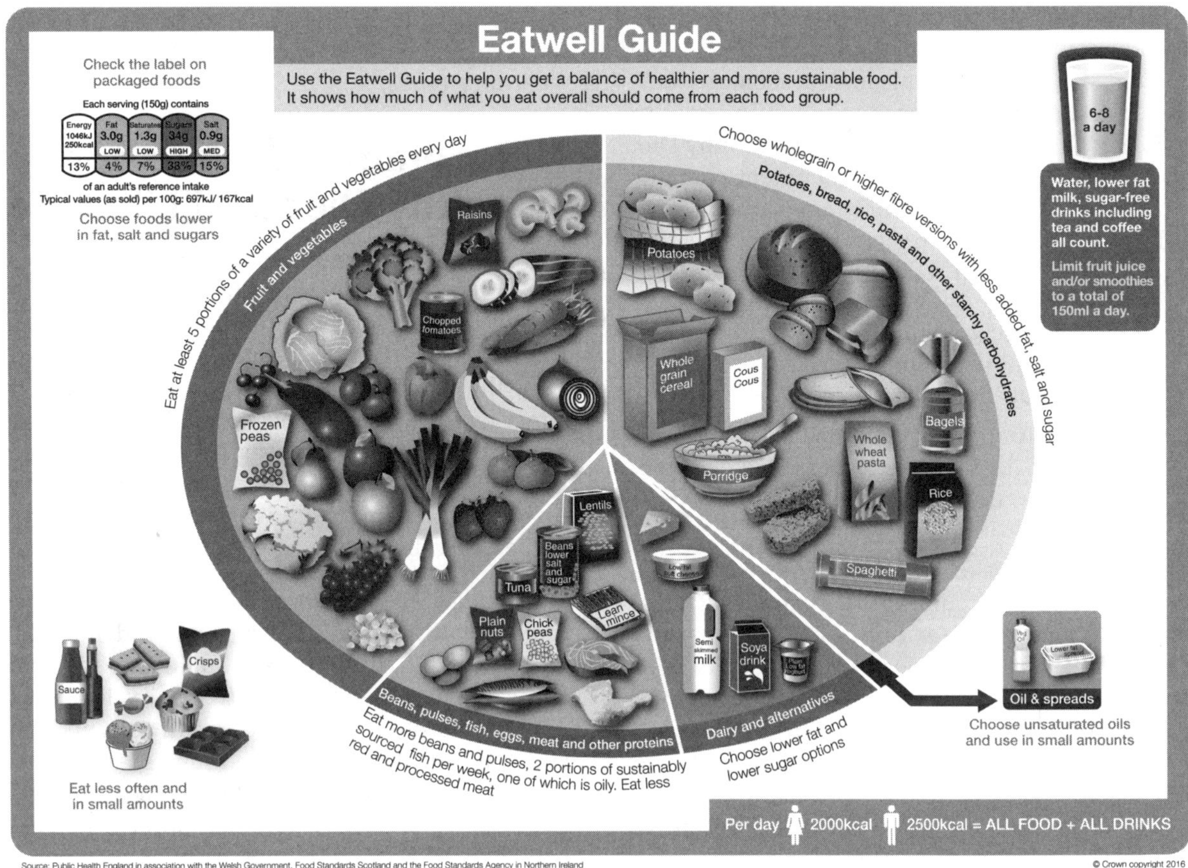

Figure 2.4 The Eatwell Guide.

as tea and coffee. Notably, fruit juice has been removed from the fruit and vegetable segment. Although fruit juice (at a maximum of 150 ml/day [5 fl oz/day]) still counts toward one of your fruit portions, the advice around drinks has been encompassed in the hydration message. Finally, an outer border featuring the energy requirements for men and women has been used to reinforce the message that all food and drinks consumed contribute to total energy intake. Consumer research revealed that the inclusion of an energy message provided adults with a useful benchmark for their own consumption.

The Australian Dietary Guidelines (2015) are based on recent scientific evidence about diet and health outcomes. As with the American and British versions, the guidelines are based on foods and food groups to make the information easier to understand and use. Canada's food guide (www.hc-sc.gc.ca/fn-an/food-guide-aliment/index-eng.php) incorporates a simple interactive eatwell plate with heathy eating tips for each food segment.

Every 10 to 15 years, new research and evidence warrant a revision of at least the major nutrient requirements and recommended intakes, which are the common foundation for all countries' food-based dietary guidelines. In the past, countries' guidelines almost exclusively focused on avoiding nutrient deficiencies, particularly in poor countries in which food quantity, quality, and variety may be severely limited. More recently, more attention has been paid to developing guidelines that consider public health and the clinical significance of intake levels (deficiency and excess) and associated disease patterns for each nutrient or food type for all age groups. The increased production of processed food, rapid urbanization, and changing lifestyles have led to a shift in dietary patterns for people in many countries. People now consume more foods that are high in calories, fats, free sugars, and sodium, and many do not eat enough fruit, vegetables, and dietary fiber such as whole grains. The exact makeup of a diverse, balanced, and healthy diet will vary depending on individual needs (e.g., age, gender, lifestyle, degree of physical activity), cultural context, locally available foods, and dietary customs, but basic principles for what constitutes a healthy diet remain the same (WHO 2015b).

Many countries that do not produce their own national guidelines rely on the WHO and the FAO to establish and disseminate information on nutrient requirements and recommended intakes. In 2015, the WHO published its updated Healthy Diet Factsheet (WHO 2015b). This document contains some practical information on how to achieve a healthy diet. According to this document, a healthy diet for adults should consist of the following:

- **Legumes** (e.g., lentils, beans), nuts, and whole grains (e.g., unprocessed maize, millet, oats, wheat, brown rice).
- At least 400 g of fruits and vegetables per day. This does *not* include potatoes, sweet potatoes, cassava, and other starchy root vegetables.
- Less than 10% of total energy intake from free sugars. This would be 50 g (about 12 level teaspoons) of sugar for a person of healthy weight who consumes about 2,000 kcal per day. Ideally, sugar intake should be less than 5% of total energy for additional health benefits. Free sugars include those added to foods or drinks by the manufacturer, cook, or consumer and those naturally present in honey, syrups, fruit juices, and fruit juice concentrates.
- Less than 30% of total energy intake from fats. Unsaturated fats such as those found in fish, avocado, nuts, and sunflower, canola, and olive oils are preferable to saturated fats (e.g., those found in fatty meat, butter, certain oils, cream, cheese, ghee, and lard). Industrial *trans* fats are not part of a healthy diet.
- Less than 5 g of salt (about 1 teaspoon) per day. Iodized salt is recommended to prevent iodine deficiency (a potential cause of hypothyroid problems).

In the first 2 years of life, optimal nutrition fosters healthy growth, improves cognitive development, and reduces the risk of the person becoming overweight or obese and developing noncommunicable diseases later in life. According to the WHO (2015b), a healthy diet for infants and children is similar to that for adults, but the following elements are also important:

- Infants should be breastfed exclusively during the first 6 months of life.
- Infants should be breastfed continuously until 2 years of age and beyond.
- From 6 months of age, breast milk should be complemented with a variety of adequate, safe, and nutrient-dense foods. Salt and sugars should not be added to complementary foods.

Recommendations for a Healthy Diet and Lifestyle

Our current recommendations for healthy eating are drawn from a variety of sources, including MyPlate, the Dietary Guidelines for Americans, the Eatwell Guide, the American Heart Association, the American Dietetic Association, and the American Diabetes Association. These guidelines are based on the latest research and may be helpful in the prevention of obesity and associated chronic diseases, including cardiovascular disease, type 2 diabetes, and cancer.

- *Follow healthy eating patterns across the life span.* Healthy eating patterns should include a variety of nutritious foods such as vegetables, fruits, grains, low-fat and fat-free dairy, lean meats and other protein foods, and healthy oils and limit saturated fats, *trans* fats, added sugars, and sodium. Healthy eating patterns can be adapted to individual taste preferences, traditions, cultures, and budgets. Specific food guidelines are addressed herein.
- *Balance food intake with physical activity to maintain a healthy weight.* Consuming moderate food portions and being physically active are important steps toward the prevention of obesity. Methods of regulating body weight will be discussed in detail in chapter 15.
- *Be physically active.* Aim to do at least 30 minutes of physical activity on most, if not all, days. The American College of Sports Medicine and the American Heart Association physical activity guidelines recommend moderate-intensity aerobic exercise for 30 minutes per day on 5 days per week or vigorously intense aerobic exercise for 20 minutes per day on 3 days per week. Moderate-intensity physical activity means working hard enough to raise the heart rate (but maintaining the ability to carry on a conversation) and break a sweat. People can also do a proportion of their regular weekly physical activity as resistance exercise by performing 8 to 12 repetitions of each of 8 to 10 strength-training exercises twice a week. Note that the 30-minute recommendation is for the average healthy adult to maintain health and reduce the risk for chronic disease (Haskell et al. 2007). To lose weight or maintain weight loss, 60 to 90 minutes of physical activity may be necessary.
- *Eat a variety of nutrient-dense foods.* Eating a variety of foods from each food group helps ensure

adequate intake of all essential nutrients. Nutrient-dense foods provide vitamins, minerals, and other substances that contribute to adequate nutrient intake and may have positive health effects. The term *nutrient dense* indicates the nutrients and other beneficial substances in a food have not been diluted by the addition solid fat, sugar, sodium, or refined starch and the foods do not contain high amounts of naturally occurring fat. Ideally, these foods also are in forms that retain naturally occurring components such as dietary fiber. When prepared with little or no added solid fat, sugar, sodium, and refined starch, all vegetables, fruits, whole grains, seafood, eggs, beans, peas, unsalted nuts and seeds, fat-free and low-fat dairy products, and lean meats and poultry are nutrient-dense foods. These foods contribute to meeting food group recommendations within desirable calorie and sodium limits.

- *Eat a diet rich in vegetables, fruits, whole grains, and high-fiber foods.* These foods will help you achieve the recommended carbohydrate and fiber intakes. In addition, these foods contain phytonutrients, which have beneficial health effects. Epidemiological studies have generally shown that whole grains (bread and cereals), legumes (beans and peas), fruits, and vegetables have significant health benefits. Eat at least five portions of fruit and vegetables daily.
- *Eat a variety of high-protein foods.* High-protein food sources include seafood, lean meat and poultry, eggs, legumes, soy products, and nuts and seeds. These foods should make up 10% to 15% of daily energy intake to ensure that protein requirements are met while avoiding excessive fat intake.
- *Incorporate dietary fats wisely.* A healthy diet is moderate in total fat and low in saturated fat, *trans* fat, and cholesterol. Apart from linoleic and α-linolenic essential fatty acids, there are no specific requirements for fat consumption. Fat is a necessary component of the diet, and many foods contain some fat. The standard recommendation is a saturated fatty acid intake below 10% of total energy intake and a cholesterol intake of 300 mg or less per day. Commercially prepared baked goods and fast foods are generally high in fat and contain *trans* fatty acids and should be avoided. Consumption of small amounts of plant oils is encouraged (e.g., canola, olive, peanut, safflower, soybean, sunflower). Healthy oils also are naturally present in nuts, seeds, seafood, olives, and avocados.
- *Cut back on beverages and foods that have high sugar content and low nutrition values.* Beverages such as soft drinks and foods with added sugar contribute significantly to energy intake but do not provide nutrients. The National Academy of Sciences says sugars should make up no more than 25% of total daily energy intake, but reducing this to 10% may be a healthier alternative. The 2015-2020 Dietary Guidelines for Americans recommend that less than 10% of daily calorie intake should come from added sugars.
- *Reduce sodium intake.* Healthy adults are advised to have a sodium intake of 2.3 g/day or less. This equates to about 1 teaspoon of salt. Most people consume about 3.4 g of sodium per day. Choose foods with low sodium and prepare foods with minimal amounts of salt.
- *Drink alcohol only in moderation.* Excessive alcohol consumption is one of the greatest health threats today, and it can add significant energy to total daily intake without adding nutrients. Current evidence suggests that light to moderate alcohol intake (one drink per day) will cause no negative health effects, except slightly increasing cancer risk for healthy adults.
- *Practice food hygiene and safety.* Food should be properly stored to avoid contamination. Perishable foods should be refrigerated, and foods should not be stored for too long (i.e., not beyond the use by date on the food label where available) Food should be cooked to a safe temperature to kill microorganisms (but note that excess grilling of meat to the point where it becomes charred can produce carcinogenic substances). To avoid microbial food-borne illness, thoroughly wash hands, food-contact surfaces, and fruits and vegetables. Meat and poultry should not be washed or rinsed. Avoid raw (unpasteurized) milk or any products made from unpasteurized milk, raw or partially cooked eggs or foods containing raw eggs, raw or undercooked meat and poultry, unpasteurized juices, and raw sprouts.
- *Avoid excessive intakes of questionable food additives and nutrition supplements.* Most food additives used in processed foods are safe, but some recommendations suggest avoiding these additives. Look for labels that do not list a lot of additives and non-nutrients. In general it may be best to avoid consumption of processed foods as much as possible, but the definition of what processed foods are is not as clearcut as often thought. Processed foods include foods that have been frozen, or dried. Not all processed foods are unhealthy (for example dried fruits, frozen vegetables) but some processed foods may contain high levels of salt, sugar, and fat and a lot of additives.

In addition, nutritional supplements are often claimed to have various positive health effects or performance benefits, but there can also be negative effects. Nutrition supplements pose risks because they are not regulated and may contain substances that are not listed on the label. Nutrition supplements will be discussed in detail in chapter 11.

Nutrition Facts Labels

Nutrition facts labels found on most packaged foods are useful tools for diet planning and nutritional assessment (see figure 2.5). They help consumers make choices by providing detailed information about the nutrient content of food and how that food fits into the overall diet. In the United States, food labeling is standardized as specified by the Nutrition Labeling and Education Act of 1990. Food labeling laws regulate about 75% of all food consumed in the United States. Labels are not found or required on unpackaged foods such as freshly baked bread, cakes, fruits, and vegetables. All packaged foods (except those produced by small businesses and those in packages too small to fit the labeling information) must be labeled. The food

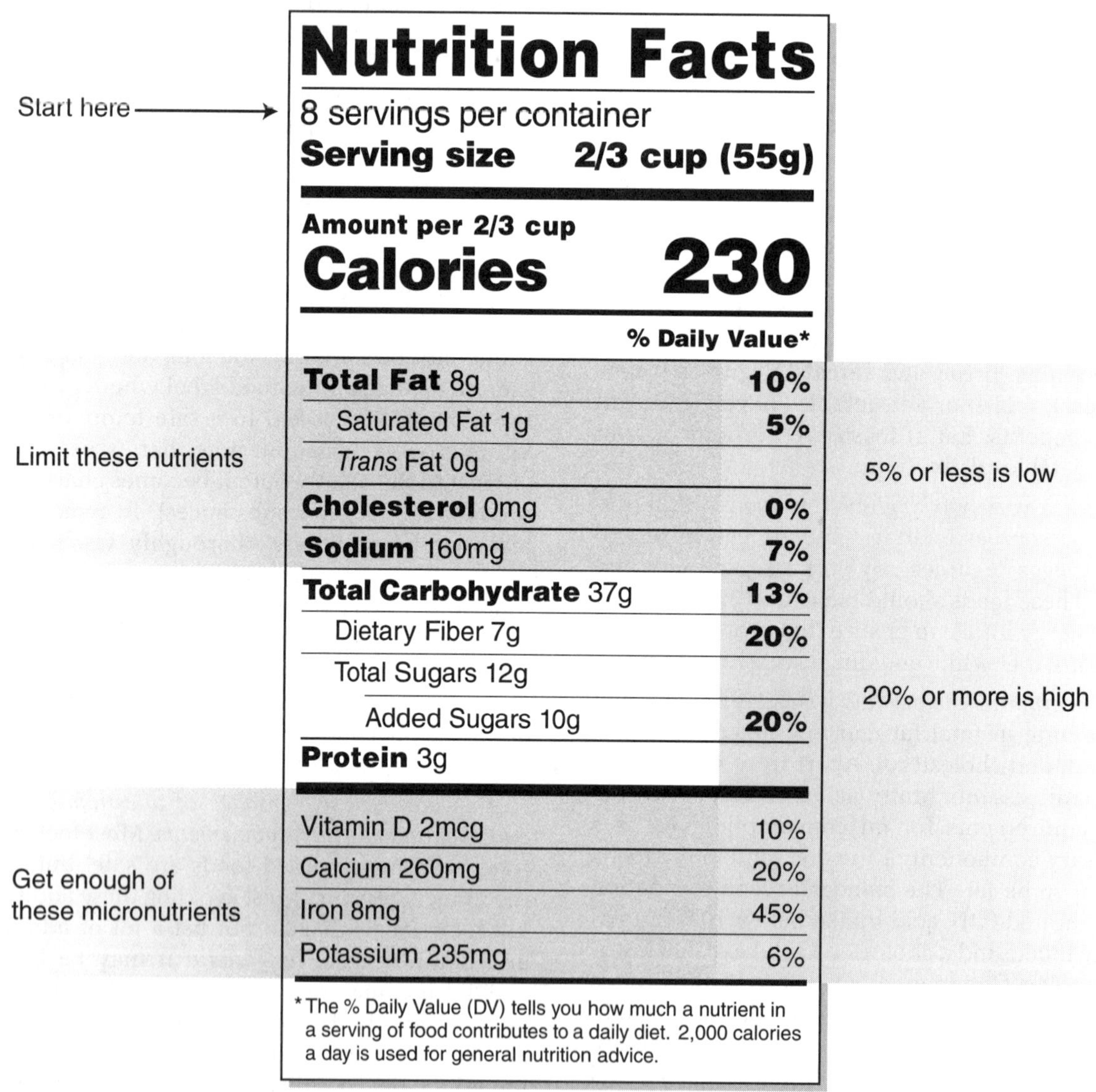

Figure 2.5 How to read a food label.

Adapted from U.S. Food & Drug Administration. https://www.fda.gov/Food/IngredientsPackagingLabeling/LabelingNutrition/ucm274593.htm#overview

label format is identical on all products so it is easy to compare foods. A broadly similar food label is used in the U.K. and Europe. In Canada, nutrition labeling is voluntary but standardized. In other parts of the world, labels are not yet standardized.

In the previous chapter the reference values (the DRVs and RDIs) that are used for reporting nutrients in nutrition facts labels were explained. Nutrition facts labels use a single term, *daily value* (DV), to designate the DRVs and RDIs. The DVs provide information about the amount of a nutrient that is present in a food and help consumers compare nutritional values of foods. They are provided for total fat, saturated fat, cholesterol, total carbohydrate, dietary fiber, sodium, potassium, and protein. Nutrition facts labels include the percentage of daily value (%DV) for each nutrient listed. The %DV for protein is not required unless a protein claim is made for the product or the product is for children under 4 years old. DVs are based on a daily energy intake of 8.4 MJ (2,000 kcal) for people aged 4 years and older. For instance, 100 ml of whole milk has 270 kJ (65 kcal) and contains 3.5 g of fat, 3.2 g of protein, 4.7 g of carbohydrate (all sugars), 120 mg of calcium, and 0.4 mg of vitamin B_{12}. In the United States, the values on food labels are expressed per serving and as a percentage of the daily value; in Europe, they are expressed per serving as well as per 100 g.

Nutrition facts labels in the United States have a top section that includes information about the product (serving size, energy content, and nutrition information). When looking at nutrition facts labels, begin with the serving size and the number of servings per package. Serving sizes are expressed in familiar terms (such as cups and pieces) and the metric amount (grams). The next line on the label indicates the calorie (energy) content followed by the amount of fat in grams and %DV. The label lists the key nutrients and the %DV for each. Nutrients for which intakes should be limited, such as total grams of fat, saturated fats, *trans* fats, cholesterol, and sodium, are listed first.

Total carbohydrate and protein are listed next. Since 2016, carbohydrate information has indicated the amount of added sugars separately from naturally occurring sugars. This was introduced because it is difficult to meet nutrition needs while staying within calorie limits if more than 10% of total daily energy comes from added sugars. The carbohydrate entry is divided into total sugars, added sugars (for which intake should be limited), and fiber (for which intake is encouraged). The nutrients are expressed in grams or milligrams per serving size but also as a percentage of daily recommended value. No %DV is provided for total sugar because no such value has been established. The %DVs are based on an 8.4 MJ (2,000 kcal) diet.

Nutrient Content and Health Claims on Food Packaging

Food packaging often contains terms that might interest consumers, such as *low fat, reduced fat, fat free, light,* and *lean*. The use of such terms is regulated, and their definitions have been established by the FDA (see table 2.2). A consumer who buys a product that is labeled low fat can be sure that it meets the established definition (in this case, less than 3 g of fat per serving).

Some food packages used to contain health claims such as "helps maintain a healthy heart" or "aids digestion." The rules on claims were extremely general, and this made it difficult for people to know what certain terms meant. Most countries now have specific rules that protect consumers from misleading claims. Any claims made about the nutritional and health benefits of a food are allowed only if they are based on good science.

For most countries, general claims about benefits to overall good health, such as "healthy" or "good for you," are allowed only if the claim has been approved by the relevant regulatory authority. General claims must be backed up by an explanation about why the food is healthy or what makes it a superfood, for example. Food packaging cannot claim that a food can treat, prevent, or cure any disease or medical condition. These claims can only be made for medicine. For example, calcium-rich products can reasonably claim to protect against osteoporosis, but no such claim is allowed on food labels. Only the claims in table 2.3 are legal in the United States. (Detailed information on health claims can be found on the FDA website.) Health claims can be used only when the food is a naturally good source (10% or more of the daily value) for one of six nutrients (vitamin A, vitamin C, protein, calcium, iron, or fiber), and the food must not contain more than 20% of the daily value for fat, saturated fat, cholesterol, or sodium. The claims must be backed up by scientific evidence (usually from epidemiological studies). In the United States, health claims must be accompanied by a disclaimer or be otherwise qualified.

TABLE 2.2 Definitions of Nutrient Content Claims

	Calories	Total fat	Sugar
Free (also zero, no, without, trivial source of, negligible source of)	Calorie free: fewer than 21 kJ (5 kcal) per reference amount* and per labeled serving	Fat free: fewer than 0.5 g of fat per reference amount and per labeled serving; for meals and main dishes**, fewer than 0.5 g per labeled serving	Sugar free: fewer than 0.5 g of sugar per reference amount and per labeled serving; for meals and main dishes, fewer than 0.5 g per labeled serving
Low (also little, few, contains a small amount of, low source of)	Low calories: no more than 167 kJ (40 kcal) per reference amount (or per 50 g if reference amount is small); for meals and main dishes, no more than 502 kJ (120 kcal) per 100 g	Low fat: no more than 3 g of fat per reference amount (and per 50 g if reference amount is small); for meals and main dishes, no more than 3 g per 100 g and not more than 30% of calories from fat	Not defined; no basis for recommended intake
Reduced or less (also lower, fewer)	Reduced calories: at least 25% fewer calories per reference amount than an appropriate reference food; reference food might not be low calorie	Reduced fat: at least 25% less fat per reference amount than an appropriate reference food; reference food might not be low fat	Reduced sugar: at least 25% less sugar per reference amount than an appropriate reference food
Additional comments	The term *light* (or *lite*) can be used if 50% or more of the calories are from fat, and the fat must be reduced by at least 50% per reference amount. If less than 50% of calories are from fat, the fat must be reduced by at least 50% or calories must be reduced by at least one-third per reference amount.	A food must have no fat for the package to say 100% fat free.	A claim that there are no added sugars is allowed if no sugar or sugar-containing ingredient is added during processing.

*The reference amount is the amount consumed in a suggested serving size. A small reference amount is 30 g (2 tablespoons) or less and is only used for dehydrated foods that are typically consumed when rehydrated with water or a diluent containing an insignificant amount of calories, total fat, or sugar). **A meal might be a complete ready meal containing, for example, some meat, pasta, vegetables, and sauce, whereas a main dish might be a starter, one part of a meal, or a dessert.

Processed Foods and Additives

The term *processed food* refers to food that is treated to extend storage life or to improve taste, nutrition, color, or texture. Processing methods include adding preservatives, colorings, or flavorings; fortifying, enriching, dehydrating, smoking, artificial ripening, drying, or freezing; and many other treatments. There is concern that the nutritional quality of food has declined in recent years because the amount of processing has increased. Modern foods contain greater amounts of refined sugar, extracted oils, and white flour. In the refinement process of their sources, nutrients are lost. For example, in the bleaching of flour, 22 known essential nutrients are lost. Artificially ripened fruit contains much smaller amounts of micronutrients than naturally ripened fruit.

Many products are completely artificial, such as synthetic fruit juices, soft drinks, and nondairy creamers. Refined or artificial products may contain few or no nutrients but have the same energy content as their natural counterparts. Thus, the **nutrient density** (the amount of essential nutrients per unit of energy) of refined or artificial products is extremely low. Food manufacturers

TABLE 2.3 Health Claims Allowed on Food Labels

Health issue	Claim
Calcium and osteoporosis	Adequate calcium intake throughout life helps maintain bone health and reduce the risk of osteoporosis. A food must contain 20% or more of the DV for calcium.
Sodium and hypertension	Diets high in sodium may increase the risk of high blood pressure in some people; hence, a diet low in sodium may protect against hypertension.
Dietary fat and cancer	Diets high in fat increase the risk of some types of cancer; hence, low-fat diets may be protective.
Saturated fat and cholesterol and risk of CHD	Diets high in saturated fat and cholesterol increase blood cholesterol and thus the risk of heart disease. A diet low in saturated fat may therefore reduce this risk.
Foods high in fiber and cancer	Diets low in fat and rich in fiber-containing grain products, fruits, and vegetables may reduce the risk of some types of cancer.
Foods high in fiber and risk of coronary heart disease	Diets low in saturated fat and cholesterol and rich in fruits, vegetables, and grain products that contain fiber, particularly soluble fiber, may reduce the risk of coronary heart disease.
Folic acid and birth defects	Adequate folic acid intake by the mother reduces the risk of birth defects of the brain or spinal cord in her baby.
Dietary sugar and dental caries	Sugar-free foods that are sweetened with sugar alcohols do not promote tooth decay and may reduce the risk of dental caries.

have tried to address this. Modern techniques used by most food manufacturers prevent major nutrient losses in processing. For example, the essential nutrient contents of frozen and canned vegetables are similar to those in fresh vegetables.

The increased use of refined sugar, oils, white flour, and salt is a significant concern because the necessary ingredients (i.e., essential nutrients) decrease while unnecessary ingredients of foods increase. Thus, foods become more energy dense and less nutrient dense.

Often food additives are used to lengthen shelf life; enhance color, texture, and taste; facilitate food preparation; and otherwise make food products more marketable. Certain additives, such as sugar, are derived from natural sources. Other additives, such as the artificial sweetener aspartame, are synthetic. Although there is a long list of additives that have been approved for use in food products, the effects of long term use and the effects of use in large amounts are sometimes not known. Consumer perception of foods that contain additives is changing and there is an increasing demand for "clean" labels (few additives). This perception is not always evidence based. For example many consumers will link artificial sweeteners with cancer but concrete evidence to support such claims has not been found. Common artificial sweeteners are listed in table 2.4 (see also chapter 15 on weight management).

The color of food is an integral part of our desire to eat it. Early civilizations recognized that people eat with their eyes as well as their palates; saffron was often used to provide a rich yellow color to various foods, and butter was colored yellow as far back as the 1300s. Today, the FDA carefully regulates all food color additives and ensures that foods with such additives are accurately labeled to indicate that the food contains these additives and are safe to eat. Food colorants are natural and synthetic. Natural colorants include beta-carotene, beet powder, carrot oil, carmine, fruit juice, paprika, riboflavin, saffron, and turmeric.

Fat Substitutes

Fat substitutes have one or more of the technical effects of fat in food but are not absorbed or metabolized as fat. The three types of fat substitutes are

TABLE 2.4 Artificial Sweeteners and Their Characteristics

Sweetener	Sweetness relative to sucrose	Characteristics	Products
Saccharin	300-500	Not metabolized in the body and is excreted in urine Fairly strong aftertaste	Used in soft drinks, tabletop sweeteners, chewing gum, canned fruit
Aspartame	180	Derived from the amino acids phenylalanine and aspartate and metabolizes back to these Contains 16 kJ/g (4 kcal/g), but adds virtually no energy Taste is quite pleasant; used to improve food taste Cannot be used in foods that need to be heated; denatures at high temperatures Limited stability in foods with low pH (e.g., soft drinks)	Sold under the brand name NutraSweet and used in a wide variety of products such as the following: • Sugar-free ice cream • Iced tea • Jams and jellies • Ice cream toppings • Fruit spreads • Sugar-free ketchup • Sugar-free cookies • Pudding
Acesulfame potassium	200	Noncaloric sweetener Not metabolized in the body and is excreted in urine	Sold under the brand name Sunnet and used in products such as the following: • Beverages (including soda, fruit juices, noncarbonated beverages, and alcohol) • Tabletop sweeteners • Dairy products • Ice cream • Desserts • Jam, jelly, and marmalade • Baked goods • Toothpaste and mouthwash
Sorbitol	0.5-0.7	Produced from sugar Contains 11 kJ/g (3 kcal/g) Excessive consumption (more than 50 g) can cause gastrointestinal problems	Used in food products like diet ("light") and diabetic drinks, sugar-free chewing gum, and candies
Sucralose	300-1,000	Discovered in 1976 and approved by the FDA in 1998 Synthesized from sucrose Absorbed only in small quantities and excreted in urine	Used in food products such as the following: • Dairy products (e.g., low-fat flavored milk, light yogurt, low-fat coffee creamer) • Cereals and cereal bars • Desserts (e.g., light pudding, light ice cream, popsicles) • Snack foods (e.g., light canned fruit, reduced calorie baked goods, candy)

carbohydrate-based fat substitutes, which use plant polysaccharides in place of fat; proteins and microparticulated proteins, which block fat absorption; and fat-based fat substitutes, which also block fat absorption.

Examples of carbohydrate-based fat replacements are corn syrup solids, dextrin, maltodextrin, modified food starch, and dietary fibers. These fat substitutes have little or no taste and contain less energy than fat. Dietary fibers such as cellulose

Sweetener	Sweetness relative to sucrose	Characteristics	Products
Xylitol	1	Contains 10 kJ/g (2 kcal/g)	Used in products such as the following: • Toothpaste • Mouthwash • Chewing gum • Peanut butter • Sugar-free candy • Sugar-free breath mints • Fruit drinks • Jellies and jams
Stevia	200	Natural sweetener made from an herbal plant extract (*Stevia rebaudiana*) High stability at low pH and high temperature Can provide long shelf life Cooking and baking resistant	Used in products such as the following: • Ice cream • Soy sauce • Chewing gum • Rice wines • Yogurts • Soft drinks • Fruit juices • Candies • Canned foods

gel, cellulose gum, guar gum, insulin, and pectin have some of the properties of fat but are minimally absorbed. A protein-based fat substitute sold under the name Simplesse is approved for use in low-temperature foods such as ice cream. It contains 4 to 8 kJ/g (1 to 2 kcal/g).

One of the most studied fat substitutes is olestra (brand name Olean). Olestra looks like fat, cooks like fat, and gives foods the rich taste and mouthfeel of fat. But unlike ordinary fats and oils, olestra is not digested or absorbed in the body, and therefore it contributes no fat or calories to the diet. In the 1990s olestra was used mainly in snack foods such as chips and crackers but lost its popularity because of its side effects (including intestinal cramping and diarrhea). Olestra is still used in some snack foods, but it is rare to find it in products today.

- Consumption of adequate amounts of essential nutrients does not guarantee the absence of potentially harmful, diet-related health effects. Diets deficient in some nonessential nutrients (e.g., fiber, phytonutrients) do not deliver what is needed for optimal functioning and health.
- Excessive intakes of some nutrients (e.g., carbohydrate, fats) or certain food subgroups (e.g., simple sugars, corn syrup, saturated fat, *trans* fatty acids) and other nonessential nutrients (e.g., alcohol, salt) can have harmful effects on health, particularly in the long term, by increasing the risk of developing chronic metabolic and cardiovascular diseases and cancer.
- There is compelling evidence that carbohydrate quantity and quality have important influences on obesity, cardiovascular disease, metabolic syndrome, and type 2 diabetes, particularly in those who have sedentary lifestyles.

- Dietary fiber is an important determinant of satiation, satiety, and weight gain, and it protects against cardiovascular disease.
- Vegetables, fruits, and grains protect against cardiovascular diseases.
- Sugar consumption is a proven cause of weight gain and obesity and is strongly associated with increased risk of cardiovascular and metabolic diseases.
- Epidemiological studies suggest that the type and quantity of fat in the diet are important factors related to the risk of cardiovascular diseases and some cancers.
- General guidelines for healthy eating include following healthy eating patterns across the life span; balancing food intake with physical activity to maintain a healthy weight; being physically active; eating a variety of nutrient-dense foods; eating a diet rich in vegetables, fruits, whole grains, and high-fiber foods; eating a variety of high-protein foods; incorporating dietary fats wisely; cutting back on high-calorie beverages and foods that have low nutrition values; reducing sodium intake; drinking alcohol only in moderation; practicing food hygiene and safety; and avoiding excessive intakes of questionable food additives and nutrition supplements.
- Dietary guidelines in several countries (e.g., United States, United Kingdom, Australia) focus on consuming recommended portions of various food groups and shifting food choices to healthier options. The overall aim is to achieve adequate intake of essential nutrients while meeting (but not exceeding) energy requirements. Most guidelines also encourage increased physical activity.
- Food labeling that includes nutrient information is now compulsory for most products in industrialized countries. Any health claims about specific foods must be backed up by scientific evidence and an explanation about why the food is healthy.
- The term *processed food* refers to food that is treated to extend storage life or to improve taste, nutrition, color, or texture. Processing methods include adding preservatives, colorings, or flavorings; fortifying, enriching, dehydrating, smoking, drying, or freezing; and many other treatments. There is concern that the nutritional quality of food has declined in recent years because the amount of processing has increased.

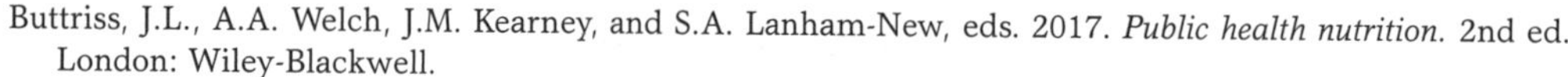

Recommended Readings

Buttriss, J.L., A.A. Welch, J.M. Kearney, and S.A. Lanham-New, eds. 2017. *Public health nutrition.* 2nd ed. London: Wiley-Blackwell.

Mann, J., and A.S. Truswell. 2002. *Essentials of human nutrition.* Oxford: Oxford University Press.

Shils, M.E., J.A. Olson, M. Shike, A.C. Ross, B. Caballero, and R.J. Cousins, eds. 2005. *Modern nutrition in health and disease.* Baltimore: Williams and Wilkins.

U.K. Government. 2016. Government dietary recommendations: The eatwell guide. www.gov.uk/government/publications/the-eatwell-guide

U.S. Department of Agriculture. 2015. *2015-2020 Dietary guidelines for Americans.* www.health.gov/DietaryGuidelines/.

Fuel Sources for Muscle and Exercise Metabolism

Objectives

After studying this chapter, you should be able to do the following:

- Describe the structure of skeletal muscle and explain the process of muscle contraction
- Describe the characteristics of the various muscle fiber types
- Describe the metabolic pathways that supply energy for muscle contraction
- Describe the nature and size of body fuel stores
- Describe the factors involved in the control of fuel mobilization and use
- Describe the metabolic responses and main causes of fatigue in moderate- and high-intensity exercise

An in-depth understanding of sport nutrition requires some knowledge of biochemistry, which usually refers to the study of events such as reactions, energy transfer, and transport processes at the subcellular and molecular levels. Those who lack a basic understanding of biochemistry and cell biology should refer to appendix A, which explains some of the basic principles. This chapter describes the sources of energy available for muscle force generation and explains how acute exercise modifies energy metabolism through intracellular effects and the action of **hormones** (for further details, see Maughan and Gleeson 2010; MacLaren and Morton 2011; and Tiidus, Tupling, and Houston 2012). The diet before exercise and feeding during exercise influence the hormonal and metabolic responses to exercise. Training also modifies the metabolic response to exercise, and training-induced adaptations encompass biochemical responses (e.g., changes in gene expression, protein content, enzyme activities in trained muscles) and physiological responses (e.g., changes in the local capillary network, maximal cardiac output, maximal oxygen uptake, $\dot{V}O_2max$). These adaptations are determined largely by the mode of exercise and the intensity, frequency, and volume of the exercise stimulus. Training-induced adaptations of skeletal muscle are also influenced to some degree by the composition and timing of nutrient intake. When ingested in sufficient amounts acutely before or during exercise or chronically during training, some dietary components can have performance-enhancing (**ergogenic**) effects. Thus, influences of diet and training on biochemical aspects of the acute response to exercise and the chronic adaptation to training are also briefly described in this chapter and are described in greater detail in the chapters that follow.

Portions of this chapter are reprinted by permission from M. Gleeson, "Biochemistry of Exercise," in *Nutrition in Sport*, edited by R.J. Maughan (Blackwell Science Ltd., 2000), 17-38.

Subcellular Skeletal Muscle Structure

Muscles are composed of long, cylindrical cells called fibers. These fibers contain the internal organelles and structures that allow muscle to contract and relax. Individual muscles are made up of many parallel fibers that may extend the entire length of the muscle. Inside the muscle fiber is the **sarcoplasm** (muscle cell cytoplasm), a red viscous fluid that contains nuclei, **mitochondria**, **myoglobin**, and about 500 threadlike 1 to 3 mm thick **myofibrils** that are continuous from end to end in the muscle fiber. The red color is caused by myoglobin, an intracellular respiratory pigment. Surrounding the myofibrils is an elaborate, baglike, membranous structure called the **sarcoplasmic reticulum**. Its interconnecting membranous tubules lie in the narrow spaces between the myofibrils and surround and run parallel to them. Energy is stored in the sarcoplasm as fat (triacylglycerol droplets), glycogen, phosphocreatine (PCr), a small pool of free amino acids (most of which are not used as an energy source), and **adenosine triphosphate (ATP)**.

The myofibrils are composed of overlapping thin and thick filaments made of protein, and the arrangement of these filaments gives skeletal muscle its striated appearance when viewed through a microscope. The thick filaments are composed of myosin molecules, each of which consists of a rodlike tail and a globular head. The latter contains **adenosine triphosphatase (ATPase)** activity sites and actin-binding sites. ATP is the energy currency of the cell. The breakdown of ATP to **adenosine diphosphate (ADP)** and inorganic phosphate (Pi) by the myosin ATPase provides the energy for muscle contraction. The thin filaments are composed of actin molecules and several regulatory proteins. Globular actin (G-actin) monomers are polymerized into long strands of fibrous actin (F-actin). Two F-actin strands twisted together in ropelike fashion form the backbone of each thin filament. Rod-shaped tropomyosin molecules spiral about the F-actin chains. The other main protein present in the thin filaments is troponin, which contains three subunits: (1) troponin-I, which binds to actin; (2) troponin-T, which binds to tropomyosin; and (3) troponin-C, which binds to calcium ions. A **sarcomere** is the smallest contractile unit, or segment, of a muscle fiber and is the region between two Z-lines (see figure 3.1).

Force Generation in Skeletal Muscle

When calcium and ATP are present in sufficient quantities, the filaments form actomyosin and shorten by sliding over each other. Sliding begins when the myosin heads of the thick filaments form **cross-bridges** (temporary linkages) that are attached to active sites on the actin subunits of the thin filaments. Each cross-bridge attaches and detaches several times during a contraction and pulls the thin filaments toward the center of the sarcomere in a ratchetlike action. When a muscle fiber contracts, its sarcomeres shorten throughout the cell, and the whole muscle fiber shortens.

The attachment of the myosin cross-bridges requires the presence of calcium ions. In the relaxed muscle, calcium is sequestered in the sarcoplasmic reticulum. Without calcium, the myosin binding sites on actin are physically blocked by the tropomyosin rods, as illustrated in figure 3.1. Electrical excitation passing as an action potential along the muscle cell membrane (**sarcolemma**) and down the T-tubules releases calcium from the sarcoplasmic reticulum into the sarcoplasm, subsequently causing activation and contraction of the filament array. The calcium ions bind to troponin, which causes a change in its shape that physically moves tropomyosin away from the myosin binding sites on the underlying actin chain.

Excitation is initiated by the arrival of a nerve impulse at the muscle membrane via the motor end plate. Activated, or cocked, myosin heads now bind to the actin, and the myosin head changes from its activated configuration to its bent shape, which causes the head to pull on the thin filament and slide it toward the center of the sarcomere. This action represents the power stroke of the cross-bridge cycle, and simultaneously ADP and Pi are released from the myosin head. As a new ATP molecule binds to the myosin head at the ATPase activity site, the myosin cross-bridge detaches from the actin. Hydrolysis of the ATP to ADP and Pi by the ATPase provides the energy required to return the myosin to its activated state, giving it the potential energy needed for the next cross-bridge cycle. ATP is the only source of energy that can be used directly not only for muscle contraction but also for other energy-requiring processes in the cell.

While the myosin is in the activated state, the ADP and Pi remain attached to the myosin head. The myosin head can attach to another actin unit farther along the thin filament, and the cross-bridge

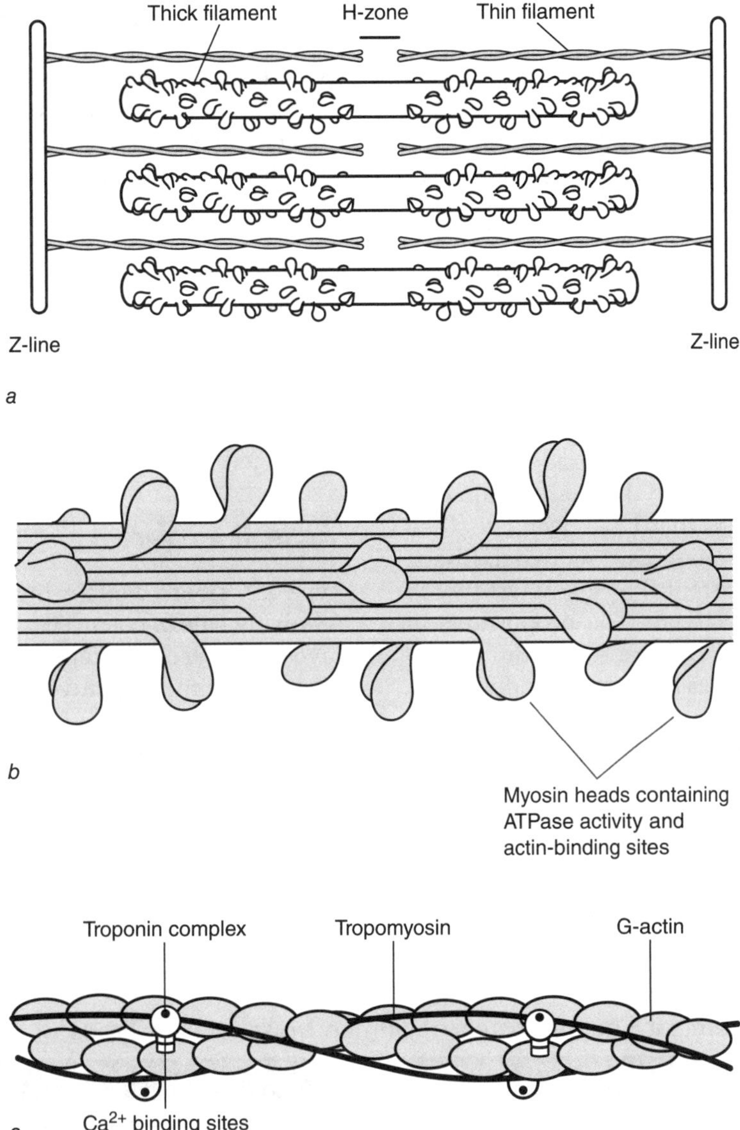

Figure 3.1 *(a)* Longitudinal cross-section of a sarcomere shows the molecular components of the myofilaments and the arrangement of the thick and thin filaments between two Z-lines in a myofibril. *(b)* The thick filaments are composed of myosin molecules. Each myosin molecule consists of a rodlike tail and a globular head. The latter contains ATPase activity sites and actin-binding sites. *(c)* The thin filaments are composed of actin molecules and the regulatory proteins tropomyosin and tropinin.

Reprinted by permission from M. Gleeson, "Biochemistry of Exercise," in *Nutrition in Sport,* edited by R.J. Maughan (Blackwell Science Ltd., 2000), 17-38.

cycle is repeated. Sliding of the filaments continues as long as calcium is present in the sarcoplasm at a concentration in excess of 10 mmol/L. Removal and sequestration of the calcium by the ATP-dependent calcium pump (ATPase) of the sarcoplasmic reticulum restore the tropomyosin inhibition of cross-bridge formation and the muscle fiber relaxes.

Fiber Types

The existence of different fiber types in skeletal muscle has long been recognized. Based on their contraction speed and metabolic characteristics, muscle fibers can be broadly classified as **type I fibers** or **type II fibers**. The physiological and biochemical bases for these differences and their functional significance have only recently been established. Much of the impetus for investigating these differences has come from the realization that success in athletic activities that require the ability to generate either high power output or great endurance is related to the proportions of the fiber types in the muscles. The muscle fibers are, however, extremely plastic (i.e., adaptable), and although the distribution of fiber type is genetically determined and not easily altered, an appropriate training program will have a major effect on the metabolic potential of the muscle regardless of the proportion of fiber types.

Human muscle fibers are commonly divided into types I, IIa, and IIX, which are analogous to animal muscle fibers that have been classified based on direct observation as slow-twitch fibers, fast-twitch fatigue-resistant fibers, and fast-twitch fatigable fibers, respectively. The proportions in which type I, IIa, and IIX are found differ substantially among muscles and among individuals. The myosin of the different fiber types exists in different molecular forms (isoforms), and the myofibrillar ATPase activity of the different isoforms displays differential **pH** sensitivity that provides the basis for the differential chemical staining and identification of fiber types. The biochemical characteristics of the three fiber types are summarized in table 3.1.

Type I Fibers

Type I fibers are small-diameter red cells that contain relatively slow-acting myosin ATPases and hence contract slowly. The red color is caused by myoglobin, which is capable of binding oxygen and releasing it only at very low partial pressures. Type I fibers have numerous energy-producing mitochondria, which are mostly located close to the periphery of the fiber, near the blood capillaries that provide a rich supply of oxygen and nutrients. Type I fibers possess a high capacity for oxidative metabolism, are extremely fatigue resistant, and are specialized for repeated contractions over prolonged periods.

Type II Fibers

Type IIX fibers contain little myoglobin and are relatively pale in color. They possess rapidly acting myosin ATPases; therefore, their contraction (and relaxation) time is relatively fast. These fibers have fewer mitochondria and a poorer capillary supply, but they have greater glycogen and phosphocreatine stores compared with the type I fibers. High glycogenolytic and glycolytic enzyme activity gives type IIX fibers a high capacity for rapid (but relatively short-lived) ATP production in the absence of oxygen (**anaerobic** capacity). Lactate and hydrogen ions accumulate quickly in these fibers, and they

TABLE 3.1 Biochemical Characteristics of Human Muscle Fiber Types

Characteristic	Type I	Type IIa	Type IIX
Nomenclature	Slow, red Fatigue resistant Oxidative	Fast, red Fatigue resistant Oxidative or glycolytic	Fast, white Fatigable Glycolytic
Capillary density	1.0	0.8	0.6
Mitochondrial density	1.0	0.7	0.4
Myoglobin content	1.0	0.6	0.3
Phosphorylase activity	1.0	2.1	3.1
PFK activity	1.0	1.8	2.3
Citrate synthase activity	1.0	0.8	0.6
SDH activity	1.0	0.7	0.4
Glycogen content	1.0	1.3	1.5
Triacylglycerol content	1.0	0.4	0.2
Phosphocreatine content	1.0	1.2	1.2
Myosin ATPase activity	1.0	>2	>2

Values of metabolic characteristics of type II fibers are shown relative to those found in type I fibers. PFK = phosphofructokinase; SDH = succinate dehydrogenase.

Reprinted by permission from M. Gleeson, "Biochemistry of Exercise," in *Nutrition in Sport*, edited by R.J. Maughan (Blackwell Science Ltd., 2000), 17-38.

fatigue rapidly. Thus, these fibers are best suited for delivering rapid, powerful contractions for brief periods. The metabolic characteristics of type IIa fibers lie between the extreme properties of type I and type IIX fibers. Type IIa fibers contain fast-acting myosin ATPases like the type IIX fibers but have an oxidative capacity more like that of type I fibers.

The differences in the activation thresholds of the motor neurons that supply the different fiber types determine the order in which fibers are recruited during exercise and in turn influence the metabolic response to exercise. During most forms of movement, an orderly hierarchy of motor unit recruitment occurs that roughly corresponds with a progression from type I to type IIa to type IIX. Light exercise uses mostly type I fibers, moderate exercise uses both type I and type IIa fibers, and severe exercise uses all fiber types.

Muscle Fiber Composition

Muscles contain a mixture of the three different fiber types, although the proportions in which the types are found differ substantially among muscles and can also differ among individuals. For example, muscles involved in maintaining posture (e.g., soleus in the leg) have a high proportion (usually >70%) of type I fibers, which is in keeping with their function of maintaining prolonged but relatively weak contractions. Type II fibers, however, predominate in muscles that produce rapid movements, such as the muscles of the hand and the eye. Muscles such as the quadriceps group in the leg contain a variable mixture of fiber types. The vastus lateralis muscle in the quadriceps muscle group of successful marathon runners has a high percentage (about 80%) of type I fibers, whereas the same muscle in elite sprinters contains a higher percentage (about 60%) of type II fibers. The fiber type composition of muscles is genetically determined and is not pliable to any significant degree by training. Hence, athletic capabilities are mostly inborn (assuming that the person realizes her or his genetic potential through appropriate nutrition and training).

Energy for Muscle Force Generation

Energy is the potential for performing work or producing force. Therefore, energy availability can be seen as a potential prerequisite for performing work or producing force. ATP is the only source of energy that can be used directly for muscle contraction and all other energy-requiring processes in the cell such as active transport across membranes and the synthesis of macromolecules from their precursors. In muscle fibers, energy from the hydrolysis of ATP by myosin ATPase activates specific sites on the contractile elements, as described previously, causing the muscle fiber to shorten. The hydrolysis of ATP yields approximately 31 kJ (7 kcal) of free energy per mole of ATP (a mole is equivalent to molecular weight in grams) degraded to ADP and Pi:

$$ATP + H_2O \rightarrow ADP + H^+ + Pi - 31 \text{ kJ per mole of ATP}$$

Active reuptake of calcium ions by the sarcoplasmic reticulum also requires ATP, as does the restoration of the membrane potential of the muscle cell through the action of the Na^+-K^+-ATPase (commonly known as the sodium pump).

The resting concentration of ATP in skeletal muscle is about 4 to 5 mmol/kg wet weight (w.w.) of muscle, which can only provide enough energy to sustain a few seconds of intense exercise. Since depletion of ATP would be fatal to the cell, the ATP concentration in the **sarcoplasm** must be maintained by resynthesis from ADP at essentially the same rate at which ATP is broken down. Three mechanisms are involved in the resynthesis of ATP for muscle force generation: (1) PCr hydrolysis; (2) **glycolysis**, which involves metabolism of **glucose-6-phosphate (G6P)** derived from muscle glycogen or blood-borne glucose and produces ATP by substrate-level phosphorylation reactions; and (3) **oxidative phosphorylation**, in which the products of carbohydrate, fat, protein, and alcohol metabolism enter the **tricarboxylic acid (TCA) cycle** in the mitochondria and are oxidized to carbon dioxide and water, which yields energy for the synthesis of ATP.

These mechanisms regenerate ATP at sufficient rates to prevent a significant fall in the intramuscular ATP concentration. PCr breakdown and glycolysis are anaerobic mechanisms that occur in the sarcoplasm. Each uses only one specific substrate for energy production: PCr and glucose-6-phosphate, respectively. The **aerobic** processes in the mitochondria use a variety of different substrates, and the sarcoplasm contains a variety of enzymes that can convert carbohydrates, fats, and proteins into usable substrate, primarily a two-carbon acetyl group linked to acetyl-CoA, which can be completely oxidized in the mitochondria with the resultant production of ATP. A general summary of the main energy sources and pathways of energy metabolism is presented in figure 3.2.

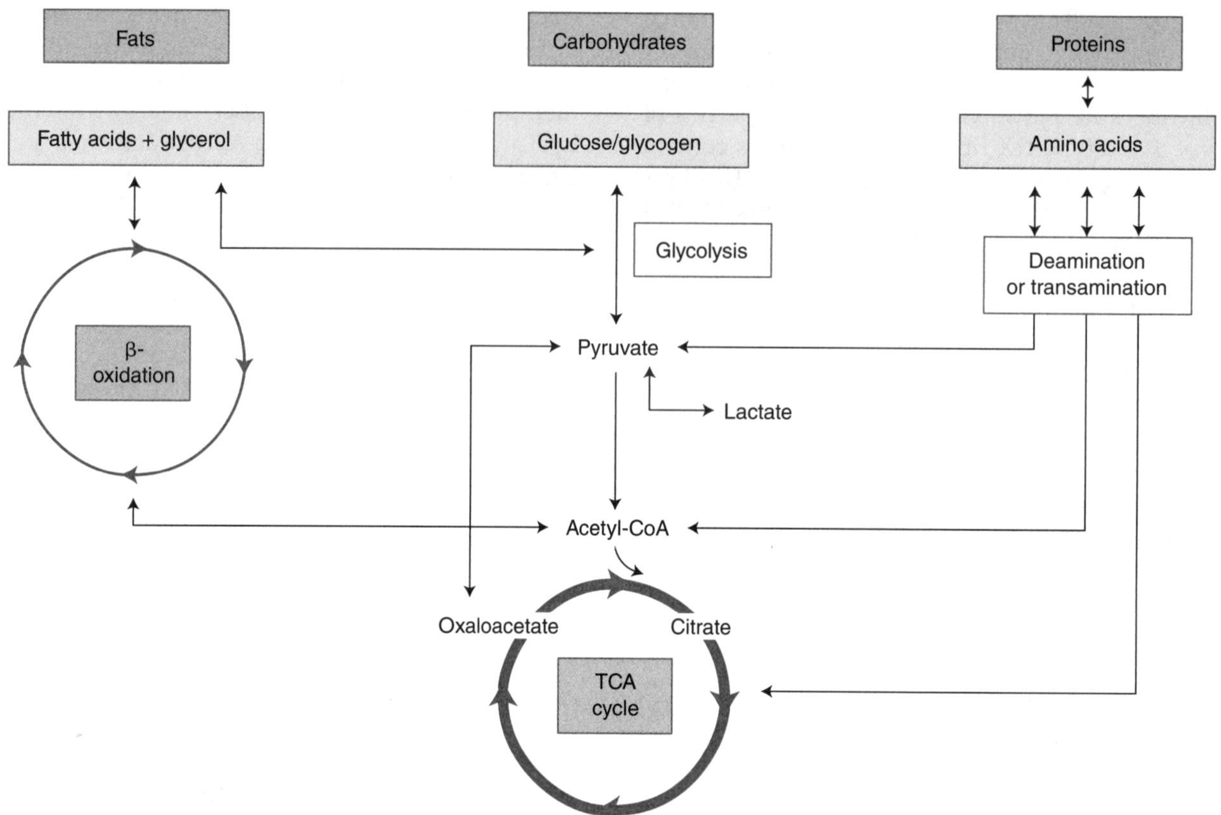

Figure 3.2 The main pathways of energy metabolism using carbohydrates, lipids, and proteins as energy sources.

Reprinted by permission from M. Gleeson, "Biochemistry of Exercise," in *Nutrition in Sport,* edited by R.J. Maughan (Blackwell Science Ltd., 2000), 17-38.

Phosphocreatine in Anaerobic Metabolism

Some of the energy for ATP resynthesis is supplied rapidly and without the need for oxygen. Within the muscle fiber, the concentration of PCr is three to four times greater than that of ATP. When PCr is broken down to creatine and Pi by the action of the enzyme creatine kinase (CK), a large amount of free energy is released (43 kJ [10 kcal] per mole of PCr):

$$ADP + PCr + H^+ \rightarrow ATP + Cr - 43 \text{ kJ per mole of PCr}$$

Because PCr has a higher free energy of hydrolysis than ATP, its phosphate is donated directly to the ADP molecule to re-form ATP. When the ATP content begins to fall during exercise, PCr is broken down, releasing energy for restoration of ATP. Note that the resynthesis of ATP through the breakdown of PCr buffers some of the hydrogen ions (H^+) formed as a result of ATP hydrolysis. This action helps to prevent a rapid acidification of the muscle sarcoplasm, which could induce premature failure of the contractile mechanism. During intense exercise, the PCr concentration falls rapidly and can be depleted within 10 to 20 seconds. However, the reactions of ATP and PCr hydrolysis are reversible, and when energy is readily available from other sources (oxidative phosphorylation), creatine and phosphate can be rejoined to form PCr:

$$ATP + Cr \rightarrow ADP + PCr$$

The PCr in muscle is immediately available at the onset of exercise and can be used to resynthesize ATP quickly. This rapid energy transfer corresponds to the ability to produce high power output (see table 3.2). The major disadvantage of this process compared with other means of regenerating ATP is its limited capacity. The total amount of energy available is small (see table 3.3). It is worth noting here that studies on dietary creatine supplementation (about 20 g/day for one

TABLE 3.2 Anaerobic Production of ATP

	Capacity (mmol ATP/kg w.w.)	Power (mmol ATP/kg w.w./s)
Phosphagen system	14-24	2.3
Glycolytic system	48-75	1.1
Combined	62-93	2.8

Values are expressed per kilogram of wet weight (w.w.) of muscle and are based on estimates of ATP provision during high-intensity exercise of the human vastus lateralis muscle.

Reprinted by permission from M. Gleeson, "Biochemistry of Exercise," in *Nutrition in Sport*, edited by R.J. Maughan (Blackwell Science Ltd., 2000), 17-38.

TABLE 3.3 ATP Resynthesis From Anaerobic and Aerobic Metabolism

	Max rate of ATP resynthesis (mmol ATP/kg w.w./s)	Delay time*
PCr breakdown	2.25	Instantaneous
Glycolysis	1.10	5-10 s
Glycogen oxidation	0.70	1-3 min
Glucose (from blood) oxidation	0.35	~90 min
Fat oxidation	0.25	>2 h

*Approximate delay time before maximal rates are attained after onset of exercise.

Reprinted by permission from M. Gleeson, "Biochemistry of Exercise," in *Nutrition in Sport*, edited by R.J. Maughan (Blackwell Science Ltd., 2000), 17-38.

week) indicate that the muscle PCr store can be increased by about 10% and the muscle creatine content can be increased by about 40%, and this can improve performance of repeated sprints (Hespel, Maughan, and Greenhaff 2006; Stephens and Greenhaff 2014). Further details can be found in chapter 11.

An additional pathway to regenerate ATP when ATP and PCr stores are depleted is through a kinase reaction that used two molecules of ADP to generate one molecule of ATP (and one molecule of adenosine monophosphate [AMP]). This reaction is catalyzed by the enzyme myokinase:

$$\text{ADP} + \text{ADP} \rightarrow \text{ATP} + \text{AMP} - 31 \text{ kJ per mole of ADP}$$

This reaction becomes important only during high-intensity exercise. Even then, the amount of energy available in the form of ATP is extremely limited, and the real importance of the reaction may be the formation of AMP, which is a potent activator of a number of enzymes involved in energy metabolism.

The total adenylate pool can decline rapidly if the AMP concentration of the cell rises during muscle force generation. This decline occurs principally by deamination of AMP to inosine monophosphate (IMP), but it also occurs by the dephosphorylation of AMP to adenosine. The loss of AMP may initially appear counterproductive because of the reduction in the total adenylate pool. But the deamination of AMP to IMP occurs only under low ATP-to-ADP ratio conditions, and, by preventing excessive accumulation of ADP and AMP, it enables the adenylate kinase reactions to continue, resulting in an increase in the ATP-to-ADP ratio and continuing muscle force generation. Furthermore, the free energy of ATP hydrolysis possibly decreases when ADP and Pi accumulate, which could further impair muscle force generation. For these reasons, adenine nucleotide loss is important to muscle function during conditions of metabolic crisis, such as during maximal exercise or in the later stages of prolonged submaximal exercise when glycogen stores become depleted.

Glycolysis in Anaerobic Metabolism

Under normal conditions, muscle does not fatigue after only a few seconds of effort, so a source of energy other than ATP and PCr must be available.

SOURCES OF ATP FOR MUSCLE FORCE GENERATION

1. PCr hydrolysis: Rapid energy release without the need for oxygen (anaerobic metabolism); occurs in the sarcoplasm.
2. Glycolysis: Energy available from the breakdown of glucose (anaerobic metabolism) through uptake from the blood, muscle glycogen breakdown, the glycolytic pathway (figure 3.3); occurs in the sarcoplasm.
3. Oxidative phosphorylation: Carbohydrates, fats, and proteins are oxidized (aerobic metabolism); occurs in the mitochondrion. See figures 3.4 through 3.8.

The source is glycolysis, which involves the breakdown of glucose (or glycogen) in a series of chemical reactions that yield pyruvate. This process does not require oxygen but does result in ATP being available to the muscle from reactions involving substrate-level phosphorylation. But the pyruvate must be removed (allowing regeneration of the oxidized form of the essential co-factor nicotinamide adenine dinucleotide [NAD^+]) for the reactions to proceed, and the rate of ATP resynthesis via these means is somewhat slower than for PCr breakdown. In low-intensity exercise, when adequate oxygen is available to the muscle, pyruvate is converted to carbon dioxide and water by oxidative metabolism in the mitochondria. In some situations when oxygen availability is limited (e.g., intense isometric exercise that occludes muscle blood flow) or the rate of formation of pyruvate is extremely high (e.g., sprinting), the pyruvate can also be removed by conversion to lactate; this reaction does not involve oxygen.

Muscle Uptake of Glucose From the Blood

A specific transporter protein, GLUT4, carries glucose molecules across the cell membrane. After the glucose molecule is inside the muscle cell, an irreversible phosphorylation (addition of a phosphate group), catalyzed by the enzyme **hexokinase**, occurs to prevent the loss of glucose from the cell. The glucose is converted to glucose-6-phosphate. Skeletal muscles lack the enzyme glucose-6-phosphatase, so they are not able to re-form free glucose following the formation of glucose-6-phosphate. Thus, the addition of a phosphate group to glucose ensures that the glucose is effectively trapped inside the cell. Note that this is an important difference between skeletal muscle and the liver. In the liver, which contains the glucose-6-phosphatase enzyme, glucose-6-phosphate can be broken down to form free glucose that can be released into the blood. In this way, the liver plays an important role in the maintenance of the blood glucose concentration, whereas muscle tissue cannot do so directly. The hexokinase reaction is an energy-consuming reaction that requires the investment of one molecule of ATP for each molecule of glucose. This reaction also ensures a concentration gradient for glucose across the cell membrane down which transport can occur. Hexokinase is inhibited by an accumulation of glucose-6-phosphate, and during high-intensity exercise, the increasing concentration of glucose-6-phosphate limits the contribution that the blood glucose can make to carbohydrate metabolism in the active muscles.

Muscle Glycogen Breakdown

If glycogen, rather than blood glucose, is the substrate for glycolysis, a single glucose molecule is split off by the enzyme glycogen phosphorylase, and the products are glucose-1-phosphate and a glycogen molecule that is one glucose residue shorter than the original. The substrates are glycogen and inorganic phosphate, so, unlike the hexokinase reaction, no breakdown of ATP occurs. Phosphorylase acts on the α-1,4 carbon bonds at the free ends of the glycogen molecule but cannot break the α-1,6 bonds forming the branch points. These bonds are hydrolyzed by the combined actions of a debranching enzyme and amylo-1,6-glucosidase, with the latter causing the release of free glucose, which is quickly phosphorylated to glucose-6-phosphate by hexokinase. Free glucose accumulates within the muscle cell only in very high-intensity exercise in which **glycogenolysis** is proceeding rapidly. Because relatively few α-1,6 bonds exist, no more than about 10% of the glucose residues appear as free glucose.

Glycolytic Pathway From Glucose-6-Phosphate to Pyruvate

The enzyme phosphoglucomutase rapidly converts the glucose-1-phosphate formed by the action of phosphorylase on glycogen to glucose-6-phosphate, which then proceeds down the glycolytic pathway (see figure 3.3). After a further phosphorylation, the glucose molecule is cleaved to form two molecules of the three-carbon sugar glyceraldehyde-3-phosphate. The second stage of glycolysis is the conversion of glyceraldehyde-3-phosphate into pyruvate, which is accompanied by the formation of ATP and reduction of nicotinamide adenine dinucleotide (NAD^+) to NADH.

The net effect of glycolysis is the conversion of one molecule of glucose to three molecules of pyruvate with the formation of two molecules of ATP and the conversion of two molecules of NAD^+ to NADH. If glycogen rather than glucose is the

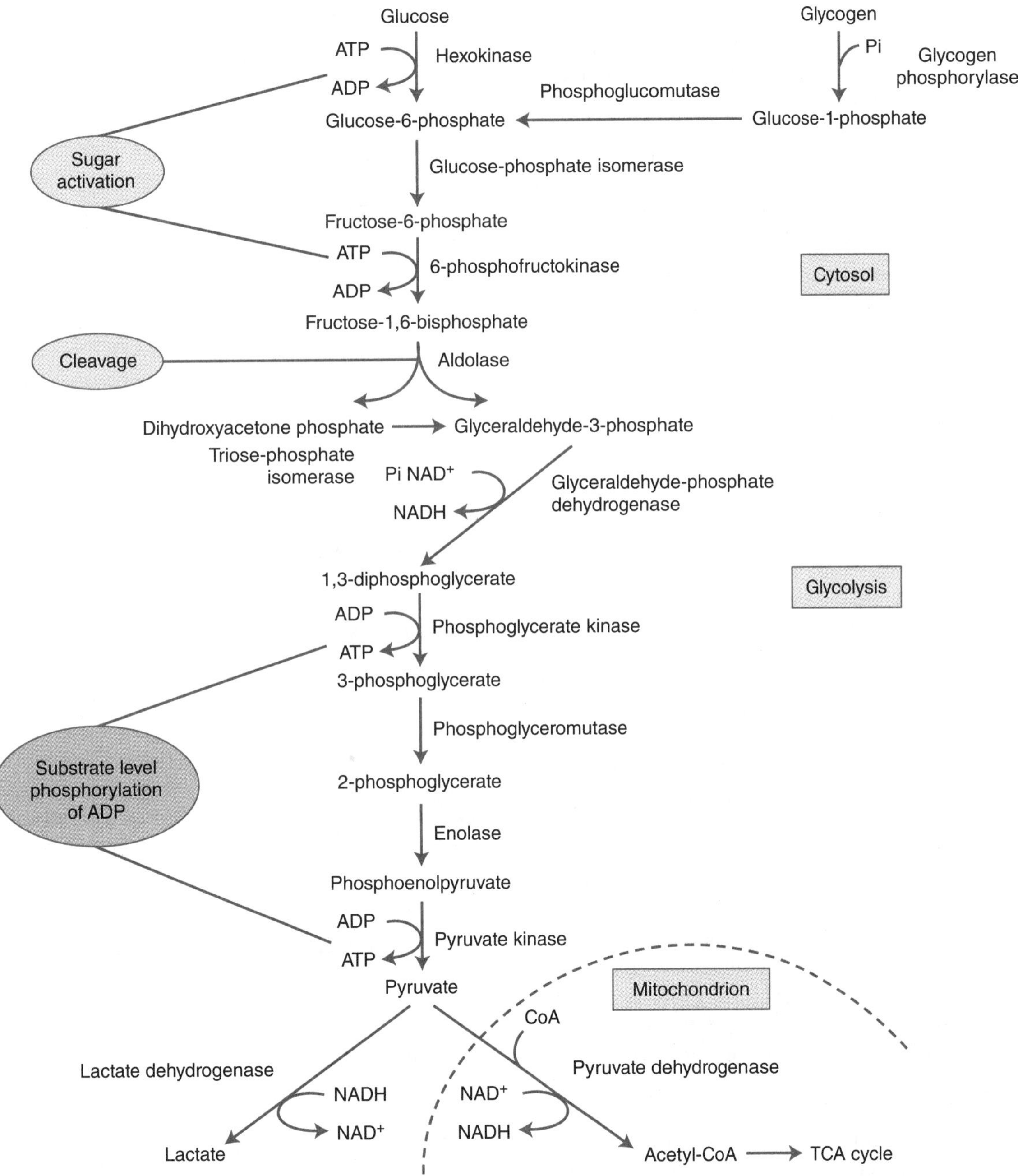

Figure 3.3 The glycolytic pathway. Glycolysis makes two molecules of ATP available for each molecule of glucose that passes through the pathway, or three molecules of ATP if muscle glycogen is the starting substrate.

Reprinted by permission from M. Gleeson, "Biochemistry of Exercise," in *Nutrition in Sport,* edited by R.J. Maughan (Blackwell Science Ltd., 2000), 17-38.

starting substrate, three molecules of ATP are produced because no initial investment of ATP is made when the first phosphorylation step occurs. Although this net energy yield appears small, the relatively large carbohydrate store available and the rapid rate at which glycolysis proceeds make energy supplied in this way crucial for the performance of intense exercise. The 800 m (0.5 mi) runner, for example, obtains about 60% of the total energy requirement from anaerobic metabolism and may convert about 100 g of carbohydrate (mostly glycogen and equivalent to about 550 mmol of glucose) to lactate in less than 2 minutes. The amount of ATP released in this way (three ATP molecules per glucose molecule degraded, about 1,667 mmol of ATP in total) far exceeds the ATP available from PCr hydrolysis. This high rate of anaerobic metabolism not only allows a faster steady-state speed than is possible with aerobic metabolism alone but also allows a faster pace in the early stages before the cardiovascular system has adjusted to the demands and before the delivery and use of oxygen have increased in response to the exercise stimulus.

The reactions of glycolysis occur in the cytoplasm of the muscle cell, and some pyruvate will escape from active muscle tissues when the rate of glycolysis is high, but most of it is further metabolized. The fate of the pyruvate produced depends not only on factors such as exercise intensity but also on the metabolic capacity of the tissue. When glycolysis proceeds rapidly, the availability of NAD^+, which is necessary as a cofactor in the glyceraldehyde-3-phosphate dehydrogenase reaction, becomes limiting. Reduction of pyruvate to lactate will regenerate NAD^+ in muscle, and this reaction can proceed in the absence of oxygen. That is not to say, however, that lactate formation occurs only in the absence of oxygen. Even at low exercise intensities, such as when walking, some lactate formation occurs. Lactate can accumulate within the muscle fibers and reach much higher concentrations than those reached by any of the glycolytic intermediates, including pyruvate. But when lactate accumulates in high concentrations, the associated hydrogen ions cause intracellular pH to fall, which inhibits some enzymes such as phosphorylase and phosphofructokinase, and the contractile mechanism begins to fail. A low pH also stimulates free nerve endings in the muscle, which causes the perception of pain. Although the negative effects of the acidosis resulting from lactate accumulation are often stressed, the energy made available by anaerobic glycolysis allows the performance of high-intensity exercise that would otherwise not be possible. The main contributors to H^+ accumulation during high-intensity exercise are ATP breakdown and the H^+ associated with lactate formation during glycolysis, although there is some debate as to the relative importance of these sources of H^+ generation.

Carbohydrate Oxidation in Aerobic Metabolism

Pyruvate may also undergo oxidative metabolism to carbon dioxide and water. This process occurs within the mitochondrion, and the pyruvate that is produced in the sarcoplasm is transported across the mitochondrial membrane by a specific carrier protein (monocarboxylic acid transporter). The three-carbon pyruvatc is converted by oxidative decarboxylation into a two-carbon acetate group, which is linked by a thioester bond to coenzyme A (CoA) to form acetyl-CoA. This reaction, in which NAD^+ is converted to NADH, is catalyzed by the pyruvate dehydrogenase enzyme complex. Acetyl-CoA is also formed from the metabolism of fatty acids (FAs) within the mitochondria in a metabolic process called **ß-oxidation**. These processes are summarized in figure 3.4. Note that this figure builds on figure 3.2 by including the products of the TCA cycle and the subcellular locations of the pathways involved.

Tricarboxylic Acid Cycle

Acetyl-CoA is oxidized to carbon dioxide in the TCA cycle (also known as the Krebs cycle and the citric acid cycle). The reactions involve a combination of acetyl-CoA with oxaloacetate to form citrate, which is a six-carbon TCA. A series of reactions lead to the sequential loss of hydrogen atoms and carbon dioxide, resulting in the regeneration of oxaloacetate:

$$\text{acetyl-CoA} + \text{ADP} + \text{Pi} + 3\ \text{NAD}^+ + \text{FAD} + 3\ \text{H}_2\text{O} \rightarrow 2\ \text{CO}_2 + \text{CoA} + \text{ATP} + 3\ \text{NADH} + 3\ \text{H}^+ + \text{FADH}_2$$

Because acetyl-CoA is also a product of FA oxidation, the final steps of oxidative degradation are common to both fat and carbohydrate. The hydrogen atoms are carried by the reduced coenzymes NADH and flavin adenine dinucleotide ($FADH_2$). These coenzymes act as carriers and donate pairs of electrons to the **electron-transport chain (ETC)**, which allows oxidative phosphorylation with the subsequent regeneration of ATP from ADP.

The reactions involved in the TCA cycle are shown in figure 3.5. The two-carbon acetate units

BUFFERS PREVENT EXCESSIVE FALLS IN PH

Processes that buffer (remove or mop up) H^+ as they start to accumulate are present in muscle. Proteins and phosphate ions act as chemical buffers because they are able to accept H^+. The monocarboxylate transporters located in the sarcolemmal membrane remove lactate and H^+ simultaneously from the muscle by cotransport into the interstitial fluid, and the expression of these transporters is increased by high-intensity interval training (Pilegaard et al. 1999). The movement of H^+ out of the muscle can be enhanced by an increase in the extracellular fluid bicarbonate concentration. This can be achieved by acute oral sodium bicarbonate loading, and ingesting a dose of approximately 0.3 g per kilogram of body weight 1 to 2 hours before exercise has been shown to improve performance in exercise that lasts 2 to 6 minutes (Hespel, Maughan, and Greenhaff 2006; Wilkes, Gledhill, and Smyth 1983). The dipeptide carnosine (which is synthesized from the amino acids histidine and ß-alanine) also plays an important role in buffering of intracellular acidosis during high-intensity exercise. The normal carnosine concentration in untrained human mixed muscle is about 4 mmol/kg w.w. but can be as high as 10 mmol/kg w.w. in 800 m runners and rowers. High carnosine concentrations are found in individuals who have high proportions of type II fibers, because these fibers are enriched with the dipeptide. Muscle carnosine content is lower in women, declines with age, and is lower in vegetarians (whose diets do not contain ß-alanine). Sprint-trained athletes display markedly high muscular carnosine, but the effect of several weeks of high-intensity training on muscle carnosine is rather small. High carnosine levels in elite sprinters are therefore either genetically determined or a result of slow adaptation to years of training. Studies have shown that the chronic oral ingestion of ß-alanine can elevate the carnosine content of human skeletal muscle by up to 80% and that such muscle carnosine loading leads to improved performance in high-intensity exercise in untrained and trained individuals (Artioli et al. 2010; Derave et al. 2010; Sale, Saunders, and Harris 2010). **ß-alanine** supplementation is now common among athletes in high-intensity sports such as middle-distance running, football, and rugby. For further details see chapter 11.

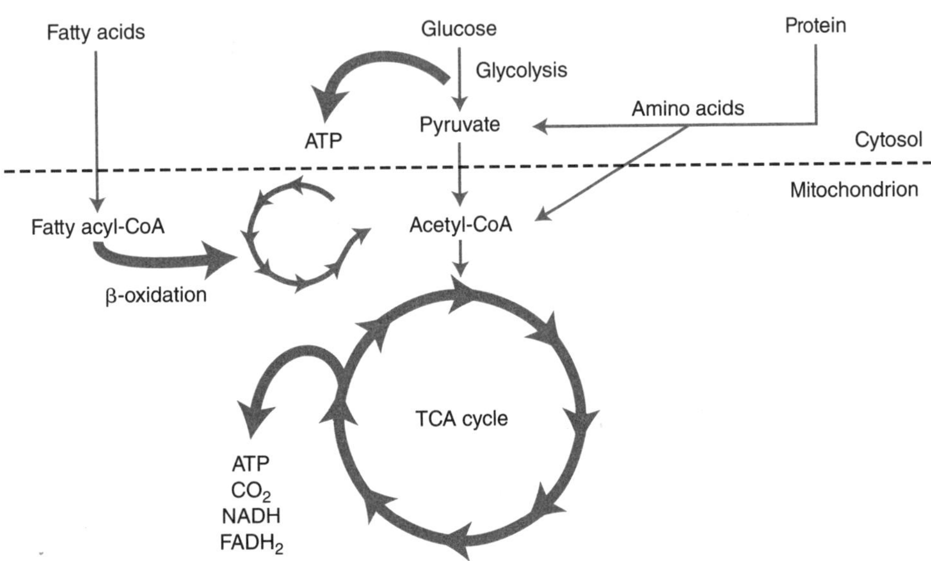

Figure 3.4 Formation of acetyl-CoA occurs from the catabolism of carbohydrates, fats, and proteins. Acetyl-CoA is oxidized in the tricarboxylic acid cycle, which generates carbon dioxide, reduced coenzymes, and ATP.

of acetyl-CoA are combined with the four-carbon oxaloactate to form six-carbon citrate. The latter undergoes two successive decarboxylations (removal of carbon dioxide) to yield four-carbon succinate, which, in subsequent reactions, is converted to oxaloacetate, completing the TCA cycle. Molecular oxygen does not participate directly in these reactions. The most important function of the TCA cycle is to generate hydrogen atoms for subsequent passage to the ETC by mcans of NADH and $FADH_2$ (see figure 3.6).

Electron-Transport Chain and Oxidative Phosphorylation

The aerobic process of electron transport and oxidative phosphorylation regenerates ATP from

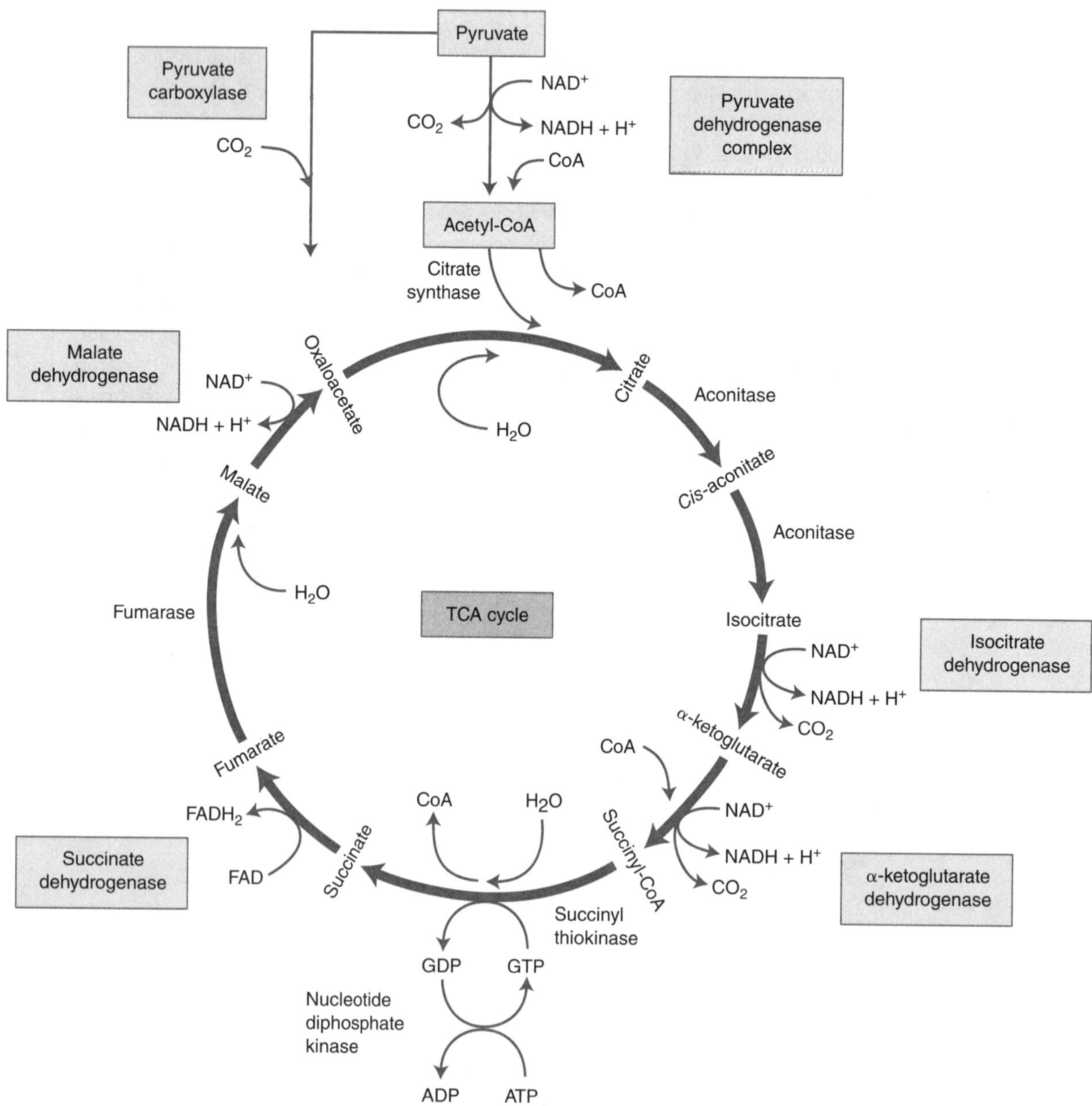

Figure 3.5 The reactions of the TCA cycle showing sites of substrate-level phosphorylation and NAD+ and FAD reduction.

Reprinted by permission from M. Gleeson, "Biochemistry of Exercise," in *Nutrition in Sport*, edited by R.J. Maughan (Blackwell Science Ltd., 2000), 17-38.

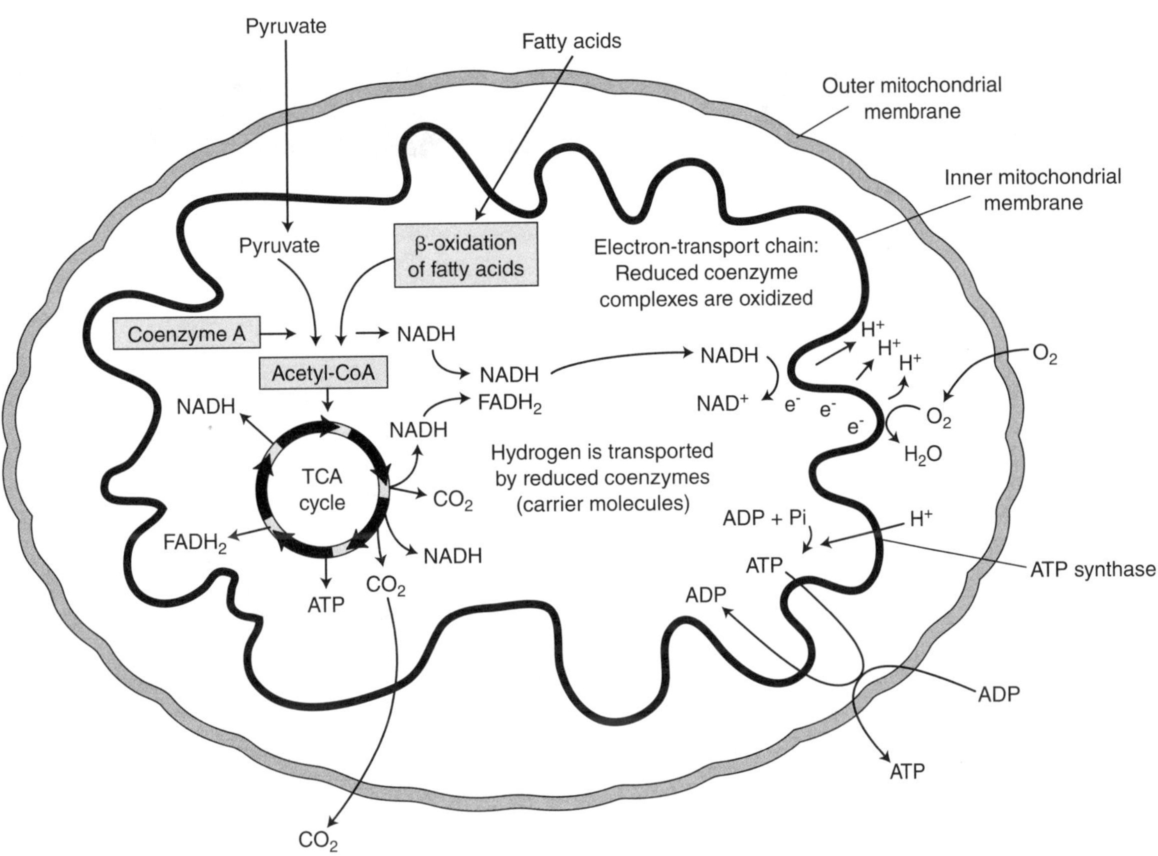

Figure 3.6 The TCA cycle generates the reduced coenzymes NADH and $FADH_2$. Oxidation of these coenzymes in the electron-transport chain releases energy that is used for the resynthesis of ATP. This process is called oxidative phosphorylation.

Reprinted by permission from M. Gleeson, "Biochemistry of Exercise," in *Nutrition in Sport*, edited by R.J. Maughan (Blackwell Science Ltd., 2000), 17-38.

ADP, thus conserving some of the chemical energy contained within the original substrates in the form of high-energy phosphates. As long as the oxygen supply is adequate and substrate is available, NAD^+ and FAD are continuously regenerated and TCA metabolism proceeds. This process cannot occur without oxygen. For each molecule of NADH that enters the ETC, three molecules of ATP are generated, and for each molecule of $FADH_2$, two molecules of ATP are formed. Thus, for each molecule of acetyl-CoA undergoing complete oxidation in the TCA cycle, a total of 12 ATP molecules are formed.

The transfer of electrons through the transport chain located on the inner mitochondrial membrane causes hydrogen ions, or protons, from the inner mitochondrial matrix to be pumped into the space between the inner and outer mitochondrial membranes. The high concentration of positively charged hydrogen ions in this outer chamber causes H^+ to flow back into the mitochondrial matrix through an ATP synthase protein complex embedded in the inner mitochondrial membrane. The flow of H^+ through this complex constitutes a proton-motive force that drives ATP synthesis. The overall reaction starting with glucose as the fuel can be summarized as follows:

$$\text{glucose} + 6\,O_2 + 38\,\text{ADP} + 38\,\text{Pi} \rightarrow 6\,CO_2 + 6\,H_2O + 38\,\text{ATP}$$

The total ATP synthesis of 38 moles per mole of glucose oxidized is primarily from oxidation of reduced coenzymes in the terminal respiratory system as shown in table 3.4.

The reactions of oxidative phosphorylation occur within the mitochondria. Glycolysis takes place in the cytoplasm, and the inner mitochondrial membrane is impermeable to NADH and to NAD^+. Without regeneration of the NAD^+ in the cytoplasm, glycolysis will stop. Therefore, a

TABLE 3.4 ATP Resynthesis in the Complete Oxidation of Glucose

Number of ATP molecules synthesized per glucose molecule oxidized	Source	
2	Substrate-level phosphorylation	In glycolysis
6	NADH	In glycolysis
24	NADH	In TCA cycle
4	$FADH_2$	In TCA cycle
2	GTP	In TCA cycle
38	Total	

mechanism must exist for the effective oxidation of the NADH formed during glycolysis. This mechanism is provided by a number of substrate shuttles that transfer reducing equivalents into the mitochondrion.

An interesting concept has developed following the finding that dietary nitrate (NO_{3^-}) supplementation can improve exercise performance via a reduction in the oxygen requirement at a given submaximal exercise intensity (Lansley, Winyard, Bailey, et al. 2011; Lansley, Winyard, Fulford, et al. 2011; Larsen et al. 2007). The effects of dietary nitrate are thought to be mediated by increased formation of nitrite (NO_{2^-}) and nitric oxide (NO). The latter may increase mitochondrial oxidative phosphorylation efficiency by increasing the phosphate/oxygen (P/O) ratio (the amount of ATP produced from the movement of two electrons through the electron transport chain, donated by reduction of an oxygen atom) ratio (i.e., more ATP is formed per amount of oxygen consumed). Skeletal muscle mitochondria harvested from muscle biopsies after nitrate supplementation display an increased P/O ratio, and the improved mitochondrial P/O ratio correlates with the reduction in oxygen cost during exercise (Larsen et al. 2011). Mechanistically, nitrate reduces the expression of ATP-ADP-translocase, a protein involved in proton conductance. Thus, it appears that dietary nitrate has profound effects on basal mitochondrial function and is able to alter the efficiency of aerobic ATP production. Nitrate is found in several plants, including beetroot, celery, cress, lettuce, rhubarb, and spinach, and a popular means of ingesting nitrate is drinking beetroot juice. Further details can be found in chapter 11.

Fat Oxidation in Aerobic Metabolism

Fat and carbohydrate are the major nutrients that provide energy for muscular contraction. Because acetyl-CoA is also a product of fat oxidation, the sequence of reactions involving the TCA cycle and oxidative phosphorylation is common to both fat and carbohydrate. Fat is mostly stored in the body as triacylglycerol (also known as triglyceride) in white adipose tissue, although skeletal muscle fibers also contain some triacylglycerol in the form of lipid droplets that are usually located close to the mitochondria. This is usually referred to as IMTG and also serves as an important energy source in submaximal exercise.

Lipolysis

To generate the two-carbon acetyl groups from fat, several metabolic steps must occur. The first step involves the breakdown of the storage form of fat, triacylglycerol, into its FA and glycerol components. This process is called **lipolysis**, and it begins with the hydrolytic removal of an FA molecule from the glycerol backbone at either position 1 or position 3. This step is catalyzed by a hormone-sensitive lipase (see figure 3.7). Insulin promotes triacylglycerol synthesis and inhibits lipolysis, whereas catecholamines (epinephrine and norepinephrine), glucagon, growth hormone, and cortisol stimulate lipolysis by activating the hormone-sensitive lipase. A specific lipase for the remaining diacylglycerol removes another FA, and another specific lipase removes the last FA from the monoacylglycerol. Thus, from each molecule of triacylglycerol, one molecule of glycerol and three molecules of FA are produced. Glycerol may diffuse, and FAs are transported out of the adipose cells and into the circulation.

The rate of lipolysis and the rate of adipose tissue blood flow influence the rate of entry of FFAs and glycerol into the circulation. During prolonged exercise at about 50% of $\dot{V}O_2max$, adipose tissue blood flow increases. During intense exercise, however, sympathetic vasoconstriction causes a fall in adipose tissue blood flow, resulting in accumulation of FA within adipose tissue and

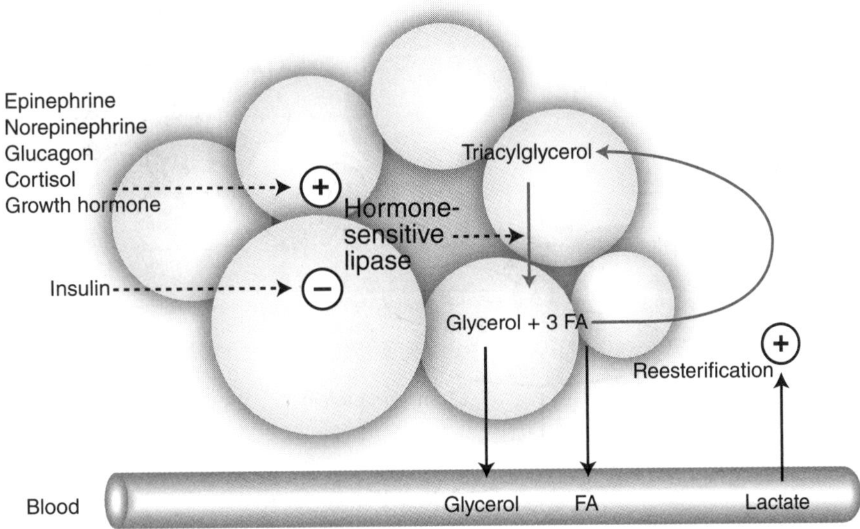

Figure 3.7 Lipolysis in adipose tissue mobilizes free fatty acids, which enter the circulation and thus become available for muscle to use as a fuel for exercise.

effectively limiting the entry of FFAs (and glycerol) into the circulation. Another factor that limits fat mobilization during high-intensity exercise is the accumulation of lactate in the blood. Lactate promotes the reesterification of FFAs back into triacylglycerol (see figure 3.7) and therefore limits the entry of FFAs into the bloodstream.

Glycerol is readily soluble in plasma and can be taken up by the liver and phosphorylated to glycerol-3-phosphate , which can be used to form triacylglycerol as described earlier or, alternately, can be oxidized to dihydroxyacetone phosphate, which can enter the glycolytic pathway or be converted to glucose. FFAs are poorly soluble in water, and most of the FAs in plasma are transported loosely bound to albumin, the most abundant protein in plasma. The normal plasma albumin concentration is about 45 g/L (approximately 0.7 mmol/L). Each albumin molecule contains three high-affinity binding sites for FAs (and seven other low-affinity binding sites) so the FA concentration in plasma rarely exceeds 2 mM. When the three high-affinity binding sites are full (at an FA concentration of 2 mM or more), the concentration of FA not bound to albumin (i.e., FFAs) increases markedly, but these nonbound FFAs form fatty-acid micelles, which are potentially damaging to tissues because of their detergent-like properties.

FA Uptake Into Muscle

The usual resting plasma concentration of FA is 0.2 to 0.4 mM. During (or shortly after) prolonged exercise, however, the plasma FA concentration may increase to about 2.0 mM. The uptake of FA by muscle is directly related to the plasma FA concentration, and, hence, the mobilization of fat stores is an important step in ensuring an adequate nutrient supply for prolonged muscular work. To be taken up by muscle, FFAs must dissociate from albumin and then pass through the endothelial lining of the blood capillary, interstitial fluid, and sarcolemma of the muscle cell. At the endothelial lining, the FA–albumin complex binds to specific albumin-binding proteins (ABPs) that allow the FAs to be released from albumin to facilitate their entry into muscle. The transport of FFAs across the sarcolemmal membrane is assisted by the plasma membrane FA-binding protein (FABPpm) on the outer side of the sarcolemma and an FA-transporter (FAT/CD36) protein (see figure 3.8).

FA transport across the sarcolemmal membrane into the muscle fiber via this carrier-mediated transport mechanism becomes saturated at a high-plasma unbound FFA concentration (approximately equivalent to 1.5 mM total FA concentration). FA uptake into muscle will occur only if the intracellular FFA concentration is less than that in the true aqueous solution in the extracellular fluid (that is, < 10 µM). The low intracellular FFA concentration is maintained by the presence of a cytoplasmic FA-binding protein (FABPc) inside the cell similar to the ones found in the cells of the small intestine and liver. Also, the rate of uptake of FFA into muscle fibers will be proportional to the difference in their concentrations inside and outside the cell until the plasma membrane transport mechanism becomes saturated. After the FFAs enter the muscle

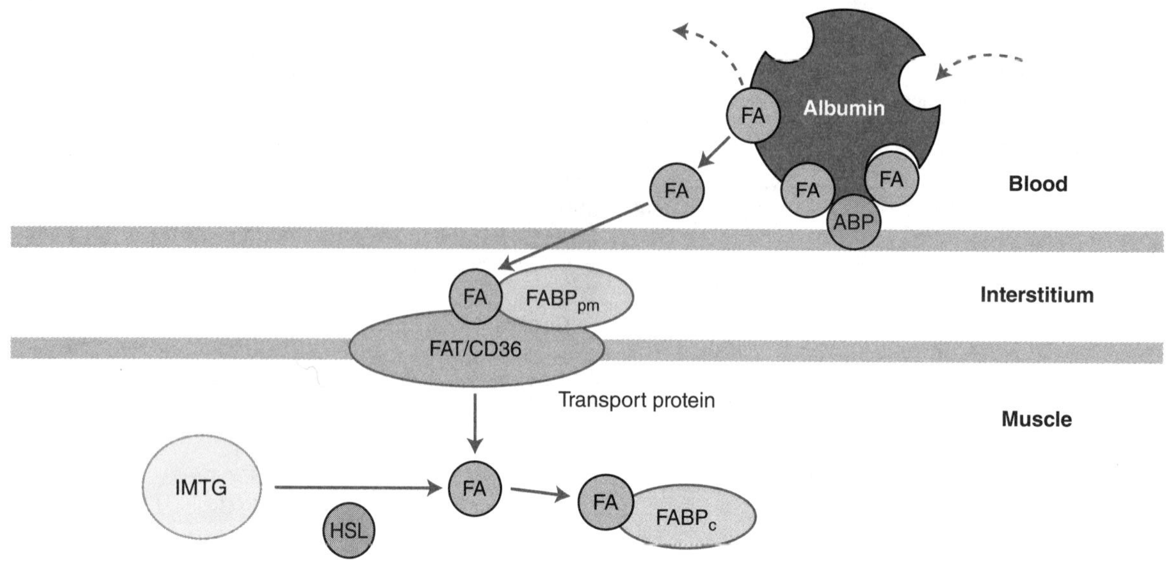

Figure 3.8 Fatty acid uptake by skeletal muscle. ABP = albumin binding protein; FABP = fatty acid binding protein.; FAT = fatty acid transporter; IMTG = intramuscular triacylglycerol; HSL = hormone-sensitive lipase.

cell, they are converted into a CoA derivative by the action of ATP-linked fatty acyl-CoA synthetase (also known as thiokinase) in preparation for ß-oxidation, the major pathway for FA breakdown. Hence, the priming (activation) of each FA molecule requires the use of one molecule of ATP:

$$RCOOH + ATP + CoA\text{-}SH \rightarrow R\text{-}C(=O)\text{-}S\text{-}CoA + AMP + PPi + H_2O$$

Intramuscular Triacylglycerols

Another source of FAs is the IMTG stores in the muscle itself. Type I muscle fibers have a higher content of IMTG than type II muscle fibers. It is now recognized that IMTG stores decrease during exercise and are used as an important source of energy. It has been shown that endurance exercise training increases the triacylglycerol content of muscle. Like adipose tissue, muscle contains a **hormone-sensitive lipase (HSL)** that is activated by ß-adrenergic stimulation and inhibited by insulin. FAs liberated from IMTGs can then be oxidized within the muscle. As with the FAs taken up by the muscle from the circulation, the FAs released following lipolysis of IMTGs are bound to FABPc and converted to fatty acyl-CoA before being transported into the mitochondria for oxidation.

ß-Oxidation of Fatty Acids

The process of ß-oxidation occurs in the mitochondria and is the sequential removal of two-carbon units from the FA chain in the form of acetyl-CoA, which can then enter the TCA cycle. Fatty acyl-CoA molecules in the muscle sarcoplasm are transported into the mitochondria through formation of an ester of the FA with **carnitine**, as illustrated in figure 3.9. The latter is synthesized in the liver and is normally abundant in tissues able to oxidize FAs. Concentrations of about 1.0 mM are found in muscle. The enzyme that regulates the transport of FA by carnitine is carnitine acyltransferase (CAT), and two forms of it exist in muscle. One form (CAT-I) is located on the outer surface of the membrane (to generate acyl-carnitine), and the other form (CAT-II) is located on the inner surface of the inner mitochondrial membrane and regenerates the acyl-CoA and free carnitine (see figure 3.10). CAT-I and CAT-II are also often referred to as carnitine palmitoyl transferase I and II (CPT I and CPT II). This transport process may be the main rate-limiting step in the use of FAs for energy production in muscle.

Carnitine has been promoted as a dietary supplement that can aid weight loss by increasing fat oxidation and can enhance endurance exercise performance by promoting fat use, thus sparing the limited glycogen stores. The evidence for this will be discussed in more detail in chapter 11.

At high exercise intensities (above about 60% of $\dot{V}O_2max$), the rate of fat oxidation cannot provide sufficient ATP for muscle contraction, and, increasingly, ATP is derived from carbohydrate oxidation and anaerobic glycolysis. Energy cannot be derived from fat through anaerobic pathways.

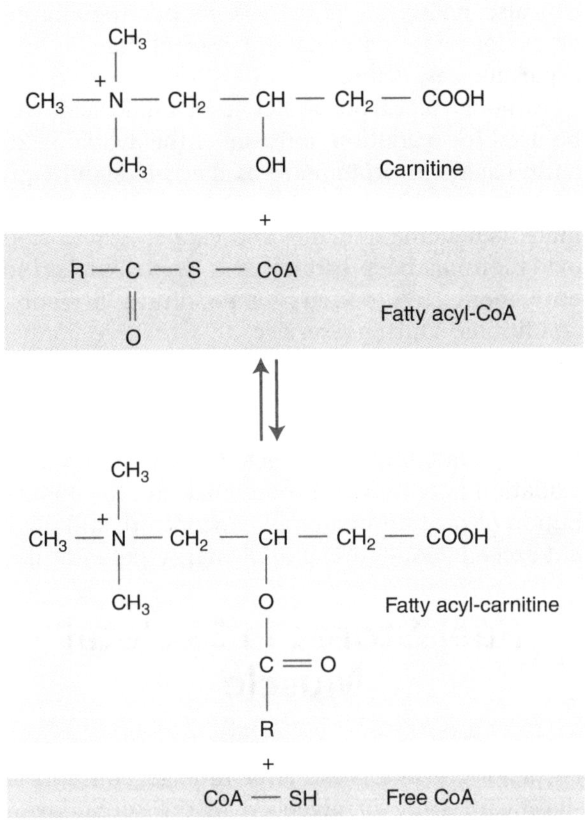

Figure 3.9 In the carnitine–fatty acyl-CoA transferase reaction, carnitine is linked to a FA molecule.

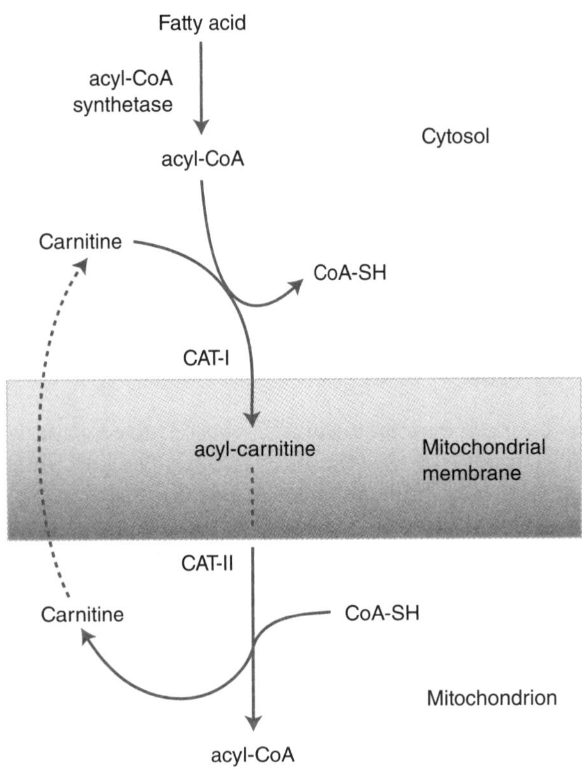

Figure 3.10 Carnitine aids the transport of long-chain FAs across the mitochondrial membrane. Inside the mitochondrion, carnitine is removed and fatty acyl-CoA is re-formed, which frees carnitine to diffuse back across the mitochondrial membrane into the cytoplasm.

After its release into the mitochondrial matrix, the fatty acyl-CoA is able to enter the ß-oxidation pathway. Carnitine acyl-transferase is inhibited by malonyl-CoA, a precursor for FA synthesis. Hence, when the ATP supply is sufficient, surplus acetyl-CoA will be diverted away from the TCA cycle to malonyl-CoA, reducing catabolism of FAs and promoting their formation and subsequent triacylglycerol synthesis.

After it is inside the mitochondria, fatty acyl-CoA is oxidized through a series of reactions catalyzed by a multienzyme complex that releases a molecule of acetyl-CoA and a fatty acyl-CoA, which is now a two-carbon unit shorter. This fatty acyl-CoA can now repeat the cycle, and the acetyl CoA formed can enter the TCA cycle. At each passage through the cycle, the FA chain loses a two-carbon fragment as acetyl-CoA and two pairs of hydrogen atoms to specific acceptors. The 16-carbon palmitic acid thus undergoes a total of seven such cycles to yield eight molecules of acetyl-CoA and 14 pairs of hydrogen atoms. The palmitic acid only needs to be primed or activated with CoA once because, at the end of each cycle, the shortened FA appears as its CoA ester. The most common FAs oxidized contain 16 (e.g., palmitic acid) or 18 (e.g., oleic acid) carbons in the acyl chain. The 14 pairs of hydrogen atoms removed during ß-oxidation of palmitic acid enter the mitochondrial respiratory chain, seven pairs in the form of the reduced flavin coenzyme of fatty acyl-CoA dehydrogenase and seven pairs in the form of NADH. The passage of electrons from $FADH_2$ to oxygen and from NADH to oxygen leads to the expected number of oxidative phosphorylations of ADP (that is, two ATP molecules from each $FADH_2$ and three ATP molecules from each NADH). Hence, a total of five molecules of ATP are formed per molecule of acetyl-CoA cleaved:

$$\text{palmitoyl-CoA} + 7\ \text{CoA} + 7\ O_2 + 35\ \text{ADP} + 35\ \text{Pi} \rightarrow 8\ \text{acetyl-CoA} + 35\ \text{ATP} + 42\ H_2O$$

The eight molecules of acetyl-CoA can enter the TCA cycle, and the following equation represents the result of their oxidation and the coupled phosphorylations:

$$8 \text{ acetyl-CoA} + 16\ O_2 + 96 \text{ ADP} + 96 \text{ Pi} \rightarrow 8 \text{ CoA} + 96 \text{ ATP} + 104\ H_2O + 16\ CO_2$$

Combining the two previous equations gives the overall equation:

$$\text{palmitoyl-CoA} + 23\ O_2 + 131 \text{ ADP} + 131 \text{ Pi} \rightarrow \text{CoA} + 16\ CO_2 + 146\ H_2O + 131 \text{ ATP}$$

Because one molecule of ATP was required initially to activate the FA, the net yield for the complete oxidation of one molecule of palmitic acid is 130 molecules of ATP.

Amino Acid Oxidation in Aerobic Metabolism

In most situations, carbohydrates and fats supply most of the energy required to regenerate ATP to fuel muscular work. Protein catabolism can provide up to 20 different amino acids, some of which may eventually be oxidized, but this normally contributes less than 5% of the energy provision for muscle contraction during physical activity. During starvation and when glycogen stores become depleted, protein catabolism may become an increasingly important source of energy for muscular work.

Before amino acids can be oxidized, the amino ($-NH_2$) group must be removed. Removal of the amino group can be achieved for some amino acids by transferring it to another molecule called a keto acid, which results in the formation of a different amino acid. This process is called transamination and is catalyzed by enzymes called aminotransferases. A good example is the transfer of the amino group from the amino acid leucine to the keto acid α-ketoglutarate which forms α-ketoisocaproate (which can be further metabolized to form acetyl-CoA) and glutamate, respectively. Each amino acid has a unique corresponding keto acid. Alternatively, the amino group can be removed from the amino acid to form free ammonia (NH_3) in a process called oxidative deamination. After the removal of the amino group from an amino acid, the remaining carbon skeleton (the keto acid) is eventually oxidized to carbon dioxide and water in the TCA cycle. The carbon skeleton of amino acids can enter the TCA cycle in several ways. Some can be converted to acetyl-CoA and enter the TCA cycle just like acetyl-CoA from carbohydrate or fat. They can also enter the TCA cycle as α-ketoglutarate or oxaloacetate as metabolites of glutamate and aspartate, respectively.

Although all carbon skeletons of amino acids can be used for oxidation, only six of the available 20 amino acids in protein are oxidized in significant amounts by muscle: asparagine, aspartate, glutamate, isoleucine, leucine, and valine. Amino acid oxidation has been estimated to contribute up to only about 15% to energy expenditure in resting conditions. During exercise, this relative contribution likely decreases to less than 5% because of an increasing importance of carbohydrate and fat as fuels. During prolonged exercise, when carbohydrate availability becomes limited, amino acid oxidation may increase somewhat, but the contribution of protein to energy expenditure still does not exceed about 10% of total energy expenditure.

Fuel Stores in Skeletal Muscle

Carbohydrate is stored in the body as the glucose polymer glycogen. Skeletal muscle contains a significant store of glycogen in the sarcoplasm. The glycogen content of skeletal muscle at rest is approximately 13 to 18 g/kg w.w. (75 to 100 mmol glucosyl units/kg w.w.). For cycling and running, a total of about 300 g of glycogen are available in the leg muscles (see figure 3.11). About 100 g of glycogen are stored in the liver of an adult human in the postabsorptive state, and this can be released into the circulation to maintain the blood glucose concentration at about 5 mmol/L (0.9 g/L). Fats are stored as triacylglycerol, mainly in white adipose tissue. Triacylglycerol molecules must be broken down by a lipase enzyme to release FA into the

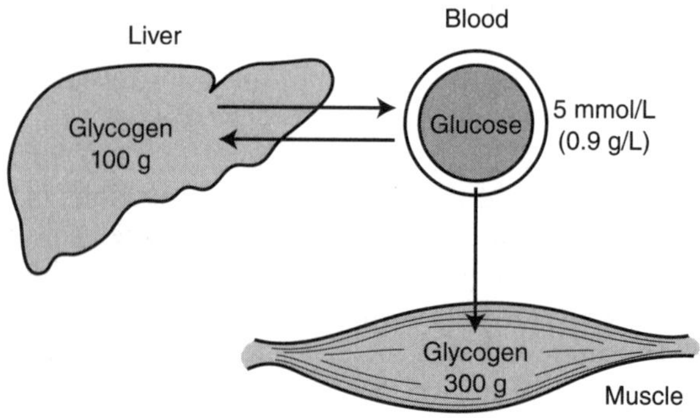

Figure 3.11 Carbohydrate availability in liver, blood, and muscle for two-legged exercise (e.g., cycling and running).

circulation for uptake by working muscle. Skeletal muscle also contains some triacylglycerol that can be used as an energy source during exercise after lipolysis. Some of this intramuscular triacylglycerol may be contained in adipose cells dispersed among the muscle fibers in the tissue, but evidence from light and electron microscopy suggests the existence of triacylglycerol droplets located close to the mitochondria within the fibers themselves.

Early studies (Havel, Pernow, and Jones 1967; Issekutz et al. 1964) of FA turnover during exercise using ^{14}C-labeled FAs showed that during prolonged exercise, plasma-derived FA could account for only about 50% of the total amount of fat oxidized, suggesting that intramuscular triacylglycerol could be providing a significant amount of the FA during prolonged exercise. Measurements of changes in intramuscular triacylglycerol content before and after exercise strongly support this view. Several studies have reported reductions of about 25% to 35% in triacylglycerol content after 1 to 2 hours of exercise at 55% to 70% of $\dot{V}O_2$max. These changes have been observed in several studies despite the unreliable nature of triacylglycerol measurement in small biopsy samples of skeletal muscle (Turcotte, Richter, and Kiens 1995).

Human skeletal muscle contains approximately 12 g/kg w.w. of triacylglycerol, and type I fibers contain more triacylglycerol than type II fibers do. Between 12 and 20 MJ (2,868-4,780 kcal) of chemical potential energy is estimated to be available for oxidation after intramuscular lipolysis. The lipolysis is probably mediated by an intracellular lipase similar to the hormone-sensitive lipase of adipose tissue; evidence suggests that catecholamines regulate the mobilization of intramuscular triacylglycerol stores.

Fat stores in the body are far larger than carbohydrate stores, and fat is a more efficient form of energy storage, releasing 37 kJ/g (9 kcal/g) compared with 16 kJ/g (4 kcal/g) from carbohydrate. Each gram of carbohydrate stored also retains about 3 g of water, which further decreases the efficiency of carbohydrate as an energy source. But the energy yield per liter of oxygen consumed during fat oxidation is about 8% to 10% less than for carbohydrate (about 19.5 kJ/L [5 kcal/L] of oxygen for fat compared with 20.9 kJ/L [5 kcal/L] of oxygen for carbohydrate). The energy cost of running a marathon is about 12,000 kJ (2,868 kcal); if this energy could be derived from the oxidation of fat alone, the total amount of fat required would be about 320 g, compared with 750 g of carbohydrate and an additional 2.3 kg of associated water. Aside from the weight that would have to be carried, this amount of carbohydrate exceeds the total amount normally stored in the liver, muscles, and blood combined. The total storage capacity for fat is extremely large, and for most practical purposes, the amount of energy stored in the form of fat far exceeds that required for any exercise task (see table 3.5).

The main problem associated with the use of fat as a fuel for exercise is the rate at which it can be taken up by muscle and oxidized to provide energy. Fat oxidation can only supply ATP at a rate sufficient to maintain exercise at an intensity of about 60% of $\dot{V}O_2$max. To generate ATP to sustain higher exercise intensities, there is an increasing reliance on carbohydrate, and at intensities above about 85% of $\dot{V}O_2$max, the oxidation of carbohydrate will be the predominant fuel with fat contributing 30% or less. Both the oxidative pathway of carbohydrate use and the anaerobic pathway of glycolysis can

TABLE 3.5 Energy Stores in the Average Man

Fuel type	Mass	Energy available	Exercise time (min)
Liver glycogen	0.10 kg (0.22 lb)	1,600 kJ (382 kcal)	20
Muscle glycogen	0.40 kg (0.88 lb)	6,400 kJ (1,530 kcal)	80
Blood glucose	0.01 kg (0.02 lb)	160 kJ (38 kcal)	2
Fat	10.5 kg (23.1 lb)	390,000 kJ (93,212 kcal)	4,900
Protein	8.5 kg (18.7 lb)	142,000 kJ (33,939 kcal)	1,800

Assumes a body mass of 70 kg (154 lb), a fat content of 15% of body mass, and a protein content of about 12% of body mass. The value for blood glucose includes the glucose content of extracellular fluid. The exercise times are the approximate times that these stores would last if they were the only source of energy available during exercise at marathon-running pace (equivalent to an energy expenditure of about 80 kJ [19 kcal]/min).

Reprinted by permission from M. Gleeson, "Biochemistry of Exercise," in *Nutrition in Sport*, edited by R.J. Maughan (Blackwell Science Ltd., 2000), 17-38.

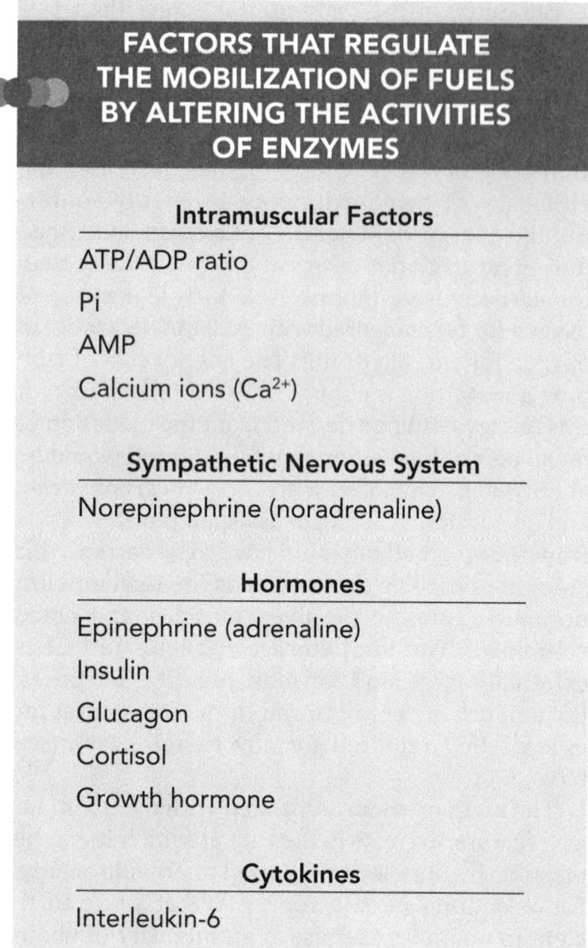

FACTORS THAT REGULATE THE MOBILIZATION OF FUELS BY ALTERING THE ACTIVITIES OF ENZYMES

Intramuscular Factors

ATP/ADP ratio

Pi

AMP

Calcium ions (Ca^{2+})

Sympathetic Nervous System

Norepinephrine (noradrenaline)

Hormones

Epinephrine (adrenaline)

Insulin

Glucagon

Cortisol

Growth hormone

Cytokines

Interleukin-6

supply ATP at a much faster rate than fat oxidation can. During most forms of submaximal exercise, a mixture of fat and carbohydrate is oxidized to provide energy for muscular contraction. Obviously, using more fat allows greater sparing of the limited carbohydrate reserves, which permits prolonged exercise.

Unlike carbohydrate (as glycogen) and fat (as triacylglycerol), protein is stored only as functionally important molecules (e.g., structural proteins, enzymes, ion channels, receptors, and contractile proteins), and the concentration of free amino acids in most extracellular and intracellular body fluids is quite low (e.g., the total free amino acid concentration in muscle sarcoplasm is about 20 mmol/L). Hence, carbohydrate and fat are the preferred fuels for exercise, and the contribution of protein to energy expenditure during even prolonged exercise does not usually exceed a maximum of about 5% to 10% of total energy expenditure.

Regulation of Energy Metabolism

Experiments in which muscle biopsies were taken before and immediately after exercise indicate that the intramuscular ATP concentration remains fairly constant (Spriet 1995a). Thus, ATP is being continuously regenerated by other energy-liberating reactions at the same rate that it is being used. This situation provides a sensitive mechanism for the control of energy metabolism within the cell. This control is exerted through changes in a number of intracellular factors, and further control is effected through the actions of the sympathetic nervous system and hormones that can also bring about changes in the activities of some enzymes involved in fuel mobilization and use (see the sidebar).

Intracellular Factors

Within the muscle fiber, several intracellular factors control the activity of key rate-limiting or flux-generating enzymes involved in energy metabolism, which allows rapid (virtually instantaneous) alteration in the rate of ATP resynthesis to occur when such an alteration is needed, such as at the onset of exercise.

The decline in cellular concentration of ATP at the onset of muscle force generation and parallel increases in ADP and AMP concentrations (i.e., a decline in the energy charge) directly stimulate anaerobic and oxidative ATP resynthesis. The relatively low concentration of ATP (and ADP) inside the cell means that any increase in the rate of hydrolysis of ATP (e.g., at the onset of exercise) produces a rapid change in the ratio of ATP to ADP (and also increases the intracellular concentration of AMP). These changes, in turn, activate enzymes that immediately stimulate the breakdown of intramuscular fuel stores to provide energy for ATP resynthesis. In this way, energy metabolism increases rapidly after the start of exercise.

ATP, ADP, and AMP are activators or inhibitors of the enzymatic reactions involved in PCr, carbohydrate, and fat degradation and use (see figure 3.12). For example, CK, the enzyme responsible for the rapid rephosphorylation of ATP at the initiation of muscle force generation, is rapidly activated by an increase in cytoplasmic ADP concentration and is inhibited by an increase in cellular ATP concentration. Similarly, glycogen phosphorylase, the

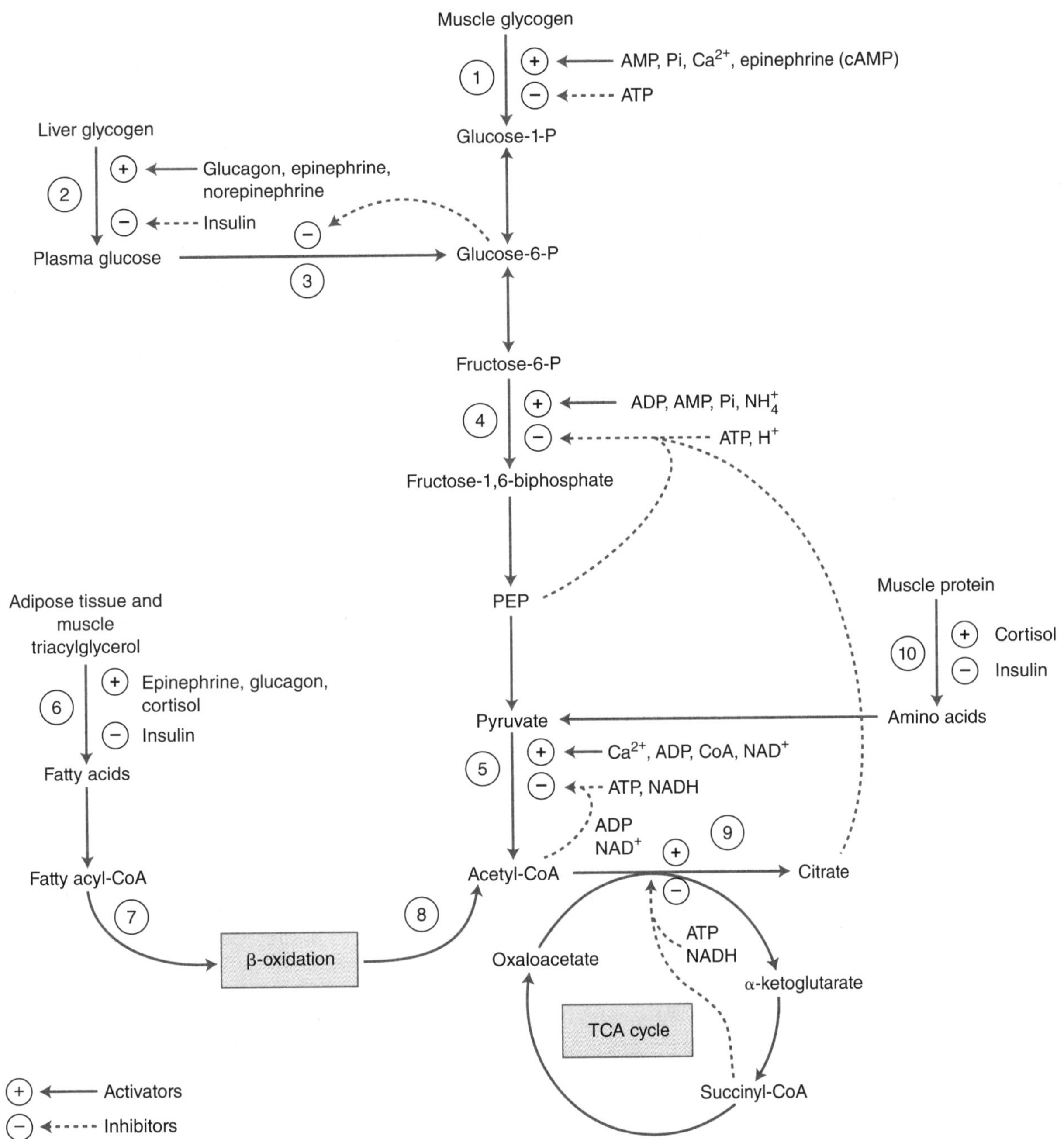

Figure 3.12 Metabolic pathways are important to energy provision during exercise. The main sites of regulation and the principal hormone and allosteric activators and inhibitors are shown. 1 and 2 = phosphorylase; 3 = hexokinase; 4 = phosphofructokinase; 5 = pyruvate dehydrogenase; 6 = hormone-sensitive lipase; 7 = carnitine acyl transferase; 8 = fatty acyl-CoA dehydrogenase; 9 = citrate synthase; 10 = proteases.

Reprinted by permission from M. Gleeson, Biochemistry of Exercise, in *Nutrition in Sport,* edited by R.J. Maughan (Blackwell Science Ltd., 2000), 17-38.

enzyme that catalyzes the conversion of glycogen to glucose-1-phosphate, is activated by increases in AMP and Pi (and calcium ion) concentration and is inhibited by an increase in ATP concentration.

The rate-limiting step in the glycolytic pathway is the conversion of fructose-6-phosphate to fructose-1,6-diphosphate, which is catalyzed by phosphofructokinase (PFK). The activity of this complex enzyme is affected by many intracellular factors, and it plays an important role in controlling flux through the pathway. The PFK reaction regulates the metabolism of glucose and glycogen. The activity of PFK is stimulated by increased concentrations of ADP, AMP, Pi, ammonia, and fructose-6-phosphate and is inhibited by ATP, H^+, citrate, phosphoglycerate, and phosphoenolpyruvate. Thus, the rate of glycolysis is stimulated when ATP and glycogen breakdown are increased at the onset of exercise. Accumulation of citrate and, thus, inhibition of PFK may occur when the rate of the TCA cycle is high and provides a means whereby the limited stores of carbohydrate are spared when the availability of FAs is high. Inhibition of PFK also causes accumulation of glucose-6-phosphate, which inhibits the activity of hexokinase and reduces the entry into the muscle of glucose, which is not needed.

Conversion of pyruvate to acetyl-CoA by the pyruvate dehydrogenase complex is the rate-limiting step in carbohydrate oxidation. It is stimulated by an increased intracellular concentration of calcium and decreased ratios of ATP to ADP, acetyl-CoA to free CoA, and NADH to NAD^+ and thus offers another site of regulation of the relative rates of fat and carbohydrate catabolism. If the rate of formation of acetyl-CoA from the ß-oxidation of FAs is high, such as after 1 to 2 hours of submaximal exercise, then this activity can reduce the amount of acetyl-CoA derived from pyruvate and cause accumulation of phosphoenolpyruvate and inhibition of PFK, thus slowing the rate of glycolysis and glycogenolysis. This process forms the basis of the glucose–fatty acid cycle proposed by Randle et al. (1963), which has for many years been accepted as the key regulatory mechanism in the control of carbohydrate and fat use by skeletal muscle. More recent work, however, has challenged this hypothesis, and it seems likely that the regulation of the integration of fat and carbohydrate catabolism in exercising skeletal muscle must reside elsewhere, such as at the level of glucose uptake into muscle, of glycogen breakdown by phosphorylase, or of the entry of FAs into the mitochondria (for further details see Hargreaves 1995 and Maughan and Gleeson 2010).

A key regulatory point in the TCA cycle is the reaction catalyzed by citrate synthase. The activity of this enzyme is inhibited by ATP, NADH, succinyl-CoA, and fatty acyl-CoA; the activity of the enzyme is also affected by citrate availability. Hence, when cellular energy levels are high, flux through the TCA cycle is relatively low but can be greatly increased when ATP and NADH use is increased, such as during exercise.

Hormones and Cytokines

Many hormones influence energy metabolism in the body (for a detailed review, see Galbo 1983). During exercise, the interaction among insulin, glucagon, and the catecholamines (epinephrine and norepinephrine) is mostly responsible for fuel substrate availability and use; cortisol and growth hormone also have some significant effects. It has been recognized that a cytokine called interleukin-6 (IL-6), which is released from active skeletal muscle during exercise, also plays a role in the regulation of fuel mobilization and metabolism. The sources, stimuli for secretion, and major actions of these various hormones and cytokines are summarized in table 3.6.

Insulin

Insulin is secreted by the ß cells of the pancreatic islets (also called the islets of Langerhans) in the pancreas. Its basic biological effects are to inhibit lipolysis and increase the uptake of glucose from the blood by the tissues (especially skeletal muscle, liver, and adipose tissue). Cellular uptake of amino acids is also stimulated by insulin.

These effects reduce the plasma glucose concentration, inhibit the release of glucose from the liver, promote the synthesis of glycogen (in liver and muscle), promote synthesis of fat and inhibit FA release (in adipose tissue), increase muscle amino acid uptake, and enhance protein synthesis. The primary stimulus for increased insulin secretion is a rise in the blood glucose concentration (e.g., after a meal). Plasma insulin concentration is usually depressed during exercise because the sympathetic nervous system and circulating catecholamines inhibit the release of insulin. However, the fall in the plasma insulin concentration during exercise does not reduce the uptake of glucose from the blood by active muscle, because the rise in intracellular calcium ion (Ca^{2+}) concentration during muscle contractions also promotes the translocation of intracellular vesicles containing GLUT4 glucose transporters into the sarcolemma (see figure 3.13).

TABLE 3.6 Roles of the Major Hormones in the Regulation of Energy Metabolism

Hormone	Source	Stimuli that activate secretion	Actions
Insulin	ß cells of the pancreatic islets	Rise in blood glucose and amino acids	Stimulates glucose uptake by liver, muscle, and adipose tissue Inhibits lipolysis Stimulates muscle amino acid uptake Inhibits protein breakdown
Glucagon	α cells of the pancreatic islets	Fall in blood glucose	Stimulates liver glycogen breakdown and gluconeogenesis
Epinephrine	Adrenal medulla	Stress and fall in blood glucose	Stimulates glycogen breakdown and lipolysis in adipose tissue
Norepinephrine	Sympathetic nerve endings	Stress and fall in blood glucose or blood pressure	Stimulates glycogen breakdown and lipolysis in adipose tissue
Cortisol	Adrenal cortex	Stress, adrenocorticotrophic hormone, IL-6	Stimulates protein breakdown and gluconeogenesis Stimulates lipolysis in adipose tissue
Growth hormone	Anterior pituitary gland	Stress	Stimulates lipolysis in adipose tissue
IL-6	Contracting skeletal muscle fibers	Increased intracellular calcium ion concentration and decreased glycogen availability	Stimulates liver glycogen breakdown Stimulates lipolysis in adipose tissue Stimulates cortisol secretion

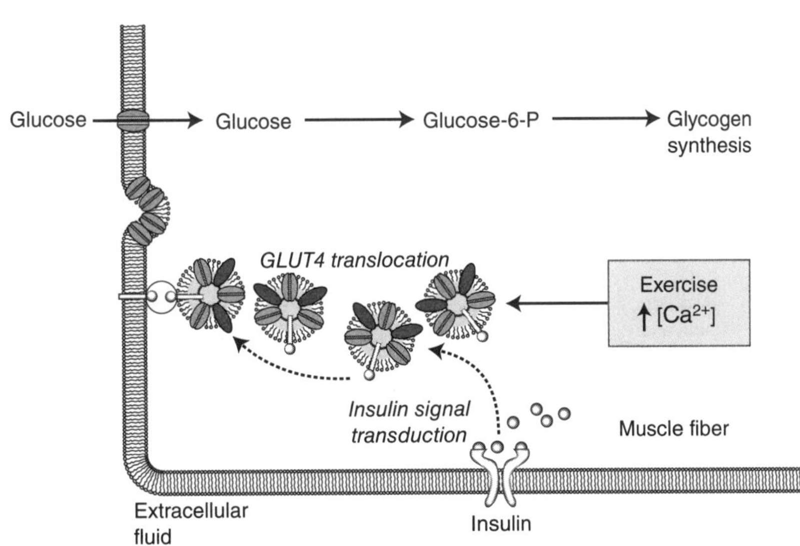

Figure 3.13 Translocation of GLUT4 glucose transporters into the sarcolemmal membrane under the influence of insulin (important during rest) and calcium ions (important during exercise).

Glucagon

Glucagon is secreted by the α cells of the pancreatic islets and exerts effects that are opposite those of insulin. It raises the blood glucose level by increasing the rate of glycogen breakdown (glycogenolysis) in the liver. It also promotes the formation of glucose from noncarbohydrate precursors (**gluconeogenesis**) in the liver. The primary stimulus for increased secretion of glucagon is a decrease in the glucose concentration in the blood. During most types of exercise, the blood glucose concentration does not fall. But during prolonged exercise, when liver glycogen stores become depleted, a drop in the blood glucose concentration (hypoglycemia) may occur.

The hormone-sensitive lipase in adipose tissue is activated by a cyclic AMP-dependent protein kinase. Binding of glucagon and epinephrine to plasma membrane receptors on adipocytes initiates the adenylate cyclase and the enzyme cascade that activates the lipase (see figure 3.14). Activation of the hormone-sensitive lipase in adipose tissue and lipoprotein lipase occurs during exercise because of the actions of epinephrine and glucagon, which are released from the adrenal medulla and pancreatic islets, respectively. FAs released from triacylglycerols in the fat storage sites are delivered by the blood to muscle tissue, and additional FAs can be provided from the breakdown of intramuscular fat depots. These FAs provide a readily usable source of energy that is liberated through the process of ß-oxidation and contribute significantly to the energy requirements of exercise.

During brief periods of light to moderate exercise, energy is derived equally from oxidation of carbohydrate and fat. If exercise is continued for an hour or more and carbohydrates become depleted, the quantity of fat used for energy gradually increases. In very prolonged exercise, fat (mainly as FAs) may supply almost 80% of total energy. This condition probably arises because of a small fall in blood glucose concentration and a subsequent increase in glucagon (and decrease in insulin) release from the pancreas. Plasma concentrations of epinephrine and cortisol also increase as exercise progresses. These hormonal changes stimulate the mobilization and subsequent use of fat stores (see figure 3.7). The uptake of FAs by working muscle rises during 1

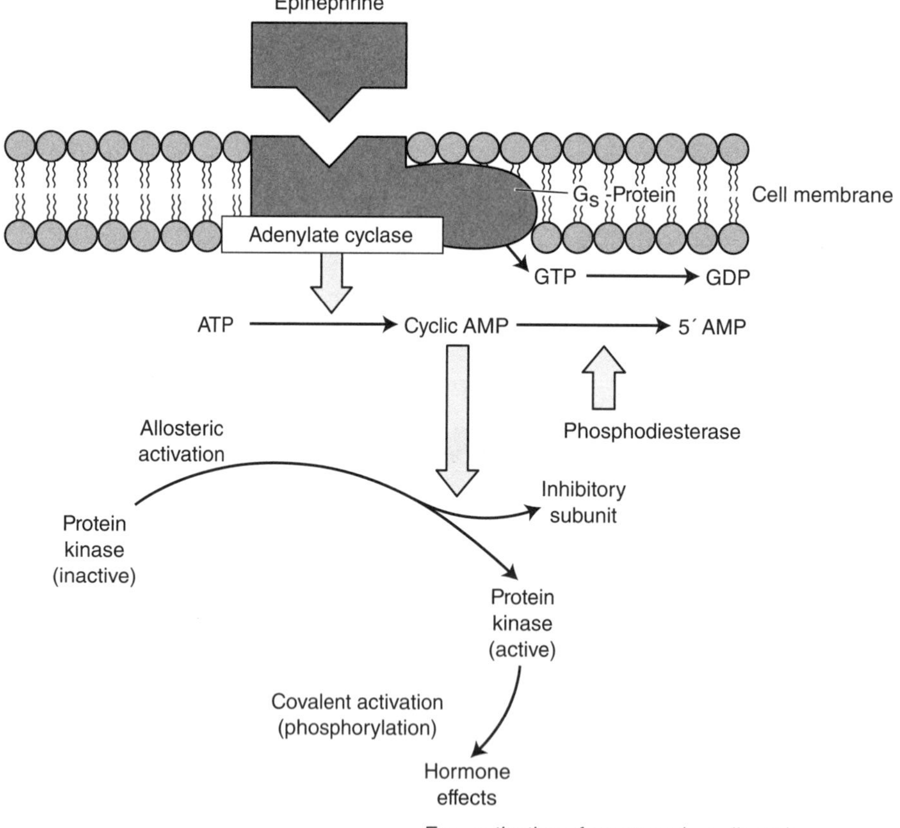

Figure 3.14 Mode of action of epinephrine (adrenaline).

to 4 hours of continuous moderate exercise. Lipolysis is stimulated by exercise, but this process occurs only gradually. Furthermore, it does not cease immediately after exercise has stopped.

The FA concentration in blood plasma reflects the balance between the FA release into the circulation (mainly from adipose tissue depots) and FA uptake by various tissues. Although the concentration of FAs in blood plasma is low (usually in the range of 0.2 to 2.0 mM), their plasma half-life is extremely short (less than 2 minutes), which indicates a rapid rate of uptake by tissues. At the onset of exercise, muscle capillaries open, facilitating FA uptake, and this process is reversed shortly after the end of exercise. Consequently, plasma FA concentrations commonly fall in the early stages of exercise and then gradually increase. At the end of exercise, when muscle uptake falls abruptly but stimulation of lipolysis continues, plasma FA concentration rises sharply, reaching up to 3 mM.

Catecholamines

The catecholamines epinephrine (adrenaline) and norepinephrine (noradrenaline) are released from the adrenal medulla. Norepinephrine is also released from sympathetic nerve endings, and leakage from such synapses appears to be the main source of the norepinephrine in blood plasma. The catecholamines have many systemic effects, including stimulation of the heart rate and contractility and alteration of blood vessel diameters. These substances also influence substrate availability, with the effects of epinephrine being more important than those of norepinephrine. Epinephrine, like glucagon, promotes glycogenolysis in liver and muscle. Epinephrine also promotes lipolysis in adipose tissue, which increases the availability of plasma FA, and inhibits insulin secretion. The primary stimulus for catecholamine secretion is the activation of the sympathetic nervous system by stressors such as exercise, hypotension, and hypoglycemia. Substantial increases in the plasma catecholamine concentration can occur within seconds of the onset of high-intensity exercise. But the relative exercise intensity must be above 50% of $\dot{V}O_2$max to elevate the plasma catecholamine concentration significantly.

Growth Hormone and Cortisol

Growth hormone, secreted from the anterior pituitary gland, also stimulates mobilization of FA from adipose tissue, and increases in plasma growth hormone concentration are related to exercise intensity. During prolonged strenuous exercise, cortisol secretion from the adrenal cortex increases. Cortisol, a steroid hormone, increases the effectiveness of catecholamines in some tissues (e.g., it promotes lipolysis in adipose tissue). But its main effects are to promote protein degradation and amino acid release from muscle and to stimulate gluconeogenesis in the liver. The primary stimulus to cortisol secretion is stress-induced release of adrenocorticotrophic hormone (ACTH) from the anterior pituitary gland. Cortisol is derived from cholesterol, and its high fat solubility allows it to diffuse across cell membranes. Cortisol receptors in the cell cytoplasm translocate the hormone to the nucleus of the cell. Interaction of the hormone-receptor complex with specific sections of DNA switches on the transcription of specific genes and thus stimulates the synthesis of new proteins in the cell (see figure 3.15). This activity is common to all the steroid hormones (e.g., testosterone, estrogen, aldosterone).

Interleukin-6

IL-6 is a cytokine (a peptide chemical messenger) produced by several different cells and tissues, although it is best known for its actions in the regulation of immune function and inflammation. It is secreted by activated monocytes and macrophages, but contracting skeletal muscle fibers also produce and release IL-6 into the circulation. Muscle secretion of IL-6 has been shown to be almost entirely responsible for the up to 100-fold rise in plasma IL-6 concentration during prolonged exercise such as marathon running. The release of IL-6 is primarily regulated by an altered intramuscular milieu in response to exercise: Changes in calcium homeostasis, impaired glucose availability (glycogen depletion), and increased formation of reactive oxygen species are all associated with exercise and are capable of activating transcription factors known to regulate IL-6 synthesis. Acute IL-6 administration to humans increases lipolysis, fat oxidation, liver glycogenolysis, and insulin-mediated glucose disposal (Pedersen and Febbraio 2008). IL-6 also has anti-inflammatory effects and may exert some of its biological effects through stimulation of cortisol secretion and inhibition of the proinflammatory cytokine tumor necrosis factor-α (Gleeson et al. 2011).

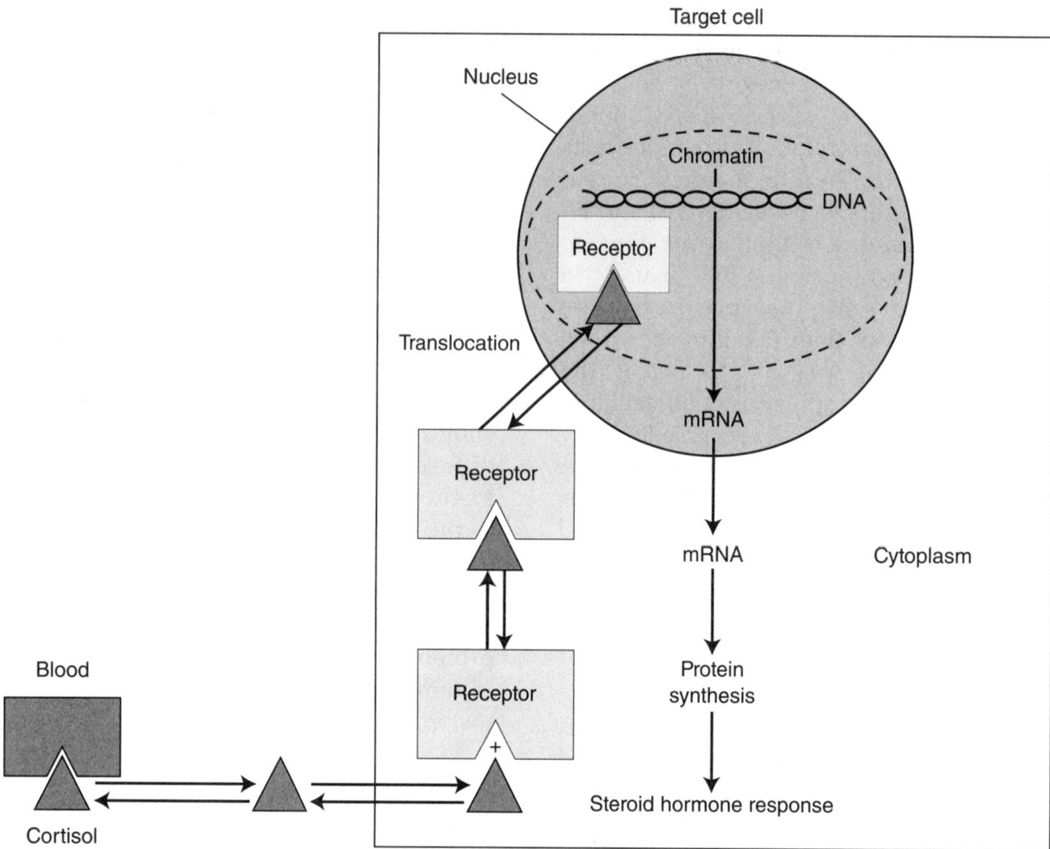

Figure 3.15 Mode of action of steroid hormones such as cortisol.

Metabolic Responses to Exercise

The most important factor influencing the metabolic response to exercise is exercise intensity. The physical fitness of the subject also modifies the metabolic response to exercise, and other factors—including exercise duration, substrate availability, nutritional status, diet, feeding during exercise, mode of exercise, previous exercise, drugs, environmental temperature, and altitude—are also important.

Causes of Fatigue in High-Intensity Exercise

ATP is the only fuel that can be used directly for skeletal muscle force generation, and the available ATP will fuel about 2 seconds of maximum-intensity exercise. Therefore, for muscle force generation to continue, ATP must be resynthesized rapidly from ADP. During high-intensity exercise, the relatively low rate of ATP resynthesis from oxidative phosphorylation stimulates rapid anaerobic energy production from PCr and glycogen hydrolysis. PCr breakdown begins at the onset of contraction to buffer the rapid accumulation of ADP from ATP hydrolysis. But the rate of PCr hydrolysis declines after only a few seconds of maximal force generation (see figure 3.16).

If high-intensity exercise is to continue beyond the first few seconds, a marked increase in the contribution from glycolysis to ATP resynthesis is necessary. Anaerobic glycolysis involves several more steps than PCr hydrolysis, although compared with oxidative phosphorylation, it is still extremely rapid. Anaerobic glycolysis starts at the onset of contraction, but unlike PCr hydrolysis, it does not reach a maximal rate until after 5 seconds of exercise, and it can be maintained at this level for several seconds during maximal muscle force generation (see figure 3.17). The mechanism or mechanisms responsible for the eventual decline in glycolysis during maximal exercise have not been determined. Exercise at an intensity equivalent to 95% to 100% of $\dot{V}O_2$max can be sustained for about 5 minutes before fatigue is experienced. Under

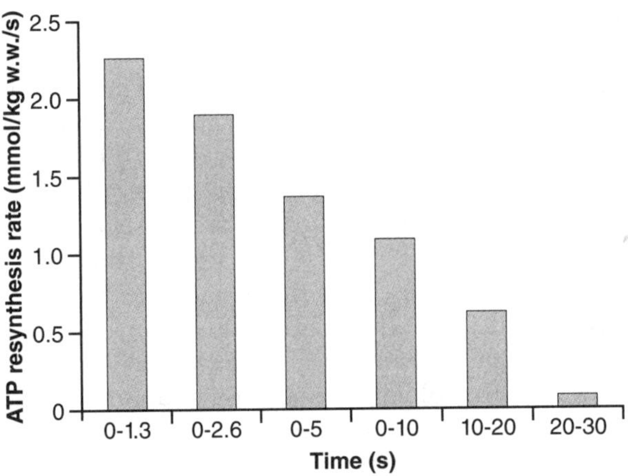

Figure 3.16 Rates of anaerobic ATP resynthesis from PCr hydrolysis during maximal isometric contraction in human skeletal muscle.

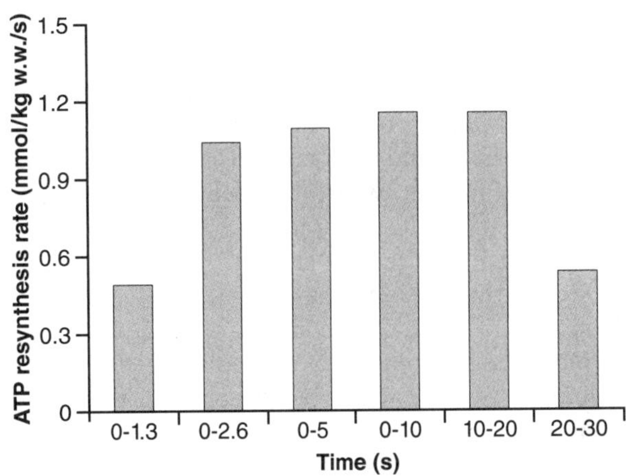

Figure 3.17 Rates of anaerobic ATP resynthesis from glycolysis during maximal isometric contraction in human skeletal muscle.

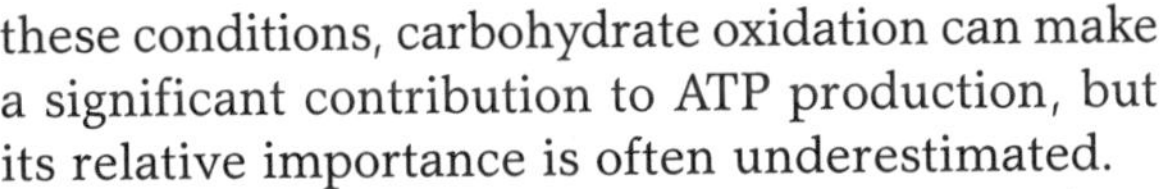
these conditions, carbohydrate oxidation can make a significant contribution to ATP production, but its relative importance is often underestimated.

Fatigue, which is the inability to maintain a given or expected force or power output, is an inevitable feature of maximal exercise. Typically, the loss of power output or force production is likely to be in the region of 40% to 60% of the maximum observed during 30 seconds of all-out exercise. Many factors contribute to fatigue, but during maximal short-duration exercise, it will be caused primarily by a gradual decline in anaerobic ATP production or an increase in ADP accumulation caused by a depletion of PCr and a fall in the rate of glycolysis.

In high-intensity exercise lasting 1 to 5 minutes, **lactic acid** accumulation may contribute to the fatigue process. At physiological pH values, lactic acid almost completely dissociates into its constituent lactate and hydrogen ions, and studies using animal muscle preparations have demonstrated that direct inhibition of force production can be achieved by increasing hydrogen and lactate ion concentrations (Green 1995). Reduced muscle pH may cause some inhibition of PFK and phosphorylase, thereby reducing the rate of ATP resynthesis from glycolysis. This development is unlikely to be important in exercising muscle, however, because the in vitro inhibition of PFK by a reduced pH is reversed in the presence of other activators such as AMP (Spriet 1991). Lactate and hydrogen ion accumulation also appear to result in muscle fatigue independent of one another, but the latter is the more commonly cited mechanism. However, although it is likely related to the fatigue process, it is unlikely that both lactate and hydrogen ion accumulation are wholly responsible for muscle fatigue. For example, studies involving human volunteers have demonstrated that muscle force generation after fatiguing exercise can recover rapidly despite also having a very low muscle pH value (Stackhouse et al. 2001). The consensus appears to be that the maintenance of force production during high-intensity exercise is pH dependent, but the initial force generation is more related to PCr availability.

One of the consequences of rapid PCr hydrolysis during high-intensity exercise is the accumulation of Pi, which inhibits muscle contraction coupling directly. Pi may act directly on the myofibrils and decrease cross-bridge force production and myofibrillar Ca^{2+} sensitivity. By acting on sarcoplasmic reticulum (SR) Ca^{2+} handling, increased Pi may also increase tetanic sarcoplasmic free Ca^{2+} concentration in early fatigue by stimulating the SR Ca^{2+} release channels, inhibiting the ATP-dependent SR Ca^{2+} uptake, and reducing tetanic sarcoplasmic free Ca^{2+} concentration in late fatigue by entering the SR, precipitating with Ca^{2+}, and thereby decreasing the Ca^{2+} available for release (Westerblad, Allen, and Lannergren 2002). However, the simultaneous PCr depletion and Pi accumulation make in vivo separation of the effect of PCr depletion from the effect of Pi accumulation difficult. This problem is further confounded by the parallel increases in hydrogen and lactate ions that occur during high-intensity exercise. All these metabolites have been independently implicated in muscle fatigue.

Calcium release by the sarcoplasmic reticulum as a consequence of muscle depolarization is essential for the activation of muscle contraction coupling. During fatiguing contractions, calcium transport slows and calcium transients become progressively smaller, which has been attributed to a reduction in calcium reuptake by the sarcoplasmic reticulum or increased calcium binding. Strong evidence that a disruption of calcium handling is responsible for fatigue comes from studies showing that the stimulation of sarcoplasmic reticulum calcium release caused by the administration of caffeine to isolated muscle can improve muscle force production even in the presence of a low muscle pH (Green 1995). Alternatively, fatigue during high-intensity exercise may be associated with an excitation-coupling failure and possibly a reduced nervous drive caused by reflex inhibition at the spinal level. In the latter hypothesis, accumulation of interstitial potassium in muscle may play a major role.

When repeated bouts of maximal exercise are performed, the rates of muscle PCr hydrolysis and lactate accumulation decline. In the case of PCr, this response is thought to occur because of incomplete PCr resynthesis during recovery between successive exercise bouts. The mechanism or mechanisms responsible for the fall in the rate of lactate accumulation are unclear.

Causes of Fatigue in Prolonged Exercise

The term *prolonged exercise* is usually used to describe exercise intensities that can be sustained for 30 to 180 minutes. Because the rate of ATP demand is relatively low compared with high-intensity exercise, PCr, carbohydrate, and fat can all contribute to energy production. The various fuel sources available to resynthesize ATP are summarized in figure 3.18. The rates of PCr degradation and lactate production during the first minutes of prolonged exercise are closely related to the intensity of exercise performed, and energy production during this period would likely be compromised without this contribution from anaerobic metabolism. After a steady state has been reached, however, carbohydrate and fat oxidation become the principal means of resynthesizing ATP. Muscle glycogen is the principal fuel during the first 30 minutes of exercise at 60% to 80% of $\dot{V}O_2$max. The rate of muscle glycogen use depends on exercise intensity (see figure 3.19).

During the early stages of exercise, fat oxidation is limited by the delay in the mobilization of FAs from adipose tissue. At rest after an overnight fast, the plasma FA concentration is about 0.3 to 0.4 mmol/L. This concentration is commonly observed to fall during the first hour of moderate-intensity exercise, and this followed by a progressive increase (see figure 3.20) as lipolysis is stimulated by the actions of catecholamines, glucagon, and cortisol. During very prolonged exercise, the plasma FA concentration can reach 1.5 to 2.0 mmol/L, and muscle uptake of blood-borne FA is proportional to the plasma FA concentration.

The glycerol released from adipose tissue cannot be used directly by muscle, which lacks the enzyme glycerol kinase. But glycerol (together with alanine and lactate) is taken up by the liver and used as a gluconeogenic precursor to help maintain liver glucose output as liver glycogen levels decline. The

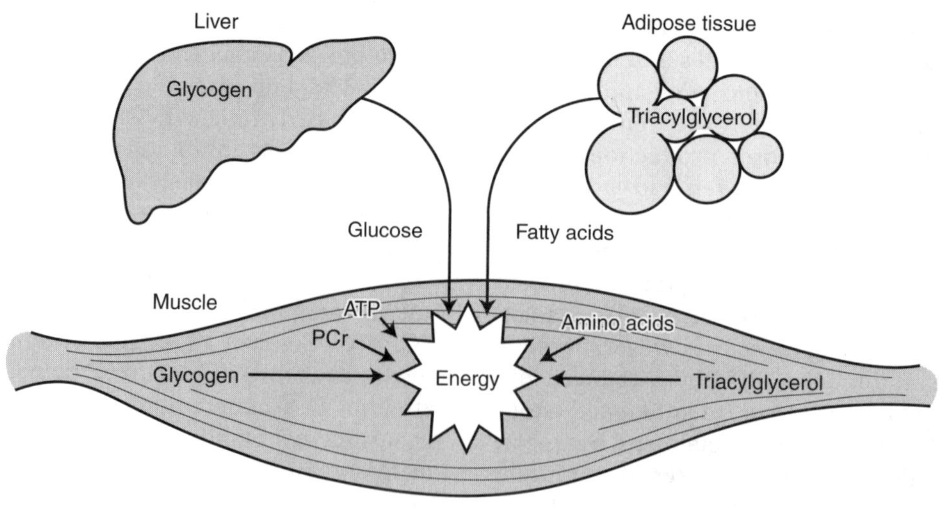

Figure 3.18 The main fuel sources available for exercise.

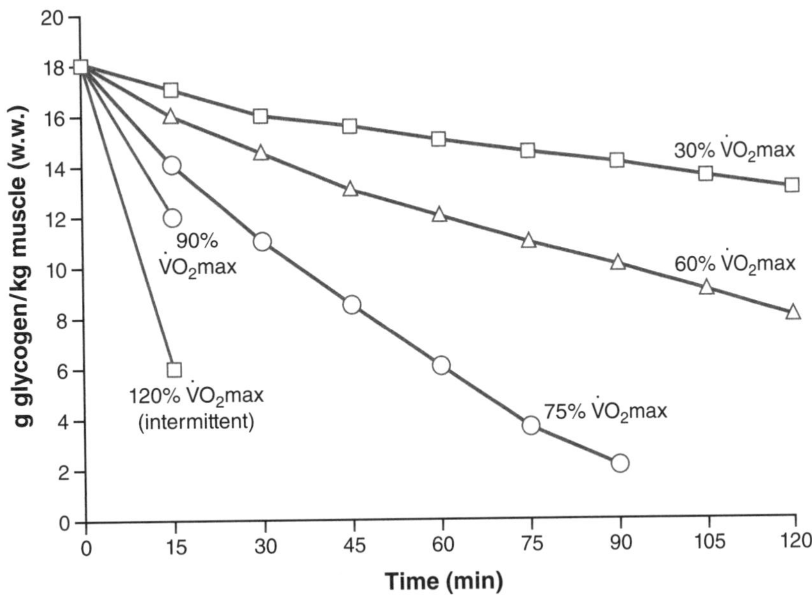

Figure 3.19 Effect of exercise intensity on rates of muscle glycogen use.

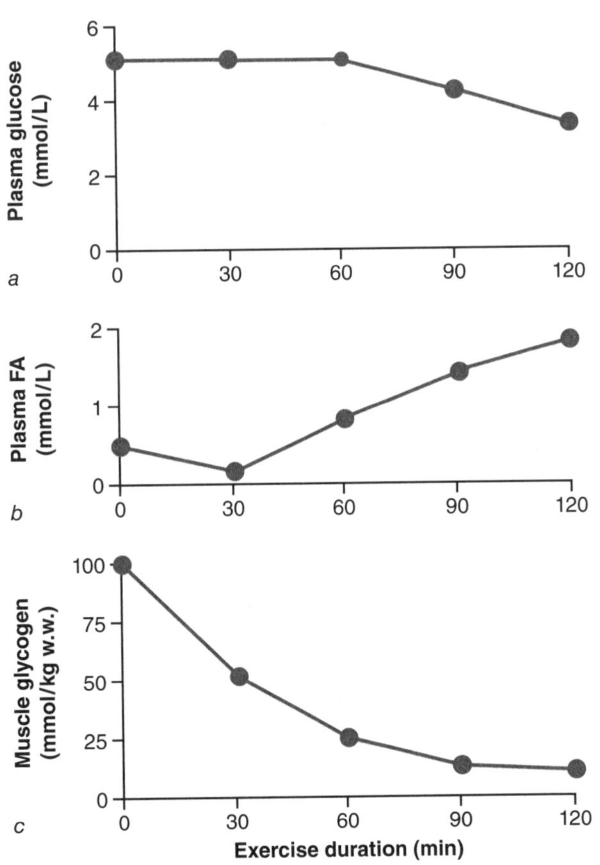

Figure 3.20 Changes in the concentrations of *(a)* plasma glucose, *(b)* plasma FAs, and *(c)* muscle glycogen during continuous exercise at an intensity equivalent to 70% of $\dot{V}O_2max$.

Reprinted by permission from M. Gleeson, Biochemistry of Exercise, in *Nutrition in Sport*, edited by R.J. Maughan (Blackwell Science Ltd., 2000), 17-38.

use of blood glucose is greater at higher work rates and increases during prolonged submaximal exercise. At an exercise intensity of 60% of $\dot{V}O_2$max, blood glucose uptake by muscle peaks after about 90 minutes (see figure 3.21). The decline in blood glucose uptake after 90 minutes is attributable to the increasing availability of plasma FA as fuel (which appears to inhibit muscle glucose uptake directly) and the depletion of liver glycogen stores.

At marathon-running pace, muscle carbohydrate stores alone can fuel about 80 minutes of exercise before depletion (see table 3.5). The simultaneous use of body fat and hepatic carbohydrate stores, however, enables ATP production to be maintained and exercise to continue. Figure 3.22 shows the contributions of fat oxidation, muscle glycogen, and blood glucose to energy expenditure during running at various speeds. At marathon-running

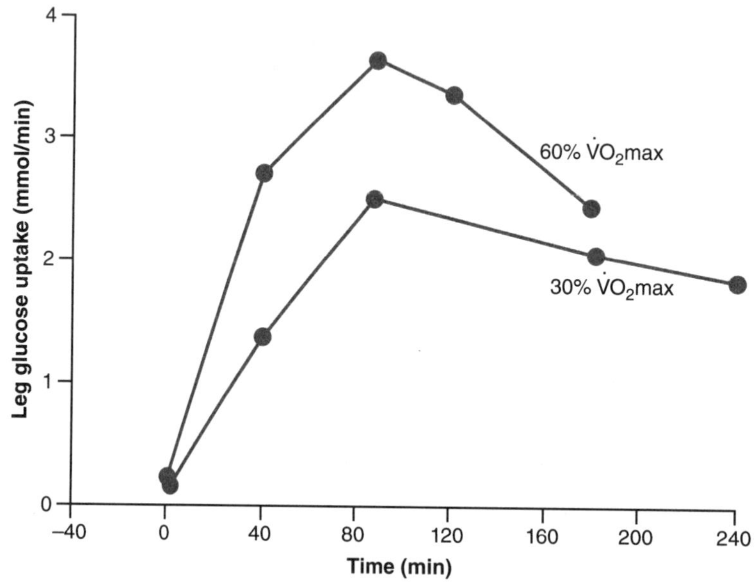

Figure 3.21 Rate of uptake of glucose from the blood by muscle during exercise at 30% of $\dot{V}O_2$max and 60% of $\dot{V}O_2$max. Peak uptake occurs after about 90 minutes of exercise.

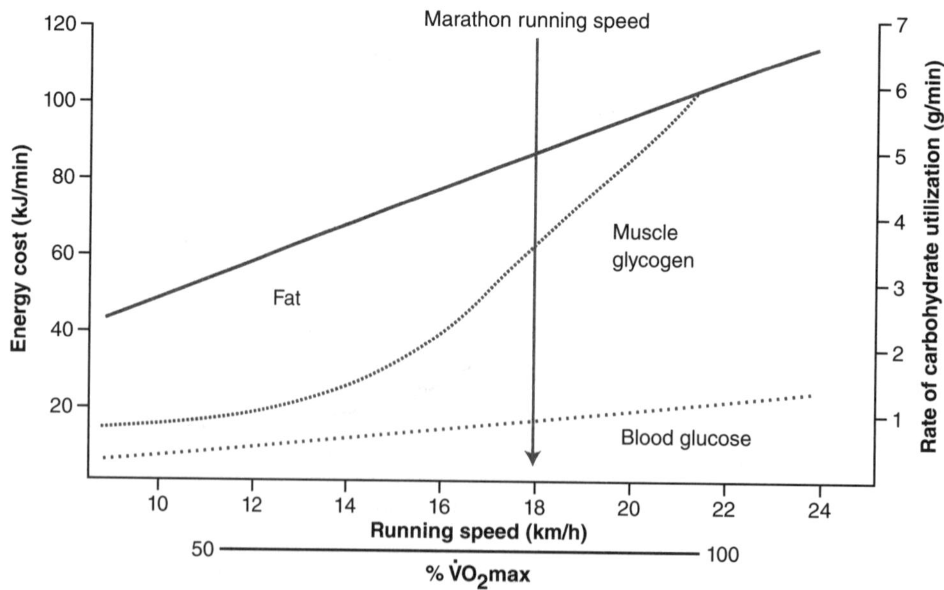

Figure 3.22 Changes in the relative contributions of the major fuel sources to ATP resynthesis during running at various speeds. At the marathon-running speed of an elite endurance athlete, the rate of carbohydrate oxidation is about 3.5 g/min.

pace, the muscle and hepatic carbohydrate stores will ultimately become depleted. At this point, ATP production becomes compromised because of the inability of fat oxidation to increase sufficiently to offset this deficit. The rate of ATP resynthesis from fat oxidation alone cannot meet the ATP requirement for exercise intensities higher than about 50% to 60% of $\dot{V}O_2$max. The factor that limits the maximal rate of fat oxidation during exercise (i.e., why it cannot increase to compensate for carbohydrate depletion) is currently unknown, but it must precede acetyl-CoA formation because from this point, fat and carbohydrate share the same fate. The limitation may reside in the rate of uptake of FA into muscle from blood or the transport of FA into the mitochondria, rather than in the rate of ß-oxidation of FA in the mitochondria.

During prolonged submaximal exercise, the main factors that influence the selection of fuel for muscular work are exercise intensity and duration. The effect of exercise duration on the contribution of different fuels during constant-load exercise at about 60% of $\dot{V}O_2$max is illustrated in figure 3.23, and the effect of exercise intensity is summarized in figure 3.24.

In sedentary people, the glycogen store in muscle is fairly resistant to change. The combination of exercise and dietary manipulation,

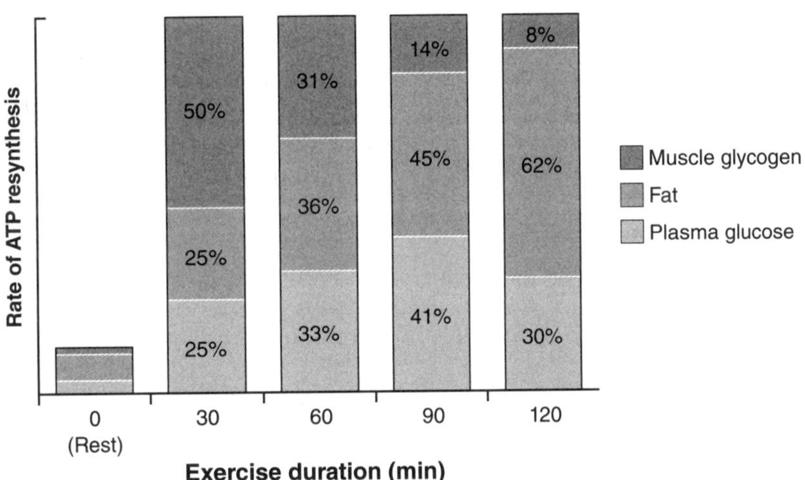

Figure 3.23 Changes in the relative contributions of the major fuel sources to ATP resynthesis during prolonged submaximal exercise at an intensity equivalent to about 60% of $\dot{V}O_2$max (approximately 10 times the resting metabolic rate).

Reprinted by permission from M. Gleeson, Biochemistry of Exercise, in *Nutrition in Sport,* edited by R.J. Maughan (Blackwell Science Ltd., 2000), 17-38.

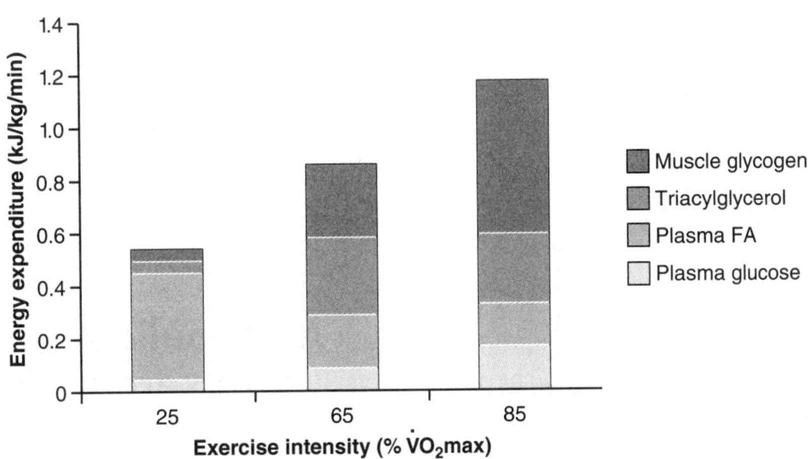

Figure 3.24 The contributions of different fuel sources to energy expenditure at three different exercise intensities.

Based on Romijn et al. (1995).

however, can have a dramatic effect on muscle glycogen storage. A clear positive relationship exists between muscle glycogen content and subsequent endurance performance. Furthermore, the ingestion of carbohydrate during prolonged exercise decreases muscle glycogen use and fat mobilization and oxidation, and it increases the rate of carbohydrate oxidation and endurance capacity. Therefore, the contribution of orally ingested carbohydrate to total ATP production under these conditions must be greater than that normally derived from fat oxidation. The precise biochemical mechanism by which muscle glycogen depletion causes fatigue is currently unresolved. However, the inability of muscle to maintain the rate of ATP synthesis in the glycogen-depleted state possibly results in ADP and Pi accumulation and consequently fatigue. Of course, a substantial fall in intramuscular ATP concentration is unlikely in this form of exercise, because very low ATP concentrations cause rigor and irreversible damage to muscle fibers. Hence, some factor other than muscle glycogen depletion—probably linked to low muscle glycogen concentrations—must act to constrain the activity of glycogen-depleted muscle before rigor can develop.

Starvation rapidly depletes the liver of carbohydrate. The rate of hepatic glucose release in resting, postabsorptive individuals is sufficient to match the carbohydrate demands of only the central nervous system. Approximately 70% of this release is derived from liver carbohydrate stores, and the remainder is derived from liver gluconeogenesis. During exercise, the rate of hepatic glucose release is related to exercise intensity. Liver carbohydrate stores contribute 90% of this release, ultimately resulting in liver glycogen depletion.

Prolonged exercise, particularly after a period of fasting or a diet low in carbohydrate, results in hypoglycemia, which may be a direct cause of fatigue. Alterations in liver rather than muscle glycogen concentrations could possibly be the more important determinant of the marked difference in exercise capacity induced by high-carbohydrate and low-carbohydrate diets. Hypoglycemia is detected by the brain and causes symptoms of tiredness and dizziness. This central fatigue could then reduce the degree of skeletal muscle recruitment by the motor cortex, causing a fall in muscle force generation. Furthermore, afferent chemoreceptor information from both the hepatic portal system (monitoring hepatic portal blood glucose concentration) and the skeletal muscle (monitoring muscle glycogenolysis) possibly feeds back to the motor cortex. These signals increase as hypoglycemia develops, and the availability of muscle glycogen declines, inducing more central fatigue and causing athletes to reduce their exercise intensity.

Thus, carbohydrate ingestion during exercise can also delay fatigue development by slowing the rate of liver glycogen depletion and helping to maintain the blood glucose concentration. Central fatigue (fatigue of the central nervous system indicated by an impaired ability to sustain maximal muscle activation during sustained contractions) is a major factor during prolonged exercise. The development of hypoglycemia contributes to this. Hyperthermia is another factor. In the heat, performance is markedly decreased, and exercise-induced hyperthermia is associated with central fatigue. Central fatigue appears to be influenced by neurotransmitter activity of the dopaminergic system, but (inhibitory) signals from thermoreceptors that detect elevated core, muscle, and skin temperatures as well as other factors all contribute to the development of fatigue.

Fatigue is a protective mechanism designed to prevent irreversible muscle damage, and—even more important—to prevent neural damage by hypoglycemia and hyperthermia. Several drugs, including amphetamines and caffeine, have been shown to be ergogenic via actions on the brain (Jones 2008) that reduce sensations of fatigue, increase alertness, and improve cognitive function; this is important for sports in which motor skills, concentration, and decision making play a role in success. However, these drugs can be hazardous in some exercise situations because they can override the protective fatigue mechanisms.

When exercise is performed with high initial muscle and liver glycogen levels, the hormonal response to exercise is attenuated compared with when exercise is performed in a carbohydrate-depleted state (see figure 3.25). Similarly, carbohydrate feeding during exercise is associated with smaller rises in the plasma concentrations of epinephrine, norepinephrine, glucagon, and cortisol. Because these hormones are involved in the stimulation of lipolysis, fat mobilization is delayed and the rate of fat oxidation is less when carbohydrate is consumed during exercise.

Metabolic Adaptations to Exercise Training

Muscle adaptations to aerobic endurance training include increases in capillary density and mitochondrial size and number. The activity of the TCA

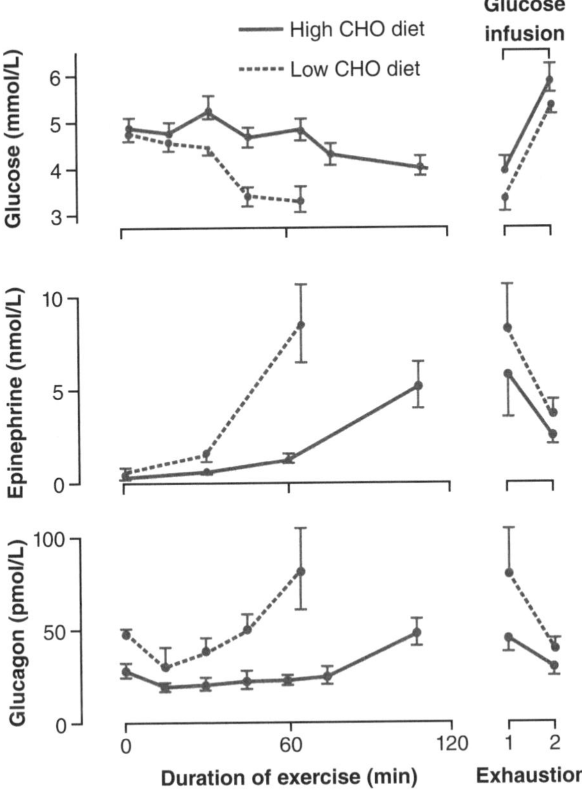

Figure 3.25 Influence of a high-carbohydrate or low-carbohydrate diet (for the preceding 3 days) on the hormonal response to prolonged exercise. Mean plasma hormone concentrations are shown for a group of seven subjects running at 70% of $\dot{V}O_2$max after 4 days on a low-carbohydrate or high-carbohydrate diet. At exhaustion (1), the subjects were encouraged to run for 10 more minutes (2) with glucose infusion.

Reprinted, by permission, from H. Galbo et al., "Exercise physiology: Humoral function," *Sport Science Review* 1, (1979): 65-93; H. Galbo et al., "The Effect of Different Diets and of Insulin on the Hormonal Response to Prolonged Exercise," *Acta Physiologica Scandanavica* 107, (1979): 19-32.

cycle and of other oxidative enzymes increases, and a concomitant increase occurs in the capacity to oxidize both fat and carbohydrate. Training adaptations in muscle affect substrate use. Endurance training also increases the relative cross-sectional area of type I fibers, increases intramuscular content of triacylglycerol, and increases the capacity to use fat as an energy source during submaximal exercise. Trained subjects also demonstrate increased reliance on intramuscular triacylglycerol as an energy source. These effects and other physiological effects of training, including increased maximum cardiac output and $\dot{V}O_2$max, improve oxygen delivery to working muscle, attenuate hormonal responses to exercise (see figure 3.26), decrease the rate of muscle glycogen and blood glucose utilization (see figure 3.27), and decrease the rate of lactate accumulation during submaximal exercise. These adaptations contribute to marked improvement in endurance capacity after training.

Alterations in substrate use with endurance training could be caused, at least in part, by less disturbance to ATP homeostasis during exercise. With increased mitochondrial oxidative capacity after training, smaller decreases in ATP and PCr and smaller increases in ADP and Pi are needed to balance the rate of ATP synthesis with the rate of ATP use. In other words, with more mitochondria, the amount of oxygen as well as the ADP and Pi required per mitochondrion will be less after training than before training. The smaller increase in ADP concentration would result in formation of less AMP by the myokinase reaction, and less IMP and ammonia would be formed by AMP deamination. Smaller increases in the concentrations of ADP, AMP, Pi, and ammonia could account for the slower rate of glycolysis and glycogenolysis in trained muscle compared with untrained muscle.

Training for strength, power, or speed has little if any effect on aerobic capacity. Heavy resistance

CHANGES IN THE METABOLIC RESPONSE TO EXERCISE FOLLOWING ENDURANCE TRAINING

- Higher relative contribution of fat oxidation (lower **respiratory exchange ratio [RER]** and **respiratory quotient [RQ]**)
- Lower rate of muscle glycogen use
- Reduced use of blood glucose by muscle
- Smaller increases in circulating hormones (e.g., epinephrine, cortisol, growth hormone)
- Smaller rise in plasma FFA concentration
- Increased FFA transporters in muscle membrane
- Increased oxidation of fat relative to carbohydrate
- Increased use of muscle triglyceride
- Reduced accumulation of muscle (and blood) lactate

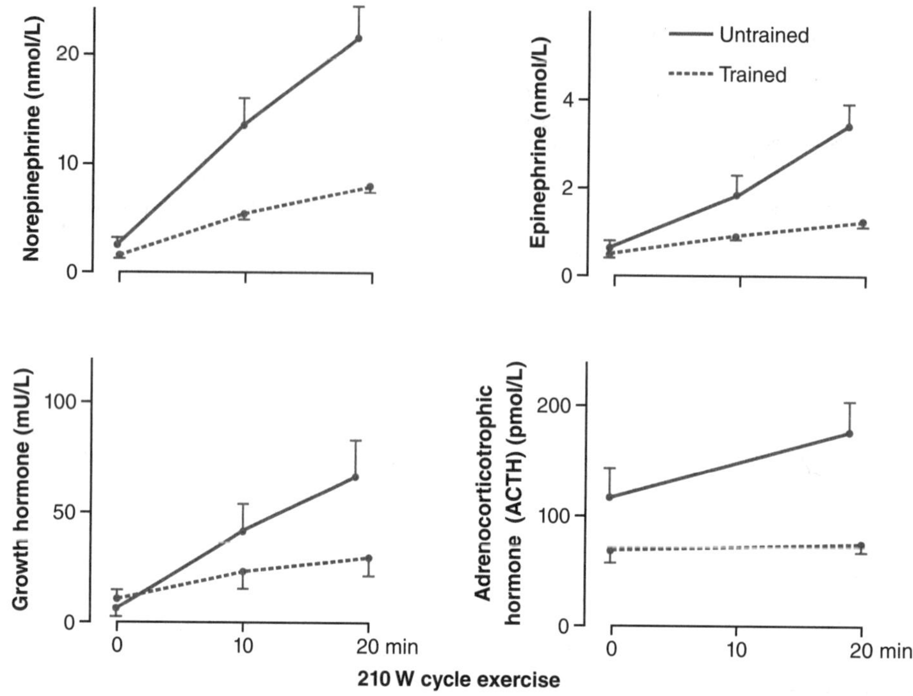

Figure 3.26 Influence of endurance training on the hormonal response to prolonged exercise.

Reprinted, by permission, from H. Galbo et al., "Exercise physiology: Humoral function," *Sport Science Review* 1, (1979): 65-93; H. Galbo et al., "The Effect of Different Diets and of Insulin on the Hormonal Response to Prolonged Exercise," *Acta Physiologica Scandanavica* 107, (1979): 19-32.

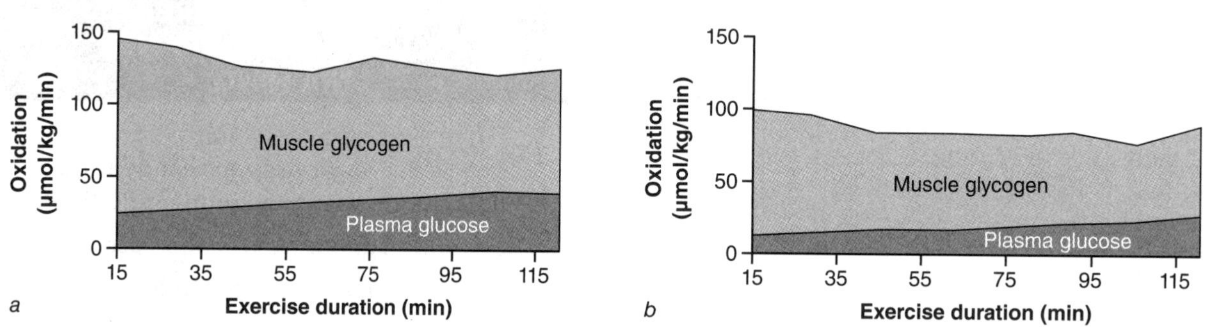

Figure 3.27 Rates of muscle glycogen and plasma glucose oxidation during 2 hours of cycling at 60% of pretraining VO_2max in *(a)* untrained men and *(b)* the same men after 12 weeks of endurance exercise training. Note the reduced rates of glycogen and glucose use following training ($P<0.05$ trained vs. untrained).

Data from Mendenhall et al. (1994).

training or sprinting brings about specific changes in the immediate (ATP and PCr) and short-term (glycolytic) energy delivery systems, increases in muscle buffering capacity, and improvements in strength or sprint performance. Several months of heavy resistance training cause hypertrophy of the muscle fibers, thus increasing total muscle mass and the possible maximum power output. Stretch, contraction, and damage to muscle fibers during exercise provide the stimuli for adaptation, which involves changes in the expression of different myosin isoforms.

Influence of Nutrition on Adaptation to Endurance Training

Interest has developed in the influence of nutrition on endurance training adaptations (Hawley et al. 2011). It is now recognized that low levels of muscle glycogen may enhance the messenger RNA (mRNA) content of some genes involved in exercise metabolism. Several studies have shown that the genes for selected metabolic enzymes, including citrate synthase, ß-hydroxyacyl-CoA-dehydrogenase, and pyruvate dehydrogenase kinase, are upregulated to a greater extent in response to exercise when exercise is performed with low pre-exercise glycogen content (Burke 2010; Hawley et al. 2011). The role of muscle glycogen could be explained by the fact that some signaling proteins, such as AMP-activated protein kinase (AMPK), possess glycogen-binding domains, and when glycogen is low, these proteins are more active toward their specific targets. Indeed, the activity of AMPK and p38 mitogen-activated protein kinase (p38 MAPK) is elevated when exercise is performed with low muscle glycogen (Burke 2010; Matsakas and Patel 2009). This may be beneficial to individuals undertaking endurance exercise training, because AMPK and p38 MAPK are believed to play a critical role in regulating mitochondrial biogenesis and endurance training adaptations. However, it is not yet known whether these exaggerated responses in a glycogen-depleted state translate into greater protein contents or higher functional activities. It is likely that signals responsive both to increased fat availability and to decreased carbohydrate availability would work in concert to determine the exact responses in gene expression in skeletal muscle. The mechanisms by which the adaptations to a high-fat, low-carbohydrate diet are mediated appear to be related to FFA activation of the family of peroxisome proliferator activator receptors (PPARs) or an insulin effect as a result of the decreased carbohydrate availability.

The level of antioxidants in the diet may also have some influence on endurance training adaptations. Reactive oxygen and nitrogen species (RONS) are involved in the modulation of cell signaling pathways and the control of several (redox-sensitive) transcription factors. Although high levels of RONS may interfere with muscle function, moderate levels of RONS are essential in the development of optimal force production in muscle (Powers and Jackson 2008; Reid 2008). These findings raise important questions concerning the possible role of free radical species as signals for wider adaptive responses in these and other tissues and question the previously held belief that tissues need protecting from damage caused by free radicals by supplementation with large doses of antioxidant nutrients. It is entirely feasible that those adaptations to stress mediated by free radicals play an important role in maintaining cell viability in tissues that are routinely subjected to repeated stresses (e.g., muscle following exercise) and that increased consumption of some antioxidant nutrients might interfere with these necessary adaptive processes. In one study, 14 men were trained for 8 weeks, and five of the men were supplemented daily with an oral dose of 1 g of vitamin C (Gomez-Cabrera et al. 2008). The administration of vitamin C significantly impaired endurance capacity. The adverse effects of vitamin C may result from its capacity to reduce the exercise-induced expression of key transcription factors involved in mitochondrial biogenesis: PPAR coactivator 1, nuclear respiratory factor 1, and mitochondrial transcription factor A. Vitamin C also prevented the exercise-induced expression of cytochrome C (a marker of mitochondrial content) and of the antioxidant enzymes superoxide dismutase and glutathione peroxidase. Thus, it seems that supplementation with large doses of antioxidants may interfere with the function of RONS and may reduce cellular adaptations to exercise training, although some studies have not supported this concept (Yfanti et al. 2010). More research needs to be done to determine the role of RONS in training, but it seems that they may not always be damaging, and their role in modulating signaling pathways may be important in adaptive processes. In in vitro and animal studies, several polyphenolic phytochemicals (e.g., epicatechins, quercetin, resveratrol) have been found to exert an exercise mimetic effect, which promotes an enhancement of mitochondrial biogenesis (Hawley et al. 2011). Further research may determine whether these non-nutritive plant compounds can influence exercise-induced adaptations in humans. Further discussion of this possibility can be found in chapter 12.

Influence of Nutrition on Adaptation to Resistance Training

The timing and composition of postexercise nutrition influences protein turnover and hence the response to a hypertrophic stimulus such as resistance training. If an athlete is fasted before a resistance training bout and remains fasted afterward, protein synthesis and degradation are elevated in the post-training period, but breakdown exceeds synthesis and results in a net loss of muscle tissue protein (Phillips 2011; Rennie 2005). The ingestion of protein or amino acids immediately after exercise can prevent this loss by promoting muscle protein synthesis and reducing breakdown such that a net gain of tissue protein occurs (see chapter 8). The supply of essential amino acids may be the limiting factor, and studies indicate that ingestion of at least 25 g of protein (containing about 10 g of essential amino acids) is needed to achieve optimal muscle tissue protein gain after a resistance exercise session (Phillips 2011). The stimulation of protein synthesis after hard exercise in combination with amino acid ingestion may last for up to 24 hours or even longer and offers athletes an opportunity to promote more effective adaptations to their training programs. Studies have established that regular ingestion of protein in close proximity to resistance training sessions results in greater muscle hypertrophy and strength gains than consumption of similar amounts of protein at other times (Burd et al. 2009; Phillips 2011). Coingestion of carbohydrate to maximize the insulin response may not be needed if the intake of protein postexercise is adequate, but it is a sensible option for the athlete who wants to maximize training adaptation and restore muscle glycogen. Research has also shown that the essential amino acid leucine plays a key role in the stimulation of muscle protein synthesis and appears to be a key activator in switching on muscle protein synthesis following resistance exercise (Phillips 2011). Thus, high-quality, rapidly digested, leucine-rich proteins such as whey protein would appear to be ideal products for stimulating muscle protein gain and promotion of hypertrophy. Further details can be found in chapter 8.

Key Points

- Skeletal muscle cells are long, striated, multinucleated fibers. Myofibers are the contractile elements composed of sarcomeres containing thin (actin) and thick (myosin) filaments arranged in a regular array. The heads of the myosin molecules form cross-bridges that bind reversibly to the actin filaments, causing the filaments to slide over each other toward the centers of the sarcomeres.
- The energy source for muscle contraction is ATP, which is continuously regenerated during exercise from phosphocreatine hydrolysis, anaerobic metabolism of glycogen or glucose, or aerobic metabolism of acetyl-CoA derived principally from the breakdown of carbohydrate or fat. The carbon skeleton of amino acids can be used as a fuel for oxidative metabolism but is not a major fuel for energy production during exercise.
- Phosphocreatine is present in the sarcoplasm of muscle at about three times the concentration of ATP. Phosphocreatine hydrolysis is initiated at the immediate onset of contraction to buffer the rapid accumulation of ADP resulting from ATP hydrolysis. The rate of phosphocreatine hydrolysis begins to decline after only a few seconds of maximal force generation. The importance of phosphocreatine to muscle energy production and function lies in the extremely rapid rate at which it can resynthesize ATP.
- Carbohydrate provides energy by anaerobic metabolism, with lactate as the end product, or by complete oxidation to carbon dioxide and water. The net effect of glycolysis is conversion of one molecule of glucose to two molecules of pyruvate. This process makes two molecules of ATP available for each molecule of glucose that is broken down. If muscle glycogen is the starting substrate, three ATP molecules are generated for each glucose residue passing down the pathway.
- Glycolysis involves the reduction of NAD^+ to NADH, which depletes the intracellular pool of NAD^+. Reduction of pyruvate to lactate allows the NAD^+ to be regenerated from NADH. The alternative pathway for NAD^+ regeneration involves conversion of pyruvate to acetyl-CoA for subsequent oxidation in the TCA cycle.

- The TCA cycle and oxidative phosphorylation occur in the mitochondria. In the aerobic resynthesis of ATP, oxygen is the final electron acceptor in the ETC, and it combines with hydrogen to form water.
- Carbohydrate stores are rapidly depleted during exercise (muscle glycogen) or during fasting (liver glycogen). Muscle glycogen stores are normally depleted after 1 to 2 hours of hard exercise. In very high-intensity exercise, muscle glycogen content falls rapidly but is not completely depleted at the point of fatigue.
- Carbohydrate is the major fuel for muscle activity in high-intensity exercise. When muscle glycogen stores are depleted, only low-intensity exercise is possible. The time that a fixed exercise intensity can be sustained is related to the size of the pre-exercise glycogen store. The size of the store depends on the pattern of exercise and diet in the previous hours and days.
- A number of hormones are involved in the integration and control of carbohydrate metabolism including (especially) insulin, which promotes carbohydrate storage, and glucagon, whose actions are generally antagonistic to those of insulin. Epinephrine and norepinephrine stimulate carbohydrate mobilization and metabolism at times of stress.
- The principal storage form of fat in the body is triacylglycerol, most of which is located in white adipose tissue. Triacylglycerol stores are also found in liver and muscle and as lipoproteins in blood. Muscles cannot oxidize triacylglycerols directly. The triacylglycerol molecules must first be broken down into their FA and glycerol components by lipolysis. This process is activated during exercise by the actions of epinephrine, glucagon, and cortisol. The principal sources of fat fuels for exercise are blood-borne FAs derived from adipose tissue and intramuscular triacylglycerol.
- Several factors influence the type of substrate used to fuel muscular work, including substrate availability, diet, intensity and duration of exercise, training status, hormones, previous exercise, and environmental conditions. Fat oxidation makes an increasing contribution to ATP regeneration as exercise duration increases. In exercise lasting several hours, fat may supply almost 80% of the total energy required.
- Endurance training increases the capacity of muscle to oxidize fat, which spares the use of muscle glycogen and blood glucose during prolonged exercise of moderate intensity. This is different from high rates of fat oxidation because glycogen is depleted after a low carbohydrate intake. In this situation, the capacity to increase fat oxidation may not be increased but the body is using the only available substrate (fat).
- Fatigue is the inability to maintain a given or expected power output or force, and it is an inevitable feature of strenuous exercise. The onset of muscle fatigue has been associated with the disruption of energy supply, product inhibition, and factors preceding cross-bridge formation. It is likely a multifactorial process.

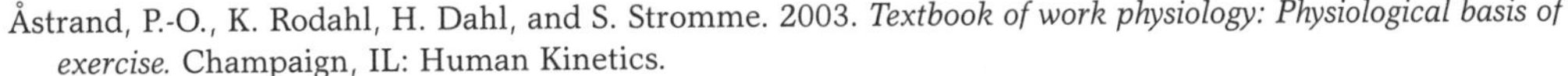

Recommended Readings

Åstrand, P.-O., K. Rodahl, H. Dahl, and S. Stromme. 2003. *Textbook of work physiology: Physiological basis of exercise.* Champaign, IL: Human Kinetics.

Bangsbo, J. 1997. Physiology of muscle fatigue during intense exercise. In *The clinical pharmacology of sport and exercise,* edited by T. Reilly and M. Orme, 123-133. Amsterdam: Elsevier.

Green, H.J. 1991. How important is endogenous muscle glycogen to fatigue in prolonged exercise? *Canadian Journal of Physiology and Pharmacology* 69:290-297.

Greenhaff, P.L., and E. Hultman. 1999. The biochemical basis of exercise. In *Basic and applied sciences for sports medicine,* edited by R.J. Maughan, 69-89. Oxford: Butterworth-Heinemann.

Hargreaves, M., and L. Spriet. 2006. *Exercise metabolism.* 2nd ed. Champaign, IL: Human Kinetics.

Komi, P.V., and J. Karlsson. 1978. Skeletal muscle fibre types, enzyme activities and physical performance in young males and females. *Acta Physiologica Scandinavica* 103:210-218.

MacLaren, D., and Morton, J. 2011. *Biochemistry for sport and exercise metabolism.* London: Wiley.

Maughan, R.J., and M. Gleeson. 2010. *The biochemical basis of sports performance.* 2nd ed. Oxford: Oxford University Press.

Sahlin, K., and S. Broberg. 1990. Adenine nucleotide depletion in human muscle during exercise: Causality and significance of AMP deamination. *International Journal of Sports Medicine* 11:S62-S67.

Saltin, B. 1985. Physiological adaptation to physical conditioning. *Acta Medica Scandinavica* 711 (Suppl): 11–24.

Sjøgaard, G. 1991. Role of exercise-induced potassium fluxes underlying muscle fatigue: A brief review. *Canadian Journal of Physiology and Pharmacology* 69:238-245.

Tiidus, P.M., A.R. Tupling, and M.E. Houston. 2012. *Biochemistry primer for exercise science.* 4th ed. Champaign, IL: Human Kinetics.

Energy

Objectives

After studying this chapter, you should be able to do the following:

- Describe what energy is and how it is expressed and give an overview of the different types of energy
- Define the terms *gross efficiency, net efficiency, delta efficiency,* and *economy*
- Describe various ways to measure energy expenditure and explain the advantages and disadvantages of each
- Describe the various components of human energy expenditure and their respective contributions to energy expenditure in active and inactive people
- Discuss the concept of energy balance and how it relates to body weight and physical performance
- Discuss the upper and lower limits of human energy expenditure and the practical problems associated with these energy expenditures

Cells need **energy** to function, muscle fibers need energy to contract, and ionic pumps in membranes need energy to transport ions across cell membranes. Although the human body has some energy reserves, most of its energy must be obtained through nutrition. During exercise, energy requirements increase and energy provision can become critical. People who have defects in energy metabolism have problems performing vigorous physical exercise. A person with McArdle's disease, for example, lacks the enzyme glycogen phosphorylase and cannot break down muscle glycogen. Hence, that person's energy provision and exercise capacity are severely impaired. In athletes, energy provision can be crucial, and energy depletion (which in most cases means carbohydrate depletion) is one of the most common contributors to fatigue. Different types of exercise and sport have different energy requirements. Therefore, athletes must adjust their food intakes accordingly. This chapter describes the energy requirements and associated practical problems for some athletes.

Forms of energy range from light energy to chemical energy. Plants use light energy in the process of photosynthesis to produce carbohydrate, fat, or protein. The energy in food is stored in the chemical bonds of various molecules. Breaking these bonds releases the energy, and it becomes available for conversion into other forms of energy. For instance, when glucose is broken down during glycolysis, chemical energy is converted to another form of chemical energy (ATP) and ultimately transformed into mechanical energy (muscle contraction).

In physiology, energy represents the capacity to do work, which is often referred to as mechanical energy. Walking, running, throwing, and jumping require the production of mechanical energy. Work (energy) is the product of force times the vertical distance covered:

$$\text{work} = \text{force} \times \text{distance, or } W = F \times d$$

If work is expressed per unit of time, the term *power* is used:

power = work / time, or P = W/t

Energy expenditure (EE) refers to energy expended (in **kilojoules [kJ]** or kilocalories [kcal]) per unit of time to produce power. During conversion of one form of energy into another, no energy is lost. This is usually referred to as the first law of thermodynamics, also known as the law of conservation of energy, which states that energy cannot be created or destroyed in an isolated system. For example, in carbohydrate and fat combustion, chemical energy is converted into mechanical energy (muscle contraction) and heat energy.

The human body is not efficient in its use of energy from the breakdown of carbohydrate and fat. During cycling exercise, for instance, only 20% of energy is converted to power. The remainder of the energy becomes heat. This heat is partly used to maintain body temperature at 37 °C (98.6 °F), but during exercise, heat production may be excessive. To prevent body temperature from rising too high, various heat-dissipating mechanisms must be activated (see chapter 9).

Energy is often expressed in **calories** (the imperial system) or **joules** (the metric system). One calorie expresses the quantity of energy (heat) needed to raise the temperature of 1 g (1 ml [0.03 fl oz.]) of water by 1 °C (1.8 °F). Thus, food containing 837 kJ (200 kcal) has enough energy potential to raise the temperature of 200 L (44 gal) of water by 1 °C. In everyday language, kilocalories are often referred to as Calories (written with a capital C). Because this may be a source of confusion, we will stick with kilojoules and kilocalories in this book.

The International System of Units (System Internationale, or SI) unit for energy is the joule, named for the British scientist Sir Prescott Joule (1818-1889). One joule of energy moves a mass of 1 g at a velocity of 1 m/s. A joule is not a large amount of energy; therefore, kilojoules are more often used. To convert calories to joules or kilocalories to kilojoules, the calorie value must be multiplied by 4.184.

When discussing energy expenditure or intake over 24 hours, megajoules (MJ) are often used to avoid large numbers. Because joules are not yet part of everyday language, both units (joules or calories) are often mentioned on food labels. When people talk about energy expended or energy content of food this is often expressed in kcal, but especially in the United States people refer to them as Calories. In this book kJ will be used, with the equivalent in kcal given in parentheses.

CONVERTING KILOCALORIES TO KILOJOULES

1 calorie (cal) = 4.184 J

1 kcal = 4.184 kJ

1 kcal = 1,000 cal =1 Cal

1 kJ = 1,000 J

1 MJ = 1,000 kJ

For example:

250 kcal = 250 × 4.184 = 1,047 kJ = 1.047 MJ

5,000 kJ = 5,000 / 4.184 = 1,194 kcal

Energetic Efficiency

The effective work performed after muscle contraction, or **efficiency**, is expressed as the percentage of total work. As already mentioned, approximately 20% of all energy produced in the human body is used to accomplish work (movement). Therefore, humans are approximately 20% efficient. Most of the remaining energy is used to maintain homeostasis and is wasted as heat. No system is 100% efficient. A gasoline engine is 20% to 30% efficient. A diesel engine is 30% to 40% efficient. An ordinary light bulb is about 20% efficient, and an energy-saving bulb is about 80% efficient. Humans are around 20% efficient, although this depends on the type of activity and how accustomed a person is to the activity. For example, a novice cyclist will not be as efficient as a well-trained and experienced cyclist; their efficiencies could be around 16% and 22%, respectively.

The precise definition of efficiency can vary. For example, **gross efficiency (GE)** is the ratio of the total work to energy expended:

GE (%) = work accomplished / energy expended × 100%

As exercise intensity increases, however, the relative proportion of the energy expended as resting metabolism decreases, which causes GE to increase with work rate. A solution for this problem is to subtract baseline energy expenditure from total energy expenditure. One way to calculate the baseline is to use **net efficiency (NE)**, where the baseline is the energy expended at rest:

NE (%) = work accomplished / (energy expended - resting energy expenditure) × 100%

The second way to calculate the baseline is to use **work efficiency (WE)**, where the baseline is the energy cost of unloaded (0 W or cycling without a chain) work (for example, unloaded cycling):

WE (%) = work accomplished / (energy expended - energy expended in unloaded condition) × 100%

Unfortunately, work efficiency is difficult or even impossible to determine reliably because of the unnatural nature of unloaded movements.

A fourth definition of efficiency is **delta efficiency (DE)**, which expresses the change in energy expended per minute relative to the change in actual work accomplished per minute:

DE (%) = delta work accomplished / delta energy expended × 100%

Delta efficiency may be the most accurate reflection of muscle efficiency, but it is more difficult to determine and is more variable. All four calculations of efficiency are commonly used in the literature, and all have their limitations.

The term **economy** is typically expressed as the oxygen uptake required to exercise at a certain intensity. For runners, it is the oxygen uptake at a speed of 16 km/h (10 mph). Efficient runners are usually better runners because they waste less energy. In other sports, such as cycling, the relationship between economy and performance does not seem to be as strong.

Measuring the Energy Content of Food

Food contains energy in the form of carbohydrate, fat, and protein, which all have energy stored within their chemical bonds. To determine the energy content of food, we use a technique called **direct calorimetry**. The food is combusted (oxidized), and the resulting heat is used as a measure of the energy content. The measurement takes place in a **bomb calorimeter** (see figure 4.1).

An accurately weighed amount of food (about 1 g) is placed in a sealed steel chamber that has high oxygen pressure. The reaction is started through ignition by an electrical current. The food burns inside the chamber and produces heat, which is transferred through the metal walls of the chamber and heats the water that surrounds it. The rise in water temperature directly reflects the energy content of the food. If the water volume surrounding the chamber is 2 L (0.5 gal) and the temperature rises by 4.0 °C (7.2 °F), the energy content of that food is 2 × 4 = 8 kcal (or 8 × 4.184 = 33.5 kJ). If the weight of the food combusted is 1.2 g, the energy content of the food is 8/1.2 = 6.7 kcal/g (27.9 kJ/g). This measure is the **gross energy value**, or total energy content, of the food, and no distinction is made between carbohydrate, fat, and protein. Although the bomb calorimeter is probably the most accurate method of determining the energy content of food, it is expensive to run, and the results tend to overestimate actual calories absorbed because not all the energy ingested can be digested or absorbed

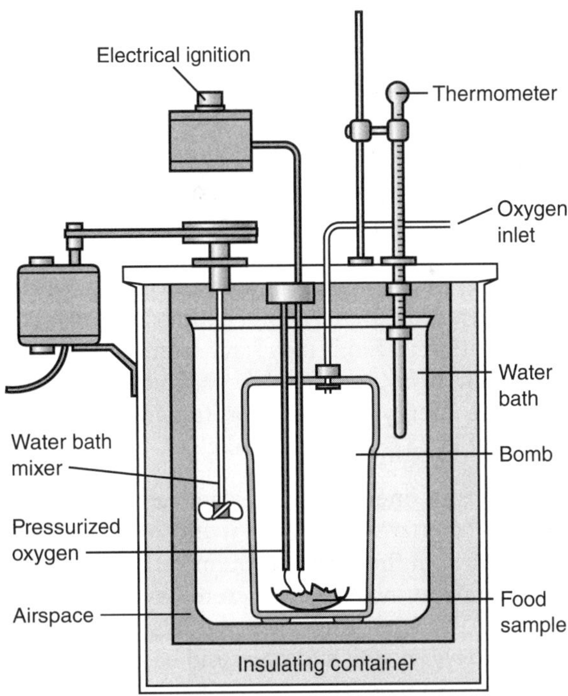

Figure 4.1 Bomb calorimeter.

Carbohydrate, fat, and protein can all provide energy but the amounts of energy they deliver are different.

- The energy content of carbohydrate depends on its type and on the arrangements of atoms within it. The combustion of glucose, for instance, gives 15.7 kJ/g (3.7 kcal/g), whereas the combustion of glycogen and starch is about 17.6 kJ/g (4.2 kcal/g). The latter figure is normally used as the energy value of carbohydrate (1 g carbohydrate = 17.6 kJ [4.2 kcal]).
- The energy content of fat also depends on the structure of the triacylglycerol or FA. A

medium-chain FA, such as octanoate (eight-carbon FA), may contain 36 kJ/g (8.6 kcal/g), whereas a long-chain FA may contain up to 40.2 kJ/g (9.6 kcal/g). The energy content of fat in the average diet is 39.3 kJ/g (9.4 kcal/g).

- The energy content of protein depends on the type of protein and the nitrogen content. Nitrogen does not provide energy; therefore, proteins with higher nitrogen densities contain less energy per gram. The nitrogen content in foods may vary from 15% (whole milk) to approximately 19% (nuts and seeds). The energy content of protein in the average diet is 23.7 kJ/g (5.7 kcal/g).

The gross energy value is not necessarily the amount of energy available if the food is eaten, particularly in the case of protein. In the body, the nitrogen in amino acids is excreted by the kidneys as urea. The urea molecule consists of nitrogen, carbon, oxygen, and hydrogen and has the formula $CO(NH_2)_2$. Some of the hydrogen atoms present in the amino acid are excreted along with nitrogen and thus cannot provide energy. About 20% of the potential energy of the amino acid will be lost. If a bomb calorimeter shows that protein contains 23.7 kJ/g (5.7 kcal/g), only 19.3 kJ/g (4.6 kcal/g) is available in the human body. This value is the net energy of food.

Sometimes food is not completely absorbed. Incomplete digestion and absorption will, of course, result in decreased availability of energy. Wilbur Olin Atwater (1844-1907), one of the pioneers in studying human energy balance (the total of energy expenditure and energy intake), determined this fact. After measuring many kinds of foods, Atwater came up with energy values for foods that accounted for differences in digestibility. Conveniently, these energy values were rounded to whole numbers. The energy contents of carbohydrate, fat, and protein were 16 kJ/g, 36 kJ/g, and 16 kJ/g (4 kcal/g, 9 kcal/g, and 4 kcal/g), respectively. These correction factors are often referred to as the **Atwater factors** or Atwater energy values.

The percentage of food energy that is absorbed is often expressed in a **coefficient of digestibility**. A coefficient of digestibility of 50 means that only half of the energy ingested is absorbed. Adding fiber to a meal generally reduces the coefficient of digestibility. Thus, a smaller amount of energy is available to the body from a food item that is high in fiber than from a food item that has identical energy but is low in fiber. Fiber causes the food to move faster through the gastrointestinal system, which leaves less time for absorption. On average, 97% of carbohydrate is completely digested and absorbed. For fat, this value is 95%, and for protein, it is 92% (see table 4.1).

The coefficient of digestibility of wheat bran protein is only 40%, and its calorie contribution is just 7.62 kJ/g (1.82 kcal/g), which is significantly less than the 16 kJ/g (4 kcal/g) estimated by Atwater. Furthermore, the coefficient of digestibility of wheat bran carbohydrate is 56%, and its calorie contribution is only 9.84 kJ/g (2.35 kcal/g), which is again far less than Atwater's estimate.

Atwater had begun to analyze the composition and energy content of food. Nowadays, many extensive databases exist; most of these have been compiled by government institutions. One of the largest and most comprehensible databases is the USDA National Nutrient Database. There is a section for USDA National Nutrient Database for Standard Reference and a USDA Branded Food Products Database (available at https://ndb.nal.usda.gov/ndb/). The United Kingdom, Australia, and other countries have their own databases that contain their own specific products. Some professional software programs combine all of these international databases to provide a very comprehensive collection of foods.

Many mobile apps can be used to record food intake and estimate intake of macronutrients and micronutrients. Often these apps use the same databases, but many apps allow users to enter their own foods and values and share these items. This means that not all values in these apps have been verified, and some nutrition information is inaccurate or incomplete. It is important to be aware of such limitations.

Measuring Energy Expenditure

The methods of measuring or estimating human energy expenditure range from direct but complex measurements of heat production (direct calorimetry) to relatively simple indirect metabolic measurements (**indirect calorimetry**) and from expensive stable isotope tracer methods (doubly labeled water) to relatively inexpensive and convenient rough estimates (heart rate monitoring and accelerometry). The following are some of the methods used to measure human energy expenditure:

- Direct calorimetry
- Indirect calorimetry
- Closed-circuit spirometry
- Open-circuit spirometry
- Douglas bag technique

TABLE 4.1 Energy Content of Nutrients and the Availability of Energy in the Body

	Energy of combustion per gram	Energy available per gram	Coefficient of digestibility
Protein			
Animal foods	23.7 kJ (5.7 kcal)	17.9 kJ (4.3 kcal)	97
Meat, fish, and poultry	23.7 kJ (5.7 kcal)	17.9 kJ (4.3 kcal)	97
Eggs	24.1 kJ (5.8 kcal)	18.3 kJ (4.4 kcal)	97
Dairy products	23.7 kJ (5.7 kcal)	17.9 kJ (4.3 kcal)	97
Plant foods	23.7 kJ (5.7 kcal)	15.7 kJ (3.7 kcal)	85
Cereals	24.3 kJ (5.8 kcal)	16.2 kJ (3.9 kcal)	85
Legumes	23.9 kJ (5.7 kcal)	14.5 kJ (3.5 kcal)	78
Vegetables	20.9 kJ (5.0 kcal)	13.0 kJ (3.1 kcal)	83
Fruits	21.8 kJ (5.2 kcal)	14.1 kJ (3.4 kcal)	83
Average protein	23.7 kJ (5.7 kcal)	17.0 kJ (4.0 kcal)	92
Fat			
Animal foods	39.3 kJ (9.4 kcal)	37.4 kJ (8.9 kcal)	95
Meat and eggs	39.8 kJ (9.5 kcal)	37.8 kJ (9.0 kcal)	95
Dairy products	38.7 kJ (9.3 kcal)	36.8 kJ (8.8 kcal)	95
Vegetable foods	38.9 kJ (9.3 kcal)	35.0 kJ (8.4 kcal)	90
Average fat	39.3 kJ (9.4 kcal)	37.4 kJ (8.9 kcal)	95
Carbohydrate			
Animal foods	16.3 kJ (3.9 kcal)	16.0 kJ (3.8 kcal)	98
Vegetable foods	17.4 kJ (4.2 kcal)	16.9 kJ (4.0 kcal)	97
Cereals	17.6 kJ (4.2 kcal)	17.2 kJ (4.1 kcal)	98
Legumes	17.6 kJ (4.2 kcal)	17.0 kJ (4.1 kcal)	97
Vegetables	17.6 kJ (4.2 kcal)	16.7 kJ (4.0 kcal)	95
Fruits	16.7 kJ (4.0 kcal)	15.1 kJ (3.6 kcal)	90
Sugars	16.5 kJ (3.9 kcal)	16.2 kJ (3.9 kcal)	98
Average carbohydrate	17.4 kJ (4.2 kcal)	16.9 kJ (4.0 kcal)	97

The coefficient of digestibility reflects the percentage of energy in a nutrient that is actually available.

Adapted from A.L. Merrill and B.K. Watt, 1973, "Energy Value of Foods: Basis and Derivation," revised, in *Agriculture Handbook 74*. U.S. Department of Agriculture.

- Breath-by-breath technique
- Portable spirometry
- Doubly labeled water
- Labeled bicarbonate
- Heart rate monitoring
- Accelerometry
- Observations, records of physical activity, activity diaries, recall

Direct Calorimetry

Ultimately, all biochemical processes in the body result in heat production. This heat production can be measured in a similar manner as the heat production from combusting food. A human calorimeter is a small, well-insulated chamber with adequate ventilation (see figure 4.2). The top of the chamber consists of a series of coils through which a known amount of water flows. The water absorbs the heat radiated by the subject in the chamber, which reflects the metabolic rate of that person.

The air is recirculated, and carbon dioxide and water are filtered out of the air before it reenters the chamber with added oxygen. This process prevents heat being lost from the chamber in the form of expired gases.

Although the direct calorimeter is based on a simple principle, the actual engineering and operation of the chamber are complicated. Specially

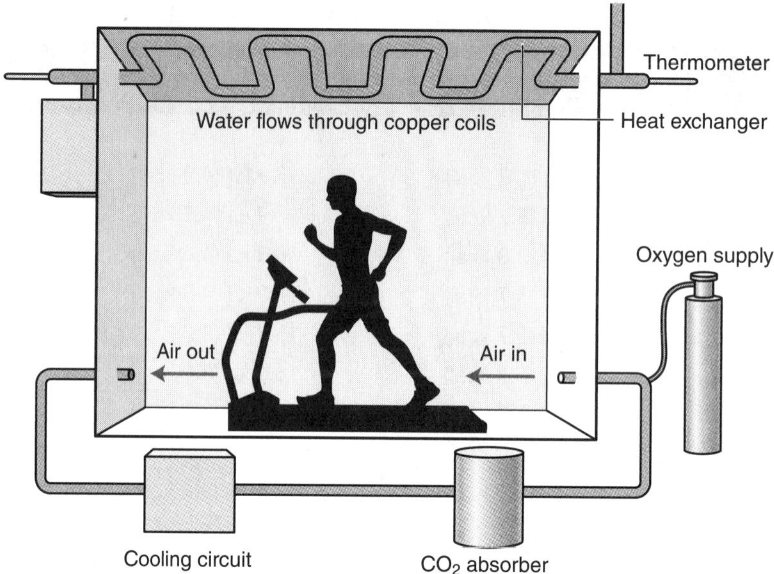

Figure 4.2 Direct calorimetry chamber.

trained personnel are required to operate the device; therefore, it is not the most popular and most common way to measure energy expenditure. An important disadvantage of the direct calorimeter is that it is unsuitable for field studies and assessment of energy expenditure in most exercise and sport situations.

Direct Calorimeter Suit

To overcome some of the practical problems of the direct calorimeter chamber, a direct calorimeter suit was developed. This suit consists of a long plastic tube through which a known amount of water flows. The tubing touches the skin and absorbs body heat. Again, the rise in water temperature is directly related to the subject's heat production and thus to the person's metabolic rate. With this suit, measurements can be conducted outside the chamber, but the suit may impair movement. The suit has been shown to be useful for walking exercise, but because it is heavy and not very flexible, it might impede more vigorous activities or faster movements. Nevertheless, the suit has been used successfully for those purposes as well.

Indirect Calorimetry

The energy for all biochemical reactions ultimately depends on the oxygen supply. The term *indirect* refers to the measurement of oxygen uptake and carbon dioxide production rather than to the measurement of heat transfer. This measurement requires a steady state carbon dioxide production and respiratory exchange ratio (RER = VCO_2/VO_2) and subjects with a normal acid-base balance. Studies with the bomb calorimeter have shown that the amount of oxygen required to combust carbohydrate, fat, and protein is directly related to the energy content. In fact, for every 1 kJ, 50 ml of oxygen are required, and for every kcal, 207 ml of oxygen are required. In other words, the energy equivalent of 1 L of oxygen is 20.2 kJ (4.8 kcal). This energy equivalent of oxygen is relatively stable and largely independent of the mixture of carbohydrate, fat, and protein oxidized. Indirect calorimetry is an accurate estimate of energy expenditure.

When $\dot{V}O_2$ is measured in liters of oxygen at STPD (standard temperature [0 °C or 32 °F], pressure [760 mm Hg], and dry) per minute, EE can be measured as follows:

$$EE\ (kJ/min) = 20.2 \times \dot{V}O_2$$

Energy expenditure can be estimated even more accurately if the respiratory exchange ratio is known because the energy equivalent for oxygen is 19.6 kJ/L (4.7 kcal/L) at an RER of 0.7 (when 100% fat is being oxidized) and rises to 20.9 kJ/L (4.9 kcal/L) at an RER of 1.0 (when carbohydrate is the only fuel being oxidized). For these calculations, the relatively small contribution of protein oxidation is ignored.

Closed-Circuit and Open-Circuit Spirometry

Oxygen uptake and carbon dioxide production can be measured using closed-circuit and open-circuit methods. The closed-circuit method is used to measure resting energy expenditure (see figure 4.3). The technique was developed in the late 1800s and is routinely used in clinical settings. The subject breathes through a mouthpiece into a spirometer that is prefilled with 100% oxygen. During each inspiration, some of the oxygen in the chamber of gas is consumed. Expired gas is passed back into the spirometer, and the carbon dioxide produced is trapped in a filter. The residual oxygen in the chamber is available for the next inspiration. As oxygen is consumed, the volume of oxygen in the spirometer decreases, and this change in volume is measured. The oxygen taken up and energy expenditure can then be calculated. Closed-circuit spirometry is a good method in resting conditions, but it is not suitable during exercise, especially high-intensity exercise. When carbon dioxide production is high, trapping the carbon dioxide may become problematic. The subject breathes through a three-way valve from and into a spirometer, which is prefilled with 100% oxygen. A recorder is connected so that the changes in volume are accurately measured.

With open-circuit spirometry (which is the most common method of estimating energy expenditure for research purposes), the subject inhales ambient air (0.03% carbon dioxide, 20.93% oxygen, and 79.04% nitrogen). Energy expenditure is calculated from the difference in oxygen and carbon dioxide content between the inspired and expired gases and the ventilation rate. Such measurements can be made in a respiration chamber by Douglas bags or online systems.

Respiration Chamber

The respiration chamber (see figure 4.4) was developed for measurement of a complete energy balance. It is comparable to the chamber used for direct calorimetry but without the coils to measure heat exchange and the insulation. Sufficient airflow into the respiration chamber prevents the chamber air from falling much below 20% oxygen, and the ventilation rate is carefully measured. Flow of air into the chamber is continuous. This flow is carefully monitored. In addition, the oxygen and carbon dioxide concentrations at the inlet and outlet of the chamber are recorded, from which oxygen uptake and carbon dioxide production can be calculated. Respiration chambers are usually designed like small hotel rooms with a bed, chair, television, radio, and telephone, and measurements can be performed over a period of several hours to several days.

The chamber is ideal for measurements of **energy balance** because food intake can be accurately controlled, and all food is prepared by the investigators and handed to the subject through

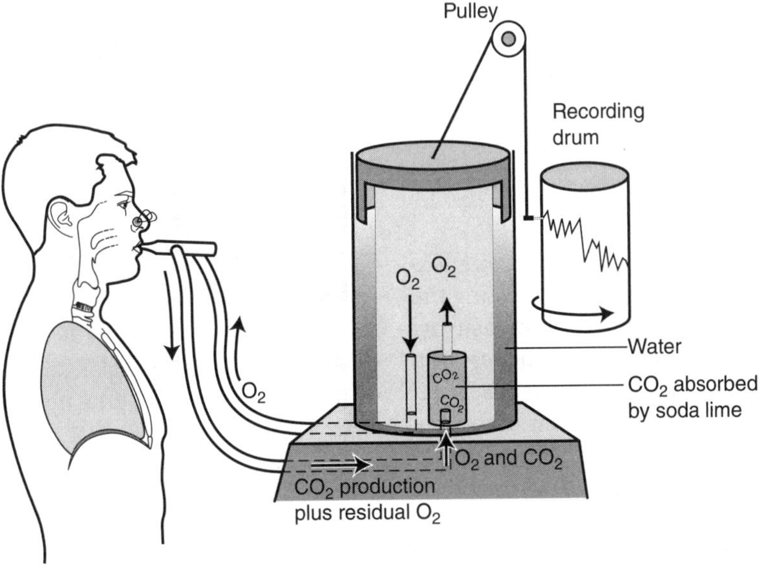

Figure 4.3 Closed-circuit spirometry.

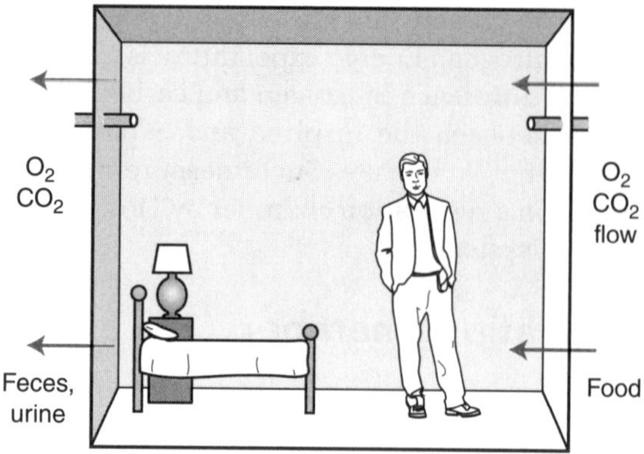

Figure 4.4 A respiration chamber.

special hatches. Urine and feces can also be collected for further analysis, which is often done when a complete energy and nitrogen balance is required.

The advantage of this technique is that, besides producing accurate information about gas exchange (and thus energy expenditure), it allows accurate control over energy intake and permits analysis of potential energy losses in feces and urine. The main disadvantages of this technique are that it requires highly trained personnel and is extremely expensive. In addition, the stay in the chamber interferes with everyday life because not all activities can be performed inside the chamber. Furthermore, most chambers are not adapted to high ventilation rates and are not suitable for vigorous exercise. Modern respiration chambers with fast-response analyzers are capable of measuring energy expenditure during very high-intensity exercise, and several studies have been performed of highly trained people performing vigorous exercise for prolonged periods.

Douglas Bag

A way to measure oxygen uptake and carbon dioxide production at the same time is by collecting the expired gases for a certain period and measuring the volume, oxygen concentration, and carbon dioxide concentration of this gas. The test subject inspires room air and expires through a mouthpiece connected to a high-flow, low-resistance valve into a large plastic bag. These Douglas bags are named after British scientist Claude Douglas (1882-1963), who was the first to use this method to measure gas exchange in humans (see figure 4.5).

After collection, the bags are closed until analysis. They are then emptied into a gas meter to measure the total volume. The ventilation rate is calculated from the duration of collection (usually 1 minute) and the volume measurement. A small sample of expired gas is collected from or in addition to the gas in the bag for analysis of oxygen and carbon dioxide concentrations. Oxygen uptake and

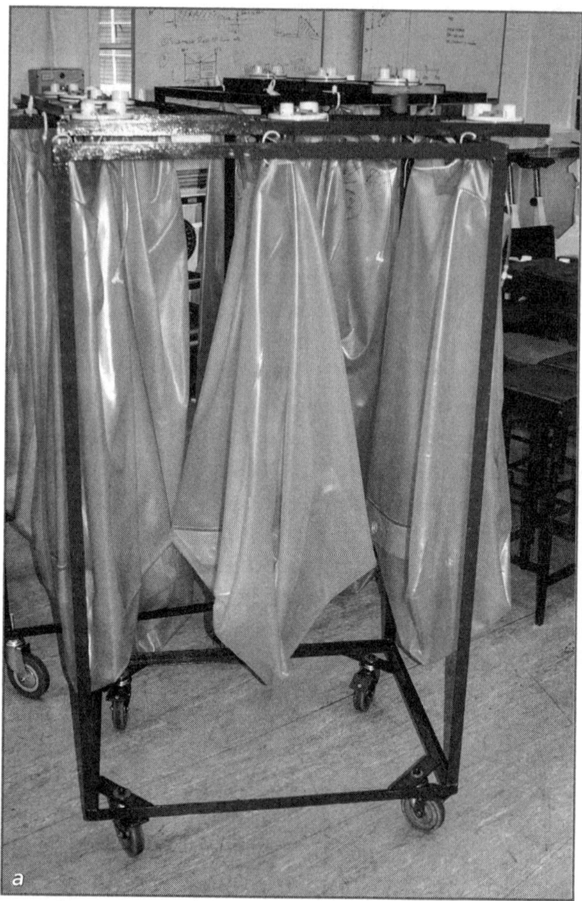

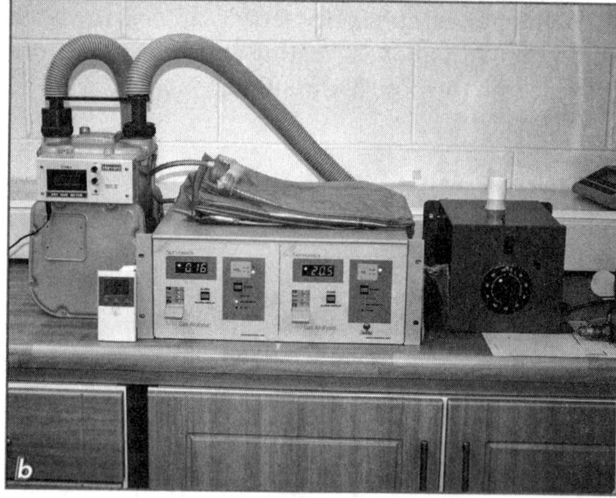

Figure 4.5 *(a)* Douglas bags and *(b)* dry gas meter (left) and oxygen and carbon dioxide analyzer (middle).

carbon dioxide production can be calculated from the difference between the inspired and expired oxygen and carbon dioxide concentrations and the ventilation rate. This relatively simple technique has been applied successfully for many years and is still used by exercise physiologists. Various versions of this technique are used, including methods in which flow is measured directly from the expired or inspired air.

Breath-by-Breath Systems

Respiratory physiologists have taken the Douglas bag technique one step further, and computers and fast-response oxygen and carbon dioxide analyzers have made it possible to develop an online breath-by-breath gas analysis system. This semiautomated or fully automated analyzer usually measures volume at the mouthpiece, and a small gas sample is collected at every expiration for analysis of oxygen and carbon dioxide concentrations (see figure 4.6). This technique enables respiratory physiologists to look at the time course of changes in various ventilatory variables. When averaged over periods of 20 seconds to several minutes, this technique gives similar values to those obtained with the Douglas bag technique. The main advantage of the breath-by-breath systems is that they can analyze every breath and are therefore able to register rapid changes and give instant feedback. Breath-by-breath systems are convenient, and most systems give an accurate estimation of energy expenditure.

The measurements are restricted to a laboratory situation, however, because the bulky, sensitive equipment is difficult to move. Recently, manufacturers have developed smaller and portable breath-by-breath systems for measurements in free-living conditions. These attempts have been reasonably successful, and in the future, smaller analyzers may replace some of the laboratory-based equipment.

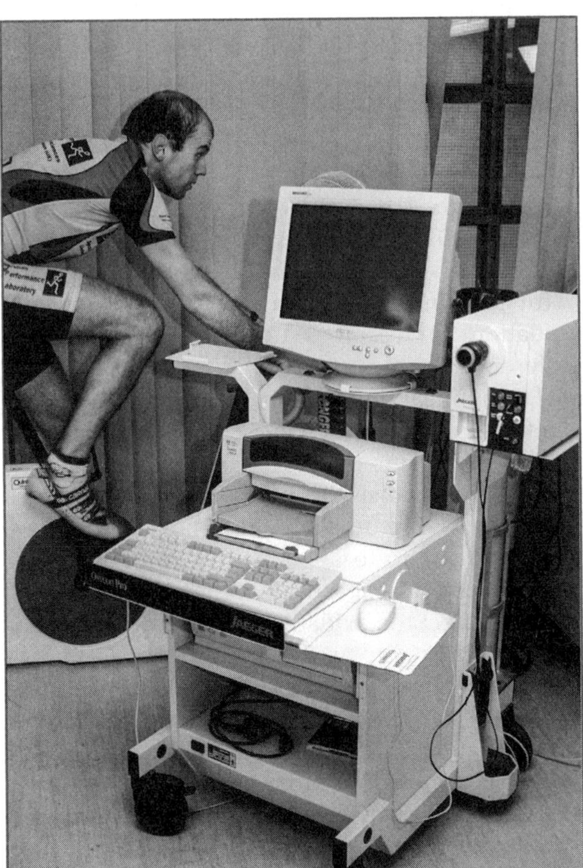

Figure 4.6 Automated breath-by-breath system.

Indirect Calorimetry and Substrate Use

Gas exchange measurements allow an estimation of the energy expenditure and the substrate mixture used. In the beginning of the 20th century, Krogh and Lindhard (1920) used the inherent differences in chemical properties of carbohydrate, fat, and protein to obtain information about fuel use. The complete oxidation of carbohydrate, fat, and protein requires different amounts of oxygen and produces different amounts of carbon dioxide. The oxidation of 1 g of glucose requires 0.746 L of oxygen and produces 0.743 L of carbon dioxide and 16 kJ (4 kcal). The oxidation of 1 g of FA (palmitic acid) requires 2.009 L of oxygen and produces 1.414 L of carbon dioxide and 40 kJ (10 kcal). The substrate used, therefore, determines the total oxygen required and the total carbon dioxide produced. The ratio of carbon dioxide production and oxygen consumption, or the respiratory quotient (RQ), provides a convenient indication of the substrate that is being used during steady-state exercise:

$$RQ = VCO_2/VO_2$$

The complete oxidation of 1 molecule of glucose (180 g) requires six molecules of oxygen and produces six molecules of carbon dioxide. The number of oxygen molecules equals the number of carbon dioxide molecules, and the RQ for carbohydrate is therefore 1:

$$C_6H_{12}O_6 + 6\ O_2 \rightarrow 6\ CO_2 + 6\ H_2O$$

$$RQ = 6\ CO_2 / 6\ O_2 = 1$$

Lipids contain significantly fewer oxygen atoms compared with carbohydrate and therefore require more oxygen in the oxidation process. Lipids can have different chemical compositions, unlike carbohydrates, for which the biochemical formula is always the same ($C_6H_{12}O_6$). The oxygen required and the carbon dioxide produced, therefore, depend somewhat on the type of lipid oxidized. Complete oxidation of 1 molecule of a typical FA (palmitic acid; 256 g) in the human body oxidizes to carbon dioxide and water using 23 molecules of oxygen. It produces 16 molecules of carbon dioxide and 16 molecules of water. The RQ of palmitic acid is therefore 0.696:

$$C_{16}H_{32}O_2 + 23\ O_2 \rightarrow 16\ CO_2 + 16\ H_2O$$

$$RQ = 16\ CO_2 / 23\ O_2 = 0.696$$

This RQ value may vary from 0.727 (octanoic acid, C8:0) to 0.686 (lignoceric acid, C24:0), depending on the chain length of the FA oxidized.

In addition to carbon, oxygen, and hydrogen, proteins (amino acids) also contain nitrogen and sometimes sulfur, which cannot be oxidized. Proteins have to be deaminated (removal of nitrogen), and nitrogen (as urea) and sulfur will be excreted in urine and feces. The remaining carbon skeleton can be oxidized to carbon dioxide and water in a similar manner to carbohydrate and fat. The oxygen required and the carbon dioxide produced depend somewhat on the type of protein. An example of the oxidation of a protein is the following:

$$\text{(albumin) } C_{72}H_{112}N_{18}O_{22}S + 77\ O_2 \rightarrow 63\ CO_2 + 38\ H_2O + SO_3 + 9\ CO(NH_2)_2 \text{ (urea)}$$

$$RQ = 63\ CO_2 / 77\ O_2 = 0.818$$

If a mixture of carbohydrate and fat is oxidized, oxygen consumption will equal the sum of oxygen required to oxidize the carbohydrate plus that required for fat. Similarly, carbon dioxide production will be the sum of carbon dioxide production from carbohydrate and carbon dioxide production from fat. If, for instance, 100 g of carbohydrate and 50 g of fat are oxidized, oxygen consumption is (100 × 0.746) + (50 × 2.009) = 175 L. Carbon dioxide production is (100 x 0.743) + (50 × 1.414) = 145 L. The RQ is 145 / 175 = 0.829.

When experiments are performed using indirect calorimetry and measures of $\dot{V}O_2$ and $\dot{V}CO_2$ are obtained, the reverse calculation is used:

$$\text{rate of carbohydrate oxidation (g/min)} \times O_2 \text{ (L/g)} + \text{rate of fat oxidation (g/min)} \times O_2 \text{ (L/g)} = \dot{V}O_2 \text{ (L/min)}$$

$$\text{rate of carbohydrate oxidation (g/min)} \times CO_2 \text{ (L/g)} + \text{rate of fat oxidation (g/min)} \times CO_2 \text{ (L/g)} = \dot{V}O_2 \text{ (L/min)}$$

Using different assumptions for the composition of fat substrate (chain length of the fatty acid) will result in different equations (see the Oxidation Rates sidebar). These calculations give two equations and two unknown variables that can be solved:

$$\text{carbohydrate oxidation (g/min)} = 4.585\ \dot{V}CO_2 - 3.226\ \dot{V}O_2$$

$$\text{fat oxidation (g/min)} = 1.695\ \dot{V}O_2 - 1.701\ \dot{V}CO_2$$

These calculations assume that protein is not an important energy fuel. In some extreme conditions, protein may contribute up to 15% to the total energy expenditure (see chapter 8). In this case, correction for protein oxidation should be made. To make this correction, urine samples are collected, and protein oxidation is estimated from the nitrogen content. One gram of nitrogen in urine represents the oxidation of 6.25 g of protein. This result is subtracted from the fat and carbohydrate oxidation rates (see the Oxidation Rates sidebar).

As mentioned previously, because the energy equivalent for oxygen is slightly different, depending on what substrate is used, measuring oxygen consumption and carbon dioxide production increases the accuracy of the estimate of energy expenditure. For instance, if $\dot{V}O_2$ is 600 L/day, $\dot{V}CO_2$ is 500 L/day, and nitrogen excretion is 25 g/day, energy expenditure is 12,068 kJ (2,884 kcal). With the simple formula (i.e., ignoring protein oxidation) the result is 12,120 kJ (2,897 kcal), a difference of only 0.2%.

The application of RQ is based on the premise that exchange of oxygen and carbon dioxide at the mouth represents the processes that occur in the tissues that oxidize the fuels. This assumption is valid at rest and during light to fairly high-intensity exercise (up to about 80%-85% of $\dot{V}O_2$max). But because RQ measured at the mouth does not always reflect the oxidation processes in cells, it is usually referred to as RER. For moderate to high exercise intensities where glycogen is an important fuel source (50%-75% $\dot{V}O_2$max) the equations in the Oxidation Rates sidebar should be used.

One common condition in which RER is different from RQ is hyperventilation. During hyperventilation, excess amounts of carbon dioxide are expired. This carbon dioxide is not derived from metabolic processes but is simply an extra excretion of body carbon dioxide stores. (Carbon dioxide is mainly stored in the form of bicarbonate in the extracellular body fluids.) Because little change occurs in $\dot{V}O_2$ during hyperventilation, the RER increases, usually above 1, and clearly no longer reflects metabolism in the cells.

Another situation in which RER differs from RQ is during strenuous exercise at intensities above 80% to 85% of $\dot{V}O_2$max. At these high exercise intensities, high glycolytic rates in the muscle result in the production and accumulation of lactic acid. The hydrogen ions associated with this acid must be buffered. The body's bicarbonate buffer system neutralizes the acidity. Hydrogen ions bind with bicarbonate ions (HCO_3^-) to form carbonic acid and subsequently water and carbon dioxide:

$$H^+ + HCO^-_3 \leftrightarrow H_2CO_3 \leftrightarrow H_2O + CO_2$$

This carbon dioxide is expired, and as a result, the RER increases rapidly and can reach values between 1 and 1.30. This increase does not reflect the metabolism in the cell; therefore, calculation of energy expenditure or substrate use based on RER and $\dot{V}O_2$ is only valid during steady-state exercise, when no accumulation of lactic acid occurs. Situations in which lipogenesis (the synthesis of fat from carbohydrate) and ketogenesis (the formation of ketone bodies) play a role are further examples of conditions in which RER may differ from RQ.

In summary, indirect calorimetry can be a very accurate and relatively easy way to measure energy expenditure. However, several assumptions have to be made, and if these assumptions are violated, the calculations of carbohydrate and fat oxidation and of energy expenditure become meaningless. One of the assumptions that is often made is that the contribution of protein is negligible. This is related to the most important assumption that all carbon dioxide produced and measured in expired gases and all oxygen extracted are used for oxidative purposes. This is not always the case. In conditions of hyperventilation and high-intensity exercise (above the lactate turning point), indirect calorimetry cannot be used to accurately measure energy expenditure or substrate use. Similarly, when rates of ketogenesis or gluconeogenesis (the new formation of glucose in the liver and kidneys) are high, figures for energy expenditure and substrate use may be distorted.

Doubly Labeled Water

The doubly labeled water technique is based on the administration of a bolus dose of two stable isotopes of water: ^2H_2O and $H_2{}^{18}O$. (For an explanation of stable isotopes, see appendix A.) These two isotopes are used as tracers, and the slightly heavier atoms ^2H and ^{18}O can be measured in various body fluids (e.g., urine). ^2H is lost from the body in water alone, and ^{18}O is lost in water and as $C^{18}O_2$ in breath. The difference between the two tracer excretion rates, therefore, represents the carbon dioxide production rate (see figure 4.7). Energy expenditure can be calculated based on the fuel mixture oxidized.

The main advantage of this technique is that it does not interfere with everyday life, and unbiased measurements of a free-living situation can be obtained. In addition, measurements can be conducted over prolonged periods, so the values can be used to estimate typical daily energy expenditure and the energy needs of a free-living person. The main disadvantages of the technique are the expense, the limited availability of the tracer, and the need for sophisticated equipment (mass spectrometer) to measure the isotopes. This method is only suitable for relatively long-term (days or weeks) estimation of energy expenditure.

OXIDATION RATES

Carbohydrate oxidation (g/min) = $4.21 \times \dot{V}CO_2 - 2.96 \times \dot{V}O_2 - 2.37 \times N$

Fat oxidation (g/min) = $1.70 \times \dot{V}O_2 - 1.70 \times \dot{V}CO_2 - 1.77 \times N$

Protein oxidation (g) = $6.25 \times N$

Energy expenditure (kJ) = $16.18 \times \dot{V}O_2 + 5.02 \times \dot{V}CO_2 - 5.99 \times N$

Energy expenditure (kcal) = $0.55 \times \dot{V}CO_2 - 4.47 \times \dot{V}O_2 - 1.43 \times N$

N is the urinary nitrogen in grams. If it is assumed that protein oxidation is negligible, then *N* should be substituted by 0.

These equations were obtained from Jeukendrup and Wallis (2005).

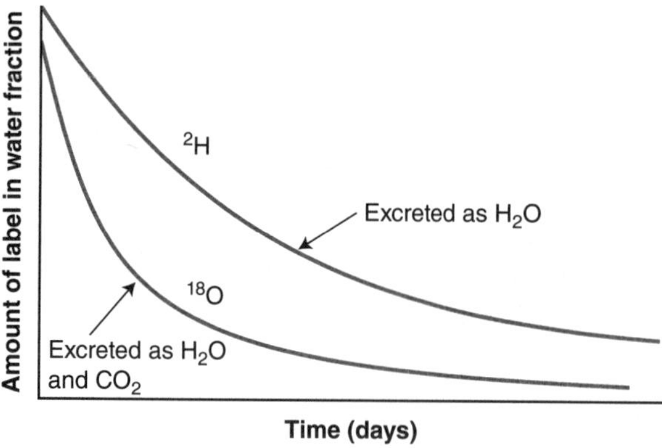

Figure 4.7 Doubly labeled water technique. Excretion of ^{2}H and ^{18}O occurs at different rates. The more rapid the drop in ^{18}O relative to the drop in ^{2}H, the higher the energy expenditure is.

Labeled Bicarbonate

Another method based on stable isotopes is the infusion of labeled bicarbonate (^{14}C or ^{13}C). When $H^{13}CO_3$ or $H^{14}CO_3$ (the latter is radioactive) is infused at a constant rate, it eventually reaches equilibrium with the body's carbon dioxide pool, after which any change in the body's carbon dioxide production will result in a change in the percentage of labeled carbon dioxide. The change in this enrichment is, therefore, a direct indication of total carbon dioxide production. This value can be used to calculate energy expenditure in a similar manner to the doubly labeled water technique. Samples are collected from expired gases, and tiny portions are needed for the analysis. Because $H^{13}CO_3$ has to be infused, this technique can be applied only for short periods (hours and, under some conditions, days). The bicarbonate labeling technique is relatively inexpensive but still requires sophisticated equipment and expertise.

Heart Rate Monitoring

To avoid some of the problems associated with the measurement of energy expenditure during free-living physical activity, various less complicated (and less accurate) methods have been developed. One of these methods is based on heart rate (HR) because of its linear relationship with oxygen uptake at submaximal exercise intensities. At very low and very high exercise intensities (supramaximal), this estimation is less reliable. To use HR for the estimation of energy expenditure, the relationship between HR and $\dot{V}O_2$ (and EE) must be determined. Measurements of oxygen uptake can then be used to calculate energy expenditure at several different HRs. The main limitation of the use of HR for measuring energy expenditure is the almost flat slope of the relationship at low levels of energy expenditure. At rest, slight movements can increase HR, but energy expenditure (i.e., oxygen consumption) remains almost the same. Emotions (e.g., anger or anxiety) may also cause HR to rise at rest with little or no change in oxygen uptake.

Although the HR method provides satisfactory estimates of average EE for a group, it is not necessarily accurate for individual subjects. For instance, Spurr et al. (1988) compared 24 hours of EE by calorimetry with EE by the HR method in 22 subjects. The maximum deviations of the values of EE between the two methods varied between +20% and −15% in individuals, but when the methods were compared statistically, no differences were found.

In addition, several factors influence the HR–$\dot{V}O_2$ relationship, including environmental conditions (temperature and humidity), altitude, body position, static (isometric) exercise, anxiety (at low work rates), and so on. Nevertheless, in some conditions, HR can provide a convenient and relatively inexpensive estimate of energy expenditure.

Accelerometer

Another way of estimating activity level is through accelerometry. Accelerometers are small devices that can be attached to the body and register all accelerations that the body makes. The number and the degree of the accelerations give an indication of activity level. Accelerometers can record accelerations along one, two, or three axes. A single-axis, or single-plane, accelerometer measures acceleration only in the vertical direction. Triaxial accelerometers measure accelerations along three axes and are likely to be more accurate. Generally, accelerometer readings (usually expressed as activity counts or in kJ [kcal]) correlate well with energy expenditure.

Simple, inexpensive pedometers that record steps taken and distance covered while walking are widely available. They usually require the owner to input normal stride length, which can be determined by measuring the distance covered when walking a given number of strides. The device can then reasonably estimate the distance covered over a long walk (e.g., 6 mi [10 km]). The distance covered on the walk can be even more accurately determined if the device includes a global positioning system (GPS) function. There is a relatively simple relationship between the distance covered (either walking or running) and the amount of energy expended. A person expends 4.184 kJ (1 kcal) per kilometer covered per kilogram of body mass, so the following equation can be used to estimate the energy expended while completing any known distance on foot.

$$\text{amount of energy expended (kcal)} = \text{distance covered (km)} \times \text{body mass (kg)}$$

or

$$\text{amount of energy expended (kJ)} = \text{distance covered (km)} \times \text{body mass (kg)} \times 4.184$$

Thus, a person who weighs 70 kg would expend 2.93 MJ (700 kcal) if he or she covered a distance of 10 km on relatively flat terrain. The amount of energy expended would be 10% to 20% higher if the person walked mostly uphill. It is the distance covered, not the pace at which it is covered, that determines the amount of energy expended. For a 70 kg (154 lb) runner, the amount of energy expended when completing a marathon race (42.2 km [26.2 mi]) is 42.2 × 70 kcal, which is 2,954 kcal or 12.4 MJ.

In the future, combined HR and accelerometer data may be used to estimate energy expenditure. Initial studies show promising results for simultaneous HR and motion measurements. Given the low weight and compactness of modern accelerometers, they offer a convenient and easy method of estimating activity level in a free-living situation.

The market for monitoring physical activity, sleep, and other behaviors has exploded in the last few years. Many consumer-wearable devices are on the market, and they have become highly popular. People use these devices and even smartphones to quantify physical activity and estimate energy expenditure. Often, these devices are referred to as fitness trackers or activity trackers. A national U.S. survey completed in 2012 indicated that 69% of adults tracked at least one health indicator for themselves, a family member, or a friend using a tracking device (Pew 2013). In this survey, 60% of adults reported tracking weight, diet, and exercise and were clearly interested in energy balance. The wearable device industry is booming and these figures will only continue to rise.

These activity monitors have also been used in various research studies. However, surprisingly little information is available about their accuracy. Many manufacturers claim the devices are highly accurate if they are worn and used as recommended. A systematic review of all available literature concluded that although the validity for steps counted was good, there was low validity for energy expenditure and sleep. There was high interdevice reliability for steps, distance, energy expenditure, and sleep for certain Fitbit models (Evenson, Goto, and Furberg 2015). So within the same device, measurements are reproducible, but this does not always mean they are also accurate (they can consistently under- or overestimate the true number of steps). Studies have shown that numbers of steps counted can be off by 9% to 36.3% (Clemes et al. 2010). Steps, however, seem to be more accurate and valid than the calculations of distance or energy expended. Device performance varies considerably, and each device has its own shortcomings. For example, the device that measured steps most accurately failed to detect standing posture and usually misclassified it as sitting. It is also clear that certain activities, such as cycling on a stationary bike, cannot be accurately picked up with these monitors.

Location of the monitor is critical; imagine brushing your teeth with a wearable monitor around your wrist. Figure 4.8 shows where these

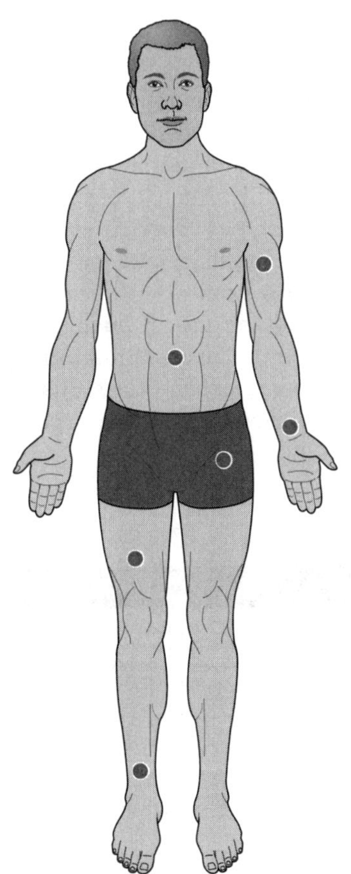

Figure 4.8 Locations where fitness or activity trackers can be worn on the body.

devices are typically worn on the body. The best placement for the devices (in terms of accuracy) has not been determined. Research tends to favor the accuracy of hip placement (Diaz et al. 2015; Storm, Heller, and Mazzà 2015), but consumers seem to prefer the wrist-worn monitors.

In summary, the research supports the usefulness of activity trackers for measuring steps, but other metrics, such as energy expenditure, may not be as accurate (Ferguson et al. 2015; Sasaki et al. 2014; Stackpool et al. 2014). There is also some uncertainty about device accuracy at different speeds, especially slow walking speeds. There are also inconsistencies in estimates of physical activity and sleep over 24 hours, which suggests that improvements are still needed (Rosenberger et al. 2016). Although the devices are affordable and very easy to use, there are many limitations, and they may not give accurate estimates of energy expenditure. In addition, more work is needed on the validation of the various devices.

Activity Records

Activity records, physical activity diaries, or physical activity recall instruments (questionnaires) are used to record activities during a 24-hour period. A rough estimation of the daily energy expenditure is obtained from this recorded information. Most of the existing questionnaires estimate the energy expenditure of only some types of activities by asking about the types of activities performed and the level or the intensity put forth or use tables similar to tables 4.2 and 4.3. They may not always be accurate and the use of such questionnaires often results in an overestimation of physical activity and energy expenditure (Busschaert et al. 2015). Nevertheless, for some purposes, average physical activity scores over a long-term period can be estimated satisfactorily using self-administered questionnaires.

Components of Energy Expenditure

Energy is needed for various processes in the body, including basal functions, digestion, absorption metabolism, and storage of food. In addition, active people expend energy during exercise. The three components of energy expenditure—resting metabolic rate, diet-induced thermogenesis, and exercise-related energy expenditure—are discussed in this section.

Resting Metabolic Rate

The largest component (60%-75%) of daily energy expenditure (average daily metabolic rate [ADMR]) in a relatively inactive person is the **resting metabolic rate (RMR)**, also referred to as resting energy expenditure (REE), which is the energy required for the maintenance of normal body functions and homeostasis in resting conditions. Factors such as sympathetic nervous system activity, thyroid hormone activity, and sodium–potassium pump activity contribute to RMR. Another measure is the **basal metabolic rate (BMR)**. This test was developed for patients with thyroid disease to measure the lowest oxygen uptake in resting thermoneutral conditions. Measurements were performed in the morning after a 12- to 18-hour fast. This measurement was inconvenient for many patients, and metabolism was affected because patients were disturbed in their sleep to obtain the measurements. Therefore, RMR has

TABLE 4.2 Energy Cost of Various Activities

Activity	kJ/min	kcal/min	Examples
Resting	4	1	Sleeping, reclining while watching TV
Very light activities	12-20	3-5	Sitting and standing activities, driving, cooking, card playing, typing
Light activities	20-28	5-7	Walking (3-5 km/h [2-3 mph]), baseball, bowling, horseback riding, golf
Moderate activities	28-36	7-9	Jogging, basketball, badminton, soccer, tennis, volleyball, walking (7-8 km/h [4-5 mph])
Strenuous activities	36-52	9-13	Running (10-13 km/h [6-8 mph]), cross-country skiing (8-10 km/h [5-6 mph])
Very strenuous activities	>52	>13	Cycling (35 km/h [22 mph]), running (faster than 14 km/h [9 mph], cross-country skiing (faster than 12 km/h [7.5 mph])

TABLE 4.3 Estimated Energy Cost of Activities in Kilojoules per Minute (Kilocalories per Minute)

	BODY WEIGHT				
Activity	**50 kg (110 lb)**	**60 kg (132 lb)**	**70 kg (154 lb)**	**80 kg (176 lb)**	**90 kg (198 lb)**
Aerobics					
Beginner	22 (5.5)	26 (6.5)	30 (7.5)	34 (8.5)	39 (9.8)
Advanced	28 (7.0)	33 (8.3)	40 (10.0)	45 (11.3)	51 (12.8)
Badminton	20 (5.0)	24 (8.0)	28 (7.0)	33 (8.3)	37 (9.3)
Ballroom dancing	11 (2.8)	13 (3.3)	15 (3.8)	17 (4.3)	19 (4.8)
Basketball	29 (7.2)	35 (8.8)	40 (10.0)	46 (11.5)	52 (13.0)
Boxing	46 (11.5)	56 (14.0)	65 (16.3)	74 (18.5)	84 (21.0)
Sparring in ring	29 (7.2)	35 (8.8)	40 (10.0)	46 (11.5)	52 (13.0)
Canoeing					
Leisure	9 (2.3)	11 (2.8)	13 (3.3)	15 (3.8)	17 (4.3)
Racing	22 (5.5)	26 (6.5)	30 (7.5)	34 (8.5)	39 (9.8)
Circuit training	22 (5.5)	26 (6.5)	30 (7.5)	34 (8.5)	40 (10.0)
Cricket					
Batting	17 (4.3)	21 (5.3)	24 (6.0)	28 (7.0)	32 (8.0)
Bowling	19 (4.8)	22 (5.5)	26 (6.5)	30 (7.5)	34 (8.5)
Cycling					
9 km/h (5.5 mph)	13 (3.3)	16 (4.0)	18 (4.5)	21 (5.3)	24 (6.0)
15 km/h (9 mph)	21 (5.3)	24 (8.0)	28 (7.0)	33 (8.3)	38 (9.5)
Racing	35 (8.8)	42 (10.5)	49 (12.3)	56 (14.0)	63 (5.8)
Football	28 (7.0)	33 (8.3)	39 (9.8)	44 (11.0)	50 (12.5)
Golf	18 (4.5)	21 (5.5)	25 (6.3)	28 (7.0)	32 (8.0)
Gymnastics	14 (3.5)	16 (4.0)	19 (4.8)	22 (5.5)	25 (6.3)
Hockey	18 (4.5)	20 (5.0)	24 (6.0)	29 (7.3)	33 (8.3)
Judo	41 (10.3)	49 (12.3)	57 (14.3)	65 (16.3)	73 (18.3)
Running					
5.5 min/km (8:51 min/mi)	40 (10.0)	49 (12.3)	57 (14.3)	65 (16.3)	73 (18.3)
5 min/km (8 min/mi)	44 (11.0)	52 (13.0)	61 (15.3)	70 (17.5)	78 (19.5)
4.5 min/km (7:14 min/mi)	48 (12.0)	55 (13.8)	65 (16.3)	75 (18.8)	85 (21.3)
4 min/km (6:26 min/mi)	54 (13.5)	65 (16.3)	76 (19.0)	87 (21.8)	98 (24.5)
Skiing					
Cross-country	35 (8.8)	42 (10.5)	49 (12.3)	56 (14.0)	63 (15.8)
Downhill (easy)	18 (4.5)	21 (5.5)	25 (6.3)	29 (7.3)	33 (8.3)
Downhill (hard)	29 (7.3)	35 (8.8)	40 (10.0)	49 (12.3)	55 (13.8)
Squash	44 (11.0)	53 (13.3)	62 (15.5)	71 (17.8)	79 (19.8)
Swimming					
Freestyle	33 (8.3)	40 (10.0)	46 (11.5)	52 (13.0)	59 (14.8)
Backstroke	36 (9.0)	43 (10.8)	49 (12.3)	56 (14.0)	63 (15.8)
Breaststroke	34 (8.5)	41 (10.3)	47 (11.8)	54 (13.5)	61 (15.3)
Table tennis	14 (3.5)	17 (4.3)	19 (4.8)	23 (5.8)	26 (6.5)
Tennis					
Social	15 (3.8)	17 (4.3)	20 (5.0)	23 (5.8)	26 (6.5)
Competitive	37 (9.3)	44 (11.0)	50 (12.5)	58 (14.5)	65 (16.3)
Volleyball	10 (2.5)	12 (3.0)	15 (3.6)	17 (4.3)	19 (4.8)
Walking					
10 min/km (16 min/mi)	21 (5.3)	26 (6.5)	30 (7.5)	35 (8.8)	39 (9.8)
8 min/km (13 min/mi)	25 (6.3)	30 (7.5)	35 (8.8)	40 (10.0)	45 (11.3)
5 min/km (8 min/mi)	44 (11.0)	52 (13.0)	61 (15.3)	70 (17.5)	78 (19.5)

All figures are approximate values.

Adapted from van Erp-Baart et al. (1989a).

ENERGY EXPENDITURE COMMON ABBREVIATIONS

ADMR = average daily metabolic rate

BMR = basal metabolic rate

RMR = resting metabolic rate

REE = resting energy expenditure

TEF = thermic effect of food

DIT = diet-induced thermogenesis

TEE = thermic effect of exercise

EEA = energy expenditure for physical activity

become the more popular measure and BMR is rarely measured. The RMR is primarily related to fat-free mass (muscle mass) and is influenced by age, gender, body composition, and genetic factors.

Different body tissues have markedly different resting energy requirements. Organs that have large metabolic demands, such as the liver, gut, brain, kidney, and heart, have the highest energy requirements per gram of tissue. In a lean adult, these organs account for approximately 75% of resting energy expenditure, although they constitute only 10% of total body weight. In contrast, resting skeletal muscle consumes only 20% of resting metabolic rate but represents approximately 40% of total body weight. Adipose tissue consumes less than 5% of resting metabolic rate but usually accounts for approximately 20% of body weight. Resting energy expenditure (REE) correlates closely with **fat-free mass (FFM)**. Although energy expenditure of metabolically active organs is responsible for a large component of REE, fat-free mass, which is composed primarily of skeletal muscle, accounts for most of the variability in energy expenditure between individuals.

RMR seems to decrease with age (2%-3% per decade), and men generally have a higher RMR than women because of their larger body size. See the sidebar for the most common abbreviations used in relation to energy expenditure.

Diet-Induced Thermogenesis

Diet-induced thermogenesis (DIT), or the thermic effect of food (TEF), is the increase in energy expenditure above RMR that occurs for several hours after ingestion of a meal. DIT is the result of digestion, absorption, metabolization, and storage of food and normally represents about 10% of total daily energy expenditure. The magnitude of DIT depends on several factors, including the energy content of the food and the size and composition of the meal. DIT also depends on the metabolic fate of the ingested substrate. The cost of storing fat in adipose tissue is approximately 3% of the energy of the ingested meal, whereas if carbohydrate is stored as glycogen, about 7% of the energy is lost. The energy cost for the synthesis and breakdown of protein is approximately 24% of the available energy. Energy expenditure can be increased up to 8 hours. The sympathetic nervous system seems to play an important role in DIT. When the effects of the sympathetic nervous system are reduced by administering a ß-adrenergic blocker (e.g., propranolol), DIT is also reduced. With increasing age there is a small decline in DIT. This might be associated with a decrease in insulin sensitivity.

Thermic Effect of Exercise

The **thermic effect of exercise (TEE)**, or energy expenditure for activity (EEA), is by far the most variable component of daily energy expenditure. It includes all energy expended above the RER and DIT. The TEE often has a voluntary component (exercise) and an involuntary component (shivering, fidgeting, or postural control). In highly trained, extremely active people, the TEE can be as much as 32 MJ/day (7,648 kcal/day). In sedentary people, the TEE may be as low as 400 kJ/day (96 kcal/day). Figure 4.9 compares the various compo-

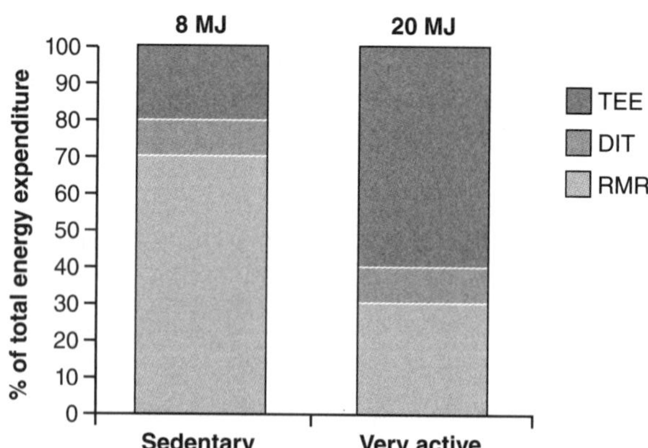

Figure 4.9 Energy expenditure and the relative contribution of its various components in a sedentary person (energy expenditure 8 MJ/day[1,912 kcal/day]) and in an athlete involved in heavy training (energy expenditure 20 MJ/day [4,780 kcal/day]).

Based on Saris et al. (1989).

nents of daily energy expenditure in a sedentary person and in an endurance athlete involved in heavy training. TEE can vary from an average of 30% of the daily energy expenditure up to 80% in extreme conditions during heavy endurance training or competition. Exercise is extremely important for the maintenance of the daily energy balance. It is not only the most variable component of 24-hour energy expenditure but also the component that can be controlled voluntarily.

Energy Balance

Energy balance refers to the balance between energy expenditure and energy intake. It can be measured on a day-to-day basis, but it probably makes more sense to measure it over a period of several days or weeks. When energy intake exceeds energy expenditure, the energy balance is positive and weight gain will occur. When energy intake is below energy expenditure, the energy balance is negative and weight loss will result. Generally, athletes are good at maintaining body weight and thus are in energy balance most of the time. Over the long term, energy balance is maintained in weight-stable individuals even though this balance may be either positive or negative on a day-to-day basis. People who want to lose weight should increase energy expenditure relative to energy intake.

In many activities in which body composition or body weight is believed to be important (gymnastics, dancing, bodybuilding, and weight category sports such as judo and boxing), participants often try to maintain a negative energy balance to lose weight. Thus, the energy intakes in these activities can be very low. At the other extreme are endurance sports such as triathlon, cycling, cross-country skiing, and ultra-endurance running, which require extremely high energy expenditures and energy intakes. In these sports, maintaining energy balance on a day-to-day basis is crucial for performance. The upper and the lower limits of energy expenditure are discussed in the following sections.

Figure 4.10 depicts the average daily energy intakes of hundreds of male and female athletes in various sports. The data show that women generally have lower energy intakes than men. Mean energy intake varied from 12.2-24.6 MJ (2,905-5,869 kcal) per day for male and 6.2-13.0 MJ (1,472-3,101 kcal) per day for female athletes. These differences may be related to body size and weight, body composition, and the number of hours spent training daily. Athletes in team sports have moderate energy intakes, whereas some endurance athletes have extremely high energy intakes.

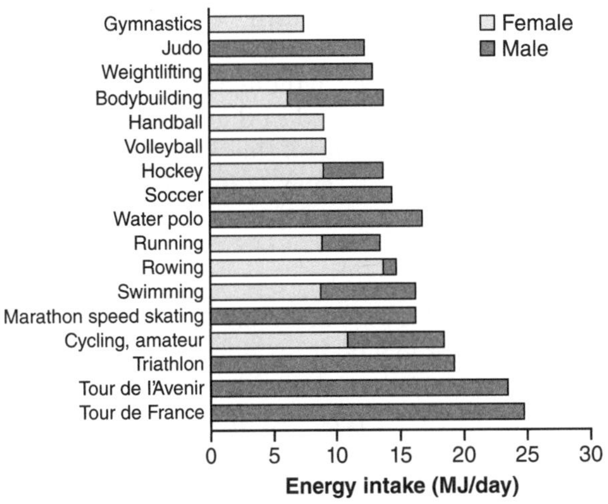

Figure 4.10 Energy intakes for female and male elite Dutch athletes in various sports.

Data from van Erp-Baart et al. (1989a).

Energy Cost of Different Activities

Some physical activities obviously require higher energy outputs than others, as shown in tables 4.2 and 4.3. But even within the same activity there can be substantial differences in energy expenditure depending the level at which it is performed. Tennis, for example, has relatively low energy expenditure if played recreationally. At this level of play, it could be classified as a light to moderate activity. Although during a game the exercise can sometimes be extremely intense and require high rates of energy expenditure in short bursts because a longer period of low-intensity activity (walking or standing) typically follows the high-intensity activity, the average energy expenditure is relatively low. Tennis played at a high level has shorter periods of rest, and the average intensity is much higher. Continuous sports such as cycling and running, which usually include little or no recovery during the activity, will generally have the highest energy expenditures.

Lower Limits of Energy Expenditure

Female gymnasts, ballet dancers, and ice dancers often have energy intakes as low as 4.2 to 8.4 MJ (1,000-2,000 kcal). In some cases, this intake is only 1.2 to 1.4 times the RMR, which is lower than sedentary people who, on average, expend 1.4 to 1.6 times the RMR, even though these athletes and dancers may be involved in 3 to 4 hours of training a day. Although not all the time gymnasts and dancers spend in the gym or in the dance studio is high-intensity training, the metabolic rate is still expected to be higher than that of the average sedentary person.

The food records of members of this group, who are striving for low body weight, may not be accurate and may underestimate true energy intakes. But even when the reported intakes are corrected for this underestimation, they are still very low. The lower limits of energy expenditure are determined by the sum of RMR, DIT, and a minimum of physical activity. DIT is directly affected by the amount of food consumed. Reducing food intake results in decreased DIT, and it may also indirectly influence the RMR. One of the problems associated with reducing energy intake to very low levels is the possibility of marginal nutrition, particularly of essential nutrients such as fat-soluble vitamins, calcium, iron, and essential FAs (see chapters 1 and 10).

Another term that is often used in this context is **energy availability** (Loucks, Kiens, and Wright 2011). Energy availability refers to dietary energy intake minus exercise energy expenditure. Energy availability is thus the amount of dietary energy available for other body functions after exercise training. When energy availability is too low, physiological mechanisms reduce the amount of energy used for cellular maintenance, thermoregulation, growth, bone development, and reproduction. Although the compensatory mechanisms tend to restore energy balance and promote survival, health may be compromised. Energy availability will be discussed in more detail in chapter 16.

Upper Limits of Energy Expenditure

Energy-related problems in endurance sports are totally different from the problems discussed in the previous section. Well-trained endurance athletes can expend more than 4.2 MJ/h (1,000 kcal/h) for prolonged periods, which results in extremely high daily energy expenditures. To maintain performance, energy stores must be replenished and energy balance must be restored, which means that these athletes must eat large amounts in periods of heavy training or competition.

Scientists have studied whether an upper limit to human energy expenditure exists. The highest values reported are from sports such as cycling, triathlon, cross-country skiing, and ultra-endurance running.

The Tour de France is a 3-week, 20-stage cycling event in which cyclists cover approximately 3,500 km (2,175 mi), including various mountain stages. On some days, the cyclists spend up to 8 hours on their bicycles. Average daily energy expenditure in the Tour de France reached values of 24 MJ (5,736 kcal) when measured in weekly intervals. The highest recorded average energy intake during the entire 3 weeks of the Tour de France was 36 MJ/day (8,604 kcal/day) (van Erp-Baart et al. 1989a) (see figure 4.11). Athletes involved in sports with such extreme daily energy expenditures must consume large quantities if they want to maintain their body weight and performance. Figure 4.11 shows that generally such consumption is possible, but on days with extremely high energy expenditures, the cyclists tend to have a negative energy balance of about 4.2 MJ (1,000 kcal).

These cyclists do not face an easy task because they must consume an enormous amount of energy (mostly in the form of carbohydrate) to maintain energy balance. This requirement can be problematic for the following reasons:

- Time for eating is limited, which makes consumption of large amounts of food during the 3- to 7-hour race difficult.

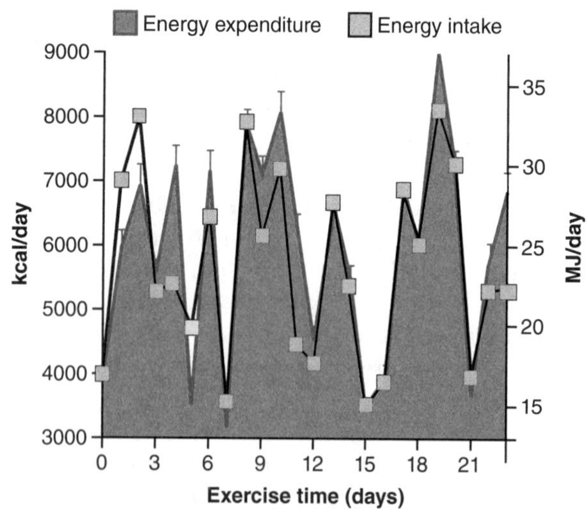

Figure 4.11 Energy balance during the Tour de France.

International Journal Sports Medicine: From W.H.M. Saris et al., "Study on Food Intake and Energy Expenditure During Extreme Sustained Exercise: The Tour de France," 1989; 10 (1 suppl): S26-S31. Reprinted by permission.

- Hunger feelings may be depressed for several hours after strenuous exercise.
- Especially during the last week of the Tour de France, gastrointestinal problems often make absorbing large quantities of food difficult or even impossible.

Nevertheless, hardly any changes in body weight occur among participants during the Tour de France, which indicates that these cyclists are indeed able to maintain energy balance (Jeukendrup, Craig, and Hawley 2000). Cyclists who do not maintain their body weight, however, might have a greater chance of dropping out.

Although eating large amounts during the race is difficult, energy intake in the form of carbohydrate solutions has been shown to be crucial (see also chapter 6). During 2 days of high-intensity cycling, when 26 MJ (6,214 kcal) of energy expenditure were not supplemented with carbohydrate during the rides, cyclists were not able to maintain energy balance (5 to 10 MJ [1,195 to 2,390 kcal] negative energy balance). When the cyclists were given a 20% carbohydrate solution during exercise from which they could drink as much as they liked, they maintained energy balance (Brouns et al. 1989b).

In some sports, even higher 24-hour energy expenditures can be reached. Using doubly labeled water, similar estimates of energy expenditure were made in Norwegian cross-country skiers during training. Energy expenditures were as high as 36 MJ/day (8,604 kcal/day) (Sjodin et al. 1994). Ironman triathletes may expend 40 MJ/day (10,000 kcal/day), and there are several reports of ultrarunners who expended 24-44 MJ/day (6,000-13,000 kcal/day) (Eden and Abernethy 1994; Rontoyannis et al. 1989). One of the highest reported records is that of Yannis Kouros, a record breaking ultrarunner who expended over 52 MJ (13,000 kcal) in 24 hours (Rontoyannis et al. 1989). For the cross-country skiers and also for Yannis Kouros, food intakes were extremely high and almost matched energy expenditure.

The greatest recorded human endurance performances occurred during the Antarctic sledding expeditions led by Robert Scott in 1911 to 1912 and Ernest Shackleton in 1914 to 1916. By man-hauling sleds for 10 hours daily for approximately 159 and 160 consecutive days, respectively, members of those expeditions would have expended almost 4,186 MJ (1,000,000 kcal) (Noakes 2007). Significant weight loss occurred because their energy intake was limited.

As mentioned, it is challenging to maintain energy balance, but there is a clear link between energy balance and performance. Sometimes periods of negative energy balance are pursued in an effort to change body composition (lower body fat for performance or aesthetic purposes) or periods of positive energy balance are pursued in an effort to gain body mass (muscle and fat, in some cases). Chapter 14 focuses on body composition, and in chapter 15, weight management is discussed in more detail.

Key Points

- All biological functions require energy. Although the human body has some energy reserves, most of the energy must be obtained through nutrition.
- Energy is the capacity to do work. The various forms of energy include light energy, chemical energy, heat energy, and electrical energy.
- Energy is often expressed in calories (imperial system) or joules (metric system); 1 calorie equals 4.184 joules.
- Efficiency describes the effective work performed after muscle contraction and is usually expressed as the percentage of total work. Humans are approximately 20% efficient.
- Gross efficiency (GE) is the ratio of the total work accomplished to the energy expended. Because resting metabolism is not accounted for, corrections have been made by subtracting baseline energy expenditure from total energy expenditure. Net efficiency, work efficiency, and delta efficiency each take resting energy expenditure into account.
- The energy content of 1 g of carbohydrate is 17.6 kJ (4.2 kcal). Fat contains between 36.0 kJ/g (8.6 kcal/g) and 40.2 kJ/g (9.6 kcal/g) (on average, about 39.3 kJ/g

[9.4 kcal/g]), and protein contains about 23.7 kJ/g (5.65 kcal/g). The coefficient of digestibility represents the proportion of consumed food that is actually digested and absorbed by the body.

- Coefficients of digestibility average about 97% for carbohydrates, 95% for lipids, and 92% for proteins. The net energy values of carbohydrate, fat, and protein are therefore 16 kJ (4 kcal), 36 kJ (9 kcal), and 16 kJ (4 kcal), respectively, and these are referred to as the Atwater energy values or Atwater factors.
- Ways to measure (or estimate) human energy expenditure include direct but complex measurements of heat production (direct calorimetry), relatively simple indirect metabolic measurements (indirect calorimetry), expensive tracer methods (doubly labeled water), and relatively inexpensive and convenient rough estimations of energy expenditure (heart rate monitoring and accelerometry).
- There are many wearable devices on the market that are used to track physical activity through step counting and estimations of energy expenditure. Although these devices are generally reliable, the accuracy of energy expenditure measurements, especially over 24 hours is questionable.
- Human energy expenditure can be divided into several components: resting metabolic rate, thermic effect of food, and exercise-related energy expenditure. RMR is the largest component (60%-75%) of the daily energy expenditure in relatively sedentary people, and the thermic effect of food represents about 10%, leaving 15% to 30% for exercise-related energy expenditure.
- Respiratory exchange measurements can be used to calculate energy expenditure and the contributions of carbohydrate and fat to energy expenditure.
- Energy balance is usually calculated over longer periods (days or weeks) and represents the difference between energy intake and energy expenditure. When energy intake exceeds energy expenditure, a positive energy balance occurs, which results in weight gain. When energy intake is below energy expenditure, a negative energy balance occurs, which results in weight loss.
- Female gymnasts, ballet dancers, and ice dancers often have energy intakes between 4.2 MJ (1,000 kcal) and 8.4 MJ (2,000 kcal). In some cases, this intake is only 1.2 to 1.4 times the resting metabolic rate. Such low energy intakes can result in nutritional deficiency.
- Cycling, triathlon, and ultra-endurance running are sports that may require energy expenditures as high as 36 MJ/day (8,600 kcal/day).

Recommended Readings

Burke, L.M. 2001. Energy needs of athletes. *Canadian Journal of Applied Physiology* 26 (Suppl): S202-S219.

Burke, L.M., A.B. Loucks, and N. Broad. 2006. Energy and carbohydrate for training and recovery. *Journal of Sports Sciences* 24 (7): 675-685.

King, N.A., P. Caudwell, M. Hopkins, N.M. Byrne, R. Colley, A.P. Hills, et al. 2007. Metabolic and behavioral compensatory responses to exercise interventions: Barriers to weight loss. *Obesity* 15 (6): 1373-1383.

Loucks, A.B., B. Kiens, and H.H. Wright. 2011. Energy availability in athletes. *Journal of Sports Sciences* 29 (Suppl 1): S7-S15.

5

Gastric Emptying, Digestion, and Absorption

Objectives

After studying this chapter, you should be able to do the following:

- Describe the functions of the gastrointestinal system and list its anatomical components and structures
- Describe the digestion processes of carbohydrate, fat, and protein
- Describe the absorption processes of carbohydrate, fat, and protein
- Describe the absorption process of water
- Describe the absorption processes of vitamins and minerals
- Describe the role of the bacterial population (microbiota) that colonizes the intestines
- Understand dietary strategies for modulating the composition or metabolic and immunological activity of the human gut microbiota
- Describe the factors that regulate gastric emptying
- State the approximate transit times within each compartment of the gastrointestinal tract
- Describe the effects of exercise on gastric emptying and absorption
- Describe the gastrointestinal problems that may occur during exercise and know which factors may augment or reduce these problems

The primary function of the **gastrointestinal** (or alimentary) **tract** is to provide the body with nutrients, water, and electrolytes from ingested food. When food moves through the gastrointestinal (GI) tract (see the sidebar Major Functions of Different Parts of the Gastrointestinal Tract), it is broken down into small units that can be absorbed in a process called **digestion**. **Absorption** (the transport of nutrients from the intestine into the blood or lymph system) takes place in various parts of the GI tract for different nutrients. Here we give an overview of the anatomy and physiology of the GI tract, the various digestion and absorption processes that take place within it, and the changes that occur during exercise.

Anatomy of the Gastrointestinal Tract

The GI tract is a long tubular structure that reaches from the mouth to the anus and includes the esophagus, stomach, small intestine, large intestine, rectum, anus, and several accessory digestive glands including the salivary glands, gallbladder, liver, and pancreas (see figure 5.1). In this 6 to 8 m (20-26 ft) tube, digestion of food and absorption of nutrients take place. The mouth, stomach, pancreas, and gallbladder have predominantly digestive functions, and most absorption occurs in the small and large intestines. After absorption, most

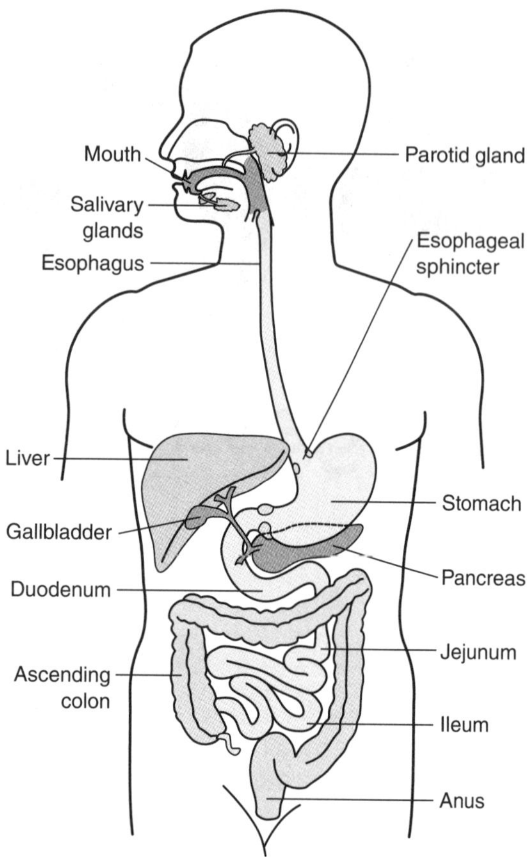

Figure 5.1 The gastrointestinal tract.

nutrients are transported to the liver, and from there they enter the main circulation.

Mouth

Chewing (or **masticating**) food is the first step of digestion. It is often referred to as **mechanical digestion**. The anterior teeth or incisors provide strong cutting action, and the posterior teeth (molars) are used for grinding. The forces applied to cut and grind the food can be as much as 25 kg on the incisors and 90 kg on the molars. Chewing food serves three major purposes. It mechanically reduces the size of the food particles, which increases the rate of **gastric emptying**. It increases the surface area of the food, which in turn increases the contact area for digestive enzymes that are released from the salivary glands and stomach (enzymatic digestion). Increasing the total surface area of the food increases the rate of digestion. Finally, it mixes the food particles with saliva and digestive enzymes. The mouth has three pairs of salivary glands: the parotid glands, the sublingual glands, and the submandibular glands (see figure 5.2). Chewing is especially important for plant material (fruits and raw vegetables) because indigestible cellulose cell walls must be mechanically destroyed to release the nutrients.

Esophagus

When the food is small and soft enough to swallow, it moves past the pharynx at the back of the mouth into the **esophagus**. The esophagus moves the food particles to the stomach. This transport process is caused by rhythmic contractions and relaxations of the esophagus. The esophagus contains an inner

MAJOR FUNCTIONS OF DIFFERENT PARTS OF THE GASTROINTESTINAL TRACT

Organ	Function
Mouth	Mechanical digestion
Salivary glands	Secretion of fluid and digestive enzymes
Stomach	Secretion of hydrochloric acid and protein-digesting enzymes (proteases)
Pancreas	Secretion of sodium bicarbonate and digestive enzymes
Liver	Secretion of bile acids
Gallbladder	Temporary storage and concentration of bile
Small intestine	Digestion of food and absorption of water, nutrients, and electrolytes
Large intestine	Absorption of electrolytes

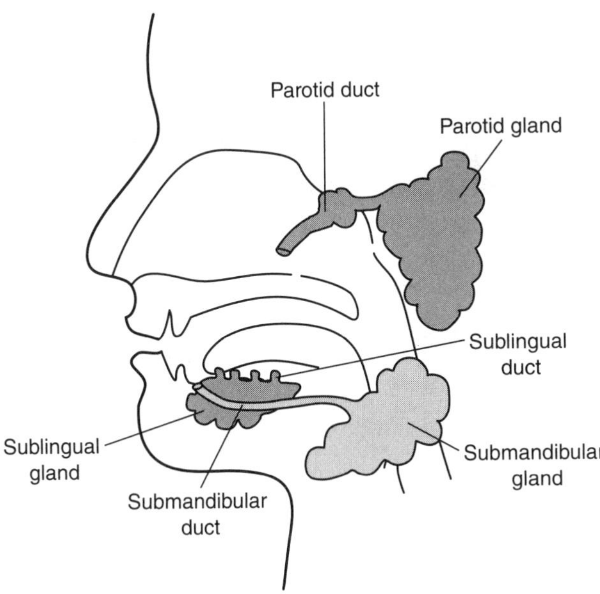

Figure 5.2 The mouth and its three pairs of salivary glands.

layer of smooth muscle that consists of circular bands and an outer layer of smooth muscle that runs longitudinally. Contraction of these muscles causes peristalsis, a squeezing action that involves progressive and recurring contractions, which mixes and moves the food to the stomach. This mechanism makes swallowing possible even when a person is hanging upside down or in space with zero gravity.

At the end of the esophagus, a valve of smooth muscle called the **esophageal sphincter** relaxes to allow food into the stomach. After some food particles have passed the esophageal sphincter, it contracts, which prevents reflux of food or fluids from the stomach into the esophagus. If the sphincter does not function properly, a person can experience some acid leaking from the stomach (heartburn). This GI problem is common among runners and cyclists.

Stomach

The stomach, which is about 20 to 25 cm (8-10 in.) long, is divided into three parts: the corpus (or body), the antrum, and the fundus (see figure 5.3). The corpus and the antrum have different physiological functions. Although the fundus is a different part of the stomach from an anatomical point of view, from a functional point of view it is considered part of the corpus. The end of the stomach is an opening to the duodenum called the **pylorus**. A circular muscular valve called the **pyloric sphincter** controls the emptying of food from the stomach into the small intestine. When this muscle relaxes, food leaves the stomach; when it contracts, food stays in the stomach. The functions of the stomach include

- storing large quantities of food until it can be accommodated in the intestine;
- mixing this food with gastric secretions to form a homogeneous, acidic, souplike liquid or paste called **chyme**; and
- regulating the emptying of chyme into the duodenum (the upper part of the small intestine) at a rate suitable for proper digestion and absorption.

Normally, food that enters the stomach forms concentric circles in the corpus and fundus so the latest food is closest to the esophagus and the oldest food is nearest to the wall of the corpus. The stomach volume is normally around 1.5 L (0.4 gal), but this volume can change from almost nothing when the stomach is empty to about 6 L (1.6 gal) when the stomach is full. The muscular tone of the stomach wall decreases as soon as food enters the stomach, which allows the stomach wall to stretch outward to accommodate more food.

The wall of the corpus contains gastric glands that secrete digestive juices. These secretions contact the food portions nearest to the stomach wall. The stomach can also contract and relax, which mixes the food into the chyme. Chyme can be a fluid or a paste, depending on the relative amounts of food and secretions and the degree of digestion. Chyme is passed down to the small intestine by a strictly controlled process of gastric emptying.

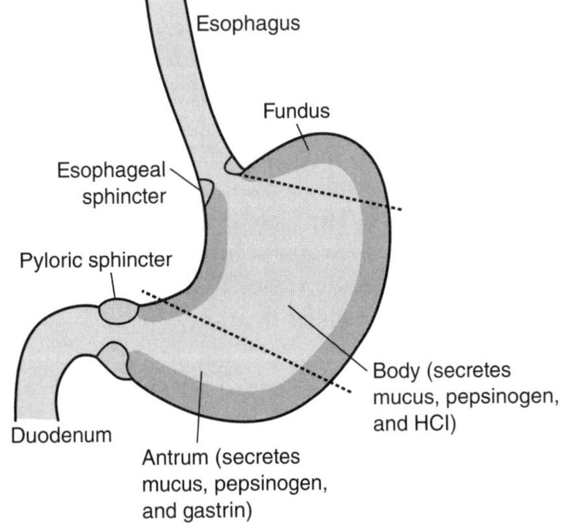

Figure 5.3 The anatomy of the stomach.

Little absorption takes place in the stomach (with the exception of some water and alcohol).

Small Intestine

The small intestine is approximately 6 to 7 m (18 ft) in length and 3 to 5 cm (1-2 in.) in diameter and is divided into the duodenum (about 25-30 cm [10-12 in.]), the jejunum (the next 2.5 m; 8 ft), and the ileum (the last 3 m; 10ft). About 95% of all absorption takes place in the duodenum and the jejunum. The intestinal mucosa of the duodenum and the jejunum contain many folds called the Kerckring folds (see figure 5.4). These folds increase the surface area of the intestine to about three times that of a similarly sized flat internal lining. These folds are covered by millions of small fingerlike structures, called villi, that project about 1 mm (0.4 in.) from the surface of the mucosa (see figure 5.5). The villi increase the total surface area of the small intestine another 10 times. The intestinal cells that form the border of the villi are covered by a **brush border** that consists of about 600 microvilli that are approximately 1 mm long. These microvilli increase the total surface area another 20 times. Therefore, the highly specialized construction of the small intestine increases absorption to 600 times what it would be in a simple tube with a flat internal surface. The total surface area of the small intestine can be as large as 250 m^2 (2,691 ft^2), which is an area larger than a tennis court.

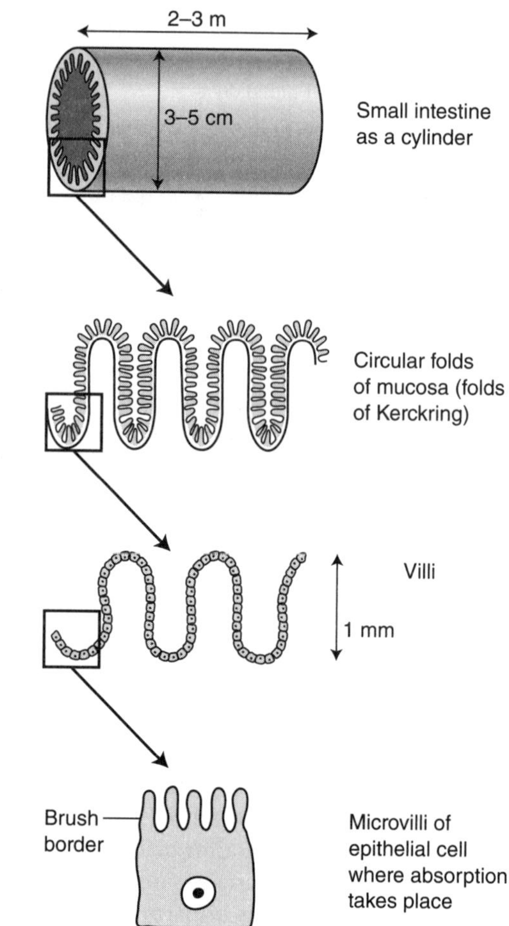

Figure 5.4 The organization of the small intestine increases the total surface area by about 600 times compared to a simple tube with a flat internal surface.

Villi

Villi are finger-shaped and highly vascularized (see figure 5.5). The wall of a villus consists of a layer of epithelial cells that each have a brush border through which absorption of nutrients takes place. Water, water-soluble particles, and electrolytes require transport or diffusion across the luminal and contraluminal membranes of the epithelial cell into the blood vessels. These nutrients are then transported to the liver through the hepatic portal vein. Each villus also contains a **lacteal** located in its central part. The lacteal transports particles that are not readily water soluble (e.g., long-chain FAs) via the lymphatic vessels. These vessels drain into large veins near the heart.

Motility and Transit Time

Depending on its composition, food spends 1 to 3 days in the GI tract before it is eliminated. The time food spends in a section of the GI tract is the **transit time**. For instance, the transit time in the small intestine is approximately 3 to 10 hours, depending on the composition of the food and its **motility** through the GI tract. The wall of the small intestine contains two layers of smooth muscle with longitudinal and circular muscle fibers that allow peristalsis and mixing contractions that push the chyme in the distal direction toward the large intestine (like squeezing toothpaste out of a tube). Mixing or segmentation contractions move the chyme back and forth to mix and break food down further. These contractions occur at a rate of 0.5 to 2.0 cm/s (0.2-0.8 in./s), with the fastest movement in the proximal intestine and the slowest movement in the distal intestine. The average speed of chyme along the small intestine is approximately 1 cm/s (0.4 in./s).

Peristalsis increases after a meal and can increase greatly after intense irritation of the intestinal mucosa such as during infectious diarrhea. Mixing, or segmentation contractions differ from

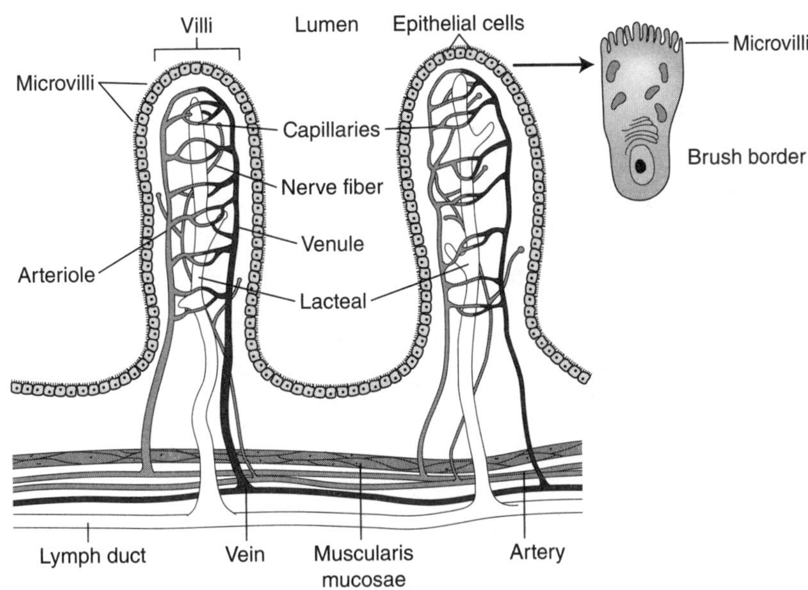

Figure 5.5 Functional organization of the villi.

peristalsis. The circular muscles contract, giving the small intestine the look of linked sausages. These intermittent contractions (8-12/min) cause the chyme to move forward and backward. The chyme moves backward before it advances. The function of these circular contractions is to mix the chyme with bile from the gallbladder, pancreatic juices, and intestinal juices. The flow of digestive juices (bile and pancreatic juice) into the second part of the duodenum is controlled by a muscular valve called the sphincter of Oddi. Because of the back and forward movement (and not just forward movement) the juices get extra time to digest the food, and the contact time and area are increased.

Gallbladder

The gallbladder is a hollow organ that sits just below the liver. It stores, concentrates, and releases bile. Bile, which is produced by liver cells, consists of water, electrolytes, **bile salts**, cholesterol, lecithin, and bilirubin. Bile facilitates the digestion and absorption of fat and is released through the hepatic duct, which joins the pancreatic duct just before entering the duodenum (see figure 5.6). The gallbladder can store approximately 30 to 60 ml (1-2 fl oz) of bile, but it secretes as much as 1,200 ml (42 fl oz) into the duodenum every day. It stores up to 12 hours of bile secretion by concentrating the bile constituents. In the gallbladder, bile is concentrated by removing water and electrolytes. Bile secretion increases after a meal, especially when the meal contains a large amount of fat. The bile salts are reabsorbed again in the intestinal mucosa of the distal ileum. They enter the portal blood and pass to the liver. In the liver, they are resecreted into the bile. In this way, 94% of the bile salts are reused. The recirculation of bile salts is called the enterohepatic circulation.

Pancreas

The pancreas is a large gland situated parallel to and just beneath the stomach (see figures 5.1 and 5.6). It secretes sodium bicarbonate to buffer the hydrochloric acid of the stomach and digestive enzymes to break down carbohydrate, protein, and fat. Pancreatic juice is mainly secreted in response to chyme in the upper portions of the small intestine. The regulatory mechanisms for sodium bicarbonate secretion and digestive enzyme secretion are different, and the secretion rates are highly dependent on the type and amount of food ingested. The concentrations of various enzymes in pancreatic juice also depend to some extent on the type of food ingested.

Ileocecal Valve

From the small intestine, chyme moves into the large intestine through the ileocecal valve (see figure 5.7). This valve prevents backflow of indigestible fecal material into the small intestine. The valve can resist pressure equal to about 50 to 60 cm (20-24 in.) of water. The distal end of the small intestine, or ileum, has a thicker muscular coat that

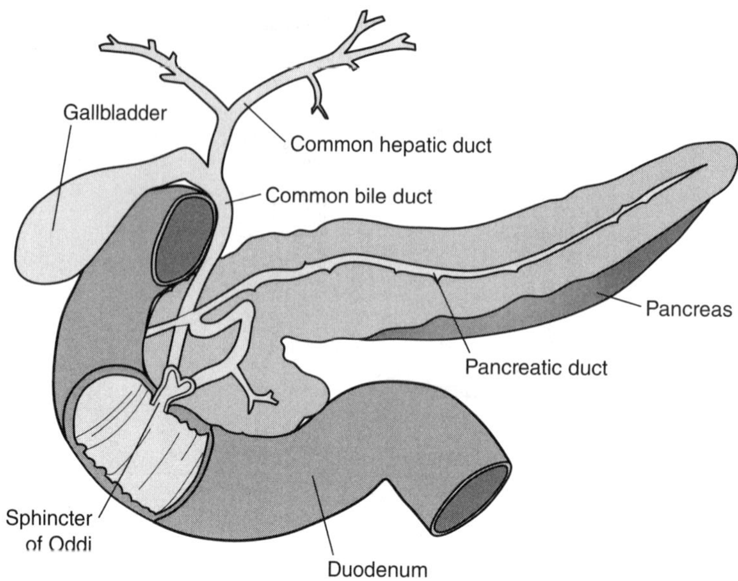

Figure 5.6 Duodenum, pancreas, and gallbladder.

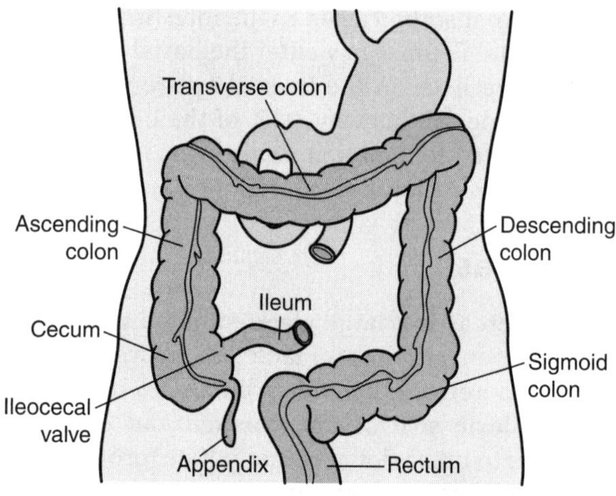

Figure 5.7 The ileocecal valve and the large intestine.

controls emptying from the ileum. Contraction of the ileocecal valve is regulated by a variety of factors including distension of the cecum (a blind pouch, open only at one end, at the beginning of the large intestine), irritating substances in the cecum, and fluidity of the chyme. An inflamed appendix (a nonfunctional part of the intestine that is short, thin, and outpouching from the cecum) restricts the emptying of the ileum. Increased fluidity of the chyme, on the other hand, increases emptying from the ileum.

Large Intestine

In the large intestine, chyme is called feces. The large intestine is approximately 1.5 m (5 ft) long and consists of the colon, the rectum, and the anal canal. The colon is divided into the ascending colon, the transverse colon, the descending colon, and the sigmoid colon (see figure 5.7). The functions of the colon are absorption of water and electrolytes from the chyme and storage of feces until they can be expelled. Absorption takes place mainly in the first part of the colon, and storage mainly occurs in the distal parts. The peristaltic movements of the colon are slower than those of the small intestine. The colon also has circular and longitudinal smooth muscle layers that move the feces toward the distal parts of the colon with rhythmic contractions. The fecal material is slowly rolled over and mixed so contact with the surface of the large intestine increases and as much water as possible is absorbed. Normally, 80 to 150 ml (3-5 fl oz) of water are present in approximately 300 ml (11 fl oz) of feces.

Regulation of the Gastrointestinal Tract

The GI tract is innervated by the sympathetic and the parasympathetic components of the autonomic nervous system. Parasympathetic stimulation stimulates motility. The vagus nerve is the source of parasympathetic activity in the esophagus, stomach, pancreas, gallbladder, small intestine, and upper section of the large intestine. The lower portion of the large intestine receives parasympathetic innervation from spinal nerves in the sacral region (the lower end of the spine). Autonomic regulation, which is extrinsic to the GI tract, is overruled by intrinsic modes of regulation. Sensory neurons in various parts of the GI tract have their cell bodies in the gut wall but are not part of the autonomic nervous system. In addition, hormonal regulation plays an important role. Endocrine glands secrete hormones into the circulation, whereas paracrine glands or cells secrete products that influence the secretion of other products by a local gland or cell. For example, **gastrin** is a hormone secreted by the stomach that increases hydrochloric acid and pepsinogen secretion in the stomach. Another example is secretin, a hormone produced by the small intestine that increases water and bicarbonate secretion by the pancreas.

Substances within the tissues of the GI tract and hormones released by organs in the GI tract affect secretion and motility. An overview of the effects of GI hormones and their functions is given in table 5.1.

Digestion

Digestion starts the moment food is ingested and may take 4 to 6 hours to complete depending on the amount of food and the types of food ingested. Specific enzymes are responsible for the digestion of different macronutrients. Digestion includes breaking down food by chewing as well as breaking it down chemically using enzymes. Processes are different for different foods and nutrients, but most foods are broken down to the smallest units of their nutrients and these can then be absorbed. Substances that cannot be digested are fermented by bacteria or expelled.

Carbohydrate Digestion

The digestion of carbohydrates starts in the mouth as saliva is added to the food. Saliva is secreted from the parotid glands, the sublingual glands, and the submandibular glands (see figure 5.2). The daily secretion of saliva normally ranges from 800 to 1,500 ml (28-53 fl oz) (on average 1,000 ml; see table 5.2). In the unstimulated state, saliva secretion rate is about 0.5 ml/min (0.02 fl oz/min, but this rate can increase up to 10 times during chewing. Saliva consists primarily of water (99.5%) derived from extracellular fluid. In addition, it contains α-amylase (also referred to as ptyalin, an enzyme responsible for the breakdown of starch into smaller units), mucoid proteins, bicarbonate, electrolytes, lysozymes (enzymes that break down proteins and attack bacteria), lingual lipase, and protein antibodies (the major secretory antibody being immunoglobulin A [IgA], which can help to destroy oral bacteria). Besides its digestive function, saliva has a protective function against invading bacteria (see chapter 13). An overview of digestive enzymes is given in table 5.3.

The mucoid proteins give saliva its viscous quality, which helps lubricate food and makes it easier to swallow. Chewing food mixes saliva with the food and increases the contact area so amylase can start breaking down the glucose chains in starches. Prolonged chewing of a cracker will cause it to taste sweeter because some starch breaks down to disaccharide sugars, such as maltose, which taste much sweeter than starch.

TABLE 5.1 Effects of Gastrointestinal Hormones

Hormone	Secreted by	Effect
Gastrin	Stomach	Stimulates hydrochloric acid production in the stomach; stimulates secretion of pepsinogen in the stomach
Secretin	Small intestine	Stimulates water and bicarbonate secretion in pancreatic juice
Cholecystokinin (CCK)	Small intestine	Stimulates secretion of enzymes in pancreatic juice, stimulates gallbladder contractions, inhibits gastric motility and secretion
Gastric inhibitory peptide (GIP)	Small intestine	Inhibits gastric motility and secretion
Glucagonlike peptide I (GLP-I)	Ileum and colon	Inhibits gastric motility and secretion
Guanylin	Ileum and colon	Removes sodium chloride and water from feces

When food is swallowed and arrives in the acid environment of the stomach, the amylase activity decreases. Carbohydrate digestion still takes place but at a much slower rate. Approximately 30% to 40% of the carbohydrate may be digested, predominantly to maltose, maltotrioses, and small oligosaccharides (see figure 5.8), in the mouth and stomach before the stomach content is completely mixed with gastric secretions.

When the carbohydrates are emptied from the stomach into the duodenum and the acid is neutralized by sodium bicarbonate from the pancreas, digestion proceeds quickly. In the duodenum, additional α-amylase will be secreted in the pancreatic juice. This α-amylase, like salivary amylase, hydrolyzes the starches into small glucose polymers (dextrins) and maltose (see figure 5.8). The hydrolysis of all starches to maltose is almost complete when the chyme enters the ileum. The disaccharides and small polysaccharides are further digested by specific enzymes located in the brush borders of intestinal epithelial cells. As soon

TABLE 5.2 Daily Secretion of Intestinal Juices

Intestinal juices	Daily volume
Saliva	1,000 ml (35 fl oz)
Gastric secretions	1,500 ml (53 fl oz)
Pancreatic secretion	1,000 ml (35 fl oz)
Bile	1,000 ml (35 fl oz)
Small intestine	2,000 ml (70 fl oz)
Large intestine	200 ml (7 fl oz)
Total	6,700 ml (235 fl oz)

TABLE 5.3 Digestive Enzymes and Their Functions

Enzyme	Site of action	Source	Substrate	Product	Optimum pH
Carbohydrates					
Salivary amylase	Mouth	Salivary glands	Starch	Maltose	6.7
Pancreatic amylase	Duodenum	Pancreatic juice	Starch	Maltose, maltotriose, and oligosaccharides	6.7-7.0
Maltase	Small intestine	Brush border	Maltose	Glucose	5.0-7.0
Sucrase	Small intestine	Brush border	Sucrose	Glucose and fructose	5.0-7.0
Lactase	Small intestine	Brush border	Lactose	Glucose and galactose	5.8-6.2
Lipids					
Lingual lipase	Mouth	Lingual salivary glands	Starch	Maltose	3.5-6.0
Pancreatic lipase	Small intestine	Pancreatic juice	Triacylglycerols	Fatty acids and monoacylglycerols	8.0
Proteins					
Pepsin	Stomach	Gastric glands	Protein	Polypeptides	1.6-2.4
Trypsin	Small intestine	Pancreatic juice	Polypeptides	Amino acids, dipeptides, and tripeptides	8.0
Chymotrypsin	Small intestine	Pancreatic juice	Polypeptides	Amino acids, dipeptides, and tripeptides	8.0
Carboxypeptidase	Small intestine	Pancreatic juice	Polypeptides	Amino acids, dipeptides, and tripeptides	8.0
Elastase	Small intestine	Pancreatic juice	Polypeptides	Amino acids, dipeptides, and tripeptides	8.5

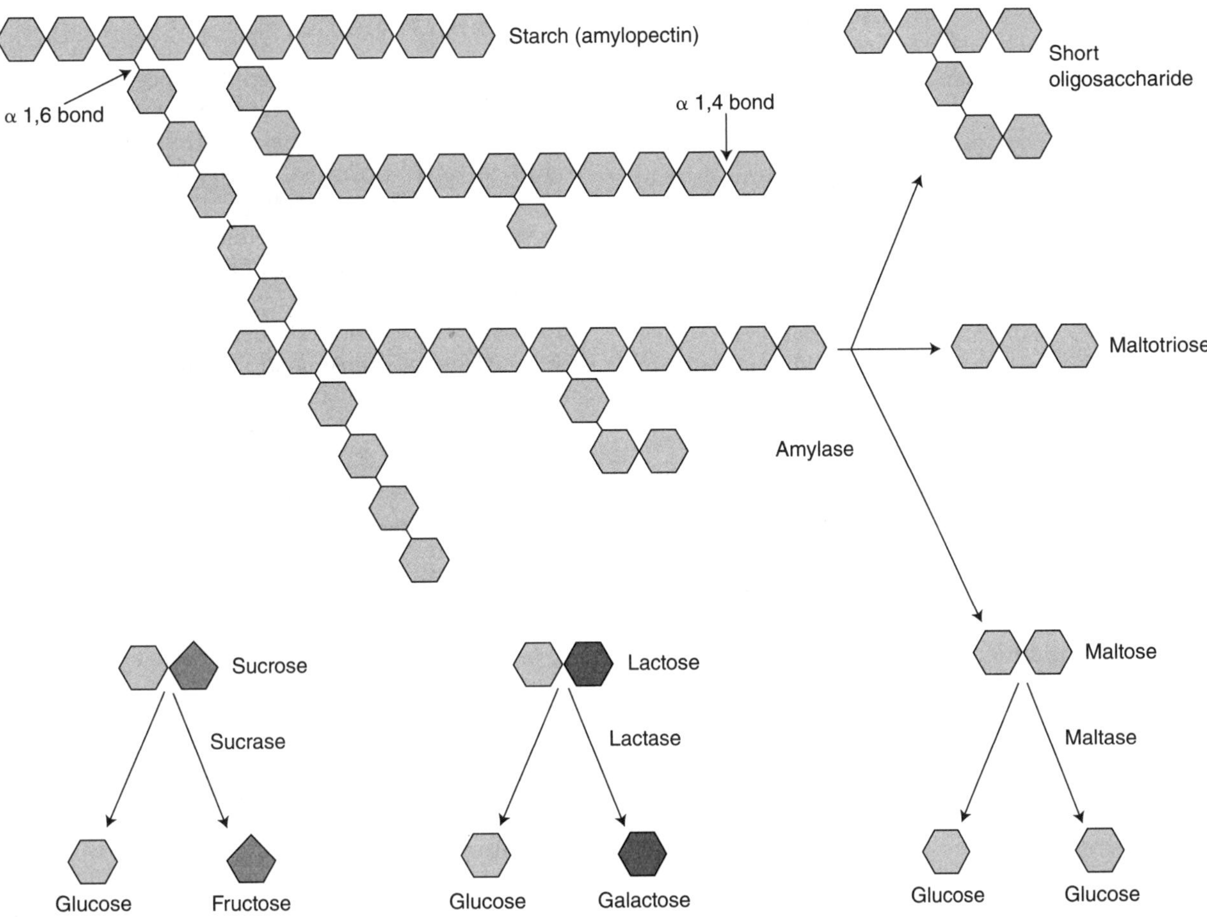

Figure 5.8 Digestion of carbohydrate. Some carbohydrates like starch have long chains of glucose molecules that are broken down by amylase into shorter units and subsequently into disaccharides and monosaccharides.

as disaccharides contact the brush border, they are digested by the enzymes lactase, sucrase, and maltase (see figure 5.8). Lactase breaks lactose down into glucose and galactose, sucrase breaks sucrose down into glucose and fructose, and maltase breaks maltose down into two glucose molecules.

Problems with the digestive process can result when a deficiency of one or more of these enzymes exists. Lactose intolerance is caused by an absence or deficiency of the intestinal enzyme lactase. When lactose, the main carbohydrate component of milk, is not digested, diarrhea and fluid loss result. In addition, bacteria in the large intestine metabolize the lactose to produce large quantities of gas, which causes bloating and pain.

Fiber, a form of dietary carbohydrate, contains cellulose, which is a structural component of plant cells that is resistant to human digestive enzymes. Cellulose can be excreted in the feces, but some of it is fermented by the bacteria in the large intestine. Similar to the way yeast ferments the sugars in grape juice to produce wine, the bacteria in the large intestine ferment cellulose to produce hydrogen and carbon dioxide gases, volatile FAs, and, in many instances, methane gas (which has an unpleasant odor). Changes in the diet or in the type of microorganisms can influence the amount of gas produced.

Peristaltic movements push undigested carbohydrates, including fibrous substances, to the colon, where more digestion occurs. Indigestible carbohydrates (predominantly cellulose) move to the rectum for expulsion though the anus.

Lipid Digestion

Digestion of lipids begins in the mouth because saliva contains small amounts of **lingual lipase**, the enzyme that splits triacylglycerols (triglycerides) into FAs and glycerol. In the stomach, this acid-stable lipase continues to hydrolyze the triacylglycerols (see figure 5.9). Hydrolysis, however, is slow because triacylglycerols are not soluble in water and therefore do not mix well with the water fraction in which lipase is found. The lingual and gastric lipases act together but mainly on the short-chain (C4-C6) and medium-chain (C8-C10) triacylglycerols, whereas most of the fat (long-chain triacylglycerols; C12-C24) is digested in the small intestine. Lingual lipase is responsible for 10% to 30% of triacylglycerol digestion. When the chyme enters the duodenum, bile is added and acts on the triacylglycerols, which by this time are organized into large lipid globules. Pancreatic lipase is secreted into the duodenum and further hydrolyzes the triacylglycerols.

After initial hydrolysis starts and the triglycerides are converted into FAs, monoglycerides and diglycerides organize themselves into small emulsion droplets. The fat-soluble part of the FA faces inward, and the water-soluble part forms the core of each droplet. When bile salts stored in the gallbladder are secreted into the duodenum, micelles are formed (see figure 5.9). Micelles are well-defined, disk-shaped structures on which phospholipids and FAs form a bilayer. The bile salts occupy the edge positions, rendering the edge of the micelle hydrophilic (i.e., more attractive to water). The bile salts emulsify the lipids into small droplets, which increases the total surface area and thus facilitates the hydrolysis of triacylglycerols by pancreatic lipase.

Protein Digestion

Protein digestion breaks down ingested proteins into simple amino acids, dipeptides, and tripeptides for absorption across the intestinal mucosa (see figure 5.10). This process, called protein hydrolysis, takes place in the stomach and the small intestine and depends on specific protein-digesting enzymes (proteases) and the acidity of the stomach. Specific cells produce and secrete hydrochloric acid into the stomach. These parietal cells secrete an isotonic 160 mM hydrochloric acid solution with a pH of about 0.8, which illustrates its extreme acidity. The pH in the stomach and of the gastric contents is typically around 2.0.

Hydrochloric acid (and the acidic ingested food) has various functions, such as

- activating the protease enzyme pepsin,
- killing many pathogenic organisms,
- increasing the absorption of iron and calcium,
- inactivating hormones of plant and animal origin, and
- breaking down food proteins and making them more vulnerable to enzyme action.

Proteases (see table 5.3) are often stored as inactive precursors, but as soon as they are released into the stomach or small intestine, they become active (and act as digestive enzymes). This mechanism prevents the digestion of the cells in which the proteases are produced and stored.

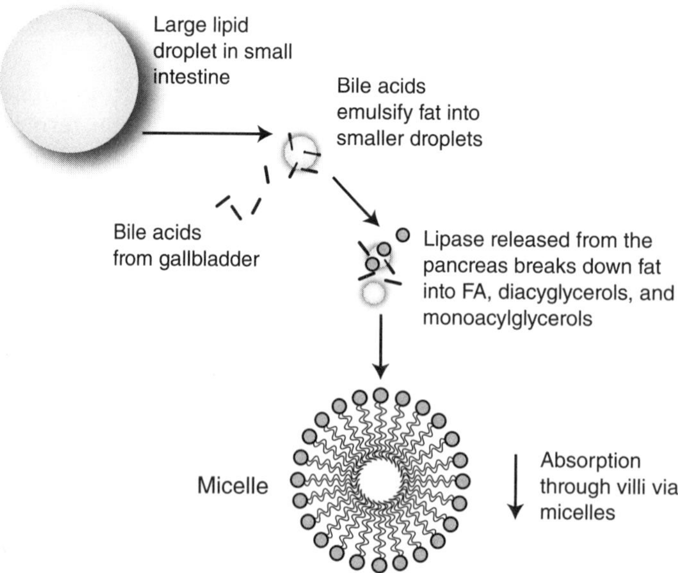

Figure 5.9 Digestion of fat.

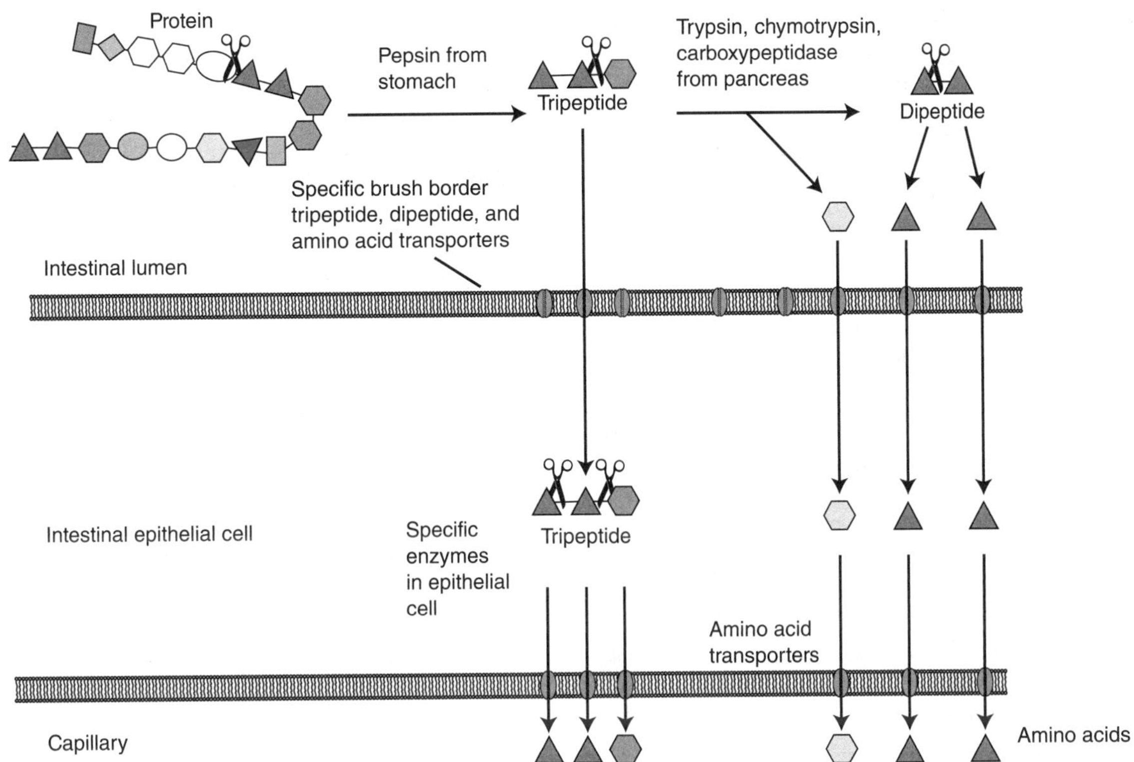

Figure 5.10 Digestion of protein.

Pepsin (an important group of proteases), which is secreted as its precursor **pepsinogen** from the cells of the stomach wall, is initially inactive. As soon as pepsinogen contacts the hydrochloric acid in the stomach, it is automatically converted into the active pepsin that breaks down protein. Pepsin degrades the collagenous connective tissue fibers of meat. After dismantling these fibers, other proteases can effectively digest the remaining animal protein. Stomach enzymes and acids attack the long, complex protein strands and hydrolyze approximately 10% to 20% of the ingested proteins. The low pH in the stomach causes denaturation of the protein, meaning that the three-dimensional structure of the protein is uncoiled and breaks into smaller polypeptide and peptide units. When the chyme passes into the small intestine, pepsin becomes inactivated by the relatively high pH in the duodenum.

Other proteases (alkaline enzymes), including trypsin, are released from the pancreas and become active to digest the remaining proteins and polypeptides. The pancreatic juice is rich in precursors of endopeptidases, carboxypeptidases, enteropeptidases, trypsinogen, and trypsin (see figure 5.10). These proteases digest the polypeptides into tripeptides, dipeptides, and single amino acids, which can be transported across the enterocyte.

Absorption

Absorption is a process whereby the digested food is transported across the wall of the intestine into the circulation (or into the lymphatic system). The intestinal tract has different transport mechanisms for different nutrients and absorption of different nutrients takes place at different speeds. Also, different transporters have different capacities for absorption. During the process of absorption there are at least two cell membranes that need to be crossed: the luminal membrane and the contraluminal membrane. These membranes may have different transport mechanisms.

Absorption of nutrients across the intestinal walls occurs either by active transport or by simple diffusion. Active transport requires energy and usually takes place against a concentration gradient or an electrical potential. Active transport often requires specialized carrier proteins. Diffusion is the movement of substances across a membrane along, rather than against, an electrochemical gradient. Simple diffusion does not require transport proteins or energy in the form of ATP, but many nutrients are transported by facilitated diffusion, which requires a protein transporter or channel.

Absorption of Carbohydrate

The major monosaccharides that result from digestion of polysaccharides and disaccharides are glucose, fructose, and galactose. These monosaccharides are absorbed by carrier-mediated transport processes. The transporters that mediate the uptake of monosaccharides in the epithelial cell (see figure 5.11) are a sodium monosaccharide cotransporter (most commonly the sodium-dependent glucose transporter [SGLT1]) and a sodium-independent facilitated-diffusion transporter with specificity for fructose (GLUT5). For each molecule of glucose, two sodium ions are transported into the epithelial cell. The sodium is then actively transported back into the gut lumen through a Na^+/K^+-ATPase pump. Galactose is the only other carbohydrate that also uses SGLT1 in the same way as glucose.

A separate monosaccharide transporter on the contraluminal side of the epithelial cell accepts all three monosaccharides (GLUT 2). The monosaccharides then enter the circulation in the hepatic portal vein, which transports them to the liver. The number of transporters and the activity of these transporters is not static and may respond to nutrient intake. For example, within a few days, increases in SGLT1 can be observed after increasing dietary carbohydrate intake. The reverse is also true: Reducing dietary carbohydrate intake will downregulate the transporters and reduce the absorptive capacity for carbohydrate.

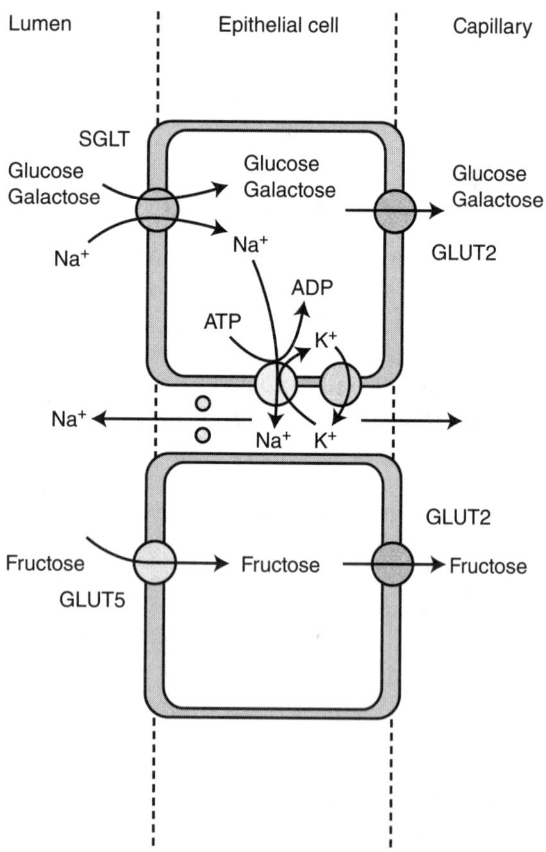

Figure 5.11 Absorption of carbohydrate.

Absorption of Fat

The monoacylglycerols and FAs incorporated into micelles are transported to the villi and move into the spaces between the microvilli. Here FAs diffuse across the membrane of the epithelium and enter the epithelial cell. The micelles then move away from the villi, incorporate new FAs, and transport them to the villi.

Micelles formed within the intestinal lumen, therefore, perform an important ferrying function. In the presence of bile salts (and, thus, micelles), fat absorption is almost complete (97%), whereas in the absence of bile, only about 50% of the FAs are absorbed.

The absorption of FAs through the epithelial membranes is by diffusion (because they are highly soluble in the lipid membranes) (see figure 5.12). In the epithelial cell, FAs are reesterified to triacylglycerols in the endoplasmic reticulum. Once formed, triacylglycerols combine with cholesterol and phospholipids to form chylomicrons (see also figure 1.4). In a chylomicron, the fatty sides of the phospholipids face toward the center, and the polar parts form the surface. Chylomicrons make possible the transport of fat in the aqueous environment of the lymph and blood plasma. These large molecules move toward the central lacteal of the villi and are slowly transported through the lymphatic system and reach the circulation in the subclavian veins.

Short-chain and medium-chain FAs are more water soluble than long-chain FAs and therefore follow a slightly different route of absorption. They enter the epithelial cell, and, without being reesterified to triacylglycerols, they directly diffuse through the contraluminal membrane into the portal blood, where they are bound to the plasma protein albumin and passed to the liver via the hepatic portal vein. So, whereas long-chain FAs reach the circulation via the (slow) lymphatic system, short- and medium-chain FAs reach the circulation directly and rapidly. The bile salts

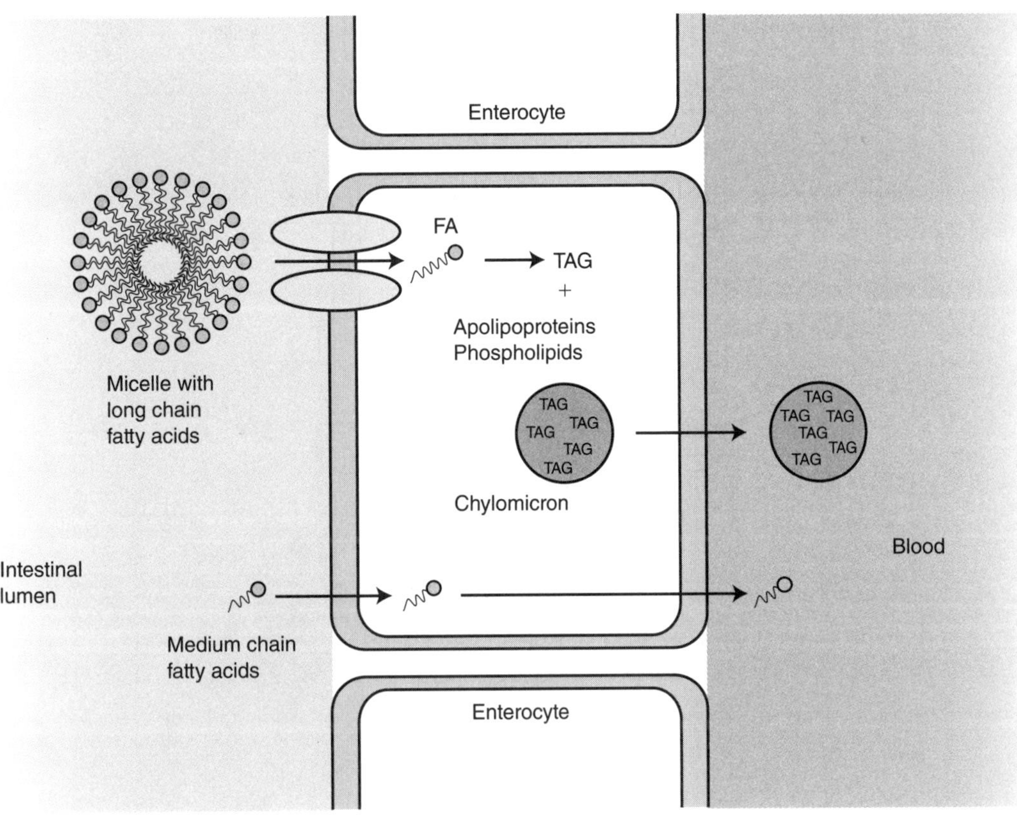

Figure 5.12 Absorption of fat.

are reabsorbed again in the intestinal mucosa of the distal ileum. They enter the portal blood and pass to the liver. In the liver, they are resecreted into the bile. In this way, 94% of the bile salts are reutilized. The recirculation of bile salts is called the enterohepatic circulation.

Absorption of Amino Acids

Amino acids, dipeptides, and tripeptides are absorbed by active transport (coupled to the transport of sodium) in the small intestine and delivered to the liver via the hepatic portal vein. Dipeptides and tripeptides that have been transported across the epithelial membrane are broken down inside the cell into their amino acid constituents by specific dipeptidases and tripeptidases (see figure 5.10).

Most amino acids are transported across the epithelium against a concentration gradient, and, therefore, carrier-mediated transport is needed (see figure 5.13). At least seven brush border–specific transport proteins have been identified. The luminal membrane usually contains sodium-dependent transport systems, whereas the contraluminal membrane transport does not require sodium. The small intestine has a large and effective capacity to absorb amino acids and small peptides. Most amino acids can use more than one transporter for absorption. Less than 1% of the ingested protein is usually found in feces. After amino acids have passed the epithelium, they are transported to the liver where they can be converted to glucose, fat, or protein, or they can be released into the bloodstream as free amino acids.

Absorption of Water

Most water absorption (99%) takes place in the small intestine, mainly in the duodenum (72%), entirely by simple diffusion. This absorption obeys the laws of osmosis (see figure 5.14). A membrane that is impermeable to solutes but permeable to water separates two compartments with the same amount of fluid but different numbers of solute particles.

Water diffuses across this membrane in both directions, but relatively more water flows toward the compartment with the lower water concentration (higher solute concentration). This net

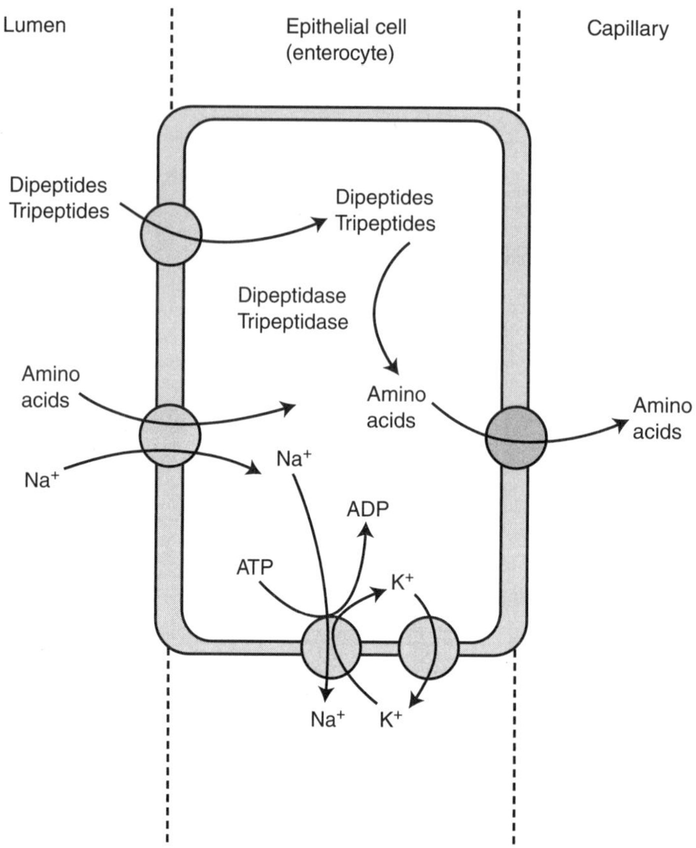

Figure 5.13 Absorption of amino acids.

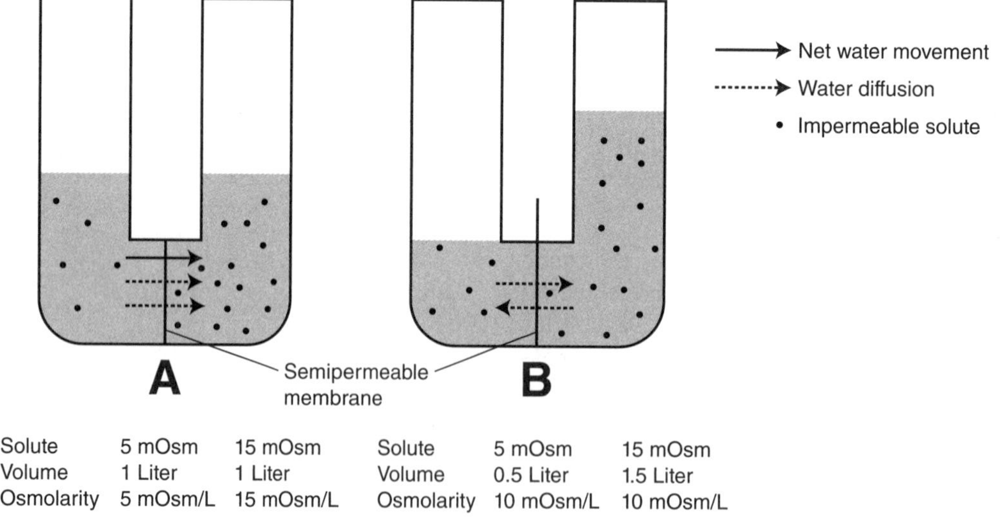

Figure 5.14 The process of osmosis.

movement of water eventually results in a similar solute concentration on both sides of the membrane. But the amount of water in the compartment with the lower water concentration increases.

The term *osmole* describes the number of solute particles, and the solute particle density is usually expressed as milliosmoles (mOsm) per unit of mass (kg) or volume (L): mOsm/kg (**osmolality**) or mOsm/L (**osmolarity**), respectively. The osmolarity of most body fluids is around 290 mOsm/L (see table 5.4). Therefore, when the osmolarity of the chyme is low (< 280 mOsm/L), water moves toward the epithelial cell and the blood plasma with higher osmolarity. If the osmolarity of the chyme is high (> 300 mOsm/L, such as in a concentrated glucose solution), water moves into the gut lumen. With the absorption of solutes (e.g., glucose and sodium), the osmotic gradient changes and pulls water into the epithelium (a process known as solvent drag).

The combined secretions of the salivary glands, stomach wall, gallbladder, pancreas, and intestine can amount to a total volume of up to 7 L (1.8 gal) per day in a sedentary adult (see table 5.2). This value may be higher for athletes who have high energy intakes.. Daily water intake can average 2 L (0.5 gal), so total daily water absorption may be as high as 9 L (2.0 gal) in a sedentary person. During exercise, especially in hot conditions when fluid losses and intakes are high, daily water absorption can easily exceed 12 L (2.6 gal). With diarrhea, absorption of water is minimal, and fluid losses can be high and, in some cases, life threatening.

TABLE 5.4 Osmolarity of Body Fluids and Commercially Available Drinks

Solution	Osmolarity (mOsm/L)
Water	10-20
Sweat	170-220
Gastric fluids	280-303
Blood serum	300
Lucozade Sport	280
Isostar	296
Gatorade	349
Powerade (UK) Powerade (U.S.)	285 381
Allsport	516
Pepsi	568
Coca-Cola	650
Fruit juice	450-690

Absorption of Vitamins

Most vitamin absorption takes place in the jejunum and the ileum and is usually a passive process (diffusion). Fat-soluble vitamins (A, D, E, and K) are absorbed with FAs. They are also incorporated into chylomicrons and transported through the lymph system into the systemic circulation to liver and other tissues. Most of the absorption of fat-soluble vitamins takes place in the small intestine.

Water-soluble vitamins are also mostly absorbed in the small intestine by diffusion. The water-soluble vitamins are not retained to any great extent by different tissues, and when large amounts are ingested, they are mostly excreted in urine. Most vitamin C is absorbed in the distal portion of the small intestine. Excess intake of vitamin C (above approximately 1,200 mg/day) decreases the efficiency of renal reabsorption of vitamin C, and much of the excess intake appears in the urine. B vitamins are often ingested as part of coenzymes in food; digestion liberates the vitamins. For example, pantothenic acid is usually present in food as part of CoA. Digestion releases the vitamin from its coenzyme, and absorption takes place. Thiamin and vitamin B_6 are mainly absorbed in the jejunum. Biotin and riboflavin are mainly absorbed in the proximal part of the small intestine. Niacin is partly absorbed in the stomach but mostly in the small intestine. Vitamin B_{12} is mainly absorbed in the ileum. Its absorption is more complex and involves binding to a specific protein (called intrinsic factor, which is secreted by the parietal cells of the gastric mucosa). Absorption of folic acid depends on the presence of the intestinal enzyme conjugase, which facilitates the absorption of folic acid in the small intestine. An overview of various vitamins and their absorption mechanisms is provided in table 5.5.

Absorption of Minerals

Minerals are not well absorbed in the human intestine, so their intake usually exceeds the requirements. Mineral absorption often depends on its chemical form. The best-known example is probably the difference in absorption between nonheme and heme iron. (Heme iron is obtained from meat; nonheme iron is obtained from plants.) About 15% of all ingested heme iron is absorbed in the small intestine, whereas only 2% to 10% of nonheme iron is absorbed. Absorption of other minerals is also relatively poor. A maximum of 35% of ingested calcium is absorbed, 20% to 30% of ingested magnesium is absorbed, 14% to 41%

TABLE 5.5 Absorption of Vitamins

Vitamin	Absorption mechanism
Vitamin C	Almost all absorption (90%) takes place in the distal portion of the small intestine.
Thiamin	Absorption occurs predominantly in the jejunum.
Riboflavin	Absorption occurs in the proximal part of the small intestine.
Niacin	Some absorption occurs in the stomach, but most occurs in the small intestine.
Pantothenic acid	This vitamin exists as part of CoA, but absorption occurs readily throughout the small intestine when the vitamin is released from CoA.
Biotin	Absorption occurs in upper one-third to one-half of the small intestine.
Folic acid	Absorption occurs in small intestine with the help of a specialized intestinal enzyme system called conjugase.
Vitamin B_6	Absorption occurs in the jejunum.
Vitamin B_{12}	Absorption occurs mainly in the ileum and requires an intrinsic factor secreted from parietal cells of the stomach.

of ingested zinc is absorbed, and less than 2% of ingested chromium is absorbed. Besides poor absorption, excretion rates in urine are also high. About 65% of absorbed phosphorus and 50% of absorbed calcium are excreted by urine. When daily mineral intake is insufficient, increased intake may result in increased retention. For example, many women in Western countries have insufficient iron and calcium intakes, and increasing the intake generally increases storage of these minerals.

Sodium is actively transported out of the epithelial cell into the portal circulation, a process that requires ATPase carrier enzymes and energy (in the form of ATP). The transport of sodium out of the epithelial cell creates a low sodium concentration in the cell, which increases diffusion of sodium from the gut lumen into the epithelial cell. About 30 g of sodium are secreted in intestinal secretions every day. Daily sodium ingestion is about 5 to 8 g. Thus, about 25 to 35 g of sodium must be reabsorbed each day, which represents a large percentage of the body sodium stores. This explains why extreme diarrhea results in large sodium losses, which can be dangerous and even life threatening.

Gut Microbiota

The term *microbiota* means the types of organisms that are present in an environmental habitat (e.g., bacteria, viruses, eukaryotes). A microbiome is a collection of different microbes and their functions or genes found in an environmental habitat. Different parts of the body have different microbiomes; for example, the skin microbiome is different from the gut microbiome, but they are all part of the human microbiome. The adult gut contains about 1 kg (2 lb) of various bacteria (colon bacilli) totaling over 100 trillion cells, which is 10 times the number of host cells in the human body. Microbiota are present in the mouth, small intestine, and large intestine (colon). The GI tract contains an immensely complex ecology of microorganisms that can include between 500 and 1,000 distinct species of bacteria. The composition and distribution of these microorganisms vary with age, state of health, and diet.

The number and type of bacteria in the GI tract vary dramatically by region. In healthy people, the stomach and proximal small intestine contain few microorganisms, largely a result of the bactericidal activity of gastric acid. One interesting testimony to the ability of gastric acid to suppress bacterial populations is seen in patients with achlorhydria, a genetic condition that prevents secretion of gastric acid. Patients with achlorhydria who are otherwise healthy may have as many as 10,000 to 100 million microorganisms per milliliter of stomach contents. The small intestine contains a very different abundance and composition of bacteria and has a much more dynamic variation compared with the colon. The population of microbes in the small intestine is shaped by its capacity for the fast import and conversion of relatively small carbohydrates and rapid adaptation to overall nutrient availability.

In sharp contrast to the stomach and the small intestine, the colon literally teems with bacteria that are predominantly strict anaerobes (bacteria that survive only in environments virtually devoid of oxygen) (see table 5.6). Between these

TABLE 5.6 Microbial Populations in the Digestive Tract of Normal Humans

	Stomach	Jejunum	Ileum	Colon
Viable bacteria per gram	0-10^3	0-10^4	10^5-10^8	10^{10}-10^{12}
pH	3.0	6.0-7.0	7.5	6.8-7.3

two extremes is a transitional zone, usually in the ileum, where moderate numbers of aerobic and anaerobic bacteria are found. The GI tract is sterile at birth, but colonization typically begins within a few hours of birth, starting in the small intestine and progressing caudally over a period of several days. In most circumstances, a mature microbiota is established by 3 to 4 weeks of age.

The bacterial populations that comprise the microbiota of the large intestine digest carbohydrates, proteins, and lipids that escape digestion and absorption in the small intestine. The nature of the colonic microbiota is largely driven by the efficient degradation of complex indigestible carbohydrates (i.e., fiber), and the bacteria are responsible for the fermentation of small amounts of cellulose. More important, however, is the production of vitamin K, vitamin B_{12}, thiamin, riboflavin, and other substances. Vitamin K is especially important because the daily vitamin K intake in foodstuffs is normally insufficient.

Five phyla of bacteria represent most of the bacteria that comprise the human gut microbiota. In the large intestines of healthy adults, the two predominant bacterial phyla are the Firmicutes (comprised mainly of Gram-positive clostridia) and Bacteroidetes (comprised mainly of Gram-negative bacteria such as the species Bacteroides fragilis). In the average healthy person, there are approximately 160 species of bacteria in the large intestine, and very few of these are shared between unrelated individuals. In contrast, the functions contributed by these species appear to be found in almost everyone's GI tract, which clearly indicates that function is more important than the actual species of bacteria that provides it. Even so, subtle differences in the gut microbiota may matter because these may influence the efficacy of a particular function, such as the amount and type of SCFAs that are synthesized by the gut-dwelling bacteria.

The gut microbes ferment the carbohydrates (mostly fiber) that reach them in the colon. Some bacteria specialize in the initial degradation of complex plant-derived polysaccharides and effectively collaborate with other species that specialize in oligosaccharide fermentation (e.g., bifidobacteria) to liberate SCFAs and gases that are used as carbon and energy sources by other species of bacteria. The efficient conversion of complex indigestible dietary carbohydrates into SCFAs not only serves other microbes in the colon but also the human host, because up to 10% of daily energy requirements come from colonic fermentation of otherwise nondigestible polysaccharides. Some of the SCFAs, including butyrate and propionate, can influence intestinal physiology and immune function, and acetate acts as a substrate for lipogenesis and gluconeogenesis (i.e., fat and sugar synthesis, respectively). Several SCFAs have been identified as factors that can regulate systemic immune function, direct appropriate immune responses to pathogens, influence the resolution of inflammation, and modify the proinflammatory cytokines produced by adipose tissue, which is a major inflammatory organ in obesity. For people who consume a typical Western diet, most of this carbohydrate fermentation occurs in the proximal part of the colon. As carbohydrate availability becomes lower as chyme moves distally, the gut microbiota switch to other substrates, notably protein or amino acids. Fermentation of amino acids produces some potentially beneficial SCFAs, but it also produces a range of potentially harmful compounds. Some of these have been suggested to play a role in gut diseases such as colon cancer or inflammatory bowel disease (IBD). Substances such as ammonia, phenols, *p*-cresol, certain amines, and hydrogen sulfide are known to play important roles in the initiation or progression of a leaky gut. This condition is characterized by an increased permeability of the gut wall, which allows bacterial pathogens and toxins to enter the circulation and results in endotoxemia, which can lead to inflammation, DNA damage, tissue injury, and cancer progression. The ingestion of plant-based foods and fiber appears to inhibit this, which highlights the importance of maintaining gut microbiome carbohydrate fermentation.

All of this leads us to conclude that the commensal microorganisms that comprise the human microbiota are not simply passengers in the host; they may drive or at least have an important influence on certain host functions as well. In germ-free rodents, the removal of the microbiota

PROBIOTICS, PREBIOTICS, AND POLYPHENOLS

A number of dietary strategies are available for modulating the composition or the metabolic and immunological activities of the human gut microbiota. **Probiotics**, **prebiotics**, and polyphenols are among the most established. Probiotics are potentially beneficial bacteria or yeasts. Probiotics are defined as live microorganisms that, when administered in adequate amounts, may confer a health benefit on the host. Probiotics can have multiple interactions with the host, including competitive inhibition of other microbes, effects on mucosal barrier function, and interaction with immune cells (particularly antigen-presenting dendritic cells). They can be found in certain foods or can be bought as supplements. Examples include strains of the bacteria genera *Bifidobacterium* and *Lactobacillus*. The most common probiotics are the latter and are commonly referred to as lactic acid bacteria (LAB). These microbes have been used in the food industry for many years. LAB are able to convert sugars (including lactose) and other carbohydrates into lactic acid. This conversion provides the characteristic sour taste of fermented dairy foods such as yogurt. By lowering the pH, it may create fewer opportunities for "bad bacteria" to grow and provide health benefits by preventing GI infections. Probiotic bacterial cultures are intended to help the body's naturally occurring gut microbiota flora (an ecology of microbes often called the "good bacteria") reestablish themselves. They are sometimes recommended after a course of antibiotics. Claims are made that probiotics strengthen the immune system and GI barrier function to help combat infections, allergies, excessive alcohol intake, stress, exposure to toxic substances, and other diseases. Indeed, there are many examples of positive results with different probiotic strains against a range of disease states in animals and humans, but it is evident that their health-promoting traits are strain-specific. There is evidence in humans that some probiotic strains can help to reduce colonic inflammation, antibiotic-induced diarrhea, some allergic conditions, and gut and respiratory infections (Olveira and González-Molero 2016). Some studies in athletes (Pyne et al. 2015) support the use of probiotics to reduce incidence and symptom severity of upper respiratory tract infections (see chapter 13 for further details).

Instead of consuming probiotics, people can eat foods that good bacteria feed on. These foods, known as prebiotics, are indigestible food fibers and complex carbohydrates that specifically stimulate the growth of good bacteria in the bowel. Examples include inulin, oligofructose, galactofructose, galacto-oligosaccharides, and xylo-oligosaccharides. It has been argued that it may be more effective to take prebiotics that boost growth of the good bacteria already present in the gut than to take supplements of live bacteria that may be destroyed by the acidity of the stomach as soon as they are swallowed. Prebiotics are found naturally in small amounts in foods such as wheat, oats, bananas, asparagus, leeks, garlic, and onions. To get an adequate daily dose, people should look for foods that have been enriched with prebiotics or consider prebiotic supplements. As with probiotics, there is some strong evidence from animal studies that prebiotics have a degree of efficacy in the prevention or treatment of several diseases (e.g., IBD, colon cancer, obesity, type 2 diabetes, cardiovascular disease), but the data in humans thus far is rather limited and firm conclusions cannot yet be made (Vitetta et al. 2014).

Polyphenols are compounds found in plants that are associated with the well-known health benefits of fruit and vegetables. Studies indicate that they can affect human physiological processes that protect against chronic diet-associated diseases (Costa et al. 2017). Many dietary polyphenols would be poorly absorbed if it were not for the actions of the gut microbiota that transform them into absorbable, biologically active compounds. Furthermore, studies show that dietary polyphenols, particularly red grape polyphenols and cocoa-derived flavanols, modulate the human gut microbiota toward a more health-promoting profile by increasing the relative abundance of *Bifidobacterium* and *Lactobacillus* species (Tomás-Barberán et al. 2016). This suggests that the ingestion of certain functional foods can modify the gut microbiome community structure and function and contribute to the health of the gut microbiota and the human body that acts as their host.

has a dramatic impact on numerous aspects of the host's ability to function normally, including resistance to infectious diseases (Chow et al. 2010). By better understanding the mechanisms and the contribution that the microbiota make to various gut-associated and other systemic diseases, it may be possible to develop novel diets, supplements, drugs, and strategies to modulate the microbiota to treat or prevent disease.

In the healthy state, the microbiota contribute nutrients and energy to the host via the fermentation of nondigestible dietary components in the large intestine and influence the host's metabolism and immune system. However, in certain situations, negative consequences of microbiota action can include acting as sources of inflammation and infection, involvement in GI diseases, and possible contributions to the development of obesity and associated metabolic disorders (OAMD), such as type 2 diabetes. Furthermore, it is now clear that diet can have a major influence on the composition of the microbiota, which should open up new possibilities for health manipulation via diet.

It has been established that there is a potential relationship between the gut microbiome and development of an obese phenotype. An increase in relative abundance of Firmicutes and a proportional decrease in Bacteroidetes were associated with the microbiota of obese mice, and this was confirmed in a human dietary intervention study demonstrating that weight loss of obese individuals was accompanied by an increase in the relative abundance of Bacteroidetes (Remely et al. 2015). Studies have identified diet, especially fat intake, as a strong modulator of the microbiota, and there is growing evidence that high fat intake, rather than obesity per se, has a direct effect on the microbiota and associated clinical parameters (Bibbò et al. 2016). Although the exact mechanisms remain obscure, the guts of people with OAMD are believed to harbor inflammation-associated microbiomes with lower potential for butyrate production and reduced bacterial diversity and gene richness. Although the main cause of OAMD is excess dietary energy intake compared with expenditure, differences in gut microbial ecology might be an important mediator and a new therapeutic target or a biomarker to predict metabolic dysfunction and obesity in later life.

Regulation of Gastric Emptying

After ingestion, food usually takes 1 to 4 hours to leave the stomach, depending on the content of the meal. Gastric motility and secretion are to some extent automatic. Contraction of the stomach increases the intragastric pressure to push the chyme through the pyloric sphincter. Such contractions are initiated by pacemaker cells in the stomach wall. Gastric emptying is further controlled by a variety of signals directly from the stomach or the duodenum (see figure 5.15). The signals are either nervous or hormonal.

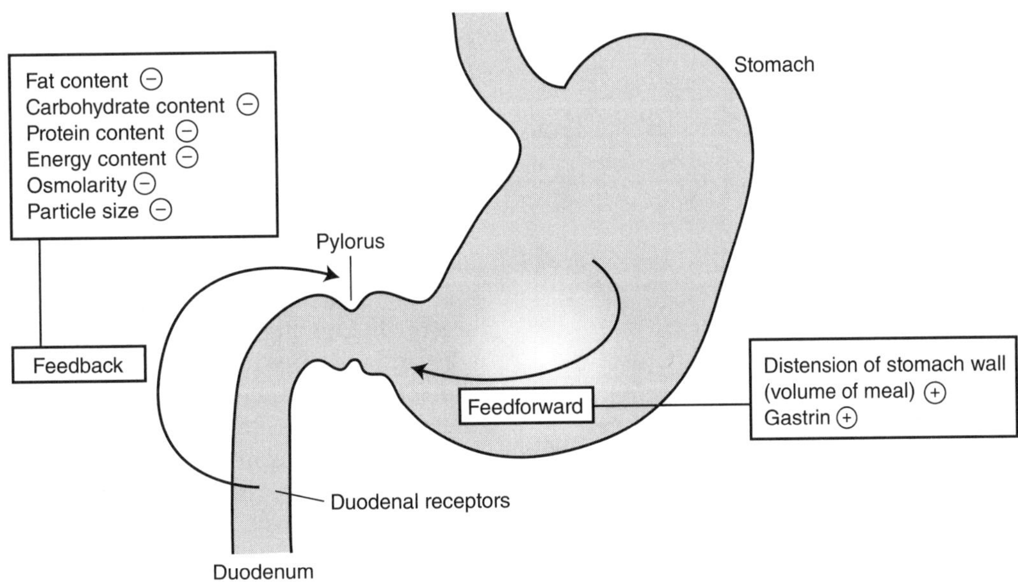

Figure 5.15 Regulation of gastric emptying by feedforward and feedback mechanisms.

The stomach signals include nervous signals caused by stretching and extension of the stomach wall and the release of the hormone gastrin by the antral mucosa. Gastrin is released in response to internal (thoughts of food and extension of the stomach) and external (sight and smell of food) stimuli. These signals from the stomach are always positive feedback signals. The increased amount of food relaxes the pyloric sphincter and increases gastric emptying. Signals from the duodenum usually provide negative feedback (i.e., inhibit gastric emptying). The duodenum contains receptors that can detect acidity, distension of the duodenum, osmolarity, and possibly carbohydrate, fat, and protein. When these receptors are stimulated, the enterogastric reflex is initiated, which increases the contraction of the pylorus. This mechanism prevents an excessive amount of chyme from being moved into the small intestine. Rapid delivery of chyme into the intestine could mean insufficient time for digestion and absorption to take place, and some nutrients would be lost in the feces. Factors that have been suggested to affect gastric emptying include the smell and sight of food, the thought of food, the volume of food, the energy density, meal or beverage temperature, osmolarity, body temperature and dehydration, type of exercise, exercise intensity, gender, and psychological stress and anxiety.

- *Volume of food.* The stomach walls can extend to accommodate larger volumes without a change in pressure. When maximal distension is reached, pressure will increase. The rate of gastric emptying of a fluid is highly dependent on the volume of the fluid in the stomach (Hunt and Donald 1954). Therefore, the rate of gastric emptying from a fluid bolus is exponential (see figure 5.16). The gastric-emptying phase is initially rapid, and when the volume is reduced, the rate of gastric emptying is reduced accordingly. The rate of gastric emptying is regulated through positive-feedback signals to the pyloric sphincter.

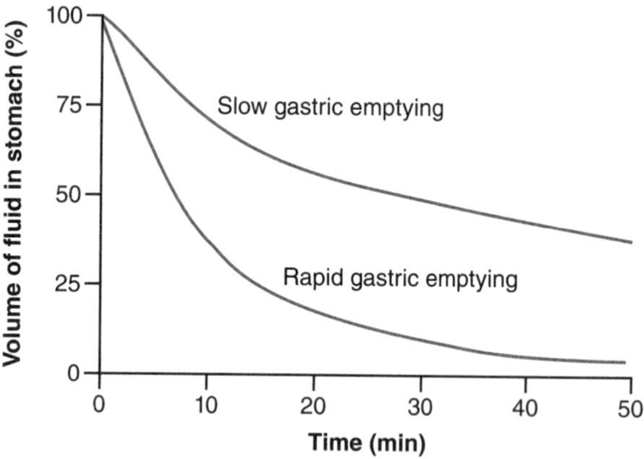

Figure 5.16 An example of a gastric-emptying curve.

- *Energy density.* Energy density has a strong effect on the rate of gastric emptying. Whether this is an effect of energy density per se or of specific nutrients is not clear. Several nutrients, such as fat, exert a strong inhibitory effect on gastric emptying. Increasing the carbohydrate or protein content of a beverage also slows gastric emptying. Carbohydrate–electrolyte solutions with 2% carbohydrate show a tendency to empty slower than water does (Vist and Maughan 1994), but solutions of 8% or more significantly inhibit gastric emptying. The energy content of the solution is more important than the osmolarity (Vist and Maughan 1995).

- *Meal or beverage temperature.* The effect of meal or beverage temperature is probably not physiologically important. Lambert et al. (1999) showed that after ingestion of a ^2H_2O-containing beverage, deuterium (^2H) accumulation in plasma was similar for drinks at varying temperatures. Gastric emptying was not different despite the differences in beverage temperature. This study reflects the findings in the literature that, generally, no effects of meal temperature have been found on the rate of gastric emptying. Some studies, however, have found a reduction in the rate of gastric emptying with very cold or very hot drinks, and gastric emptying may be influenced by beverage temperature when the intragastric temperature is much higher or lower than body temperature.

- *Osmolarity.* Osmolarity has always been considered an important factor in controlling the rate of gastric emptying. Increased beverage osmolarity not only increases gastric secretions but also increases intestinal secretions. Osmolarity is therefore an important factor to consider when selecting a beverage for ingestion during exercise. Higher osmolarity may reduce gastric emptying and decrease water absorption. In addition, osmolarity and the concentration of simple carbohydrates are related. A high-energy or high-carbohydrate content is usually related to high osmolarity, and the effects of concentration and osmolarity are therefore difficult to distinguish. Studies suggest that although osmolarity reduces the rate of gastric emptying, this factor is not important in beverages with osmolarities in the range of 200 to 400 mOsm/L (Brouns et al. 1995). This range is typical for most sports drinks (see table 5.4).

Osmolarity might be more important in beverages with extremely high osmolarities (> 500 mOsm/L).

- *Body temperature and dehydration.* Studies in hot conditions have shown that dehydration and hyperthermia can slow gastric emptying (Neufer, Young, and Sawka 1989; Rehrer et al. 1990). Because subjects in these studies became dehydrated and hyperthermic at the same time, determining whether dehydration, hyperthermia, or a combination of the two was responsible for the reduced gastric-emptying rate is not possible.
- *Type of exercise and exercise intensity.* Below 80% of $\dot{V}O_2$max, the rate of gastric emptying does not seem to be affected by exercise intensity. Above 80% of $\dot{V}O_2$max, there may be a reduction in fluid and nutrient delivery to the small intestine (Costill and Saltin 1974; Sole and Noakes 1989). From a practical point of view, however, this reduction may not be important because exercise intensities of greater than 80% of $\dot{V}O_2$max generally cannot be sustained long enough to cause a limitation in fluid or carbohydrate delivery. Eating and drinking at these high intensities are problematic anyway because of exercise-induced hyperventilation. Gastric emptying of liquids is slowed during brief, intermittent, high-intensity exercise compared with rest or steady-state moderate exercise (Leiper, Prentice, et al. 2001). Gastric emptying measured after a five-a-side indoor soccer match decreased even though the average intensity of the activity was only 54% to 63% of $\dot{V}O_2$max (Leiper, Broad, and Maughan 2001). The relatively short bouts of very high-intensity exercise were clearly enough to reduce gastric emptying.
- *Gender.* Women have slower gastric-emptying rates than men, although rates seem to increase somewhat during ovulation (Notivol et al. 1984). Women are reportedly more prone to GI complaints after prolonged endurance exercise (Prado de Oliveira, Burini, and Jeukendrup 2014). This finding could be related to a slower rate of gastric emptying.
- *Psychological stress.* Stress affects GI motility and the rate of gastric emptying. This reduction in the rate of gastric emptying is usually related to changes in circulating hormone concentrations because of stress. Some of these hormones (e.g., epinephrine) reduce blood flow to the GI tract.

There are considerable differences in the rate of gastric emptying between individuals. Some people empty 70% to 80% of a solution in 15 minutes, whereas others empty only 20% to 30% of that same solution in 15 minutes. The reasons for these individual differences are not known, but diet has been suggested as an important factor. The GI tract might adapt to the intake of certain nutrients, and a high habitual fat intake may result in a high gastric-emptying rate of fat (Jeukendrup 2017b). Whatever the mechanisms, these observations highlight the importance of individual fluid intake recommendations.

Gastrointestinal Problems During and After Exercise

GI complaints are common among endurance athletes. An estimated 30% to 50% of distance runners experience intestinal problems related to exercise (Prado de Oliveira, Burini, and Jeukendrup 2014). Bill Rogers, the legend who won the Boston Marathon and the New York City Marathon four times each between 1975 and 1980, said "More marathons are won or lost in the porta-toilets than at the dinner table" (Prado de Oliveira, Burini, and Jeukendrup 2014). This comment illustrates the magnitude of the problem for endurance athletes and for long-distance runners in particular.

The most common complaints include nausea, gastroesophageal reflux (or heartburn), abdominal pains, loose stool, diarrhea or bloody diarrhea, and vomiting. The complaints are normally divided into two categories: symptoms of the upper intestinal tract and symptoms of the lower intestinal tract (see the sidebar Frequently Reported Gastrointestinal and Related Problems). Several symptoms are not classified as either upper or lower GI problems but might be related to the GI tract (e.g., stitch).

Of the 471 marathoners who completed a survey, 83% reported suffering from GI problems occasionally or frequently during or after running, 53% reported the urge to defecate, and 38% reported diarrhea. Women were more likely than men to experience these problems. Among 155 mountain marathoners, 24% had intestinal symptoms and two dropped out because of GI troubles (Riddoch and Trinick 1988).

A study by Keeffe et al. (1984) surveyed 1,700 participants after a marathon race. Lower GI symptoms such as diarrhea, abdominal cramps, urge to defecate, flatulence, and GI bleeding were found to be more common than upper GI symptoms such as nausea, vomiting, heartburn, bloating, and side ache (stitch). The most common symptom was the urge to defecate (36%-39% of the participants) during and immediately after running. Bowel movements (35%) and diarrhea (19%) were reported frequently and immediately after running. During the race,

GASTROINTESTINAL AND RELATED PROBLEMS FREQUENTLY REPORTED BY ATHLETES

Upper GI Symptoms

- Heartburn
- Bloating
- Vomiting

Lower GI Symptoms

- Urge to defecate
- Loose stool
- Diarrhea
- Bleeding

Related Symptoms

- Nausea
- Dizziness
- Side ache (stitch)
- Urge to urinate

some runners (16%-18%) had to stop to defecate, and some runners (8%-10%) had to stop because of diarrhea. Bloody bowel movements were reported by 1% to 2% of the participants. Similar results were obtained by Jeukendrup, Vet-Joop, et al. (2000), who found that 93% of the participants of a long-distance triathlon reported at least one symptom of GI discomfort; 29% had symptoms serious enough to affect performance.

Lower GI symptoms are more often observed in women than in men, and some symptoms are more frequently reported by younger participants. Problems seem to occur more frequently during running than during activities such as cycling or swimming, possibly because of the vertical movements of the gut during running. People with preexisting GI issues (such as reflux, lactose intolerance, or irritable bowel syndrome) are more likely to get GI symptoms during competition.

Causes of Gastrointestinal Problems

The causes of GI symptoms are not completely understood. The symptoms are difficult to investigate because they are often specific to race situations and cannot be simulated in a laboratory. Nevertheless, some laboratory studies have been performed, and field studies have correlated the symptoms with nutritional intake and other factors. From these studies, several potential causes and contributors have been identified. These can be divided into three categories: (1) physiological, (2) mechanical, and (3) nutritional.

Physiological Causes

Physiological causes of GI symptoms include reduced blood flow and increased anxiety (especially before competition). During exercise, blood flow is preferentially redirected to the working muscles, and blood flow to the gut can be reduced by as much as 80%. The low blood supply can compromise gut function and result in commonly experienced GI symptoms such as cramping. In severe cases, it can result in ischemic colitis (injury of the large intestine due to inadequate blood supply). These cases have been reported after prolonged exercise in the heat during which dehydration likely occurred, and this may have further reduced blood flow to the intestine by reducing total blood volume. With training, a decrease in blood flow during exercise may become less pronounced, but no clear evidence shows that less fit people are more prone to symptomatic ischemia. Anxiety has an effect on hormone secretion, which in turn can affect gut motility, resulting in incomplete absorption and loose stool.

Mechanical Causes

The mechanical causes of GI problems are related to impact or posture. GI bleeding is common among runners, and this is thought to be a result of the repetitive high-impact mechanics of running and subsequent damage to the intestinal lining. This repetitive gastric jostling is also thought to contribute to lower GI symptoms such as flatulence, diarrhea, and urgency. Estimates of the incidence of occult blood (blood in feces) after a race range from 8% to 85% mostly because of the wide range of race distances in various studies. The longer the distance, the greater the incidence. As many as 16% of runners in one study reported having bloody diarrhea on at least one occasion after a race or hard run. The mechanical trauma suffered by the gut from the repetitive impact of running in combination with gut ischemia is probably the cause of the bleeding. Presence of bloody bowel movements after endurance events raises the possibility of ischemic colitis and hemorrhagic gastritis.

Posture can also have an effect on GI symptoms. For example, in a cyclist, upper GI symptoms are more prevalent possibly because of increased pressure on the abdomen due to the cycling position, specifically when in the aero position. Swallowing air as a result of increased respiration and drinking from water bottles can also result in mild to moderate stomach distress.

Nutritional Causes

Nutrition can also have a strong influence on GI distress. Fiber, fat, protein, and fructose have all been associated with a greater risk of developing GI symptoms. Dehydration, possibly because of inadequate fluid intake, may also exacerbate the symptoms. A study by Rehrer, van Kemenade, et al. (1992) demonstrated a link between nutritional practices and GI complaints during a half-Ironman triathlon. GI problems were more likely to occur with the ingestion of fiber, fat, protein, and concentrated carbohydrate solutions during the triathlon. Beverages with high osmolarities (>500 mOsm/L) were responsible for some of the reported complaints. The intake of dairy products may also be linked to the occurrence of GI distress. Mild lactose intolerance is common and could result in increased bowel activity and mild diarrhea (Noakes 1986). Although some risk factors have been identified, it is still unclear why some people seem to be more prone to develop GI problems than others. To minimize GI distress, all these risk factors must be taken into account. Milk products and fiber as well as high fat and protein intakes must be avoided 24 hours before competition and during exercise. A detailed discussion of preventative measures follows.

Prevention of Gastrointestinal Problems

To help prevent GI distress, a few guidelines should be considered. Although these suggestions are based on limited research (Prado de Oliveira, Burini, and Jeukendrup 2014), anecdotally they seem to be effective. These guidelines are especially for competition as this is where most gastrointestinal problems are seen, but many could also be applied to training if this is where the issues occur.

- *Avoid products that contain lactose, because even mild lactose intolerance can cause problems during exercise.* Avoid milk completely or drink lactose-free milk. Soy, rice, and almond milks generally do not contain lactose.
- *Avoid high-fiber foods the day of or even in the days before competition.* For the athlete in training, a diet with adequate fiber will help keep the bowel regular. Fiber before race day is different. Fiber is not digestible, so any fiber that is eaten essentially passes through the intestinal tract. Increased bowel movements during exercise are not desirable, will accelerate fluid loss, and may result in unnecessary gas production that might cause GI discomfort (e.g., cramping). Especially for people who are prone to develop GI symptoms, a low-fiber diet the day before (or even a couple of days before) competition is recommended. Choose processed white foods such as regular pasta, white rice, and plain bagels instead of whole-grain bread, high-fiber cereals, and brown rice. Check food labels for fiber content. Most fruits and vegetables are high in fiber, but zucchini, tomatoes, olives, grapes, and grapefruit all have less than 1 g of fiber per serving.
- *Avoid aspirin and nonsteroidal anti-inflammatory drugs (NSAIDs) such as ibuprofen.* Athletes commonly use aspirin and NSAIDs, but they have been shown to increase intestinal permeability and may increase the incidence of GI complaints. The use of NSAIDs in the 24 hours before competition is discouraged.
- *Avoid high-fructose foods (especially drinks that exclusively contain fructose as the carbohydrate component).* Fructose is found in fruit and in most processed sweets (candy, cookies, and so forth) in the form of high-fructose corn syrup. Some fruit juices are almost exclusively fructose. Fructose is absorbed by the intestines more slowly, and fructose is much less tolerated than glucose (and may lead to cramping, loose stool, and diarrhea). In chapter 6, we will discuss how fructose in combination with glucose may not cause problems and may even be better tolerated.

- *Avoid dehydration.* Dehydration can exacerbate GI symptoms. Start races well hydrated (see chapter 9 for further details).
- *Practice new nutrition strategies.* Experiment with prerace and race-day nutrition plans many times before race day to figure out what does and does not work and to reduce the chances that GI issues will ruin the race.
- *Train with carbohydrate intake during exercise, and make sure carbohydrate intake in the weeks leading up to an important event is relatively high.* This so called train-high approach may increase the gut's capacity to absorb carbohydrate during exercise; therefore, it might reduce the residual volume in the intestine and reduce the risk of GI discomfort or problems.

Key Points

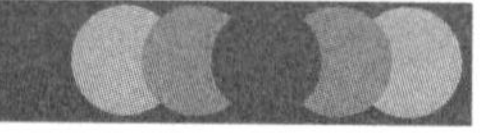

- The primary function of the gastrointestinal (or alimentary) tract, a 6 to 8 m (20-26 ft) tube that reaches from the mouth to the anus, is to provide the body with nutrients.
- Chewing food makes the food particles smaller and increases the surface area of the food. This increases the contact area for digestive enzymes. Chewing also mixes the food particles with saliva and digestive enzymes.
- In the stomach, food is mixed with gastric secretions (hydrochloric acid and digestive enzymes).
- Pancreatic juices and bile are added to the chyme in the duodenum to digest carbohydrate, fat, and protein. Specialized enzymes split these macronutrients into the smallest subunits for absorption. Bile is added to emulsify lipid droplets and facilitate digestion and absorption.
- About 90% to 95% of all absorption takes place in the duodenum and jejunum (the first parts of the small intestine).
- The large intestine is a storage place for undigested food residues, and the final water and electrolyte absorption occur there.
- The microbiota in the large intestine digest and ferment carbohydrates, proteins, and lipids that escape digestion and absorption in the small intestine. The bacteria are also responsible for fermenting small amounts of cellulose and producing vitamin K.
- Dietary or supplemented probiotics, prebiotics, and polyphenols can modulate the composition or the metabolic and immunological activity of the human gut microbiota, which can have some positive benefits for health.
- Gastric emptying is influenced by volume of food, energy density, osmolarity, dehydration, and psychological stress and, to a lesser degree, by exercise intensity, meal temperature, and gender.
- Gastrointestinal problems are common, mainly among endurance athletes, and their incidence is increased by physiological, mechanical, and nutrition factors.

Recommended Readings

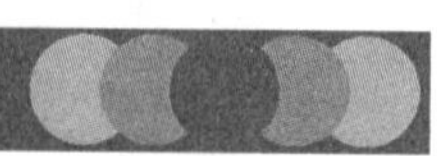

Brouns, F., and E. Beckers. 1993. Is the gut an athletic organ? Digestion, absorption and exercise. *Sports Medicine* 15:242-257.

Guyton, A.C., and J.E. Hall. 2005. *Textbook of medical physiology.* Philadelphia: Saunders.

de Oliveira, E.P., R.C. Burini, and A. Jeukendrup. 2014. Gastrointestinal complaints during exercise: Prevalence, etiology, and nutritional recommendations. *Sports Medicine* 44 (Suppl 1): S79-S85.

Carbohydrate

Objectives

After studying this chapter, you should be able to do the following:

- Describe the main biochemical pathways involved in carbohydrate metabolism
- Describe the changes that occur in carbohydrate metabolism at different intensities of exercise
- Describe how blood glucose concentrations are maintained and regulated
- Describe the metabolic and performance effects of carbohydrate ingestion 3 to 4 hours before exercise
- Describe the metabolic and performance effects of carbohydrate ingestion 1 hour before exercise
- Describe the metabolic and performance effects of carbohydrate ingestion during exercise
- Describe the mechanisms involved in glycogen synthesis
- Give generally accepted guidelines for carbohydrate intake before and during exercise
- Give generally accepted guidelines for carbohydrate intake to improve recovery in the short term and long term
- Describe the dietary requirements for carbohydrate in a variety of sports

One hundred years ago, beef was believed to be the most important component of an athlete's diet, but now pasta, bread, and rice seem to form the central part of an athlete's diet. Athletes are often advised to eat a high-carbohydrate diet, consume carbohydrate before exercise, ensure adequate carbohydrate intake during exercise, and replenish carbohydrate stores as soon as possible after exercise. More recently, it has been suggested that a low-carbohydrate approach may work for athletes, but, as we will see in the next two chapters, the foundation of that is rather thin, and it may only be appropriate for certain activities.

Since the beginning of the 20th century, carbohydrate intake has been known to be related to exercise performance. The availability of carbohydrate as a substrate for skeletal muscle contraction and the central nervous system (e.g., the brain) is important for endurance exercise performance. Carbohydrate availability may influence not only the performance of prolonged exercise but also the performance of intermittent-intensity and high-intensity exercise. Because carbohydrate is the most important fuel for the central nervous system, various cognitive tasks and motor skills that play a crucial role in skill sports may also be affected by carbohydrate availability.

Various strategies have been developed over the past 30 years to optimize carbohydrate availability and athletic performance. Generally, this can be achieved through carbohydrate intake before exercise to replenish muscle and liver glycogen stores and carbohydrate intake during exercise to maintain blood glucose levels and high rates of glucose oxidation derived from the plasma. In this chapter, the effects of carbohydrate on exercise metabolism and performance are explained. The results of some classic experimental studies

CARBOHYDRATE INTAKE AND DENTAL HEALTH

Much has been written in the popular press about the potential negative effects of sports drinks on dental health. Frequent intake of acidic drinks (pH 3-4) during training and competition could lead to dental erosion, which is characterized by painless chemical dissolution of the dental hard tissue not involving bacterial action. Although numerous factors can cause enamel erosion, the acidic properties of acidic drinks (soft drinks, sports drinks, fruit juices) such as pH, type of acid, and buffering capacity are among the principal factors in the etiology of enamel erosion. Manufacturers are looking into ways to reduce enamel erosion by increasing the pH of beverages or adding calcium. One study showed that a sports drink was as erosive as orange juice but that a modified drink with a higher pH and calcium had an erosive effect equal to water (Venables et al. 2005).

are discussed along with practical implications that arise from this work. We specifically address carbohydrate intake in the days before competition (or training), carbohydrate intake in the hours before competition, carbohydrate intake during competition or training, and carbohydrate intake after training or competition.

First, we start with a short history of the role of carbohydrate in sports nutrition, beginning with the first studies that investigated the role of carbohydrate in the body and the effects of carbohydrate on exercise performance.

History

Krogh and Lindhard (1920) were probably the first investigators to recognize the importance of carbohydrate as a fuel during exercise. In their study, subjects consumed a high-fat diet (bacon, butter, cream, eggs, and cabbage) for 3 days and then ate a high-carbohydrate diet (potatoes, flour, bread, cake, marmalade, and sugar) for 3 days. The subjects performed a 2-hour exercise test and reported various symptoms of fatigue when they consumed the high-fat diet. When they consumed the high-carbohydrate diet, the exercise was reported to be easy. The investigators also demonstrated that after several days of a low-carbohydrate, high-fat diet, the average RER during 2 hours of cycling declined to 0.80 compared with 0.85 to 0.90 when a mixed diet was consumed. Conversely, when subjects ate a high-carbohydrate, low-fat diet, RER increased to 0.95.

Important observations were also made by Levine, Gordon, and Derick (1924). They measured blood glucose in some of the participants of the 1923 Boston Marathon and observed that in most runners, glucose concentrations declined markedly after the race. These investigators suggested that low blood glucose levels were a cause of fatigue. To test that hypothesis, they encouraged several participants in the same marathon 1 year later to consume carbohydrate (in the form of candy) during the race. This practice, in combination with consuming a high-carbohydrate diet before the race, prevented hypoglycemia (low blood glucose) and significantly improved running performance (i.e., time to complete the race).

The importance of carbohydrate for improving exercise capacity was further demonstrated by Dill, Edwards, and Talbott (1932). These investigators let their dogs, Joe and Sally, run without feeding them carbohydrate. The dogs became hypoglycemic and fatigued after 4 to 6 hours. When the test was repeated with the only difference being that the dogs were fed carbohydrate during exercise, the dogs ran for 17 to 23 hours.

Christensen (1932) showed that with increasing exercise intensity, the proportion of carbohydrate use increased. A group of Scandinavian scientists (Bergstrom et al. 1966, 1967a) expanded this work in the late 1960s by reintroducing the muscle **biopsy** technique. These studies indicated the critical role of muscle glycogen. The improved performance after a high-carbohydrate diet was linked with the higher muscle glycogen concentrations observed after such a diet. A high-carbohydrate diet (approximately 70% of dietary energy from carbohydrate) elevated muscle glycogen stores and seemed to enhance endurance capacity compared with normal-carbohydrate (about 50%) and low-carbohydrate (about 10%) diets. These observations led to the recommendations to **carboload** (i.e., eat a high-carbohydrate diet) before competition (Costill and Miller 1980; Sherman and Costill 1984).

In the 1980s, the effects of carbohydrate intake during exercise on exercise performance and metabolism were further investigated (Coyle and Coggan 1984; Coyle et al. 1986). Costill et al. (1973) were the first to study the contributions of ingested carbohydrate to total energy expenditure, and in the following years, studies were conducted using isotopic tracers (e.g., ^{14}C-glucose or ^{13}C-glucose) to investigate differences in oxidation rates and metabolism of different types of carbohydrate, different amounts of carbohydrate, different feeding schedules, and other factors that influence the efficacy of carbohydrate ingestion (Jeukendrup 2004). Although Costill et al. (1973) concluded that ingested carbohydrate was not oxidized to any major extent, later studies have convincingly shown that ingested carbohydrate is an important energy source during prolonged exercise.

MUSCLE GLYCOGEN UNITS

In the literature, muscle glycogen is expressed in various ways. The units used most frequently are millimole glycosyl (glucose) units per kilogram of dry mass or per kilogram of wet mass. To express the results per kilogram of dry mass, the muscle biopsy sample must be freeze dried. All the water is removed by placing the frozen biopsy sample in a freeze dryer. Muscle contains approximately 75% to 80% water, and to convert values from wet mass to dry mass the concentration is usually multiplied by 4.5.

Role of Carbohydrate

As discussed in chapter 1, carbohydrate plays many roles in the human body, but one of its main functions is to provide energy for the contracting muscle. Glycogen, the storage form of carbohydrate, is found mainly in muscle and the liver.

Muscle Glycogen

Muscle glycogen is a readily available energy source for the working muscle. The glycogen content of skeletal muscle at rest is approximately 65-90 mmol glucosyl units/kg w.w. [see the sidebar Muscle Glycogen Units]), which equates to 300 to 400 g of carbohydrate. (This can be up to 900 g in extreme cases in athletes with a large muscle mass.) The rate at which muscle glycogen is oxidized depends largely on exercise intensity. At low to moderate exercise intensity, most of the energy can be obtained from oxidative phosphorylation of acetyl-CoA derived from both carbohydrate and fat. As the exercise intensity increases to high levels, the oxidation of carbohydrate and fat cannot by itself meet the energy requirements. Muscle glycogen becomes the most important substrate because anaerobic energy delivery (ATP resynthesis from glycolysis) is mostly derived from the breakdown of muscle glycogen. Figure 6.1 shows the effects of exercise intensity on muscle glycogen breakdown and liver glucose output. At very high exercise intensity, muscle glycogen is broken down very rapidly and becomes nearly depleted in a relatively short time when this type of exercise is performed intermittently.

Liver Glycogen

The main role of glycogen in the liver is to maintain a constant blood glucose level. Glucose is the main (and in normal circumstances, the only) fuel used by the brain. The liver is often referred to as the glucoregulator or glucostat—the organ responsible for the regulation of the blood glucose concentration. An average liver weighs approximately 1.5 kg (3 lb), and approximately 80 to 110 g of glycogen are stored in the liver of an adult human in the postabsorptive state. Glycogen is broken down in the liver to glucose and then released into the circulatory system. The kidneys also store some glycogen and release glucose into the blood, but from a quantitative point of view, the kidneys are far less important than the liver. In this book, the terms *liver glucose output* or **hepatic glucose output** are used for the release of glucose from the liver and kidneys. This release is also often called **endogenous** glucose production. Glycogen that is broken down in the muscle is not released as glucose into the circulation because muscle lacks the enzyme G6P (the enzyme that removes a phosphate group from G6P) (figure 6.2). After glucose has been phosphorylated in the muscle cell by the enzyme hexokinase (the enzyme that attaches a phosphate group to glucose), it cannot be dephosphorylated (see chapter 3). Because a phosphorylated glucose molecule cannot be transported out of the cell, G6P is trapped within the muscle cell. The glucose will therefore be stored or oxidized within the muscle.

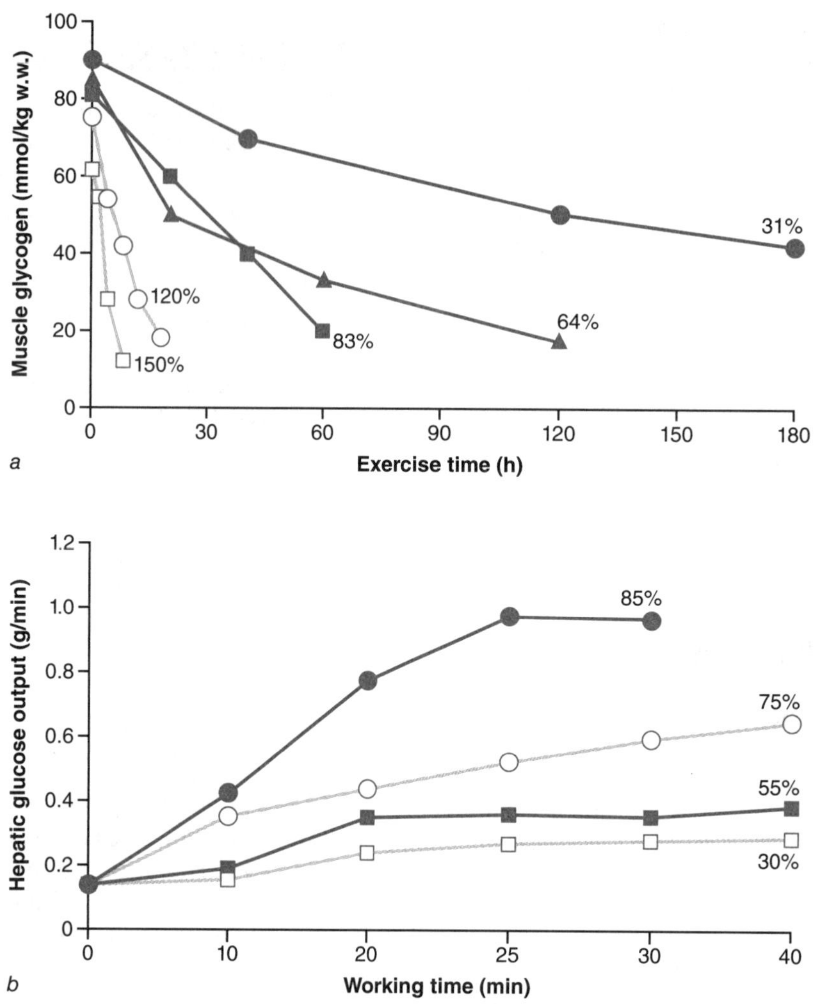

Figure 6.1 The effects of exercise intensity (shown as a percentage of $\dot{V}O_2max$) on *(a)* muscle glycogen breakdown and *(b)* liver glucose output.

Data from Gollick, Peel, and Saltin (1974).

The liver has a much higher concentration of glycogen (per kilogram of tissue) than muscle does; however, due to its mass, muscle contains more glycogen than the liver (in absolute terms, 300-600 g versus 80-110 g). After an overnight fast, the liver glycogen content can be reduced to low levels (< 20 g) because tissues such as the brain use glucose at a rate of about 0.1 g/min in resting conditions. During exercise, the rate of glucose use by tissues other than muscle does not change much (about 0.1 g/min).

Circulation (of blood) can be regarded as a sink (see figure 6.3) from which various tissues, especially exercising muscle, can tap glucose. An extremely precise mechanism, however, regulates the blood glucose concentration in this sink at 4.0 to 4.5 mmol/L. (This is equivalent to a plasma glucose concentration of 5-6 mmol/L because the concentration of free glucose inside the red blood cells is somewhat less than that in the plasma; see the sidebar Differences Between Whole Blood, Plasma, and Serum). Note that 5.55 mmol/L equates to 1 g of glucose per liter. When the blood glucose concentration drops, the liver releases glucose. If the demand for glucose is less, the liver produces less glucose or takes up glucose from the bloodstream to synthesize glycogen. After a meal, for instance, when a large amount of glucose enters the liver through the hepatic portal vein, the liver uses this glucose to synthesize glycogen. Despite the changes in glucose flux, both after feeding and during exercise (or fasting), normoglycemia is usually nicely maintained.

Liver glycogen plays an important role in regulating the blood glucose concentration at rest and during exercise. Although this has been known for many years, the exact role of the liver during exercise is still not completely understood because

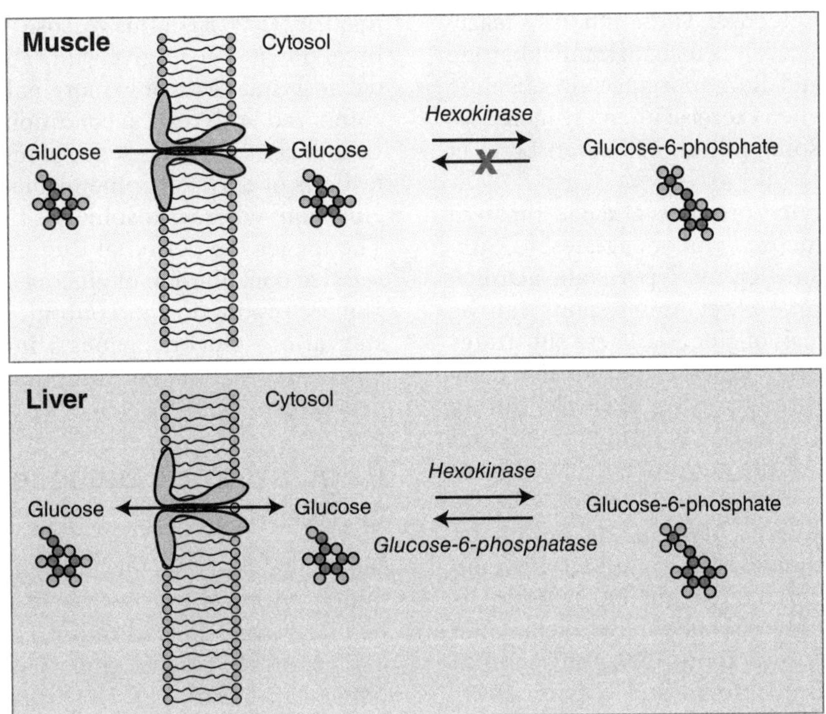

Figure 6.2 Glucose enters the cytosol of the cell by facilitated transport. In the cell it is phosphorylated by hexokinase, and after it is phosphorylated, glucose cannot leave the cell. The exceptions are liver and kidney cells. Liver and kidney cells have an enzyme called glucose-6-phosphatase that reverses the glucokinase reaction.

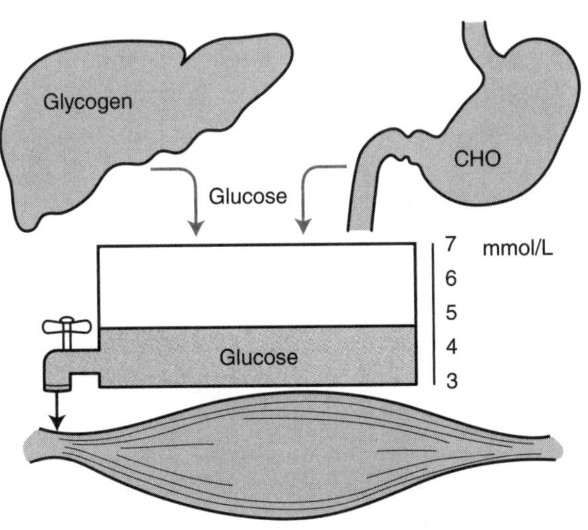

Figure 6.3 The bloodstream can be regarded as a sink in which the blood glucose concentration is accurately controlled. During exercise, muscle glucose uptake increases dramatically. To prevent the blood glucose concentration from dropping, the liver must produce glucose at an equally high rate.

liver glycogen is notoriously difficult to measure. Although some studies using liver biopsies were performed in the 1960s, limited information is available about liver glycogen synthesis after exercise and its potential effect on performance. A noninvasive technique that has been used to address this problem is nuclear magnetic resonance (NMR) imaging. Using ^{13}C-NMR, Casey et al. (2000) measured liver glycogen concentrations after exercise and during 4 hours of recovery. They observed that liver glycogen resynthesis was evident after glucose and sucrose ingestion but not after water ingestion. Relatively small amounts of carbohydrate were ingested (1 g/kg of body weight), and these amounts were sufficient to initiate postexercise liver glycogen resynthesis. More recently, studies have demonstrated that liver glycogen is more readily replenished with fructose, galactose, or sucrose than with glucose (Decombaz et al. 2011; Fuchs et al. 2016), although the practical implications of these findings remain uncertain (Gonzalez 2016).

Early studies in Scandinavia using liver biopsies showed that liver glycogen is decreased by about 50% after 1 hour of exercise at 75% of $\dot{V}O_2max$ (Nilsson and Hultman 1973). Later studies have used stable isotopes to indirectly measure the oxidation of liver glucose. These studies clearly show that liver glycogen is a significant substrate during exercise, and its importance (in absolute terms) increases when exercise intensity increases (Gonzales 2016; Romijn et al. 1993; van Loon et al. 2001).

The liver can also produce glucose through newly formed glucose (gluconeogenesis). Substrates such as lactate, glycerol, pyruvate, alanine, glutamine, and some other amino acids can be used for the synthesis of glucose. These substrates are usually formed in other organs of the body and transported to the liver. For example, during exercise, most of the lactate is formed in skeletal muscle, and most of the glycerol is from adipose tissue.

In resting conditions, the glucose output by the liver is approximately 150 mg/min (0.8 mmol/min. About 60% of this output (90 mg/min) is derived from liver glycogenolysis (the breakdown of liver glycogen), and about 40% (60 mg/min) is gluconeogenesis (Hultman and Nilsson 1971; Nilsson and Hultman 1973). During exercise, the liver glucose output increases dramatically. During high-intensity exercise (>75% of $\dot{V}O_2max$), liver glucose output increases to about 1 g/min, and the majority (>90%) of this glucose is derived from the breakdown of liver glycogen. The rate of gluconeogenesis increases only marginally during exercise compared with resting conditions. Gluconeogenesis increases in the presence of high plasma concentrations of cortisol, epinephrine (adrenaline), and glucagon, whereas insulin has the opposite effect. The longer the period of exercise, the greater the relative contribution of gluconeogenesis is to liver glucose production and output. During periods of starvation, gluconeogenesis increases, whereas after carbohydrate consumption gluconeogenesis decreases.

Regulation of Glucose Concentration

Blood glucose concentrations are normally maintained within a narrow range (a normal resting blood glucose concentration is usually between 4-4.5 mmol/L; plasma glucose concentrations are between 5-6 mmol/L). Hormones play a key role in this regulation. In resting conditions, **insulin** is the most important glucoregulatory hormone. It increases the uptake of glucose into various tissues. After a meal, plasma insulin concentra-

DIFFERENCES BETWEEN WHOLE BLOOD, PLASMA, AND SERUM

Blood refers to the red liquid in the arteries and veins. It is composed of cells (red blood cells, or erythrocytes; white blood cells, or leukocytes; and cell fragments called platelets, or thrombocytes) that are suspended in a fluid called plasma. The plasma contains proteins, lipoproteins, electrolytes, and small organic molecules such as glucose, fatty acids, glycerol, lactate, and amino acids, but by weight it is about 93% water.

In a blood sample, plasma can be separated from the cellular components by centrifugation if an anticoagulant (a substance that prevents the activation of clot formation) is added to the blood sample soon after it is collected. Typical anticoagulants that can be used include heparin, oxalate, citrate, and ethylene-diamine-tetraacetate (EDTA). If an anticoagulant is not added, the blood will clot within a matter of minutes. Centrifuging the clotted blood will separate the cellular elements and the insoluble clotting protein fibrin from the fluid; this fluid is called serum.

Hence, the difference between plasma and serum is that plasma has an anticoagulant in it and still contains soluble fibrinogen, whereas serum does not. Substances such as glucose can be measured in whole blood (after lysing all the blood cells), plasma, or serum, but the glucose concentrations measured in each will be a little different because the concentration of free glucose inside the red blood cells is somewhat less than in the plasma. This means that whole blood will have a lower glucose concentration than plasma or serum. The concentration of most substances in plasma is pretty much the same as in serum if the blood is not left too long to clot before centrifugation takes place. If left at room temperature, blood cell metabolism will use up glucose at a rate of about 0.5 mmol/L/h. In this situation, the serum glucose concentration will be less than in plasma if the latter was obtained by centrifugation immediately after blood sampling.

tions increase, and as a result, glucose uptake by muscle, liver, and other tissues increases. Insulin promotes not only the uptake but also the storage of the glucose. Glycogen synthase activity increases, and glycogen phosphorylase (the enzyme responsible for the breakdown of glycogen) decreases. Glucagon is the most important counteractive hormone. Secretion of glucagon causes the breakdown of liver glycogen and the release of glucose into the circulation. Several other hormones may have a role in the regulation of blood glucose concentrations, including growth hormone, cortisol, somatostatin, and catecholamines.

During exercise, catecholamine release reduces the secretion of insulin by the pancreas, and plasma insulin concentrations can decrease to extremely low levels. Muscle glucose uptake is enhanced by contraction-stimulated glucose transport. As mentioned previously, however, despite dramatically increased glucose uptake by the muscle during exercise, blood glucose levels are well maintained in most conditions.

But a mismatch between glucose uptake and glucose production by the liver occurs during high-intensity exercise. At an intensity of approximately 80% of $\dot{V}O_2$max or more, the liver produces glucose at a higher rate than it is taken up by the muscle. This increased hepatic glucose release is most likely caused by neural feedforward mechanisms and results in slightly elevated blood glucose concentration compared with rest. Another situation in which a mismatch occurs is during the later stages of prolonged exercise. As liver glycogen becomes depleted, the rate of glucose production may become insufficient to compensate for the glucose uptake by the muscle and other tissues. As a result, hypoglycemia develops, and blood glucose levels sometimes drop below 3 mmol/L.

Hypoglycemia

If blood glucose concentrations drop below a critical level (often 3 mmol/L), the rate of glucose uptake by the brain is insufficient to meet its metabolic requirements, and symptoms of hypoglycemia result. Hypoglycemia is characterized by a variety of symptoms, including dizziness, nausea, cold sweat, reduced mental alertness and ability to concentrate, loss of motor skill, increased heart rate, excessive hunger, and disorientation. Hypoglycemia is a common problem in exercise and sport and can be treated by simply consuming carbohydrate. Hypoglycemia has received considerable attention because preexercise carbohydrate feeding seems to induce **reactive hypoglycemia** (also referred to as rebound hypoglycemia). Although the symptoms of hypoglycemia that may occur during prolonged exercise are identical to those resulting from rebound hypoglycemia, the cause is very different. This topic is discussed in more detail in the section Carbohydrate Intake 30 Minutes to 60 Minutes Before Exercise.

Carbohydrate Use and Replenishment During Periods of Intense Training

Athletes often train (or compete) on consecutive days, and in these cases, rapid replenishment of muscle glycogen can be crucial. Costill et al. (1971) reported that in subjects running 16 km (10 mi) on 3 consecutive days, a diet that contains only moderate amounts of carbohydrate (40%-50%) may not be enough to fully restore muscle glycogen (see figure 6.4). A marked decrease in muscle glycogen occurred immediately after the run, and although some glycogen was synthesized before

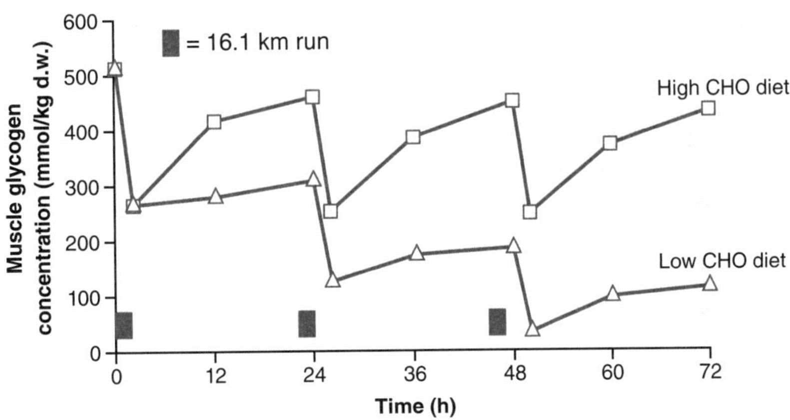

Figure 6.4 Muscle glycogen concentration after repeated bouts of running.
Data from Costill, Bowers, Barman, K. Sparks (1971).

the run the next day, the starting muscle glycogen concentrations were lower. After 3 days of running, the muscle glycogen concentration had dropped considerably.

Sherman et al. (1993) fed subjects a diet containing either 5 or 10 g of carbohydrate per kilogram of body weight per day during 7 days of training. The diet containing 5 g of carbohydrate resulted in a decline in muscle glycogen concentration in the first 5 days, which was then maintained for the remainder of the study. With the high-carbohydrate diet (10 g per kilogram of body weight per day), muscle glycogen concentrations were maintained despite daily training.

In another study, well-trained cyclists exercised 2 hours per day at 65% of $\dot{V}O_2max$ (Coyle et al. 2001). They ingested 581, 718, or 901 g of carbohydrate. These high carbohydrate intakes made maintaining high muscle glycogen concentrations possible (120 mmol/kg w.w., 155 mmol/kg w.w., and 185 mmol/kg w.w., respectively). The amount of glycogen stored in the muscles is, therefore, highly dependent on the amount of carbohydrate ingested between exercise bouts performed on consecutive days. Well-trained athletes seem to be more capable of rapidly restoring muscle glycogen than untrained or less trained individuals.

A higher carbohydrate intake can also reduce some symptoms of overreaching (an early stage of overtraining), such as changes in mood state and feelings of fatigue, but it cannot completely prevent them. Achten et al. (2004) observed such an effect in runners who increased their training volume and intensity and controlled their carbohydrate intake at either 5.4 or 8.5 g per kilogram of body weight per day.

Unless large amounts of carbohydrate are ingested, muscle glycogen does not normalize on a day-to-day basis (Costill et al. 1971). But just how much carbohydrate must we eat to replenish glycogen stores within 24 hours? Costill et al. (1981) suggested that increasing carbohydrate intake from 150 to 650 g results in a proportional increase in muscle glycogen. Intakes greater than 600 g/24 h, however, were suggested not to result in a further increase in glycogen resynthesis. More recent studies seem to suggest that with daily exercise, an almost linear increase in glycogen storage occurs in relation to carbohydrate intake (Coyle et al. 2001). These findings and others have led sport nutrition experts to recommend increasing carbohydrate intake depending on activity level. Recommendations may be as low as 5 g/kg on easy training days and as high as 10 to 12 g per kilogram of body weight per day when training consists of >4 to 5 hours of hard training daily.

What does a high-carbohydrate diet look like? For some time (from the 1980s until well into the 21st century), carbohydrate recommendations were expressed as a percentage of daily energy intake. The typical intake in a Western diet is around 50% to 60% carbohydrate. An intake of 70% was often recommended to athletes. However, whether a carbohydrate intake of 70% of total energy intake is high depends on the person's total energy intake. It is possible to have an intake of 70% carbohydrate but still have a relatively low carbohydrate intake. Guidelines expressed

CARBOHYDRATE TYPE

The amount of carbohydrate ingested may be the most important factor in stimulating glycogen resynthesis after exercise, but the type of carbohydrate may also play a role. One study investigated the effects of the glycemic index on muscle glycogen resynthesis. Subjects performed a bout of exercise that depleted their glycogen stores on two occasions and received a diet of high-glycemic index carbohydrate on one occasion and a diet of low-glycemic index carbohydrate on the other (Coyle et al. 2001). The total carbohydrate intake over 24 hours was 10 g per kilogram of body weight. The increase in muscle glycogen was more than 50% greater when the high-glycemic index carbohydrate was consumed. Therefore, high-glycemic index foods may be important for complete muscle glycogen resynthesis in a short period of time (8-24 hours). The higher insulin responses of the high-glycemic index meals are likely responsible for the increased glycogen synthesis. Jozsi et al. (1996) compared two forms of starch (100% amylose and 100% amylopectin) with maltodextrins and glucose and reported slower glycogen resynthesis with the amylose starch compared with the other carbohydrate types. If there is more recovery time, the carbohydrate type may be less important.

in percentages have muddled the advice given to athletes. For example, a 50% carbohydrate diet may contain a large amount of carbohydrate for a triathlete or cyclist who expends and consumes 25 MJ/day (5,975 kcal/day) but only a small amount of carbohydrate for a middle-distance runner who has an intake of 8.4 MJ/day (2,000 kcal/day). A more sensible expression of carbohydrate intake is grams per kilogram of body weight per day. All modern guidelines express carbohydrate intake in grams per kilogram of body weight.

Recommendations for Carbohydrate Intake

Modern carbohydrate intake recommendations are not one size fits all. Carbohydrate intake should be a function of carbohydrate use or needs. According to the new ACSM guidelines, "individualized recommendations for daily intakes of carbohydrate should be made in consideration of the athlete's training/competition program and the relative importance of undertaking it with high or low carbohydrate according to the priority of promoting the performance of high-quality exercise versus enhancing the training stimulus or adaptation, respectively" (Thomas, Erdman, and Burke 2016). Therefore, intake should be periodized according to specific goals. In a recent review article (Jeukendrup 2017b), the importance of periodizing carbohydrate intake along with various other aspects of nutrition was discussed. We will discuss this more in chapters 12 and 17.

The following carbohydrate intake recommendations are based on the International Olympic Committee's consensus on sport nutrition (Burke et al. 2004, 2011; Jeukendrup 2011). These recommendations are generally supported by strong evidence, but they are also general and should be tailored to account for total energy needs, specific training needs, and feedback from training performance. These recommendations should enable athletes to restore muscle glycogen within 24 hours, although they may become depleted in a training session.

- Depending on the exercise intensity and duration, consume 5 to 12 g per kilogram of body weight per day (see the sidebar Postexercise Carbohydrate Intake Recommendations).
- Choose nutrient-rich carbohydrate foods and add other foods to recovery meals and snacks to provide a good source of protein and other nutrients. These nutrients may assist in other recovery processes and, in the case of protein, may promote additional glycogen recovery when carbohydrate intake is suboptimal or when frequent snacking is not possible.
- Consume a sports drink to provide a convenient source of carbohydrate in the first hour after exercise when appetite is suppressed. Carbohydrate solutions have the advantage of providing fluid that helps to restore fluid balance (see chapter 9).
- When the period between exercise sessions is less than 8 hours, begin carbohydrate intake as soon as is practical after the first workout to maximize the effective recovery time between sessions. Meeting carbohydrate intake targets as a series of snacks during the early recovery phase may offer some advantages.
- During longer recovery periods (24 hours), organize the pattern and timing of carbohydrate-rich meals and snacks according to what is practical and comfortable for your situation. Glycogen synthesis is the same whether liquid or solid forms of carbohydrate are consumed.
- Carbohydrate-rich foods with a moderate to high glycemic index (see table 6.1) provide a readily available source of carbohydrate for muscle glycogen synthesis and should be the major carbohydrate choices in recovery meals.
- Adequate energy intake is important for optimal glycogen recovery; the restrained eating practices of some athletes, particularly women, make it difficult to meet carbohydrate intake targets and optimize glycogen storage.
- When it is important to train hard or with high intensity, daily carbohydrate intakes should match the fuel needs of training and glycogen restoration.
- Targets for daily carbohydrate intake are usually based on body mass (or proxy for the volume of active muscle) and exercise load. Guidelines can be suggested but need to be fine-tuned according to overall dietary goals and feedback from training.
- Guidelines for carbohydrate intake should not be provided in terms of percentage contributions to total dietary energy intake.

POSTEXERCISE CARBOHYDRATE INTAKE RECOMMENDATIONS

Immediately (0-4 hours) after exercise	1.0 to 1.2 g of carbohydrate per kilogram of body weight per hour, ingested at frequent intervals
Low-intensity or skill-based activities	3 to 5 g of carbohydrate per kilogram of body weight per day
Moderate exercise program (i.e., 1 hour/day)	5 to 7 g of carbohydrate per kilogram of body weight per day
Endurance program (i.e., moderate- to high-intensity exercise 1-3 hours/day)	6 to 10 g of carbohydrate per kilogram of body weight per day
Extreme commitment (i.e., moderate- to high-intensity exercise >4-5 hours/day)	10 to 12 g of carbohydrate per kilogram of body weight per day

These general recommendations should be fine-tuned based on total energy needs, specific training needs, and feedback from training performance. Timing of intake may be chosen to promote speedy refueling or to provide fuel intake around training sessions in the day. Otherwise, as long as total fuel needs are provided, the pattern of intake can be guided by convenience and personal choice. Protein- and nutrient-rich carbohydrate foods or meal combinations will allow the athlete to meet other acute or chronic sport nutrition goals.

- When carbohydrate intake is suboptimal for refueling, adding protein to a meal or snack will enhance glycogen storage.
- Early refueling may be enhanced by a higher carbohydrate intake, especially when consumed in frequent small feedings.
- Although there are small differences in glycogen storage across the menstrual cycle, women can store glycogen as effectively as men if they consume adequate carbohydrate and energy.
- Athletes should follow sensible practices regarding alcohol intake at all times, but particularly in the recovery period after exercise.

Carbohydrate Intake in the Days Before Competition

Carbohydrate can play an important role in preparing for competition. Carbohydrate intake in the days before competition mainly replenishes muscle glycogen stores, whereas carbohydrate intake in the hours before competition optimizes liver glycogen stores. Because carbohydrate intake in the days before competition has distinctly different effects from carbohydrate intake immediately before competition, these issues will be discussed separately.

It is important to achieve high muscle glycogen concentration at the start of an endurance event; this is why in the late 1960s researchers started to experiment with different exercise and nutrition regimens to achieve this.

Scandinavian researchers discovered that muscle glycogen could be "supercompensated" by changes in diet and exercise (Bergstrom and Hultman 1967b). In a series of studies, they developed a "**supercompensation**" protocol, which resulted in extremely high muscle glycogen concentrations. This diet and exercise regimen started with a glycogen-depleting exercise bout (see figure 6.5). A week before the important event, the athlete would complete a glycogen-depleting bout of exercise (an extremely hard workout). Then they would not train until the day of the event or in some cases perform one more workout 4 days before the event. The glycogen-depleting bout of exercise was followed by 3 days of a high-protein, high-fat diet, after which the subjects were placed on a high-carbohydrate diet for 3 days. In the original study, a control group followed the same exercise protocol, but their diets were in the reverse order. This study revealed that the subjects who received

TABLE 6.1 Foods With High, Moderate, and Low Glycemic Index

Glycemic index (glycemic load)	Food, serving size, carbohydrate	Glycemic index (glycemic load)	Food, serving size, carbohydrate	Glycemic index (glycemic load)	Food, serving size, carbohydrate
High glycemic index (>70)		**Moderate glycemic index (55-70)**		**Low glycemic index (<55)**	
102 (23)	Pancakes, buckwheat, 80 g (2.8 oz), 23 g	**69** (24)	Bagel, white, 70 g (2.5 oz), 35 g	**54** (11)	Potato crisps/chips, 50g (1.8 oz), 21 g
95 (40)	Lucozade (original), 250 ml (8.5 fl oz), 42 g	**67** (17)	Doughnut, 47 g (1.7 oz), 23 g	**52** (17)	Sweet corn, 150 g (5.3 oz), 32 g
92 (8)	Scones, 25 g (0.9 oz), 9 g	**67** (17)	Croissant, 57 g (2 oz), 23 g	**52** (16)	Cookies, chocolate, 45 g (1.6 oz), 30 g
88 (23)	Rice bubbles/pops, 30 g (1.1 oz), 26 g	**66** (5)	Beer, 250 ml (8.5 fl oz), 8 g	**52** (12)	Banana, 120 g (4.2 oz), 24 g
86 (26)	Baked potato, 150 g (5.3 oz), 27 g	**65** (9)	Couscous, 150 g (5.3 oz), 14 g	**51** (15)	Porridge (wheat and oat), 250 g (8.8 oz), 30 g
83 (16)	Pretzels, 30 g (1.1 oz), 20 g	**64** (28)	Raisins, 60 g (2.1 oz), 44 g	**50** (13)	Orange juice, 250 ml (8.5 fl oz), 26 g
82 (17)	Puffed rice cakes, 25 g (0.9 oz), 21 g	**63** (16)	Coca-Cola, 250 ml (8.5 fl oz), 26 g	**49** (10)	Muesli, 30 g (1.1 oz), 20 g
81 (21)	Cornflakes (cereal), 30g (1.1 oz), 26 g	**62** (26)	Baguette with butter and jam, 70 g (2.5 oz), 41 g	**49** (24)	Spaghetti, white, boiled, 180 g (6.3 oz), 48 g
80 (22)	Jelly beans, 30 g (1.1 oz), 28 g	**60** (7)	Bread, white, toasted, 30 g (1.1 oz), 15 g	**48** (7)	Baked beans, 150 g (5.3 oz), 15 g
78 (12)	Typical sports beverage, 250 ml (8.5 fl oz), 15 g	**59** (10)	Digestives (cookies), 25 g (0.9 oz), 16 g	**47** (3)	Carrots, 80 g (2.8 oz), 6 g
75 (11)	Bread, white, wheat flour, 30 g (1.1 oz), 15 g	**57** (6)	Ice cream, regular, 50 g (1.8 oz), 10 g	**46** (8)	Grapes, 120 g (4.2 oz), 18 g
75 (12)	Weetabix (cereal), 30 g (1.1 oz), 22 g	**57** (22)	Blueberry muffin, 70 g (2.5 oz), 39 g	**44** (9)	All-Bran (cereal), 30 g (1.1 oz), 20 g
75 (16)	Boiled potato, 150 g (5.3 oz), 28 g	**57** (9)	Fruit loaf, 30 g (1.1 oz), 18 g	**40** (15)	Rice noodles, boiled, 180 g (6.3 oz), 39 g
74 (21)	Cheerios (cereal), 30 g (1.1 oz), 20 g	**56** (24)	Power bar, chocolate, 65g (2.3 oz), 42 g	**38** (6)	Apple, 120 g (4.2 oz), 15 g
73 (15)	Iced cupcake, 38 g (1.3 oz), 26 g	**56** (23)	Long-grain rice, boiled 150 g (5.3 oz), 42 g	**36** (9)	Pizza, margherita, 100 g (3.5 oz), 24 g
72 (9)	Popcorn, 20 g (0.7 oz), 12 g	**55** (19)	Snickers bar, 60 g (2.1 oz), 35 g	**31** (4)	Milk, full fat, 250 ml (8.5 fl oz), 12 g
72 (30)	Rice, white, boiled, 150 g (5.3 oz), 42 g	**55** (10)	Honey, 25 g (0.9 oz), 18 g	**30** (5)	Lentils, 150 g (5.3 oz), 17 g
72 (4)	Watermelon, 120 g (4.2 oz), 6 g	**55** (9)	Fruit cocktail, canned, 120 g (4.2 oz), 16 g	**15** (1)	Tomato, spinach, broccoli, asparagus, 150 g (5.3 oz), 6 g

Glycemic index is in bold font and glycemic load is in parentheses.

Data from Atkinson, Foster-Powell, and Brand-Miller (2008); Henry et al. (2005); Diogenes GI Database (2010).

the high-protein, high-fat diet followed by the high-carbohydrate diet had higher rates of muscle glycogen resynthesis. The authors therefore concluded that a period of carbohydrate deprivation further stimulated glycogen resynthesis when carbohydrates were given after exercise.

Several top athletes have successfully used the supercompensation protocol, including the

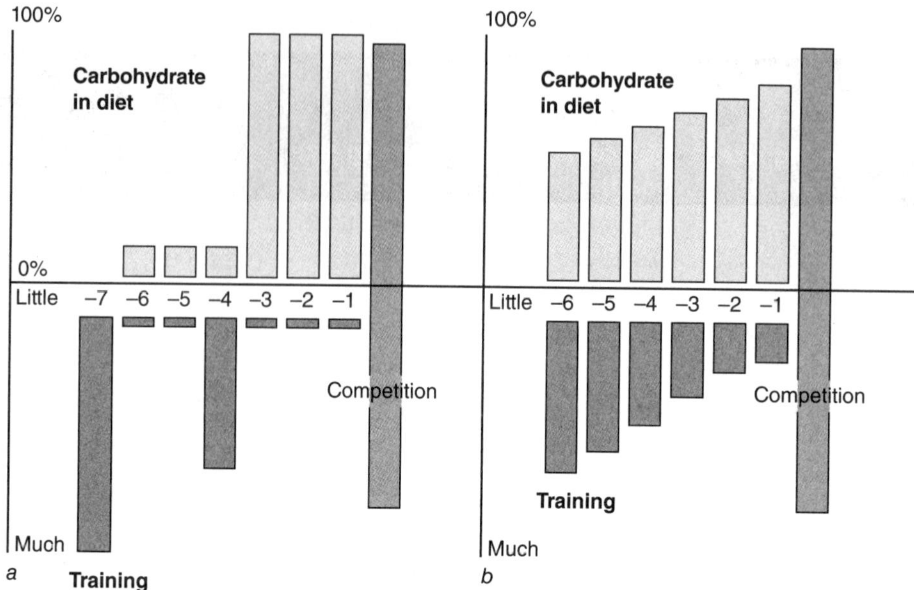

Figure 6.5 *(a)* The classical supercompensation protocols consisted of a glycogen-depleting exercise bout followed by 3 days of a high-protein, high-fat diet and another exhausting exercise bout on day 4 followed by a 3-day high-carbohydrate diet. *(b)* A more moderate protocol was later suggested to be almost as effective.

legendary British runner Ron Hill. Many marathon runners use this method to optimize their performance. Although the supercompensation protocol has been effective in increasing muscle glycogen to very high concentrations, it also has the following important potential disadvantages:

- Hypoglycemia during the low-carbohydrate period
- Practical problems (difficulty in preparing extreme diets)
- GI problems (especially on the low-carbohydrate diet)
- Poor recovery when no carbohydrate is ingested
- Tenseness during a week without training
- Increased risk of injury
- Mood disturbances (lethargy and irritability) during the low-carbohydrate period

The main problem may be the incidence of GI problems when using this regimen. Diarrhea has often been reported on the days when the high-protein, high-fat diet is consumed. During the first 3 days, athletes may also experience hypoglycemia, and they may not recover well from the exhausting exercise bout when no carbohydrate is ingested. Also, the fact that athletes cannot prepare as normal and train daily in the week before an event is not ideal, because the worst punishment for most athletes seems to be asking them to avoid training. These factors may also affect mental preparation for an event.

Because of the numerous disadvantages of the classical supercompensation protocol, studies have focused on a more moderate supercompensation protocol that can achieve similar results. Sherman et al. (1981) studied three types of muscle glycogen supercompensation regimens in runners. The subjects slowly reduced their training over a 6-day period from 90 minutes of running at 75% of $\dot{V}O_2$max to complete rest on the last day. During each reduction, they ingested one of the following three diets:

1. A mixed diet with 50% carbohydrate
2. A low-carbohydrate diet (25% carbohydrate) for the first 3 days followed by 3 days of a high-carbohydrate diet (70%) (classical supercompensation protocol)
3. A mixed diet for the first 3 days (50% carbohydrate) followed by 3 days of a high-carbohydrate diet (70%) (moderate supercompensation protocol)

The classical protocol resulted in very high muscle glycogen stores (211 mmol/kg w.w.), which confirmed the results of earlier studies. But the moderate approach produced similar muscle glycogen levels (204 mmol/kg w.w.). Therefore, a normal training taper in conjunction with a moderate- to high-carbohydrate diet proved just as effective as the classical supercompensation protocol. A slightly modified and commonly applied strategy of the moderate supercompensation protocol is depicted in figure 6.5*b*. Because it does not have the disadvantages of the classical protocol, the moderate supercompensation protocol is the preferred regimen.

More recently, various glycogen-loading protocols have been used successfully. In one study, endurance-trained athletes performed very-high-intensity exercise for only 2 minutes (cycling for 150 seconds at 130% of $\dot{V}O_2$max followed by 30 seconds of all-out cycling) and then consumed a very-high-carbohydrate diet (Fairchild et al. 2002). This protocol resulted in very high muscle glycogen concentrations 24 hours later (198 mmol/kg w.w.). Studies seem to show that an exhausting bout of exercise is not necessary to achieve very high (supercompensated) glycogen stores (Bussau et al. 2002; Coyle et al. 2001). Note that after glycogen stores are high, they will stay high for several days if limited exercise is performed.

Some studies suggested that women have a reduced ability to synthesize glycogen (Tarnopolsky et al. 1995), but this may have been a result of the smaller amount of carbohydrate the female subjects ingested. When men and women consume a comparable amount of carbohydrate (expressed in grams per kilogram of fat-free mass [FFM]), no differences in glycogen loading are observed (McLay et al. 2007; Tarnopolsky et al. 1997). In addition, it has been suggested that glycogen loading might be affected by menstrual cycle phase, but a study found no differences in the ability to synthesize glycogen in different phases of the menstrual cycle (McLay et al. 2007).

Carbohydrate loading increases time to exhaustion (endurance capacity) by about 20% on average and reduces the time required to complete a set task (e.g., time trial, endurance performance) by 2% to 3% (Hawley et al. 1997). Available studies seem to suggest that the duration of exercise has to be at least 90 minutes before performance benefits occur. Carbohydrate loading seems to have no effect on sprint performance and high-intensity exercise up to about 30 minutes compared with normal diets (about 50% carbohydrate). This finding is expected, because at these high intensities, glycogen depletion is probably not the performance-limiting factor. But several days on a very-low-carbohydrate diet (< 10%) after a prolonged cycle ride to exhaustion has been shown to impair endurance capacity at 100% of $\dot{V}O_2$max (Maughan, Greenhaff, et al. 1997).

IS GLYCOGEN LOADING NECESSARY?

It is clear that glycogen plays an important role, and low glycogen stores at the start of exercise will most likely result in reduced exercise capacity and performance during prolonged exercise. There is no question that glycogen stores should be high at the start of exercise, but is higher better? The answer may be no. Once you have achieved high levels of glycogen, extra glycogen may not be more beneficial because rates of glycogen breakdown during exercise will also increase. The rates of glycogenolysis are directly related to glycogen concentration. This means that if you start with extremely high glycogen concentrations, you will break down glycogen very rapidly at the start of exercise. It is likely that 30 to 60 minutes into the exercise, glycogen concentrations would be similar whether you started with high or very high glycogen stores. Glycogen loading is not needed for relatively short events (<30 minutes), but longer events could benefit.

Carbohydrate loading has also been reported to improve performance in team sports involving high-intensity intermittent exercise and skills, such as soccer and hockey (Balsom et al. 1999), although this result has not always been confirmed. A study was performed in elite Swedish soccer players who played two matches 3 days apart (Saltin 1973). Between the matches, one group consumed a high-carbohydrate diet and the other consumed a normal diet. Before the second match, muscle glycogen concentrations were 50% lower in the group that consumed the normal diet. At halftime (after 45 minutes), muscle glycogen was virtually depleted in this group, whereas the high-carbohydrate group still had some glycogen left (see table 6.2). This glycogen status was related to the distance covered during the match, which was significantly lower with the control diet and low

TABLE 6.2 Diet and Performance in Soccer

	MUSCLE GLYCOGEN CONCENTRATION (G/KG W.W.)			
	Before	**Halftime**	**End**	
High-carbohydrate diet	15	4	1	
Normal diet	7	1	0	
	DISTANCE COVERED			
	First half	**Second half**	**Walk (%)**	**Sprint (%)**
High-carbohydrate diet	6,100 m (3.8 mi)	5,900 m (3.7 mi)	27	24
Normal diet	5,600 m (3.5 mi)	4,100 m (2.5 mi)	50	15

Adapted from Saltin (1973).

muscle glycogen concentrations. The players also spent less time sprinting and thus were believed to have impaired running performance.

Several strategies can optimize muscle glycogen, and they do not have to be complicated. Approaches are similar for men and women. Essentially, carbohydrate intake should be high in the days before the event and muscle activity should be limited.

Supercompensation in Practice

Although muscle glycogen is important in most endurance sports, supercompensation strategies are not always applicable. In some sports, supercompensation strategies are impractical or impossible given the time frame and the rules of the sport. In cycling, for instance, stage races consist of several days of consecutive competition. Although a supercompensation regimen could be followed before the first stage, the nature of the sport does not allow the athletes to prepare for a week or more of daily hard exercise. Similar problems occur in sports in which there are consecutive competitions within 1 to 5 days. The supercompensation protocol does, however, seem suitable for marathon running and triathlon competing.

Muscle glycogen supercompensation is not of great importance to athletes involved in events that are short and explosive. Muscle glycogen availability is not usually responsible for fatigue during high-intensity exercise (>95% of $\dot{V}O_2max$) if the preexercise glycogen store is not depleted below 25 mmol/kg w.w. Even so, athletes involved in high-intensity training do need to consume sufficient carbohydrate in their diets. Diets very low in carbohydrate can compromise exercise performance at intensities around 95% to 100% of maximum oxygen uptake (Maughan, Greenhaff, et al. 1997).

Note that every gram of carbohydrate is stored with approximately 3 g of water, which means that storage of 500 g (8,000 kJ [1,912 kcal]) of carbohydrate is accompanied by an increase in body mass of approximately 2 kg (4 lb). In some sports or disciplines (especially weight-bearing activities), this increase in body mass may not be desirable.

Carbohydrate Intake in Practice

Although the recommendations are generally to consume fairly large amounts of carbohydrate, what do athletes actually do? In-depth discussion of the many reports of athletes' dietary intakes is beyond the scope of this book, so we will summarize the findings. The interested reader is referred to an excellent publication (Burke 2001) in which this topic is discussed in detail. The conclusion drawn in this publication is that most male athletes achieve a dietary intake of 5 to 7 g of carbohydrate per kilogram of body weight per day for regular training needs and 7 to 10 g of carbohydrate per kilogram of body weight per day during periods of increased training or competition. Female athletes, particularly endurance runners, are less likely to achieve their specific carbohydrate intake targets because they sometimes try to reduce their energy intake to achieve or maintain low levels of body fat without paying enough attention to carbohydrate intake.

Carbohydrate Intake in the Hours Before Exercise

Athletes should have the last fairly large meal 3 to 5 hours before competition. This meal (usually breakfast) can be important after an overnight fast when the liver is almost depleted of glycogen. The advantages of a meal in the hours before exercise are related to the increased carbohydrate availability in muscle and the liver. In the 3 to 5 hours before exercise, some carbohydrate is incorporated into muscle glycogen. Carbohydrate intake in the last hour before competition will not affect muscle glycogen but will affect liver glycogen and increase th[illegible]delivery of carbohydrate to the muscle during e[illegible]

[illegible]hydrate-rich meal (contain-[illegible] of carbohydrate) [illegible]scle gly-[illegible] [illegible]as [illegible]as, [illegible]an [illegible]car-[illegible]ergy

[illegible]h skim [illegible]l oz) of

[illegible] or honey

[illegible]ight stir fry [illegible] or chicken, [illegible] and 250 ml

[illegible]rved in research [illegible]ncreases in pre-exe[illegible]eplenishing liver glycogen lev[illegible]e important. Liver glycogen concentratio[illegible]stantially reduced after an overnight fast. Ingestion of carbohydrate increases these reserves and, together with any ongoing absorption of the ingested carbohydrate, contributes to the maintenance of blood glucose concentrations during the subsequent exercise bout. Plasma glucose and insulin concentrations return to basal levels within 30 to 60 minutes after ingestion. Ingestion of carbohydrate in the hours before exercise has three important effects:

1. Transient fall in plasma glucose with the onset of exercise
2. Increased carbohydrate oxidation and accelerated glycogen breakdown
3. Blunting of FA mobilization and fat oxidation

The effects on FA mobilization can persist for a long time after carbohydrate ingestion. Montain et al. (1991) showed a blunting of FA mobilization 6 hours after ingestion of a carbohydrate meal.

These metabolic changes, however, do not appear to be detrimental to exercise performance because increased carbohydrate availability compensates for the greater carbohydrate use. No differences in exercise performance were observed after ingestion of meals that produced marked differences in plasma glucose and insulin levels (Wee et al. 1999). From a practical perspective, if access to carbohydrate during exercise is limited or nonexistent, ingestion of 200 to 300 g of carbohydrate 3 to 4 hours before exercise may be an effective strategy for enhancing carbohydrate availability during the subsequent exercise period.

Carbohydrate Intake 30 to 60 Minutes Before Exercise

The ingestion of carbohydrate in the hour before exercise results in a large rise in plasma glucose and insulin. With the onset of exercise, however, a rapid fall in blood glucose occurs. This phenomenon is called rebound or reactive hypoglycemia. Until a few years ago, athletes were often advised not to consume carbohydrate in the hour before exercise because this was thought to induce hypoglycemia and negatively affect performance. This view has gradually changed.

A combination of several metabolic events causes the fall in blood glucose. First, hyperinsulinemia stimulates glucose uptake, and contractile activity further stimulates muscle glucose uptake. The exercise-induced increase in the normal liver glucose output is inhibited by carbohydrate ingestion (Marmy-Conus et al. 1996). Enhanced uptake and oxidation of blood glucose by skeletal muscle may account for the increased carbohydrate oxidation after preexercise carbohydrate ingestion. In addition, in some studies, an increase in muscle glycogen degradation has been observed.

The increase in plasma FA with exercise is attenuated after preexercise carbohydrate ingestion because of insulin-mediated inhibition of lipolysis (Horowitz et al. 1997). Even small increases in plasma insulin (e.g., after fructose ingestion) can result in a marked reduction of lipolysis. Fat oxidation is reduced not only because of the lower plasma FA availability (Horowitz et al. 1997) but also because of inhibition of fat oxidation in skeletal muscle. Artificially increased plasma FA availability did not completely return fat oxidation to levels seen during exercise in the fasted state (Horowitz et al. 1997). Some evidence indicates that the hyperinsulinemia and hyperglycemia reduce the uptake of FA into the mitochondria (Coyle et al. 1997).

Factors that determine the glycemic response during exercise include

- the combined stimulatory effects of insulin and contractile activity on muscle glucose uptake,
- the balance of inhibitory and stimulatory effects of insulin and catecholamines on liver glucose output, and
- the magnitude of ongoing intestinal absorption of glucose from the ingested carbohydrate.

Because the metabolic effects of preexercise carbohydrate ingestion are a consequence of hyperglycemia and hyperinsulinemia, interest has developed in strategies that minimize the changes in plasma glucose and insulin before exercise. These strategies include the ingestion of fructose or carbohydrate types other than glucose that have a lower **glycemic index** (see the Glycemic Index sidebar for an explanation), varying the carbohydrate load or the ingestion schedule, the addition of fat, and the inclusion of warm-up exercise in the preexercise period. In general, although these various interventions do modify the metabolic response to exercise, blunting the preexercise glycemic and insulinemic responses appears to offer no advantage for exercise performance.

The metabolic alterations associated with ingestion of carbohydrate in the 30 to 60 minutes before exercise have the potential to influence exercise performance. The increase in muscle glycogenolysis and suppression of fat metabolism could possibly result in earlier onset of fatigue during exercise as suggested in a study by Foster, Costill, and Fink (1979). Indeed, this early study reported a reduction in exercise performance. Since then, however, the overwhelming majority of more than 100 studies have shown either unchanged or enhanced endurance exercise performance after ingestion of carbohydrate in the hour before exercise and no study has been able to confirm the findings of decreased performance.

Interestingly, a series of studies (Jentjens and Jeukendrup 2003; Moseley, Lancaster, and Jeukendrup 2003) demonstrated that certain individuals may develop hypoglycemia when carbohydrate is ingested in the hour before exercise, although this was not a predictor of performance. The causes of hypoglycemia in this situation are different from the causes of hypoglycemia after prolonged exercise when endogenous carbohydrate stores become depleted. Hypoglycemia seemed to be more prevalent when the carbohydrate was ingested 75 minutes before exercise compared with 45 minutes, and when it was ingested 15 minutes before exercise, few people developed hypoglycemia (Moseley, Lancaster, and Jeukendrup 2003). Hypoglycemia can be completely prevented when carbohydrate is taken 5 minutes before exercise or during a warm-up. This is because there is not enough time for insulin to increase significantly, so the insulin concentrations are still low at the onset of exercise.

More and more products are advertised as slow carbohydrates or slow-release carbohydrates. Essentially, these are low glycemic index carbohydrates and usually carbohydrates that are slowly absorbed. The idea that these reach the bloodstream slowly and don't cause a spike in blood glucose and insulin is appealing to the customer. However, it must be noted that such products have not been shown to have any performance benefits. Recent reviews concluded that there was no clear benefit to consuming a low glycemic index preexercise meal for endurance performance (Burdon et al. 2016; Jeukendrup and Killer 2010).

In conclusion, despite the well-documented metabolic effects of preexercise carbohydrate ingestion, little evidence appears to support the practice of avoiding carbohydrate ingestion in the hour before exercise if sufficient carbohydrate is ingested. Some people, however, may be more prone to develop hypoglycemia; therefore, it is recommended to determine individual practice based on experience with various preexercise carbohydrate ingestion protocols (Jeukendrup and Killer 2010). Finally, when carbohydrate is ingested during prolonged exercise, the potential negative effects of the preexercise carbohydrate feedings are reduced. When a high-GI food is ingested before exercise, it has little or no effect on metabolism and performance if carbohydrate is ingested during exercise (Burke et al. 1998).

Carbohydrate Intake During Exercise

Convincing evidence from numerous studies indicates that carbohydrate feeding during exercise of about 45 minutes or longer (Jeukendrup 2004, 2008, 2011, 2014; Jeukendrup et al. 1997) can improve endurance capacity and performance. A critical review of performance studies (Stellingwerff and Cox 2014) reported that of the 61 published performance studies (n = 679 subjects), 82% showed statistically significant performance benefits (n = 50 studies) and 18% showed no change

GLYCEMIC INDEX

The glycemic index refers to the increase in blood glucose and insulin in response to a standard amount of food. It is determined by a test in which the blood glucose concentration is measured in response to a meal. Specifically, the area under the blood glucose concentration curve is calculated. The GI is usually based on the ingestion of 50 g of carbohydrate and measurements of blood glucose over a 2-hour period. The greater the glucose response is and the greater the area under the curve is, the greater the GI of a food is. A greater GI indicates rapid absorption and delivery of the carbohydrate into the circulation. The GI is calculated using the following formula:

GI = area under the glucose curve of test food / area under the glucose curve of reference food × 100

The reference food, which is usually glucose or white bread, has a glycemic index of 100. Foods are generally divided into low-GI foods, moderate-GI foods, and high-GI foods. Low-GI foods have a GI of 55 or less, moderate-GI foods have a GI between 56 and 70, and high-GI foods have a GI of 71 or higher. Consumption of apples or lentils, for example, results in a slow and small rise of blood glucose concentration, whereas consumption of white bread or potatoes results in a rapid rise in blood glucose concentration. Apples and lentils, therefore, are classified as low-GI foods, and bread and potatoes are classified as high-GI foods. A list of some high-GI, moderate-GI, and low-GI foods is given in table 6.1.

The use of the GI as a tool is controversial, mainly because the GI for any given food might vary considerably between individuals. The glycemic index tables usually provide an average value that is not necessarily useful in controlling blood glucose concentration. The GI of foods is also sometimes confusing. In general, foods with large amounts of refined sugar (simple carbohydrates) have a high GI, and sugars with high fiber content and complex carbohydrates have a lower GI. Some complex carbohydrates (starches), however, can have a high GI. On the other hand, adding relatively small amounts of fat to a high-GI carbohydrate can lower the GI of the food substantially. Therefore, the GI must be interpreted and used with caution. It can probably be a useful tool if its limitations and pitfalls are well understood.

The **glycemic load (GL)** is a relatively new way to assess the effect of carbohydrate consumption that takes the GI into account but gives a fuller picture than GI does alone. A GI value indicates only how rapidly a carbohydrate appears as glucose in the circulation but does not take into account the amount of the food that is normally consumed. For example, the carbohydrate in watermelon has a high GI, but there is not a lot of it, so the GL of watermelon is relatively low. The GL is calculated by multiplying the GI by the amount of carbohydrate (g) in one serving and dividing by 100. For example, a carrot weighing 60 g (2 oz) contains only 4 g of carbohydrate. To get 50 g, a person would have to eat about 750 g (26 oz) of carrots. GL takes the GI value and multiplies it by the actual amount of carbohydrate in a serving. A GL is low if it is between 1 and 10, medium if it is between 11 and 19, and high if it is 20 or higher. Foods that have a low GL almost always have a low GI. Foods with an intermediate or high GL range from a very low to a very high GI.

compared with a placebo. No studies reported negative effects.

Studies have also addressed questions of which carbohydrates are most effective, what feeding schedule is the most effective, and what amount of carbohydrate consumption is optimal. Other studies have looked at factors that could influence the oxidation of ingested carbohydrate, such as muscle glycogen levels, diet, and exercise intensity. Mechanisms by which carbohydrate feeding during exercise may improve endurance performance include the following:

• *Maintaining blood glucose and high levels of carbohydrate oxidation.* Coyle et al. (1986) demonstrated that carbohydrate feeding during exercise at 70% of $\dot{V}O_2max$ prevented the drop in blood glucose that was observed when water (placebo) was ingested. In the placebo trials, the glucose concentration started to drop after 1 hour of exercise and reached extremely low concentrations (2.5 mmol/L) at exhaustion after 3 hours. With carbohydrate feeding, glucose concentrations were maintained above 3 mmol/L, and subjects continued to exercise for 4 hours at the same intensity. Total-carbohydrate oxidation rates followed a similar pattern. A drop in carbohydrate oxidation occurred after about 1.5 hours of exercise with placebo, and high rates of carbohydrate oxidation were maintained with carbohydrate feeding. When subjects ingested only water and exercised to exhaustion, they were able to continue again when glucose was ingested or infused intravenously. These studies showed the importance of plasma glucose as a substrate during exercise.

• *Glycogen sparing in the liver and possibly muscle.* Carbohydrate feedings during exercise spare liver glycogen (Jeukendrup et al. 1999), and Tsintzas and Williams (1998) discussed a potential muscle glycogen sparing effect. Generally, muscle glycogen sparing is not found during cycling (Jeukendrup et al. 1999), but it may be important during running (Tsintzas et al. 1995).

• *Promoting glycogen synthesis during exercise.* After intermittent exercise, muscle glycogen concentrations were higher when carbohydrate was ingested than when water was ingested (Yaspelkis et al. 1993). This finding could indicate reduced muscle glycogen breakdown. But the ingested carbohydrate was possibly used to synthesize muscle glycogen during the low-intensity exercise periods (Keizer, Kuipers, and van Kranenburg 1987).

• *Affecting motor skills.* There have been few attempts to study the effect of carbohydrate drinks on motor skills. One such study investigated 13 trained tennis players and observed that when players ingested carbohydrate during a 2-hour training session (Vergauwen, Brouns, and Hespel 1998), stroke quality improved during the final stages of prolonged play. This effect was most noticeable when the situations required fast running speed, rapid movement, and explosiveness.

• *Affecting the central nervous system.* Carbohydrate may also have central nervous system effects. Although direct evidence for such effects is lacking, the brain can sense changes in the composition of the mouth and stomach contents. For example, taste can influence mood and may influence perception of effort. An interesting observation provides support for a central nervous system effect: When a hypoglycemic person bites a candy bar, that person's symptoms almost immediately decrease, and the person feels better again long before the carbohydrate reaches the systemic circulation and the brain. The central nervous system effect may also explain why some studies report positive effects of carbohydrate during exercise on performance lasting approximately 1 hour (Jeukendrup et al. 1997). During such short-duration exercise, only a small amount of the carbohydrate becomes available as a substrate. Most of the ingested carbohydrate is still in the stomach or intestine. These observations resulted in the development of the carbohydrate-sensing theories that will be discussed in the next section. Studies in which athletes rinsed their mouths with carbohydrate (but did not ingest any) during 1-hour time trials showed performance improvements similar to those that occurred when the athletes ingested the carbohydrate (Carter, Jeukendrup, and Jones 2004). Others (Pottier et al. 2010) recently confirmed these findings.

The Carbohydrate Mouth Rinse Phenomenon

One hour of sustained or intermittent high-intensity exercise is not limited by the availability of muscle glycogen stores given adequate nutritional preparation. Therefore, evidence of enhanced performance when carbohydrate is consumed during a variety of such exercise protocols has been perplexing. Findings of a lack of improvement in the performance of a 1-hour cycling time trial protocol with glucose infusion but benefits from carbohydrate ingestion (Carter, Jeukendrup, and Jones 2004) created an intriguing hypothesis that the central nervous system might sense the presence of carbohydrate via receptors in the mouth and oral space, thereby promoting an enhanced sense of well-being and improved pacing. This theory was subsequently confirmed by observations that simply rinsing the mouth with a carbohydrate solution can also enhance performance of the cycling bout (Carter, Jeukendrup, and Jones 2004). A number of studies have now investigated this phenomenon, including several in which brain imaging technology (fMRI) tracked changes in various areas of the brain related to carbohydrate mouth sensing (Chambers, Bridges, and Jones 2009). In these studies, both sweet and nonsweet carbohydrates were shown to activate regions in the brain associated with reward and motor control. There is robust evidence that in situations when a high power output is required over durations of about 45 to 75 minutes, mouth rinsing or ingesting very small amounts of carbohydrate play a nonmetabolic role in enhancing performance by about 2% to 3% (figure 6.6). Not all studies have reported this effect though, possibly because a carbohydrate-rich preevent meal is associated with a dampening of the effect (Jeukendrup and Chambers 2013a).

Mouth rinse studies were initiated to study the mechanisms, not to develop a new strategy whereby athletes rinse their mouths with a carbohydrate solution and then spit it out. Ingesting the carbohydrate solution works just as well. There may be a few situations in which a mouth rinse can be practical, such as when an athlete cannot ingest any carbohydrate because of stomach problems or when energy intake needs to be restricted. Whether the central nervous system effects of glucose feeding are mediated by sensory detection of glucose or perception of sweetness is not known, but studies with placebo solutions containing artificial sweeteners with identical taste to glucose solutions suggest that sweetness is not the key factor (Jeukendrup 2013a, 2014). Brain imaging studies also show that increased brain activity is specific to carbohydrates.

Feeding Strategies and Exogenous Carbohydrate Oxidation

During prolonged exercise, it is the actual delivery of energy to the muscle that seems to be responsible for the beneficial effects of carbohydrate intake on performance. A greater contribution of **exogenous** (external) fuel sources (carbohydrate) spares endogenous (internal) sources, and the notion that a greater contribution from exogenous sources increases endurance capacity is enticing. The contribution of exogenous substrates can be measured using stable (or radioactive) isotopic tracers. The principle of this technique is simple: The ingested substrate (e.g., glucose) is labeled, and the label can be measured in expired gas after the substrate has been oxidized. The more the ingested substrate has been oxidized, the more of the label (tracer) will be recovered in the expired gas. Knowing the amount of tracer ingested, the

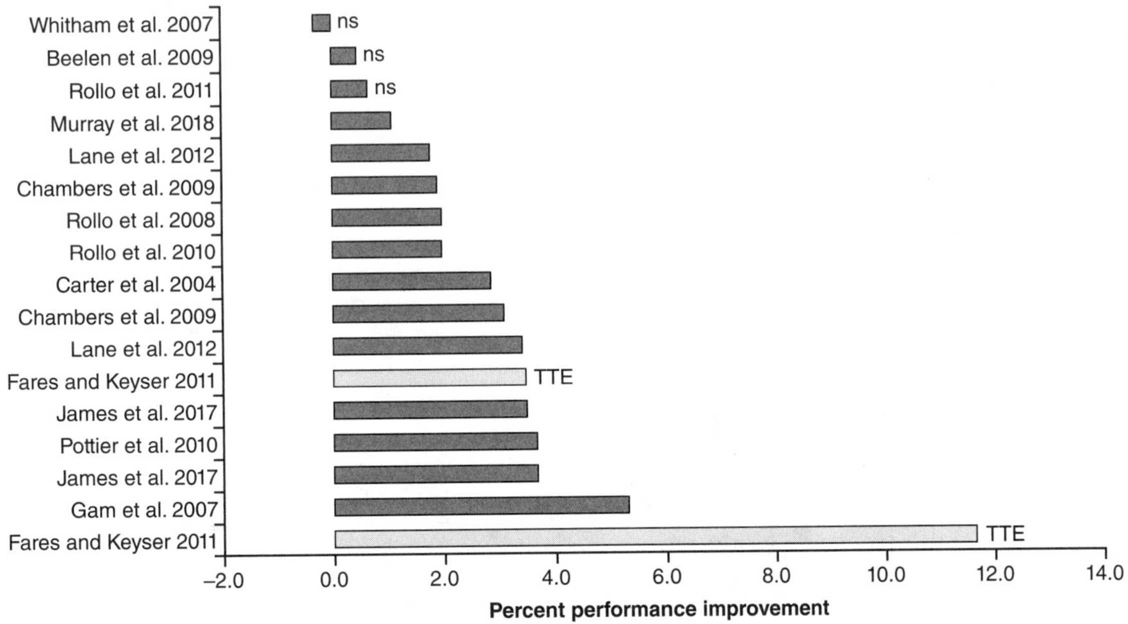

Fig 6.6 Overview of carbohydrate mouth rinse studies. The gray bars indicate time to exhaustion tests as opposed to time trials. The magnitude of performance change is influenced by the type of performance test (i.e., time to exhaustion gives exaggerated changes; time trials provide more realistic estimates of the effects as they are typically more representative of real sporting events). ns = nonsignificant; TTE = time to exhaustion.

amount of tracer in the expired gas, and the total carbon dioxide production allows the calculation of exogenous substrate oxidation rates.

The typical pattern of exogenous glucose oxidation rates is shown in figure 6.7. The labeled carbon dioxide starts to appear 5 minutes after ingestion of the labeled carbohydrate. During the first 75 to 90 minutes of exercise, **exogenous carbohydrate oxidation** continues to rise as more and more carbohydrate is emptied from the stomach and absorbed in the intestine. After 75 to 90 minutes a leveling off occurs, and the exogenous carbohydrate oxidation rate reaches its maximum value and does not increase further. Several factors have been suggested to influence exogenous carbohydrate oxidation, including feeding schedule, type and amount of carbohydrate ingested, and exercise intensity.

Timing of Intake

The timing of carbohydrate feedings seems to have relatively little effect on exogenous carbohydrate oxidation rates. Studies in which a large bolus (100 g) of a carbohydrate in solution was given produced exogenous carbohydrate oxidation rates similar to those in studies in which 100 g of carbohydrate was ingested at regular intervals (Jeukendrup 2004).

Amount of Carbohydrate

From a practical point of view, the amount of carbohydrate that needs to be ingested to attain optimal performance is important. The optimal amount is likely to be the amount that results in maximal exogenous oxidation rates without causing GI problems. Rehrer, Wagenmakers, et al. (1992) studied the oxidation of different amounts of carbohydrate ingested during 80 minutes of cycling exercise at 70% of $\dot{V}O_2max$. Subjects received either a 4.5% glucose solution (a total of 58 g glucose during 80 minutes of exercise) or a 17% glucose solution (220 g during 80 minutes of exercise). Total exogenous carbohydrate oxidation was measured and found to be slightly higher with the larger carbohydrate dose (42 g versus 32 g in 80 minutes). So, even though the amount of carbohydrate ingested was increased almost fourfold, the oxidation rate was barely affected. Jeukendrup et al. (1999) investigated the oxidation rates of carbohydrate intakes up to 3.00 g/min and found oxidation rates of up to 0.94 g/min at the end of 120 minutes of cycling exercise.

The results from a large number of studies (discussed in Jeukendrup and Jentjens 2000) were used to construct figure 6.8. The peak exogenous carbohydrate oxidation rates are plotted against the rate of ingestion. The maximal rate at which a single ingested carbohydrate can be oxidized is about around 1.0 g/min. The horizontal line depicts the absolute maximum just below 1.1 g/min. The dotted line represents the line of identity where the rate of carbohydrate ingestion equals the rate of exogenous carbohydrate oxidation. This graph suggests that oxidation of orally ingested carbo-

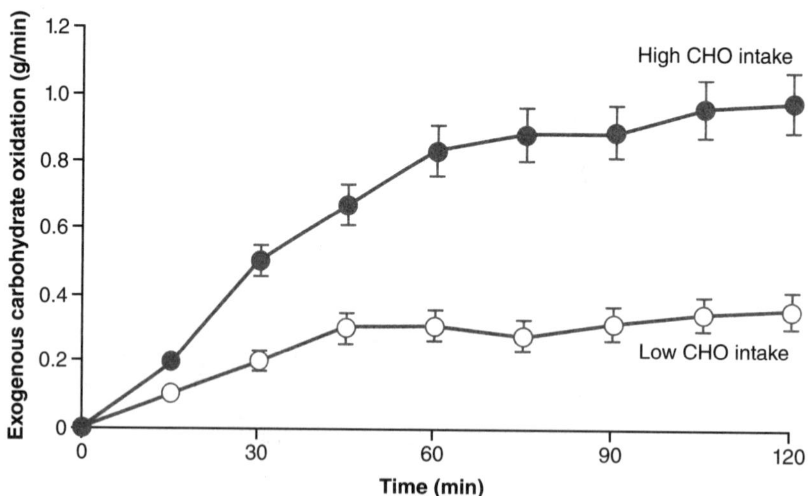

Figure 6.7 Exogenous carbohydrate oxidation during exercise. The curve shows the typical pattern of the oxidation of carbohydrate ingested at regular intervals.

Reprinted by permission from A.E. Jeukendrup and R. Jentjens, "Oxidation of Carbohydrate Feedings During Prolonged Exercise: Current Thoughts, Guidelines, and Directions for Future Research," *Sports Medicine* 29, no. 6 (2000): 407-424. Reproduced with permission from Adis, A Wolters Kluwer business (Copyright Adis Data Information BV 1994. All rights reserved.)

hydrate may already be optimal at ingestion rates around 1.2 g/min. Thus, athletes should ensure a carbohydrate intake of about 70 g/h to optimize exogenous carbohydrate oxidation. Ingesting more than this amount of a single carbohydrate does not result in higher carbohydrate oxidation rates and is more likely to cause GI discomfort. This amount of carbohydrate can be found in the following sources:

- 3 medium bananas
- 2 rice cakes
- 1 L sports drink
- 600 ml (20 fl oz) cola drink
- 1.5 energy bars
- 2 to 3 energy gels
- 120 to 150 g sweets or chews

It is possible, however, to deliver more carbohydrate by combining different types of carbohydrates. This will be discussed in more detail next. Studies have shown that with the appropriate combination of carbohydrate, oxidation rates can be increased significantly. Studies have even shown dose-response relationships with ingestion and performance (Smith et al. 2013; Vandenbogaerde and Hopkins 2011).

Type of Carbohydrate

Studies have compared the oxidation rates of various types of carbohydrate to the oxidation of ingested glucose during exercise (Jeukendrup 2004, 2008, 2011, 2014; Jeukendrup, Craig, and Hawley 2000). Glucose is oxidized at relatively high rates (up to about 1 g/min). The other two monosaccharides, fructose and galactose, are oxidized at much lower rates because they have to be converted into glucose in the liver before they can be metabolized. They are, therefore, a relatively slow energy source.

The oxidation rates of maltose, sucrose, and glucose polymers (maltodextrins) are comparable to those of glucose. Starches with a relatively large amount of amylopectin are rapidly digested and absorbed, whereas those with high amylose content have relatively slow rates of hydrolysis. Ingested amylopectin is oxidized at very high rates (similar to glucose), whereas amylose is oxidized at very low rates. Carbohydrates are divided into two categories according to the rate at which they are oxidized: a higher rate group (about 1 g/min) and a lower rate group (about 0.6 g/min). These two categories are listed in the sidebar Oxidation Rates of Ingested Carbohydrate During Exercise together with some mixtures of carbohydrates that can result in the highest oxidation rates (> 1 g/min).

Shi et al. (1995) suggested that the inclusion of two or three different carbohydrates (glucose, fructose, and sucrose) in a drink may increase water and carbohydrate absorption despite the increased osmolality. This effect is attributed to the separate transport mechanisms across the intestinal wall for glucose, fructose, and sucrose.

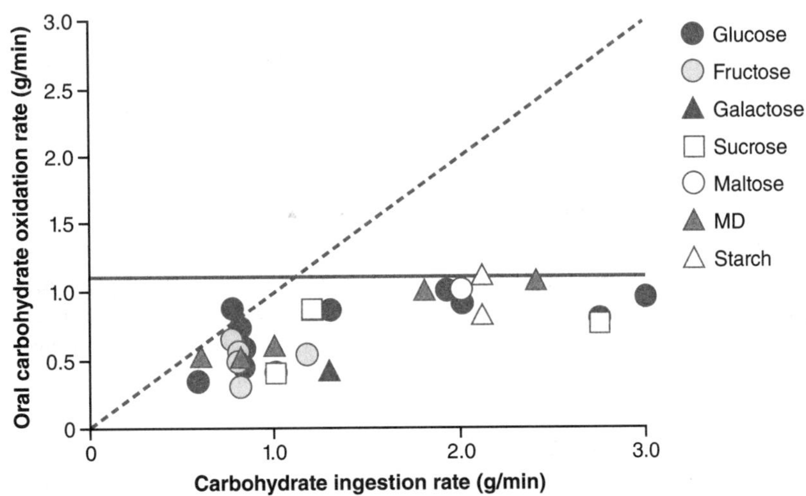

Figure 6.8 Maximal exogenous carbohydrate oxidation versus the rate of ingestion. MD = maltodextrin.

Reprinted by permission from A.E. Jeukendrup and R. Jentjens, "Oxidation of Carbohydrate Feedings During Prolonged Exercise: Current Thoughts, Guidelines, and Directions for Future Research," *Sports Medicine* 29, no. 6 (2000): 407-424. Reproduced with permission from Adis, A Wolters Kluwer business (Copyright Adis Data Information BV 1994. All rights reserved.)

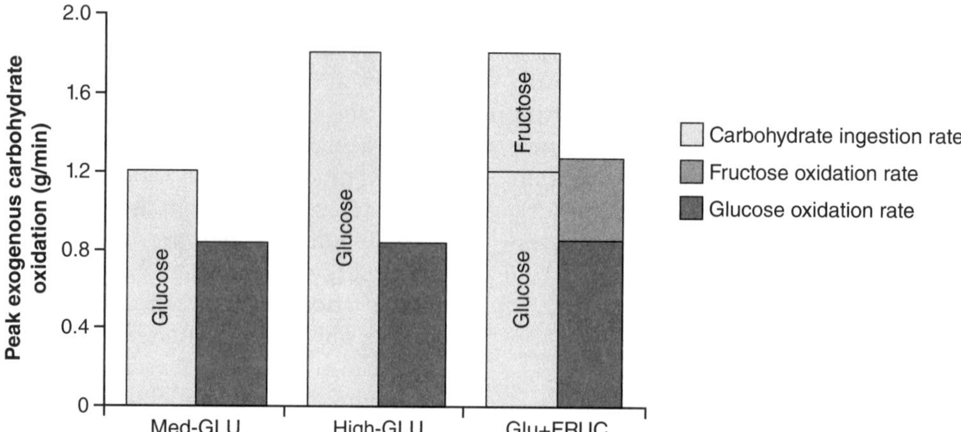

Figure 6.9 The oxidation rate of glucose plus fructose in a combined drink is higher than the oxidation rate of similar amounts of either glucose or fructose alone. FRUC = fructose; GLU = glucose.

Reprinted by permission from A.E. Jeukendrup and R. Jentjens, "Oxidation of Carbohydrate Feedings During Prolonged Exercise: Current Thoughts, Guidelines, and Directions for Future Research," *Sports Medicine* 29, no. 6 (2000): 407-424. Reproduced with permission from Adis, A Wolters Kluwer business (Copyright Adis Data Information BV 1994. All rights reserved.)

The monosaccharides glucose and galactose are transported across the luminal membrane by a glucose transporter called SGLT1 (see chapter 5) and fructose is transported by GLUT5. Interestingly, fructose absorption from a certain amount of the disaccharide sucrose is more rapid than the absorption of the same amount of fructose. If a combination of glucose and fructose is ingested, more carbohydrate will be absorbed and made available for oxidation. Ingestion of relatively large amounts of glucose and fructose can result in exogenous carbohydrate oxidation rates well over 1 g/min (Jeukendrup 2004, 2008) (see figure 6.9).

To ingest 50 g of carbohydrate, a person can ingest 1 L of a sports drink, two carbohydrate gels (typically 25 g each), or one to two energy bars. The solid and semisolid food is more energy dense and easier to carry during sporting events, but solid food may have a slowing effect on gastric emptying, especially when the food contains fiber and fat. Few studies have compared the efficacy of drinks versus gels and energy bars. Personal preference and tolerance are probably the main factors when choosing between these carbohydrate sources.

Exercise Intensity

With increasing exercise intensity, the active muscle mass becomes more dependent on carbohydrate as a source of energy. Both increased muscle glycogenolysis and increased plasma glucose oxidation contribute to the increased energy demands (Romijn et al. 1993). Therefore, exogenous carbohydrate oxidation increases with increasing exercise intensity. Indeed, Pirnay et al. (1982) reported lower exogenous carbohydrate oxidation rates at low exercise intensity compared with moderate intensity, but exogenous carbohydrate oxidation tended to level off between 51% and 64% of $\dot{V}O_2$max. When exercise intensity increased from 60% to 75% of $\dot{V}O_2$max, exogenous carbohydrate oxidation rates leveled off or even decreased (Pirnay et al. 1995).

Lower exogenous carbohydrate oxidation rates are possibly observed only at very low exercise intensities when the reliance on carbohydrate as an energy source is minimal. In this situation, part of the ingested carbohydrate may be directed toward nonoxidative glucose disposal (storage in the liver or muscle) rather than toward oxidation. Studies with carbohydrate ingestion during intermittent exercise have suggested that during low-intensity exercise, glycogen can be resynthesized (Kuipers et al. 1989).

Thus, at exercise intensities below 50% of $\dot{V}O_2$max, exogenous carbohydrate oxidation increases with increasing total carbohydrate oxidation rates. Usually above approximately 60% of $\dot{V}O_2$max, oxidation rates will not increase further.

Limitations to Exogenous Carbohydrate Oxidation

As discussed earlier, exogenous carbohydrate oxidation seems to be limited to rates of 1 to 1.1 g/min (see figure 6.7). This finding is supported by most of the studies that use radioactive or stable

OXIDATION RATES OF INGESTED CARBOHYDRATE DURING EXERCISE

Slowly Oxidized Carbohydrates (up to 0.6 g/min)

Fructose (a sugar found in honey, fruits, and so on)

Galactose (a sugar found in sugar beets)

Isomaltulose (a sugar found in honey and sugarcane)

Trehalose (a sugar found in fungi, some plants, and invertebrate animals)

Amylose (from starch breakdown)

Rapidly Oxidized Carbohydrates (about 1 g/min)

Glucose (a sugar formed by the breakdown of starch)

Sucrose (table sugar—glucose plus fructose)

Maltose (two glucose molecules)

Maltodextrins (from starch breakdown)

Amylopectin (from starch breakdown)

Very Rapidly Oxidized Carbohydrate Mixes (>1 g/min)

Glucose and fructose (with at least 60 g/h from glucose)

Maltodextrin and fructose (with at least 60 g/h from maltodextrin)

Glucose, sucrose, and fructose (with at least 60 g/h from glucose and sucrose)

isotopes to quantify exogenous carbohydrate oxidation during exercise. Understanding the causes of this limitation is important so strategies can be developed to make the exogenous supply of fuel more effective.

The following factors could limit the oxidation of ingested carbohydrate:

- Gastric emptying
- Digestion of the carbohydrate
- Intestinal carbohydrate absorption
- Retention of carbohydrate by the liver
- Glucose uptake by the muscle
- Metabolism in the muscle (glycolysis, TCA cycle, and oxidative phosphorylation)

One of the possible limiting factors could be the rate of gastric emptying (see figure 6.10). Some studies, however, indicate that gastric emptying is unlikely to affect exogenous carbohydrate oxidation rates (Rehrer, Wagenmarkers, et al. 1992; Saris et al. 1993). Because in these studies only a small percentage (32%-48%) of the carbohydrate delivered to the intestine was oxidized, gastric emptying was determined not to be limiting exogenous carbohydrate oxidation.

Another potential limiting factor is the rate of absorption of carbohydrate into the systemic circulation from the small intestine. Studies using a triple-lumen technique have measured glucose absorption and estimated whole-body intestinal absorption rates of a 6% glucose–electrolyte solution (Duchman et al. 1997). The estimated maximal absorption rate of the intestine ranged from 1.2 to 1.7 g/min. Studies using stable isotopes have observed a reduction in the glucose output by the liver when carbohydrate is ingested. When very large amounts of glucose are ingested, hepatic glucose output can be blocked completely (Jeukendrup et al. 1999). At low to moderate ingestion rates, no net storage of glucose occurs in the liver. Instead, all ingested glucose appears in the bloodstream. The glucose output from the liver can vary from nothing to approximately 1 g/min when no carbohydrate is ingested, the intensity of exercise is high enough (>60% of $\dot{V}O_2$max), and the duration is long enough (>1 hour).

Glucose that appeared in the bloodstream was taken up at rates similar to its rate of appearance (Ra), and 90% to 95% of this glucose was oxidized during exercise. When a larger dose of carbohydrate was ingested (3 g/min), the rate of appearance of glucose from the intestine was one-third the rate

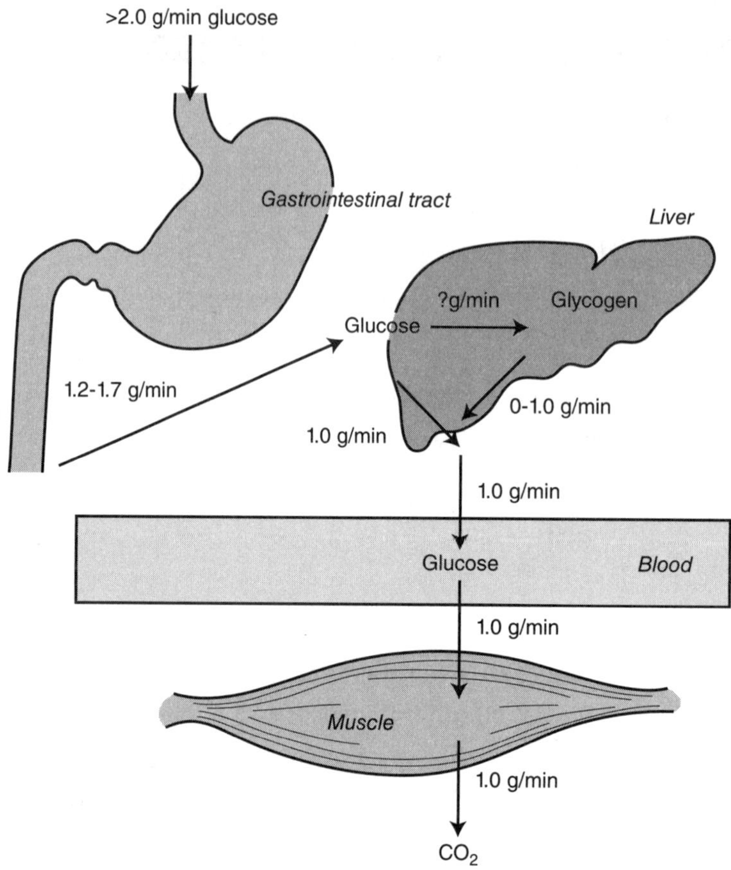

Figure 6.10 Gastric emptying of glucose, absorption, and uptake in skeletal muscle. Glucose travels from the gut after ingestion to the muscle. The suggested maximal flux at each of the stages is indicated. It is unknown how much glucose is directed toward liver glycogen storage.

Reprinted by permission from L.P.G. Jentjens and A.E. Jeukendrup, "Glycogen Resynthesis After Exercise," *Sports Medicine* 33, no. 2 (2003): 117-144. Reproduced with permission from Adis, A Wolters Kluwer business (Copyright Adis Data Information BV 2003. All rights reserved.)

of carbohydrate ingestion (0.96-1.04 g/min). Thus, only part of the ingested carbohydrate entered the systemic circulation. A large proportion of the glucose that appeared in the blood was taken up by tissues (presumably mainly by the muscle), however, and 90% to 95% was oxidized. Therefore, entrance into the systemic circulation is a limiting factor for exogenous glucose oxidation rather than intramuscular factors. Hawley et al. (1994) bypassed both intestinal absorption and hepatic glucose uptake by infusing glucose into the circulation of subjects exercising at 70% of $\dot{V}O_2$max. When large amounts of glucose were infused and subjects were hyperglycemic (10 mmol/L), blood glucose oxidation rates increased substantially above 1 g/min.

Exogenous carbohydrate oxidation is limited by the rate of digestion, absorption, and subsequent release of glucose into the systemic circulation. During high-intensity exercise (i.e., >80% of $\dot{V}O_2$max), reduced blood flow to the gut may result in decreased absorption of glucose and water (Brouns and Becker 1993) and hence a low rate of absorption relative to the rate of ingestion. Taken together, this information suggests that intestinal absorption is a contributing factor in limiting the oxidation of ingested carbohydrate at rates higher than 1.1 g/min, but it may not be the sole factor. The liver may also play an additional important role. Hepatic glucose output is highly regulated, and the glucose output derived from the intestine and from hepatic glycogenolysis and gluconeogenesis possibly does not exceed 1.1 g/min, even though the maximal rate of glucose absorption is slightly higher than this rate. If supply from the intestine is too large (>1.0 g/min), glycogen synthesis may be stimulated in the liver.

Multiple Transportable Carbohydrates

It has been suggested that by feeding a single carbohydrate source (e.g., glucose, fructose, or maltodextrins) at high rates, the specific transporter proteins that aid in absorbing that carbohydrate from the intestine become saturated. After these transporters are saturated, feeding more of that carbohydrate will not result in greater intestinal absorption and increased oxidation rates. Shi et al. (1995) suggested that the ingestion of carbohydrates that use different transporters might increase total carbohydrate absorption. Subsequently, a series of studies was conducted at the University of Birmingham in the United Kingdom using different combinations of carbohydrates to determine their effects on exogenous carbohydrate oxidation during exercise. In the first study, subjects ingested a drink containing glucose and fructose (Jentjens, Moseley, et al. 2004). Glucose was ingested at a rate of 1.2 g/min and fructose at a rate of 0.6 g/min. In the control trials, the subjects ingested glucose at a rate of 1.2 g/min and 1.8 g/min (matching glucose intake or energy intake). It was found that the ingestion of glucose at a rate of 1.2 g/min resulted in oxidation rates of about 0.8 g/min. Ingesting glucose at 1.8 g/min did not increase the oxidation rate. But after ingesting glucose plus fructose, the rate of total exogenous carbohydrate oxidation increased to 1.23 g/min, an increase in oxidation of 45% compared with a similar amount of glucose. In subsequent studies, different combinations and amounts of carbohydrates were evaluated in an attempt to determine the maximal rate of oxidation of mixtures of exogenous carbohydrates (Jentjens and Jeukendrup 2005; Jentjens, Moseley, et al. 2004; Jentjens, Shaw, et al. 2005; Jentjens et al. 2006; Jentjens, Venables, and Jeukendrup 2004b; Jeukendrup et al. 2005; Wallis et al. 2005). Very high oxidation rates were observed with combinations of glucose plus fructose, maltodextrins plus fructose, and glucose plus sucrose plus fructose. The highest rates were observed with a mixture of glucose and fructose ingested at a rate of 2.4 g/min. With this feeding regimen, exogenous carbohydrate oxidation peaked at 1.75 g/min, a rate 75% greater than what was previously thought to be the absolute maximum.

In subsequent studies, subjects ingested more practical but still quite large amounts of carbohydrate (1.5 g/min). It was observed that the subjects' ratings of perceived exertion (RPE) tended to be lower with the mixture of glucose and fructose compared with glucose alone (Jeukendrup et al. 2006). More recently, it was demonstrated that a glucose and fructose blend of carbohydrate can improve performance significantly more than a glucose-only drink can (Currell and Jeukendrup 2008a). This finding was supported by a number of other studies (see Jeukendrup 2014).

The term *oxidation efficiency* was introduced to describe the percentage of the ingested carbohydrate that is oxidized (Jeukendrup and Jentjens 2000). High oxidation efficiency means that smaller amounts of carbohydrate remain in the GI tract, thereby reducing the risk of causing the GI discomfort that is frequently reported during prolonged exercise. Therefore, compared with a single source of carbohydrate, ingesting multiple carbohydrate sources results in a smaller amount of carbohydrate remaining in the intestine, and

CAFFEINE AND EXOGENOUS CARBOHYDRATE OXIDATION

The main factor that limits the oxidation of carbohydrate from a drink seems to be absorption. In a study (van Nieuwenhoven et al. 2000), it was suggested that caffeine might increase glucose absorption. This notion led to the idea that caffeine added to a carbohydrate drink may not only increase absorption but also result in greater delivery of carbohydrate to the muscle and higher exogenous carbohydrate oxidation rates. Yeo et al. (2005) tested this hypothesis and found that exogenous carbohydrate oxidation increased by 17% when relatively large amounts of caffeine were added. Therefore, caffeine may not only have a direct effect on exercise performance (see chapter 11) but also may aid the absorption and oxidation of carbohydrate. The exact dose of carbohydrate and caffeine required is still unclear because a follow-up study with a lower dose of caffeine did not find a significant increase in the exogenous carbohydrate oxidation rate, although time-trial performance was improved compared with carbohydrate alone or a placebo (Hulston and Jeukendrup 2008). More information on caffeine can be found in chapter 11.

osmotic shifts and malabsorption may be reduced. This probably means that drinks with multiple transportable carbohydrates are less likely to cause GI discomfort. This finding has occurred consistently in studies that have attempted to evaluate GI discomfort during exercise (Jeukendrup 2008). Subjects tended to feel less bloated with the glucose plus fructose drinks compared with drinking glucose-only solutions. A further advantage of the carbohydrate blend (glucose plus fructose) is that fluid delivery seems to be improved compared with glucose-only drinks (Jeukendrup 2013b).

Metabolic Effects of Carbohydrate Intake

The metabolic effects of carbohydrate intake during exercise depend on various factors, including the amount ingested, the timing of the intake, and the intensity and duration of exercise. Generally, carbohydrate ingestion early in exercise has large effects on insulin response, fat mobilization, and substrate use, whereas ingestion late in exercise has relatively little effect. If carbohydrate is ingested at the onset of exercise, plasma insulin concentrations rise in the first minutes of exercise and lipolysis is suppressed. FA availability is lowered, and this condition may partly explain the lower fat oxidation rates observed in this situation. Carbohydrate intake during exercise also inhibits fat oxidation by hindering the transport of FA into the mitochondria.

When carbohydrate is ingested later in exercise, the already-raised catecholamine levels blunt the insulin response, and hence fat oxidation is less affected. Similarly, when a small amount of carbohydrate is ingested during exercise, the effect on the plasma insulin concentration is also small, whereas larger intakes result in an increased insulin response. Exercise intensity may be important as well. Studies suggest that the suppressive effect of carbohydrate feeding on fat metabolism is greater at low exercise intensity than at high exercise intensity.

Intake Recommendations

The amount of carbohydrate that should be ingested during exercise depends on a number of factors. First, it depends on the goal. If performance is the main goal, one might consider carbohydrate intake during exercise. If the goal is recovery, improving muscle adaptations, increasing fat metabolism, or weight loss, carbohydrate intake is not required or desirable. Second, the type of exercise needs to be suited for carbohydrate intake. If the rules of the sport don't allow carbohydrate intake or if carbohydrate or glycogen use during exercise is limited, there may not be a chance or a need for carbohydrate intake. The third and most important factor seems to be duration of exercise. Figure 6.11 shows the recommendations for carbohydrate intake as a function of time. There is no evidence that events shorter than 30 minutes

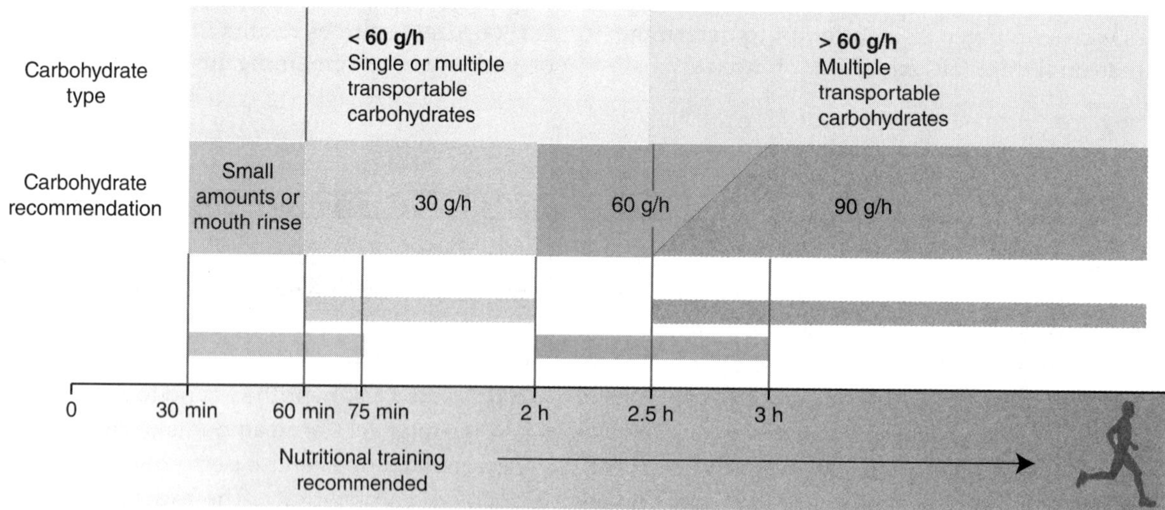

Figure 6.11 Carbohydrate intake recommendations during exercise as a function of duration of exercise. If the absolute exercise intensity is low, these figures may need to be adjusted downward. It is recommended to train with higher intakes if such intakes are targeted at events, and intakes greater than 60 g/h would have to come from multiple transportable carbohydrates.

will benefit from carbohydrate intake. Events that involve about 1 hour of all-out exercise (range 30-75 minutes) may benefit from a carbohydrate mouth rinse or very small amounts of carbohydrate. When exercise duration increases, carbohydrate intake should increase as well. Moderate amounts (approximately 30 g/h) should be ingested for exercise that lasts up to about 2 hours. After 2 hours, larger amounts are advised (up to 60 g/h), and when the duration exceeds 2.5 to 3 hours for some events (long endurance events) and for some athletes (those that are able to sustain high absolute exercise intensities), intakes of up to 90 g/h could be considered. Any intake higher than 60 to 70 g/h should be from multiple transportable carbohydrate sources, and any intake over about 60 g/h should be practiced regularly in training. It is possible to mix and match various carbohydrate sources (liquid, gels, and solids) as long as fiber, fat, and protein intakes during exercise are relatively low (they can all slow down gastric emptying and absorption of carbohydrate).

To help athletes plan their nutrition, computer software has been developed (www.fuelthecore.com) that helps to put these recommendations into practice. The software accounts for the recommendations discussed as well as personal preferences, weather conditions, and a number of other factors.

Carbohydrate Intake After Exercise

The main purpose of carbohydrate intake after physical activity is to replenish depleted stores of liver and muscle glycogen. The replenishment of muscle glycogen is directly related to recovery of endurance capacity, and glycogen loading or carboloading between training sessions has become common practice among endurance athletes.

Regulation of Glucose Uptake and Glycogen Synthesis

Glucose uptake in the muscle is through facilitated diffusion by the glucose transporter **GLUT4**, which is largely responsible for transporting glucose across the sarcolemma. GLUT4 is normally stored in intracellular vesicles but can translocate to the cell membrane, merge with the cell membrane, and allow increased transport of glucose into the cell (see figure 6.12). Both muscle contraction (through Ca^{2+} ions) and insulin secretion will stimulate the translocation of GLUT4 and hence glucose transport into the cell.

After its transport across the sarcolemma, glucose is phosphorylated to G6P by the enzyme hexokinase (see figure 6.12). G6P is next converted to glucose-1-phosphate (G1P) by the enzyme phosphoglucomutase, and G1P is combined with uridine triphosphate (UDP) to form uridine diphosphate-glucose and pyrophosphate (PPi) in a reaction catalyzed by 1-phosphate uridyltransferase. UDP is a carrier of glucose units and takes the glucose molecule to the terminal glucose residue of a preexisting glycogen molecule. UDP-glucose can be considered an activated glucose molecule. The UDP-glucose then forms an α-1,4 glycosidic bond, a reaction catalyzed by glycogen synthase, which results in one long, straight chain of glucose molecules. Branch points (α-1,6 glycosidic bond), however, are introduced into the glycogen structure by a branching enzyme. When the length of a chain is about 12 glucose residues, the branching enzyme detaches a chain about seven residues long and reattaches it to a neighboring chain by an α-1,6 glycosidic bond. Branching results in the formation of a large but compact glycogen molecule.

The rate of glycogen synthesis depends on

- the availability of glucose;
- the transport of glucose into the cell, which in turn depends on prior exercise (exercise stimulates glucose uptake for 1-2 hours postexercise and increases insulin sensitivity), insulin concentration (high insulin stimulates glucose uptake), and muscle glycogen content (low muscle glycogen stimulates glucose uptake); and
- the activity of enzymes (in particular glycogen synthase), which also depends on insulin concentration (high insulin stimulates glycogen synthesis).

As a result of the changing activity of these enzymes and the effectiveness of these transport mechanisms, two phases can be distinguished in the process of glycogen synthesis after exercise. These phases are the initial insulin-independent, or rapid, phase and the insulin-dependent, or slow, phase.

Rapid Phase of Glycogen Synthesis After Exercise

The rate-limiting enzyme for glycogen resynthesis after exercise, glycogen synthase, exists in an inactive D-form and an active I-form. More glycogen synthase is present in the active I-form when muscle glycogen concentrations are low. As glycogen stores are replenished, more glycogen synthase

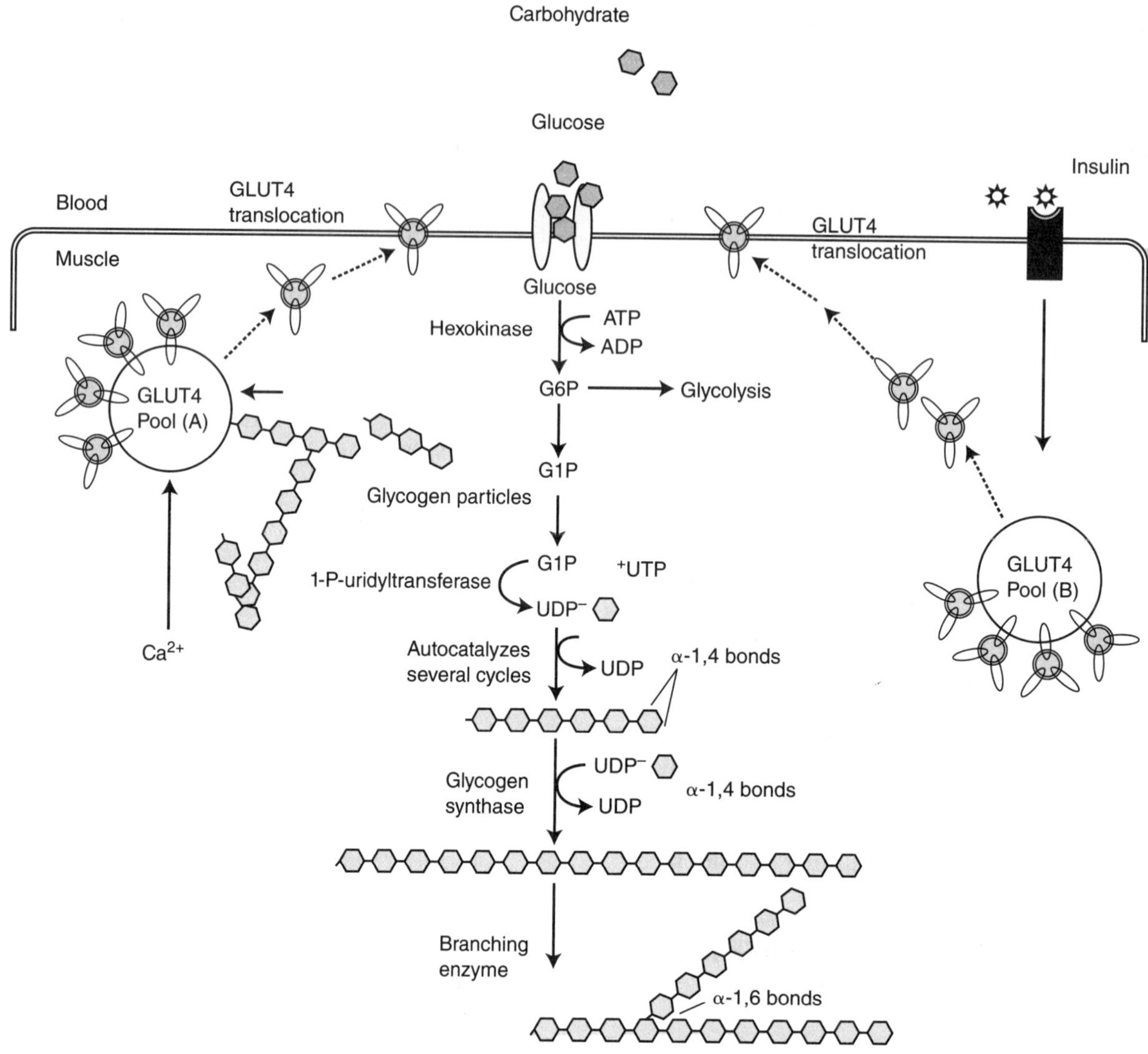

Figure 6.12 Mechanisms of glucose transport into the muscle and the synthesis of glycogen.

Reprinted by permission from L.P.G. Jentjens and A.E. Jeukendrup, "Glycogen Resynthesis After Exercise," *Sports Medicine* 33, no. 2 (2003): 117-144. Reproduced with permission from Adis, A Wolters Kluwer business (Copyright Adis Data Information BV 2003. All rights reserved.)

is transformed back into the D-form. Exercise activates glycogen synthase (immediately after exercise, as much as 80% of all glycogen synthase may be in the active I-form), but glycogen can be formed only if the substrate (UDP-glucose) is available. Another important factor in glycogen resynthesis, therefore, is the availability of glucose, which is mainly dependent on glucose transport across the sarcolemma. During exercise and in the first hour after exercise, an abundance of GLUT4 is available at the cell membrane, and glucose uptake into the muscle is facilitated. This exercise-induced effect on glucose transport lasts only a few hours in the absence of insulin. The increase in the permeability of the sarcolemma for glucose after exercise seems to be directly related to the amount of glycogen in the muscle. When muscle glycogen concentrations are very low, the enhanced glucose uptake may last longer. With high muscle glycogen concentrations, the effect is rapidly reversed.

Slow Phase of Glycogen Synthesis After Exercise

When the effect of the exercise-induced increase in glucose transport wears off, glycogen resynthesis occurs at a much slower rate. The rate at which glycogen synthesis occurs during the slow phase depends largely on the circulating insulin concentration, which increases GLUT4 translocation to the cell membrane and increases glucose transport into the muscle cell.

In addition, muscle contraction increases insulin sensitivity, and this effect may last for several hours. This increased insulin sensitivity after exercise is thought to be an important component of the slow phase of glycogen synthesis. The glycogen synthase activity decreases during this phase as muscle glycogen is restored.

After it is inside, the muscle cell glucose is directed toward muscle glycogen rather than oxidation. This effect is mediated by an increased glycogen synthase activity. An increase in the amount of GLUT4 present in the cell may also contribute to higher glycogen synthesis rates (Ren et al. 1994). After exercise, a rapid increase in GLUT4 expression may occur, resulting in increased synthesis of this protein, which in turn results in a proportional increase in insulin-stimulated glucose uptake and glycogen synthesis.

Postexercise Feeding and Rapid Recovery

A high rate of glycogen synthesis in the hours after exercise depends on the availability of substrate. In the absence of carbohydrate ingestion, glycogen resynthesis rates are extremely low despite increased insulin sensitivity, increased glycogen synthase activity, and increased permeability of the sarcolemma to glucose (Ivy, Katz, et al. 1988). Often, the time available to recover between successive athletic competitions or training sessions is short. In such cases, rapid glycogen synthesis is even more important. Although muscle glycogen concentrations are unlikely to be completely restored to preexercise levels, all methods of carbohydrate supplementation that maximize glycogen restoration may benefit performance. Five factors have been recognized as potentially important in promoting restoration of muscle glycogen stores: (1) timing of carbohydrate intake, (2) rate of carbohydrate ingestion, (3) the type of carbohydrate ingested, (4) the ingestion of protein and carbohydrate after exercise, and (5) the intake of caffeine.

Timing of Carbohydrate Intake

The timing of carbohydrate intake can have an important effect on the rate of muscle glycogen synthesis after exercise (Ivy, Lee, et al. 1988). When carbohydrate intake is delayed until 2 hours after exercise, muscle glycogen concentration after 4 hours is 45% lower compared with ingestion of the same amount of carbohydrate immediately after exercise. Average glycogen resynthesis rates in the 2 hours after ingestion are 3 to 4 mmol/kg w.w./h when carbohydrate is ingested after 2 hours and 5 to 6 mmol/kg w.w./h when it is ingested immediately after exercise (see figure 6.13). When carbohydrate intake is delayed until after the rapid phase, less glucose is taken up and stored as glycogen, primarily because of decreasing insulin sensitivity after the first few hours after exercise. A substantial intake of carbohydrate immediately after exercise seems to prevent this developing insulin resistance quite effectively.

Rate of Carbohydrate Ingestion

When no carbohydrate is ingested after exercise, the rate of muscle glycogen synthesis is extremely low (1-2 mmol/kg w.w./h) (Ivy, Lee, et al. 1988). The ingestion of carbohydrate, especially in the first hours after exercise, results in enhanced muscle glycogen restoration, and glycogen is generally synthesized at a rate between 4.5 and 11 mmol/kg w.w./h. In figure 6.14, the results of a large number of studies performed in various laboratories have been compiled. The rate of muscle glycogen synthesis plotted against the ingestion rate shows that, with an increase in intake, an increase in synthesis also occurs in the first 3 to 5 hours after exercise. This graph shows a trend toward a higher glycogen synthesis rate when more carbohydrate is ingested, up to intakes of about 1.4 g/min, which is higher than previously suggested (Blom et al. 1987). At a given rate of carbohydrate intake, large

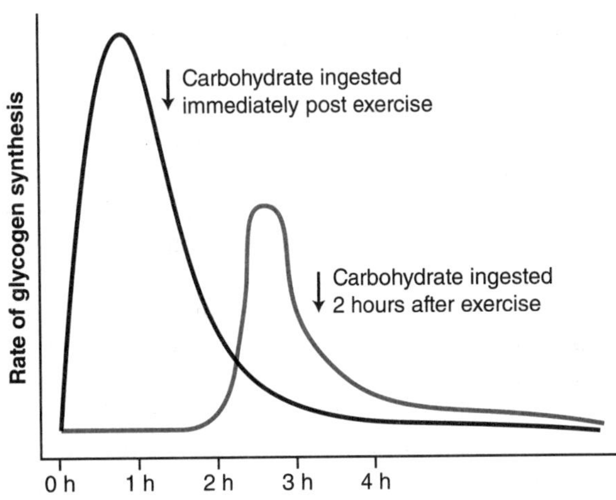

Figure 6.13 Effect of timing on muscle glycogen resynthesis.

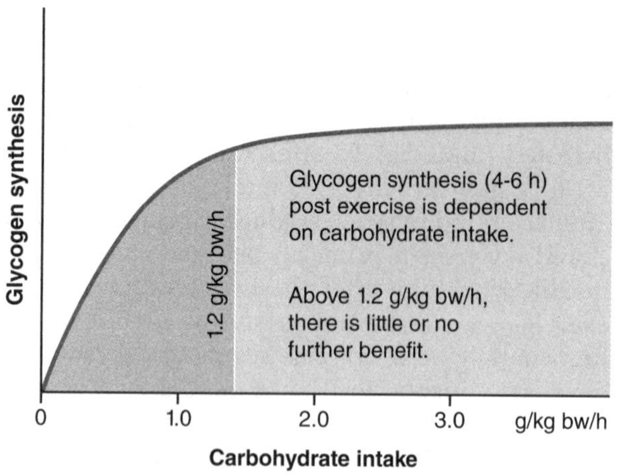

Figure 6.14 Muscle glycogen resynthesis after exercise as a function of carbohydrate intake.
© Asker Jeukendrup. www.mysportscience.com.

variability exists in the rate of glycogen synthesis, which probably indicates that other factors, such as timing, type of carbohydrate ingested, and training, are also important.

Type of Carbohydrate Ingested

Ingestion of different types of carbohydrate has different effects on glycogen synthesis. Blom et al. (1987) demonstrated that fructose ingestion resulted in lower rates of muscle glycogen synthesis after exercise compared with glucose or sucrose ingestion. Fructose must be converted to glucose in the liver before it can be used for glycogen synthesis in the muscle. Because this process takes time, glycogen synthesis occurs at a lower rate compared with a directly available carbohydrate source such as glucose. Other studies confirmed that glycogen synthesis from fructose occurs at only 50% of the rate of glycogen synthesis from glucose. In the study by Blom et al. (1987), sucrose intake resulted in muscle glycogen levels 4 hours after exercise that were similar to those that occurred after glucose intake.

Glycogen synthesis depends on the GI of the meal consumed after exercise. After 6 hours of recovery, muscle glycogen is more restored with a high-GI meal compared with a low-GI meal. Thus, the absorption rate and the availability of glucose seem to be important factors for glycogen synthesis. Low-GI foods result in lower glycogen resynthesis in the first hours after exercise.

Because the delivery of carbohydrate seems to be a factor and because combinations of multiple transportable carbohydrates such as glucose and fructose have been shown to increase absorption and delivery to the muscle during exercise, it is possible that these carbohydrate mixtures can also increase muscle glycogen synthesis after exercise. But it was recently observed that a combination of glucose and fructose ingested at relatively high rates did not improve glycogen synthesis compared with the ingestion of glucose only. It is possible that the fructose is preferentially stored in the liver postexercise and therefore does not reach the muscle. Note, however, that the glucose–fructose mix did not result in less glycogen synthesis.

Protein and Carbohydrate Ingestion After Exercise

Certain amino acids have a potent effect on the secretion of insulin. The effects of adding amino acids and proteins to a carbohydrate solution have been investigated to optimize glycogen synthesis. Zawadzki, Yaspelkis, and Ivy (1992) compared glycogen resynthesis rates after ingestion of carbohydrate, protein, or carbohydrate plus protein. As expected, little glycogen was stored when protein alone was ingested. Glycogen storage increased when carbohydrate was ingested, but interestingly, glycogen storage increased further when carbohydrate was ingested with protein.

The increased glycogen synthesis also coincided with higher insulin levels. Van Loon et al. (2000) used a protein hydrolysate and amino acid mixture (0.8 g of carbohydrate per kilogram of body weight per hour and 0.4 g of protein–amino acid per kilogram of body weight per hour) that had previously been shown to result in a marked insulin response in combination with carbohydrate. When subjects ingested carbohydrate and this protein–amino acid mixture, they had higher glycogen resynthesis rates than when they ingested only carbohydrate. In this study, subjects also ingested an isoenergetic carbohydrate solution. Despite a larger insulin response with the added protein, glycogen resynthesis was highest with the isoenergetic amount of carbohydrate (see figure 6.13). These results suggest that insulin is an important factor, but the main limiting factor is the availability of carbohydrate. When a protein–amino acid mixture (0.4 g per kilogram of body weight per hour) was added to a large amount of carbohydrate (1.2 g per kilogram of body weight per hour), insulin concentrations increased, but the increase did not further increase glycogen resynthesis (Jentjens et al. 2001). These studies are summarized in figure 6.15. The maximal capacity to store muscle glycogen is likely reached, and, therefore, no additional effect of elevated insulin concentration is found. Thus, to achieve rapid

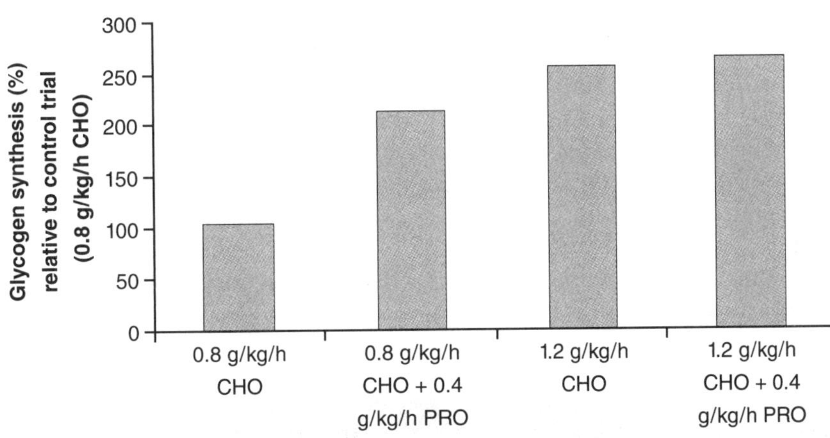

Figure 6.15 The rate of muscle glycogen synthesis after ingestion of various carbohydrate and carbohydrate–protein beverages. The synthesis rate for a drink that contains 0.8 g of carbohydrate per kilogram of body weight per hour is set at 100%, and all other synthesis rates are expressed relative to this baseline. PRO = protein.

muscle glycogen replenishment, ingesting an adequate amount of carbohydrate is more important than adding protein or amino acid mixtures to a recovery meal or drink.

Eccentric Exercise, Muscle Damage, and Glycogen Resynthesis

It has been known for some time that eccentric exercise and muscle damage can slow the rate of muscle glycogen resynthesis after exercise. Although the exact mechanisms are unknown, it is thought that this type of activity, perhaps through damage or inflammation, reduces GLUT4 translocation to the cell membrane and reduces glucose uptake. This is completely in line with observations in soccer players that glycogen restoration took longer than would be expected even when players consumed a high-carbohydrate diet. Studies have also demonstrated that a higher carbohydrate intake can compensate for some of the compromised glycogen resynthesis. Therefore, in sports with eccentric and damaging exercise, it may be even more important to follow carbohydrate intake guidelines.

CAFFEINE AND GLYCOGEN RESTORATION

Caffeine has been shown to reduce insulin-stimulated glucose uptake and has therefore been claimed to impair glucose metabolism. Caffeine ingestion before an oral glucose tolerance test or a hyperinsulinemic euglycemic clamp results in significant impairment in insulin-mediated glucose disposal and carbohydrate storage. Although caffeine ingestion exerts a negative effect on skeletal muscle glucose disposal in resting humans, exercise appears to diminish such effects. As discussed earlier, the coingestion of caffeine with carbohydrate during exercise increased glucose delivery to the muscle and oxidation (Yeo et al. 2005). If caffeine can increase the delivery of glucose during exercise, it might do the same following exercise, which could increase muscle glycogen synthesis. In a study by Pedersen et al. (2008), caffeine was added to a carbohydrate drink and given to subjects during a 4-hour recovery period from exhaustive, glycogen-depleting exercise. Glycogen restoration was greatest with caffeine. A follow-up study by Beelen et al. (2009) showed that coingestion of caffeine does not further accelerate postexercise muscle glycogen synthesis when ample amounts of carbohydrate (1.2 g per kilogram of body weight per hour) are ingested. Although evidence is thin, these initial results seem promising.

Solid Versus Liquid

Few studies have investigated the effect of solid versus liquid carbohydrate foods on glycogen synthesis in the early hours after exercise. Keizer, Kuipers, van Kranenburg, and Geurten (1987) demonstrated that glycogen synthesis rates were similar after consumption of a liquid or a solid carbohydrate meal. Several other studies confirmed these findings and therefore, research indicates that there is no difference in glycogen synthesis with solid or liquid feedings. In the studies mentioned previously, the investigators used a high-GI carbohydrate that probably resulted in rapid delivery of glucose. Low-GI solid meals are likely to result in lower rates of glycogen synthesis compared with carbohydrate solutions. For further reading about glycogen synthesis after exercise, see reviews by Burke, van Loon, and Hawley (2017), Jentjens and Jeukendrup (2003), Ivy (1998), and Ivy and Kuo (1998).

Key Points

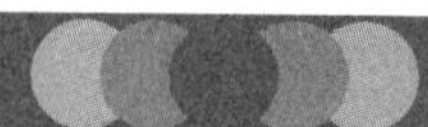

- Muscle glycogen is a readily available energy source for the working muscle. The glycogen content of skeletal muscle at rest is approximately 65-90 mmol glucosyl units/kg w.w., which is about 300 to 600 g of carbohydrate.
- The main role of glycogen in the liver is to maintain a constant blood glucose level. An average liver weighs approximately 1.5 kg (3 lb), and approximately 80 to 110 g of glycogen is stored in the liver of an adult human in the postabsorptive state.
- In resting conditions, the glucose output of the liver is approximately 150 mg/min, of which 60% is derived from the breakdown of liver glycogen and 40% is from gluconeogenesis. During exercise, the liver glucose output increases dramatically, up to about 1 g/min, and most of this glucose (>90%) is derived from the breakdown of liver glycogen.
- The classical supercompensation protocol results in very high muscle glycogen stores, but a moderate approach results in similar muscle glycogen levels without the disadvantages of the classical protocol; therefore, this is the preferred regimen.
- The brain is highly dependent on glucose as a fuel. As blood glucose concentrations drop, hypoglycemia may develop, which results in dizziness, nausea, cold sweat, reduced mental alertness and ability to concentrate, loss of motor skill, increased heart rate, excessive hunger, and disorientation.
- The primary role of carbohydrate in the days leading up to competition is to replenish muscle glycogen stores fully.
- Carbohydrate loading increases time to exhaustion (endurance capacity) by about 20% on average and reduces time required to complete a set task (e.g., time trial, endurance performance) by 2% to 3%.
- In the 3 to 5 hours before exercise, some carbohydrate may be incorporated into muscle glycogen, but most will be stored as liver glycogen.
- Carbohydrate intake in the hours before exercise results in a transient fall in plasma glucose with the onset of exercise, increases carbohydrate oxidation and accelerates glycogen breakdown, and results in a blunting of fatty acid mobilization and fat oxidation.
- Carbohydrate feeding during exercise of about 45 minutes or longer is believed to improve endurance capacity and performance. The mechanisms may be the maintenance of blood glucose levels and high carbohydrate oxidation rates, glycogen sparing, or central nervous system effects.
- During exercise between 30 and 75 minutes, a mouth rinse with a carbohydrate solution may have performance-enhancing effects through central nervous system effects.
- Oxidation of ingested carbohydrate during exercise depends on the type of carbohydrate, the amount ingested, and the exercise intensity, but the maximum oxidation rate seems to be about 1 g/min.

- Recommendations for carbohydrate intake during exercise are dependent on exercise duration and, to some degree, intensity.
- Multiple transportable carbohydrates (e.g., glucose and fructose) in a beverage can increase oxidation rates during exercise.
- Two phases can be distinguished in the process of glycogen synthesis after exercise: the initial insulin-independent, or rapid, phase and the insulin-dependent, or slow, phase.
- Restoration of muscle glycogen stores after exercise may depend on the timing of carbohydrate intake, the rate of carbohydrate ingestion, the type of carbohydrate consumed, and the addition of other macronutrients (e.g., protein).
- As a general guideline, the recommended carbohydrate ingestion during periods of moderate training intensity is 5 to 7 g per kilogram of body weight per day and 7 to 10 g per kilogram of body weight per day when training is increased. For endurance athletes who are involved in extreme training programs, increasing carbohydrate intake to 10 to 13 g per kilogram of body weight per day when exercising daily is generally recommended.

Recommended Readings

Burke, L.M., J.A. Hawley, S. Wong, and A.E. Jeukendrup. 2011. Carbohydrates for training and competition. *Journal of Sports Sciences* 29 (Suppl 1): S17-S27.

Gonzalez, J.T., C.J. Fuchs, J.A. Betts, and L.J. van Loon. 2016. Liver glycogen metabolism during and after prolonged endurance-type exercise. *American Journal of Physiology-Endocrinology and Metabolism* 311 (3): E543-E553.

Hargreaves, M., J.A. Hawley, and A.E. Jeukendrup. 2004. Pre-exercise carbohydrate and fat ingestion: Effects on metabolism and performance. *Journal of Sports Sciences* 22:31–38.

Hawley, J.A., E.J. Schabort, T.D. Noakes, and S.C. Dennis. 1997. Carbohydrate loading and exercise performance: An update. *Sports Medicine* 24:73-81.

Ivy, J. 1998. Glycogen resynthesis after exercise: Effect of carbohydrate intake. *International Journal of Sports Medicine* 19:S142-S145.

Ivy, J.L., and C.-H. Kuo. 1998. Regulation of GLUT4 protein and glycogen synthase during muscle glycogen synthesis after exercise. *Acta Physiologica Scandinavica* 162:295-304.

Jentjens, L.P.G., and A.E. Jeukendrup. 2003. Glycogen resynthesis after exercise. *Sports Medicine* 33 (2): 117-144.

Jeukendrup, A. 2013. The new carbohydrate intake recommendations. *Nestle Nutrition Institute Workshop Series* 75: 63-71.

Jeukendrup, A. 2014. A step towards personalized sports nutrition: Carbohydrate intake during exercise. *Sports Medicine* 44 (Suppl 1): S25-S33.

Jeukendrup, A. 2017. Training the gut for athletes. *Sports Medicine* 47 (Suppl 1): 101-110.

Jeukendrup, A.E. 2004. Carbohydrate intake during exercise and performance. *Nutrition* 20:669-677.

Jeukendrup, A.E. 2008. Carbohydrate feeding during exercise. *European Journal of Sport Science* 8:77-86.

Jeukendrup, A.E. 2011. Nutrition for endurance sports: Marathon, triathlon, and road cycling. *Journal of Sports Sciences* 29 (Suppl 1): S91-S99.

Jeukendrup, A.E. 2013. Oral carbohydrate rinse: Placebo or beneficial? *Current Sports Medicine Reports* 12 (4): 222-227.

Jeukendrup, A.E., and R. Jentjens. 2000. Oxidation of carbohydrate feedings during prolonged exercise: Current thoughts, guidelines and directions for future research. *Sports Medicine* 29 (6): 407-424.

Jeukendrup, A.E., and S.C. Killer. 2010. The myths surrounding pre-exercise carbohydrate feeding. *Annals of Nutrition and Metabolism* 57 (Suppl 2): 18-25.

Maughan, R.J., and M. Gleeson. 2010. *The biochemical basis of sports performance.* Oxford: Oxford University Press.

Stellingwerff, T., and G.R. Cox. 2014. Systematic review: Carbohydrate supplementation on exercise performance or capacity of varying durations. *Applied Physiology Nutrition and Metabolism* 39 (9): 998-1011.

Thomas, D.T., K.A. Erdman, and L.M. Burke. 2016. American College of Sports Medicine joint position statement: Nutrition and athletic performance. *Medicine and Science in Sports and Exercise* 48 (3): 543-568.

Fat

Objectives

After studying this chapter, you should be able to do the following:

- Describe the main biochemical pathways in fat metabolism
- Describe the changes that occur in fat metabolism at different intensities of exercise
- Discuss the factors that limit fat oxidation
- Describe the interactions between carbohydrate and fat metabolism at rest and in response to exercise
- Describe the metabolic and performance effects of fat intake 3 to 4 hours before exercise
- Describe the metabolic and performance effects of short-term high-fat diets
- Describe the metabolic and performance effects of long-term high-fat diets

Dietary fat is frequently undervalued as a contributor to the health and performance of athletes. Fat is an extremely important fuel for endurance exercise (along with carbohydrate), and some fat intake is required for optimal health. Dietary fat provides the essential fatty acids (EFAs) that cannot be synthesized in the body.

The fat stores of the body are very large compared to carbohydrate stores. In some forms of exercise (e.g., prolonged cycling or running), carbohydrate depletion is a possible cause of fatigue, and depletion and can occur within 1 to 2 hours of strenuous exercise (see chapter 6). The total amount of energy stored as glycogen in the muscles and liver has been estimated to be 8,000 kJ (1,912 kcal). Fat stores can contain more than 50 times the amount of energy contained in carbohydrate stores. A person with a body mass of 80 kg (176 lb) and 15% body fat has 12 kg (26 lb) of fat (see table 7.1). Most of this fat is stored in subcutaneous adipose tissue, but some fat can also be found in muscle as **intramuscular triacylglycerol (IMTG)**. In theory, fat stores could provide sufficient energy for a person to run at least 1,300 km (808 miles).

Because carbohydrate stores are small but important and fat stores are large, endurance athletes would like to tap into their fat stores as much as possible and save the carbohydrate for later in a competition. Researchers, coaches, and athletes have tried to devise nutritional strategies to enhance fat metabolism, spare carbohydrate stores, and thereby improve endurance performance. Understanding the effects of various nutritional strategies requires an understanding of fat metabolism and the factors that regulate fat oxidation during exercise. This chapter describes fat metabolism in detail and discusses various ways in which researchers and athletes have tried to enhance fat metabolism by nutritional manipulation. Finally, the effects of both low-fat and high-fat diets on metabolism, exercise performance, and health are discussed.

TABLE 7.1 Availability of Substrates in the Human Body

Substrate	Weight	Energy
Carbohydrates		
Plasma glucose	0.01 kg (0.02 lb)	160 kJ (38 kcal)
Liver glycogen	0.1 kg (0.2 lb)	1,600 kJ (382 kcal)
Muscle glycogen	0.4 kg (0.9 lb)	6,400 kJ (1,530 kcal)
Total (approximately)	0.5 kg (1.1 lb)	8,000 kJ (1,912 kcal)
Fat		
Plasma fatty acid	0.0004 kg (0.0009 lb)	16 kJ (4 kcal)
Plasma triacylglycerols	0.004 kg (0.009 lb)	160 kJ (38 kcal)
Adipose tissue	12.0 kg (26.5 lb)	430,000 kJ (102,772 kcal)
Intramuscular triacylglycerols	0.3 kg (0.7 lb)	11,000 kJ (2,629 kcal)
Total (approximately)	12.3 kg (27.1 lb)	442,000 kJ (105,641 kcal)

Values given are estimates for a male non-athlete who weighs 80 kg (176 lb) and has 15% body fat who might be leaner and have more stored glycogen. The amount of protein in the body is not mentioned, but it would be about 10 kg (22 lb [167,440 kJ or 40,019 kcal]) and mainly located in the muscles.

Adapted from Jeukendrup et al. (1998).

Fat Metabolism During Exercise

FAs that are oxidized in the mitochondria of skeletal muscle during exercise are derived from various sources. The main two sources are adipose tissue and muscle triacylglycerols (delivered in chylomicrons and VLDL). A third fuel, plasma triacylglycerol, may also be used, but the importance of this fuel is subject to debate. Figure 7.1 gives an overview of the fat substrates and their journey to the muscle. Triacylglycerols in adipose tissue are split into FAs and glycerol. The glycerol is released into the circulation along with some of the FAs. A small percentage of FAs are not released into the circulation but are used to form new triacylglycerols within the adipose tissue; this process is called **reesterification.** The released FAs are transported to the other tissues and can be taken up by skeletal muscle during exercise. Glycerol is transported to the liver, where it serves as a gluconeogenic substrate to form new glucose.

Besides the FAs in plasma, two other sources of FAs for oxidation in skeletal muscle are available: circulating triacylglycerols and intramuscular triacylglycerols. Circulating triacylglycerols (for example in a very low-density lipoprotein [VLDL]) can temporarily bind to the enzyme lipoprotein lipase (LPL), which splits off FAs that can then be taken up by the muscle. A source of fat exists inside the muscle in the form of intramuscular triacylglycerol. Intramuscular triacylglycerols are split by an HSL, and FAs are transported into the mitochondria for oxidation in the same way that FAs from plasma and plasma triacylglycerol are used.

Limits to Fat Oxidation

Despite the fact that humans have large fat stores, in many situations using these large amounts of fat as a fuel seems impossible. Why can fat not be oxidized at higher rates in some conditions? Is it because the FAs cannot be mobilized? To find the factor that causes this limitation, we examine all the steps that are important in the process of fat oxidation from the mobilization of FAs to the transport and oxidation of FAs in the mitochondrion.

The steps that could potentially limit fat oxidation are

- lipolysis (the breakdown of triacylglycerols to FAs and glycerol),
- removal of FAs from the fat cell,
- transport of fat by the bloodstream,
- transport of FAs into the muscle cell,
- transport of FAs into the mitochondria, and
- oxidation of FAs in the ß-oxidation pathway and TCA cycle.

Lipolysis in Adipocytes

Most FAs are stored in the form of triacylglycerols in subcutaneous adipose tissue. Before these FAs

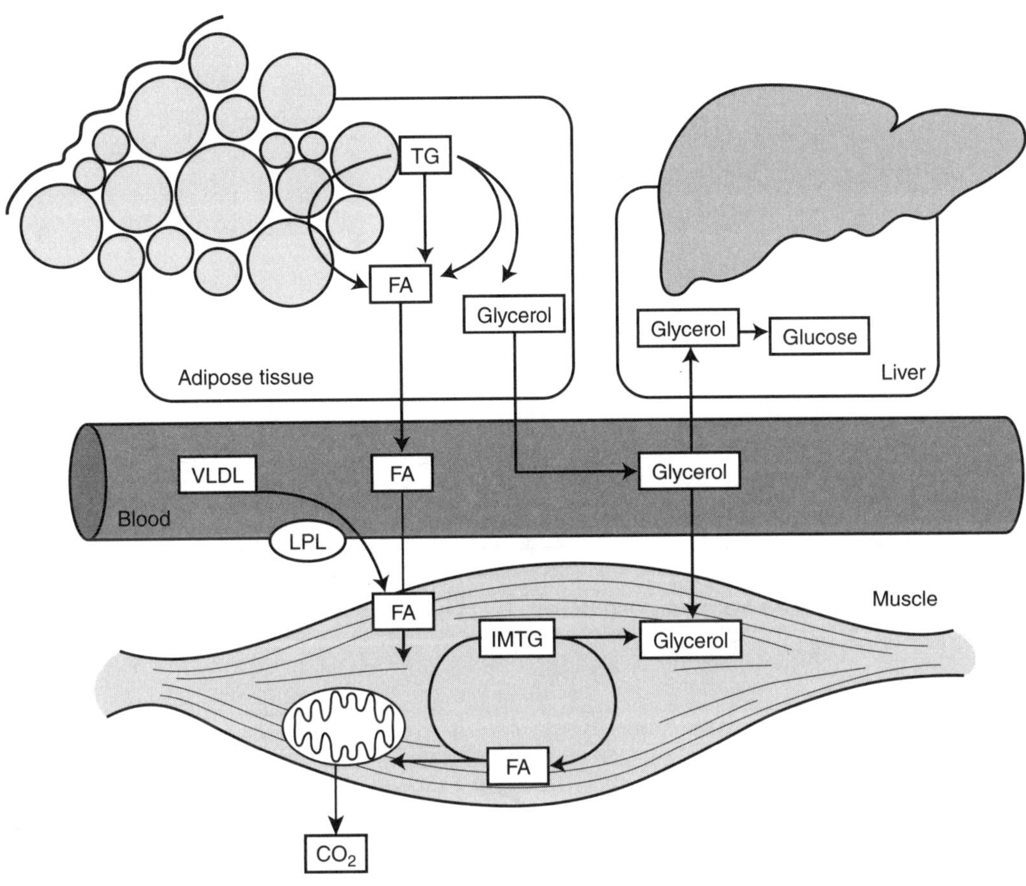

Figure 7.1 Overview of fat metabolism and the main organs involved. TG = triacylglycerol; FA = fatty acid; IMTG = intramuscular triacylglycerol; LPL = lipoprotein lipase; VLDL = very low-density lipoprotein.

are oxidized, they must be mobilized and transported to the site of oxidation. The **adipocyte** contains lipases that break down triacylglycerols. Upon stimulation by the sympathetic nervous system (SNS), HSL splits triacylglycerols into FAs and glycerol and, as its name implies, is regulated by hormones (see figure 7.2). Adipocytes also contain triacylglycerol lipase and enzymes that split off the first FAs, which results in the formation of a diacylglycerol (DAG). HSL may be translocated to the triacylglycerol in the cell and subsequently activated. Conversion of the inactive form of HSL into the active form mainly depends on the sympathetic nervous system and circulating epinephrine. Norepinephrine is released from nerve endings of the sympathetic nervous system, whereas epinephrine is produced in the adrenal medulla, especially during high-intensity exercise. The effects are mediated through adrenergic receptors found on the adipocyte membrane. Insulin is probably the most important counter-regulatory hormone, and its secretion from the pancreatic islets is usually suppressed in the presence of elevated concentrations of epinephrine.

When lipolysis is stimulated, the glycerol released by this reaction diffuses freely into the blood. The adipocyte cannot reuse it, because the enzyme **glycerokinase**, which is required to phosphorylate the glycerol before reesterification with FAs, is only present in extremely low concentrations. Therefore, almost all the glycerol produced by lipolysis is released into the plasma, and the measurement of glycerol in the blood is often used as a measure of lipolysis. FAs released by lipolysis are either reesterified within the adipocyte or transported into the bloodstream for use in other tissues (see figure 7.3).

At rest, approximately 70% of all FAs released during lipolysis are reesterified (Wolfe et al. 1990). During exercise, reesterification is suppressed, which results in increased availability of FAs in the adipocyte. The availability of FAs increases even more because lipolysis is stimulated by ß-adrenoreceptors during exercise. Catecholamines

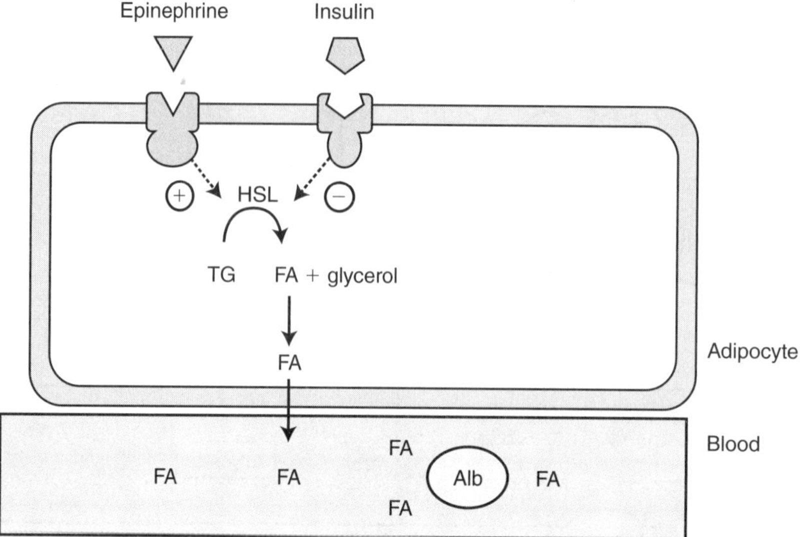

Figure 7.2 Mobilization of FAs from adipose tissue. TG = triacylglycerol; HSL = hormone-sensitive lipase; Alb = albumin.

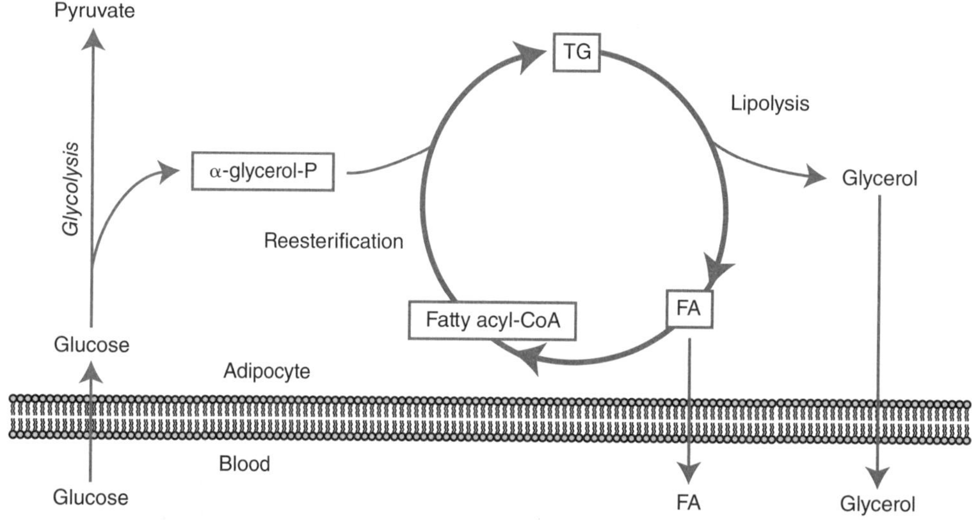

Figure 7.3 Lipolysis of triacylglycerol and reesterification of FAs.

International Journal of Sports Medicine: From A.E. Jeukendrup et al., "Fat Metabolism During Exercise. Part I. Fatty Acid Mobilization and Muscle Metabolism," 1998; 19(4): 231-244.

released from the adrenal gland stimulate lipolysis during exercise.

Lipolysis is usually in excess of the demand for FAs at rest and during exercise. Reesterification is therefore believed to play an important role in regulating FA mobilization. Reesterification depends on the rate at which FAs are removed from the adipocyte by the blood, the rate of glycerol-3-phosphate production, and the activity of triacylglycerol synthesizing enzymes. Because glycerol cannot be recycled to any major extent in human adipocytes (or myocytes), the backbone for a triacylglycerol molecule is derived from glycerol-3-phosphate, an intermediate of the glycolytic pathway.

FAs are not soluble in the aqueous environment of the adipocyte cytoplasm. Therefore, they are bound to FABPs that transport the FAs to the cell membrane. At least during low-intensity to moderate-intensity exercise, the increase in lipolysis and the reduction in esterification of FAs result in a substantially increased level of FAs in the blood (Romijn et al. 1993; Wolfe et al. 1990).

Removal of FAs and Transport in the Blood

The removal of FAs from the adipocyte into the bloodstream depends on several factors, the most important of which are blood flow to the adipose tissue, the albumin concentration in the blood, and the number of free binding sites for FAs on the albumin molecule. Albumin is the most abundant protein in plasma, and one of its functions is as a carrier protein that transports FAs. When it arrives at the target tissue (e.g., muscle) it binds to specific ABPs. Binding to this protein then aids the release of FAs from albumin and their uptake.

A typical plasma albumin concentration is around 0.7 mmol/L (which is equivalent to 45 g/L), and albumin has at least three high-affinity binding sites for FAs, which provide a large capacity to bind FAs. Therefore, most FAs in the blood are bound to albumin (>99.9%), and only those dissolved in the plasma water (<0.1%) circulate freely. Under most conditions, only a fraction of the total number of binding sites of albumin are occupied. At rest, in the postabsorptive state, the plasma FA concentration is about 0.2 to 0.4 mmol/L. However, during prolonged exercise, the FA concentration in the blood can rise to about 2 mmol/L. At this concentration, the maximum capacity of albumin to bind FAs may be reached. When the FA concentration rises further, the percentage of unbound FAs increases, which is believed to be toxic for cells because of detergent-like properties of unbound FAs. These extremely high FA levels, however, are unusual, and the body seems to have protective mechanisms to prevent rises much above 2 mmol/L. One of these mechanisms could be increased incorporation of FAs into plasma triacylglycerol. During every pass through the liver, a fraction of the FAs is extracted from the circulation and incorporated into VLDL particles.

Plasma Lipoproteins

Triacylglycerols bound to lipoproteins (VLDLs and chylomicrons) are another potential source of FAs (Havel, Pernow, and Jones 1967). The enzyme LPL in the vascular wall hydrolyzes some of the triacylglycerols in circulating lipoproteins passing through the capillary bed. As a result, FAs are released, and the muscle takes them up to use for oxidation. But the FA uptake from plasma lipoprotein triacylglycerols occurs slowly and accounts for less than 3% of the energy expenditure during prolonged exercise (Havel, Pernow, and Jones 1967). Therefore, it is generally believed that plasma triacylglycerols contribute only minimally to energy production during exercise. Some interesting observations need further investigation. For instance, LPL activity increases significantly after training and after consumption of a high-fat diet; in both situations, fat oxidation increases markedly. In addition, acute exercise also stimulates LPL activity.

Transport of FAs Into the Muscle Cell

For a long time, the transport of FAs into the muscle cell was believed to be a passive process. This belief was based on early observations that FA uptake increased linearly with FA concentration. Recently, however, specific carrier proteins have been identified (see figure 7.4). In the sarcolemma, at least two proteins are involved in the transport of FAs across the membrane: a specific FABPpm and an FA transporter (FAT/CD36) protein. These proteins are likely to be responsible for the transport of most FAs across the sarcolemma. Animal studies indicate that the transporters become saturated at plasma FA concentrations around 1.5 mmol/L. FAT/CD36 can translocate from intracellular vesicles to the cell membrane in a similar manner as the GLUT4 protein, which indicates that FA transport can also be regulated acutely (Bonen et al. 1999; van Oort et al. 2008). Muscle contraction increases plasma membrane FAT/CD36 and decreases the concentration of FAT/CD36 in the sarcoplasm (cytoplasm of muscle cells). Along with a higher density of FAT/CD36 at the cell membrane, increased FA transport into the cell was observed. It appears that muscle contraction increases the translocation of the FAT/CD36 to the cell membrane, but the exact mechanism is currently not known. Similar factors that result in GLUT4 translocation might also be responsible for the translocation of FAT/CD36.

In the sarcoplasm, the FAs are bound to another specific cytoplasmic FA-binding protein (FABPc). FABPc is thought to be responsible for the transport of FAs from the sarcolemma to the mitochondria.

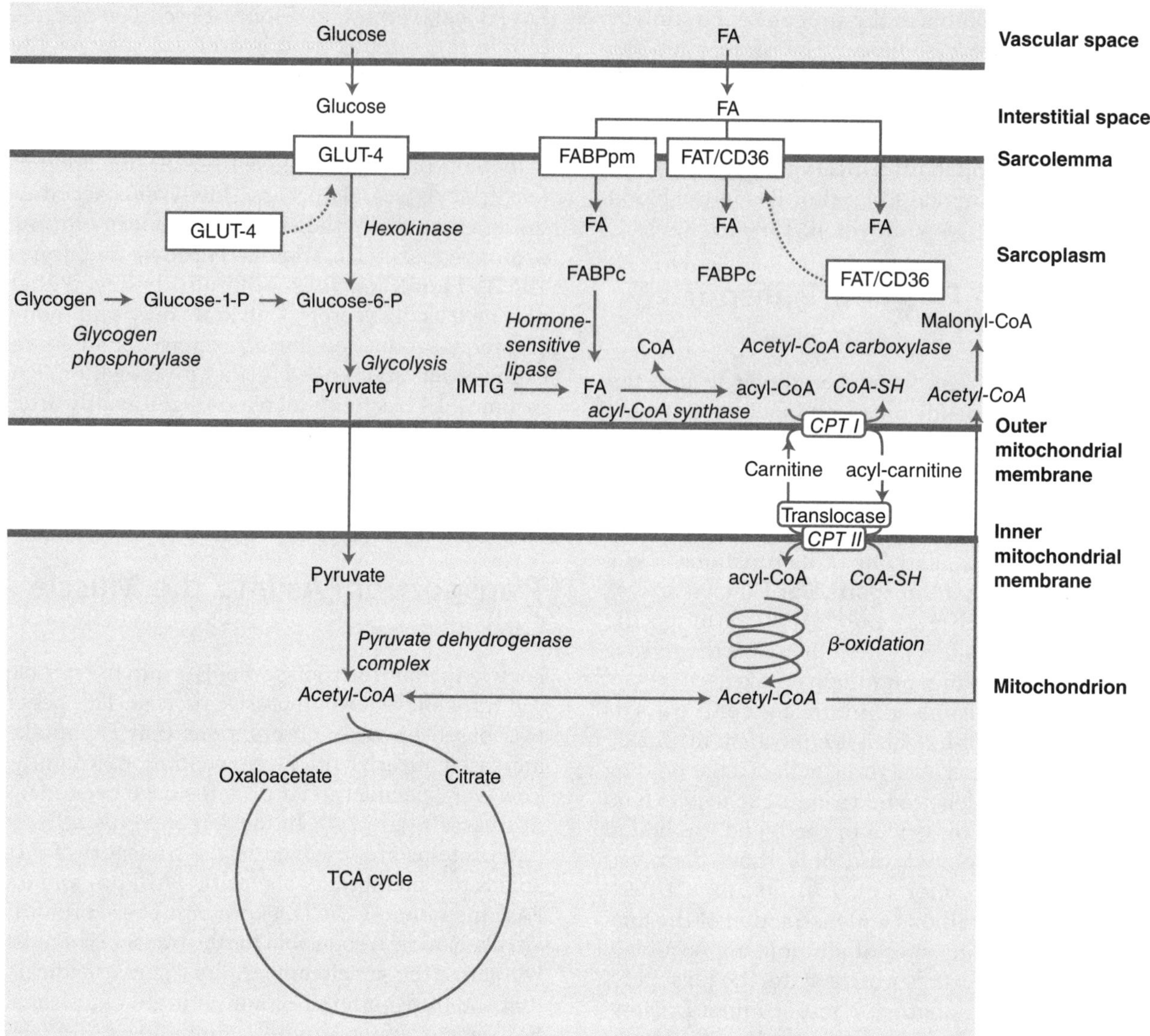

Figure 7.4 Presentation of the transport of glucose and FAs from the blood into the mitochondria. CoA-SH = free coenzyme A; CPT I = carnitine palmitoyl transferase I; CPT II = carnitine palmitoyl transferase II; FABP = fatty acid binding protein; IMTG = intramuscular triacylglycerol.

From A.E. Jeukendrup, "Regulation of Skeletal Muscle Fat Metabolism," *New York Academy of Sciences* 2002; 967: 1-19.

At present, little is known about the roles of these FA-binding proteins and transporters, and whether they are a limiting factor for fat oxidation is unknown.

Intramuscular Triacylglycerols

Another source of FAs is the IMTG stores in the muscle itself. Type I muscle fibers have a higher content of IMTG than type II muscle fibers. IMTG stores, usually located adjacent to the mitochondria as lipid droplets (see figure 7.5), have been recognized as an important energy source during exercise. Studies in which muscle samples were investigated under a microscope revealed that the size of these lipid droplets decreases during exercise. Also, indirect measures of IMTG breakdown provide evidence for its use during exercise. The location of the droplets seems to be important as well. In trained muscle, the lipid droplets are believed to be located next to the mitochondria, whereas in untrained muscle, the lipid droplets may not be so intricately linked with the mitochondria and may be dispersed throughout the cytoplasm. It has been shown that exercise training increases the number of intramuscular triacylglycerols next to

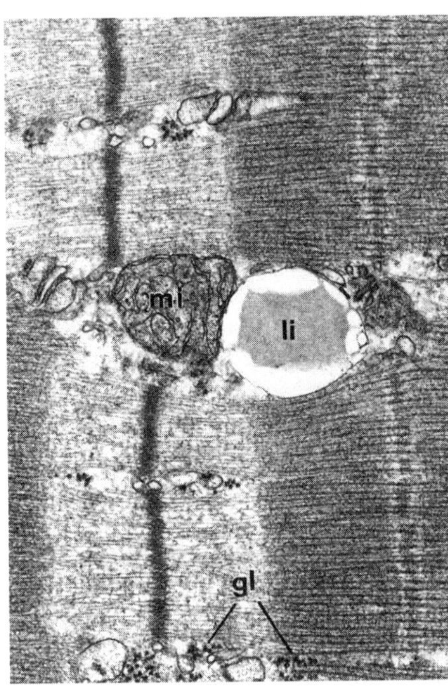

Figure 7.5 An electromyograph of skeletal muscle showing intramuscular triacylglycerols. A large lipid droplet (li) is located adjacent to the mitochondria (mi). Compare the enormous stores of lipid with the small stores of glycogen (gl) in this muscle.

International Journal of Sports Medicine: From A.E. Jeukendrup et al., "Fat Metabolism During Exercise. Part I. Fatty Acid Mobilization and Muscle Metabolism," 1998; 19(4): 231-244.

the mitochondria (Devries et al. 2007). Like adipose tissue, muscle contains an HSL that is activated by ß-adrenergic stimulation and inhibited by insulin. FAs liberated from IMTGs may be released into the blood, reesterified, or oxidized within the muscle. Because the lipid droplets are located close to the mitochondria, at least in trained muscle, most of the FAs released after lipolysis are assumed to be oxidized. The FAs released are bound to FABPc until they are transported into the mitochondria.

Transport of FAs Into the Mitochondria

FAs in the cytoplasm may be activated by the enzyme acyl-CoA synthetase or thiokinase to form an acyl-CoA complex (often referred to as an activated FA) (see figure 7.6). This acyl-CoA complex is used for the synthesis of IMTGs or it is bound to carnitine under the influence of the enzyme CPT I (which is also known as carnitine acyl transferase I or CAT-I), which is located at the outside of the outer mitochondrial membrane.

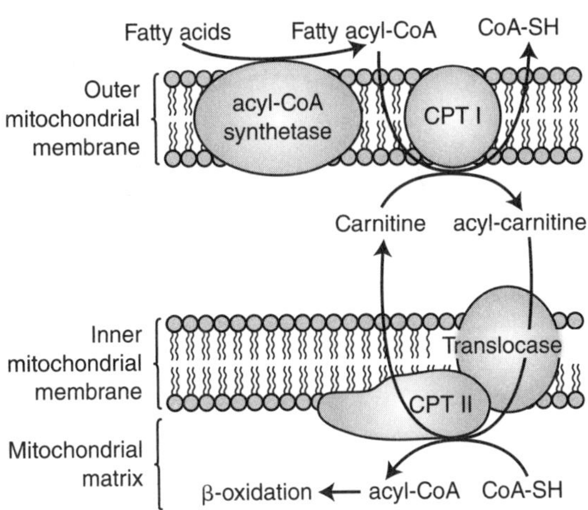

Figure 7.6 Transport of FAs into the mitochondria.

The bonding between carnitine and the activated FA is the first step in the transport of the FA into the mitochondria. As carnitine binds to the FA, free CoA is released. The fatty acyl-carnitine complex is transported with a translocase and reconverted into fatty acyl-CoA at the matrix side of the inner mitochondrial membrane by the enzyme CPT II. The carnitine that is released diffuses back across the mitochondrial membrane into the cytoplasm and thus becomes available again for the transport of other FAs. Fatty acyl-carnitine crosses the inner membrane in a one-to-one exchange with a molecule of free carnitine. Although SCFAs and MCFAs are believed to diffuse freely into the mitochondrial matrix, carrier proteins with a specific maximum affinity for short-chain or medium-chain acyl-CoA transport at least some of these FAs. In addition, it has recently been discovered that FAT/CD36 is involved in the transport of fatty acids across the mitochondria. FAT/CD36 is translocated to the mitochondrial membrane before it can transport FA across.

ß-Oxidation

After it is in the mitochondrial matrix, the fatty acyl-CoA is subjected to ß-oxidation, a series of reactions that splits a two-carbon acetyl-CoA molecule of the multiple-carbon FA chain (see figure 7.7). The ß-oxidation pathway uses oxygen and generates some ATP through substrate-level phosphorylation. The acetyl-CoA is then oxidized in the TCA cycle. The complete oxidation of FAs in the mitochondria depends on several factors, including the activity of enzymes of the ß-oxidation pathway, the concentration of TCA-cycle intermediates and

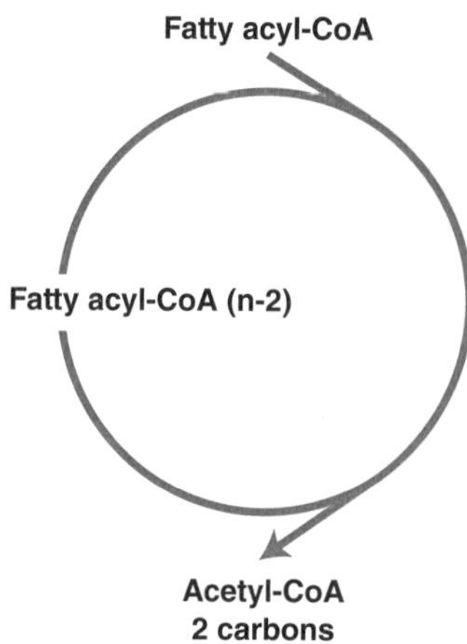

Figure 7.7 The ß-oxidation process.

activity of enzymes in the TCA cycle (these factors determine the total TCA-cycle activity), and the presence of oxygen.

Fat as a Fuel During Exercise

Carbohydrate and fat are always oxidized as a mixture, and whether carbohydrate or fat is the predominant fuel depends on a variety of factors, including the intensity and duration of exercise, the level of aerobic fitness, diet, and carbohydrate intake before or during exercise.

Popular literature, especially, refers to switching from carbohydrate to fat as a fuel; often this is used in the context of endurance exercise: "and after a while, you switch from carbohydrate to fat." This is incorrect. There is no switch, and the two substrates are always used simultaneously. Depending on the conditions and availability, one substrate may contribute more than the other. During prolonged exercise, fat oxidation will increase as carbohydrate sources become depleted. The changes in fat metabolism that occur in the transition from rest to exercise and the various factors that influence fat mobilization and oxidation are discussed in the following sections.

Fat Use at Rest and During Exercise

After an overnight fast (after the effects of insulin from the last meal have worn off), most of the energy requirement is covered by the oxidation of FAs derived from adipose tissue. The rate of lipolysis in adipose tissue depends mostly on the circulating concentrations of hormones (epinephrine stimulates lipolysis, and insulin inhibits lipolysis). Most of the FAs liberated after lipolysis seem to be reesterified within the adipocyte. Some FAs enter the bloodstream, but only about half of them are oxidized. Resting plasma FA concentrations are typically between 0.2 and 0.4 mmol/L.

When exercise is initiated, the rate of lipolysis and the rate of FA release from adipose tissue increase. During moderate-intensity exercise, lipolysis increases approximately threefold mainly because of an increased ß-adrenergic stimulation (by catecholamines). In addition, during moderate-intensity exercise, blood flow to adipose tissue is doubled and the rate of reesterification is halved. Blood flow in skeletal muscle increases dramatically, and, therefore, the delivery of FAs to the muscle increases.

During the first 15 minutes of exercise, plasma FA concentrations usually decrease because the rate of FA uptake by the muscle exceeds the rate of FA appearance from lipolysis. Thereafter, the rate of appearance exceeds the use by muscle, and plasma FA concentrations increase. The rise in FA depends on the exercise intensity. During moderate-intensity exercise, FA concentrations may reach 1 mmol/L within 60 minutes of exercise, but at higher exercise intensities, the rise in plasma FAs is small or may even be absent.

Fat Oxidation and Exercise Duration

Fat oxidation increases as exercise duration increases. Edwards, Margaria, and Dill (1934) reported fat oxidation rates of over 1 g/min after 6 hours of running. Christensen and Hansen (1939) observed that the contribution of fat could increase to levels as high as 90% of energy expenditure when a fatty meal was consumed, leading to fat oxidation rates of 1.5 g/min. The mechanism of this increased fat oxidation as exercise duration increases is not entirely clear, but it seems to be linked to the decrease in muscle glycogen stores.

Fat Oxidation and Exercise Intensity

Fat oxidation is usually the predominant fuel at low exercise intensities, whereas during high exercise intensities, carbohydrates are the major fuel. In absolute terms, fat oxidation increases as the exercise intensity increases from low to moderate, although the percentage contribution of fat may actually decrease (see figure 7.8). The increased fat oxidation is a direct result of the increased energy expenditure. At higher exercise intensities (>75% of $\dot{V}O_2max$) fat oxidation is inhibited, and the relative and absolute rates of fat oxidation decrease to negligible values. Achten et al. (2002, 2003) studied this relationship over a wide range of exercise intensities in a group of trained subjects and found that, on average, the highest rates of fat oxidation were observed at 62% to 63% of $\dot{V}O_2max$.

During exercise at 25% of $\dot{V}O_2max$, most of the fat oxidized is derived from plasma FAs and only small amounts come from IMTGs (Romijn et al. 1993) (see figure 7.9). During moderate-intensity exercise (65% of $\dot{V}O_2max$), however, the contribution of plasma FAs declines and the contribution of IMTGs increases and provides about half of the FAs used for total fat oxidation (Romijn et al. 1993). Training also decreases the contribution of

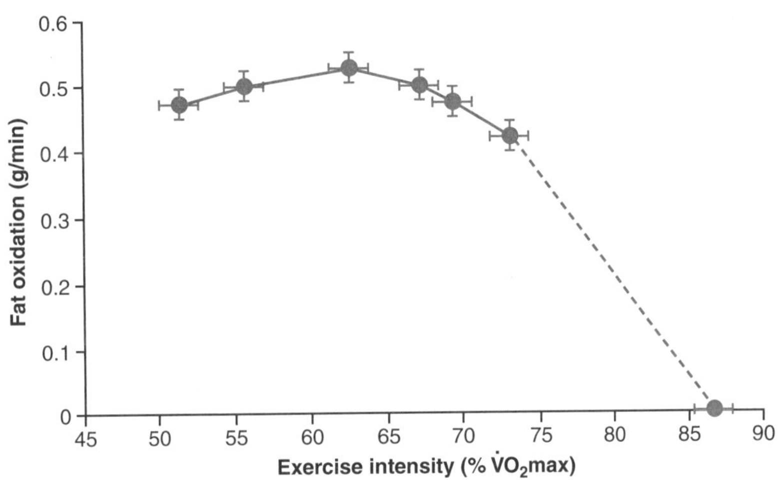

Figure 7.8 Fat oxidation as a function of exercise intensity.

International Journal of Sports Medicine: From J. Achten and A.G. Jeukendrup. "Maximal Fat Oxidation During Exercise in Trained Men," 2003; 24(8): 603-608.

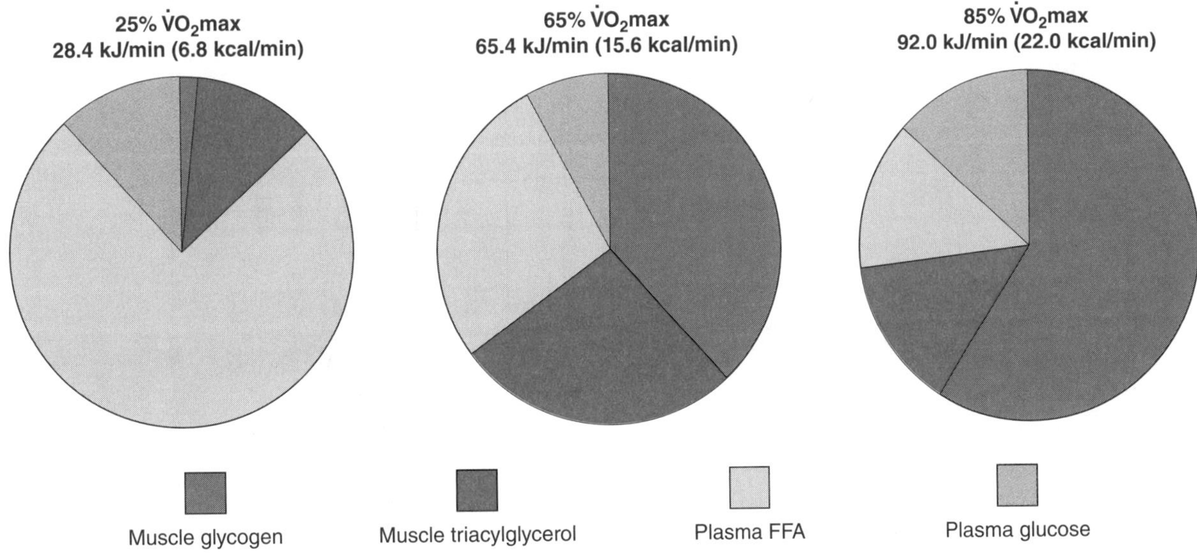

Figure 7.9 Substrate use at different exercise intensities.

Data from Romijn et al. (1993).

plasma FAs, despite a dramatic increase in total fat oxidation. This decrease in plasma FA oxidation is accounted for by a marked increase in the contribution of muscle triacylglycerols to energy expenditure.

When the exercise intensity is further increased, fat oxidation decreases, although the rate of lipolysis is still high. The blood flow to the adipose tissue may decrease (because of sympathetic vasoconstriction), which may result in decreased removal of FAs from adipose tissue. During high-intensity exercise, lactate accumulation may also increase the rate of reesterification of FAs. As a result, plasma FA concentrations are usually low during intense exercise. This decreased availability of FAs can only partially explain the reduced fat oxidation observed in these conditions. When Romijn et al. (1995) restored FA concentrations to levels observed at moderate exercise intensities by infusing triacylglycerols (Intralipid) and heparin, fat oxidation increased only slightly and was still lower than at moderate intensities (see the sidebar and figure 7.10). Therefore, an additional mechanism in the muscle must be responsible for the decreased fat oxidation observed during high-intensity exercise.

TRIACYLGLYCEROL AND HEPARIN INFUSION

To increase plasma FA concentrations for experimental purposes, researchers have used infusions of triacylglycerol and heparin. Because FAs are not soluble in water (plasma), they cannot be infused directly. Therefore, a lipid emulsion (often Intralipid) is used in combination with a heparin injection. Heparin releases LPL from the capillaries. After LPL becomes freely available in the circulation, it starts to break down the plasma triacylglycerol, and FA concentrations rise rapidly. The amount of heparin needs to be titrated carefully, because introducing too much heparin could result in extremely high (toxic) levels of FAs in the circulation. Furthermore, heparin is an anticoagulant and prevents the blood from clotting when an injury occurs; therefore, it must always be used with extreme care.

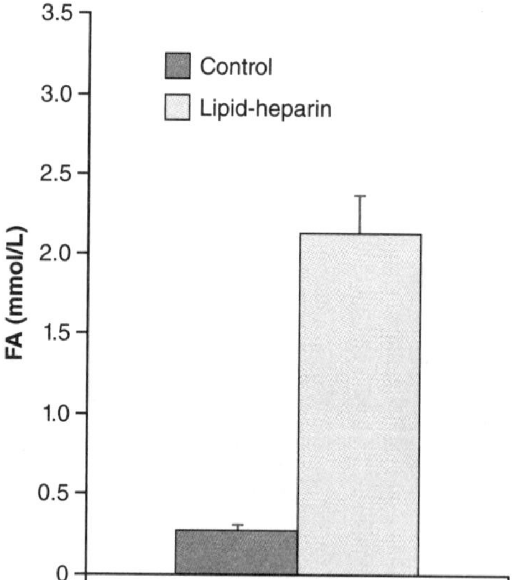

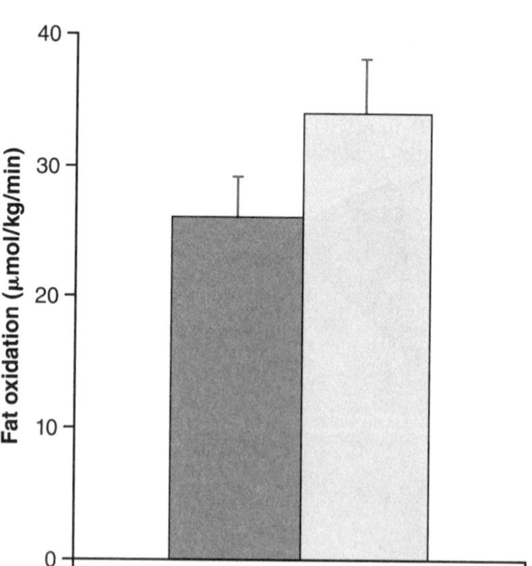

Figure 7.10 FA concentrations are usually low at high exercise intensities (>85% of $\dot{V}O_2$max), which could explain the relatively low oxidation rates of fat compared with moderate exercise intensities. When lipid and heparin are infused, high plasma FA concentrations are achieved but do not restore fat oxidation to the levels observed at moderate exercise intensities (65% of $\dot{V}O_2$max).

Data from Romijn et al. (1995).

Sidossis et al. (1997) and Coyle et al. (1997) suggested that the decreased fat oxidation is related to the transport of FAs into the mitochondria. They observed that during high-intensity exercise, the oxidation of LCFAs is impaired, whereas the oxidation of medium-chain FAs is unaffected. Because the medium-chain FAs are less dependent on transport mechanisms into the mitochondria, these data provide evidence that carnitine-dependent FA transport is a limiting factor.

Fat Oxidation and Aerobic Capacity

Endurance training affects substrate use and exercise capacity. Studies involving animals and humans have established a marked adaptive increase in oxidative potential in response to increased regular physical activity (Holloszy and Booth 1976; Holloszy and Coyle 1984). A consequence and probably a contributing factor to the enhanced exercise capacity after endurance training is the metabolic shift to greater use of fat and a concomitant sparing of glycogen. The contribution of fat to total energy expenditure increases after training at relative and absolute exercise intensities. The adaptations that contribute to stimulation of fat oxidation in trained subjects include

- increased mitochondrial density and an increased number of oxidative enzymes in trained muscle, which increases the capacity to oxidize fat;
- increased capillary density, which enhances FA delivery to the muscle;
- increased FABP concentrations, which may facilitate uptake of FAs across the sarcolemma; and
- increased CPT concentration, which facilitates the transport of FAs into the mitochondria.

One factor that does not seem to be influenced by training is lipolysis in adipose tissue (Klein, Coyle, and Wolfe 1994) (see figure 7.11). After training, the rate of lipolysis at the same absolute exercise intensity does not seem to be affected. At the same relative exercise intensity, the rate of lipolysis increases after training (Klein et al. 1996). Increased lipolysis of IMTG likely contributes to this increased whole-body lipolysis.

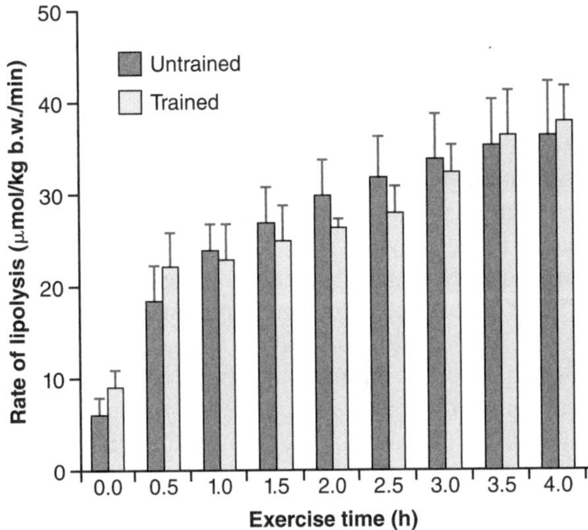

Figure 7.11 Whole-body lipolysis in trained and untrained subjects.

Data in Klein, Coyle, and Wolfe (1994).

Fat Oxidation and Diet

Diet also has marked effects on fat oxidation. Generally, a high-carbohydrate, low-fat diet reduces fat oxidation, whereas a high-fat, low-carbohydrate diet increases fat oxidation. Some scientists have argued that the results seen in most of these studies are the effects of the last meal, which is known to influence substrate use. But Burke et al. (1999) showed that a high-fat, low-carbohydrate diet had a similar effect on substrate use even after a day on a high-carbohydrate diet. The results indicate that some chronic effects of diet cannot be directly explained by substrate availability. In the study by Burke et al. (1999), for example, subjects consumed a high-fat diet or a high-carbohydrate diet for 5 days and then a high-carbohydrate diet for 1 day. The 1-day high-carbohydrate intake replenished glycogen stores in both conditions, and muscle glycogen concentrations were identical, but large differences existed in substrate use between the two diets.

The RER changed from 0.90 to 0.82 after 5 days on a high-fat diet. After consuming a high-carbohydrate diet for 1 day, RER was still lower compared with baseline values (0.87). Because these changes were not caused by alterations in muscle glycogen availability, they are likely related to metabolic adaptations in the muscle.

Chronic diets can have marked effects on metabolism. These effects seem only partly related to the effects of diets on substrate availability. Adaptations at the muscular level, which result in changes in substrate use in response to a diet, may occur within a period as short as 5 days.

Response to Carbohydrate Feeding

The fastest way to alter fat metabolism during exercise is probably by carbohydrate feeding. Carbohydrate increases the plasma insulin concentration, which reduces lipolysis and causes a marked reduction in FA availability. In a study by Horowitz et al. (1997), carbohydrate was ingested 1 hour before exercise, and lipolysis and fat oxidation were reduced. Plasma FA concentrations decreased to extremely low levels during exercise. But when Intralipid was infused and heparin was injected to increase the plasma FA concentrations, fat oxidation was only partially restored. These findings indicate that reduced availability of FAs is indeed a factor that limits fat oxidation, but because increasing the plasma FA concentrations does not completely restore fat oxidation, other factors must play a role as well. These factors must be located inside the muscle itself.

When a large amount of glucose is ingested 1 hour before exercise, plasma insulin levels are very high at the start of exercise, whereas plasma FA and glycerol concentrations are very low (Coyle et al. 1997). This circumstance results in a 30% reduction in fat oxidation compared with no carbohydrate intake. In a study by Coyle et al. (1997), trace amounts of labeled medium-chain or long-chain FAs were infused, and the oxidation rates of these FAs were determined. The oxidation of long-chain FAs appeared to be reduced, whereas the oxidation of medium-chain FAs appeared to be unaffected (see figure 7.12). Because medium-chain FAs are not as dependent on transport mechanisms into the mitochondria but the long-chain FAs are highly dependent on this mechanism, these results provide evidence that this transport is an important regulatory step. Although the exact mechanisms are still unclear, carbohydrate feeding before exercise reduces fat oxidation by reducing lipolysis and plasma FA availability and exerts an inhibitory effect on carnitine-dependent FA transport into the mitochondria.

Regulation of Carbohydrate and Fat Metabolism

In all situations, carbohydrate and fat together constitute most, if not all, of the energy provision. The percentage contribution of these two fuels, however, varies depending on the factors discussed previously. The rate of carbohydrate use during prolonged strenuous exercise is closely related to the energy needs of the working muscle. In con-

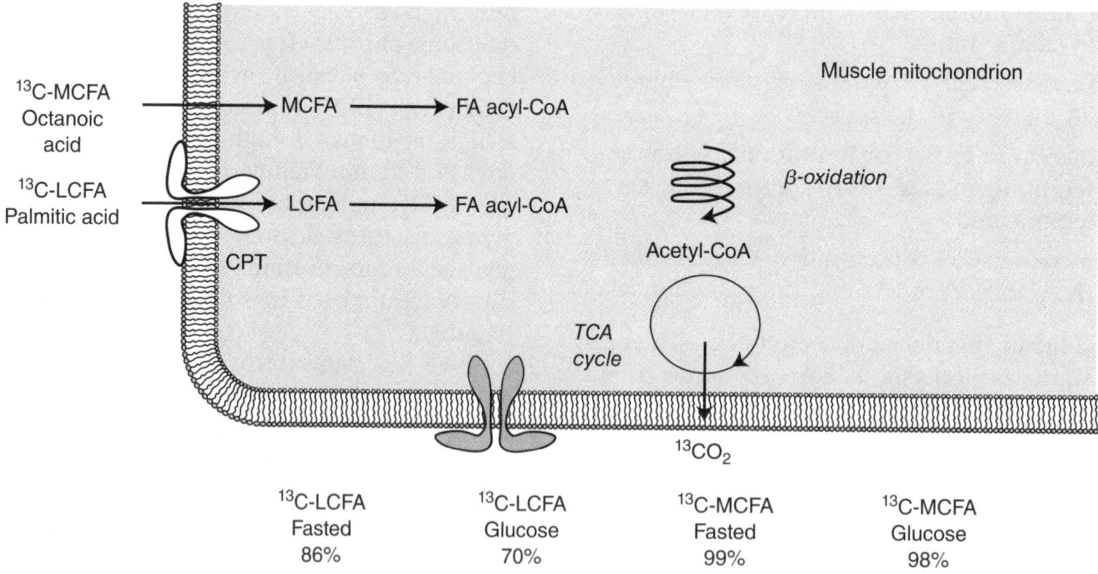

Figure 7.12 Oxidation of MCFAs and LCFAs in the mitochondria during fasted and fed conditions (glucose). Glucose intake reduced the oxidation of LCFAs but not MCFAs. Because LCFAs use a transport protein to enter the mitochondria and MCFAs are less dependent on this protein, glucose availability possibly regulates the entry of FA into the mitochondria.

Data from Coyle et al. (1997).

trast, fat use during exercise is not tightly regulated. No mechanisms closely match the metabolism of FAs to energy expenditure. Fat oxidation is therefore mainly influenced by fat availability and the rate of carbohydrate use.

Some evidence suggests that increases in plasma FA concentration can cause a decrease in the rate of muscle glycogen breakdown. This action could theoretically be beneficial, because muscle glycogen depletion is one of the prime causes of fatigue. Researchers have artificially elevated plasma FA concentrations by raising plasma triacylglycerol concentrations through a fat meal or intravenous infusion of triacylglycerol (Intralipid) followed, in both cases, by a heparin injection; heparin activates lipoprotein lipase, an endothelial enzyme that breaks down blood triacylglycerol into fatty acids and glycerol. Using this method, it has been repeatedly shown that an increase in FA concentration can reduce carbohydrate dependence.

In a study by Costill et al. (1977), Intralipid was infused and heparin was injected during exercise at 70% of $\dot{V}O_2$max. After 60 minutes, a muscle biopsy was taken and muscle glycogen was measured before and after the exercise bout. Muscle glycogen breakdown decreased with the elevated plasma FA concentrations (see figure 7.13). Similar results were obtained when a fat feeding was given in combination with heparin infusion (Vukovich et al. 1993). Although elevating FA levels seems to reduce muscle glycogen breakdown during exercise, the mechanisms are still incompletely understood.

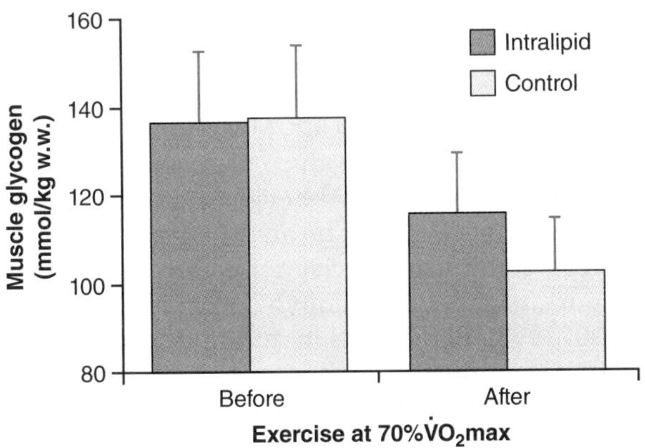

Figure 7.13 Glycogen sparing with increased FA availability. This increased availability of FAs was achieved by infusing a triacylglycerol emulsion with heparin.

Data from Costill et al. (1997).

The classical glucose–FA cycle, or Randle cycle, was originally thought to explain this interaction between carbohydrate and fat metabolism (see figure 7.14). This theory states that with an increase in plasma FA concentration uptake of FAs increases, and these FAs undergo ß-oxidation in the mitochondria, in which they are broken down to acetyl-CoA. An increasing concentration of acetyl-CoA (or an increased acetyl-CoA-to-CoA ratio) inhibits the pyruvate dehydrogenase complex that breaks down pyruvate to acetyl-CoA. In addition, increased formation of acetyl-CoA from FA oxidation in the mitochondria increases muscle citrate levels, and after diffusing into the sarcoplasm, citrate could inhibit phosphofructokinase, the rate-limiting enzyme in glycolysis. The effect of increased acetyl-CoA and citrate levels is, therefore, a reduction in the rate of glycolysis. This reduced rate of glycolysis, in turn, may cause accumulation of G6P in the muscle sarcoplasm, which inhibits hexokinase activity and thus reduces muscle glucose uptake.

With increased fat availability the disturbance in the cellular homeostasis declines. Increasing FA availability decreases intramuscular Pi and AMP accumulation during exercise, possibly because of a greater accumulation of mitochondrial reduced nicotinamide adenine dinucleotide (NADH) (Dyck et al. 1993, 1996). Pi and AMP are indicators of the energy charge of the cell; high concentrations indicate low energy status, and low concentrations reflect ample energy availability. Because Pi and AMP are known to stimulate the enzyme glycogen phosphorylase, the reduction in Pi and AMP levels may be at least partially responsible for reduced muscle glycogen breakdown.

Some studies offer an alternative explanation for reduced muscle glycogen breakdown after elevation of plasma FA concentrations. When studied in more detail, the plasma FA concentrations appear significantly elevated (by infusion of triacylglycerol and injection of heparin) compared with the control condition. The FA concentrations in the control condition, however, were below 0.2 mmol/L. Conceivably, these FA levels are too low to provide the muscle with sufficient fat substrate. As a result, muscle glycogen breakdown may have been increased in the control condition. Therefore, the observed sparing of glycogen with the high FA concentrations could have been caused by increased breakdown of glycogen in the control condition. Blocking lipolysis and reducing FA availability by giving nicotinic acid or a derivative increases muscle glycogen breakdown during exercise.

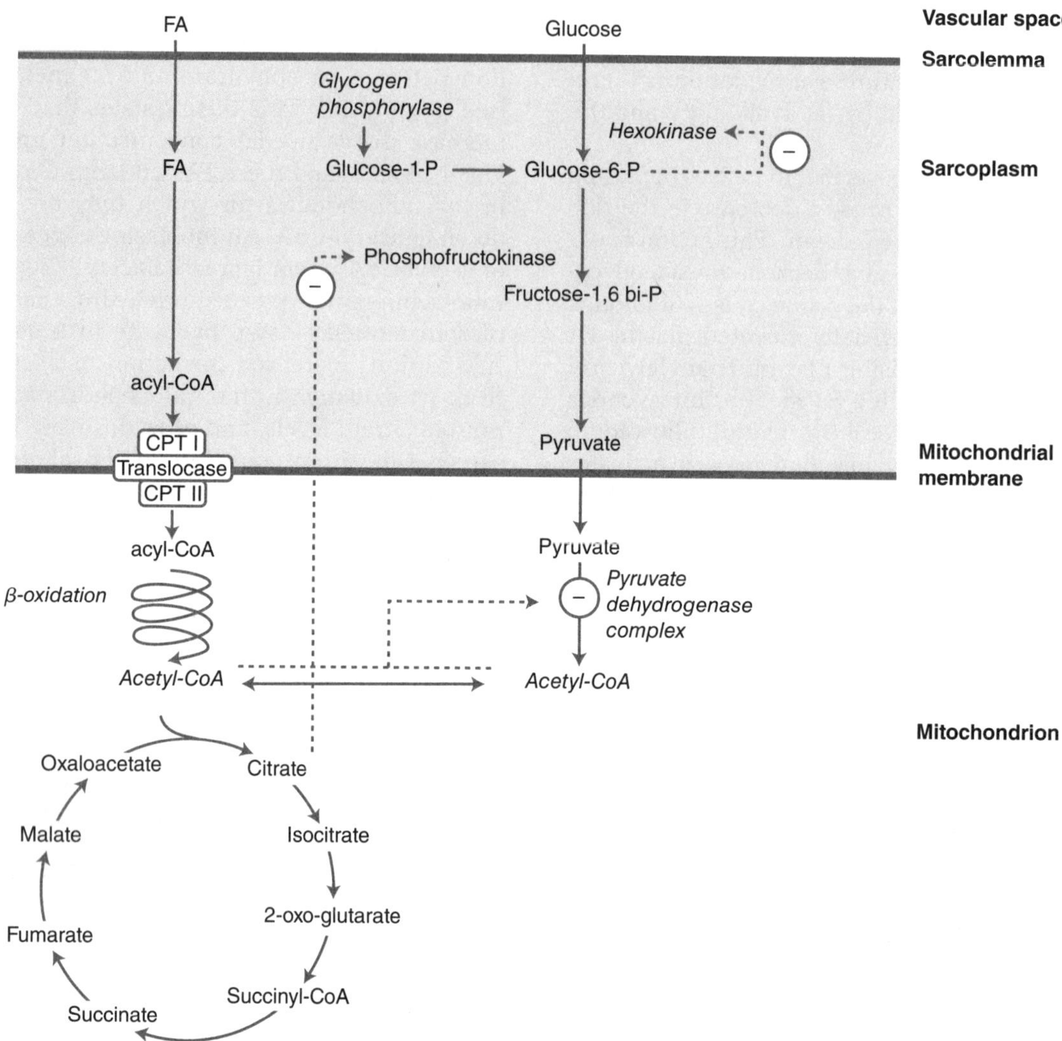

Figure 7.14 Glucose–FA cycle.

Reprinted by permission from A.E. Jeukendrup, "Regulation of Metabolism in Skeletal Muscle," *New York Academy of Sciences* 967 (2002): 217-235.

A more recent theory about the regulation of carbohydrate and fat metabolism proposes that fat does not regulate carbohydrate metabolism but rather that carbohydrate regulates fat metabolism. An increase in the rate of glycolysis decreases fat oxidation. Figure 7.15 shows some of the factors that regulate carbohydrate and fat metabolism.

Regulation of fat metabolism involves the transport of FAs into the mitochondria, which is controlled mainly by the activity of CPT I. CPT I is regulated by several factors, including the malonyl-CoA (a precursor of FA synthesis) concentration. The high rate of glycogenolysis during high-intensity exercise increases the amount of acetyl-CoA in the muscle cell, and some of this acetyl-CoA is converted to malonyl-CoA by the enzyme acetyl-CoA carboxylase (ACC). Malonyl-CoA inhibits CPT I and could thus reduce the transport of FAs into the mitochondria. Although evidence suggests that malonyl-CoA may be an important regulator at rest, studies in exercising humans indicate no important role of malonyl-CoA (Odland et al. 1996, 1998). Reductions in intramuscular pH that may occur during high-intensity exercise may also inhibit CPT I and hence FA transport into the mitochondria (Starritt et al. 2000).

Another explanation is that reduced free carnitine concentration plays a role. When glycogenolysis accelerates, acetyl-CoA accumulates during intense exercise, and some of this acetyl-CoA is bound to carnitine. As a result, the free carnitine concentration drops, and less carnitine is available

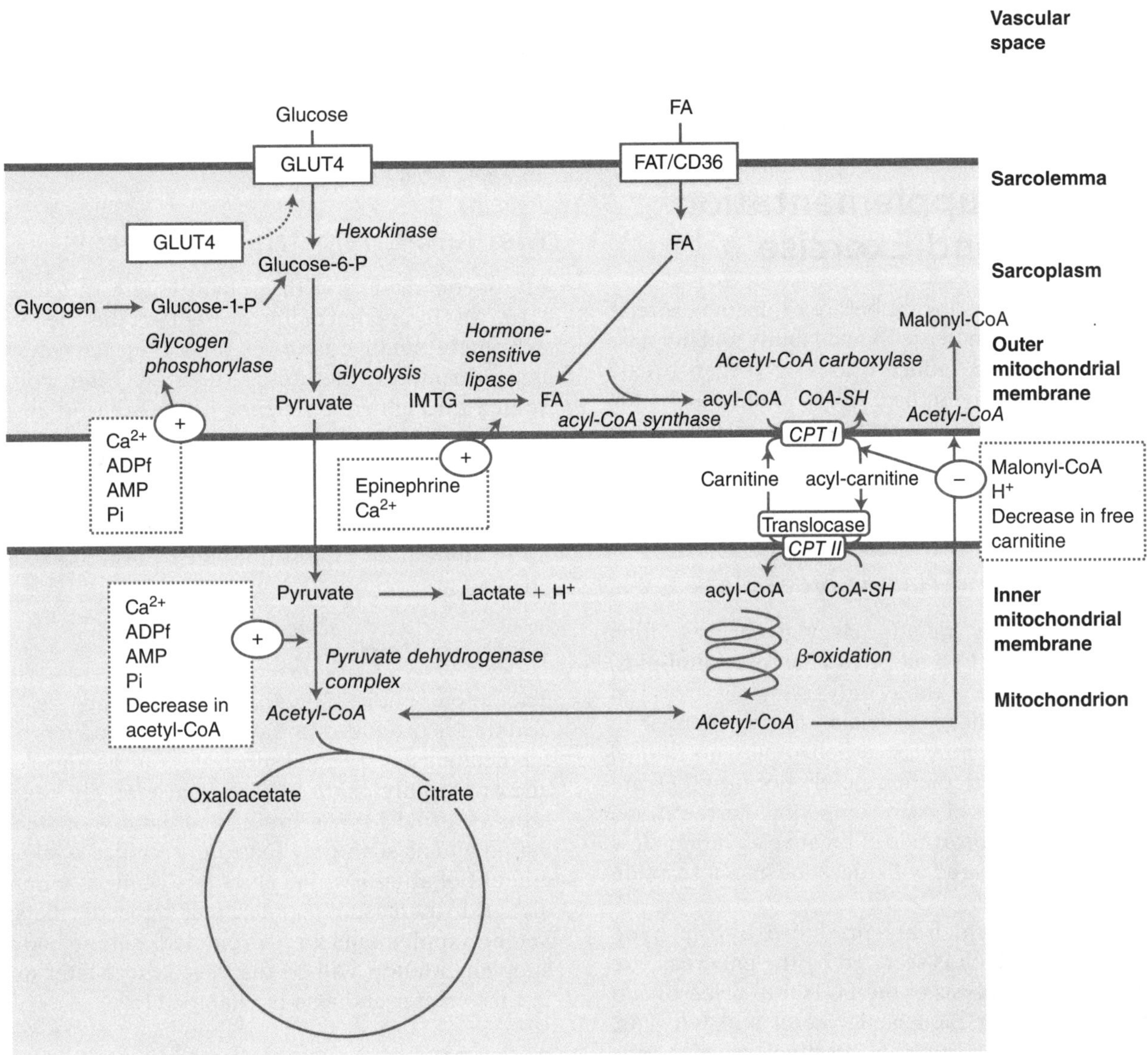

Figure 7.15 Glucose FA cycle reversed. An increase in glycolysis can reduce the FA transport into the mitochondria. CPT I = carnitine palmitoyl transferase I; CPT II = carnitine palmitoyl transferase II; ADPf = free ADP.

Reprinted by permission from A.E. Jeukendrup, "Regulation of Metabolism in Skeletal Muscle," *New York Academy of Sciences* 967 (2002): 217-235.

to transport FAs into the mitochondria (Greenhaff and Timmons 1998a). It also has been proposed that pyruvate-derived acetyl-CoA competes with the FA-derived acetyl-CoA for entrance into the TCA cycle. Currently, it is thought that the most important factor in reducing fat metabolism during high-exercise intensity is the high rates of glycolysis that result in increased acetyl-CoA production, thereby reducing the availability of free carnitine (Jeppesen and Kiens 2012; Jordy and Kiens 2014) and therefore limiting the amounts of FA that can enter the mitochondria.

The rate of carbohydrate use during prolonged strenuous exercise is closely related to the energy needs of the working muscle. In contrast, fat use during exercise is not tightly regulated. No mechanisms closely match the metabolism of FAs to energy expenditure. Fat oxidation is, therefore, mainly influenced by fat availability and the rate of carbohydrate use. The importance of each of these factors may depend on the situation. For example, carbohydrate use may be a more important factor during exercise, whereas the availability of FAs may be more important at rest. The regulation of carbohydrate and fat metabolism during exercise is discussed in more detail in a number of review articles (Jeppesen and Kiens 2012; Jeukendrup 2002; Jordy and Kiens 2014; van Hall 2015).

Fat Supplementation and Exercise

The effects of eating fat before or during exercise as a method to increase FA availability and increase fat oxidation to reduce muscle glycogen breakdown have been studied. Initial studies looked at fatty meals that consisted mainly of long-chain triacylglycerols (LCTs); later studies also looked at alternative lipid fuels such as medium-chain triacylglycerols (MCTs).

Long-Chain Triacylglycerols

Nutritional fats include triacylglycerols (which contain mostly C16 and C18 FAs), phospholipids, and cholesterol; of these, only triacylglycerols can contribute to energy provision during exercise to any extent. In contrast to carbohydrates, nutritional fats reach the circulation slowly because they are potent inhibitors of gastric emptying. Furthermore, digestion and absorption of fat are also rather slow processes compared with digestion and absorption of carbohydrate.

Bile salts, which are produced by the liver, and lipase, which is secreted by the pancreas, are needed for lipolysis of the LCTs into glycerol and three LCFAs or monoacylglycerol and two FAs. The FAs diffuse into the intestinal mucosa cells and are reesterified in the cytoplasm to form LCTs. These LCTs are encapsulated by a coat of proteins, and the resulting LCT-protein complex is called a chylomicron, which is far more water soluble than isolated LCTs. These chylomicrons are then released in the lymphatic system, which ultimately drains in the systemic circulation. Exogenous LCTs enter the systemic circulation much more slowly than carbohydrates do, because carbohydrates are absorbed as glucose (or, to minor extents, as fructose or galactose) and directly enter the main circulation through the portal vein. Long-chain dietary FAs typically enter the blood 3 to 4 hours after ingestion.

The fact that these LCFAs enter the circulation in chylomicrons is also important, and the rate of breakdown of chylomicron-bound triacylglycerols by muscle is generally believed to be relatively low. The primary role of these triacylglycerols in chylomicrons may be the replenishment of IMTG stores after exercise (Oscai, Essig, and Palmer 1990). Therefore, the intake of fat during exercise should be avoided. Many so-called sports bars or energy bars contain relatively large amounts of fat, so food labels should be checked when choosing an energy bar.

Medium-Chain Triacylglycerols

MCTs contain FAs with a chain length of C8 or C10. MCTs are normally present in the diet in extremely small quantities, and they have few natural sources; therefore, MCTs are often consumed through supplements. MCTs are sold as a supplement to replace normal fat because MCTs are not stored in the body and could therefore help athletes lose body fat. MCT supplements are popular among bodybuilders and have been used as an alternative fuel source during exercise (see chapter 11).

Ketone Bodies

The ketone bodies ß-hydroxybutyrate and acetoacetate are produced in the body as byproducts of fat metabolism, are good substrates for the muscle, and are rapidly oxidized. They have largely been seen as a fuel for the brain in situations of starvation and as such they have not received a large amount of attention. Recently this changed when alongside increasing popularity of ketogenic diets, ketone supplements were promoted. Ketone body supplementation will be discussed more later on in this chapter and also in chapter 11.

Fish Oil

Fish oil is a natural source of long-chain omega-3 FAs. It contains DHA and EPA. Fish oil is said to improve membrane characteristics and improve membrane function when more of these omega-3 FAs are incorporated into the lipid bilayer of the membrane (see chapter 11).

Effects of Diet on Fat Metabolism and Performance

Another strategy that has been used to increase fat oxidation and reduce reliance on carbohydrate stores involves longer-term manipulations of the diet that last days or weeks. These methods included **fasting** and high-fat, low-carbohydrate diets.

Fasting

Fasting has been proposed as a way to increase fat use, spare muscle glycogen, and improve exercise performance. In rats, short-term fasting increases plasma epinephrine and norepinephrine concentrations, stimulates lipolysis, and increases the concentration of circulating plasma FAs. These effects increase fat oxidation and spare muscle glycogen, which leads to a similar (Koubi et al. 1991) or even an increased running time to exhaustion in rats (Dohm et al. 1983). In humans, fasting also results in increased concentration of circulating catecholamines, increased lipolysis, increased concentration of plasma FAs (Dohm et al. 1986), and decreased glucose turnover (Knapik et al. 1988). Muscle glycogen concentrations, however, are unaffected by fasting for 24 hours when no strenuous exercise is performed (Knapik et al. 1988; Loy et al. 1986). Although fasting has been reported to have no effect on endurance capacity at low exercise intensities (45% of $\dot{V}O_2$max), decreases in performance have been observed for exercise intensities between 50% and 100% of $\dot{V}O_2$max. The observed decreased performance was not reversible by carbohydrate ingestion during exercise (Riley et al. 1988).

Some investigators have argued that the effects observed in most of these studies were seen because, in the control situation, the last meal was provided 3 hours before the exercise to exhaustion. The effects, therefore, result from the improvement in endurance capacity after feeding rather than from decreased performance after fasting. But the studies that compared a prolonged fast (>24 hours) to a 12-hour fast also reported decreased performance (Knapik et al. 1988; Maughan and Gleeson 1988; Zinker, Britz, and Brooks 1990), and thus the conclusion that fasting decreases endurance capacity seems justified. The mechanism remains unclear, although certainly liver glycogen stores are substantially depleted after a 24-hour fast. Thus, euglycemia may not be as well maintained during exercise. Some degree of metabolic acidosis may also be observed after prolonged fasting. When hepatic glycogen stores are exhausted (e.g., after 12 to 24 hours of total fasting), the liver produces ketone bodies (acetoacetate, ß-hydroxybutyrate, and acetone) to provide an energy substrate for peripheral tissues. These keto acids lower blood pH, although the acidosis is usually only mild.

Short-Term High-Fat Diet

Christensen and Hansen (1939) showed that short-term exposure to a high-fat diet resulted in impaired fatigue resistance. Short term in this context is days rather than weeks (many studies have used dietary intervention periods of 1-3 days). After muscle biopsy techniques were redeveloped, a high-fat, low-carbohydrate diet was shown to result in decreased muscle glycogen levels, and this was the main factor causing lack of fatigue resistance during prolonged exercise (Bergstrom and Hultman 1967b; Hultman 1967). Plasma FA concentrations increase at rest and increase more rapidly when a low-carbohydrate diet is consumed (Conlee et al. 1990; Martin, Robinson, and Robertshaw 1978; Maughan et al. 1978). These changes in plasma FA concentrations are attributed to changes in the rate of lipolysis. After consumption of a low-carbohydrate diet, both plasma FAs and plasma glycerol concentrations increase.

Jansson and Kaijser (1982) reported that the uptake of FAs by the muscle during 25 minutes of cycling at 65% of $\dot{V}O_2$max was 82% higher in subjects who received a low-carbohydrate diet (5%) for 5 days compared with subjects who received a high-carbohydrate diet (75%) for 5 days. Plasma FAs contributed 24% and 14%, respectively, to energy expenditure. Increased FA concentrations in the blood after a period of carbohydrate restriction lead to increased ketogenesis with elevated plasma levels of ß-hydroxybutyrate and acetoacetate. After a few days of high-fat feeding, the ketone body production increases fivefold (Fery and Balasse 1983), and the arterial concentration of ketone bodies may increase 10- to 20-fold (Fery and Balasse 1983). During the first phase of light to moderate exercise, ketone body concentrations usually decline, and after 30 to 90 minutes, they increase again (Fery and Balasse 1983; Knapik et al. 1988; Zinker, Britz, and Brooks 1990). But the observed plasma concentrations under those conditions are still higher after a high-fat diet compared with those associated with a low-fat diet. Carbohydrate-restricted diets may also lead to increased breakdown of muscle triacylglycerols. There is a substantial body of evidence that short-term high-fat, low-carbohydrate diets will result in impaired performance or endurance capacity, and this is mostly because of a reduction in muscle and liver glycogen stores, poor recovery, and increases in ratings of perceived exertion.

Long-Term High-Fat Diet

Longer-term (weeks not days) dietary interventions are thought to result in adaptations that will restore exercise tolerance. It has been suggested that a 3- to 4-day alteration in dietary composition is an insufficient time to induce an adaptive response to the changed diet. A high-fat diet over a prolonged period, however, may result in decreased use of carbohydrates and increased contribution of fat to energy metabolism. In rats, adaptation to a high-fat diet leads to considerable improvements in endurance capacity (Miller, Bryce, and Conlee 1984; Simi et al. 1991) (see figure 7.16). These adaptations can be attributed to the increased number of oxidative enzymes and decreased degradation of liver glycogen during exercise (Simi et al. 1991). The results suggest that after adaptation to a high-fat diet, the capacity to oxidize FAs instead of carbohydrates increases because of an adaptation of the oxidative enzymes in the muscle cell. These adaptations are much like the adaptations that occur after endurance training.

One of the first studies that investigated the effects of prolonged high-fat diets on humans was conducted by Phinney et al. (1980). They investigated exercise performance in obese subjects who followed a high-fat diet (a ketogenic diet in which 90% of energy intake was from fat) for 6 weeks. Before and after the diet, subjects exercised at 75% of $\dot{V}O_2max$ until exhaustion. Subjects were able to exercise as long on the high-fat diet as they did on their normal diet, but after the high-fat diet, fat became the main substrate. The results of this study, however, may have been influenced by the fact that these subjects were not in energy balance and lost 11 kg (24 lb) of body mass. So, although no differences were seen in absolute $\dot{V}O_2max$ before and after the dietary period, considerable differences were apparent in relative exercise intensity.

The observed improvement in performance may have been an artifact rather than a positive effect of the adaptation period. Therefore, Phinney and colleagues (Phinney, Bistrian, Evans, et al. 1983; Phinney, Bistrian, Wolfe, and Blackburn 1983) conducted a follow-up study in which trained subjects were studied before and after a 4-week high-fat diet (< 20 g/day of carbohydrates). The diet reduced the preexercise muscle glycogen concentration by 50%, but no difference in the average time to exhaustion at 62% to 64% of $\dot{V}O_2max$ before and after the diet was found. The results are difficult to interpret, however, because of the large variability of the subjects' times to exhaustion. One subject exercised 57% longer, whereas other subjects showed no improvement or even had decreased times to exhaustion. In addition, exercise intensity was relatively low and subjects' reliance on carbohydrates during exercise at 62% to 64% of $\dot{V}O_2max$ was low. In such a situation, reduced carbohydrate stores may not be limiting. At higher exercise intensities, performance may have been impaired. Nevertheless, it is remarkable that performance did not decline in all subjects even though muscle glycogen levels measured before exercise decreased by almost 50% and fat oxidation during exercise increased markedly. These observations have been attributed to enzymatic adaptations (including a 44% increase in carnitine palmitoyl transferase activity and a 46% decrease in hexokinase activity) (Phinney, Bistrian, Evans, et al. 1983). In subsequent studies, maintained or improved performance was seen at relatively low exercise intensities (60%-65% of $\dot{V}O_2max$), which are far below the intensities observed during competition. How these results translate into practical applications in training and competition for most athletes is unclear.

Eating large amounts of fat has been associated with the development of obesity and cardiovascular disease. Whether this association is true for athletes is not known. Few studies have described the effects of high-fat diets on cardiovascular risk factors in athletes who train regularly. Pendergast et al. (1996) reported no changes in plasma LDL, HDL, or total cholesterol levels in male and female runners with diets in the range of 17% to 40% fat. Although the risk of obesity and cardiovascular disease increases with the consumption of high-fat diets in sedentary people, regular exercise or endurance training seems to attenuate these risks (Sarna and Kaprio 1994). Exposure to high-fat diets has also been associated with insulin resistance, which has traditionally been linked to an effect of the IMTG pools on glucose uptake (Pan et al. 1997). This observation was made in obese subjects, however, and whether these results can

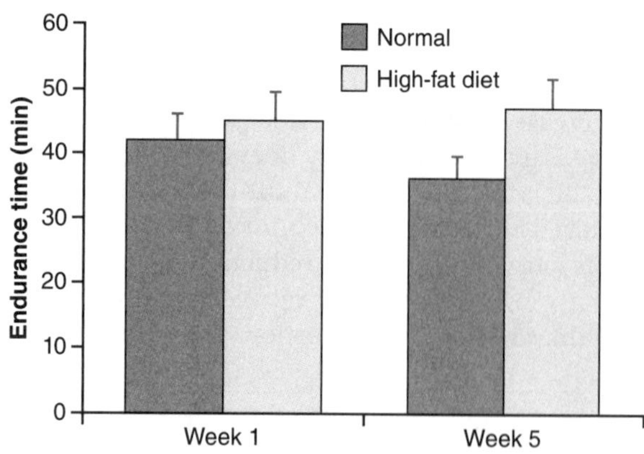

Figure 7.16 Running performance with high-fat diets in rats.

Data from Miller, Bryce, and Conlee (1984).

be extrapolated to athletes is not clear, especially because athletes seem to have larger IMTG stores and increased insulin sensitivity.

Although chronic high-fat diets induce persistent enzymatic adaptations in skeletal muscle that favor fat oxidation, the effects on performance may not be visible because muscle glycogen levels are suboptimal. A period of adaptation to a high-fat diet followed by acute carbohydrate feeding might theoretically induce the enzymatic adaptations in the muscle while also optimizing preexercise glycogen stores. If the high glycogen levels are accompanied by a slightly lower rate of glycogenolysis, an improvement in exercise capacity is expected. In rats, after 3 to 8 weeks of adaptation to a high-fat diet (0%-25% carbohydrate) followed by 3 days of carbohydrate feeding (70% carbohydrate), muscle and liver glycogen were restored to extremely high levels.

In humans, Helge, Wulff, and Kiens (1998) studied trained subjects who, after 7 weeks of adaptation to a high-fat diet (62% fat, 21% carbohydrate), changed to a high-carbohydrate diet (65% carbohydrate, 20% fat) for 1 week (see figure 7.17). A control group followed a high-carbohydrate diet for 8 weeks. Although exercise times to exhaustion increased from week 7 to week 8 in the subjects who received the high-fat diet followed by the high-carbohydrate diet, their performance was inferior to those in the group that received the high-carbohydrate diet for 8 weeks. Because switching to a high-carbohydrate diet after 7 weeks of a high-fat diet did not reverse the negative effects, these authors concluded that the negative performance effects of 7 weeks of a high-fat diet are caused not by a lack of carbohydrate as a fuel but rather by suboptimal adaptations to the training (i.e., improvements in endurance capacity were smaller compared with the group that consumed the high-carbohydrate diet).

In another study by Burke et al. (1999), trained cyclists received a high-fat diet for a relatively short period (5 days) followed by carbohydrate loading on day 6. On day 7, substrate oxidation during exercise was measured, and a performance ride followed. No significant performance improvement was observed. The potential benefits of an adaptation period to a high-fat diet followed by a period of carbohydrate loading are not clear. A fat-adaptation period beyond 4 weeks may decrease exercise performance, which cannot be reversed by a week on a high-carbohydrate diet.

Although the hypothesis that chronic high-fat diets may increase the capacity to oxidize fat and improve exercise performance during competition is attractive, little evidence indicates that it is true. The available studies suggest a positive effect on performance but they were conducted at exercise intensities lower than typical intensities during competition and were performed in relatively untrained individuals. Very few studies have investigated the effects of high-fat diets on high-level performers.

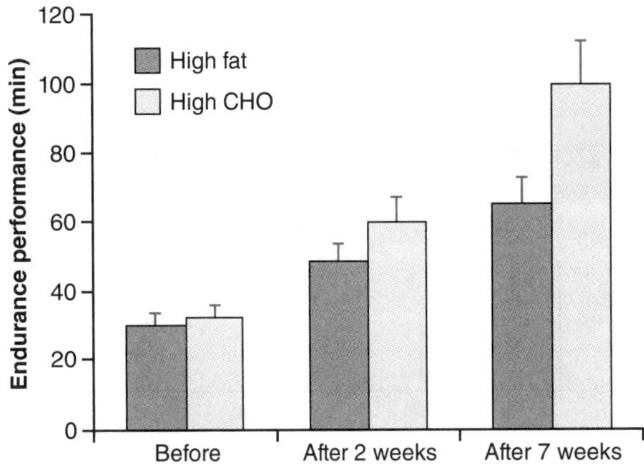

Figure 7.17 High-fat diets and performance improvements during training in humans.
Data from Helge, Wulff, and Kiens (1998).

In a study in elite racewalkers, Burke et al. (2017) compared three different 3-week dietary interventions. One group received a traditional high-carbohydrate diet, the second group received an isoenergetic diet that involved periodized nutrition with a carbohydrate intake to alternate between low and high carbohydrate availability, and the third group received an isoenergetic, very low-carbohydrate, high-fat (LCHF) diet of less than 50 g of carbohydrate per day. Subjects trained throughout the 3-week period and performance was measured at the beginning and at the end of the 3-week period. No differences were observed between the high-carbohydrate and periodized nutrition groups, but the LCHF group performed significantly worse during a 10 km (0.6 mi) race-walk compared with the other groups (figure 7.18). The researchers also reported greater fat oxidation and lower exercise economy (greater oxygen use for the same intensity) with the LCHF diet.

Often, increases in fat oxidation are seen as a positive adaptation, and they are sometimes interpreted as synonymous to improvements in performance. However, increases in fat oxidation can also be the result of depletion of carbohydrate stores or an inability to use carbohydrate (e.g., in McArdle's disease, in which muscle glycogen

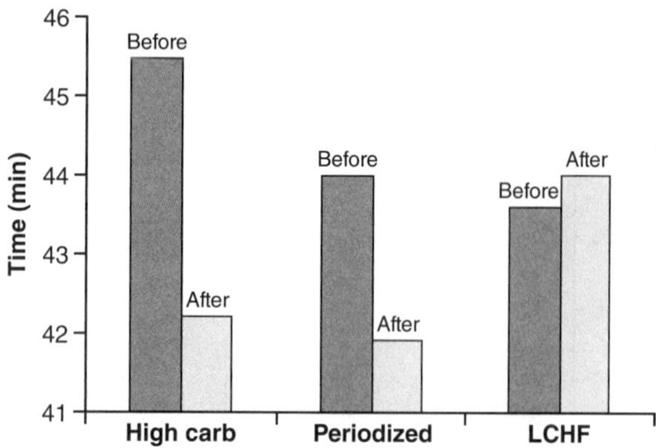

Figure 7.18 Performance in racewalkers on high-fat or high-carbohydrate diets.

Reprinted from www.mysportscience.com; Data from Burke et al. (2007).

phosphorylase is deficient). In these cases, improved fat oxidation is linked with a decrease in performance. Stellingwerff et al. (2006) found that one of the adaptations to several days on a high-fat diet was a reduction in pyruvate dehydrogenase activation. This finding could indicate that the increase in fat oxidation is at least partly caused by a reduction in the ability to oxidize carbohydrate because pyruvate dehydrogenase is a key enzyme in carbohydrate metabolism that catalyzes the conversion of pyruvate to acetyl-CoA in the mitochondrion and controls the entry of substrate into the TCA cycle.

Additional well-controlled studies are needed to clarify the importance of the effect of dietary carbohydrate and fat content on athletic performance. In the absence of evidence of a performance benefit and with a lack of information about possible negative effects of high-fat diets for athletes, caution should be exercised when recommending a high-fat diet to athletes.

The Ketogenic Diet

The ketogenic diet is an extreme form of high-fat diet. Carbohydrate is severely restricted to an intake of less than 20 g/day. Severe carbohydrate restriction will deprive the brain of glucose, and after a few days, ketogenesis will produce ketone bodies as an alternative energy source for the brain. Some have argued that these ketone bodies are a good substrate for the muscle and they may also serve as signaling molecules that promote adaptation. This is an attractive theory, but evidence so far is lacking. The only study that has investigated a truly ketogenic diet in endurance-trained athletes so far is by Phinney, Bistrian, Evans, et al. (1983). This study, which only included 5 subjects, showed no performance benefits and raised several questions with respect to methodology and interpretation. A change in substrate use was observed that favored fat metabolism, but this did not result in improved performance. Sometimes a study by Volek et al. (2016) is quoted as evidence that a ketogenic diet works for athletes. In this cross-sectional study, two groups of trained athletes were compared: one that habitually followed a self-selected ketogenic diet and one that followed a self-selected high-carbohydrate diet. As one would expect, the group that ate more fat and less carbohydrate had higher rates of fat oxidation during exercise. This study provides little new information and gives us no clues with respect to effects on performance.

Ketogenic diet advocates dismiss the results of studies that suggest negative effects based on two primary arguments: (1) The studies were not long enough for keto adaptation to occur, and (2) the carbohydrate restriction was not severe enough. Although the second argument might be valid in some cases, the first argument is problematic because keto adaptation is never defined and adaptations are clearly measurable even after a few days. If we don't understand what keto adaptation really means, it will never be possible to prove or disprove the idea. Without evidence for improvements in performance and without evidence of other beneficial effects, it is difficult to see why athletes would adopt such a ketogenic diet that is highly disruptive to the training process in the short term. There is a real need for longer duration studies and a clear definition of keto adaptation.

Ketone bodies are another way to administer fat energy, and they can be ingested as ketone salts or ketone esters. Most ketone supplements contain ketone salts, which have one major disadvantage: When larger amounts of ketone salts are ingested, significant amounts of sodium or potassium (or other electrolytes) are also ingested, and this can cause GI distress. Therefore, ketone monoesters such as (R)-3-hydroxybutyl (R)-3-hydroxybutyrate were developed as an oral source of ketones to increase the amount of ketones that can be delivered without adding large amounts of salt (Cox et al. 2016). These esters are expensive. Although emerging studies suggest that ketone esters increase fat oxidation and performance in rats (Murray et al. 2016) and have performance benefits in cyclists, more studies, especially human studies, are needed before such practices can be recommended to athletes. Most supplements on the market sold as "ketones" contain very small

LOW-CARBOHYDRATE, HIGH-FAT DIETS

High-fat diets, LCHF diets, and ketogenic diets are talked about a lot. They have replaced Atkins, South Beach, and other popular low-carbohydrate diets. The messages regarding their use for weight loss or exercise performance are often confusing for two reasons. First, it is not always clear what is meant by a high-fat diet. There is no uniform definition (even in the scientific literature). It is sometimes defined as 60% fat (i.e., fat provides 60% of total dietary energy intake), 80% fat, less than 5% carbohydrate, less than 20 g carbohydrate, and so on. If a Tour de France rider eats a 60% fat diet (which would be classed as a high-fat diet) on the day of a long mountain stage, he can still have a high-carbohydrate diet (>8 g/kg of carbohydrate) because of his high total daily energy intake. So would this be classed as a high carbohydrate- or a high-fat diet? A LCHF diet (which usually has a carbohydrate content varying between 50-400 g/day) is likely to have effects that differ from a diet that restricts carbohydrate intake to less than 20 g/day. It is crucial that the term *high-fat diet* is defined clearly to have meaningful discussions about the topic. Because carbohydrate, not fat, is the dominant driver of metabolism, it is important to express diets according to their carbohydrate content (i.e., percentage of total energy intake and, more important, in grams per day or grams per kilogram of body weight per day).

Second, the people being discussed and their reasons for following a particular type of diet are not always comparable. We cannot use data from a sedentary population with obesity and insulin resistance to predict what is going to happen with performance in elite athletes. These are distinctly different discussions. A weight loss discussion is different from a performance discussion. An elite athlete is different from a diabetic patient. The discussions need to be clearly separated, and the arguments used should not confuse the different aspects. The context of the discussion should always be clear and focused.

amounts of ketone salts that will have no physiological effects. Evidence regarding the use of exogenous ketone esters is discussed in chapter 11.

High-Fat Diets and Health

Athletes probably do not need to be warned against high-fat diets if they are in energy balance and do not overeat. The same applies to high-carbohydrate diets. Some studies have examined the influence of high-fat diets on risk factors for cardiovascular disease in well-trained athletes. Pendergast et al. (1996) reported no effect of fat content of the diet in the range of 17% to 40% of total energy intake on circulating levels of HDL, LDL, and total cholesterol in endurance runners. Although high-fat diets are known to increase the risk of obesity and cardiovascular disease in sedentary people, engaging in regular endurance exercise training appears to markedly reduce these risks. Humans evolved on a range of high-carbohydrate and high-fat diets and thrived on both; they had to eat whatever was available based on location and season. The problem with modern diets is not macronutrient composition but excess intakes that lead to a positive energy balance and weight gain. This is a complex problem that has arisen because society is engineered to minimize physical activity and access to food is made as easy as possible. It is easier to overeat and be underactive. Athletes who are training and do not overeat can be healthy on high-carbohydrate or high-fat diets, but evidence seems to indicate that performance can suffer with lower carbohydrate diets.

Supplements That Increase Fat Oxidation

Several nutritional supplements claim to increase fat oxidation, increase fat loss and lean body mass, and promote weight loss. The following supplements have been associated with fat oxidation:

- Caffeine
- Pyruvate
- Carnitine
- Vanadium (vanadyl sulfate)
- Chromium
- Yohimbine
- Dihydroxyacetone

- Green tea or green tea extracts
- Epigallocatechin gallate (EGCG)
- Fucoxanthin

Caffeine is thought to stimulate lipolysis and the mobilization of FAs. Carnitine is believed to help transport FAs into the mitochondria. Pyruvate and dihydroxyacetone are often sold as supplements to increase fat oxidation. Similarly, the trace elements chromium and vanadium are claimed to promote fat oxidation and promote weight loss. (For other supplements and more detail see chapter 11.)

Key Points

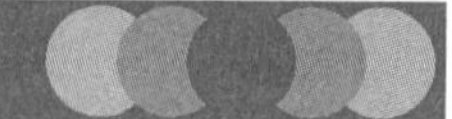

- In contrast to carbohydrate stores, fat stores are large in humans and are regarded as practically unlimited. The stores of fat are located mainly in adipose tissue, but significant amounts also exist as IMTGs.
- The steps that could potentially limit fat oxidation are lipolysis, removal of FAs from the fat cell, transport of fat by the bloodstream, transport of FAs into the muscle cell, transport of FAs into the mitochondria, or oxidation of FAs in the ß-oxidation pathway and TCA cycle.
- Most FAs are stored in the form of triacylglycerols in subcutaneous adipose tissue, and FAs are released along with glycerol after the breakdown of triacylglycerols (lipolysis) by the enzyme hormone-sensitive lipase.
- Most FAs in the blood (>99.9%) are bound to albumin.
- Transporter proteins (FAT/CD36) have been identified that are likely responsible for most of the transport of FAs across the sarcolemma. After they are in the muscle cell, FAs are bound to FA-binding proteins.
- In the muscle, FAs are stored as IMTGs, which can provide important fuel during exercise.
- The enzyme CPT I plays a crucial role in the transport of FAs into the mitochondria.
- Carbohydrate and fat are always oxidized as a mixture, and the relative contribution of these two substrates depends on exercise intensity and duration, the level of aerobic fitness, diet, and carbohydrate intake before and during exercise.
- In absolute terms, fat oxidation increases as exercise intensity increases from low to moderate levels, although the percentage contribution of fat may actually decrease. At higher intensities of exercise (>75% of $\dot{V}O_2max$), fat oxidation is inhibited, and the relative and absolute rates of fat oxidation decrease to negligible values. In trained people, the maximal rates of fat oxidation are observed at 62% to 63% of $\dot{V}O_2max$.
- Diet has marked effects on fat oxidation. Generally, a high-carbohydrate, low-fat diet reduces fat oxidation, whereas a high-fat, low-carbohydrate diet increases fat oxidation.
- Carbohydrate feeding before exercise reduces fat oxidation by reducing lipolysis and plasma FA availability and by inhibiting the carnitine-dependent FA transport into the mitochondria.
- The rate of carbohydrate use during prolonged strenuous exercise is closely related to the energy needs of the working muscle. In contrast, fat use during exercise is not tightly regulated. No mechanisms exist that closely match the metabolism of FAs to energy expenditure. Fat oxidation is therefore mainly influenced by fat availability and the rate of carbohydrate use.
- Ingestion of long-chain triacylglycerols during exercise is not desirable because they slow gastric emptying, appear only slowly in the systemic circulation, and enter the systemic circulation in chylomicrons, which are believed to be an insignificant fuel source during exercise.

- Medium-chain triacylglycerols are rapidly emptied from the stomach, absorbed, and oxidized, but the ingestion of large amounts of MCTs results in gastrointestinal distress. When ingested in smaller amounts, MCTs do not appear to have the positive effects on performance that are often claimed.
- Fasting increases the availability of lipid substrates and results in increased oxidation of FAs at rest and during exercise. Because the liver glycogen stores are not maintained, however, fatigue resistance and exercise performance are impaired.
- High-fat diets for 3 to 5 days increase the availability of lipid substrates but reduce the storage of glycogen. As a result, fat oxidation increases during exercise, but fatigue resistance and exercise performance are compromised.
- Although the hypothesis that chronic high-fat diets may increase the capacity to oxidize fat and improve exercise performance during competition is attractive, little evidence indicates that the hypothesis is true.

Recommended Readings

Hawley, J.A., F. Brouns, and A. Jeukendrup. 1998. Strategies to enhance fat utilization during exercise. *Sports Medicine* 26:241-257.

Jeukendrup, A.E. 1999. Dietary fat and physical performance. *Current Opinion in Clinical Nutrition Metabolic Care* 2:521-526.

Jeukendrup, A.E. 2002. Regulation of skeletal muscle fat metabolism. *Annals of the New York Academy of Science* 967:217-235.

Jeukendrup, A.E. 2003. Modulation of carbohydrate and fat utilization by diet, exercise and environment. *Biochemical Society Transactions* 31:270-273.

Jeukendrup, A.E., W.H.M. Saris, and A.J.M. Wagenmakers. 1998. Fat metabolism during exercise: A review. Part I: Fatty acid mobilization and muscle metabolism. *International Journal of Sports Medicine* 19:231-244.

Jeukendrup, A.E., W.H.M. Saris, and A.J.M. Wagenmakers. 1998. Fat metabolism during exercise: A review. Part II: Regulation of metabolism and the effects of training. *International Journal of Sports Medicine* 19:293-302.

Jeukendrup, A.E., W.H.M. Saris, and A.J.M. Wagenmakers. 1998. Fat metabolism during exercise: A review. Part III: Effects of nutritional interventions. *International Journal of Sports Medicine* 19:371-379.

Van der Vusse, G.J., and R.S. Reneman. 1996. Lipid metabolism in muscle. In *Handbook of physiology*, edited by L.B. Rowell and J.T. Shephard, section 12. New York: Oxford University Press.

Protein and Amino Acids

Objectives

After studying this chapter, you should be able to do the following:

- Give a general description of amino acids and name the most abundant amino acids
- Give a general description of protein and amino acid metabolism
- Describe the effects of training on body proteins
- List the techniques available to study protein metabolism and discuss the advantages and disadvantages of these techniques
- Discuss the contribution of protein to energy expenditure at rest and during exercise
- Discuss the effects of exercise, feeding, and the timing and composition of meals on protein synthesis and breakdown
- Describe the recommendations for protein intake generally given for strength and endurance athletes
- Discuss strategies to maximize anabolic potential and training adaptation in relation to exercise and protein intake
- Discuss the need for protein supplementation in athletes
- Describe the potential health hazards of excess protein intake
- Discuss the effects of ingesting single amino acids

Debate has long raged over how much dietary protein is required for optimal athletic performance. Because muscle plays a crucial role in exercise performance and contains the largest proportion of the protein in a human body (about 40%), this controversy is not surprising. Body proteins are continually turning over; that is, they are constantly being synthesized and degraded to maintain optimal function. Proteins turn over at different rates ranging from minutes to days. Despite the mass of protein in muscle, however, its rate of protein turnover accounts for only 25% to 35% of total protein turnover in the body. Muscle proteins turn over quite slowly compared with, for example, blood proteins. The most abundant proteins in muscle are the contractile proteins actin and myosin. Together they account for approximately 80% to 90% of all muscle protein. Both the structural proteins that make up the myofibrils and the proteins that act as **enzymes** within a muscle cell change as an adaptation to exercise training. Indeed, muscle mass, muscle protein content, and muscle protein composition change in response to training (see chapter 12). The type of training has an important influence on protein turnover and adaptive responses. Endurance training has little effect on muscle mass or total protein content (although mitochondrial protein content is increased), whereas resistance training has the potential to increase muscle mass and total protein content, which results in increased strength when dietary protein intake is adequate. Certain dietary strategies, which are discussed in detail in this chapter, can maximize this anabolic potential.

Interest in protein consumption is high among amateur and professional athletes. Therefore, the fact that meat, which contains high-quality protein (high biological value), is a popular protein source for athletes (especially strength athletes) is not surprising. This preference for meat probably dates to ancient Greece, where athletes preparing for the Olympic Games consumed large quantities of meat. Nowadays, **whey protein**, which is derived from milk, has become a popular supplement for those who want to gain lean body mass (i.e., skeletal muscle). The reasons for this are explained in this chapter.

There is a strong belief, especially among strength athletes, that a large protein intake or the ingestion of certain protein or amino acid supplements increases muscle mass and strength. Despite the long history of protein use in sport, debate continues even over questions such as whether protein requirements are greater for athletes. Protein and amino acid metabolism is complex, and many organs and tissues are involved. Thus, no uniform opinion exists about what should be measured as an endpoint. For example, the effectiveness of protein intake or supplements could be assessed by measuring performance, muscle mass, or strength, or it could be measured by the **nitrogen balance** (which is essentially the balance of protein because nitrogen in the diet comes exclusively from protein) over several days or by short-term methods that incorporate labeled amino acids into muscle proteins.

The use of different techniques to estimate protein turnover may give different results. Therefore, the principles of the techniques and their limitations must be understood. This chapter discusses the various techniques available to investigate protein metabolism. Then, a brief overview of protein and amino acid metabolism is given. Subsequently, protein metabolism during and following exercise and dietary protein needs for endurance and strength-training athletes are examined. Finally, the effects of supplementing the diet with various individual amino acids are discussed.

Amino Acids

Both muscle and milk contain all the naturally occurring amino acids, and thus meat and dairy products are valuable foods (both have high biological value, and dairy sources have higher values). The most abundant amino acids in muscle are the three **branched-chain amino acids (BCAAs)**, **leucine**, valine, and isoleucine, which together account for 20% of the total amino acids found in muscle protein. Both meat and dairy protein have high BCAA content.

Amino Acid Transport

The concentrations of amino acids in muscle and in blood differ, which suggests that maintaining these concentration gradients is important. Because concentration gradients of amino acids differ, different transporters move individual or groups of amino acids across membranes. Amino acid transporters are membrane-bound proteins that recognize specific amino acid shapes and chemical properties (e.g., neutral, basic, anionic). The transporters are divided into sodium-dependent and sodium-independent carriers. Generally, the sodium-dependent transporters maintain a larger gradient than the sodium-independent transporters. Note that all these transporters are facilitative and usually coupled to cotransport with sodium and thus are not directly energy dependent. To date, some transporter proteins have been identified, but many more are yet to be discovered.

Amino Acid Metabolism

The metabolism of most amino acids is linked to the metabolism of other amino acids, and some amino acids can be synthesized from other amino acids. This feature is especially important in conditions of limited dietary protein intake or when metabolic requirements increase. Some amino acids are essential and are not synthesized in the body, whereas others can be synthesized in the body (nonessential amino acids) as described in chapter 1.

Amino acids are involved in a variety of biochemical and physiological processes, some of which are common to all and some of which are highly specific to certain amino acids. Amino acids are constantly incorporated into proteins (**protein synthesis**), and proteins are constantly broken down (**protein degradation** or breakdown). This constant turnover of proteins is summarized in figure 8.1. The vast majority of the amino acids in the body are incorporated into tissue proteins, but a small pool of free amino acids also exists (about 120 g of free amino acids are present in the skeletal muscle of an adult). Amino acids are constantly extracted from the free amino acid pool for synthesis of various proteins, and breakdown of protein makes amino acids available for the free amino acid pool.

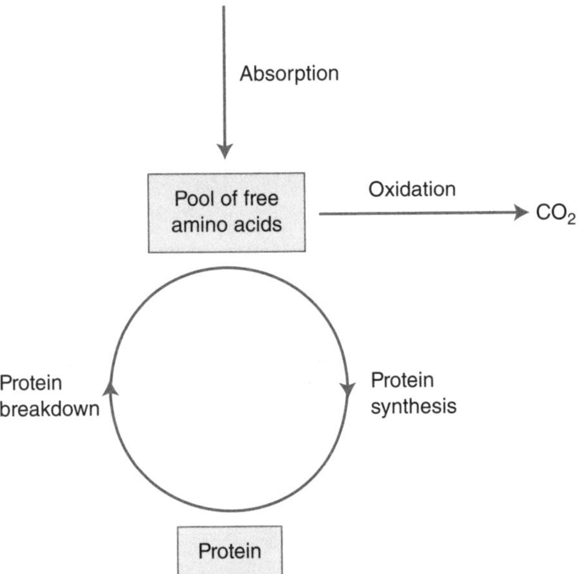

Figure 8.1 Protein metabolism. Amino acids enter the free amino acid pool from the diet (absorption) or from breakdown of protein. Amino acids leave the free amino acid pool for protein synthesis or oxidation to carbon dioxide.

Protein Breakdown

The breakdown of protein serves three main purposes:

1. It degrades potentially damaged proteins to prevent a decline in their function. Note that there is usually a net replacement of these degraded proteins (see figure 8.1).
2. It provides energy when some of its individual amino acids are converted into acetyl-CoA or TCA-cycle intermediates and are oxidized in the mitochondria.
3. Individual amino acids can be used for the synthesis of other compounds, including neurotransmitters (e.g., **serotonin**), hormones (e.g., epinephrine), purines and pyrimidines (components of DNA and RNA), creatine, carnitine, carnosine, glutathione, and other peptides and proteins.

This breakdown of protein and incorporation of the amino acids into a new protein links protein degradation with protein synthesis. Amino acids can also be incorporated into compounds that are not proteins. In this case, the body loses protein. For example, some amino acids are converted into glucose (gluconeogenesis), ketones (**ketogenesis**), or fat (lipogenesis) and subsequently stored in adipose tissue.

Some, but not all, of the 20 different amino acids found in protein are oxidized in the mitochondria for ATP resynthesis (see chapter 3) although this contribution to energy metabolism is always far less than that from carbohydrate and fat oxidation except possibly in the cases of extreme carbohydrate depletion and starvation. Before amino acids can be oxidized, the amino group must be removed. Removal of the amino group can be achieved for some amino acids by transferring it to another molecule called a **keto acid**, which results in the formation of a different amino acid. This process, called **transamination**, is catalyzed by enzymes called aminotransferases. A good example is the transfer of the amino group from the amino acid leucine to the keto acid α-ketoglutarate to form α-ketoisocaproate (which can be further metabolized to form acetyl-CoA) and **glutamate**, respectively, as illustrated in the following equation:

$$\text{L-leucine} + \alpha\text{-ketoglutarate} \rightarrow \alpha\text{-ketoisocaproate} + \text{L-glutamate}$$

Each amino acid has its own unique corresponding keto acid. Alternatively, the amino group can be removed from the amino acid to form free **ammonia (NH3)**, in a process called oxidative **deamination**. One example is the breakdown of asparagine to form aspartate and ammonia. Because free ammonia is a toxic substance, it is used either to form **glutamine** from glutamate or alanine from pyruvate within the muscle. These amino acids and some free ammonia can be transported to the liver, where they are converted to urea (with the carbon skeletons of the two amino acids being used to form glucose). Urea is then transported via the circulation to the kidneys where it is incorporated into urine and eventually excreted by the body. Smaller amounts of ammonia and urea can also be excreted via sweat.

After the removal of the amino group from an amino acid, the remaining carbon skeleton (the keto acid) is eventually oxidized to carbon dioxide in the TCA cycle. The carbon skeleton of amino acids can enter the TCA cycle in several ways. Some can be converted to acetyl-CoA and enter the TCA cycle just like acetyl-CoA from carbohydrate or fat. They can also enter the TCA cycle as α-ketoglutarate or oxaloacetate as metabolites of glutamate and aspartate, respectively (see figure 8.2).

Some amino acids can serve as glucogenic or lipogenic (ketogenic) precursors. The amino acids that can be converted into α-ketoglutarate,

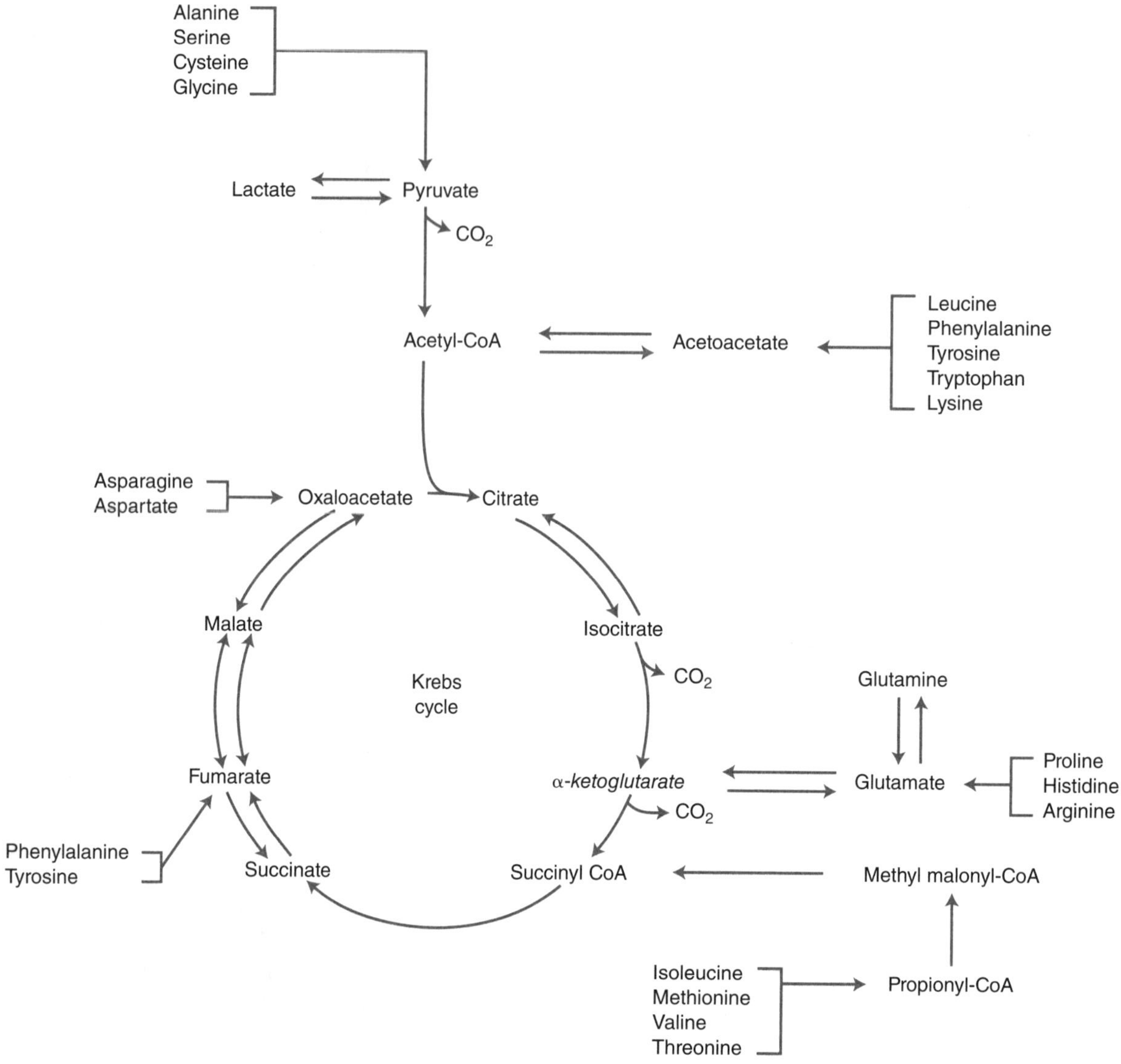

Figure 8.2 Interactions between amino acids and the TCA cycle.

oxaloacetate, or pyruvate can also be used for the synthesis of glucose in the liver (gluconeogenesis). Amino acids or keto acids that are eventually broken down to acetyl-CoA can also be used in the synthesis of FAs. Acetyl-CoA units can be used in an elongation process to form longer FAs by adding on to the hydrocarbon chain of the 16-carbon FA palmitate. The following are examples of some common aminotransferase reactions:

L-glutamate + oxaloacetate → α-ketoglutarate + L-aspartate

L-alanine + α-ketoglutarate → pyruvate + L-glutamate

Several amino acids undergo reversible transamination. These amino acids include alanine, aspartate, glutamate, and the BCAAs—leucine, isoleucine, and valine. The BCAAs are the only essential amino acids that can undergo transamination. Transamination is usually rapid, and the main limiting factor is that these processes sometimes take place in different tissues. Amino acids thus have to be transported by the circulation. Glutamate serves a central role in these transamination reactions because several amino acids can undergo transamination with glutamate (see the sidebar).

Most of the nitrogen from amino acid degradation is transferred to α-ketoglutarate to form glutamate and subsequently glutamine; these two amino acids are the most abundant free amino acids in muscle. Although all carbon skeletons of amino acids can potentially be used for oxidation, only 6 of the available 20 amino acids in protein are oxidized in significant amounts by muscle: asparagine, aspartate, glutamate, isoleucine, leucine, and valine. An outline of the pathways involved in degradation of the various amino acids is provided in table 8.1.

Amino Acid Synthesis

The discussion of synthesis of amino acids is limited to the nonessential amino acids because the essential amino acids cannot be synthesized in the body. Figure 8.3 provides a summary of the synthetic pathways of nonessential amino acids. Again, glutamate plays a central role. Glutamate serves as the donor of nitrogen in the synthesis of

AMINO ACIDS THAT CAN UNDERGO TRANSAMINATION WITH GLUTAMATE

- Leucine
- Valine
- Isoleucine
- Alanine
- Aspartate
- Glutamine
- Ammonia + α-ketoglutarate

TABLE 8.1 Pathways of Amino Acid Degradation

Metabolic pathway	Important enzymes	Nitrogen end product	Carbon end product
AMINO ACIDS CONVERTED TO OTHER AMINO ACIDS			
Asparagine	Asparaginase	Aspartate + ammonia	
Glutamine	Glutaminase	Glutamate + ammonia	
Arginine	Arginase	Ornithine + urea	
Phenylalanine	Phenylalanine hydroxylase	Tyrosine	
Proline		Glutamate	
Cysteine		Taurine	
TRANSAMINATION TO FORM GLUTAMATE			
Alanine		Glutamate	Pyruvate
Aspartate		Glutamate	Oxaloacetate
Leucine		Glutamate	Ketones
Isoleucine		Glutamate	Succinate
Valine		Glutamate	Succinate
Ornithine		Two glutamates	α-ketoglutarate
Tyrosine		Glutamate	Ketone + fumarate
Cysteine		Glutamate	Ketone + SO^{2-}_4 (sulfate)
OTHER PATHWAYS			
Serine	Serine dehydratase	Ammonia	Pyruvate
Threonine	Threonine dehydratase	Ammonia	Ketobutyrate
Histidine	Histidase	Ammonia	Urocanate
Tryptophan		Ammonia	Kynurenine
Glycine		Ammonia	Carbon dioxide
Methionine		Ammonia	Ketobutyrate
Lysine		Two glutamates	Acetate

Data from Matthews (1999).

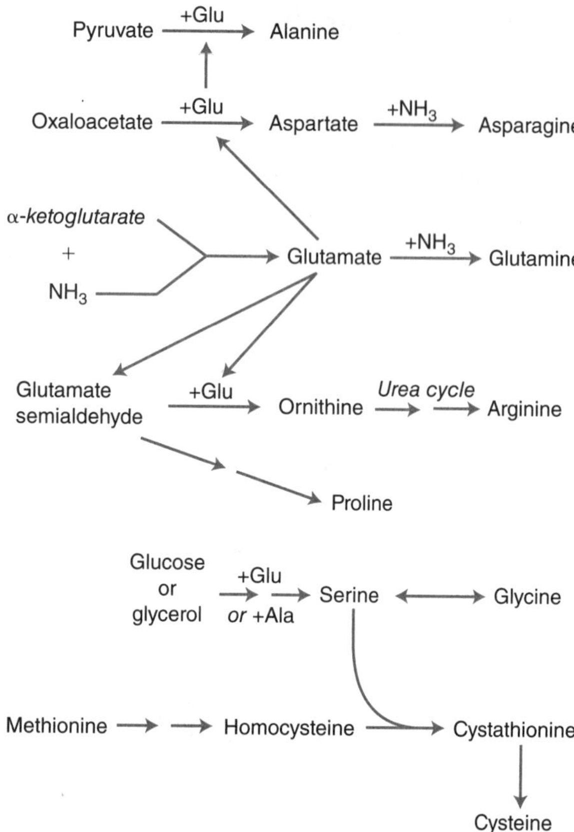

Figure 8.3 Synthetic pathways of the nonessential amino acids. Glu = glutamate; Ala = alanine.
Data from Matthews (1999).

many amino acids, which occurs by transferring ammonia to a carbon skeleton precursor (keto acid) from the TCA cycle, from another nonessential amino acid, or from an essential amino acid.

Synthesis of amino acids by the transfer of ammonia to a carbon skeleton precursor from the TCA cycle is rarely limited because of the ample availability of the substrates (carbon skeleton precursors and ammonia). On the other hand, synthesis of amino acids from other amino acids can sometimes be limited because of limited dietary supply. Cysteine and tyrosine are special cases because they are synthesized from essential amino acids and are therefore indirectly dependent on adequate protein (and thus amino acid) intake.

Incorporation of Amino Acids Into Protein

Different proteins are synthesized and degraded at different rates. Generally, the proteins that have a regulatory function (such as enzymes) or that act as signals (hormones) have a relatively rapid rate of turnover (minutes, hours, or days). The structural proteins, such as collagen and contractile proteins (actin and myosin), have a relatively slow turnover (days, weeks, or months). In humans who are weight stable and are not gaining or losing muscle mass, the overall synthesis and degradation of proteins must be in balance. This also means that the amount of nitrogen consumed in the diet equals the amount of nitrogen excreted in urine, feces, and other routes.

Protein turnover is several times greater than protein intake, as is illustrated in figure 8.4 for a healthy 70 kg (154 lb) person. A normal daily protein intake is approximately 90 g. In this example, the intake of protein provides only about 25% of the amino acids that enter the free amino acid pool each day (340 g). Most of the amino acids that appear in and disappear from the free amino acid pool are derived from proteins in the gut, kidneys, and liver. Although this is a relatively small portion of the total mass of protein, it represents about two-thirds of the total protein turnover because of the rapid turnover in these tissues. Muscle has a relatively slow protein turnover and provides most of the remainder. Various techniques are used to study protein metabolism, including nitrogen balance. These techniques are reviewed later in this chapter.

Incorporation of Amino Acids Into Other Compounds

Amino acids are used for the synthesis of amino acid–like compounds. A list of the most important products is provided in table 8.2. The amino acids glutamate, tyrosine, and tryptophan, for example, are precursors of neurotransmitters. Glutamate is a special amino acid in this respect because it is not only a precursor of neurotransmitters but also is itself a neurotransmitter. Tyrosine is the precursor of catecholamines (dopamine, epinephrine, and norepinephrine), and tryptophan is the precursor of serotonin (5-hydroxytryptamine). The roles of amino acids as precursors of creatine and carnitine synthesis are discussed in detail in chapter 11.

Techniques to Study Protein and Amino Acid Metabolism

The following is a list of currently available techniques to study protein metabolism. These techniques range from simple techniques, such as the measurement of urea in urine, to complex

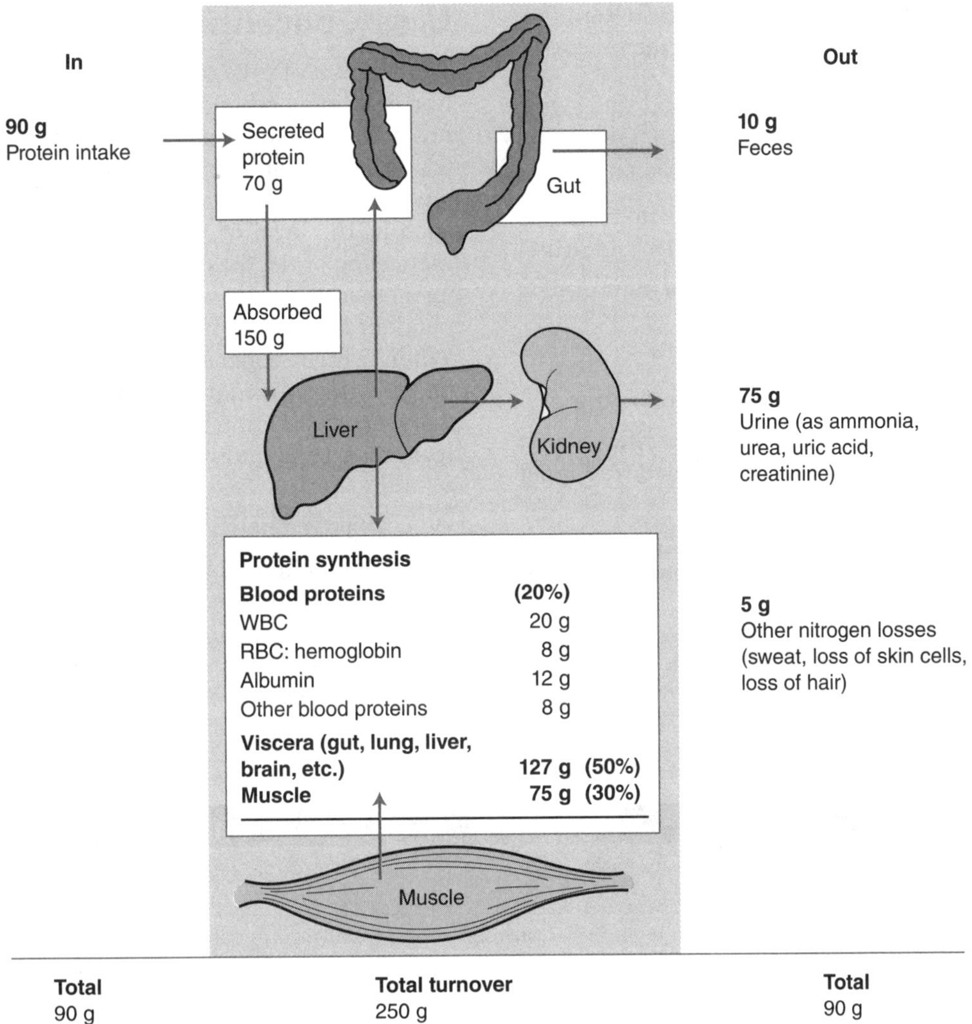

Figure 8.4 Daily protein balance in humans. RBC = red blood cells; WBC = white blood cells.

Data from Matthews (1999).

TABLE 8.2 Products Synthesized From Amino Acids

Product	Synthesized from	Product	Synthesized from
Creatine	Arginine Glycine Methionine	Pyrimidines	Aspartate Glutamine
Glutathione	Cysteine Taurine Glutamine	Histamine Carnitine	Histidine Lysine
Neurotransmitters	Glutamate Tyrosine Tryptophan	Choline Serine	Methionine
Purines	Aspartate Glutamine Glycine	Triiodothyronine (T3) Tetraiodothyronine (T4) Epinephrine Norepinephrine	Tyrosine

techniques that involve expensive and sophisticated equipment and more invasive techniques.

- Urea concentration in urine, blood, and sweat
- 3-methylhistidine in urine and blood (indication of myofibrillar protein breakdown)
- Nitrogen balance (nitrogen intake minus nitrogen excretion in sweat, feces, and urine)
- Arteriovenous measurements of amino acids across a tissue bed
- Radiolabeled isotopes
- Stable isotopes, including the following:
  - Tracer incorporation into a specific protein (protein synthesis), often called fractional synthetic rate (FSR)
  - Tracer release from a specific protein (protein breakdown), often called fractional breakdown rate (FBR)

An overview of these techniques, including their strengths and weaknesses, is given in table 8.3.

Urea Concentration in Urine

The amount of urea excreted in urine is an indication of whole-body protein breakdown, but it does not provide detailed information and gives only a rough indication of protein breakdown. The urinary urea concentration depends on many factors, such as the level of hydration and the diet (e.g., increasing or decreasing protein intake will result in increased or decreased urea production independent of changes in tissue protein breakdown). When urine is collected over 24 hours, the results become slightly more meaningful because total daily urea excretion can be determined, but the results are still highly dependent on protein intake.

Nitrogen Balance

Most experts in various countries have used nitrogen balance studies to determine the recommended dietary intakes for protein. Subjects are fed a diet with a certain level of protein intake, and for a time (3-14 days), urine and feces are collected

TABLE 8.3 Methods for Estimating Protein Metabolism

Method	Advantages	Disadvantages and limitations
Urea concentration in urine and sweat	Easy; relatively inexpensive	Only rough estimate; heavily affected by diet (protein intake)
3-methylhistidine in urine	Simple measure of myofibrillar protein breakdown	Only rough estimate of myofibrillar protein breakdown; requires strict control of meat intake; does not provide information about actual changes in muscle mass
Nitrogen balance (nitrogen intake minus nitrogen excretion in sweat and urine)	Accurate method when used over relatively long periods (e.g., a week or more)	Difficult and time consuming; tends to overestimate nitrogen retention; usually ignores nitrogen loss in sweat; highly dependent on subject compliance; gives no insight into metabolic pathways
Arteriovenous measurements of amino acids across a tissue bed	Gives information about net exchange of amino acids across a tissue; net uptake of essential amino acids related to rate of protein synthesis	Invasive; can have high variability depending on blood flow measurement
Radiolabeled isotopes	Relatively inexpensive; relatively easy to measure; small amounts of tracer needed	Potential health risk because they are radioactive
Stable isotopes	No health risk	Relatively expensive; sophisticated equipment needed for analyses
Tracer incorporation into a specific protein (protein synthesis)	Gives direct information about protein synthesis in a tissue	Invasive (tissue biopsies needed); relatively expensive; sophisticated equipment needed for analyses
FSR and FBR	No health risk (uses stable isotopes)	Short-term measurement; does not provide information about actual changes in muscle mass; relatively expensive; sophisticated equipment needed for analyses

over 24-hour periods. The nitrogen intake (protein intake) and nitrogen excretion are measured as accurately as possible. A week or more may be required before collection reflects the adaptations to a particular diet.

Nitrogen excretion can be measured from urine, feces, and sweat. Nitrogen is detectable in feces because not all protein is completely absorbed, and some of the nitrogen secreted (often in the form of cells from the GI tract itself) into the GI tract is not reabsorbed. When nitrogen balance is measured in exercising subjects, nitrogen excretion in sweat is substantial and must be included in the measurements. Nitrogen is excreted mainly in the form of urea (about 90%) but also in creatinine, ammonia, uric acid, and other nitrogen-containing compounds. Urinary nitrogen is often the only measure taken and assumptions are made for the excretion in sweat and feces, but nitrogen excretion may be underestimated when using this measure alone.

When nitrogen intake exceeds excretion, a person is in positive nitrogen balance and must be retaining nitrogen (i.e., protein). When nitrogen excretion exceeds nitrogen intake, a person is in negative nitrogen balance, and thus nitrogen or protein loss is occurring. The latter situation cannot continue for a long time. The body uses protein, and because it does not contain large stores of protein, the breakdown and atrophy of tissues and organs will occur. Only when nitrogen intake matches nitrogen excretion is a person in nitrogen balance.

Although the estimation of nitrogen balance is an often-used technique, it is not easy to apply, and it has been criticized for numerous reasons. The technique is time consuming and involves several (usually 5-7) 24-hour periods of urine collection. It is labor intensive for the investigators. Its success is highly dependent on subject compliance. This technique also tends to underestimate nitrogen excretion and thus overestimate nitrogen retention, and it gives only a measure of the net nitrogen balance; it does not provide any insight into the metabolic pathways involved in changes in protein metabolism. Furthermore, nitrogen balance measurements, especially at high protein intakes, often result in physiologically impossible estimates of positive nitrogen balance. For example, in some studies, weightlifters who ate approximately 2.5 g protein per kilogram of body weight per day had positive nitrogen balances of about 17 g/day. That number would represent about 110 kg (243 lb) of lean tissue gained in 1 year! Clearly, this number cannot possibly be correct, and the methodology must be in error. Nevertheless, done properly and with the appropriate understanding of the limitations, important information may be gleaned from nitrogen balance studies.

3-Methylhistidine Excretion

Another method of estimating protein metabolism is the measurement of 3-methylhistidine or N-methylhistidine excretion in the urine. When proteins are degraded, 3-methylhistidine cannot be recycled within the muscle and is excreted in the urine. The amount of 3-methylhistidine in urine is, therefore, a measure of contractile protein breakdown. Diet can confound the results of this relatively simple technique. Meat and fish contain relatively large amounts of 3-methylhistidine and could cause erroneous results. The measurement of 3-methylhistidine is, therefore, meaningful only when the diet is strictly controlled, usually by eliminating meat. The urinary 3-methylhistidine is also highly dependent on the renal clearance rate. Thus, 3-methylhistidine excretion is often expressed relative to creatinine excretion to allow corrections for renal clearance and individual differences in muscle mass. The technique has several limitations but is regarded as a relatively easy and noninvasive way to get an idea of muscle protein breakdown.

Arteriovenous Differences

Nitrogen balance can also be determined across a specific organ. When arterial and venous blood across a certain tissue is sampled, the difference in the amino acid concentration gives information about the net exchange of specific amino acids. The arterial blood delivers amino acids to a tissue, and some of these amino acids are taken up and used for protein synthesis. The venous blood contains amino acids from protein breakdown. Depending on the tissue of interest, measuring arteriovenous (AV) differences can be more or less invasive. For example, **AV differences** from tissues such as the gut, liver, and brain are difficult to obtain in humans, but AV differences across an arm or leg muscle are relatively easy to obtain. Recently, techniques have been developed to sample across adipose tissue. Independent of the tissue sampled, measurements of AV differences always require a medically qualified person with good skills.

The AV differences provide a measure of net uptake and release of amino acids by a tissue. The

COMMONLY USED STABLE AND RADIOLABELED ISOTOPES IN METABOLIC RESEARCH

Common stable	Rare stable	Radioactive
^{1}H	^{2}H (0.02%)	^{3}H
^{12}C	^{13}C (1.1%)	^{14}C
^{14}N	^{15}N (0.37%)	^{13}N*
^{16}O	^{18}O (0.04%)	^{17}O*

* Indicates no long-lived radioisotopes for these elements.

most valuable information is obtained from amino acids that are not metabolized. For example, the AV differences of phenylalanine, tyrosine, and lysine (which are not metabolized in the muscle) are assumed to reflect the differences between net amino acid uptake from protein synthesis and the release of amino acids from muscle protein breakdown. The most often used amino acid is phenylalanine because it may give the best representation of overall amino acid metabolism. The assumption is that the amino acid measured reflects overall amino acid metabolism, but this may not always be the case because different amino acids may behave differently. Furthermore, the AV difference measurements reflect the balance across the leg (or arm) and would thus represent metabolism not only in skeletal muscle but also in bone, skin, and adipose tissue. This method measures the uptake of amino acids into tissues but does not measure incorporation into a protein, and the method does not provide information about specific metabolic pathways in that tissue. Adding a tracer improves the value of the measurement and allows for firmer conclusions about metabolic pathways that play a role in the tissue. AV differences of 3-methylhistidine across a muscle may be used as specific markers of contractile protein breakdown.

Tracer Methods

Labeled tracers are used to follow amino acids in the body. These tracers have properties identical to the amino acid or metabolite they are meant to trace. They are, however, distinguishable because they either emit radiation (radioactive isotopes) or are slightly heavier (stable isotopes). Radioactively labeled tracers such as ^{3}H (hydrogen) and ^{14}C (carbon) have been used most often in the past, but many laboratories now use stable isotopic tracers because, unlike radioisotopes, they do not pose a health risk. Stable isotopes have a different number of neutrons and, therefore, a different molecular mass. The difference in mass can be detected with mass spectrometry.

Stable isotopes occur naturally, and most elements have one abundant mass and up to three less abundant masses. For example, the abundant mass for hydrogen is ^{1}H, and the less abundant mass is ^{2}H. For carbon the abundant and less abundant isotopes are ^{12}C and ^{13}C, respectively. The sidebar lists some common stable isotopes and their abundance.

Most tracer techniques are based on the principle of dilution. A tracer is infused at a constant rate, and after an isotopic steady state is achieved (the appearance of tracer is equal to its disappearance), the dilution of the tracer gives information about release of the amino acid of interest. This principle can be illustrated by a simple analogy. If you want to know the amount of water in a bucket, you can add a known amount of dye. After mixing the dye with the water, a sample of the mixture can be taken and the concentration of the dye can be determined. From the dilution of the dye, the amount of water in the bucket can be calculated. This calculation is accurate, of course, only if the exact amount of dye is known, mixing with the water is complete, and the concentration of the dye can be determined after mixing. Similar measurements can be made in a dynamic system if the dye is infused at a known constant rate. For example, a dye could be used to calculate the flow of water through a stream. The same principle can be applied by infusing a tracer into the human circulation. Several variations of this technique exist to study whole-body protein metabolism or the metabolism of specific amino acids. Here we discuss only the principles. The interested reader should refer to other literature to learn more about stable and radioactive tracers (Matthews 1999; Wolfe 1992).

Methods have been developed to calculate the FSR and FBR. These techniques, which use isotopic tracers, calculate the relative rate of protein breakdown and synthesis. By studying the incorporation of a labeled amino acid into a tissue, information can be obtained about the rates of protein synthesis. It is possible to get a measure of protein synthesis for that tissue (e.g., mixed muscle protein synthesis), or if different protein fractions are extracted, it is possible to look at protein synthesis in those specific fractions (e.g., myofibrillar proteins or mitochondrial proteins). Modern techniques even make it possible to study and quantify the amounts of messenger RNA (mRNA) for specific proteins and the rate of synthesis of specific proteins, but a description of these techniques is beyond the scope of this book. Although the techniques to study protein metabolism in humans are constantly being improved, all methods have their limitations, and no agreement has been reached on which method is best. Nevertheless, the available information allows us to draw some conclusions about exercise and protein requirements.

In the past decade, a new minimally invasive technique using stable isotopes has been developed (Elango et al. 2012) called the indicator amino acid oxidation (IAAO) method. This was developed as an alternative to the traditional nitrogen balance technique as a means to assess the individual amino acid and protein recommendations in a variety of populations. The short dietary adaptation period (~ 1 day) required for the IAAO method relative to nitrogen balance technique (5-7 days) allows for a greater number of test dietary protein intakes to be assessed for each individual participant. The IAAO method is based on the concept that when one essential amino acid (EAA) is deficient for protein synthesis, then the excess of all other EAA, including the indicator amino acid, will be oxidized. In this method ^{13}C-phenylalanine is used as the indicator amino acid to determine whole body phenylalanine flux, $^{13}CO_2$ excretion, and phenylalanine oxidation. With increasing intakes of the limiting amino acid, IAAO will decrease, reflecting increasing incorporation into protein. Once the requirement for the limiting amino acid is met there will be no further change in the indicator oxidation. The IAAO method has been systematically applied to determine most EAA requirements in adults and it has also been applied to determine the metabolic availability of amino acids from dietary proteins and to determine total protein requirements. Due to its noninvasive nature, the IAAO method has also been used to determine requirements for amino acids in neonates and children and in disease, and recently it has been applied to determine the protein requirements of athletes (Kato et al. 2016).

Protein Requirements for Exercise

The protein requirements and the recommendations for protein intake for athletes have not been without controversy. Generally, scientists seem to be divided into two camps: those who believe that participation in exercise and sport increases the nutritional requirement for protein and those who believe that protein requirements for athletes and exercising people are no different from the requirements for sedentary people. Evidence has been found for both arguments. Although this issue may be scientifically relevant, from a practical perspective, the requirement for protein—as most often defined—may not be relevant to most athletes. The scientists who believe that protein requirements are greater for athletes and exercising people offer two explanations:

1. Amino acids may be oxidized during exercise.
2. Increased protein synthesis is necessary to repair damage and forms the basis of training adaptations.

Acute endurance exercise results in increased oxidation of the BCAAs leucine, isoleucine, and valine. Because these are essential amino acids that cannot be synthesized within the body, the implication is that they come from increased breakdown of proteins. Dietary protein requirements thus increase. Several studies using the nitrogen balance technique confirm that the dietary protein requirements for athletes involved in prolonged endurance training are higher than those for sedentary individuals (Houltham and Rowlands 2014; Tarnopolsky 2004). Based on nitrogen balance, it can be estimated that protein contributes about 5% to 15% to energy expenditure at rest. During exercise, in relative terms, more amino acids may be oxidized. In relative terms, however, protein as a fuel is not important because of the much greater increase of carbohydrate and fat oxidation. Therefore, during prolonged exercise, the relative contribution of protein to energy expenditure is usually much lower than it is at rest; it is usually well below 5% of total energy expenditure. Only in extreme conditions when carbohydrate availability is limited (e.g., after a few hours of strenuous exercise that results in liver and muscle glycogen depletion) can the contribution of protein increase up to about 10% of total energy expenditure. Nevertheless, it could be argued that the oxidation of the essential amino acids leucine, isoleucine, and valine is increased and, therefore, the requirements are increased. The counterarguments are that leucine oxidation does not represent overall total protein oxidation and grossly overestimates protein oxidation. For example, one study by Koopman and colleagues (2004) found an increase in leucine oxidation during prolonged endurance exercise but no change in phenylalanine oxidation, confirming that not all amino acids are oxidized to the same degree and suggesting that leucine oxidation overestimates protein oxidation. Furthermore, the oxidized amino acids do not appear to be derived from degradation of myofibrillar proteins (Kasperek and Snider 1989). Finally, several nitrogen balance studies have not found differences or even improved nitrogen and leucine balances in active people (el-Khoury et al. 1997; Moore et al. 2007).

After resistance exercise, muscle protein turnover increases because of an acceleration of protein synthesis and degradation. Muscle protein breakdown increases after resistance exercise but to a smaller degree than muscle protein synthesis provided that dietary protein intake is adequate. When amino acid availability is limiting (i.e., in the fasted state), the rate of muscle protein breakdown exceeds that of muscle protein synthesis and net tissue protein gain does not occur. The elevations in protein degradation and synthesis are transient but are still present at 3 and 24 hours after exercise, although protein turnover returns to baseline levels after 48 hours. These results seem to apply to resistance exercise or dynamic exercise at a relatively high intensity. Low-intensity to moderate-intensity dynamic endurance exercise does not seem to have the same effects on muscle protein turnover, although studies have shown that endurance exercise may result in increased protein oxidation, especially during the later stages of very prolonged exercise and in conditions of glycogen depletion (Koopman et al. 2004).

Some studies have shown that the body adapts to training by becoming more efficient with protein (Butterfield and Calloway 1984; Phillips et al. 1999). Protein turnover decreases after training, and less net protein degradation occurs. In other words, after training, athletes become more efficient and waste less protein (Butterfield and Calloway 1984). Another study has demonstrated that BCAA oxidation at the same relative workload is the same in untrained and trained individuals (Lamont, McCullough, and Kalhan 1999). Although the protein requirement may increase initially, after adaptation to the training, this increase seems to disappear. This finding has been used as an argument that protein requirements are not greater in athletes.

Recommendations for Endurance Athletes

Although most researchers agree that exercise increases protein oxidation to some extent and this increased oxidation is accompanied by increased nitrogen losses, controversy persists over whether athletes have to eat more protein than less active people do. Nitrogen balance studies (Houltham and Rowlands 2014; Tarnopolsky 2004) show that endurance athletes need to eat about 1.2 to 1.4 g of protein per kilogram of body weight per day to maintain nitrogen balance. Furthermore, the more recent application of the IAAO technique to endurance athletes (Kato et al. 2016) has indicated that the metabolic demand for protein on a high volume training day is greater than current recommendations for athletes based primarily on nitrogen balance methodology (1.6-1.8 vs 1.2-1.4 g protein per kg body weight per day, respectively). Several research groups claim that evidence supports the contention that athletes should eat more protein, whereas others believe that the evidence is insufficient to make such a statement. One interesting observation is that training seems to have a protein-sparing effect. The better trained a person is, the lower the protein breakdown and oxidation are during exercise. The research groups that advocate increased protein intake for endurance athletes usually recommend an intake of 1.2 to 1.68 g of protein per kilogram of body weight per day (as opposed to the recommended intake of 0.8 g of protein per kilogram of body weight per day for the average person). Protein requirements for endurance athletes to achieve nitrogen balance are likely somewhere around 1.2 g per kilogram of body weight per day (Bolster et al. 2005) but could be as high as 1.6 g in individuals who engage in intense exercise (Houltham and Rowlands 2014; Kato et al. 2016; Tarnopolsky 2004). However, these amounts do not necessarily represent the optimal protein intake, which could

(1) support an athlete's ability to repair and replace any damaged proteins (due potentially to oxidative stress or mechanical damage); (2)

adaptively "remodel" proteins in muscle, bone, tendon, and ligaments to better withstand the mechanical stress imposed by athletic training and competition; (3) maintain optimal function of all metabolic pathways in which amino acids are participatory intermediates (which includes being oxidative fuels); (4) support increments in lean mass, if desired; (5) support an optimally functioning immune system; and (6) support the optimal rate of production of all plasma proteins required for optimal physiological function. If the protein "requirements" of athletes were sufficient to support all of the aforementioned processes, then the intake would not be a requirement to prevent deficiency but rather an intake that is "optimal" and would provide an adaptive advantage for athletes. (Phillips 2012)

Even if protein requirements are increased, athletes have no problem achieving the elevated dietary protein intakes needed to maintain nitrogen balance. As an extreme example, we can look at the Tour de France. Cyclists in this event compete for 3 to 7 hours per day, and maintaining energy balance is often problematic (Jeukendrup, Craig, and Hawley 2000). Nevertheless, the athletes seem to have no problems maintaining nitrogen balance (Brouns et al. 1989). With greater food intake, the intake of protein automatically increases because many food products contain at least some protein. A study by van Erp-Baart et al. (1989a) showed a linear relationship between energy intake and protein intake. Tour de France cyclists consumed 12% of their daily energy intake (26 MJ [6,214 kcal]) in the form of protein, and they easily met the suggested increased requirements (about 2.5 g per kilogram of body weight per day). These results demonstrate that if energy intake matches energy expenditure on a daily basis, endurance athletes do not need to supplement their diets with protein. In reality, the timing of intake and the quality of protein may be more important factors than the amount.

Recommendations for Strength Athletes

Unlike endurance exercise, resistance exercise does not increase the rate of leucine oxidation to any major degree. The suggested increased dietary protein requirements are related to increased need for amino acids as precursors for proteins being synthesized, resulting in increased muscle bulk (hypertrophy).

As with endurance exercise, the question of whether strength athletes have increased protein requirements is controversial. Nitrogen balance studies suggest that resistance athletes need about 1.5 g per kilogram of body weight per day, but these studies have been criticized because they were generally of short duration and a steady-state situation may not be established in such

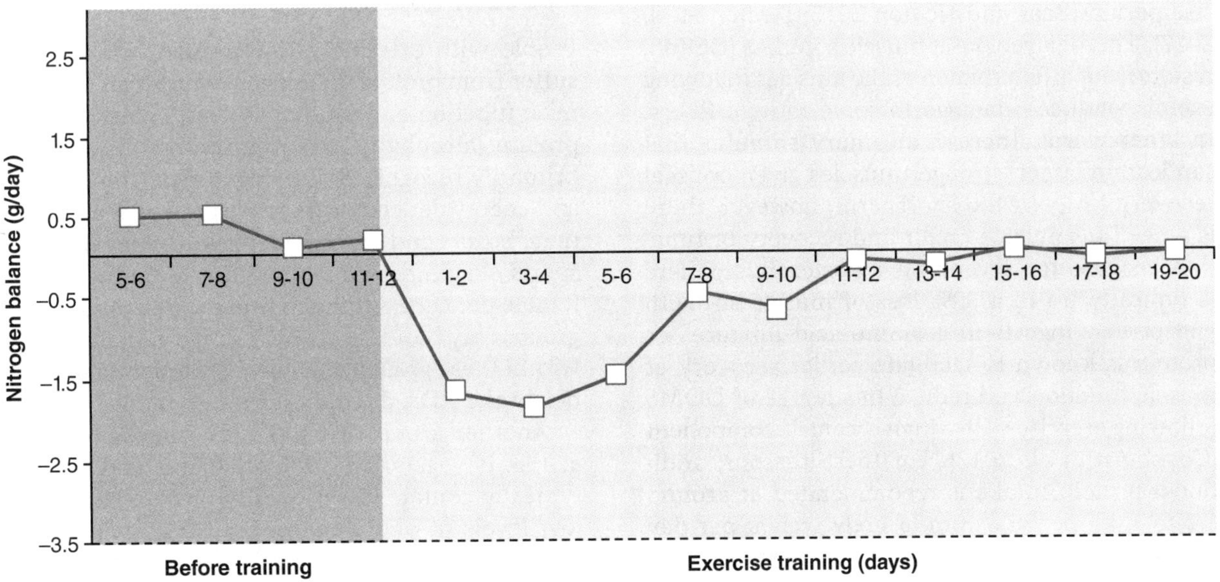

Figure 8.5 Nitrogen balance in response to exercise training.

Adapted from I. Gontzea, R. Sutzeescu, and S. Dumitrache, "The Influence of Adaptation to Physical Effort on Nitrogen Balance in Man," *Nutrition Report International* 11, no. 3 (1975): 231-236.

circumstances (Rennie and Tipton 2000). Gontzea, Sutzeescu, and Dumitrachc (1975) showed that the negative nitrogen balance used by many to indicate increased protein needs disappears after approximately 12 days of training (see figure 8.5). Note, however, that this study examined cycling exercise training rather than resistance training. The protein requirements, therefore, may be only temporarily elevated, but with a further increase in training load, the protein requirement is likely to increase again. The recommendation for protein intake for strength athletes is often 1.6 to 1.7 g per kilogram of body weight per day. Again, people seem to be able to meet this requirement easily with a normal diet, so they do not need extra protein intake. Protein supplements are often used, but they are not necessary to meet the recommended protein intake.

Recommendations for Game Players

Games such as football, rugby, and soccer can be thought of as a series of intermittent sprints separated by periods of less intense running or walking and that contain a substantial number of high-load, lengthening contractions with an eccentric bias when decelerating from fast running and jumping. What this means is that playing these games is similar to a very heavy resistance exercise bout that uses a lot of eccentric or plyometric movements (activities in which the muscle is lengthened during its activation) and generally results in sensations of muscle soreness in the 12- to 72-hour postexercise period (Baar and Heaton 2015; Heaton et al. 2017). This delayed onset muscle soreness (DOMS) results from inflammation of the muscles following exercise-induced damage to some muscle fibers. In other words, there is an injury stimulus that can lead to larger, stronger muscles given optimal recovery time. In the short term, however, there is a need for muscle repair and recovery of function because for several days postexercise, there is typically up to a 30% loss of muscle strength and power. Ingestion of amino acid mixtures or protein is known to facilitate earlier recovery of muscle function and reduce the degree of DOMS following exercise with a high eccentric component (Cockburn et al. 2012). For these reasons, additional protein intake is recommended at around 1.2 to 1.4 g per kilogram of body weight per day with emphasis on dietary protein ingestion in the immediate post-training or postgame period (Baar and Heaton 2015) for reasons that will be explained later in this chapter.

Reported Protein Intake by Athletes

The literature contains several reports of protein intake by athletes in a variety of sports. These intakes are usually self-reported but generally give a good indication of nutritional habits and can reveal whether the athlete is achieving the recommended protein intake. In a study by van Erp-Baart et al. (1989b), protein intake in a variety of elite athletes was investigated. The lowest recorded intake was in a group of field hockey players, but their intake was still over 1.0 g per kilogram of body weight per day. The highest intakes were recorded for endurance cyclists, who consumed almost 3 g per kilogram of body weight per day, and bodybuilders, who consumed 2.5 g per kilogram of body weight per day. Some reports describe intakes below 0.8 g per kilogram of body weight per day in gymnasts and runners and well above 3.0 g per kilogram of body weight per day in weightlifters and bodybuilders. Because most athletes have protein intakes that exceed the daily recommendations (0.8-1.6 g per kilogram of body weight per day, depending on their activity level), the whole discussion about how much protein an athlete needs on a daily basis is rather academic. As previously indicated, factors such as the protein timing and type may be more important (this will be discussed in the Timing of Protein Intake and Type of Protein sections).

Athletes at Risk of Insufficient Protein Intake

People with extremely low protein intakes may suffer from protein deficiency, which can compromise function and ultimately lead to loss of body protein (atrophy). Certain groups of athletes are primarily recognized as being at risk from protein and energy deficiency: female runners, male wrestlers, boxers and other athletes in weight category sports, ski jumpers, male and female gymnasts, and female dancers. Although protein intake for these groups may be adequate on average, certain people within these groups may have protein intakes well below the RDA due to low energy intake.

Another group that has been suggested to be at risk is vegetarian athletes. Plant food sources typically contain lower-quality proteins that have low levels of one or more essential amino acids (for a definition of high- and low-quality proteins, see chapter 1). In addition, the digestibility of plant protein can be low compared with animal protein. Although some concern exists that vegetarian athletes may struggle to meet the protein requirements, the evidence for this is lacking, and adequate protein intake seems possible through a balanced vegetarian diet.

Training and Protein Metabolism

Long-term muscle health and functional capacity largely depends on avoiding dietary protein deficiency, maintaining **protein balance**, being physically active, and the ability to rapidly increase protein turnover in response to damage (Hwee et al. 2014). Increasing protein turnover (i.e., increasing the rate of both protein synthesis and breakdown) is essential for repair of muscle fibers damaged during exercise, particularly eccentric muscle actions. Following damaging exercise, protein breakdown is proportional to protein synthesis (Phillips et al. 1997), and the amino acids made available following protein degradation can be recycled by athletes for muscle protein synthesis (Phillips et al. 1999), resulting in larger and stronger muscles when protein turnover is high (Heaton et al. 2017; Hwee et al. 2014)

Training can have profound effects on protein turnover, muscle morphology, and function. Different types of training have distinct effects. For example, strength training results in muscle hypertrophy, increased muscle mass, and likely maintained, or slightly increased, mitochondrial mass (Tang, Hartman, and Phillips 2006). Endurance training has no effect on muscle mass, but the mitochondrial density inside the muscle fibers increases dramatically. Exercise training is often a combination of strength and endurance, and the improvements in either depend on the relative intensity and the strength required to complete the training sessions. Whatever the adaptation, protein synthesis is required and must occur in the recovery phase between training sessions. Both forms of exercise have been shown to stimulate exercise-specific rises in muscle protein synthesis, and over time this results in changes in muscle mass or mitochondrial mass. Resistance exercise stimulates a rise in myofibrillar protein synthesis, whereas endurance training stimulates a rise in muscle mitochondrial protein synthesis (Wilkinson et al. 2006).

The remodeling of the muscle protein components (i.e., increasing or decreasing the amounts of different proteins and total protein in the muscle fibers) is the underlying mechanism of skeletal muscle plasticity in response to different loading patterns such as immobilization, which leads to atrophy, and resistance exercise (e.g., weightlifting), which leads to hypertrophy. The imbalances between muscle protein synthesis and muscle protein breakdown in adults determine whether a net gain (hypertrophy) or loss (atrophy) of muscle fiber protein occurs. For most adults aged 20 to 50 years, muscle mass remains constant and thus muscle protein synthesis equals muscle protein breakdown. Beyond the fifth decade of life, however, muscle loss begins to occur and muscle mass slowly declines in a process called sarcopenia. This age-related loss of muscle protein can be limited through regular resistance exercise, which can promote increases in muscle protein synthesis.

Repeated elevations in muscle protein synthesis with resistance exercise training create periods of positive net protein balance that add up to create hypertrophy. An increase in muscle mass results in greater strength. In the elderly, this can help preserve the ability to perform everyday functions, such as walking upstairs and getting up from an armchair or the toilet, and can reduce the risk of falls. For the athlete, it can result in increased force generation, power, and sprint speed, which increase the chances of success in sporting events. The balance between muscle protein synthesis and muscle protein breakdown in all people is influenced by exercise training and diet and has an effect on dietary protein requirements. In chapter 12, the underlying mechanisms that explain specific training adaptations will be explained in detail.

Effect of Protein Intake on Protein Synthesis

Nutrition always plays an important role in establishing training adaptations. In the hours after exercise, protein synthesis may exceed protein degradation but only after feeding. If feeding is delayed by several hours, net protein balance remains negative and no muscle hypertrophy occurs (Rennie and Tipton 2000). In fact, a combination of resistance exercise and protein consumption, usually as amino acids or protein ingested following resistance exercise, results in a synergistic stimulation of muscle protein synthesis (Phillips 2013). Critically, the stimulation of muscle protein synthesis is thought to be a key process in the acute, exercise-induced, small increase in muscle size that eventually adds up when exercise is repeated regularly to yield hypertrophy. Agreement between short-term

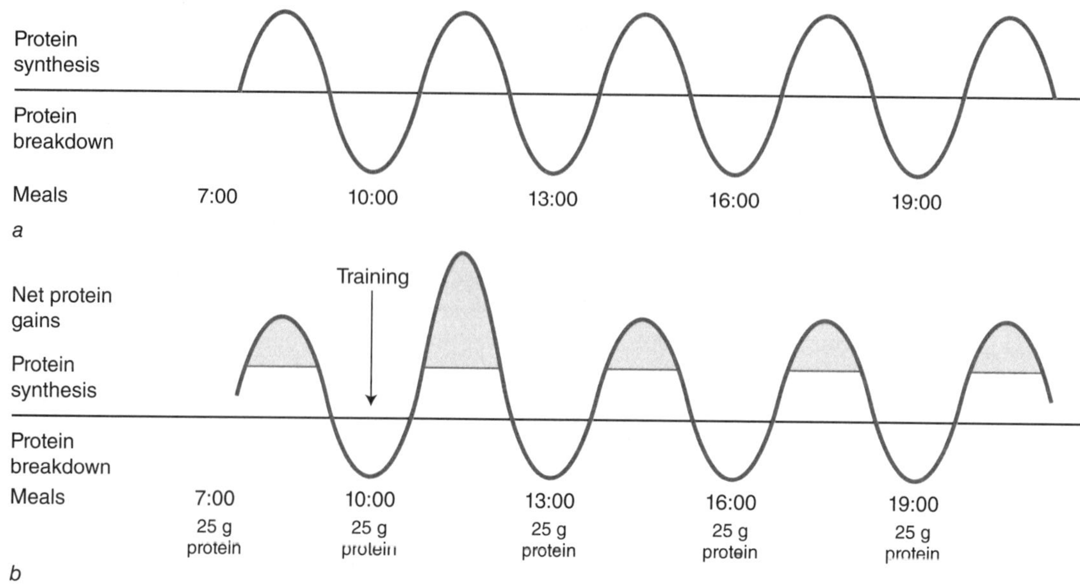

Figure 8.6 Protein synthesis and breakdown in response to training and regular protein intake throughout the day. It is possible to increase net protein synthesis (in blue) *(a)* at rest with regular meals containing 10-20 g protein and *(b)* with 25 grams of protein intake every 3 hours, but the strongest stimulus comes from a combination of training (exercise) and protein intake.

changes in muscle net protein balance (i.e., muscle protein synthesis minus muscle protein breakdown) and long-term gains in muscle mass has been observed in studies that have varied nutrient provision (Hartman et al. 2007; Wilkinson et al. 2007) and resistance exercise training regimens (Mitchell et al. 2012). Importantly, it appears that the meal-to-meal fluctuations in muscle protein synthesis are far more influential in determining gains in and losses of skeletal muscle mass. Thus, in a dynamic sense, undulations in muscle protein synthesis and small changes in muscle protein breakdown determine net muscle protein balance (see figure 8.6). Therefore, the suggestion is often made that the timing of protein intake is crucial. Key factors that affect protein synthesis are the coingestion of other nutrients, the amount of protein, the timing of protein intake, and the type of protein.

In resting conditions, higher amino acid concentrations in plasma have a stimulatory effect on protein synthesis (Bennet et al. 1990; Bennet and Rennie 1991). Immediately after exercise, this effect of increased availability of amino acids on protein synthesis is exaggerated compared with the resting condition (Biolo et al. 1997). Amino acids and exercise thus seem to have an additive effect on net protein synthesis. Note, however, that in these studies, amino acids were infused and plasma amino acid concentrations were elevated to extremely high levels (much higher than those observed after oral ingestion of amino acid mixtures or protein). Intravenous infusion is not a practical method for athletes, and infused amino acids bypass the liver. The liver normally extracts between 20% and 90% of all amino acids after absorption from the gut (a phenomenon known as first-pass splanchnic extraction). Therefore, whether similar effects are to be expected after oral ingestion of amino acids is not clear. A follow-up study investigated this question (Tipton et al. 1999). In this study, a relatively large amount of amino acids was ingested after resistance exercise. Following exercise, muscle protein balance was negative after placebo ingestion, but when amino acids were ingested, the net balance was positive mainly because of increased muscle protein synthesis. From this study and a limited number of other studies, one can conclude that ingestion of amino acids or protein after exercise enhances net protein synthesis.

Coingestion of Other Nutrients

Feeding a mixed diet not only provides substrates but also results in a favorable hormonal milieu for protein synthesis. Increased availability of glucose and amino acids also results in increased plasma insulin concentrations, which, in turn, may cause a reduction of protein breakdown and a small increase in protein synthesis (Bennet and Rennie 1991; Biolo et al. 1999).

Carbohydrate ingestion per se may not have an effect on protein synthesis after exercise, but carbohydrate ingestion elevates plasma insulin concentrations and thereby may reduce the breakdown of protein that normally occurs with resistance exercise. Insulin inhibits protein breakdown and also promotes amino acid (and glucose) uptake by some tissues, including skeletal muscle. The combined ingestion of protein and carbohydrate seems to be preferred after exercise, at least for situations where the amount of protein ingested is quite small (most studies reporting this effect fed their subjects only about 6 to 12 g of protein or amino acids after exercise together with 30 to 100 g carbohydrate). The protein delivers the substrate (amino acids), and carbohydrate further increases the anabolic hormonal milieu required for net protein synthesis.

In a study by Miller et al. (2003), volunteers performed leg resistance exercise and then ingested one of three drinks—amino acids (about 6 g) only, carbohydrate (about 35 g) only, or the amino acids and carbohydrate combined—at 1 and 2 hours postexercise. Total net uptake of phenylalanine across the leg over 3 hours was greatest in response to amino acids and carbohydrate combined and least in carbohydrate alone. Stimulation of net uptake with amino acids and carbohydrate combined was due to increased muscle protein synthesis (figure 8.7). In the control (carbohydrate only) condition, a net protein breakdown was observed, confirming that hyperinsulinemia alone (i.e., in the absence of ingested amino acids) does not stimulate protein synthesis. These results suggest that the ingestion of a relatively small amount of amino acids with a larger amount of carbohydrate can increase net muscle protein synthesis in the hours after resistance exercise. Similar data is available for endurance exercise (Howarth et al. 2009), and the coingestion of carbohydrate and protein in the 2 hours following exhaustive exercise was shown to improve time to exhaustion during strenuous steady state cycling exercise 18 hours later compared to an isocaloric amount of carbohydrate during the first 2 hours post exercise (Rustad et al. 2016). In many of the earlier studies the dose of amino acids was suboptimal for the maximum rate of postexercise protein synthesis. When 20 g of amino acids or protein are ingested after exercise, there is a larger increase in protein synthesis compared with 0 or 6 g, and the addition of large amounts of carbohydrate to 20 g of protein does not further increase net protein synthesis (Koopman et al. 2007).

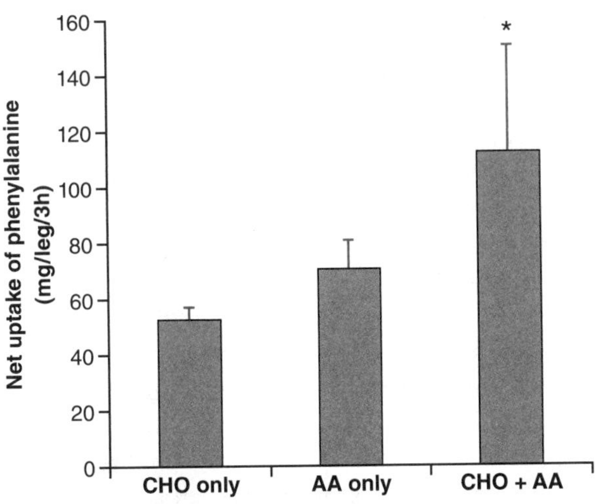

Figure 8.7 Protein synthesis over 3 hours after a bout of resistance exercise as measured by the area under the curve for net uptake of phenylalanine. Protein synthesis seems the lowest with carbohydrate, followed by amino acids only. The combined effect of carbohydrate and amino acids, however, is significantly greater than the individual effects of carbohydrate or protein. AA = amino acids; CHO = carbohydrate.

Adapted from Miller et al. (2003).

Fat also seems to have an effect on protein synthesis. This was discovered in a study that was probably the first to investigate protein synthesis in response to an intact food (Elliot et al. 2006). After a bout of resistance exercise, subjects consumed either fat-free milk or whole milk. Both milk drinks stimulated protein synthesis, but the greatest effect was seen with whole milk. The explanation for this is not immediately clear, but it was suggested that the fat in the whole milk delayed the delivery of the amino acids and provided a more sustained supply of amino acids for protein synthesis. More research is needed to look into the effects of added fat on protein synthesis. In fact, more research is needed to understand the effects of normal meals that contain carbohydrate, fiber, fat, protein, and other nutrients. Most studies have been performed using pure forms of protein in isolated form rather than food form. Therefore, we will need to understand the behavior of protein when ingested in and with normal foods.

Amount of Protein

Although the question about daily protein intake may be rather academic and have little practical relevance because most athletes exceed even the highest recommendations, it is important to understand the amount of protein needed in each meal to optimize protein synthesis. A study by Bohe et al.

CARBOHYDRATE AND PROTEIN DURING OR AFTER EXERCISE

The excitement about adding protein to carbohydrate drinks stems from a small number of studies that suggested that adding a small amount of protein (about 2% whey protein or about 20 g/L) to a carbohydrate drink produced improvements in endurance capacity compared with a carbohydrate drink alone (Ivy et al. 2003; Saunders, Kane, and Todd 2004; Saunders, Luden, and Herrick 2007; Saunders et al. 2009). It has been speculated that increased endurance capacity with carbohydrate and protein may be due to increased protein oxidation when muscle glycogen is depleted (Koopman et al. 2005) or to attenuations in central fatigue (Blomstrand et al. 1991). None of these explanations seems plausible, and evidence is lacking. The few studies that reported positive effects have been criticized, and others have not been able to show any performance effects. In a study by van Essen and Gibala (2006), athletes performed an 80 km (50 mi) cycling time trial on three occasions and drank either a 6% carbohydrate blend, a 6% carbohydrate and 2% whey-protein blend, or a sweetened placebo. All the subjects consumed the solutions at a rate of 1 L/h (0.3 gal/h). The average performance time was identical for the carbohydrate and carbohydrate plus protein trials (roughly 135 minutes) and both were significantly faster (by approximately 4%) than the placebo trial (141 minutes). This study demonstrated that when athletes ingested a carbohydrate during exercise at a rate considered optimal for carbohydrate delivery, protein provided no additional performance benefit during an event that simulated real-life competition. A recent meta-analysis of the effects of protein in combination with carbohydrate supplements acutely ingested during exercise on endurance performance (11 studies) or ingestion during and after exercise to affect subsequent endurance exercise performance (15 studies) came to essentially the same conclusion (McLellan, Pasakios, and Lieberman 2014): When carbohydrate is delivered at optimal rates during or after endurance exercise, protein supplements have no performance-enhancing effect. Therefore, there is currently no convincing evidence to advise athletes to ingest protein during endurance exercise.

The ingestion of protein, protein hydrolysates, or a mixture of amino acids (in particular BCAA) is often associated with faster recovery and reductions in muscle damage and soreness after exercise (Saunders 2011), especially after eccentric exercise (in which the muscle is activated while it is lengthening; this occurs with squat jumping, bench stepping, downhill running, and lowering of weights). Most studies that have examined the influence of carbohydrate and protein coingestion on recovery from exercise-induced muscle damage provided carbohydrate postexercise in combination with protein (often as milk-based beverages). Some of these studies demonstrated that carbohydrate and protein coingestion can reduce postexercise plasma creatine kinase (CK, a marker of muscle damage) and, to a limited extent, attenuate muscle soreness and hasten the recovery of muscle function in the days following a damaging bout of eccentric exercise (Cockburn et al. 2012; Rankin, Stevenson, and Cockburn 2015). It has also been suggested that greater reductions in postexercise CK found for carbohydrate plus protein beverages may help prolong endurance capacity during a second exercise test. Although evidence is accumulating that protein somehow affects muscle soreness postexercise, mechanisms are unclear. It is generally assumed that the well-established acute benefits of protein supplementation on postexercise muscle **anabolism** facilitate muscle fiber repair and the recovery of muscle function and performance. When protein supplements are provided, however, acute changes in postexercise protein synthesis and anabolic intracellular signaling do not consistently result in measurable reductions in muscle damage and enhanced recovery of muscle function (Pasiakos, Lieberman, and McLellan 2014). More research is needed to study the effects of carbohydrate and protein intake on recovery from exercise.

(2003) may provide some initial information. In this study, extracellular, rather than intracellular, amino acid concentrations determined the rate of protein synthesis. The results showed that there appears to be a plateau above which protein synthesis is not further stimulated, and more recent studies have examined how much ingested protein is required to attain this plateau. Although it is difficult to determine exactly what amino acid intake is required to achieve this plateau, the amounts appear to be relatively small. Studies suggest that 20 to 25 g of protein or 8 to 10 g of essential amino acids are required to reach this plateau (Moore et al. 2009; Symons et al. 2009; Witard et al. 2014). Ingesting higher amounts of protein (e.g., 40 g) does not further stimulate muscle protein synthesis after resistance exercise (Moore et al. 2009; Witard et al. 2014) for healthy young men regardless of training status, as illustrated in figure 8.8 (Witard et al. 2014). Similar results have been reported using whole food (lean minced beef) in young men and women; a moderate amount (30 g protein) was just as effective as a much higher amount (90 g protein) for stimulating muscle protein synthesis (Symons et al. 2009).

Protein consumed in excess of 25 to 30 g is oxidized at a higher rate (Moore et al. 2009; Witard et al. 2014) and results in increased urea production (Witard et al. 2014), which indicates there is a limit to the quantity of amino acids that can be used for muscle protein synthesis. This has been called the muscle full effect (Atherton et al. 2010). From a regression analysis of dose–response studies, Moore et al. (2015) refined the estimate for protein to a dose that is expressed per kg of body weight. They concluded that the dose of protein beyond which there was no further increase in muscle protein synthesis in young men was 0.325 g per kilogram of body weight per meal. To account for interindividual variability, they proposed the addition of two standard deviations to this estimate, yielding an optimal dose of protein of 0.4 g per kilogram of body weight per meal. The amounts of various foods that contain 25 g protein and the quality of the protein (see chapter 1) they contain is shown in table 8.4. Published ACSM guidelines (American College of Sports Medicine 2015) on protein intake for optimal muscle maintenance are based on these data.

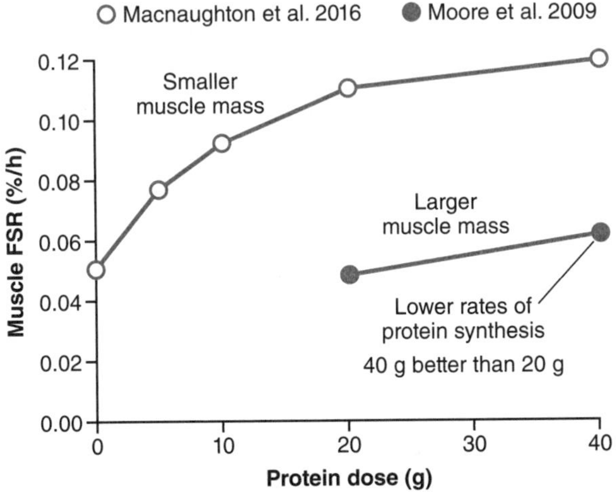

Figure 8.8 Muscle fractional synthetic rate in two studies. When a smaller muscle mass was used, FSR was higher but plateaued after about 20 g of ingested protein. Training a larger muscle mass resulted in lower FSR values, but doubling protein intake modestly further increased FSR.

Data from Moore et al. (2009), Macnaughton et al. (2016), and Mysportscience.

Recently, it was suggested that larger amounts of protein may be needed for optimal adaptations to resistance exercise training when large muscle groups are involved. Macnaughton et al. (2016) argued that in previous studies, smaller muscle groups were trained, but when a larger muscle mass is involved (as would be the case for most athletes and most practical situations), larger amounts of protein may be required. When these researchers performed a study in which volunteers trained a larger muscle mass, there were two main observations. First, protein synthesis rates were lower than previous studies, possibly because the same amount of protein now had to be shared with a larger amount of muscle. Second, they observed that ingesting 40 g of protein resulted in greater protein synthesis than 20 g of protein, in contrast to previous studies. This is the only study currently in the literature that makes this suggestion, and more studies are probably needed to distill new guidelines from it.

Timing of Protein Intake

The timing of food intake after exercise is important to the balance between protein synthesis and protein degradation. Studies have investigated protein ingestion immediately after exercise, 1 or 3 hours after exercise, or before exercise. In one study by Tipton et al. (2001), volunteers ingested 6 g of essential amino acids plus 35 g of carbohydrate immediately before and immediately after completion of an intense leg resistance exercise bout. Amino acid uptake seemed to be greater when the nutrients were ingested before the exercise bout than immediately afterward, but the anabolic

TABLE 8.4 Protein Content and Quality of Foods

Food	Average protein content (g/100 g)	Amount that contains 25 g protein	Protein quality (PDCAAS)*
Cooked meats			
Beef	32	78 g (2.8 oz)	0.92
Pork	32	78 g (2.8 oz)	0.90
Chicken	31	81 g (2.9 oz)	0.91
Turkey	31	81 g (2.9 oz)	0.90
Lamb	30	83 g (2.9 oz)	0.90
Ham	25	100 g (3.5 oz)	0.90
Cooked fish			
Tuna	30	83 g (2.9 oz)	0.90
Salmon	27	93 g (3.3 oz)	1.00
Sardine	25	100 g (3.5 oz)	0.98
White fish	23	110 g (3.9 oz)	1.00
Dairy			
Cheddar cheese	27	93 g (3.3 oz)	1.00
Feta cheese	15	160 g (5.6 oz)	1.00
Cottage cheese	12	210 g (7.4 oz)	1.00
Goat's milk	7	350 ml (12 fl oz)	1.00
Yogurt	6	430 g (15.2 oz)	0.95
Cow's milk	3.5	700 ml (24 fl oz)	1.00
Boiled vegetables			
Soybeans	17	147 g (5.2 oz)	0.91
Chickpeas	9	280 g (9.9 oz)	0.78
Peas	8	300 g (10.6 oz)	0.50
Kidney beans	5	500 g (17.6 oz)	0.68
Corn	3	830 g (29.3 oz)	0.42
Other			
Whey protein isolate	80	32 g (1.1 oz)	1.00
Soy protein isolate	80	32 g (1.1 oz)	1.00
Peanuts (dry roasted)	24	105 g (3.7 oz)	0.62
Tofu	16	155 g (5.5 oz)	0.93
Quorn mince	15	160 g (5.6 oz)	0.91
Egg (boiled)	12	210 g (3 eggs)	1.00
Cereals (e.g., granola)	11	230 g (8.1 oz)	0.59
Bread	10	250 g (8.8 oz; 8 slices)	0.60
Rice	7	350 g (12.3 oz)	0.47
Soy milk	6	420 ml (14 fl oz)	0.94

*The protein digestibility corrected amino acid score (PDCAAS) is a method of evaluating protein quality based on the amino acid requirements of humans and their ability to digest the protein in question. The PDCAAS rating was adopted by the FDA and the FAO and WHO in 1993 as the preferred best method to determine protein quality. The maximum score of 1.00 means that after digestion of the protein, it provides, per unit of protein, 100% or more of the essential amino acids required. See chapter 1 for further details.

response was similar in magnitude for both preexercise and postexercise feeding. Thjs study suggested that the anabolic response to exercise and amino acid and carbohydrate ingestion is greater with preexercise ingestion versus immediately postexercise, and it was suggested that the observed differences were likely related to the delivery of amino acids to the muscle. Free amino acids ingested before exercise may result in increased amino acid delivery (because of increased blood flow to active muscles during the exercise session) and lead to superior amino acid uptake compared with amino acids ingested after exercise. However, this study was performed with essential amino acids. When some of these studies were repeated with whey protein (and no carbohydrate), the difference between feeding before a bout of resistance exercise and after was not evident (Tipton et al. 2007). The current consensus is that ingesting protein soon after exercise (within approximately 1 hour after exercise), which is more practical than preexercise protein consumption, is the best way to increase net protein synthesis postexercise.

It has been known for some time that resistance exercise alone results in an elevation in muscle protein synthesis for at least 48 hours and in muscle protein breakdown for 24 hours (Phillips et al. 1997); thus, even in the basal fasted state, there is a subsequent increase in the turnover of muscle proteins. In this situation, however, muscle protein breakdown exceeds muscle protein synthesis, so no net tissue protein accretion occurs. Resistance exercise essentially primes the muscle to be more responsive, in terms of an increased muscle protein synthesis response to aminoacidemia (elevated plasma amino acid concentration), following ingestion of a protein-containing meal. This increased sensitivity lasts for at least 24 hours (Burd et al. 2011) and possibly up to 48 hours but diminishes over time. Therefore, it is most advantageous to ingest protein to generate a large increase in the plasma amino acid concentration in the postexercise period. It has also been suggested that preexercise protein ingestion may prime the system and offer some advantage over a postexercise supplementation strategy. However, ingesting 20 g of protein either before or 1 hour after 10 sets of knee extensor exercises resulted in similar rates of amino acid uptake (Tipton et al. 2007). In other studies, there was no benefit shown with preexercise amino acid feeding (Burke, Hawley, et al. 2012; Fujita et al. 2009), so the general scientific consensus now is that it is optimal to ingest protein soon after a bout of resistance exercise. Moreover, it is possible that a feeding-induced aminoacidemia before or during exercise may blunt the subsequent postexercise muscle protein synthesis response to amino acids due to an overlap in the aminoacidemic responses and the muscle full effect (Atherton et al. 2010). A recent meta-analysis examining protein timing and hypertrophy concluded that ingestion of a protein supplement shortly after resistance exercise positively influenced hypertrophy (Schoenfeld, Aragon, and Krieger 2013) but that the amount of total protein intake was the strongest predictor of muscular hypertrophy and timing did not influence it. However, total intake and timing can probably not be uncoupled that easily, because when total intake increased it is likely that protein content of all meals increased, and as a result of this more meals will have a protein quantity that is sufficient to stimulate protein synthesis. So the timing of meals and the protein content of meals throughout the day may be very important.

The importance of timing and amount of protein ingestion over the course of a day needed to optimize training adaptation is becoming clearer as well. In one study, an intermittent pattern of whey protein ingestion (20 g every 3 hours during a 12-hour recovery period) following a bout of resistance exercise was found to be more effective than ingestion of large boluses (40 g every 6 hours) or a pulse (10 g every 1.5 hours) protocol for stimulating muscle protein synthesis (Areta et al. 2013). These results agree with the muscle full effect described previously in this chapter. However, it should be noted that many studies that have examined the effect of protein feeding on muscle protein synthesis provided oral amino acid mixtures or protein in an isolated form (i.e., not accompanied by other macronutrients). In real life, people eat meals composed of a mixture of macronutrients (i.e., protein, carbohydrate, fat). The macronutrient composition and form of meal intake may influence the meal-induced rise in the plasma amino acid concentration and subsequent muscle and whole-body protein synthesis (Burke, Winter, et al. 2012). Future studies need to examine the influence of mixed macronutrient meals on rates of muscle protein synthesis and muscle protein breakdown over longer periods of time.

The postexercise period should be relaxing as well as a time for rehydration (to restore fluid and electrolyte losses), refueling (to restore glycogen), and repair and remodeling (tissue repair and adaptation to the training stimulus); this is known as the 4Rs. The appropriate amounts of fluid, electrolytes, carbohydrate, and protein should be ingested to accomplish the goals defined by the 4Rs.

Eating just before bedtime has been suggested as a good time to provide dietary protein that can be directed toward remodeling muscle proteins. A study by Res et al. (2012) in which healthy male subjects ingested 40 g (equivalent to 0.6 g per kilogram of body weight) of protein before bedtime showed that muscle protein synthesis (MPS) was stimulated and net protein balance was improved overnight. Recently, a 12-week progressive resistance exercise training study showed that a presleep beverage that contained 27.5 g protein, 15 g carbohydrate, and 0.1 g fat augmented muscle mass, muscle fiber area, and strength gains compared with a noncaloric placebo beverage (Snijders et al. 2015). The placebo control group in this study did not receive a protein supplement, which resulted in a 0.6 g per kilogram of body weight difference in daily total protein intakes, which could have conferred an advantage to the protein beverage group regardless of when the protein was consumed.

In summary, it seems that the timing of protein intake throughout the day is an important variable to consider in optimizing skeletal muscle recovery and hypertrophy. It appears optimal to ingest protein in the postexercise period, though the purported anabolic window for protein ingestion lasts at least 24 hours (Burd et al. 2011), and therefore the timing of protein ingestion in relation to exercise does not have as drastic an effect on outcomes as was previously thought (Schoenfeld, Aragon, and Krieger 2013). It is also important to ingest protein in sufficient doses (about 0.4 g per kilogram of body weight per meal) throughout the day (Areta et al. 2013). In addition to this, ingesting a large dose of protein (0.6 g per kilogram of body weight) before bedtime appears to augment acute overnight muscle protein synthesis (Res et al. 2012) and chronic skeletal muscle adaptations (Snijders et al. 2015).

Type of Protein

Because the delivery of amino acids is important, digestive properties of proteins influence the anabolic response at rest and after exercise. Proteins are often classified as fast or slow (in regard to the speed at which they can be digested and their amino acids absorbed following ingestion). The interest in fast and slow proteins started with a series of studies by Boirie et al. (1997). Their comparison of fast and slow proteins involved comparing protein supplements that contained whey with those that contained casein or soy protein, which are the three most commonly consumed isolated protein sources. Casein and whey are derived from whole milk, and soy is derived from plants. About 80% of milk protein is casein. The remaining 20% is whey. Whey and soy are considered fast proteins because the body digests and absorbs them relatively rapidly, which results in a rapid aminoacidemia. Casein, on the other hand, is a slow protein; it takes the body longer to break down and absorb it. Casein seems to clot in the stomach, which slows gastric emptying. Casein intake also results in the release of peptides from the stomach during digestion, which also slows gastric emptying. Whey, soy, and casein vary in their effects on the rate at which proteins are synthesized and broken down. Similar to how foods differ in their effect on blood glucose concentrations, different sources of protein may be digested and absorbed at different rates.

In a series of studies it was found that milk protein results in greater rates of protein synthesis and a greater increase in muscle mass in weightlifters compared with soy protein (Hartman et al. 2007; Wilkinson et al. 2007). Although milk protein seems to be preferred to soy protein, it is difficult to recommend which source of protein would be optimal for protein accretion. The anabolic response postexercise depends not only on the type of protein but also on the timing of intake and the ingestion of other nutrients as previously explained. A protein that is optimal in one condition is not necessarily optimal in all conditions.

Fast proteins such as whey and soy induce a larger but more transient rise in muscle protein synthesis than casein (Reitelseder et al. 2011; Tang et al. 2009). Whole-body protein synthesis is stimulated more with whey protein and is suppressed with casein (Boirie et al. 1997). After ingestion of isolated casein, soy, and whey protein (all providing 10 g of essential amino acids), the rise in muscle protein synthesis over the following 3 hours was found to be greatest with whey protein both at rest and following resistance exercise (Tang et al. 2009). Interestingly, soy protein had higher muscle protein synthesis than casein in resting conditions and after exercise (Tang et al. 2009). Thus, it appears that at least up to 3 hours after a bout of resistance exercise, the most effective protein source is whey.

Another factor that determines the anabolic response is the amount of the amino acid leucine, which acts as a signaling molecule to stimulate translation-initiation pathways, which results in increased rates of protein synthesis (Tipton et al. 1999). These effects will be discussed in more detail in chapter 12, because they may have an essential role in the underlying mechanisms of training adaptations.

Leucine stimulates the **mammalian target of rapamycin complex-1 (mTOR)**, a key signaling protein, and triggers a rise in muscle protein synthesis (Phillips 2016). Therefore, ingested proteins with a high leucine content would be advantageous in triggering a rise in muscle protein synthesis. Thus, protein quality (reflected in leucine content, essential amino acid content, and protein digestibility) has an effect on changes in muscle protein synthesis, which could ultimately affect skeletal muscle mass. Whey protein contains 10 g of leucine per 100 g, which is more leucine per gram than casein (8.2 g/100 g) or soy (5.9 g/100 g). Foods that are relatively high in leucine are shown in table 8.5. Following ingestion of protein with a relatively high leucine content, such as whey, the rapid and relatively large aminoacidemia may increase essential amino acid (and specifically leucine) delivery to the muscle to a certain threshold that triggers a stimulation of muscle protein synthesis and the associated anabolic pathways (figure 8.9). Indeed, the importance of leucine in promoting the muscle anabolic response to postexercise feeding was highlighted in a study by Reidy et al. (2013) in which a dairy-soy protein mixture (1:2:1 ratio of whey, casein, and soy) was shown to be as effective as whey protein alone in stimulating muscle protein synthesis when the leucine content was matched. Another study (Churchward-Venne et al. 2014) reported that participants who ingested 6.25 g of whey protein combined with 5 g leucine had just as large an increase in muscle protein synthesis after resistance exercise as when they consumed 25 g of whey protein despite the lower protein and total amino acid dose. The leucine threshold amount that triggers the stimulation of

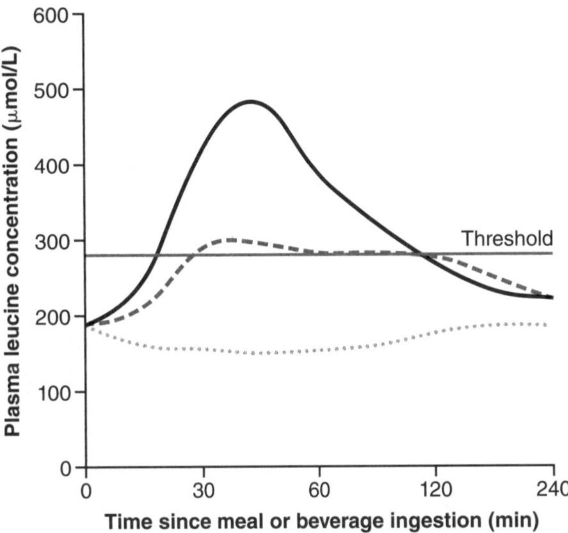

Figure 8.9 The leucine trigger concept. Leucine triggers a rise in muscle protein synthesis; therefore, more rapidly digested proteins (solid line) that contain a relatively high proportion of leucine (e.g., whey) are most effective in promoting increases in muscle protein synthesis. Proteins that are more slowly digested (dashed line) and/or have lower leucine content (e.g., casein) do not increase protein synthesis to the same extent. The dotted line represents ingestion of a meal or beverage that does not contain protein.

Based on Phillips (2013); Boirie et al. (1997); Pennings et al. (2011); Reitelseder et al. (2011).

TABLE 8.5 Leucine Content of Various Foods

Food	Amount needed to supply 3 g leucine	Leucine content (g/419 kJ [100 kcal])
Whey protein isolate	25 g (0.9 oz)	2.90
Soy protein isolate	37 g (1.3 oz)	2.00
Greek yogurt	300 g (10.6 oz)	1.75
Chicken breast	170 g (6 oz)	1.70
Lean beef	170 g (6 oz)	1.30
Cheese	105 g (3.7 oz)	1.09
Egg	4 large eggs	0.94
Skim milk	900 ml (30 fl oz)	0.93
Kidney beans	525 g (18.5 oz)	0.65
Tofu	600 g (21.2 oz)	0.44
Raw peanuts	180 g (6.3 oz)	0.29
Bread	770 g (27.2 oz; 14 slices)	0.07

PRACTICAL RECOMMENDATIONS TO MAXIMIZE HYPERTROPHY WITH RESISTANCE EXERCISE TRAINING AND NUTRITION

- Engage in regular training bouts of high load resistance training.
- Lift heavier loads over longer durations to stimulate greater improvements in muscular strength.
- Lift to the point of contraction failure.
- Maintain energy balance.
- Use the postexercise period as a time for the 4Rs (rehydration, refueling, repair, and remodeling).
- Ingest protein in the postexercise period in a sufficient dose (about 0.4 g per kilogram of body weight) and up to three other meals throughout the day including a large dose of protein (about 0.6 g per kilogram of body weight) before bedtime to augment acute overnight muscle protein synthesis and chronic skeletal muscle adaptations. Try to achieve a total dietary protein intake of 1.4 to 1.6 g per kilogram of body weight per day. Eating fewer meals with more protein is not a better alternative.
- For the postexercise meal, choose rapidly digested, high-quality proteins with a high leucine content, such as whey, skim milk, and eggs.
- For other meals, choose mostly lean, high-quality proteins that contain all the essential amino acids in approximately equal proportions (e.g., animal sources including beef, ham, lamb, poultry, fish; supplement with soy, beans, cheese, nuts, and bread).

muscle protein synthesis appears to be about 3 g of leucine per meal (Churchward-Venne et al. 2014), which may be the main factor in determining the recommended amount of protein per meal.

It should also be noted that the addition of the two other BCAAs, isoleucine and valine, does not further improve MPS (Churchward-Venne et al. 2014), so it makes sense to supplement only with leucine (or to consume dietary proteins that are known to have a high leucine content). All three BCAAs share the same transporter, and consumption of a mixture of BCAAs would be expected to result in antagonism for uptake from the gut and into the muscle and thus be less effective than leucine alone in stimulating muscle protein synthesis. Despite the continued popularity of BCAA supplements among athletes, there is very little evidence for their efficacy in promoting muscle protein synthesis or gains in muscle mass, and current advice is to ingest intact dietary proteins that have a high leucine content and are rapidly digested. The slower and more protracted aminoacidemia accompanying the ingestion of casein may be more effective at sustaining muscle protein synthesis and possibly at attenuating negative net protein balance during sleep or over longer periods of time, but this requires confirmation by future studies (Morton, McGlory, and Phillips 2015). As research continues, it is likely that we will be able to make clearer recommendations in the years to come.

Amino Acids as Ergogenic Aids

In the past, the body's amino acid needs were primarily met by ingestion of whole proteins. Over the past few years, however, the supplementation of individual amino acids has become increasingly popular. Technological advances have made it possible to manufacture food-grade, ultrapure amino acids. The individual amino acids, called free-form amino acids, are mostly produced by bacterial fermentation. Scientific studies have focused on the pharmacologic and metabolic interactions of free-form amino acids. Considerable progress has been made in clinical nutrition, where individual amino acids are used to reduce nitrogen losses and improve organ functions in traumatized and critically ill patients. Individual amino acids also are marketed as supplements for athletes and healthy people. Intake of separate amino acids is often claimed to improve exercise performance, stimulate hormone release, and improve immune function, among other positive effects. Here we review the facts and fallacies of these claims, which are summarized in table 8.6.

TABLE 8.6 Manufacturers' Claims for Amino Acids

Amino acid	Claim
Arginine	Improves immune function, increases tissue creatine levels, increases release of insulin and growth hormone, leads to fewer gastrointestinal problems, improves performance
Aspartate	Improves energy metabolism in muscle, reduces amount of fatigue-causing metabolites, improves endurance performance
Glutamine	Improves immune function (fewer colds), hastens recovery after exercise, improves performance, leads to fewer gastrointestinal problems
Ornithine	Increases growth hormone and insulin release, stimulates protein synthesis, reduces protein breakdown, improves performance
BCAAs	Provide fuel for working muscle, reduce fatigue, improve endurance, reduce muscle protein breakdown
Tyrosine	Increases blood concentration of catecholamines, improves fuel mobilization and metabolism during exercise
Tryptophan	Increases the release of growth hormone, improves sleep, decreases sensations of pain, improves performance
Taurine	Delays fatigue, improves performance, facilitates faster recovery, leads to less muscle damage and pain, leads to fewer gastrointestinal problems, scavenges free radicals
Glycine	Increases phosphocreatine synthesis, improves sprint performance, increases strength

Arginine

Infusion of some amino acids into the blood can stimulate the release of growth hormone from the pituitary gland. Arginine is not the only amino acid that can have such an effect. Other amino acids that may stimulate the release of hormones from endocrine glands include lysine and ornithine. The intravenous administration of arginine to adults in a dose of 30 g in 30 minutes caused a marked increase in the secretion of human pituitary growth hormone (Knopf et al. 1966). Intravenous and oral arginine administration also resulted in a marked insulin release from the ß cells of the pancreas (Dupre et al. 1968). The finding that arginine increases the secretion of anabolic hormones such as human growth hormone and insulin has made it a popular supplement among bodybuilders and strength athletes. But the amount of arginine present in sport nutritional supplements is often rather small (between 1 and 2 g/day) compared to intravenous doses that have been shown to have potent secretagogic actions (30 g/30 minutes). Well-controlled (double-blind, crossover) studies (Fogelholm, Naveri, et al. 1993; Lambert et al. 1993) failed to show an effect of oral L-arginine supplementation taken in low quantities on the plasma concentrations of growth hormone and insulin (measured over a 24-hour period) in male competitive weightlifters and bodybuilders. Note also that the growth hormone responses can be obtained through exercise. The response that can be obtained by ingesting relatively large amounts of arginine is still smaller than what can be obtained through 60 minutes of moderate-intensity exercise. Finally, the oral ingestion of large doses of arginine can cause severe gastrointestinal discomfort and is therefore not practical.

In summary, although arginine infused in large quantities can have anabolic properties, oral ingestion of tolerable doses (i.e., amounts that do not cause gastrointestinal problems) do not result in increased secretion of human growth hormone and insulin. Large increases in insulin secretion can be obtained by ingestion of carbohydrate, and much larger increases in plasma growth hormone are observed during exercise than with even large doses of arginine and other individual amino acids.

Aspartate

Aspartate is often claimed to improve aerobic exercise performance. Aspartate, a precursor for TCA-cycle intermediates, reduces plasma ammonia accumulation during exercise. Because ammonia formation is associated with fatigue, aspartate supplementation could theoretically be ergogenic.

In a study by Maughan and Sadler (1983), eight subjects cycled to exhaustion at 75% to 80% of $\dot{V}O_2max$ after ingestion of 6 g of aspartate (as magnesium and potassium salts) or placebo over 24 hours. No effect of aspartate supplementation was observed on plasma ammonia concentration or exercise time to exhaustion.

Branched-Chain Amino Acids

The three BCAAs—leucine, isoleucine, and valine—are not synthesized in the body. Yet they are oxidized during exercise, and they must therefore be replenished by the diet. In the late 1970s, BCAAs were suggested to be the third fuel for skeletal muscle after carbohydrate and fat (Goldberg and Chang 1978). BCAAs are sometimes supplied to athletes in energy drinks to provide extra fuel. The following are some claims that have been made about BCAAs:

- BCAAs are fuels during exercise.
- BCAAs spare glycogen.
- BCAA supplementation can increase protein synthesis following exercise.
- BCAAs can reduce net protein breakdown in muscle during exercise.
- BCAAs reduce muscle damage.
- BCAAs reduce muscle soreness.
- BCAAs reduce fatigue.
- BCAAs enhance performance.
- BCAAs improve immune function (prevent immunodepression).

Despite the lack of strong evidence for the efficacy of BCAA supplements, athletes continue to use them. Normal food alternatives are available, however, and are almost certainly less expensive. For example, a typical BCAA supplement sold in tablet form contains 100 mg of valine, 50 mg of isoleucine, and 100 mg of leucine. A chicken breast (100 g [3.5 oz]) contains approximately 470 mg of valine, 375 mg of isoleucine, and 656 mg of leucine, or the equivalent of about seven BCAA tablets. Peanuts contain even more BCAAs; 60 g (2 oz) contain the equivalent of 11 tablets.

It has also been argued that taking BCAAs could be counterproductive because leucine, isoleucine, and valine compete with each other for transport. If the main goal is to increase leucine, providing isoleucine and valine at the same time may reduce leucine availability.

Fuel Source and Glycogen Sparing

As mentioned earlier, a study by Goldberg and Chang (1978) suggested that BCAAs can act as a fuel during exercise in addition to carbohydrate and fat. More recently, however, the activities of the enzymes involved in the oxidation of BCAAs were shown to be too low to allow a major contribution of BCAAs to energy expenditure (Wagenmakers et al. 1989). Detailed studies with a ^{13}C-labeled BCAA (^{13}C-leucine) showed that the oxidation of BCAAs increases only two- to threefold during exercise, whereas the oxidation of carbohydrate and fat increases 10-fold to 20-fold (Knapik et al. 1991). Also, carbohydrate ingestion during exercise can prevent the increase in BCAA oxidation. A related claim is that BCAAs can spare glycogen because they are used as a fuel instead of muscle glycogen. Studies, however, have clearly demonstrated no glycogen sparing during exercise with BCAA ingestion. Therefore, BCAAs do not seem to play an important role as a fuel during exercise, and, from this point of view, the supplementation of BCAAs during exercise is unnecessary.

Protein Breakdown

The claims that BCAAs reduce protein breakdown are mainly based on early in vitro studies that showed that adding BCAAs to an incubation or perfusion medium stimulated tissue protein synthesis and inhibited protein degradation. Several in vivo studies in healthy individuals (Frexes-Steed et al. 1992; Nair et al. 1992) failed to confirm the positive effect on protein balance that had been observed in vitro. No BCAA supplementation studies to date have demonstrated improved nitrogen balance during or after exercise, although one study found that BCAA supplementation during exercise decreased negative net balance across the leg during exercise (MacLean, Graham, and Saltin 1994).

Protein Synthesis

It is claimed that BCAAs increase muscle mass. Resistance exercise increases muscle protein synthesis by stimulation of signaling pathways inside the muscle cells that have been contracted. But without increased availability of amino acids from ingestion of protein or amino acids in food or in supplements, positive protein balance will not occur. Therefore, increased amino acid intake is necessary for two reasons: to stimulate the signaling pathways and to provide building blocks.

BCAAs, particularly leucine, are able to stimulate the signaling pathways and protein synthesis. To date, however, no studies have examined the effects of leucine or BCAA ingestion on protein synthesis following exercise. It is likely, however, that BCAAs stimulate the signals in muscle, but this increased signaling would result in increased synthesis only if sufficient building blocks (other amino acids) are provided. One study demonstrated that the addition of protein to carbohydrates following resistance exercise increases MPS (Koopman et al. 2005). When extra leucine was added to the carbohydrate–protein mixture, however, protein did not increase further. Muscle protein synthesis was likely already fully stimulated by the combination of exercise and protein, so extra leucine could not increase it any more. In summary, although leucine can theoretically help signaling and protein synthesis, in reality it is unlikely that leucine ingestion will be effective when given in isolation (without other amino acids). The same would be true for BCAAs.

Central Fatigue Hypothesis

The central fatigue hypothesis, illustrated in figure 8.10, was proposed in 1987 as a mechanism that contributed significantly to the development of fatigue during prolonged exercise (Newsholme, Acworth, and Blomstrand 1987). This hypothesis predicts that, during exercise, FAs are mobilized from adipose tissue and are transported by the blood to the muscles to serve as fuel. Because the rate of mobilization is greater than the rate of uptake by the muscle, the blood FA concentration increases. Both FAs and the amino acid tryptophan bind to albumin and compete for the same binding sites. Tryptophan is prevented from binding to albumin by the increasing FA concentration, and, therefore, the free tryptophan (fTRP) concentration and the fTRP-to-BCAA ratio in the blood rises. Experimental studies in humans have confirmed that these events occur. The central fatigue hypothesis predicts that the increase in the fTRP-to-BCAA ratio results in increased fTRP transport across the blood–brain barrier, because BCAA and fTRP compete for carrier-mediated entry into the central nervous system by the large neutral amino acid (LNAA) transporter (Chaouloff et al. 1986; Hargreaves and Pardridge 1988). After it is taken up, tryptophan is converted to serotonin, leading to a local increase of this neurotransmitter (Hargreaves and Pardridge 1988).

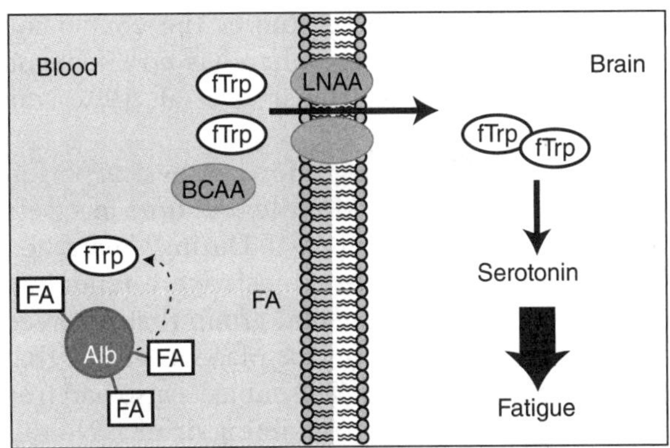

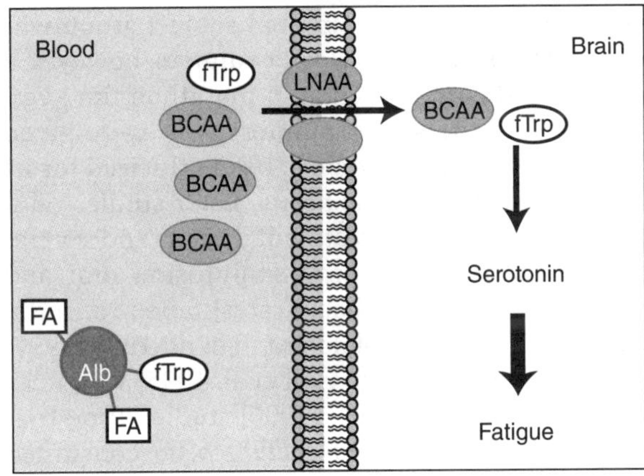

Figure 8.10 Central fatigue hypothesis.

Serotonin plays a role in the onset of sleep and is a determinant of mood and aggression. Therefore, the increase in serotoninergic activity might subsequently lead to central fatigue and force athletes to stop exercise or reduce exercise intensity. Of course, the assumption that increased fTRP uptake leads to increased serotonin synthesis and activity of serotoninergic pathways (i.e., increased synaptic serotonin release) is a large leap of faith.

The central fatigue hypothesis also predicts that ingestion of BCAA will raise the plasma BCAA concentration and hence reduce transport of fTRP into the brain. Subsequent reduced formation of serotonin may alleviate sensations of fatigue and in turn improve endurance exercise performance. If the central fatigue hypothesis is correct and the ingestion of BCAAs reduces the exercise-induced increase of brain fTRP uptake and thereby delays fatigue, the opposite must also be true; that is, ingestion of tryptophan before exercise should reduce the time to exhaustion. A few studies have investigated the effect of ingesting supplemental tryptophan in human subjects before or during exercise, and from these studies the conclusion must be drawn that tryptophan has no effects on exercise performance (Stensrud et al. 1992; van Hall et al. 1995).

The effect of BCAA ingestion on physical performance was investigated for the first time in a field test by Blomstrand et al. (1991). During a marathon in Stockholm, 193 male subjects were randomly divided into an experimental group that received BCAA in plain water and a placebo group that received flavored water. The subjects also had free access to carbohydrate-containing drinks. No difference was observed in the marathon times of the two groups. When the original subject group was divided into faster and slower runners, however, a small significant reduction in marathon time was observed in the slower runners who were given BCAAs. This study has since been criticized for its design and statistical analysis. Later studies with various exercise and treatment designs and several forms of BCAA administration (infusion, oral, and with and without carbohydrates) failed to find a performance effect (Blomstrand et al. 1995, 1997; Madsen et al. 1996; van Hall et al. 1995; Varnier et al. 1994). Van Hall et al. (1995) studied time-trial performance in trained cyclists who consumed control beverages that contained carbohydrate only (6% w/v sucrose) or 6% w/v sucrose supplemented with either a low dose of BCAA (6 g/L) or a high dose of BCAA (18 g/L) during exercise and reported no differences in time-trial performance (mean time to exhaustion was 122 ± 3 minutes).

Muscle Damage and Soreness

BCAAs are often associated with reductions in muscle damage and soreness after eccentric exercise. Indeed, studies have shown some effect of acute or chronic BCAA supplementation on markers of muscle damage in the blood after endurance cycling exercise. Studies have consistently found reductions in muscle soreness, but no studies have found any differences in muscle function. Note that all these studies were performed in untrained, unaccustomed subjects. This finding suggests that the importance of BCAA supplementation may be limited to decreasing muscle soreness in untrained individuals.

Glutamine

Glutamine is a naturally occurring nonessential amino acid (it can be synthesized in the body). Glutamine is important as a constituent of proteins and as a means of nitrogen transport between tissues. It is also important in acid–base regulation and as a precursor of the antioxidant glutathione. Glutamine is the most abundant free amino acid in human muscle and plasma. Its alleged effects can be classified as anabolic and immunostimulatory. Relying somewhat on an uncritical evaluation of the scientific literature, various manufacturers and suppliers claim that glutamine supplements have the following beneficial effects:

- More rapid water absorption from the gut
- Improved intracellular fluid retention (i.e., a volumizing effect)
- Improved gut barrier function and reduced risk of endotoxemia
- Nutritional support for immune system and prevention of infection
- Stimulation of muscle protein synthesis and muscle tissue growth
- Stimulation of muscle glycogen resynthesis
- Reduction in muscle soreness and improved muscle tissue repair
- Enhanced buffering capacity and improved high-intensity exercise performance

The normal daily intake of glutamine from dietary protein is about 3 to 6 g/day (assuming a daily protein intake of 0.8 to 1.6 g per kilogram of body weight for a 70 kg [154 lb] person). Researchers who examined the effects of glutamine on the postexercise decline in plasma glutamine concentration reported that a dose of about 0.1 g per kilogram of body weight must be given every 30 minutes over a 2- to 3-hour period to prevent a fall in the plasma glutamine concentration (Nieman and Pedersen 2000).

Glutamine is used at high rates by white blood cells (particularly lymphocytes) to provide energy and optimal conditions for nucleotide biosynthesis and, hence, cell proliferation (Ardawi and Newsholme 1994). Indeed, glutamine is considered important, if not essential, to lymphocytes and other rapidly dividing cells, including the gut mucosa and bone marrow stem cells. Prolonged exercise is associated with a fall in the intramuscular and plasma concentration of glutamine, and this decrease in glutamine availability has been hypothesized to impair immune function (Parry-Billings et al. 1992). Periods of heavy training are associated with a chronic reduction in plasma glutamine levels, and this reduction may be partly responsible for the immunodepression apparent in many endurance athletes (Parry-Billings et al. 1992). The intramuscular concentration of glutamine is related to the rate of net protein synthesis (Rennie et al. 1989), and some evidence also indicates a role for glutamine in promoting glycogen synthesis (Bowtell et al. 1999). But the mechanisms underlying these alleged anabolic effects of glutamine remain to be elucidated.

Fluid Absorption

Water transport from the gut into the circulation is promoted by the presence of glucose and sodium in drinks. Water movement is determined by osmotic gradients, and the cotransport of sodium and glucose into the gut epithelial cells is accompanied by the osmotic movement of water molecules in the same direction. Glutamine is transported into gut epithelial cells by both sodium-dependent and sodium-independent mechanisms, and the addition of glutamine to oral rehydration solutions increases the rate of fluid absorption above that of ingested water alone (Silva et al. 1998). The potential benefits of adding glutamine to commercially available sports drinks have not been adequately tested, however, and any additional benefit in terms of increased rate of fluid absorption and retention is likely to be small. Placebo-controlled studies that have investigated the effects of glutamine supplementation on extracellular buffering capacity and high-intensity exercise performance have not found any beneficial effect (Phillips 2007). Glutamine is not included in commercial sports drinks mainly because of its relative instability in solution.

Muscle Protein Balance

Research indicates that resistance exercise reduces the extent of protein catabolism, but an anabolic (muscle growth) response requires an intake of essential amino acids (dietary protein) in the recovery period after exercise (Borsheim et al. 2002). In one study, glutamine ingested in addition to carbohydrate and essential amino acids appeared to suppress a rise in whole-body proteolysis during the later stages of recovery (Wilkinson et al. 2006). The functional significance of this is yet to be elucidated. In general, if ingested protein contains all eight essential amino acids, taking supplements of individual nonessential amino acids is unlikely to provide any additional benefit. There is no evidence that glutamine alone will stimulate protein synthesis or reduce protein breakdown.

Muscle Glycogen Synthesis

Some evidence exists for an effect of glutamine supplements in promoting glycogen synthesis in the first few hours of recovery after exercise (Bowtell et al. 1999). More recent work, however, suggests that the addition of glutamine to a beverage containing carbohydrate and essential amino acids has no effect on postexercise muscle glycogen resynthesis (Wilkinson et al. 2006). Therefore, at present, limited evidence is available to substantiate claims that glutamine accelerates muscle glycogen synthesis.

Muscle Damage and Soreness

Several scientists have suggested that exogenous provision of glutamine supplements may prevent muscle damage, muscle soreness, and the impairment of immune function after endurance exercise. Eccentric exercise-induced muscle damage, however, does not affect the plasma glutamine concentration (Walsh et al. 1998), and no scientific evidence supports a beneficial effect of oral glutamine supplementation on muscle repair after exercise-induced damage. No evidence supports reduced muscle soreness when glutamine is consumed compared with a placebo.

Immune System

Prolonged exercise at 50% to 70% of $\dot{V}O_2max$ causes a 10% to 30% fall in plasma glutamine concentration that may last for several hours during recovery (Castell et al. 1997; Parry-Billings et al. 1992; Walsh et al. 1998). This fall in plasma glutamine coincides with the theory that there is a window of opportunity for infection after prolonged exercise when an athlete is more susceptible to infections (Walsh et al. 1998).

One study showed that an oral glutamine supplement (5 g in 330 ml [12 fl oz] water) consumed immediately after and 2 hours after a marathon reduced the incidence of upper respiratory tract infection in the 7 days after the race (Castell, Poortmans, and Newsholme 1996). But in this study, plasma glutamine concentrations were not measured, and the amount of glutamine ingested was unlikely to have prevented a reduction in plasma glutamine concentrations. A number of review articles (Gleeson 2008; Gleeson and Bishop 2000b; Nieman and Pedersen 2000) concluded, however, that glutamine supplementation during exercise has no effect on various indices of immune function, and studies failed to find any beneficial effects.

A larger dose of glutamine (0.1 g per kilogram of body weight) than that given by Castell, Poortmans, and Newsholme (1996) ingested at 0, 30, 60, and 90 minutes after a marathon race prevented a fall in the plasma glutamine concentration but did not prevent a fall in a number of markers of immune function (Gleeson 2008; Gleeson and Bishop 2000b; Nieman and Pedersen 2000). Similarly, maintaining the plasma glutamine concentration by consuming glutamine in drinks taken both during and after a prolonged bout of cycling did not affect a number of important indicators of immune function (Gleeson 2008; Gleeson and Bishop 2000b; Nieman and Pedersen 2000). Unlike the feeding of carbohydrate during exercise, glutamine supplements seem not to affect the immune function perturbations that have been examined to date (see chapter 13 for further details).

Glutamine is thought to be relatively safe and well tolerated by most people, although administration to people with kidney disorders is not recommended. No adverse reactions to short-term glutamine supplementation have been reported, and no information is available on long-term use exceeding 1 g/day. Excessive doses may cause gastrointestinal problems.

Glycine

Glycine is a nonessential amino acid that is involved in the synthesis of phosphocreatine. Therefore, it has been theorized to have ergogenic properties. Early studies indicated improvements in strength after glycine (or gelatin that contains about 25% glycine) supplementation, but these studies were poorly designed. Thus, the effects of glycine remain unconfirmed.

Ornithine

Ornithine is a nonprotein amino acid that has been suggested to stimulate growth hormone release from the pituitary gland (Evain-Brion et al. 1982) and insulin release from the pancreas. Growth hormone release after infusion of ornithine was even higher than that observed after arginine infusion. Most ornithine supplements, however, contain 1 to 2 g of ornithine, and this dosage does not affect the 24-hour hormone profile (Fogelholm, Naveri, et al. 1993). Therefore, ornithine supplementation does not seem to increase growth hormone release or increase muscle mass or strength. Although ornithine is often claimed to increase the secretion of insulin from the pancreas, a study in bodybuilders in which the effects of ornithine supplementation on insulin release were investigated failed to show any effect (Bucci et al. 1992).

Taurine

Taurine is a nonprotein amino acid and a derivative of cysteine. Taurine has recently become a popular ingredient of many sports drinks. The concentrations of taurine in the brain, heart, and muscle are high, but its role is poorly understood. It has been suggested to act as a membrane stabilizer, an antioxidant, and a neuromodulator. Taurine plays an undefined role in calcium currents in cells, influences ionic conductance in excitable membranes, and plays a role in the regulation of cell volume. Many of the proposed effects remain largely unexplored, particularly in humans. The potential role for taurine within human skeletal muscle has yet to be identified, despite a high intramuscular content (50-60 mmol/kg of dry muscle) in relation to plasma (30-60 mmol/L in plasma) and an absence of taurine in protein within skeletal muscle. A recent study found that 7 days of taurine supplementation did not alter skeletal muscle taurine content or carbohydrate and fat oxidation during exercise. Its value as a nutrition supplement is still unclear.

Tyrosine

Oral doses of tyrosine (5-10 g) result in increases in circulating concentrations of epinephrine, norepinephrine, and dopamine—hormones that are heavily involved in the regulation of body function during physical stress and exercise. Both dopamine and norepinephrine are synthesized from the nonessential amino acid tyrosine through a shared metabolic pathway. Increased intake of tyrosine may increase transport across the blood–brain barrier, and the increased delivery of tyrosine into the central nervous system may result in increased brain dopamine and norepinephrine synthesis, although this relationship may not be straightforward. Most tyrosine supplements on the market contain only very small amounts of tyrosine (less than 100 mg), whereas much larger doses are probably required to alter hormone levels. Tyrosine has been examined in animal models and human studies (mostly in military settings) and appears to prevent the substantial decline in various aspects of cognitive performance and mood associated with many kinds of acute stress (Jongkees et al. 2015; Lieberman 2003). For example, Banderet and Lieberman (1989) found that vigilance, choice reaction time, pattern recognition, coding, and complex behaviors, such as map and compass reading, were all improved by tyrosine administration when volunteers were exposed to the combination of cold and high altitude (hypoxia). Tyrosine supplementation does appear to consistently attenuate losses in cognitive function when individuals are exposed to extreme and challenging environments. Currently, the balance of evidence does not support performance-enhancing effects of tyrosine in situations that would be encountered in sports. Since many sporting situations are highly dependent on effective decision-making and the successful execution of fine and gross motor skills, the improved maintenance of cognitive function would be desirable, despite no apparent benefit to physical performance. Some have warned about regular supplementation of large amounts (5-10 g) and have suggested this could have adverse health effects in the long term because it affects sympathetic nervous system activity. Caffeine can also limit declines in cognitive function during exercise (Hogervorst et al. 2008) and may be a more suitable and safer alternative.

Tryptophan

Tryptophan has been suggested as a way to stimulate the release of growth hormone. The most common proposed ergogenic effect, however, is based on another function. Tryptophan is the precursor of serotonin, a neurotransmitter in the brain that may induce sleepiness, decrease aggression, and elicit a mellow mood. Serotonin has also been suggested to decrease the perception of pain. Segura and Ventura (1988) hypothesized that tryptophan supplementation increases serotonin levels and the tolerance of pain and thereby improves exercise performance. They studied 12 subjects during running to exhaustion at 80% of $\dot{V}O_2$max with ingestion of tryptophan or placebo. Tryptophan was supplemented in four doses of 300 mg in the 24 hours before the endurance test, and the last doses were ingested 1 hour before the test (total tryptophan ingestion was 1,200 mg). The investigators observed a 49% improvement in endurance capacity and decreased ratings of perceived exertion after tryptophan ingestion. Because a 49% performance improvement seemed somewhat unrealistic, several other investigators have challenged the results of this study (Stensrud et al. 1992; van Hall et al. 1995).

In a study by Stensrud et al. (1992), 49 well-trained male runners were exercised to exhaustion at 100% of $\dot{V}O_2$max, and no significant effect of tryptophan supplementation on endurance time was found. A very well-controlled study by van Hall et al. (1995) of eight cyclists who were given tryptophan supplements found no effect on time to exhaustion at 70% of $\dot{V}O_2$max.

Both tryptophan and BCAAs have been suggested as supplements to reduce central fatigue. Yet the BCAAs and tryptophan have opposite effects. Whereas some claim that tryptophan reduces central fatigue (Segura and Ventura 1988), others have associated it with the development of central fatigue (Newsholme, Blomstrand, and Ekblom 1992). Tryptophan could also exert some negative effects, including blocking gluconeogenesis and decreased mental alertness. Based on these studies, tryptophan does not seem to be ergogenic and may even be ergolytic in prolonged exercise.

Protein Intake and Health Risks

Excessive protein intake (more than 3 g per kilogram of body weight per day) has been claimed to have various negative effects, including kidney damage, increased blood lipoprotein levels (which has been associated with arteriosclerosis), and dehydration. The latter may occur because of increased nitrogen excretion in urine, which results in increased urinary volume and dehydration. Athletes consuming a high-protein diet should therefore increase their fluid intake to prevent dehydration. The recommended protein intakes for athletes (1.2-1.8 g per kilogram of body weight per day) and up to approximately 2 g per kilogram of body weight per day are not harmful. Perhaps the main risk of increased protein intakes for athletes is the necessary reduction of carbohydrate (or fat) intake if energy levels are maintained. It is not possible to keep energy intake constant while increasing protein intake without lowering carbohydrate or fat intake. This risk is probably more important for endurance athletes, but it may also be a consideration for strength athletes who fancy extremely high protein intakes. Clear evidence shows that low glycogen levels before a training session impair intracellular signaling that leads to increased muscle protein synthesis.

No evidence demonstrates that intake of individual amino acids has any added nutritional value compared with the intake of proteins containing those amino acids. A possible advantage of the intake of individual amino acids is that larger amounts can be ingested. Purified amino acids were developed for clinical use in intravenous infusion of patients for adequate protein nutrition (particularly when oral consumption is compromised). Individual amino acids are also used as food additives to enhance the protein balance in case the diet is deficient in certain amino acids.

In 1989, an epidemic in the United States of the eosinophilia-myalgia syndrome (EMS), a neuromuscular disorder characterized by weakness, fever, edema, rashes, bone pain, and various other symptoms, was attributed to excessive intake of L-tryptophan. L-tryptophan has been classified as a neurotoxin and was banned for a while in the United States. It was later discovered that the EMS outbreak was caused by a contaminated batch of tryptophan, and in 2001, L-tryptophan was again sold in its original form.

Key Points

- Amino acids are constantly incorporated into proteins (protein synthesis), and proteins are constantly broken down (protein breakdown or degradation) to amino acids. This protein turnover is several times greater than the actual dietary requirement for protein. Some amino acids are essential and are not synthesized in the body, whereas others are nonessential and can be synthesized in the body.
- Muscle contains 40% of the total protein in the human body and accounts for 25% to 35% of all protein turnover in the body. The contractile proteins actin and myosin are the most abundant proteins in muscle and together account for 80% to 90% of all muscle protein.
- Training has marked effects on body proteins. Both the structural proteins that make up the myofibrils and the proteins that act as enzymes within a muscle cell change as an adaptation to exercise training. Muscle mass, muscle protein composition, and muscle protein content all change in response to training.
- Methods of studying protein metabolism include nitrogen excretion (urea and 3-methylhistidine), nitrogen balance, arteriovenous balance studies, and tracer methods. All methods available to measure protein turnover in humans have their limitations, and no method has been identified as the best one. Nonetheless, with consideration of their limitations, we can learn a great deal about protein metabolism and nutrition from studies that employ these methods.
- Amino acids have many metabolic functions. They can be used to synthesize other amino acids, can be incorporated into proteins or other compounds (i.e., FAs and glucose), or can be oxidized in the TCA cycle.
- The BCAAs are the most abundant amino acids in skeletal muscle and together account for 20% of all amino acids in muscle. Glutamine is the most abundant free amino acid in muscle and plasma.
- Protein (or, more accurately, amino acid) oxidation has been estimated to contribute up to about 15% of energy expenditure in resting conditions. During exercise, this relative contribution likely decreases because of an increasing importance of carbohydrate and fat as fuels. During prolonged exercise, when carbohydrate availability becomes limited, amino acid oxidation may increase somewhat, but the contribution of protein to energy expenditure decreases to a maximum of about 10% of total energy expenditure.
- In the hours after exercise, protein synthesis and breakdown increase. Protein synthesis increases more than breakdown does, but it will exceed protein degradation only after feeding of a source of amino acids. The balance between muscle protein synthesis and breakdown determines whether the tissue protein content remains constant, increases (hypertrophy), or decreases (atrophy).

- Muscle protein gain in response to resistance exercise training is influenced by the training load and the amount, timing, and type of protein ingested in the following 24- to 48-hour period. Optimal adaptation to the training occurs when meals containing 0.4 g protein per kilogram of body weight are consumed shortly after a training session and at regular intervals throughout the day totaling about 1.6 to 1.7 g per kilogram of body weight per day. Included within this total amount should be a dose of about 0.6 g per kilogram of body weight before bedtime, which appears to augment acute overnight muscle protein synthesis and chronic skeletal muscle adaptations.
- In order to optimize protein synthesis, athletes should ingest a high-quality protein (20-25 g or 0.4 g per kilogram of body weight) with 8 to 10 g of essential amino acids and at least 3 g of leucine at regular (3-4 hour) intervals.
- Proteins that are rapidly digested and absorbed and that have a high leucine content are most effective at generating increases in protein synthesis. The addition of carbohydrate to the postexercise meal will only increase rates of protein synthesis when the amount of protein ingested is less than optimal (<0.4 g protein per kilogram of body weight).
- The recommended protein intake for strength athletes is generally 1.6 to 1.7 g per kilogram of body weight per day, which is about twice the recommended value for the general population. The recommended protein intake for endurance athletes is usually 1.2 to 1.8 g per kilogram of body weight per day, although in extreme situations the amount may rise to as much as 2.5 g per kilogram of body weight per day.
- Most athletes consume ample protein to support their training needs even if the higher recommended intakes are accepted. With increased food intake, the intake of protein automatically increases because many food products contain at least some protein. The relationship between energy intake and protein intake is linear.
- In healthy people with no indication of kidney issues, there is no evidence that moderately high protein intakes of up to 2 g per kilogram of body weight per day are dangerous. For most athletes, the biggest danger of high protein intake is that it often comes at the cost of carbohydrate intake.
- Arginine infused in large quantities can have anabolic properties in patients, but oral ingestion of tolerable amounts does not result in increased secretion of human growth hormone and insulin.
- BCAAs are among the most popular nutrition supplements. The evidence for the manufacturers' claims, however, is not convincing.

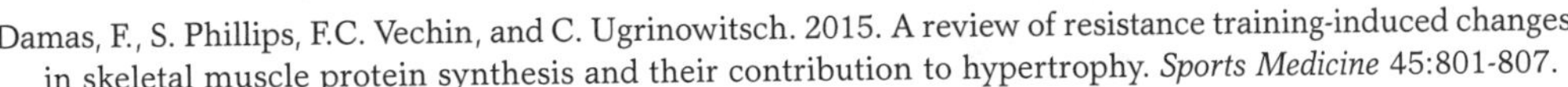

Recommended Readings

Damas, F., S. Phillips, F.C. Vechin, and C. Ugrinowitsch. 2015. A review of resistance training-induced changes in skeletal muscle protein synthesis and their contribution to hypertrophy. *Sports Medicine* 45:801-807.

Heaton, L.E., J.K. Davis, E.S. Rawson, R.P. Nuccio, O.C. Witard, W. Stein, K. Baar, J.M. Carter, and L.B. Baker. 2017. Selected in-season nutritional strategies to enhance recovery for team sport athletes: A practical overview. *Sports Medicine* 47:2201-2218.

Morton, R.W., C. McGlory, and S.M. Phillips. 2015. Nutritional interventions to augment resistance training-induced skeletal muscle hypertrophy. *Frontiers in Physiology* 6 (245): 1-9.

Phillips, S.M. 2012. Dietary protein requirements and adaptive advantages in athletes. *British Journal of Nutrition* 108 (Suppl 2): S158-S167.

Phillips, S.M. 2013. Protein consumption and resistance exercise: Maximizing anabolic potential. *Sport Science Exchange* 26 (107): 1-5.

Phillips, S.M. 2016. The impact of protein quality on the promotion of resistance exercise-induced changes in muscle mass. *Nutrition and Metabolism* 13:64.

Rennie, M.J., and K.D. Tipton. 2000. Protein and amino acid metabolism during and after exercise and the effects of nutrition. *Annual Review of Nutrition* 20:457-483.

Tarnopolsky, M.A. 1999. Protein and physical performance. *Current Opinion in Clinical Nutrition Metabolic Care* 2:533-537.

Tarnopolsky, M.A. 2004. Protein requirements for endurance athletes. *Nutrition* 20:662-668.

Tipton, K.D., and A.A. Ferrando. 2008. Improving muscle mass: Response of muscle metabolism to exercise, nutrition and anabolic agents. *Essays in Biochemistry* 44:85-98.

Tipton, K.D., and O.C. Witard. 2007. Protein requirements and recommendations for athletes: Relevance of ivory tower arguments for practical recommendations. *Clinics in Sports Medicine* 26:17-36.

Tipton, K.D., and R.R. Wolfe. 2004. Protein and amino acids for athletes. *Journal of Sports Sciences* 22:65-79.

Wagenmakers, A.J. 1998. Protein and amino acid metabolism in human muscle. *Advances in Experimental Medicine and Biology* 441:307-319.

9

Water Requirements and Fluid Balance

Objectives

After studying this chapter, you should be able to do the following:

- Describe how body temperature is regulated at rest and during exercise
- Describe the effect of dehydration on exercise performance
- Describe the effects of fluid intake before and during exercise on exercise performance
- Describe fluid intake strategies that help ensure the fluid requirements of athletes are met
- Describe the composition of drinks that are suitable for consumption by athletes during and after exercise

Most athletes and coaches are aware that **dehydration**, which is a reduction in the body's water content, impairs exercise performance. Nevertheless, athletes do not always follow appropriate strategies to prevent or limit dehydration during training and competition. Others overdo it and may suffer from the consequences of **overhydration**. The **hydration** status of the body is determined by the balance between water intake and water loss. As with all nutrients, regular and sufficient water intake is required to maintain health and physical performance. Lack of water intake causes deficiency symptoms, and failure to drink water for more than a few days can result in death. Overconsumption of water also has associated symptoms.

In most people, water accounts for 50% to 60% of body mass. Lean body tissues (e.g., muscle, heart, liver) contain about 75% water by mass, whereas adipose tissue contains only about 5% water by mass, because the bulk of the adipocytes are filled with triacylglycerol fat. The fat content of the body, therefore, largely determines the normal body-water content. A healthy, lean, young man who weighs 70 kg (154 lb) has a body-water content of about 42 L (11 gal) or 60% of body weight. A healthy, lean, young woman who weighs 70 kg has a total body-water content of about 35 L (9 gal) or about 50% of body weight (see table 9.1 and the illustration below it). The water content of the female body is less than that of the male body because the female body is lighter and contains a higher proportion of fat (see table 9.1). Body water is distributed among various body fluid compartments as shown in table 9.2.

TABLE 9.1 Fat Content and Volumes of Body Fluid Compartments* in Adults and Infants

Body fluid	Infants	Adult men	Adult women
Plasma	4	5	4
Interstitial fluid	26	15	11
Intracellular fluid	45	40	35
Total	75	60	50
Fat	5	18	25

*Expressed as percentage of body mass.

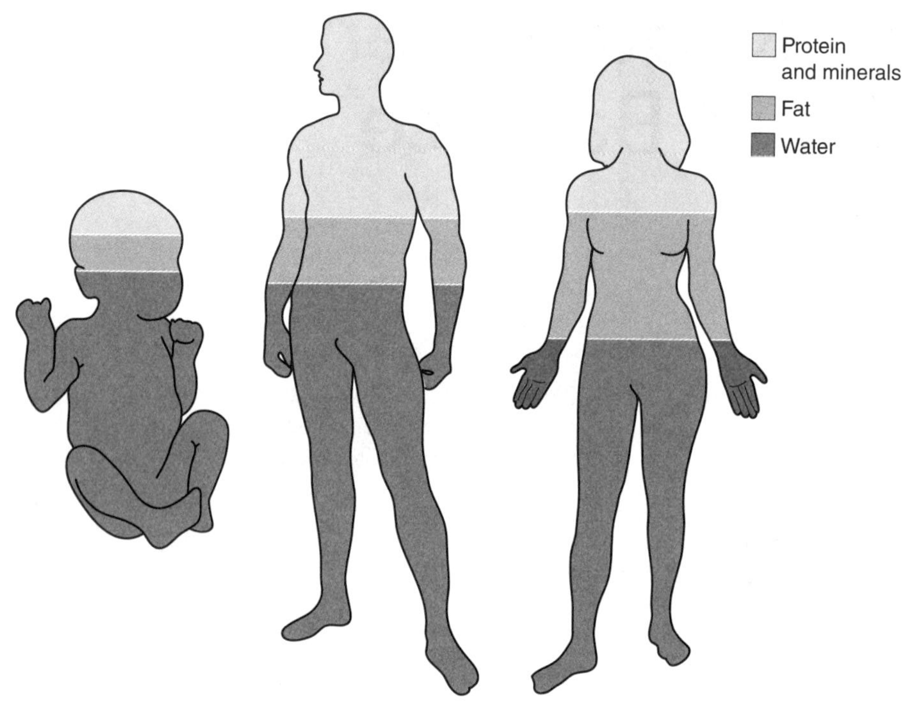

TABLE 9.2 Distribution of Body Water in a Young 70 kg (154 lb) Man

Body fluid	Volume L (gal)	Body mass	Total body water (%)
Intracellular fluid	28 (6.2)	40	62.5
Extracellular fluid	14 (3.1)	20	37.5
Interstitial fluid	10.5 (2.3)	15	30
Blood plasma	3.5 (0.8)	5	7.5

Total body-water volume is 42 L (11 gal) or 60% of body mass.

An important route of water (and electrolyte) loss from the body is through sweating, which is the body's principal means of preventing an excessive rise in body temperature (**hyperthermia**) during exercise in the heat. Some understanding of the regulation of body temperature is, therefore, fundamental to the discussion of fluid balance in the body and the formulation of drinks intended for consumption during and after exercise. This chapter begins with a brief overview of heat production and **thermoregulation** during exercise. The chapter then considers the effects of dehydration on exercise performance and discusses the need for water and electrolyte consumption by athletes.

Thermoregulation and Exercise in the Heat

Increased muscular activity during exercise increases heat production in the body because of the inefficiency of the metabolic reactions that provide energy for muscle force development. Thermoregulation concerns the mechanisms that prevent excessive rises in body temperature.

Heat Production During Exercise

For every liter of oxygen consumed during exercise, approximately 16 kJ (4 kcal) of heat are produced and only about 4 kJ (1 kcal) are used to perform mechanical work. For an athlete consuming oxygen at a rate of 4 L/min during exercise, the rate of heat production in the body is about 16,000 × 4 / 60 = 800 J/s, or watts (W), or 16 × 4 × 60 / 1,000 = 3.84 MJ/h (918 kcal/h). Only a small proportion of the heat produced in active skeletal muscle is lost from the overlying skin. Most of the heat is passed to the body core by the convective flow of venous blood returning to the heart. The rate of temperature increase in the belly of the quadriceps muscle group is close to 1 °C/min (1.8 °F/min) during the initial moments of high-intensity cycling (Saltin, Gagge, and Stolwijk 1968). This rate of heat storage cannot persist, because the muscle contractile proteins and enzymes would be inactivated by heat-induced denaturation within 10 minutes. Thus, most of the heat generated in the muscle is transferred to the body core. Increases in body core temperature are sensed by thermoreceptors located in the **hypothalamus**. This area of the brain also receives sensory input from skin thermoreceptors and integrates this information to produce appropriate reflex effector responses—increasing blood flow to the skin and initiating sweating—to increase heat loss and limit further rises in body temperature.

Heat Storage During Exercise

During exercise at a constant work rate, heat production increases in a square-wave fashion. The set point of the hypothalamic thermostat does not change during exercise, but some heat storage does occur. When heat loss from the body equals heat production, the rise in body temperature plateaus. During high-intensity exercise, however, particularly in an environment with a high ambient temperature and high humidity, core temperature continues to rise.

During exercise at an intensity equivalent to about 80% to 90% of $\dot{V}O_2max$, heat production in a fit person may exceed 1,000 W (resting heat production is about 70 W), which could potentially increase body temperature by 1 °C (1.8 °F) every 4 to 5 minutes if no changes occur in the body's heat-dissipating mechanisms. This estimate is based on the specific heat capacity of human tissues, which is 3.47 kJ/kg/°C (0.46 kcal/kg/°F) for lean tissue and 1.73 kJ/kg/°C (0.23 kcal/kg/°F) for fat. For a man who weighs 70 kg (154 lb) and has 15% body fat, the specific heat capacity of the body is (3.47 × 0.85) + (1.73 × 0.15) = 3.21 kJ/kg/°C (0.43 kcal/kg/°F). Using this value, we can calculate that at a rate of body heat production of 1,000 W, in 1 minute 1,000 J/s × 60 s = 60,000 J or 60 kJ (14.3 kcal) of heat energy is produced, which raises the body temperature of this 70 kg man by 60 kJ / (70 kg × 3.21 kJ/kg/°C) = 0.27 °C (0.49 °F). Thus, within 12 to 15 minutes, core body temperature could approach dangerous levels or exercise will end because of the symptoms of fatigue that occur from this degree of hyperthermia. It is generally accepted that heat stress alone will impair aerobic exercise performance.

Problems of hyperthermia and heat injury are not restricted to prolonged exercise in a hot environment. Heat production is directly proportional to exercise intensity, so extremely strenuous exercise, even in a cool environment, can cause a substantial rise in body temperature.

The absolute body temperature at the end of exercise depends on the starting body temperature. A vigorous warm-up causes a rise in body temperature and results in a higher final body temperature. Originally, it was thought that there was a critical body core temperature (sensed by the hypothalamus) beyond which exercise would not be sustainable (González-Alonso et al. 1999; Walters et al. 2000). This was suggested to be a protective mechanism against denaturation of body proteins and damage to internal organs.

It was thought that when body temperature rises to about 39.5 °C (103 °F), central fatigue (i.e., fatigue in the brain rather than in the working muscles) ensues, so a high starting temperature is undesirable for athletes who are exercising in a hot environment. Such large increases in body temperature during exercise tend not to occur in individuals who run at a slower pace (e.g., those who run a marathon in 4-6 hours) but are common in the faster, highly motivated athletes. It has now become clear that it is the interplay of multiple

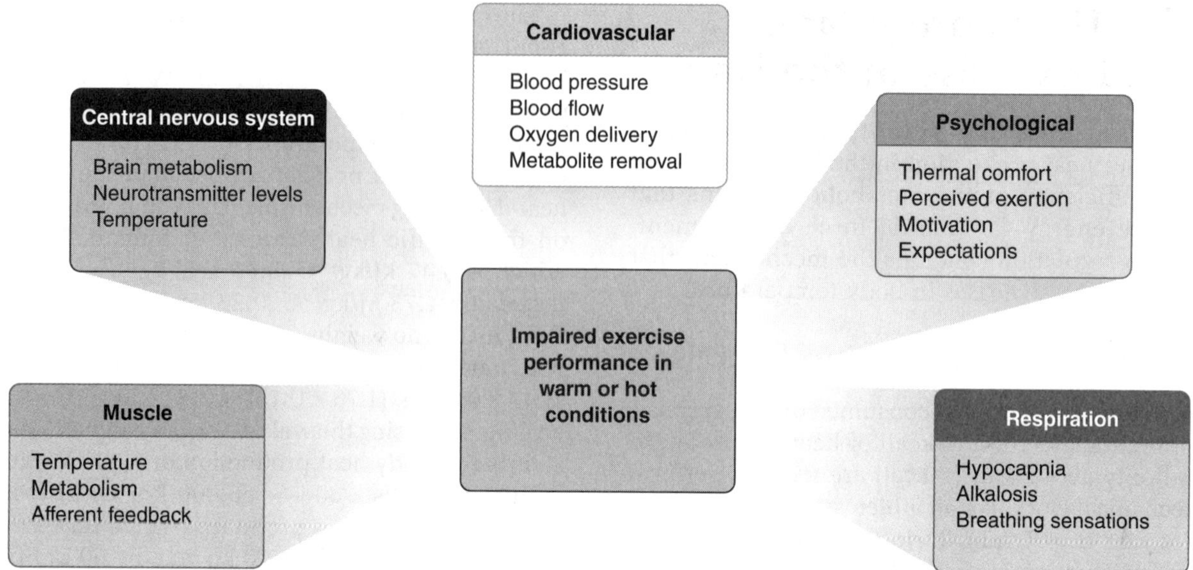

Figure 9.1 Factors that affect performance in the heat. Previously it was believed that core temperature was the main factor affecting performance in the heat, but it has become clear that skin temperature and other factors play an important role, too.

Reprinted from www.mysportscience.com; Based on Nybo, Rasmussen, and Sawka (2014).

factors, rather than only the core temperature, that is responsible for performance decrements in the heat (Nybo, Rasmussen, and Sawka 2014) (figure 9.1) and **hypohydration** exacerbates these negative effects.

The normal body temperature range is 36 to 38 °C (96.8-100.4°F), but it can rise to 38 to 40 °C (100.4-104 °F) during exercise. Further increases are commonly associated with heat exhaustion and occasionally with heatstroke, which is a life-threatening disorder characterized by lack of consciousness after exertion and by clinical symptoms of damage to the brain, liver, and kidneys (Gleeson 1998; Sutton and Bar-Or 1980). The elevated core temperature associated with exercise is caused by the temporary imbalance between the rates of heat production and dissipation during the early stages of exercise and the rapidity with which the heat-dissipating mechanisms respond to an increase in core and skin temperature.

Environmental Heat Stress and Heat Loss by Evaporation of Sweat

Environmental heat stress is determined by the ambient temperature, relative humidity, wind velocity, and solar **radiation** (directly from the sun and reflected from the ground) (see figure 9.2). During exercise, the working muscles produce heat at a high rate and body temperature rises. If the skin is hotter than the surroundings, heat is lost from the skin by physical transfer (evaporation of sweat, **convection**, and **conduction**) to the environment. If the environment is hotter than the skin, heat is gained by convection and conduction. If the environment is saturated with water vapor (i.e., relative humidity = 100%), **evaporation** of sweat does not occur and the body does not lose heat. Relative humidity is important because high humidity severely compromises the evaporative loss of sweat, and sweat must evaporate from the body surface to exert a cooling effect.

Evaporation of 1 L (0.3 gal) of water from the skin will remove 2.4 MJ (573 kcal) of heat from the body. The sweat rate during exercise must be at least 1.6 L/h (0.42 gal/h) if all the heat produced is to be dissipated by evaporative loss alone. At such high sweat rates, some of the sweat rolls off the skin; because this has virtually no cooling effect, the sweat rate probably has to be closer to 2 L/h (0.5 gal/h). A reduction in skin blood flow and sweat rate as the body becomes progressively dehydrated and high humidity limit evaporative loss of sweat, which leads to further rises in core temperature and results in fatigue and possible heat injury to body tissues. The latter is potentially fatal.

A useful index of environmental heat stress is the wet bulb globe temperature (WBGT), which is calculated as follows:

$$WBGT = 0.7\ TWB + 0.2\ TBG + 0.1\ TDB$$

where TWB is the temperature (in °C) of a wet-bulb thermometer, TBG is the temperature of a black-globe thermometer, and TDB is the temperature of a dry-bulb thermometer. Note the 70% bias toward the TWB, which recognizes the greater relative importance of environmental humidity. Some typical environmental scenarios and physiological responses to exercise in various environmental conditions are shown in table 9.3.

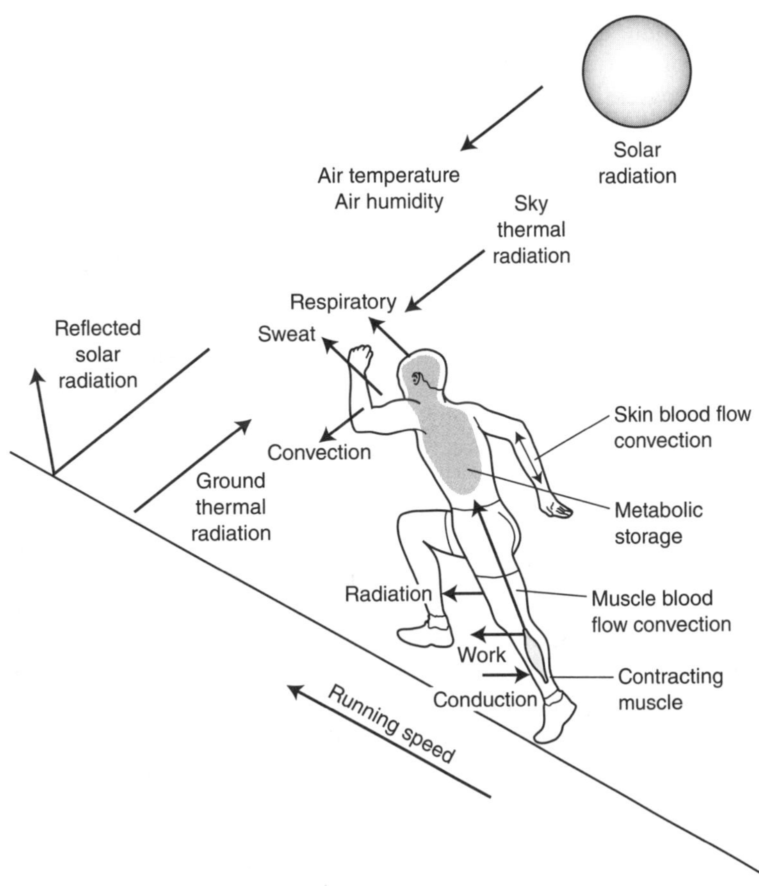

Figure 9.2 Sources of body heat gain and heat loss mechanisms.

TABLE 9.3 Sweat Loss and Heart Rates After 60 Minutes of Exercise

Ambient temperature	Humidity (%)	Sweat loss	Core temperature	Heart rate (beats/min)
13 °C (55 °F)	7	0.8 L (0.2 gal)	38.0 °C (100.4 °F)	140
18 °C (64 °F)	50	1.2 L (0.3 gal)	38.3 °C (100.9 °F)	143
25 °C (77 °F)	50	1.4 L (0.4 gal)	38.7 °C (101.6 °F)	145
30 °C (86 °F)	30	2.1 L (0.6 gal)	39.3 °C (102.7 °F)	148
30 °C (86 °F)	90	2.8 L (0.7 gal)	39.5 °C (103.1 °F)	150
35 °C (95° F)	30	3.0 L (0.8 gal)	39.9 °C (103.8 °F)	153

Exercise was performed at about 60% to 70% of $\dot{V}O_2max$ under various environmental conditions.

Heat loss through the evaporation of sweat is largely determined by the water vapor pressure (humidity) of the air close to the body surface. The local humidity may be high if inappropriate, poorly ventilated clothing is worn because it reduces the convective flow of air over the skin surface. Sweat drips off the skin rather than evaporates, and heat loss by this route is severely restricted. If exercise continues at the same intensity, body core temperature rises further, a higher sweat rate is induced, and the athlete dehydrates more rapidly. This dehydration poses further problems for the athlete because progressive dehydration impairs the ability to sweat and, consequently, to thermoregulate. At any given exercise intensity, body temperature rises faster in the dehydrated state, and this condition is commonly accompanied by a higher heart rate during exercise, as shown in figure 9.3. Dehydration equivalent to the loss of only 2% of body mass (i.e., the loss of about 1.5 L [0.4 gal] of water for a typical 70 kg [154 lb] male athlete) is sufficient to cause significant impairment in exercise performance (Armstrong, Costill, and Fink 1985; Craig and Cummings 1966; Maughan 1991; Sawka and Pandolf 1990).

During exercise in hot conditions, there is a redirection of blood flow to the skin for heat dissipation. As the environmental temperature and humidity increase, skin temperature also increases. Core temperature is mostly dependent on exercise intensity and heat production and less dependent on the environment. Warm or hot skin means that there is greater skin blood flow and cutaneous venous compliance. This results in increased strain on the cardiovascular system because more blood needs to be circulated or it needs to be circulated faster to maintain blood pressure (this is often referred to as relative hypovolemia). If hypohydration occurs and the absolute plasma volume decreases (absolute hypovolemia), this may act as an extra strain on the cardiovascular system. The combination of relative and absolute hypovolemia determines how much the cardiovascular system is compromised and how much performance is affected. Performance is less affected if an athlete is dehydrated in a cool environment compared with a hot environment. It has been suggested that when skin temperature exceeds 27 °C (81 °F), hypohydration impairs performance by an additional 1% for every 1 °C (1.8 °F) increase in skin temperature (Sawka, Cheuvront, and Kenefick 2015).

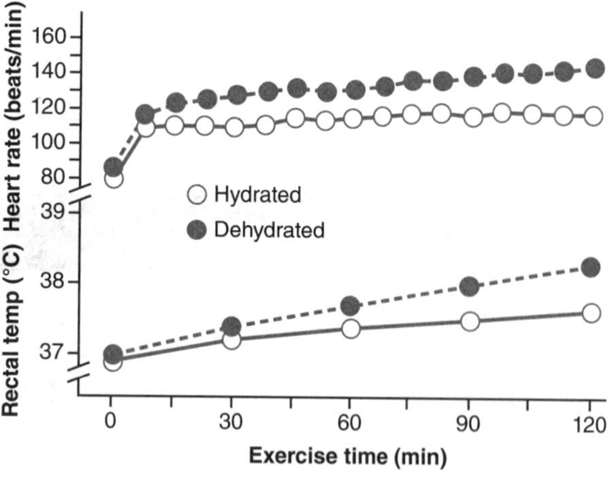

Figure 9.3 Effect of dehydration on heart rate and rectal temperature during 2 hours of cycling.

Heat Loss by Radiation and Convection

The other crucial effector mechanism in thermoregulation during exercise in the heat is increased blood flow through the skin capillaries. This mechanism allows increased heat loss from the body core to the environment by radiation and convection. Radiation is the transfer of energy waves by emission from one object and absorption by another. Convection is the exchange of heat between a solid medium (e.g., the human body) and one that moves (e.g., air or water). The rate of heat transfer away from the body core is the product of the skin blood flow and the temperature difference between the core and the skin.

High skin blood flow alone may not be sufficient to remove heat from the body core during exercise in hot, humid conditions when the skin temperature rises because of the inability to evaporate sweat. The effectiveness of this route of heat loss also depends largely on the amount of body surface available for heat exchange and the temperature gradient between the body surface and the surrounding atmosphere. When ambient temperature is close to body temperature, heat loss by the skin blood flow is minimal. The body then depends almost entirely on evaporative cooling. Inappropriate clothing impairs convection and radiation of heat from the body surface, so total heat dissipation will decrease to a critically low level.

Regulation of Body Temperature

Sensory information about body temperature is input to the central controller by nerves emanating from deep-body and peripheral thermoreceptors. The latter, located in the skin, provide advance warning of environmental heat input. Central thermoreceptors, located in the hypothalamus, are sensitive to changes in internal core temperature and effectively monitor the temperature of blood flowing to the brain. Input from these receptors is more important than input from the peripheral receptors in eliciting appropriate effector responses designed to limit increases in body temperature. The central thermal controller, or "thermostat," located in the preoptic anterior hypothalamus also receives nonthermal sensory inputs that can modulate the homeostatic regulation of body temperature.

These other inputs include nervous signals from **osmoreceptors** and pressure receptors, so changes in plasma osmolarity and blood volume are capable of affecting sweating and cutaneous vasodilation responses to rises in core temperature. These effects are summarized in figure 9.4. Some hormones (e.g., estrogen) and cytokines (e.g., interleukin-1, interleukin-6) are also capable of influencing thermoregulatory responses. Interleukin-6, also known as endogenous pyrogen, is secreted from macrophages and is responsible for raising the set-point temperature of the hypothalamic thermostat, causing a rise in core temperature during fever. The influence of other sensory inputs also appears to take place at the level of the hypothalamic neurons and is mediated by neurotransmitters, including dopamine, 5-hydroxytryptamine (5-HT or serotonin), norepinephrine (noradrenaline), and acetylcholine.

Exercise Training, Acclimatization, and Temperature Regulation

Exercise training improves temperature regulation during exercise at the same absolute work rate. To obtain thermoregulatory benefits from training, people must adequately stimulate thermoregulatory effector responses (i.e., sweating and increased skin blood flow). In other words, they must exercise at a sufficiently high intensity. Improvements in thermoregulatory responses to exercise have consistently been seen in studies in which subjects exercised at 70% to 100% of

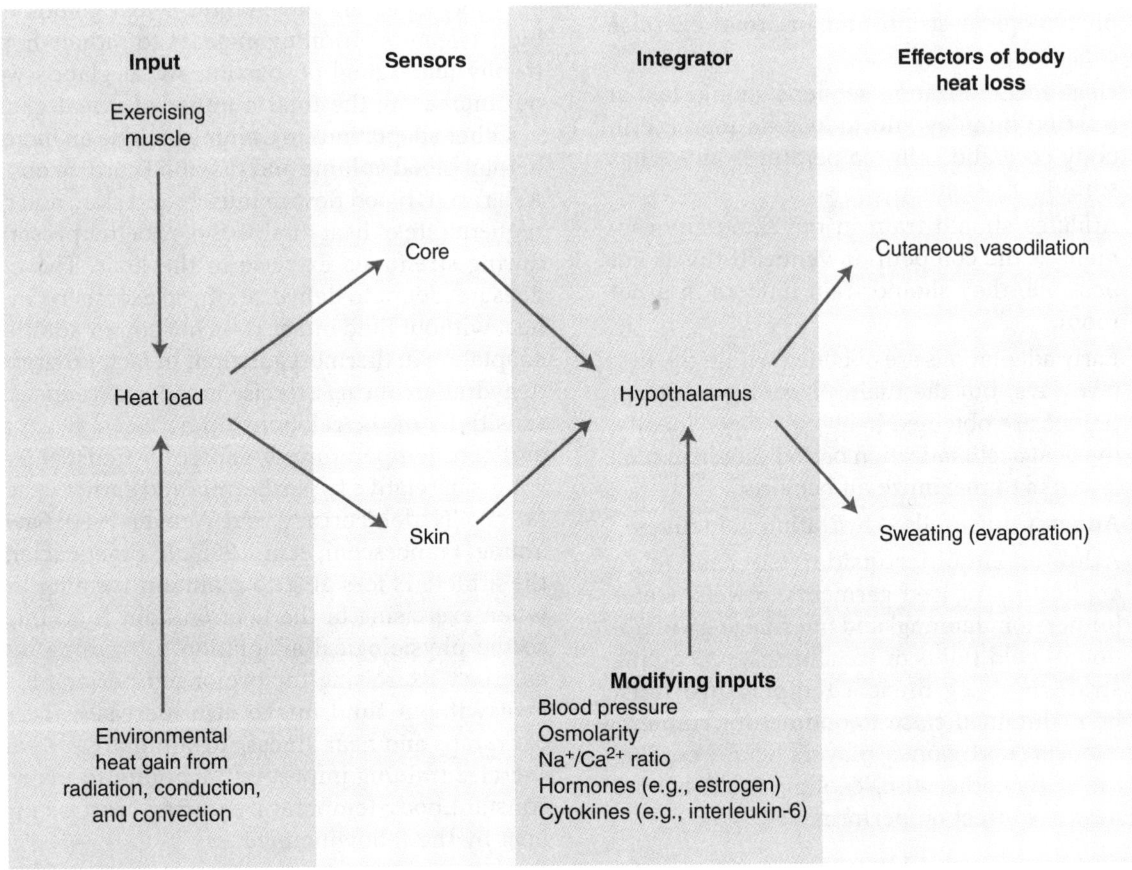

Figure 9.4 Summary of thermoregulation during exercise in the heat.

$\dot{V}O_2max$ and increased their body temperature above 39 °C (102.2 °F). Studies in which subjects exercised at lower intensities (typically 35% to 60% of $\dot{V}O_2max$) have commonly shown little or no thermoregulatory benefit in response to training.

Most serious athletes regularly exercise at intensities above 70% of $\dot{V}O_2max$; this training allows them to achieve thermal equilibrium during exercise at 25% to 35% of $\dot{V}O_2max$ in desert heat conditions, but this exercise intensity is considerably lower than the usual race pace in hot conditions. Appropriate training, however, increases tolerance to exercise in hot conditions, and acclimation to warm environments (achieved by exercising in hot environments) confers further benefits in the ability to regulate body temperature during exercise in the heat at higher exercise intensities (Greenleaf 1979).

According to a consensus document (Racinais et al. 2015), general recommendations for heat acclimation include the following:

- Athletes who are planning to compete in hot ambient conditions should acclimatize to the heat (through repeated training in the heat) to obtain biological adaptations that lower physiological strain and improve exercise capacity in the heat.
- Heat acclimatization sessions should last at least 60 min/day and induce an increase in body core and skin temperatures as well as stimulate sweating.
- Athletes should train in the same environment as the competition venue. If this is not possible, they should train indoors in a hot room.
- Early adaptations are obtained within the first few days, but the main physiological adaptations are obtained in about 7 days. Ideally, the heat acclimatization period should exceed 2 weeks to maximize all benefits.
- Athletes must follow hydration guidelines.
- Athletes should consider external (e.g., application of iced garments, towels, water immersion, fanning) and internal (e.g., ingestion of cold fluids or ice slurries) precooling strategies. Leg muscle temperature must be maintained close to optimal for runners, cyclists, and games players while cooling the body; otherwise, cooling could have a negative effect on performance.

Marathon runners exhibit a lower resting body temperature and have a lower sweating (and shivering) threshold. This is an indication that the hypothalamic set-point temperature (normally 37°C or 98.4°F) of endurance athletes seems to decrease as a result of training. Endurance athletes have also been reported to have lower resting metabolic rates in thermoneutral conditions and lower skin temperatures. This effect appears to mimic the insulative hypothermia reported in Australian aborigines who sleep in the cold desert; skin and core temperatures drop, reducing the temperature gradient between the body surface and the environment, which reduces heat loss and conserves energy. Heat and cold **acclimatization** are not mutually exclusive and can occur simultaneously in the same person.

Exercise training improves thermoregulation in the heat through earlier onset of sweat secretion and by increasing the total amount of sweat that can be produced. Thus, training increases the sensitivity of the relationship between sweat rate and core temperature and decreases the internal temperature threshold for sweating. Sweat rates can vary markedly between individuals (up to a maximum of about 3 L/h [0.8 gal/h]), even at the same relative exercise intensity (Maughan 1991), but evidence suggests that individuals characterized as heavy sweaters have larger sweat glands than light sweaters. Training appears to induce hypertrophy (enlarging) of existing sweat glands without increasing the total number of sweat glands.

Other adaptations to training include an increase in total blood volume and maximal cardiac output. As a result, blood flow in muscle and skin, and consequent rate of heat dissipation, is better preserved during strenuous exercise in the heat. The body does not adapt to dehydration, so exercising in the heat without fluid intake does not confer additional adaptation in thermoregulation. In fact, progressive dehydration during exercise in the heat reduces the sensitivity of the relationship between sweat rate and core temperature as shown in figure 9.5 and results in relative hyperthermia and earlier onset of fatigue (Nadel, Fortney, and Wenger 1980; Sawka, Young, Francesconi, et al. 1985). In practical terms, the athlete is less able to maintain training loads when exercising in the heat without fluid intake, so the physiological adaptation to training is not as great. Exercising for prolonged periods in the heat without fluid intake also increases the risk of cramps and heat illness. To summarize, aerobic exercise training improves the ability to maintain constant body temperature during exercise in the heat by the following means:

- Increased blood volume
- Increased capacity for skin blood flow

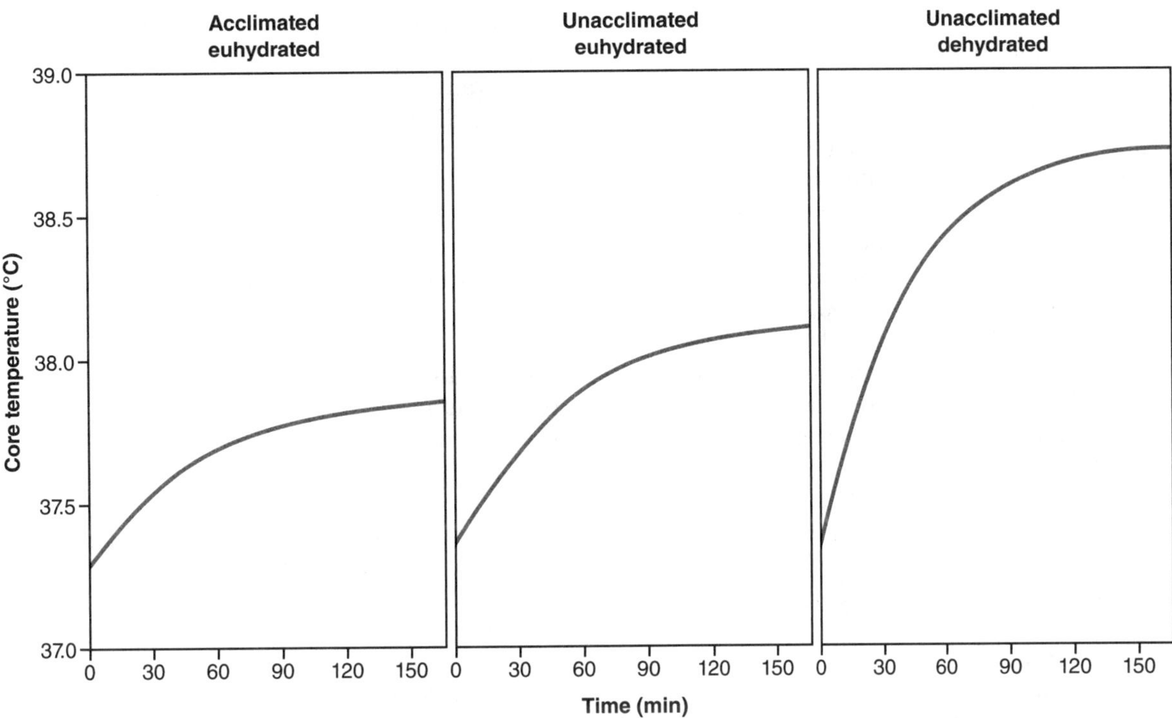

Figure 9.5 Core temperature responses during exercise in the heat when acclimated and euhydrated, unacclimated and euhydrated, or unacclimated and dehydrated. Core temperature especially rises during exercise when an unacclimated person is dehydrated.

Based on Sawka and Montain (2000).

- Increased size of sweat glands
- Lower set-point core temperature for onset of sweating (i.e., earlier onset of sweating)
- Increased sweat rate (increased sensitivity of the relationship between sweat rate and core temperature)

Effects of Dehydration on Exercise Performance

Fatigue toward the end of a prolonged sporting event is likely to be multifactorial, but dehydration (as well as carbohydrate depletion) can contribute. There has been a lot of debate about the precise effects of dehydration on exercise performance. Numerous studies report that dehydration impairs aerobic performance when exercise is performed in warm or hot environments and body water deficits exceed about 2% of body mass. Some studies of cycling, however, suggest that dehydration up to 4% body mass does not alter performance under ecologically valid conditions (i.e., in "real world" conditions rather than artificial experimental settings) (Cheung et al. 2015). For example, wind cooling on a cycle ergometer in a laboratory is much less than it is when road cycling outdoors.

Several studies have reported that sweat losses in excess of 5% of body weight can decrease the capacity for work by about 30% (Armstrong, Costill, and Fink 1985; Craig and Cummings 1966; Maughan 1991; Sawka and Pandolf 1990). These results exaggerate the importance of fluid intake for exercise performance (particularly by companies manufacturing and selling sports drinks). The figure of 30% refers to the reduction in time to exhaustion measurements and not to actual performance (time to complete a certain distance as fast as possible). The effects on performance would be much smaller, perhaps only about 2%. Many of the previously mentioned studies induced dehydration in their subjects prior to a performance test, which is different from a competitive situation. Studies in which subjects start the exercise in a euhydrated state and develop dehydration during exercise have been less consistent in reporting decreased exercise performance (Goulet 2011). There is ongoing debate about the level of dehydration at which performance is affected and how large the negative effect is, and these things depend on many factors, including the environmental conditions, the intensity and the duration of the exercise, the level of hydration at the onset of exercise, and individual differences.

Many studies of the performance effects of dehydration are potentially limited by methodology. For example, it is difficult to blind subjects to the treatment; if subjects are dehydrated, they generally know. Therefore, the subjects' expectations of the outcome might affect the outcome measures. Studies that used intravenous rehydration to blind subjects to the treatment found no effects of dehydration (Cheung et al. 2015), which suggests that previous studies may have been confounded by the lack of blinding. Physiological effects of infusions, however, are different from those of drinking, so although these studies are interesting, they do not answer the question of whether dehydration affects performance. James et al. (2017) performed a study in which fluids were administered through a nasogastric tube, which allowed blinding and maintaining normal physiological responses. The investigators concluded that exercise performance in the heat is impaired by hypohydration (2.4% loss of body mass) even when the subjects are blinded to the intervention. A follow-up to this small study using larger numbers of trained athletes could better establish what effects dehydration has on exercise performance.

Sprint athletes are generally less concerned than endurance athletes about the effects of dehydration. The capacity to perform high-intensity exercise, which results in exhaustion within a few minutes, can be affected by prior dehydration if this results in a loss of 2.5% or more of body weight (Sawka et al. 1985). Although sprint events offer little opportunity for sweat loss, athletes who travel to compete in hot climates are likely to experience acute dehydration that persists for several days and may be serious enough to have a detrimental effect on performance in competition. Even in cool laboratory conditions, maximal aerobic power ($\dot{V}O_2$max) decreases by about 5% when people experience fluid losses equivalent to 3% of body mass or more (Pinchan et al. 1988). In hot conditions, similar water deficits can cause a larger decrease in $\dot{V}O_2$max.

In their meta-analysis, Savoie et al. (2015) concluded that, as a whole, upper- and lower-body muscle strength falls by 5.5% with hypohydration. Anaerobic power is significantly decreased with hypohydration, but anaerobic capacity and vertical jumping ability are not. The authors concluded that hypohydration impairs non-body-weight-dependent muscle performance in a practically relevant manner. Athletes in some sports might benefit from the reduced weight as a result of dehydration. For example, the energy and oxygen cost of distance running (in kJ/km and mL of oxygen/km, respectively) depends mostly on running speed, and losing weight will improve running economy. The importance of this effect was exemplified when Haile Gebrselassie set a world record for the marathon (2:03:59) on a cool (14-18 °C), dry, sunny day in 2008, losing almost 10% of his body mass in the process. He drank relatively little during the race but tolerated his discomfort during running and became dehydrated. Whether this dehydration affected his performance cannot be established. While it's likely that drinking more would have reduced his discomfort, doing so could have negatively affected his performance. The loss of some of his body mass through sweating benefited his running economy, and this effect, at least in relatively cool conditions, may more than compensate for the potentially detrimental effects of dehydration on performance. In sports in which jumping is important or performance is body-weight dependent, analyses need to be performed to determine whether hypohydration may be of benefit because of a lower weight or may decrease performance because of its effects on the brain and physiology.

One study investigated the capacity of eight subjects to perform treadmill walking (at 25% of $\dot{V}O_2$max and a target time of 140 minutes) in very hot, dry conditions (49 °C [120 °F], 20% relative humidity) when they were euhydrated and when they were dehydrated by a 3%, 5%, or 7% loss of body mass (Sawka, Young, Francesconi, et al. 1985). All eight subjects were able to complete 140 minutes walking when euhydrated and 3% dehydrated. Seven subjects completed the walk when 5% dehydrated. When they were dehydrated by 7%, six subjects stopped walking after an average of 64 minutes. Thus, even during relatively low-intensity exercise, dehydration clearly increases the incidence of exhaustion from heat strain. Sawka et al. (1992) had subjects walk to exhaustion at 47% of $\dot{V}O_2$max in the same environmental conditions as their previous study. Subjects were euhydrated and dehydrated to a loss of 8% of each person's total body water. Dehydration reduced exercise endurance time from 121 minutes to 55 minutes. Dehydration also appeared to reduce the core temperature that a person could tolerate, because core temperature at exhaustion was about 0.4 °C (0.7 °F) lower in the dehydrated state. The main reasons dehydration has an adverse effect on exercise performance can be summarized as follows:

- Reduction in blood volume
- Decreased skin blood flow
- Decreased sweat rate
- Decreased heat dissipation
- Increased core temperature
- Increased rate of muscle glycogen use

Reduced maximal cardiac output (i.e., the highest pumping capacity of the heart that can be achieved during exercise) is the most likely physiological mechanism whereby dehydration decreases a person's $\dot{V}O_2max$ and impairs work capacity in fatiguing exercise of an incremental nature. Dehydration causes a fall in plasma volume at rest and during exercise, and decreased blood volume increases blood thickness (viscosity), lowers central venous pressure, and reduces venous return of blood to the heart. During maximal exercise, these changes can decrease the filling of the heart during diastole (the phase of the cardiac cycle when the heart is relaxed and is filling with blood before the next contraction), hence reducing stroke volume and cardiac output. Also, during exercise in the heat, the opening of the skin blood vessels reduces the proportion of the cardiac output available to the working muscles.

Even for euhydrated people, climatic heat stress alone decreases $\dot{V}O_2max$ by about 7%. Thus, environmental heat stress and dehydration can act independently to limit cardiac output and blood delivery to the active muscles during high-intensity exercise. Dehydration also impairs the body's ability to lose heat. Both sweat rate and skin blood flow are lower at the same core temperature for the dehydrated state compared with the euhydrated state (Nadel et al. 1979; Nadel, Fortney, and Wenger 1980; Sawka and Wenger 1988). Body temperature rises faster during exercise when the body is dehydrated. The reduced sweating response in the dehydrated state is probably mediated through the effects of a fall in blood volume (**hypovolemia**) and elevated plasma osmolarity (i.e., dissolved salt concentration) (see figure 9.5).

Dehydration not only elevates core temperature responses but also negates the thermoregulatory advantages conferred by high aerobic fitness and heat acclimatization. The effects of dehydration (5% loss of body weight) on core temperature responses in the same people when unacclimated and when acclimated to heat are shown in figure 9.5. Heat acclimation lowered core temperature responses when subjects were euhydrated. When they were dehydrated, however, similar core temperature responses were observed in unacclimated and acclimated states (Pinchan et al. 1988).

A person's ability to tolerate heat strain appears to be impaired when dehydrated, and a critical temperature for experiencing central fatigue is near 39.0 °C (102.2 °F) when the person is dehydrated by more than about 5% of body mass (Sawka et al. 1992). Skin temperature is another important factor. The larger rise in core temperature during exercise in the dehydrated state is associated with a bigger catecholamine response, and these effects may lead to increased rates of glycogen breakdown in the exercising muscle, which in turn may contribute to earlier onset of fatigue in prolonged exercise. Although it is well established that hypohydration (reduced total body water) impairs endurance exercise performance, the influence of hypohydration on muscular strength, power, and very high-intensity endurance (maximal activities lasting >30 seconds but <2 minutes) is poorly understood because of the inconsistent results reported in the literature. Several subtle methodological choices that exacerbate or attenuate the apparent effects of hypohydration explain much of this variability (Judelson et al. 2007). After accounting for these factors, hypohydration appears to attenuate strength, power, and high-intensity endurance by approximately 2%, 3%, and 10%, respectively, suggesting that alterations in total body water affect some aspect of force generation. Although the mechanisms are not well understood, the physiological demands of strength, power, and high-intensity endurance suggest alterations in cardiovascular, metabolic, or buffering function are responsible for the performance impairment associated with hypohydration. On the other hand, hypohydration might directly affect some component of the neuromuscular system, but this possibility awaits thorough evaluation. Hypohydration is, therefore, an important factor to consider when attempting to maximize intense muscular performance in athletic, military, and industrial settings.

Dehydration is associated with a reduced gastric emptying rate of ingested fluids during exercise in the heat. For example, one study reported a 20% to 25% reduction in gastric emptying when subjects were dehydrated by 5% of body mass (Neufer, Young, and Sawka 1989).

Fluid consumption should begin during the early stages of exercise in the heat not only to minimize the degree of dehydration but also to maximize the bioavailability of ingested fluids. Dehydration poses a serious health risk in that it increases the risk of cramps, heat exhaustion, and life-threatening heatstroke (Sutton and Bar-Or 1980).

Mechanisms of Heat Illness

Heat injury is most common during exhaustive exercise in a hot, humid environment, particularly if the person is dehydrated. These problems affect not only highly trained athletes but also sport participants who are not well trained. In fact, individuals with less training have less-effective thermoregulation during exercise, don't work as economically, use more carbohydrate for muscular work, and take longer to recover from exhausting exercise than do highly trained people.

During the initial stages of exercise in a hot environment, sweating begins and the skin blood vessels dilate, causing increased heat loss from the body. But as central blood volume and pressure fall, sympathetic nervous activity increases and the skin blood vessels constrict. A more powerful constriction of the blood vessels supplying the abdominal organs leads to cellular hypoxia in the region of the gastrointestinal tract, liver, and kidneys. Cellular hypoxia leads to the production of reactive oxygen species (ROS), including superoxide anion, hydrogen peroxide, hydroxyl radical, peroxynitrite, and nitric oxide (NO). The latter is a potent blood vessel dilator, and although its production can be viewed as protective (i.e., helping to conserve some blood flow through the capillary beds of the abdominal organs), ultimately the ROS may cause damage through their actions on membranes. The ROS cause peroxidation of lipids in cellular membranes, making them leaky. In the gastrointestinal tract, this action allows the passage of bacterial toxins (endotoxins) from the gut into the systemic circulation, which leads to endotoxemia (blood poisoning) and a drastic fall in blood pressure (hypotension). Increased levels of NO probably contribute to the development of hypotension. The consequences for the athlete can be heat syncope (fainting) and organ injury (see figure 9.6).

Animal studies have shown a disappearance of manganese-superoxide dismutase (Mn-SOD), an important antioxidant enzyme that deactivates ROS, after 2 hours of heat exposure and a later

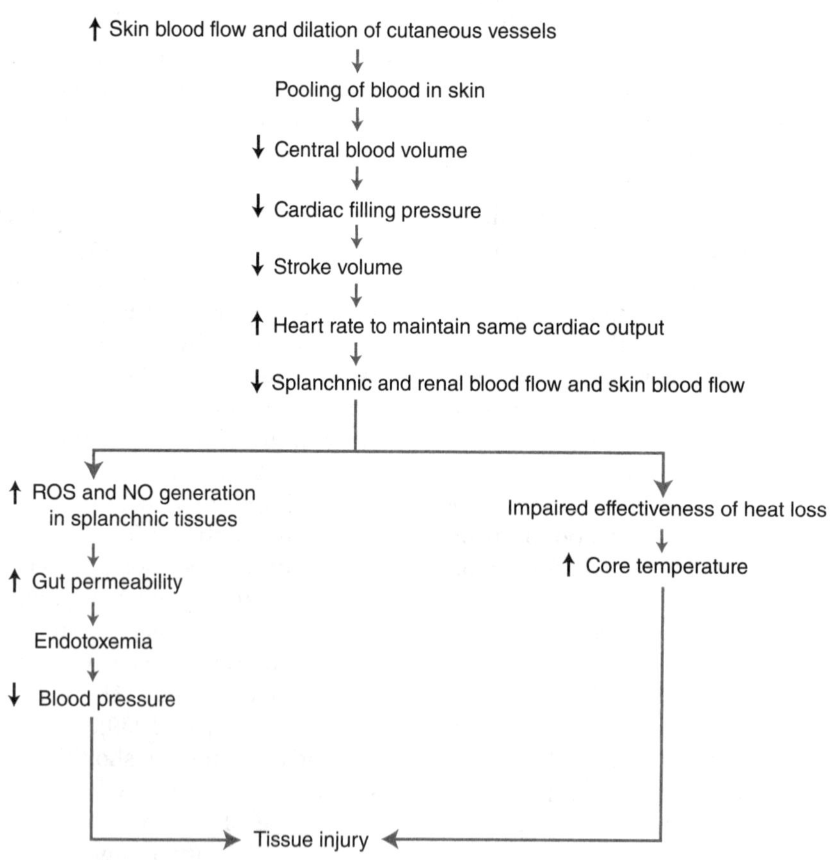

Figure 9.6 Potential mechanisms of heat-stress injury.

induction of Mn-SOD in the liver cells of animals exposed to elevated core temperatures (41 °C [106 °F]) over a 24-hour period. Increased levels of hemoglobin, NO, semiquinone radical (a marker of mitochondrial oxidative stress), and ceruloplasmin (a copper-binding protein with antioxidant properties) have been found in the hepatic portal vein after exposure to heat stress.

A doubling of hepatic portal blood endotoxin levels has also been reported within 24 hours of the onset of heat exposure. Thus, ROS generation appears to increase within abdominal tissues during heat exposure. Antioxidant status is compromised within the first few hours but gradually recovers and is enhanced after 24 hours of heat exposure. ROS generation probably increases most in areas of high metabolic activity and in areas that have greatest potential for reduction in blood flow.

This ischemia–reperfusion mechanism involving the gastrointestinal tract may play a role in the vascular dysfunction and tissue injury associated with heat stress. Further studies are warranted about the possible benefits of antioxidant supplementation in people who regularly experience high body temperatures, such as athletes who train and compete in hot, humid climates.

Although it is dramatically underreported, heat-related pathology contributes to significant morbidity as well as occasional mortality in athletic, elderly, and disabled populations and in children. Among U.S. high school athletes, heat illness is the third-leading cause of death (Coris, Ramirez, and Van Durme 2004). Significant risk factors for heat illness include dehydration, hot and humid climate, obesity, low physical fitness, lack of acclimatization, previous history of heatstroke, sleep deprivation, medications (especially diuretics or antidepressants), sweat gland dysfunction, and upper respiratory or gastrointestinal illness. Many of these risk factors can be addressed with education and awareness of people at risk. Dehydration, with fluid loss occasionally as high as 6% to 10% of body weight, appears to be one of the most common risk factors for heat illness in people who exercise in the heat. Core body temperature has been shown to rise an additional 0.15 to 0.2 °C (0.27 to 0.36 °F) for every 1% of body weight lost during exercise. Identifying athletes at risk, limiting environmental exposure, and monitoring closely for signs and symptoms are all important components of preventing heat illness. Monitoring hydration status and promoting appropriate drinking strategies may be the most important factors in preventing severe heat illness.

Effects of Fluid Intake on Exercise Performance

Oral fluid ingestion during exercise helps restore plasma volume to near preexercise levels and prevents the adverse effects of dehydration on muscle strength, endurance, and coordination. Elevating blood volume just before exercise by various **hyperhydration** strategies has been suggested to be effective in enhancing exercise performance, but only a few studies have directly investigated this possibility.

Preexercise Hyperhydration

Because even mild dehydration has debilitating effects on exercise performance, hyperhydration (greater than normal body water content) has been hypothesized to improve thermoregulation by expanding blood volume and reducing plasma osmolarity, thereby improving heat dissipation and exercise performance. Although some studies report higher sweating rates, lower core temperatures, and lower heart rates during exercise after hyperhydration, several of these studies used control conditions that represented dehydration rather than **euhydration**, calling results into question. But the findings generally support the notion that hyperhydration reduces the thermal and cardiovascular strain of exercise. Relatively few studies have directly investigated the effects of hyperhydration on exercise performance, but one well-controlled study reported that expansion of blood volume by 450 to 500 ml (15-17 fl oz) improved cycling time-trial performance by 10% (81 minutes compared with 90 minutes).

Temporary hyperhydration is induced in test subjects by having them drink large volumes of water or water-electrolyte solutions for 1 to 3 hours before exercise. Much of the fluid overload is rapidly excreted, however, so expansion of body water and blood volume is only transient. Studies in which the blood volume was directly expanded by infusion reported decreased cardiovascular strain during exercise but yielded conflicting results on sweat loss, heat dissipation, and exercise performance. Some studies that limited the rise in plasma osmolarity during exercise reported improved heat dissipation but did not address the question of whether it affects exercise performance.

Greater fluid retention is achieved if glycerol is added to fluids consumed before exercise. When glycerol is consumed orally, it is rapidly absorbed primarily in the small intestine and soon becomes evenly distributed among all fluid compartments, with the exception of the cerebrospinal fluid and aqueous humour. The increased osmotic gradient induced by the elevated body fluid glycerol content enhances water absorption in the kidney tubules (nephrons), which results in a degree of hyperhydration. The magnitude of the rise in the plasma glycerol concentration is directly related to the dose of glycerol ingested. When the plasma glycerol concentration exceeds the renal threshold for glycerol reabsorption it results in urinary glycerol excretion. Thus, in order to maintain hyperhydration, additional glycerol needs to be ingested at regular intervals (Nelson and Robergs 2007).

One study reported a higher sweating rate and lower core temperature when subjects exercised in the heat after hyperhydrating with glycerol (1 g [0.4 oz] per kilogram of body weight) and water (21.4 ml [0.7 fl oz] per kilogram of body weight) compared with an equal volume of water alone (Lyons et al. 1990). Other studies, however, report no thermoregulatory advantage during exercise after glycerol solution–induced hyperhydration (Inder et al. 1998; Latzka et al. 1997, 1998). In these studies, the volume of water consumed (500 ml [17 fl oz]) may have been too small. In a study by Murray et al. (1991), no indications of hyperhydration were found. Generally, however, the ingestion of 1 g/kg b.m. of glycerol with 1 to 2 L (0.3-0.5 gal) of water seems to protect against heat stress and thus may have some health benefits for people who exercise in hot conditions. One study examined the effect of ingesting a large bolus of water (20 ml [0.7 fl oz] per kilogram of body weight) with or without added glycerol (1 g per kilogram of body weight) 2 hours before 90 minutes of submaximal cycling (98% of lactate threshold) in dry, hot conditions (35 °C [95 °F], 30% relative humidity) followed by a 15-minute time trial (Anderson et al. 2001). Although preexercise glycerol ingestion did not affect skin temperature, muscle temperature, circulating catecholamine, or muscle metabolic responses to the steady state exercise, heart and core temperature were lower than with the ingestion of water alone. Furthermore, time-trial performance (total work performed) improved significantly by 5%. In subsequent studies, this finding could not be confirmed, although those studies reported indications of improved thermoregulation. Why one study provides favorable results and another does not is unclear. Possible explanations may include subject characteristics, environmental factors, research design, whether fluids with or without glycerol were given during exercise, the rate at which fluids were initially given to induce hyperhydration, the time between peak hyperhydration and peak plasma glycerol concentration and the start of the exercise, the weight-specific glycerol dose (i.e., grams per kilogram of body mass), and the concentration of glycerol in the administered beverage (e.g., 5%, 10%, 20%) or perhaps the intensity, mode, and nature of the exercise test (e.g., time to exhaustion at a fixed work rate, time trial). What is clear is that glycerol has the capacity to enhance fluid retention. In so doing, glycerol hyperhydration may give a performance advantage by offsetting dehydration during subsequent exercise. In 2010, glycerol was prohibited as an ergogenic aid by the World Anti-Doping Agency (WADA) due to the potential for its plasma expansion properties to have masking effects (i.e., diluting the presence of other banned substances that might be present in the blood). In 2018, however, glycerol was removed from the WADA prohibited list. This decision was based on the results of scientific articles published after 2012 that particularly addressed the ability of glycerol to influence the athlete's plasma volume and parameters of the Athlete Biological Passport (ABP), where the magnitude of glycerol-derived effects was regarded as minimal. For more information on glycerol, see chapter 11.

Fluid Intake During Exercise

During exercise, especially in a hot environment, dehydration can be avoided only by matching fluid consumption with sweat loss. Achieving this goal, however, is difficult for the following reasons:

- Sweat rates during strenuous exercise in the heat can be around 2 to 3 L/h (0.5-0.8 gal/h). A volume of ingested fluid in the stomach of more than about 1 L (0.3 gal) feels uncomfortable for most people when exercising, so achieving fluid intake that matches sweat loss during exercise is often not practical.
- Sweat rates vary widely among individuals under the same ambient conditions. (Figure 9.7 shows the sweat rates of people competing in a marathon race in Scotland.) Hence, it is difficult to prescribe the specific amount a person should ingest without knowing the person's sweat rate under the prevailing weather conditions.
- Thirst is not an accurate indicator of body-water requirements or the degree of dehydration. In general, the sensation of thirst is not perceived until a person has lost at least

2% of body weight through sweating. As already mentioned, even this mild degree of dehydration is sufficient to impair exercise performance. Numerous studies show that ad libitum intake of water during exercise in the heat results in incomplete replacement of body-water losses (observed values of fluid intakes and losses are shown in table 9.4).

- The rules or practicalities of specific sports may limit the opportunities for drinking during competition.

Because relatively mild dehydration and small decreases in plasma volume can impair endurance exercise capacity, athletes should try to minimize the extent of dehydration by ingesting fluids during exercise. Regular water intake during prolonged exercise is effective in improving exercise capacity (time to exhaustion; see figures 9.8 and 9.9) and exercise performance (time to complete a given amount of work; see figure 9.10) in thermoneutral and hot ambient conditions (Fallowfield et al. 1996; Maughan et al. 1987).

Fluid intake during prolonged exercise offers the opportunity to ingest some fuel as well. The addition of carbohydrate to some drinks consumed during exercise has an additional independent effect in improving exercise performance (see figures 9.9 and 9.10; see also chapter 6) (Below et al. 1995). Too much added carbohydrate in a sports drink decreases the amount of water that can be absorbed. In this situation, water is drawn out of the interstitial fluid and plasma into the lumen of the small intestine by osmosis. The ingestion of a concentrated (16.5% carbohydrate) glucose solution that is hypertonic with respect to plasma delays the restoration of plasma volume during exercise compared with the ingestion of a more dilute (3.6% carbohydrate) hypotonic glucose–electrolyte drink (Maughan et al. 1987).

As long as the fluid remains hypotonic with respect to plasma, the uptake of water from the

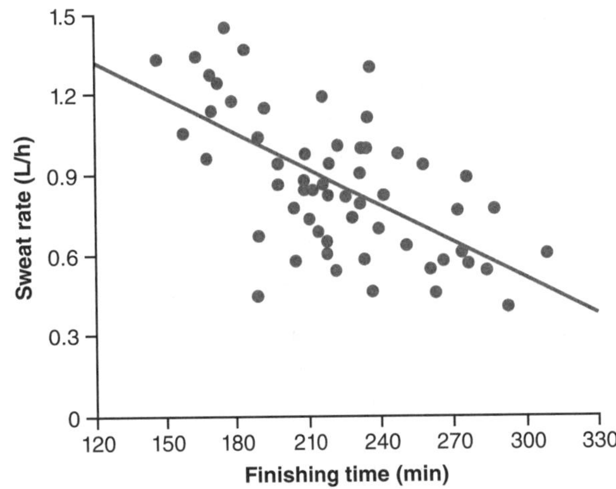

Figure 9.7 Sweat rates for subjects who competed in a marathon race held in cool (about 12 °C [54 °F]) conditions. The sweat rate was related to running speed, but a large variation existed between individuals, even those running at the same speed.

Data from Maughan et al. (1987).

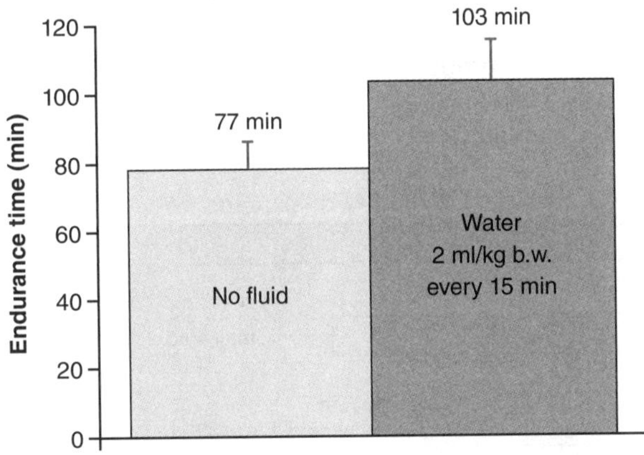

Figure 9.8 Effect of water intake on running endurance capacity in an ambient temperature of 20 °C (68 °F) .

Data from Fallowfield et al. (1996).

TABLE 9.4 Fluid Losses and Intakes of Athletes

Sport	Ambient temperature	Sweat loss per hour	Fluid intake per hour
Marathon running	15-20 °C (59-68 °F)	800-1,200 ml (27-41 fl oz)	500 ml (17 fl oz)
Soccer	10 °C (50 °F) 25 °C (77 °F)	1,000 ml (34 fl oz) 1,200 ml (41 fl oz)	350 ml (12 fl oz) 500 ml (17 fl oz)
Basketball	20-25 °C (68-77 °F)	1,600 ml (54 fl oz)	1,080 ml (37 fl oz)
Rowing	10 °C (50 °F) 30 °C (86 °F)	1,165 ml (39 fl oz) 1,980 ml (67 fl oz)	580 ml (20 fl oz) 960 ml (32 fl oz)
Cycling	30 °C (86 °F)	2,000 ml (68 fl oz)	800 ml (27 fl oz)

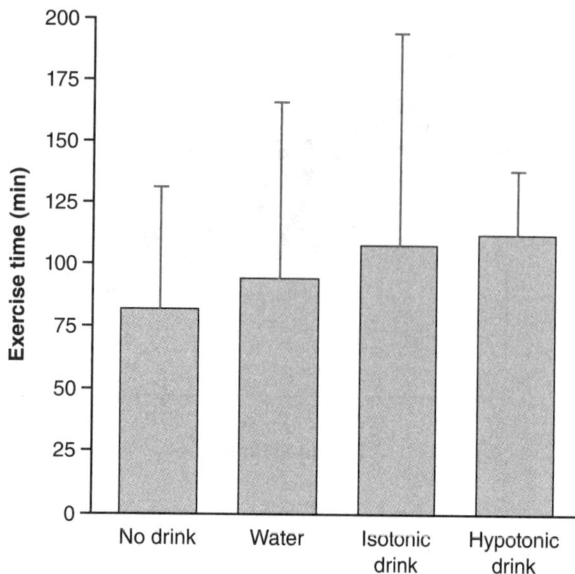

Figure 9.9 Effects of ingestion of different drinks on exercise capacity during a cycle ergometer test to exhaustion at 70% of $\dot{V}O_2$max. Ingestion of water resulted in a longer time to exhaustion than in the no-drink trial, but ingestion of the two dilute carbohydrate–electrolyte drinks resulted in the longest endurance times.

Data from Maughan et al. (1987).

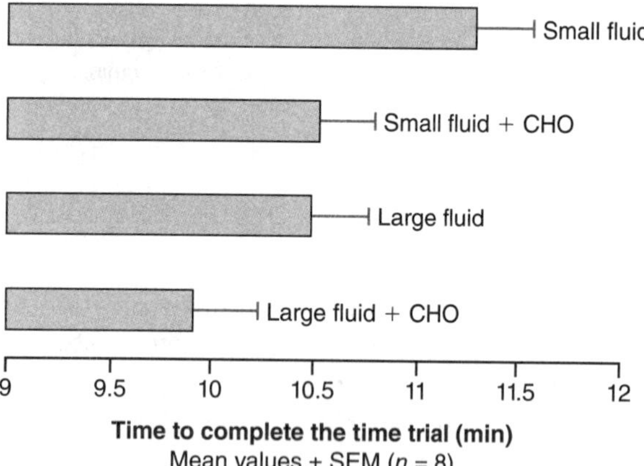

Figure 9.10 Effect of carbohydrate and fluid ingestion on a cycling time trial performed at the end of a prolonged exercise test at 31 °C (88 °F) in which either a small (200 ml [7 fl oz]) or a large (1,330 ml [45 fl oz]) fluid volume with either zero carbohydrate or a large amount (79 g) of carbohydrate was given. Ingestion of water and carbohydrate has independent and additive effects on improving exercise performance.

Data from Below et al. (1995).

small intestine is not adversely affected. In fact, the presence of small amounts of glucose and sodium tends to cause a slight increase in the rate of water absorption compared with pure water (Maughan and Murray 2000). Sodium and other electrolytes are added to sports drinks not to replace electrolytes lost through sweating but to provide the following benefits:

- Increase palatability
- Maintain thirst (and therefore promote drinking)
- Prevent hyponatremia (low serum sodium concentration, which can occur when people ingest far more water than required)
- Increase the rate of water uptake
- Increase the retention of fluid

Replacement of the electrolytes lost in sweat can normally wait until the postexercise recovery period. Fluid intake during strenuous exercise of less than 30 minutes offers no advantage. Gastric emptying is inhibited at high work rates, and insignificant amounts of fluid are absorbed during exercise of such short duration. For exercise that lasts longer than 1 hour or for exercise in hot or humid conditions, consumption of carbohydrate–electrolyte sports drinks is warranted. These drinks supply fluid together with carbohydrate that helps maintain blood glucose and high levels of carbohydrate oxidation. The electrolyte (sodium) content partly offsets salt losses in sweat, but perhaps more important, it maintains the desire to drink.

Sweat-loss rates during exercise depend on exercise intensity, duration, and environmental conditions but vary considerably among individuals. Some people may lose up to 3 L/h (0.8 gal/h) of sweat during strenuous activity in a warm environment (see figure 9.11) (Sawka and Pandolf 1990), and even at low ambient temperatures of about 12 °C (54 °F), sweat loss can exceed 1 L/h (0.3 gal/h) (Maughan 1985). Because the electrolyte composition of sweat is hypotonic to plasma (in other words, the total concentration of dissolved anions and cations is considerably lower in sweat than in plasma; see table 9.5), the replacement of water rather than electrolytes is the priority during exercise. Plasma volume falls by up to 20% during exercise, and most of the fall is related to the relative exercise intensity. Typically, at work rates equivalent to 60% to 80% of the maximal oxygen uptake, plasma volume falls acutely by about 10% to 15% because of the increased capillary hydrostatic pressure and osmotic uptake of water into

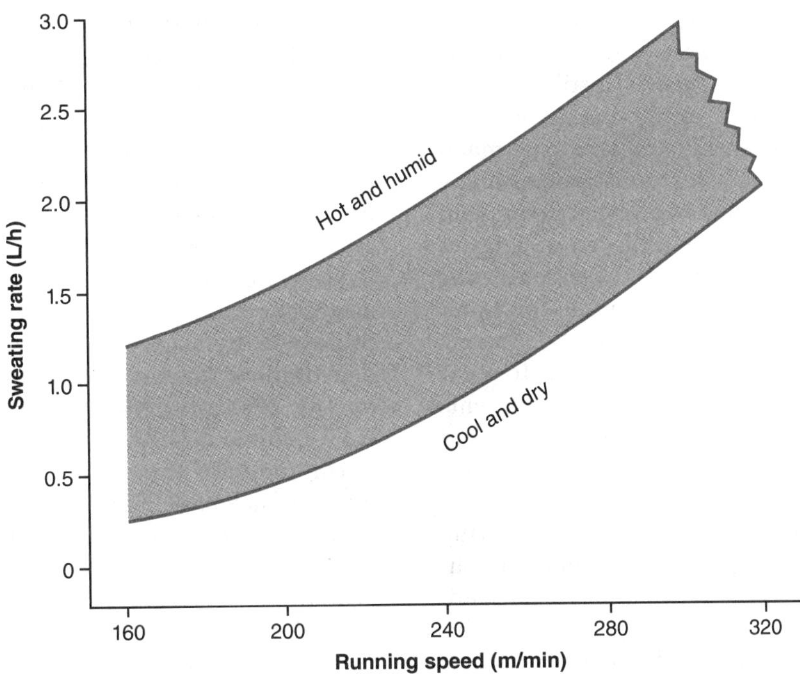

Figure 9.11 Approximate hourly sweating rates as a function of environmental conditions and running speed.

Reprinted by permission from M.N. Sawka and K.B. Pandolf, "Effects of Body Water Loss on Physiological Function and Exercise Performance," in *Perspectives in Exercise Science and Sports Medicine*, Vol. 3, edited by C.V. Gisolfi and D.R. Lamb (Traverse City, MI: Cooper Publishing, 1990), 1-38.

TABLE 9.5 Concentrations of Electrolytes in Sweat, Plasma, and Intracellular Water

Electrolyte	Sweat (mmol/L)	Plasma (mmol/L)	Intracellular water (mmol/L)
Cations			
Sodium	20-80	130-155	10
Potassium	4-8	3.2-5.5	150
Calcium	0.1-1.0	2.1-2.9	0.01
Magnesium	0.1-0.2	0.7-1.5	15
Anions			
Chloride	20-60	96-110	8
Bicarbonate	1-35	23-28	10
Phosphate	0.1-0.2	0.7-1.6	65
Sulfate	0.1-2.0	0.3-0.9	10

active skeletal muscle tissue. Without fluid intake, particularly in a warm, humid environment, further falls in plasma volume and increases in plasma osmolarity occur because of the loss of hypotonic sweat as exercise proceeds.

As mentioned previously, the decrease in plasma volume that accompanies dehydration may be of particular importance in influencing work capacity. Blood flow to the muscles must be maintained at a high level to supply oxygen and fuel substrates (glucose and fatty acids), but high blood flow to the skin is also necessary to convect heat to the body surface where it can be dissipated. When the ambient temperature is high and plasma volume decreases through sweat loss during prolonged exercise (as shown in figure 9.12), skin blood flow is likely to be compromised (Costill and Fink 1974), thereby allowing central venous pressure and blood flow to the working muscle to be maintained but reducing heat loss and causing body temperature to rise to dangerous levels. To prevent dehydration, water must be replaced at a faster rate. Metabolic water production increases during exercise but not enough to compensate for water loss through sweating. Oral fluid ingestion during exercise helps restore plasma volume to near preexercise levels (see figure 9.12) and prevents the adverse effects of dehydration on thermal and cardiovascular strain, muscle strength, endurance, and coordination.

One study compared time to exhaustion during cycling at 60% of $\dot{V}O_2$max in warm ambient conditions (30 °C [86 °F]) when six subjects were given either no drink, 500 ml (17 fl oz) of a 15% carbohydrate-electrolyte drink immediately before exercise and 125 ml (4 fl oz.) of the same drink every 10 minutes throughout exercise, or 500 ml of a 2% carbohydrate-electrolyte drink immediately before exercise and 250 ml (8 fl oz.) of the same drink every 10 minutes throughout exercise (Galloway and Maughan 2000). With no drink, subjects fatigued after 71 minutes (median range 39-97 minutes). With the 15% carbohydrate-electrolyte drink, they could continue for longer times (median 84 minutes, range 63-145 minutes). But the best performance was achieved with the 2% carbohydrate-electrolyte drink (median 118 minutes, range 83-168 minutes). The median core temperature at exhaustion was the same in all three trials (39.5 °C [103 °F]). A significant fall in plasma volume occurred within the first 15 minutes of exercise on all trials. Subsequently, plasma volume remained below resting values on the no-drink and the 15% carbohydrate-electrolyte trials, but on the 2% carbohydrate-electrolyte trial, plasma volume was gradually restored during exercise.

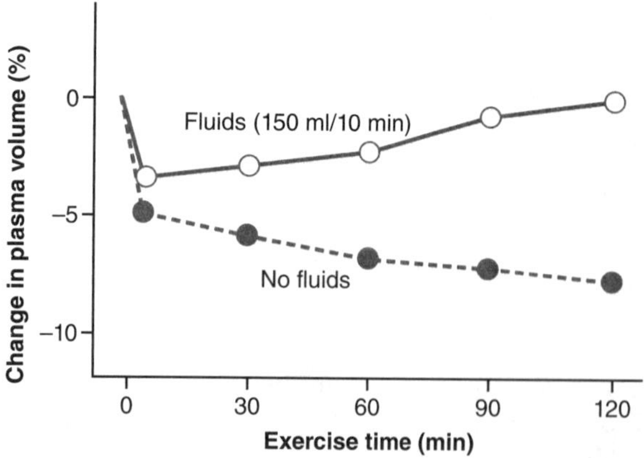

Figure 9.12 Changes in plasma volume during exercise in the heat with and without regular fluid ingestion.

Data from Costill and Fink (1974).

Gonzalez-Alonso et al. (1998) showed that exercising-limb perfusion may decrease during prolonged exercise combined with heat stress and dehydration. The maintenance of plasma volume on the 2% carbohydrate-electrolyte trial may have resulted in better perfusion of active muscles during exercise and may have resulted in better maintenance of cellular hydration.

Ingestion of relatively cool fluid may have an additional small benefit during exercise in the heat, because the additional volume of fluid in the body after drinking adds to the body's heat-storage capacity. The improvement in heat-storage capacity can be calculated based on the specific heat capacity of water, which is 4.184 kJ/kg/°C (0.555 kcal/kg/°F). For example, the ingestion of 2 L (0.5 gal) of fluid at 10 °C (50 °F) increases heat-storage capacity by $4.184 \times 2 \times (37 - 10)$ kJ = 226 kJ (54 kcal).

In the study by Galloway and Maughan (2000), subjects ingested fluids cooled to 14 °C (57 °F). The investigators calculated that the extra fluid consumed on the 2% carbohydrate-electrolyte treatment (2.3 L [0.6 gal]) could have produced an 8-minute improvement in performance because of its effect in increasing body heat-storage capacity compared with the no-drink treatment.

Daily Water Balance

The typical daily water balance for a sedentary person who lives in a cool or temperate climate (ambient temperature 10 to 20 °C [50 to 68 °F]) is shown in figure 9.13. Variable amounts of water are lost from the body through sweating in response to the requirement for thermoregulation, but for a sedentary person in cool conditions, evaporative loss of water through the skin amounts to only about 600 ml/day (20 fl oz/day). Additional water is lost in the feces (about 100 ml/day [3 fl oz/day]) and urine. Normally, about 800 to 1,600 ml (27-54 fl oz) of urine is produced each day. The kidneys can regulate the amount of water lost in urine, but even in severe dehydration some urine is produced to maintain fluid flow through the kidney tubules (nephrons) and excrete toxic nitrogenous wastes such as ammonia and urea. Urinary water loss is not usually less than 800 ml/day (27 fl oz/day).

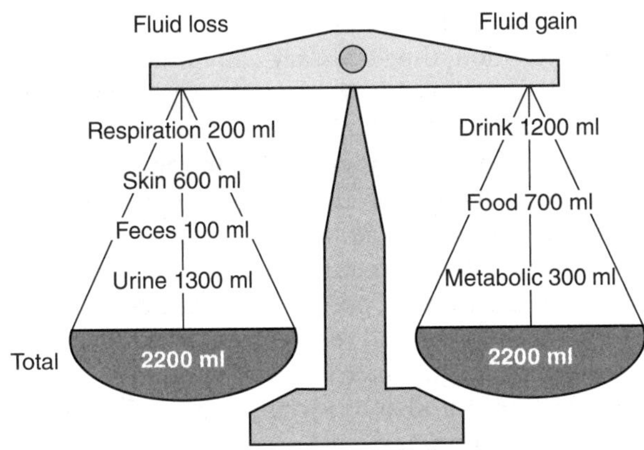

Figure 9.13 Daily water balance for a sedentary adult.

Environmental conditions affect a person's water requirements by altering the losses that occur by the various routes. Water losses may be two to three times greater for a sedentary person who lives in a hot climate compared with a sedentary person who lives in a temperate climate. These higher rates of water loss are not caused exclusively by increased sweating; they may also be incurred by a marked increase in transcutaneous and respiratory water losses. These routes of water loss are heavily influenced by the humidity of the ambient air, which may be a more important factor than the ambient temperature. Respiratory water losses are greater when the relative humidity (RH) of the ambient air is low because air breathed out of the body is fully saturated with water vapor (RH = 100%). Although these losses are small for a sedentary person in a moist, warm environment (about 200 ml/day [7 fl oz/day]), they may increase approximately twofold in low-humidity conditions (RH = 0%-20%) and may rise up to 1,500 ml/day (51 fl oz/day) during periods of hard training in cold, dry air at altitude.

Water intake comes from drinks and food; some foods (especially plant material) have high water content. Water in food, in fact, makes a major contribution to total water intake. Water is also produced internally (metabolic water) from the catabolism of carbohydrate, fat, and protein. For example, in the complete oxidation of one molecule of glucose, six molecules of carbon dioxide and six molecules of water are produced. In a sedentary individual, metabolic water production amounts to about 300 ml/day (10 fl oz/day), although most of this water is lost in expired gas, because oxidizing fuel in the body generates carbon dioxide, which stimulates breathing and hence increases respiratory water loss. Although an athlete increases his or her metabolic water production because of the increased rate of fuel catabolism during exercise, this increase, again, is offset by the obligatory increase in lung ventilation and respiratory evaporative water loss.

The body's water balance is under tight regulation and involves nervous and hormonal factors that respond to a number of inputs. The osmolarity of the blood plasma is maintained within tight limits around 290 mOsmol/L. A rise or fall in the plasma osmolarity is sufficient to alter kidney function from maximum water conservation to maximum water excretion. Because sodium is the major electrolyte in the extracellular fluids (accounting for 50% of plasma osmolarity), the maintenance of osmotic balance is closely coupled to the intake and excretion of sodium and water. Even small reductions in plasma osmolarity invoke a marked increase in urine output (diuresis), and this increase is normally sufficient to prevent fluid overload when large volumes of water or low-electrolyte drinks, such as beer, are consumed. But some cases of **hyponatremia** (low plasma sodium concentration) have been reported, usually in people who have ingested excessively large volumes of plain water or low-electrolyte drinks in a relatively short time.

The subjective sensation of thirst initiates the desire to drink and is therefore a key factor in the regulation of fluid intake. Although the kidneys can effectively conserve water or electrolytes by reducing the rate of loss, they cannot restore a fluid deficit. Only consumption of fluid can correct this imbalance. The sensation of thirst is mainly evoked by the detection of elevated plasma osmolarity (and, to a lesser extent, by reductions in blood volume and pressure) by osmoreceptors located in the hypothalamus of the brain. The thirst sensation results in a profound desire to drink and an increase in the secretion of antidiuretic hormone (ADH) from the posterior pituitary gland, which acts on the kidneys to reduce urine excretion. Other factors that promote thirst are learned responses such as dryness of the mouth or throat, salty tastes, and feeling hot. Thirst is quickly alleviated by drinking fluid, and alleviation can occur before a significant amount of the fluid is absorbed in the gut. This effect suggests a role for sensory receptors in the mouth and stomach. Distension of the stomach wall appears to reduce the perception of thirst and may result in premature cessation of fluid ingestion. Thus, the absence of the sensation of thirst cannot be used as an indicator that fluid balance (euhydration) is established; the perception of thirst is often not present until a significant degree of dehydration has occurred.

An electrolyte imbalance commonly called water intoxication, which results from hyponatremia (low plasma sodium) caused by excessive water consumption, is occasionally reported in endurance athletes. This condition appears to be most common among slow runners in marathon and ultramarathon races and probably arises because of the loss of sodium in sweat coupled with extremely high intakes (8-10 L [2-3 gal]) of water (Noakes et al. 1985). The symptoms of hyponatremia are similar to those of dehydration and include mental confusion, weakness, and fainting. Therefore, this condition can be misdiagnosed when it occurs in people who participate in endurance races. The usual treatment for dehydration is administration of fluid intravenously and orally. If this treatment is given to a hyponatremic individual, the consequences can be fatal. The normal plasma sodium concentration is around 140 to 144 mmol/L. Symptomatic hyponatremia can occur when the plasma sodium concentration rapidly drops to 130 mmol/L or less. The longer that it remains low, the greater the risk is of developing swelling of the brain (the clinical term is dilutional encephalopathy) and accumulating extracellular fluid in the lungs (pulmonary edema). When plasma sodium falls well below 120 mmol/L, the risk of brain seizure, coma, and death increases. In long-distance events, symptomatic hyponatremia is more likely to occur in small, lean people who run slowly, sweat less, and ingest large volumes of water or hypotonic fluids before, during, and even after the event. People with genes for cystic fibrosis tend to be more prone to salt depletion and therefore may be at higher risk for developing exercise-associated hyponatremia. Women generally have lower sweating rates than men and are thus at higher risk for developing exercise-associated hyponatremia.

In one study, the fluid requirements for American footballers performing two-a-day training sessions in a hot, humid environment were compared with cross country runners in the same conditions (Godek, Bartolozzi, and Godek 2005). Sweating rates during exercise were determined in morning and afternoon practices or runs from the change in body weight adjusted for fluids consumed and urine produced. Overall sweat rate was higher in the footballers than in the cross country runners (2.14 vs. 1.77 L/h [0.6 vs. 0.5 gal/h]). Daily sweat losses were substantially higher in the footballers (9.4 vs. 3.5 L [2.5 vs. 0.9 gal]), but the footballers consumed much larger volumes of fluid during morning and afternoon training sessions. For complete hydration, the necessary daily fluid consumption calculated as 130% of daily sweat loss in the footballers was 12.2 L (3.2 gal) compared with 4.6 L (1.2 gal) in the runners. Consuming such large volumes of hypotonic fluid may promote sodium dilution unless care is taken to ensure adequate electrolyte replacement. Thus, footballers and others (e.g., military personnel in hot conditions) whose fluid losses and replacement needs are high require careful guidance not only to avoid excessive dehydration but also to promote safe rehydration and avoid hyponatremia.

Fluid Requirements for Athletes

Athletes must be fully hydrated before they train or compete because the body cannot adapt to dehydration. Training quality will suffer if an athlete becomes dehydrated during training, and performance quality will suffer if an athlete becomes dehydrated during competition.

Ensuring Adequate Hydration Before Exercise

An adequately hydrated state can be ensured by high fluid intake in the last few days before competition. A useful check is to observe the color of the urine. It should be pale in color, although this simple test cannot be reliably used if the athlete is taking vitamin supplements, because some of the excreted water-soluble B vitamins add a yellowish hue to urine. A clearer indication of hydration status is obtained by measuring urine osmolality. (Note that the units of osmolality are Osmol/kg, whereas osmolarity is expressed as Osmol/L.) This measurement can be done quickly and simply using a portable osmometer. A urine osmolality of over 900 mOsmol/kg indicates that the athlete is relatively dehydrated; values of 100 to 300 mOsmol/kg indicate that the athlete is well hydrated. Measuring the athlete's body weight after rising and voiding each morning may also prove useful. A sudden drop in body mass on any given day is likely to indicate dehydration. Approximate fluid intake requirements in liters per day in hot, dry conditions are shown in figure 9.14. The fluid intake requirement (to maintain water balance or euhydration) increases as ambient temperature increases and as daily energy expenditure increases.

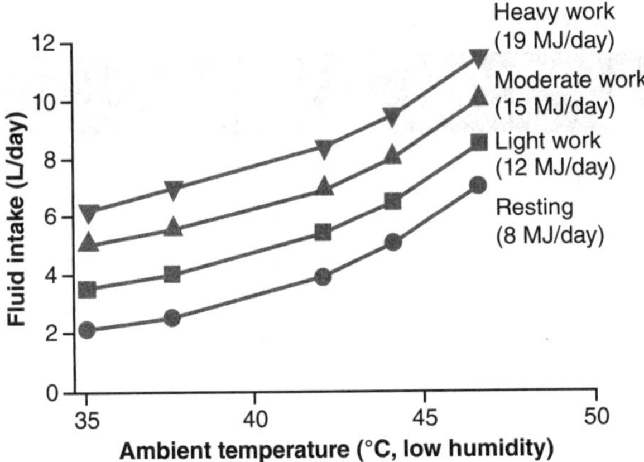

Figure 9.14 Approximate daily fluid intake requirements for people at rest or performing various amounts of physical work while living in different ambient temperatures.

Adapted from Sawka and Montain (2000).

Ensuring Hydration During Exercise

Relying on feeling thirsty as the signal to drink is unreliable because a considerable degree of dehydration (certainly sufficient to impair athletic performance) can occur before the desire for fluid intake is evident. Ideally, athletes should consume enough fluids during activity that body weight remains fairly constant before and after exercise. Guidelines for the amount of fluid to be consumed before, during, and after exercise can only be general because of the large variation in individual sweating responses. The American and Canadian Dietetic Associations recommend that approximately 500 ml (17 fl oz) of fluid be consumed 2 hours before exertion and another 500 ml (17 fl oz) be consumed about 15 minutes before prolonged exercise. In hot and humid environments, frequent consumption (every 15-20 minutes) of small volumes (120-180 ml [4-6 fl oz]) of fluid are recommended throughout exertion. Detailed recommendations on fluid replacement strategies during and following exercise have been given in the ACSM position stand on exercise and fluid replacement (American College of Sports Medicine 2007). Athletes should become accustomed to consuming fluid at regular intervals (with or without thirst) during training sessions so they do not experience discomfort during competition. For most persons exercising for 30 to 60 minutes in moderate temperatures, an appropriate beverage is cool water.

Composition of Sports Drinks During Exercise

Fluid ingestion during exercise supplies exogenous fuel substrate (usually carbohydrate), helps maintain plasma volume, and prevents dehydration, but the availability of ingested fluids may be limited by the rate of gastric emptying or intestinal absorption. Gastric emptying of fluids is slowed by the addition of carbohydrate or other macronutrients that increase the osmolarity of the solution ingested. Hence, with increasing glucose concentration in the fluid ingested, the rate of fluid volume delivery to the small intestine decreases, although the rate of glucose delivery increases.

Water absorption in the small intestine is by osmosis and is promoted by the coupled transport of glucose and sodium. Hence, the composition of fluids to be used during exercise depends on the relative needs to replace water and provide fuel substrate. Where rehydration is the main priority (e.g., for prolonged exercise in the heat), the solution should contain some carbohydrate as glucose or glucose polymers (20-60 g/L) and sodium (20-60 mmol/L) and should not exceed isotonicity (290 mOsmol/L). Most commercially available sports drinks contain 60 to 80 g/L of carbohydrate (predominantly as glucose, glucose polymers, or both, although some drinks may also contain fructose or sucrose) and 20 to 25 mmol/L of sodium. Table 9.6 compares the compositions of several commercially available drinks that athletes commonly consume during training or competition. In cool environments, where substrate provision to maintain endurance performance is more important, a concentrated solution that incorporates large amounts of glucose polymers in concentrations of 550 to 800 mmol/L glucosyl units (100 to 150 g/L) is recommended. To minimize the limitation imposed by the rate of gastric emptying, the osmolarity of the beverage should be minimized by providing the glucose in the form of glucose polymers, and the volume of fluid in the stomach should be kept as high as is comfortable by frequent ingestion of small amounts of fluid. Athletes should drink water when ingesting carbohydrate gels or solid foods to reduce the carbohydrate concentration and osmolality of the stomach contents.

The importance of practicing drinking during training is often neglected. This practice will accustom athletes to the feeling of exercising with fluid in the stomach. It also provides the opportunity to experiment with different volumes and flavorings to determine how much fluid intake

TABLE 9.6 Compositions of Commonly Consumed Sport Drinks

Drink	Carbohydrate (g/L)	Sodium (mmol/L)	Potassium (mmol/L)	Osmolality (mOsmol/kg)
Coca-Cola	105	3	0	650
Allsport	80	10	6	516
Gatorade	60	18	3	349
Isostar	65	24	4	296
Lucozade Sport	64	23	4	280
Lucozade	180	0	0	658
Powerade (UK)	60	24	4	285
Powerade (U.S.)	80	5	4	381

Some drink bottles show carbohydrate content as a percentage or a percentage of weight/volume (w/v), which is equivalent to g/100 ml; for example, in the table, Lucozade Sport's carbohydrate content is 64 g/L, which is 6.4 g/100 ml or 6.4%. Sodium content may be given in milligrams (mg), which can be obtained from the table by multiplying the sodium concentration in mmol/L by 23 (the atomic mass of sodium). For example, Lucozade Sport's sodium content is 23 mmol/L, which is 529 mg/L. Thus, a 500 ml (17 fl oz) bottle of Lucozade Sport contains 265 mg of sodium.

athletes can tolerate and which formulations suit them best. Measuring fluid consumption and body mass changes before and after training gives an idea of the athlete's sweat rate under different environmental conditions. This information will help determine the athlete's requirements for fluid intake during competition. Practicing race nutrition and doing this regularly as part of training the gut is discussed in chapter 17. Gastric emptying and absorption are discussed in chapter 5.

The ideal drink for fluid replacement during exercise is one that tastes good to the athlete, does not cause gastrointestinal discomfort when consumed in large volumes (this rules out all carbonated drinks), promotes rapid gastric emptying and fluid absorption to help maintain extracellular fluid volume, and provides energy in the form of carbohydrate for the working muscles. Exercising subjects prefer cool, pleasantly flavored, sweetened beverages, and the presence of sodium in the drinks seems to promote their consumption, probably by maintaining thirst.

Drinking to Thirst Versus Drinking With a Plan

Thirst develops when a person is already dehydrated, and when dehydration occurs, gastric emptying and absorption are affected. Therefore, it is important to use the early parts of competition to drink and fuel when the gastrointestinal system is not yet compromised. When people drink according to how thirsty they feel, voluntary dehydration commonly occurs. This is not a problem as long as dehydration is not excessive. As discussed earlier in this chapter, there is some debate about what *excessive* means. It is generally agreed that dehydration of 2% of body mass has little or no effect on performance if the athlete was well hydrated at the start of exercise. There is a good rationale for this number. A body-water deficit greater than 2% exceeds two standard deviations in normal day-to-day body mass variability and also seems to represent a threshold where alterations in fluid regulation occur. Whether exercise performance is affected by 2% dehydration depends on a number of factors, and it is unlikely that performance will be affected in cool conditions, but it may be affected in hot conditions. When exercise is performed in hot conditions and cooling is very dependent on sweating, it may be wise to prevent dehydration beyond 2% to 3%. In cooler conditions, larger sweat losses may be tolerated (3-4%). There are examples of great performances with athletes dehydrating more than 4% (mainly in cool conditions), but it is likely that these athletes were accustomed to dehydration or, for reasons that are not completely understood, are more resistant to the negative effects of dehydration.

Drinking according to thirst works for many athletes and especially slower athletes. Their sweat rates will be relatively low and there is more time to drink. For high-level athletes, this is a little different. It is probably wise to start drinking earlier to prevent excessive dehydration.

Also, during a race or competition, an athlete cannot always drink when thirsty. In some sports water is available all the time, but in other sports the rules prevent athletes from drinking even when they are thirsty or water may not be available (no feed stations) at times when they are feeing thirsty. Therefore, athletes must be a little more deliberate and conscious about their hydration strategies if they are serious about maximizing performance, particularly in hot weather.

The other thing to keep in mind is that fueling and hydrating are tightly linked for most people. For example, a marathon runner needs to drink to ensure adequate consumption and absorption of calories from gels or sports drinks. Unless it's a really hot day, most people are going have a harder time keeping up with their calorie needs than their fluid needs; if they take care of the former, the latter may take care of itself.

It never hurts to do regular measurements of weight loss over time in different environmental conditions so sweat rates can be calculated. All that is required to get a reasonable estimate is a scale; measure body weight before and after a known duration of exercise and correct for any fluid (or solids) consumed.

Rehydration After Exercise

Replacement of water and electrolytes in the postexercise recovery period may be of crucial importance when repeated bouts of exercise must be performed and rehydration must be maximized in the time available. As previously mentioned, dehydration is associated with impaired thermoregulation, increased cardiovascular strain, and the loss of the thermoregulatory advantages conferred by heat acclimation and high aerobic fitness. With progressive dehydration, losses of intracellular and extracellular fluid volume occur. Loss of intracellular volume may have important implications for recovery from exercise given the emerging evidence of a role for cell volume in the regulation of cell metabolism. Reduced intracellular volume reduces rates of glycogen and protein synthesis, whereas high cell volume stimulates these processes.

The main factors that influence the effectiveness of postexercise rehydration are the volume and composition of the fluid consumed. Plain water is not the ideal rehydration beverage when rapid and complete restoration of body fluid balance is necessary and when all intake is in liquid form. Ingestion of water alone causes a rapid fall in plasma sodium concentration and in plasma osmolarity. These changes reduce the stimulation to drink (thirst) and increase urine output, both of which delay the rehydration process. Plasma volume is more rapidly and completely restored if some sodium chloride (77 mmol/L or 0.45 g/L) is added to the water consumed (Nose et al. 1988). This sodium concentration is similar to the upper limit of the sodium concentration found in sweat but is considerably higher than the sodium concentration of many commercially available sports drinks, which usually contain 10 to 25 mmol/L (see table 9.6). Optimal rehydration after exercise can be achieved only if the sodium lost in sweat is replaced along with the water.

Shirreffs et al. (1996) showed that if an adequate volume of fluid is consumed, euhydration is achieved when sodium intake is greater than sodium loss. Ingesting a beverage that contains sodium not only promotes rapid fluid absorption in the small intestine but also allows the plasma sodium concentration to remain elevated during the rehydration period and helps maintain thirst while delaying stimulation of urine production. Sodium is the major cation in extracellular fluid. The inclusion of potassium in the beverage consumed after exercise would be expected to enhance the replacement of intracellular water and thus promote rehydration, but currently little experimental evidence supports this expectation. The rehydration drink should also contain carbohydrate (glucose or glucose polymers) because the presence of some glucose also stimulates fluid absorption in the gut and improves beverage taste. After exercise, the uptake of glucose into the muscle for glycogen resynthesis should also promote intracellular rehydration.

Fluid Consumption After Exercise

For a person undertaking regular exercise, any fluid deficit incurred during one exercise session can potentially compromise the next exercise session if adequate fluid replacement does not occur. Fluid replacement after exercise can frequently be thought of as hydration before the next exercise bout. Until recently, athletes were generally encouraged to consume a volume of fluid equivalent to their sweat loss incurred during exercise to rehydrate adequately in the postexercise recovery period. In other words, they were to consume about 1 L (0.3 gal) of fluid for every kilogram lost during an exercise session. This amount is insufficient because it does not take into account the obligatory urine losses that are incurred after beverage consumption over a period of hours. Existing data indicate that ingestion of 150% or more of weight loss (i.e., 1.5 L [0.4 gal] of fluid consumed during recovery for every kilogram of weight lost during exercise) may be required to achieve normal hydration within 6 hours after exercise (see figure

SELECTED RECOMMENDATIONS ON EXERCISE AND FLUID REPLACEMENT

The following recommendations are taken from the American College of Sports Medicine position stand on exercise and fluid replacement (2007).

Adequate fluid replacement helps maintain hydration and therefore promotes the health, safety, and optimal physical performance of people who participate in regular physical activity. The following are general recommendations on the amount and composition of fluids that should be ingested in preparation for, during, and after exercise or athletic competition:

- People should consume nutritionally balanced diets and drink adequate fluids during the 24-hour period before an event, especially during the period that includes the meal before exercise, to promote proper hydration before exercise or competition.
- People should drink about 6 to 8 ml (0.2-0.3 fl oz) of fluid per kilogram of body weight about 2 hours before exercise to allow sufficient time for fluid absorption and to allow time for excretion of excess ingested water. Consuming beverages that contain sodium or drinking beverages while eating salted snacks or small meals can help stimulate thirst and retain needed fluids.
- During exercise, athletes should start drinking early and at regular intervals in an attempt to consume fluids at a rate sufficient to prevent excessive dehydration (reductions from baseline body weight greater than 2%). Because people vary considerably in their rates of sweating (and, of course, sweating rate depends greatly on environmental conditions and exercise intensity), athletes should develop customized fluid replacement programs to achieve this goal. The routine measurement of preexercise and postexercise body weight is useful for determining sweat rates and establishing appropriate customized fluid replacement programs.
- Ingested fluids should be cooler than the ambient temperature (between 15 and 22 °C [59 and 72 °F]) and flavored to enhance palatability and promote fluid replacement. Fluids should be readily available and served in containers that allow adequate volumes to be ingested with ease and with minimal interruption of exercise.
- Addition of proper amounts of carbohydrates or electrolytes to a fluid replacement solution is recommended for exercise events longer than 1 hour because such additives do not significantly impair water delivery to the body and can enhance performance. For exercise of less than 1 hour, little evidence exists of physiological or physical performance differences resulting from consuming a carbohydrate–electrolyte drink compared with consuming plain water.
- During intense exercise lasting longer than 1 hour, carbohydrates should be ingested at a rate of 30 to 60 g/h to maintain oxidation of carbohydrate and delay fatigue. This rate of carbohydrate delivery can be achieved without compromising fluid delivery by drinking 600 to 1,200 ml/h (20-41 fl oz/h) of solutions that contain 4% to 8% carbohydrates (g/100 ml). The carbohydrates can be sugars (glucose or sucrose) or starch (e.g., maltodextrins).
- Inclusion of sodium (500-700 mg/L of water) in the rehydration solution ingested during exercise lasting longer than 1 hour is recommended because it may enhance palatability, promote fluid retention, and possibly prevent hyponatremia in certain people who drink excessive quantities of fluid. Little physiological evidence suggests the need for sodium in an oral rehydration solution for enhancing intestinal water absorption as long as sodium is sufficiently available from the previous meal.
- After exercise, in situations in which people need rapid and complete recovery from excessive dehydration, 1.5 L (0.4 gal) of fluid should be consumed for each kilogram of body weight lost. Consuming beverages with sodium will help the attainment of rapid and complete recovery of hydration status by stimulating thirst and fluid retention.

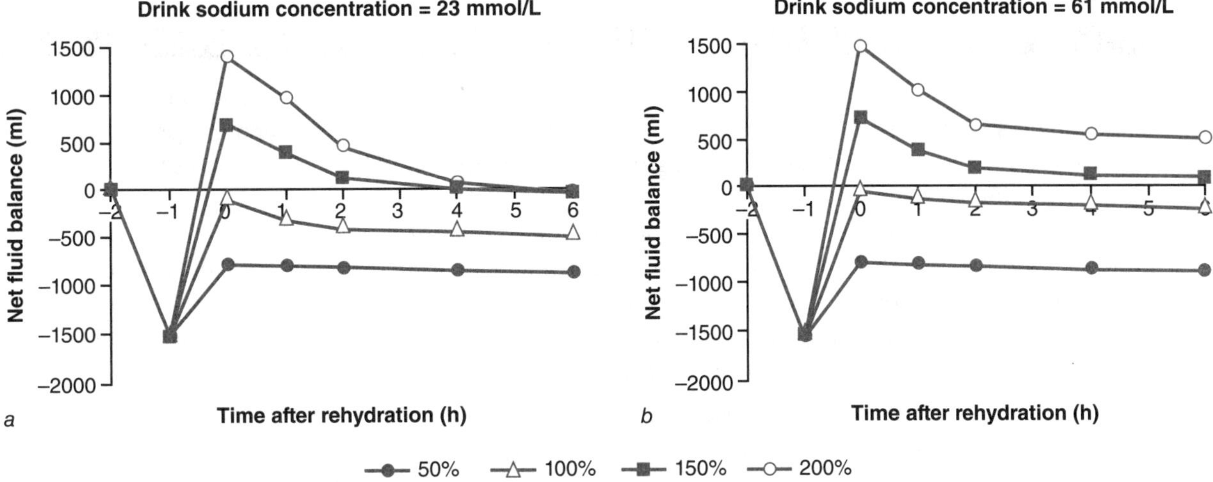

Figure 9.15 Net fluid balance plotted against time after dehydration (loss of 1,500 ml [51 fl oz] of body water) induced by mild exercise in a hot environment. Zero net fluid balance represents euhydration. Drink volume ingested was half of (50%), equal to (100%), one-and-a-half times (150%), and twice (200%) the sweat loss. The drink sodium concentration was either *(a)* 23 mmol/L or *(b)* 61 mmol/L. Mild dehydration was present 6 hours after rehydration when a large volume of the low-sodium drink (23 mmol/L) was consumed, but with the same volume, hyperhydration was achieved with the high-sodium drink (61 mmol/L).
Adapted from Shirreffs et al. (1996).

9.15) (Shirreffs et al. 1996; Shirreffs and Maughan 1998, 2000)). The American College of Sports Medicine (2007) guidelines on fluid ingestion before, during, and after exercise are shown in the sidebar.

Intake of caffeine and alcohol in the postexercise recovery period is generally discouraged because of the diuretic actions of these beverages. The diuretic effect of alcohol appears to be blunted, however, when it is consumed by persons who are moderately dehydrated after exercise in a warm environment (Shirreffs and Maughan 1997). If shandy (a mixture of beer and lemonade) is consumed in the postexercise period, then (as expected) urinary output increases with increasing alcohol intake. But this increase only approaches statistical significance (compared with lemonade alone) when alcohol content is around 4% w/v. This concentration of alcohol in the rehydration drink is also associated with a slower rate of recovery of plasma volume, as shown in figure 9.16, whereas drinks containing 1% and 2% alcohol seem just as effective as lemonade alone.

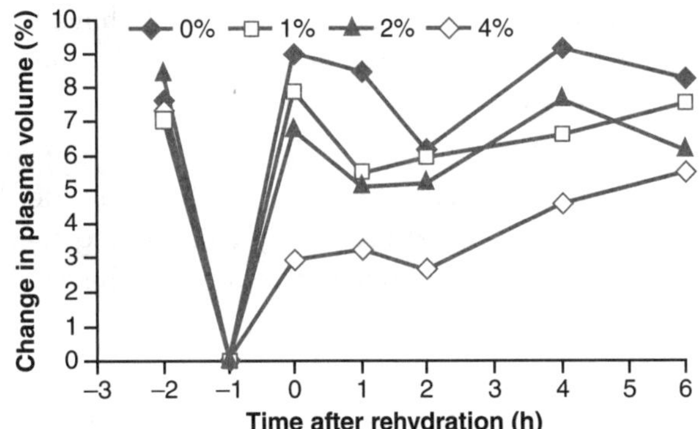

Figure 9.16 Percentage change in plasma volume with dehydration equivalent to 2% of body weight followed by rehydration with drinks containing 0%, 1%, 2%, and 4% (w/v) alcohol in a volume equivalent to one-and-a-half times the sweat loss. Note that plasma volume restoration was delayed with the 4% alcohol drink.
Data from Shirreffs and Maughan (1997).

DEVELOPING A CUSTOMIZED FLUID INGESTION STRATEGY

The routine measurement of body weight in kilograms before and after exercise is useful for determining sweat rates and establishing appropriate customized fluid replacement programs. The following example illustrates how a customized fluid ingestion strategy can be established for a 70 kg (154 lb) male athlete:

- Recommendation before exercise: Drink about 6 to 8 ml (0.2-0.3 fl oz) of fluid per kilogram of body weight about 2 hours before exercise. Application: To achieve this, a 70 kg athlete would need to drink 420 to 560 ml (15-19 fl oz). If the fluid ingested is water, body fluid retention will be improved if a salty snack (e.g., pretzels) is eaten at the same time. Alternately, a carbohydrate–electrolyte beverage could be ingested.
- Recommendation during exercise: Customize fluid ingestion during exercise according to estimated sweat loss. Approximate sweat loss during exercise under known environmental conditions could be determined from training sessions. Application: For example, body weight is measured just before a training session begins and found to be 70.38 kg (155.16 lb), and it is 68.75 kg (151.57 lb) at the end of the 90-minute session. The athlete drank 350 ml (12 fl oz) of sports drink during the session (this volume could be estimated from weighing a drink bottle before and after the session or using a graduated drink bottle). Assuming that all weight lost during the session was from sweat, which is not unreasonable because only a small amount of weight would be lost as carbon dioxide and water in breathing, the change in body weight was 70.38 - 68.75 = 1.63 kg (155.16 – 151.57 = 3.59 lb). We need to correct this for the additional weight of the 350 ml fluid that was ingested, which was 0.35 kg (0.77 lb; it can be assumed that the density of the drink was 1 g/ml or 1 kg/L [0.04 oz/0.03 fl oz]). Thus, actual weight loss if no fluid had been ingested would have been 1.63 kg + 0.35 kg = 1.98 kg (3.59 lb + 0.77 lb = 4.36 lb). This amount of weight was lost in 90 minutes (1.5 hours), so the estimated sweating rate was 1.98 kg/1.5 h or 1.32 L/h.
- Recommendation after exercise: For rapid and complete recovery from excessive dehydration, consume 1.5 L (0.4 gal) of fluid per kilogram of body weight lost. Application: In our example, actual body weight loss during exercise was 1.63 kg. Therefore, 1.63 × 1.5 = 2.45 L (86 fl oz.) of fluid should be consumed in the first hour or so after exercise to restore hydration status.

In most circumstances, athletes should consume solid foods and drink between exercise bouts unless food intake is likely to result in gastrointestinal disturbances. In one study, the same fluid volume consumed as a meal-plus-water combination compared with a sports drink alone resulted in a smaller volume of urine produced and hence greater fluid retention (Maughan, Leiper, and Shirreffs 1996). The greater efficacy of the meal-plus-water treatment in restoring whole-body fluid balance was probably a consequence of its greater total sodium and potassium content. In exercise situations in which sweat losses are large, total sodium and chloride losses are high. For example, the loss of 10 L (2.6 gal) of sweat, with a sodium concentration of 50 mmol/L, amounts to a loss of about 29 g of sodium chloride.

Obviously, food intake can be important in restoring these salt losses because most commercial sports drinks do not contain more than about 25 mmol/L (0.58 g/L) of sodium. Rehydration after exercise can be achieved only if sweat electrolyte losses and water are replaced. One problem is that drinks with high-sodium content (i.e., 40-80 mmol/L) are unpalatable to some people, which results in reduced consumption. On the other hand, drinks with low-sodium content (e.g., most soft drinks) are much less effective for rehydration, and they reduce the stimulus to drink.

Key Points

- High rates of sweat secretion are necessary during hard exercise to limit the rise in body temperature that would otherwise occur. If the exercise is prolonged, body-temperature increase leads to progressive dehydration and loss of electrolytes.
- A body temperature of 36 to 38 °C (96.8-100.4 °F) is considered the normal range at rest, and it may increase to 38 to 40 °C (100.4-104 °F) during exercise. When body temperature rises to 39.5 °C (103 °F), central fatigue ensues. Further increases are commonly associated with heat exhaustion and occasionally with life-threatening heatstroke, which is characterized by lack of consciousness after exertion and by clinical symptoms of organ damage.
- Some people may lose up to 2 to 3 L/h (0.5-0.8 gal/h) of sweat during strenuous activity in a hot environment. Even at low ambient temperatures of about 10 °C (50 °F), sweat loss can exceed 1 L/h (0.3 gal/h).
- Because the electrolyte composition of sweat is hypotonic to plasma, the replacement of water rather than electrolytes is the priority during exercise.
- Fatigue toward the end of a prolonged event may result as much from the effects of dehydration as from substrate depletion. Exercise performance is impaired when a person becomes dehydrated by as little as 2% of body weight, and losses in excess of 5% of body weight can decrease the capacity for work by about 30%. Some evidence indicates that lower levels of dehydration can also impair performance during relatively short-duration, intermittent exercise.
- Dehydration during physical activity in the heat provokes greater performance decrements than similar activity in cooler conditions; this is thought to be due, at least in part, to greater cardiovascular and thermoregulatory strain associated with heat exposure. Although additional research is needed to produce greater understanding of the effect of low-level dehydration on physical performance, we can generalize that when performance is at stake, being well hydrated is better than being dehydrated.
- Oral fluid ingestion during exercise helps restore plasma volume to near preexercise levels and prevents the adverse effects of dehydration on muscle strength, endurance, and coordination. Dehydration also poses a serious health risk because it increases the risk of cramps, heat exhaustion, and life-threatening heatstroke.
- Relying on feeling thirsty as the signal to drink is unreliable because a considerable degree of dehydration (sufficient to impair athletic performance) can occur before the desire for fluid intake is evident. Ideally, athletes should consume adequate fluids during activity so body weight remains fairly constant before and after exercise.
- The composition of drinks to be taken during exercise should suit individual circumstances. Where rehydration is the main priority (e.g., for prolonged exercise in the heat), the solution should contain some carbohydrate as glucose or glucose polymers (20-60 g/L) and sodium (20-60 mmol/L) and should not exceed isotonicity (290 mOsmol/L).
- Optimal rehydration after exercise can be achieved only if the sodium lost in sweat is replaced along with the water. Plasma volume is more rapidly and completely restored in the postexercise period if some sodium chloride is added to the water consumed. A volume equivalent to at least one-and-a-half times the sweat loss must be consumed to ensure that complete rehydration is achieved at the end of a 6-hour recovery period after exercise.

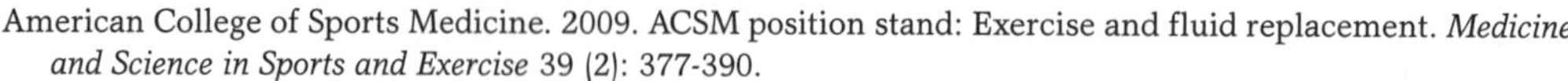

Recommended Readings

American College of Sports Medicine. 2009. ACSM position stand: Exercise and fluid replacement. *Medicine and Science in Sports and Exercise* 39 (2): 377-390.

Armstrong, L.E. 2000. *Performing in extreme environments.* Champaign, IL: Human Kinetics.

Baker, L.B., and A.E. Jeukendrup. 2014. Optimal composition of fluid-replacement beverages. *Comparative Physiology* 4 (2): 575-620.

Coris, E.E., A.M. Ramirez, and D.J. Van Durme. 2004. Heat illness in athletes: The dangerous combination of heat, humidity and exercise. *Sports Medicine* 34 (1): 9-16.

Judelson, D.A., C.M. Maresh, J.M. Anderson, et al. 2007. Hydration and muscular performance: Does fluid balance affect strength, power and high-intensity endurance? *Sports Medicine* 37 (10): 907-921.

Maughan, R.J. 2000. Water and electrolyte loss and replacement in exercise. In *Nutrition in sport,* edited by R.J. Maughan, 226-240. Oxford: Blackwell Science.

Maughan, R.J., and L.M. Burke, eds. 2002. *Handbook of sports medicine and sciences: Sport nutrition.* Oxford: Blackwell Science.

Maughan, R.J., and R. Murray, eds. 2000. *Sports drinks: Basic science and practical aspects.* Boca Raton, FL: CRC Press.

Maughan, R.J., and E.R. Nadel. 2000. Temperature regulation and fluid and electrolyte balance. In *Nutrition in sport,* edited by R.J. Maughan, 203-215. Oxford: Blackwell Science.

Nelson, J.L., and R.A. Robergs. 2007. Exploring the potential ergogenic effects of glycerol hyperhydration. *Sports Medicine* 37 (11): 981-1000.

Sawka, M.N., S.N. Cheuvront, and R.W. Kenefick. 2012. High skin temperature and hypohydration impair aerobic performance. *Experimental Physiology* 97 (3): 327-332.

Sawka, M.N., S.N. Cheuvront, and R.W. Kenefick. 2015. Hypohydration and human performance: Impact of environment and physiological mechanisms. *Sports Medicine* 45 (Suppl 1): S51-S60.

Sawka, M.N., W.A. Latzka, and S.J. Montain. 2000. Effects of dehydration and rehydration on performance. In *Nutrition in sport,* edited by R.J. Maughan, 216-225. Oxford: Blackwell Science.

Shirreffs, S.M., L.E. Armstrong, and S.N. Cheuvront. 2004. Fluid and electrolyte needs for preparation and recovery from training and competition. *Journal of Sports Sciences* 22 (1): 57-63.

Shirreffs, S.M., and R.J. Maughan. 2000. Rehydration and recovery of fluid balance after exercise. *Exercise and Sport Sciences Reviews* 28:27-32.

10

Vitamins and Minerals

Objectives

After studying this chapter, you should be able to do the following:

- Describe the vitamins and minerals that are required to maintain a healthy body
- Describe some of the major dietary sources of essential micronutrients
- Describe the role of micronutrients in growth and repair of body tissues, in metabolism as cofactors for enzymes, in oxygen transport, in immune function, and in defense against free radicals
- Describe the effects of exercise training on micronutrient requirements
- Describe groups of athletes who may be at risk for micronutrient deficiencies
- Describe some of the consequences of micronutrient deficiency and excess

Besides consuming the macronutrients (i.e., carbohydrate, fat, and protein), humans must consume relatively small amounts of certain micronutrients (i.e., organic vitamins and inorganic minerals) in the diet to maintain health. In addition to being found in foods, micronutrients are available individually or in a variety of combined preparations referred to as supplements. Many top athletes consume large quantities of vitamin and mineral supplements in the mistaken belief that they will help prevent infection or injury, speed recovery, or improve athletic performance. Some minerals are likely to do more harm than good. Although vitamin and mineral supplementation may improve the nutritional status of people who consume marginal amounts of micronutrients from food and may improve performance in athletes with deficiencies, no evidence indicates that doses that exceed the RDA improve performance.

This chapter discusses the micronutrient requirements of athletes and the problems associated with inadequate or excessive intakes. Emphasis is on the vitamins and minerals that are important for athletic performance. Rather than dealing with the role and requirement for each individual vitamin and mineral, this chapter describes some of the important roles for which various vitamins and minerals are needed (e.g., in forming the building blocks of body tissues, as cofactors in enzyme catalyzed metabolic reactions, for oxygen transport and oxidative metabolism, and as **antioxidants**). This approach should help the reader understand

- why micronutrients are an essential component of the diet,
- why the requirement for some micronutrients may be greater in athletes,
- which groups of athletes are most at risk for inadequate micronutrient intake, and
- the scientific basis of advice given to athletes regarding their intake of vitamin and mineral supplements.

Any sustained deficiency of an essential vitamin or mineral results in ill health, and an unhealthy athlete is extremely unlikely to perform to the best of his or her potential. Several micronutrients are important for the maintenance of immune function, and this important role is discussed in detail in chapter 13.

Water-Soluble and Fat-Soluble Vitamins

Vitamins are organic compounds that are needed in small quantities in the diet. They are essential for specific metabolic reactions in the body and for promoting normal growth and development. With the exception of vitamin D (which can be synthesized in the presence of sunlight), vitamin K, and small quantities of selected B vitamins (which can be produced by the bacterial microflora of the gastrointestinal tract), vitamins are not produced by the human body and must be consumed in the diet.

Although vitamins do not directly contribute to the energy supply, they play an important role in energy metabolism as reusable coenzymes in many metabolic reactions. Many vitamins, particularly from the B group, are cofactors in the pathways of energy metabolism, including glycolysis, the ß-oxidation of FAs, the tricarboxylic acid cycle, and the electron-transport chain. A deficiency of some of the B-group vitamins that act as cofactors of enzymes in carbohydrate (e.g., vitamins B_1, B_3, B_6), fat (e.g., vitamin B_2, thiamin, pantothenic acid, biotin), and protein (e.g., pyridoxine) metabolism causes premature fatigue and inability to maintain a heavy training program.

Other vitamins play a role in **heme** synthesis and red and white blood cell production (e.g., folic acid, vitamin B_{12}) or assist in the formation of bones, connective tissue, and cartilage (e.g., vitamins C and D). Several vitamins, including A, C, and E, act as antioxidants and help protect the body tissues against the potentially damaging effects of **free radicals**.

Thirteen different compounds are now considered vitamins, and they are classified either as water soluble or fat soluble. The water-soluble vitamins—C, B_1, B_2, B_3, B_6, pantothenic acid, and biotin—are involved in mitochondrial energy metabolism. Folic acid and vitamin B_{12} are mainly involved in nucleic acid synthesis and hence are important for maintaining healthy populations of rapidly dividing cells in the body (e.g., red blood cells, immune cells, the gut mucosa). Of the fat-soluble vitamins—A, D, E, and K—only vitamin E has a probable role in energy metabolism. Vitamins A, C, and E have antioxidant properties. Vitamin K is required for the addition of sugar residues to proteins to form glycoproteins such as the blood-clotting factors. Tables 10.1 and 10.2 summarize the major roles of the vitamins and the main effects of dietary deficiency or excess.

Vitamin deficiencies inhibit body function and impair health. Indeed, most of the vitamins were first recognized by the deficiency symptoms and illnesses that arose when intake was inadequate (e.g., scurvy in vitamin C–deficient sailors; rickets in vitamin D–deficient children). Although marginal deficiencies of vitamins may have only a small effect on otherwise healthy, young, sedentary people, such deficiencies may crucially affect athletic performance in elite athletes. The margins between winning and coming in second can be minuscule in many sports, and a deficiency that impairs performance by only 1% could easily affect the outcome of a competitive event.

TABLE 10.1 Major Functions of Fat-Soluble Vitamins and the Effects of Dietary Deficiency or Excess

Vitamin	Major roles in body	Effects of deficiency	Effects of excess
A (retinol)	Maintains epithelial tissues in skin, mucous membranes, and visual pigments of eye; promotes bone development and immune function	Night blindness, infections, impaired growth, impaired wound healing	Nausea, headache, fatigue, liver damage, joint pains, peeling skin, abnormal fetal development in pregnancy
D (calciferol)	Increases calcium absorption in gut and promotes bone formation; important for muscle and immune function	Weak bones (rickets in children and osteomalacia in adults), suboptimal muscle function, increased susceptibility to infections	Nausea, loss of appetite, irritability, joint pains, calcification of soft tissues (e.g., kidneys)
E (α-tocopherol)	Defends against free radicals; protects cell membranes	Hemolysis, anemia	Headache, fatigue, diarrhea
K (menadione)	Forms blood-clotting factors	Bleeding, hemorrhage	Thrombosis, vomiting

TABLE 10.2 Major Functions of Water-Soluble Vitamins and the Effects of Dietary Deficiency or Excess

Vitamin	Major roles in body	Effects of deficiency	Effects of excess
B_1 (thiamin)	Forms coenzyme with thiamin pyrophosphate; promotes carbohydrate metabolism and central nervous system function	Loss of appetite, apathy, depression, beriberi, pain in calf muscles	No toxic effects
B_2 (riboflavin)	Forms coenzymes with FAD and FMN; promotes carbohydrate and fat oxidation; maintains healthy skin	Dermatitis, lip and tongue sores, damage to cornea of eyes	No toxic effects
B_3 (niacin)	Forms coenzymes with NAD and NADP; promotes anaerobic glycolysis, carbohydrate and fat oxidation, and fat synthesis; maintains healthy skin	Weakness, loss of appetite, skin lesions, gut and skin problems, pellagra	Headache, nausea, skin irritation, liver damage, inhibition of lipolysis
B_6 (pyridoxine)	Forms coenzyme with pyridoxal phosphate; promotes protein metabolism, formation of hemoglobin and red blood cells, glycogenolysis, and gluconeogenesis	Irritability, convulsions, anemia, dermatitis, tongue sores	Loss of nerve sensation, abnormal gait
B_{12} (cobalamin)	Forms coenzyme for DNA and RNA; promotes formation of red and white blood cells; maintains nerve, gut, and skin tissue	Pernicious anemia, fatigue, nerve damage, paralysis, infections	No toxic effects
Folic acid	Forms coenzyme for DNA and RNA; promotes formation of hemoglobin and red and white blood cells; maintains gut tissue	Anemia, fatigue, diarrhea, gut disorders, infections	No toxic effects
Biotin	Forms coenzyme for carbon dioxide transfer; promotes carbohydrate, fat, and protein metabolism	Nausea, fatigue, skin rashes	No toxic effects
Pantothenic acid	Forms CoA for energy metabolism; promotes carbohydrate and fat oxidation and fat synthesis	Nausea, fatigue, depression, loss of appetite	No toxic effects
C (ascorbic acid)	Antioxidant; promotes collagen formation, development of connective tissue, catecholamine and steroid synthesis, and iron absorption	Weakness, slow wound healing, infections, bleeding gums, anemia, scurvy	No toxic effects in smaller doses (<1,000 mg/day); diarrhea, kidney stones, and iron overload in larger doses

FAD = Flavin adenine dinucleotide; FMN = flavin mononucleotide; NAD = nicotinamide adenine dinucleotide; NADP = nicotinamide adenine dinucleotide phosphate.

Recommended Intakes of Vitamins

Each vitamin has a minimal requirement that covers only the basic needs and is sufficient to prevent clinical deficiency and ensuing disease symptoms. The EAR is higher, and it ensures a safety margin. As discussed in chapter 1, the EAR represents the amount of a nutrient deemed sufficient to meet the needs of the average individual in a certain age and gender group. The recommended dietary allowance (RDA) or recommended daily intake of any particular vitamin is defined as the intake required to meet the known nutritional needs of more than 97.5% of healthy people. For some vitamins, including biotin, pantothenic acid, and vitamin D, scientific evidence is currently insufficient to estimate an EAR, and in these cases an AI has been set. People should use the AI as a goal for intake if no RDA exists.

The EAR is normally distributed, and the RDA recommendation is set so it covers 97.5% of all healthy people with an ordinary (normal) diet. This coverage is achieved by adding two standard deviations to the average daily requirement. Thus, individuals who consume less than the RDA of a nutrient are not necessarily deficient in that nutrient, but the more the actual intake lies below the RDA, the greater the risk of a deficiency state that is detrimental to the person's health.

Tables 10.3 and 10.4 show the amounts of vitamins normally required in the adult diet (recommended dietary allowance [RDA] or adequate intake [AI] and the major food sources from which they are obtained.

Recommended Intakes of Vitamins for Athletes

When determining RDAs, the data used often did not include athletes, or the activity levels of the subjects were not reported. Therefore, the RDAs may not be an accurate means of evaluating the nutritional needs of those who engage in regular strenuous exercise. The RDAs are calculated from population-based data. Metabolic, environmental, and genetic factors as well as age, gender, and body mass can make individual nutrient requirements different from these estimated needs.

Although physical activity may increase the requirement for some vitamins (e.g., vitamins C, B_2, and possibly B_6, A, and E), this increased requirement typically can be met by consuming a balanced high-carbohydrate, moderate-protein, low-fat diet. As shown for vitamin B_1 and vitamin C in figure 10.1, vitamin intakes in athletes are correlated with energy intakes up to 20 MJ/day (4,780 kcal/day). Thus, if energy intake matches the energy requirement and athletes consume a reasonably balanced diet, they get all the vitamins (with the possible exception of vitamin D) that they need from food without any need for supplements.

Individuals at risk for low vitamin intake are those who consume a low-energy or unbalanced diet. When energy intake is high (>20 MJ/day [>4,780 kcal/day]), athletes tend to consume a large number of in-between meals and high-energy sports drinks that are often composed mainly of refined carbohydrate and are low in protein and micronutrients; consequently, the nutrient density for vitamins drops. Vegetarian athletes obviously

TABLE 10.3 Major Sources of Fat-Soluble Vitamins

Vitamin	Sources	RDA or AI
A	Liver, fish, dairy products**, eggs, margarine; formed in body from provitamin A (carotenoids) found in carrots, dark green leafy vegetables, tomatoes, oranges	0.9 mg (M)*** 0.7 mg (F)
D	Liver, fish, eggs, fortified dairy products, oils, margarine; formed by action of sunlight on the skin	15 µg* (M, F)
E	Liver, eggs, whole-grain cereal products, vegetable oils, seed oils, margarine, butter	15 mg (M, F)
K	Liver, eggs, green leafy vegetables, cheese, butter; formed in large intestine by bacteria	120 µg* (M) 90 µg* (F)

*Denotes AI values; other values are RDAs. M = male; F = female.

**Dairy products include milk, cream, butter, and cheese.

***RDA for vitamin A is 0.9 mg of retinol or 5.4 mg of beta-carotene for men; 80% of these values for women.

TABLE 10.4 Major Sources of Water-Soluble Vitamins

Vitamin	Sources	RDA or AI
B_1	Whole-grain cereal products, fortified breads, pulses, potatoes, legumes, nuts, pork, ham, liver	1.2 mg (M) 1.1 mg (F)
B_2	Dairy products**, meat, liver, eggs, green leafy vegetables, beans	1.3 mg (M) 1.1 mg (F)
B_3	Meat, liver, poultry, fish, whole-grain cereal products, lentils, nuts; formed in the body from the essential amino acid tryptophan	16 mg (M) 14 mg (F)
B_6	Meat, liver, poultry, fish, whole-grain cereal products, potatoes, legumes, green leafy vegetables, dairy products**, bananas, nuts	1.3 mg (M, F)
B_{12}	Meat, fish, shellfish, poultry, liver, eggs, dairy products**, fortified breakfast cereals	2.4 µg (M, F)
Folic acid	Meat, liver, green leafy vegetables, whole-grain cereal products, potatoes, legumes, nuts, fruit	400 µg (M, F)
Biotin	Meat, milk, egg yolk, whole-grain cereal products, legumes, most vegetables	30 µg* (M, F)
Pantothenic acid	Liver, meat, dairy products**, eggs, whole-grain cereal products, legumes, most vegetables	5 mg* (M, F)
C	Citrus fruits, green leafy vegetables, broccoli, potatoes, peppers, strawberries	90 mg (M) 75 mg (F)

*Denotes AI values; other values are RDAs. M = male; F = female.

**Dairy products include milk, cream, butter, and cheese.

have problems obtaining sufficient intakes of some vitamins, particularly vitamin B_{12}, for which the only natural dietary source is meat. Fortunately, in Western countries, milk and several breakfast cereals are fortified with vitamin B_{12}, so this potential problem can be overcome by appropriate food selection and vitamin supplementation. An important and unique issue with vitamin D is that, unlike all the other fat- and water-soluble vitamins, it (specifically vitamin D_3 or cholecalciferol) can be synthesized in the skin from cholesterol when exposure from sunlight ultraviolet B (UVB) radiation is adequate. Evidence indicates the synthesis of vitamin D from sunlight exposure is regulated by a negative feedback loop that prevents toxicity, but because of uncertainty about the cancer risk from overexposure to sunlight, no recommendations are currently issued by national bodies regarding the amount of sunlight exposure required to meet vitamin D requirements. Accordingly, the RDA of

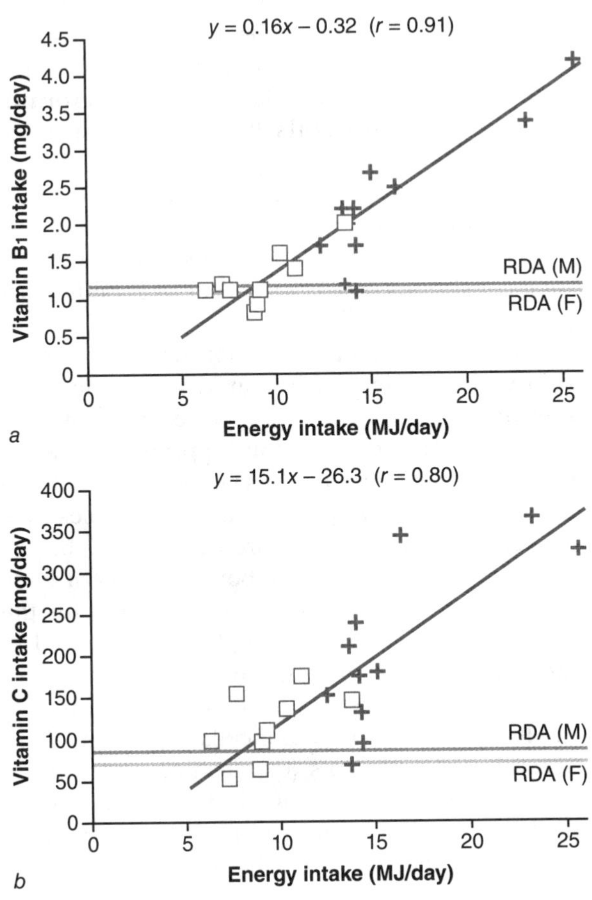

Figure 10.1 The relationship between mean intake of dietary energy and *(a)* vitamin B_1 and *(b)* vitamin C intake in male (crosses) and female (squares) athletes. Each point represents a mean value for a group.

Data from van Erp-Baart (1989a); Fogelholm (1994a).

vitamin D for adults (5 μg or 200 IU in the European Union and 15 μg or 600 IU in the United States) assumes that no synthesis occurs and all of a person's vitamin D is from food intake, although that will rarely occur in practice. Recent studies indicate that in the winter months, many people (including athletes) can become deficient in vitamin D (He et al. 2016).

Vitamin losses in sweat are negligible, and no increased vitamin excretion in urine and feces of athletes is evident. Temporary increases in the plasma concentrations of some vitamins (e.g., vitamin C [as shown in figure 10.2], vitamin E, and vitamin B_6, as pyridoxal 5′-phosphate) have been reported after an acute bout of exercise, which may reflect a redistribution of labile pools of these vitamins. In general, however, vitamin turnover seems to be remarkably unaffected by exercise.

Physical training may increase vitamin B_2 and vitamin B_6 requirements, which may be a consequence of increased retention of these vitamins in skeletal muscle. Adaptations to regular prolonged exercise include an increased number of mitochondria in skeletal muscles and increased oxidative enzyme activity, which might explain the increased retention of vitamins that are cofactors in energy metabolism within the muscle. Because of the increased free-radical production during exercise compared with the resting state, an increased intake of antioxidant vitamins (C, E, and beta-carotene) may be desirable for those who engage in regular physical activity. A free radical is an atom or molecule that possess at least one unpaired electron in its outer orbit. The free radicals produced by oxidation in the mitochondria include superoxide ($\cdot O_2^-$), hydroxyl ($\cdot OH$), and nitric oxide ($\cdot NO$). These radical species are highly reactive and directly target lipid membrane structures by lipid peroxidation, causing membrane instability and increased permeability. Free radicals can also cause oxidative damage to proteins including enzymes and DNA.

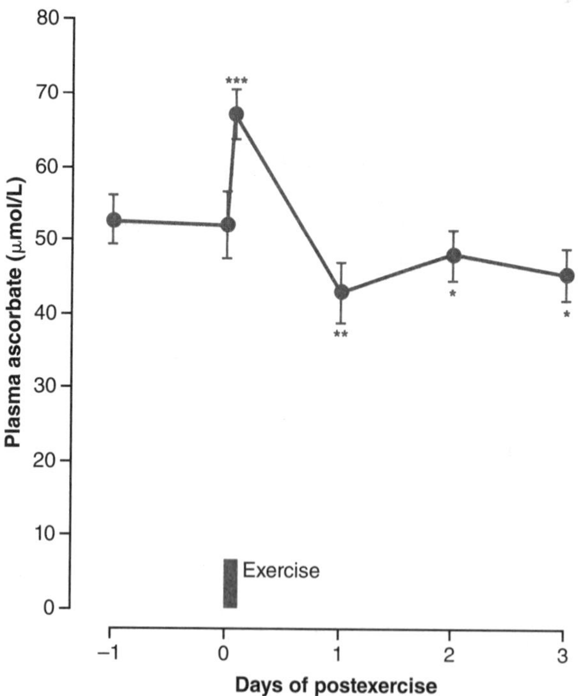

Figure 10.2 The effect of running a 21 km (13 mi) road race on the plasma concentration of vitamin C (ascorbate). Data are means ± SEM from nine subjects. Statistical significance of differences of means compared with the immediately preexercise value on day 0: $*P < 0.05$, $**P < 0.01$, $***P < 0.001$.

Reproduced by permission from M. Gleeson, J.D. Robertson, and R.J. Maughan, *Clinical Science* 73, (1987): 501-505. Copyright © The Biochemical Society and the Medical Research Society.

Macrominerals and Microminerals

A mineral is an inorganic compound found in nature, and the term is usually reserved for solid compounds. In nutrition, the term *mineral* usually refers to the dietary constituents essential to life processes. Minerals are classified as **macrominerals** or **microminerals** (trace elements) based on the extent of their occurrence in the body and the amounts needed in the diet. The seven macrominerals are potassium, sodium, chloride, calcium, magnesium, phosphorus, and sulfur, and each constitutes at least 0.01% of total body mass (see table 10.5).

Inadequate mineral nutrition has been associated with a variety of human diseases including **anemia**, cancer, diabetes, hypertension, osteoporosis, and tooth decay. Thus, appropriate dietary intake of essential minerals is necessary for optimal health and physical performance (see tables 10.6 and 10.7). Some minerals are the building blocks for body tissues including bones and teeth (e.g., calcium, phosphorus), some are essential for the normal function of enzymes that are involved in the regulation of metabolism (e.g., magnesium, copper, zinc), and some have an essential role in the functioning of immune cells (e.g., iron, zinc). Several other minerals (e.g., sodium, potassium, chloride) exist as ions or electrolytes dissolved in the intracellular and extracellular fluids. Like vitamins, minerals cannot be used as a source of energy.

TABLE 10.5 Adult Total Body Content and Body Fluid Concentrations of Macrominerals

				BODY FLUID CONCENTRATION (MG/L)		
Macromineral	**Symbol**	**Atomic weight**	**Total amount in body (mg)**	**Plasma**	**Sweat**	**Urine**
Calcium	Ca	40	1,500,000	85-105	0-40	100-180
Chloride	Cl	35.5	75,000	3,400-3,900	700-2,100	5,000-7,500
Magnesium	Mg	24	25,000	16-30	4-15	60-100
Potassium	K	39	180,000	130-220	160-320	800-3,200
Phosphorus	P	31	850,000	20-50	3-6	20-1,100
Sodium	Na	23	65,000	3,000-3,500	460-1,840	2,500-5,000

Electrolyte concentrations in interstitial fluid are virtually identical to those in plasma.

TABLE 10.6 Major Functions of Macrominerals and the Effects of Dietary Deficiency or Excess

Macromineral	Major roles in the body	Effects of deficiency	Effects of excess
Calcium	Promotes bone and teeth formation, muscle contraction, membrane potentials, and nerve impulse transmission; regulates enzyme activity	Osteoporosis, brittle bones, impaired muscle contraction, muscle cramps	Impaired trace metal absorption, cardiac arrhythmia, constipation, kidney stones, calcification of soft tissue
Chloride	Promotes nerve impulse conduction and hydrochloric acid formation in the stomach	Convulsions*	Hypertension**
Magnesium	Promotes protein synthesis and metalloenzyme, ATPases, and 2,3-diphosphoglycerate (DPG) formation; bone component	Muscle weakness, fatigue, apathy, muscle tremor, cramps	Nausea, vomiting, diarrhea
Potassium	Promotes membrane potential, nerve impulse generation, muscle contraction, acid–base balance	Hypokalemia, muscle cramps, apathy, loss of appetite, irregular heartbeat	Hyperkalemia, cardiac arrhythmia, cardiac failure
Phosphorus	Promotes bone formation; buffer in muscle contraction; component of ATP, PCr, NADP, DNA, RNA, and cell membranes	Osteoporosis, brittle bones, muscle weakness, muscle cramps	Impaired iron, zinc, and copper absorption; impaired calcium metabolism
Sodium	Promotes blood volume homeostasis, nerve impulse generation, muscle contraction, acid–base balance	Hyponatremia, dizziness, coma, muscle cramps, nausea, vomiting, loss of appetite, seizures	Hypertension, nausea
Sulfur	Acid–base balance; liver function	Unknown and extremely unlikely to occur	Unknown

*In rare instances, chloride deficiency can be caused by excess vomiting.

**In conjunction with excess sodium.

Recommended Intakes of Minerals

At least 20 mineral elements are known to be essential for humans, and 14 trace elements have been identified as essential for maintenance of health. Besides those listed in table 10.7, trace amounts of arsenic, nickel, silicon, tin, and vanadium may also be essential, but deficiencies or excesses (because of dietary sources) for these micronutrients are extremely rare. Deficiencies of one or more of the trace elements result in symptoms of disease, and many deficiencies are also associated with immune dysfunction and increased incidence of infection (see table 10.7).

The RDA has been established for seven minerals, and the AI is available for five others (see tables 10.8 and 10.9). Estimated mineral requirements have been proposed for potassium, sodium, and chloride. Each of the trace elements (e.g., iron, zinc, copper, chromium, selenium) constitutes less than 0.01% of total body mass (see table 10.10) and is needed in a quantity of less than 100 mg/day.

TABLE 10.7 Major Functions of Microminerals (Trace Elements) and the Effects of Dietary Deficiency or Excess

Micromineral	Major roles in body	Effects of deficiency	Effects of excess
Chromium	Augments insulin action	Glucose intolerance, impaired lipid metabolism	Rare toxic effects
Cobalt	Forms component of vitamin B_{12} needed for red blood cell development	Pernicious anemia	Nausea, vomiting, death
Copper	Promotes normal iron absorption, oxidative metabolism, connective tissue formation, hemoglobin synthesis; forms cofactor with superoxide dismutase	Anemia, impaired immune function, bone demineralization	Nausea, vomiting
Fluorine	Promotes bone and teeth formation	Dental caries	Discolored teeth, inhibited glycolysis in high doses
Iodine	Forms component of thyroid hormones T3 and T4	Goiter, reduced metabolic rate	Depressed thyroid gland activity
Iron	Transports oxygen as hemoglobin and myoglobin; forms cytochromes and metalloenzymes; promotes immune function	Anemia, fatigue, increased infections	Hemochromatosis, liver cirrhosis, heart disease, increased infections
Manganese	Forms cofactor with energy metabolism enzymes; promotes bone formation and fat synthesis	Poor growth	Weakness, confusion
Molybdenum	Forms cofactor with riboflavin in carbohydrate and fat metabolism enzymes	No deficiency effects	Rare toxic effects
Selenium	Forms cofactor with glutathione peroxidase	Cardiomyopathy, cancer, heart disease, impaired immune function, erythrocyte fragility	Nausea, vomiting, fatigue, hair loss
Zinc	Forms metalloenzymes; promotes protein synthesis, immune function, tissue repair, energy metabolism, and antioxidant activity	Impaired growth, impaired healing, increased infections, anorexia	Impaired absorption of iron and copper, increased HDL to LDL cholesterol ratio, anemia, nausea, vomiting, impaired immunity

TABLE 10.8 Sources and Recommended Daily Allowances or Adequate Intakes of Macrominerals for Adults 19 to 50 Years of Age

Macromineral	Sources	RDA or AI	Percent absorbed***
Calcium	Dairy products**, egg yolk, beans, peas, dark green vegetables, cauliflower	1,000 mg* (M, F)	30-40
Chloride	Meat, fish, bread, canned foods, table salt, beans, milk	2,300 mg* (M, F)	90-99
Magnesium	Seafood, nuts, green leafy vegetables, fruit, whole-grain products, milk, yogurt	420 mg (M) 320 mg (F)	25-60
Potassium	Meat, fish, milk, yogurt, fruit, vegetables, bread	4,700 mg* (M, F)	90-99
Phosphorus	Meat, eggs, fish, milk, cheese, beans, peas, whole-grain products, soft drinks	700 mg (M, F)	80-90
Sodium	Meat, fish, bread, canned foods, table salt, sauces, pickles	1,500 mg* (M, F)	90-99

*Denotes AI values; other values are RDAs. M = male; F = female. **Dairy products include milk, cream, butter, and cheese. ***This is the portion of the ingested amount that is absorbed; the remainder is excreted in the feces.

TABLE 10.9 Sources and Recommended Daily Allowances or Adequate Intakes of Microminerals for Adults 19 to 50 Years of Age

Micromineral	Sources	RDA or AI	Percent absorbed***
Chromium	Liver, kidney, meat, oysters, cheese, whole-grain products, beer, asparagus, mushrooms, nuts, stainless steel cookware	35 µg* (M) 25 µg* (F)	<1
Cobalt	Meat, liver, milk	As part of vitamin B_{12}	Unknown
Copper	Liver, kidney, shellfish, meat, fish, poultry, eggs, bran cereals, nuts, legumes, broccoli, bananas, avocados, chocolate	0.9 mg (M, F)	20-50
Fluorine	Milk, egg yolk, seafood, drinking water	4 mg* (M) 3 mg* (F)	Unknown
Iodine	Iodized salt, seafood, vegetables	150 µg (M, F)	Unknown
Iron	Liver, kidney, eggs, red meat, seafood, oysters, bread, flour, molasses, dried legumes, nuts, leafy green vegetables, broccoli, figs, raisins, cocoa	8 mg (M) 18 mg (F)	10-30 (heme iron) 2-10 (nonheme iron)
Manganese	Whole grains, peas, beans, leafy vegetables, bananas	2.3 mg* (M) 1.8 mg*(F)	Unknown
Molybdenum	Liver, kidney, whole-grain products, peas, beans	45 µg (M, F)	Unknown
Selenium	Meat, liver, kidney, poultry, fish, dairy products**, seafood, whole grains, nuts from selenium-rich soil	55 µg (M, F)	Unknown
Zinc	Oysters, shellfish, beef, liver, poultry, dairy products, whole grains, vegetables, asparagus, spinach	11 mg (M) 8 mg (F)	20-50

*Denotes AI values; other values are RDAs. M = male; F = female. **Dairy products include milk, cream, butter, and cheese. ***This is the portion of the ingested amount that is absorbed (where known); the remainder is excreted in the feces.

TABLE 10.10 Adult Total Body Content and Body Fluid Concentrations of Microminerals (Trace Elements)

				BODY FLUID CONCENTRATION (MG/L)		
Micromineral	**Symbol**	**Atomic weight**	**Total amount in body (mg)**	**Plasma**	**Sweat**	**Urine**
Chromium	Cr	52	6			
Cobalt	Co	59	<1			
Copper	Cu	64	100	0.7-1.7	0.2-0.6	0.03-0.04
Fluorine	F	19	2,500			
Iodine	I	127	11			
Iron	Fe	56	5,000	0.4-1.4	0.3-0.4	0.1-0.15
Manganese	Mn	55	12			
Molybdenum	Mo	96	9			
Selenium	Se	79	13			
Zinc	Zn	65	2,000	0.7-1.3	0.7-1.3	0.2-0.5

Electrolyte concentrations in interstitial fluid are virtually identical to those in plasma. *Values are only shown when the concentration of the mineral is greater than 0.1 mg/L.

Critical Micronutrient Functions

Micronutrients not only form the building blocks of tissues but also function as antioxidants and perform or are associated with a variety of functions that are essential to the maintenance of life and health including oxygen transport, enzyme-catalyzed reactions, immunity, muscle contraction, and nerve impulse conduction.

Micronutrients Form the Building Blocks of Tissues

Although vitamins are not structural components in body tissues, several minerals including calcium, phosphorus, and fluorine are, particularly in bones and teeth. Vitamin D is required for the normal absorption of dietary calcium, and deficiency of this vitamin is associated with brittle bones. Vitamin C is required for normal production of collagen and hence is important for the maintenance of healthy connective tissue and cartilage.

The mineral in bone is calcium phosphate crystalline salts in the form of hydroxyapatite. Bone matrix is a mixture of collagen fibers, which resist pulling forces, and solid hydroxyapatite crystals, which resist compression. Bone tissue is not metabolically inert. Even in adults, bone undergoes continuous turnover and remodeling of the matrix with simultaneous release and uptake of calcium. The cells involved in bone formation are osteoblasts, and the cells responsible for breakdown (demineralization) are osteoclasts (see figure 10.3). When the rate of demineralization exceeds the rate of bone formation, osteoporosis, which is a weakening of the bone structure, occurs.

The hormones calcitonin and parathyroid hormone (PTH) are principally involved in the regulation of calcium metabolism in bone tissue. Their main actions are shown in figure 10.3. Calcitonin is released from the thyroid gland and stimulates bone formation when the plasma concentration of calcium rises. PTH stimulates bone demineralization when calcium levels in blood are low. PTH and ultraviolet radiation from sunlight also stimulate production in the skin of the active form of vitamin D, which promotes the uptake of calcium in the small intestine. Studies indicate that during the winter months, athletes who live at latitudes above 35° N do not get sufficient sunlight to synthesize vitamin D_3 in their skin and consequently may develop inadequate or deficient vitamin D status (Owens, Fraser, and Close 2015). This is a particular concern for bone health in growing adolescents and infection risk in adults. Vitamin D is mainly obtained through exposure of the skin to UVB through sunlight, and a small amount typically comes from the diet. Vitamin D needs to be hydroxylated twice to achieve the biologically active form 1, 25 dihydroxy vitamin

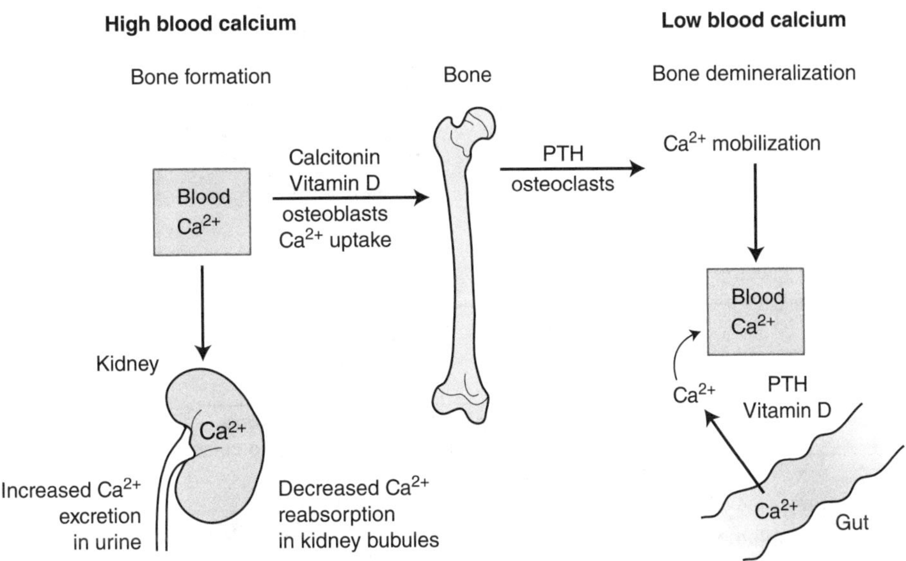

Figure 10.3 Bone formation and demineralization in calcium homeostasis.

D (1, 25(OH)$_2$D). The endogenously synthesized vitamin D_3 and diet-derived D_2 and D_3 are first hydroxylated in the liver into 25(OH)D (calcidiol or calcifediol) by the enzyme 25-hydroxylase (figure 10.4). The main storage form of vitamin D, 25(OH)D, is found in muscles and adipose tissue, and 25(OH)D is the major circulating metabolite of vitamin D with a half-life of 2 to 3 weeks. Therefore, the total plasma concentration of 25(OH)D is considered to be the primary indicator of vitamin D status (Bendik et al. 2014). In the second hydroxylation, 25(OH)D is converted in the kidney to the biologically active form, 1, 25(OH)$_2$D (calcitriol or calciferol), by 1-α-hydroxylase, an enzyme that is stimulated by PTH when serum calcium and phosphate concentrations fall below their normal physiological ranges of 2.1 to 2.6 mmol/L and 1.0 to 1.5 mmol/L, respectively. Then, 1, 25(OH)$_2$D is released into the circulation from the kidney, which is considered as a vital endocrine source of hormone. Some cells other than kidney cells also express 1-α-hydroxylase and have the enzymatic machinery to convert 25(OH)D to 1, 25(OH)$_2$D in nonrenal compartments including epithelial cells and some cells of the acquired immune system (T lymphocytes, monocytes, macrophages, and dendritic cells) as illustrated in figure 10.4. These cells also secrete 1, 25(OH)$_2$D locally to exert paracrine effects on other immune cells including those involved in innate immunity (neutrophils and natural killer cells). The actions of 1, 25(OH)$_2$D on immune cells are generally stimulatory and activate antimicrobial activity.

Importantly, 1, 25(OH)$_2$D limits its own activity in a negative feedback loop by inducing 24-hydroxylase, which converts 1, 25(OH)$_2$D into the biologically inactive metabolite 1, 24, 25(OH)$_3$D. In addition, 1, 25(OH)$_2$D inhibits the expression of renal 1-α-hydroxylase, which reduces the likelihood of hypercalcemia by preventing excessive vitamin D signaling, thus maintaining bone health, and it exerts its biological actions by acting as a modulator of more than 900 genes (Aranow 2011). Circulating 11, 25(OH)$_2$D passes through the plasma membrane of target cells and binds to the vitamin D receptor (VDR) in the cytoplasm, which activates its other function as a transcription factor. Binding of 1, 25(OH)$_2$D to the VDR activates transcription by linkage with the retinoid X receptor (RXR), which translocates to the nucleus, where it binds to vitamin D response elements located in the regulatory regions of 1, 25(OH)$_2$D target genes and then induces expression of the vitamin D responsive genes, which include the gut and bone calcium ion transporters (Aranow 2011).

Calcium intake influences the development of osteoporosis. Among different groups of athletes, calcium intake is closely related to total energy intake (see figure 10.5). Other factors that influence the development of osteoporosis are estrogen levels, alcohol and caffeine intakes, family history, female gender, and the amount and type of physical activity (Aulin 2000). In the prevention of osteoporosis, emphasis should be on maximizing the body's stores of calcium at an early age and minimizing calcium loss. A calcium intake of 1,000 to 1,300 mg/day is recommended to protect against

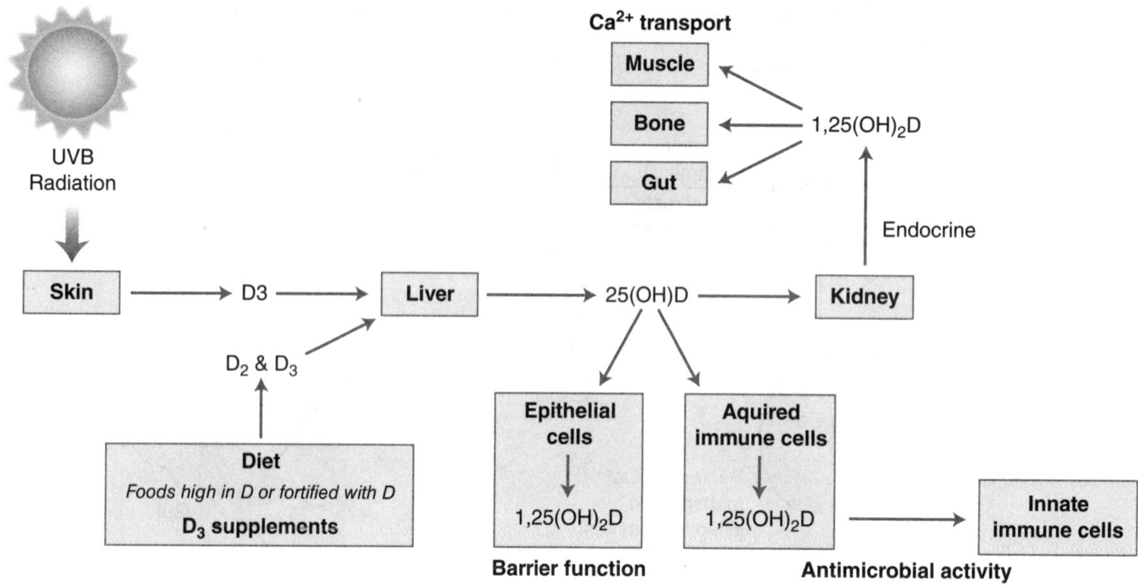

Figure 10.4 A summary of vitamin D metabolism and actions in the body illustrating how vitamin D can influence acquired and innate immunity.

Adapted from He et al. (2016).

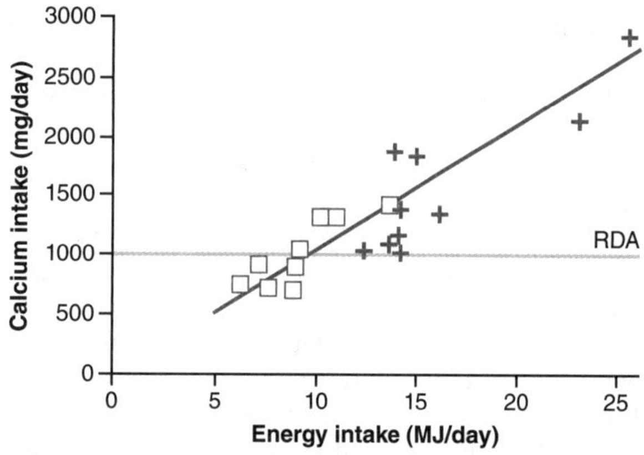

Figure 10.5 The relationship between mean intake of dietary energy and calcium intake in male (crosses) and female (squares) athletes. Each point represents a mean value for a group.

Data from van Erp-Baart (1989a).

the development of osteoporosis. The performance of regular weight-bearing activity promotes the deposition of calcium in bone.

Calcium status is difficult to assess since there are no serum markers of acute calcium intake. Given the fundamental role of calcium as a signal for skeletal muscle and cardiac contraction it is not surprising that serum calcium concentration is tightly regulated within a narrow range regardless of acute calcium intake. Adequate dietary intake of calcium is essential; however, this presents many problems since dietary intake assessment is required and the calcium content of foods is highly variable. Given the rise in vegan athletes, the assessment of calcium intake is particularly important. Calcium may also be lost through sweat and particular attention should therefore be given to athletes training or competing in hot environments. If supplements are to be used, calcium carbonate and calcium citrate are well absorbed, although it has been suggested that calcium absorption plateaus at about 500 mg; therefore, intake should be spread throughout the day rather than in one big dose.

Several groups of athletes can be identified as possibly having insufficient dietary intake of minerals and calcium (see table 10.11), and an insufficient intake of calcium increases the risk of osteoporosis. The absence of menstruation (amenorrhea) or infrequent menstruation (oligomenorrhea), which are commonly associated with low levels of body fat, low energy intake, and high physical activity (especially gymnastics, swimming, and long-distance running), are associated with a high risk of early osteoporosis because of the chronically low plasma estrogen levels (Aulin 2000). This condition, which forms part of the female athlete triad syndrome (also known as relative energy deficiency in sports) and can be precipitated by eating disorders, is discussed in detail in chapter 16. The steroid hormone estrogen promotes bone

TABLE 10.11 Risk Factors for Marginal Mineral Nutrition in Athletes

Conditions and causes	Sports
Low body weight: chronically low energy intake to achieve low body weight	Gymnastics, horse racing, ballet, ice dancing, dancing
Making competition weight: drastic weight-loss regimens to achieve desired weight category	Weight-class sports (rowing, wrestling, boxing, judo)
Low fat: drastic weight-loss regimens to achieve low body fat	Bodybuilding
Vegetarian diets	Endurance events
Training in hot, humid conditions	Endurance events

formation in women; in men, the hormone testosterone assumes this role. In young female athletes, amenorrhea may hinder bone growth at a time when bone should be forming at its maximum rate. Side effects, such as the increased risk of stress fractures, could hinder athletic performance and cause potentially debilitating problems later in life. When amenorrhea is present, increasing the consumption of calcium to 120% of the RDA appears to help maintain bone density and aid in proper development (Aulin 2000).

Nutrition guidance should be given to low-body-weight amenorrheic women. Weight-conscious athletes (e.g., gymnasts) may markedly reduce their consumption of dairy products to decrease their intake of dietary fat. Because the main sources of calcium are milk, butter, and cheese, their intake of calcium may fall considerably below the RDA. Most low-fat dairy products (e.g., skim milk) contain similar amounts of calcium as full-fat dairy products, so athletes should be encouraged to include low-fat dairy products in their diets to preserve calcium intake.

Phosphorus, in the form of phosphate salts, is the other major inorganic constituent of bones and teeth. The adult male body contains about 850 g of phosphorus, of which 80% is found in bone. Phosphorus is also found as a component of nucleic acids (DNA and RNA) and phospholipids, which form the lipid bilayer of cell membranes. The RDA for adolescents and young adults (aged 9-18 years) is 1,250 mg of phosphorus; for persons older than 19 years, the requirement is 700 mg. Phosphorus deficiency is rare because many food items contain substantial amounts of it.

Fluorine is necessary for the normal formation of healthy bones and teeth, and it protects against dental caries (tooth decay by oral bacteria). Frequent intakes of soft drinks and carbohydrate, particularly sugars, depress the pH in the mouth and cause a net demineralization of the teeth. Sugars in the mouth are metabolized to organic acids by bacteria in plaque. Given the relatively high intake of sugary foods and sports drinks by athletes, good oral hygiene and plaque control are important. The RDA for fluorine is 3 to 4 mg/day, and this trace element is found in milk, egg yolk, and seafood. Several toothpastes and mouth rinses contain fluorine (as sodium fluoride), and in some countries, including the United States, fluoride is added to drinking water. Excess intake of fluoride is poisonous because of its inhibitory effects on a number of enzymes, including some of the enzymes of glycolysis.

Several other trace elements have been suggested to be capable of increasing lean body mass. Boron supplementation has been reported to increase the serum estrogen and testosterone concentrations in postmenopausal women; subsequent studies found no effect on serum testosterone, lean body mass, or muscle strength in male athletes who took boron supplements. Chromium is also claimed to increase lean body mass through potentiating insulin action. Insulin promotes glucose and amino acid uptake into muscle and stimulates muscle protein synthesis. Most studies, however, show that chromium supplements are not effective in increasing lean body mass, and chromium supplementation is accompanied by increased urinary excretion of chromium. Chromium stores are unlikely to be inadequate in people who consume a well-balanced diet, because chromium is widely available in fruits, vegetables, cereals, and organ meats.

Vanadium appears to increase tissue sensitivity to insulin in individuals suffering from type 2 (non-insulin-dependent) diabetes, but to date, no studies have established whether vanadium compounds exhibit insulin-like actions such as promoting muscle protein and glycogen synthesis. A study showed no effect of vanadium on insulin sensitivity in healthy people assessed by an oral glucose tolerance test (Jentjens and Jeukendrup 2002). (See chapter 11 for details of studies that have investigated the effects of boron, chromium, and vanadium supplementation.)

Micronutrients as Antioxidants

Antioxidants prevent or limit the actions of free radicals usually by removing their unpaired electron and thus converting them into something far less reactive. Vitamins with antioxidant properties (including vitamins C, E, and beta-carotene [provitamin A]) may be required in increased quantities in athletes to inactivate the products of exercise-induced increased free-radical formation and **lipid peroxidation**. Free radicals damage membranes, proteins, and DNA. Damage to DNA could result in mutations that cause cancer. Several minerals (including selenium, copper, and manganese) are components of antioxidant enzymes involved in the defense against free radicals. Increased intake of antioxidant vitamins and other antioxidant compounds has been suggested to reduce the extent of exercise-induced muscle damage. Current evidence is not convincing, however, so more studies of the effects of antioxidants on exercise-induced muscle soreness and damage are needed.

Antioxidant Protection Against Exercise-Induced Skeletal Muscle Damage

Unaccustomed exercise or muscle activity that involves eccentric actions (lengthening of the muscle during activation) can damage some of the myofibers. Such exercises include downhill running, bench stepping, and lowering of weights. The consequences of exercise-induced muscle damage include muscle pain, soreness, and stiffness; reduced range of motion; higher than normal blood lactate concentration and perceived exertion during exercise; and loss of strength and reduced maximal dynamic power output that can last 5 to 10 days. Exercise-induced muscle damage also impairs the restoration of muscle glycogen stores. Damaged muscle has an impaired ability to take up glucose from the blood, which is required to resynthesize glycogen in the muscle. This condition results in decreased endurance performance in subsequent exercise bouts.

A practical index of muscle damage in athletes who perform heavy training is elevated muscle proteins (e.g., myoglobin, CK, lactate dehydrogenase) in the blood plasma. The damaged muscle tissue causes an initial activation of the immune system as white blood cells are attracted to the damaged muscles to begin breakdown of damaged fibers and initiate the repair process. This process involves the production of free-radical **reactive oxygen species (ROS)** by the invading leukocytes. Growing evidence indicates that ROS are an underlying cause of disrupted muscle homeostasis, muscle soreness, and elevated CK activity in eccentric type exercise. ROS can also cause oxidative damage to DNA and proteins, including enzymes.

Reactive Oxygen Species and Other Free Radicals

In normal cellular metabolism, small amounts of ROS are produced during the aerobic process by which humans and animals derive energy from the mitochondria. In the electron-transport chain located on the inner mitochondrial membrane, most of the oxygen consumed by cells is reduced by cytochrome oxidase to yield water (and energy that is used to resynthesize ATP from ADP and Pi). But a small proportion, estimated to be about 0.15% of the total oxygen consumed at rest (Powers and Jackson 2008), can be used in an alternate pathway for the univalent reduction of oxygen; thus, ROS are produced. Note that earlier studies suggested that this proportion was as high as 3% to 5% of the total oxygen consumed (more than 10-fold higher than the current accepted value) (St-Pierre et al. 2002). One free-radical molecule can start a destructive process by removing electrons from stable compounds, such as polyunsaturated FAs, and forming large numbers of ROS, thereby transforming stable compounds into highly reactive free radicals.

Additional sources of ROS and other free radicals are ultraviolet light, alcohol, cigarette smoke, high-fat diets, and the respiratory burst of white blood cells, such as neutrophils and monocytes, that are capable of ingesting foreign material, including bacteria. The generation of ROS by the neutrophil respiratory burst is an essential mechanism of the host defense mechanism of the immune system for killing bacteria and clearing away damaged tissue. But these ROS can also initiate damaging chain reactions, such as lipid peroxidation, and the subsequent release of large numbers of ROS. In addition to the production of free radicals by the mitochondrial respiratory chain during whole-body eccentric exercise, invading neutrophils and monocytes are thought to be important sources of oxidative stress. Several inflammatory diseases have been associated with increased generation of ROS by monocytes. Migration of neutrophils into damaged muscle tissue occurs within the first hour after eccentric exercise and is followed by infiltration of monocytes and macrophages, reaching a maximum at 24 to 72 hours after exercise.

Increases in the free iron concentration of body fluids (caused, for example, by hemolysis or ischemia followed by reperfusion) may amplify ROS toxicity by increasing the generation of the highly reactive hydroxyl radical. Ferric iron (Fe^{3+}) ions can stimulate free-radical reactions by breaking down lipid peroxides to chain-breaking alkoxyl radicals, and ferrous (Fe^{2+}) ions can react with hydrogen peroxide (H_2O_2) to produce ·OH and other highly reactive species in what is called a Fenton reaction:

$$Fe^{2+} + H_2O_2 \rightarrow Fe^{3+} + \cdot OH + OH^-$$

The hydroxyl radical can also be formed through the Haber-Weiss reaction:

$$Fe^{2+} + H_2O_2 + \cdot O_2^- \rightarrow Fe^{3+} + \cdot OH + OH^- + O_2$$

This potential is one of the reasons that iron supplements should not be recommended indiscriminately. Free radicals have been implicated in the etiology of various diseases, including cancer and coronary heart disease, and an excess of iron could potentiate their adverse effects. Excess iron intake may also increase the risk of hemochromatosis.

Reactive Oxygen Species Production by Exercising Muscle

The first serious studies of the generation and potential roles of ROS during exercise were carried out in the late 1970s. During the ensuing years, a great deal of research has been undertaken to try to understand the nature and sources of the species generated, the factors influencing their generation, their effects on muscle and other cells, and how these effects might be manipulated. An assumption that has underpinned much of the work since the early studies is that the species generated are essentially by-products of metabolism and are damaging to cells and tissues. Note that even the earliest studies in the area attempted to scavenge the species generated and look for potential functional benefits of such interventions. Unsurprisingly, early studies were also characterized by limitations in the analytical methods available to detect free-radical species. Nonspecific approaches—for example, the analysis of lipid peroxides such as malondialdehyde or thiobarbituric acid reactive species (TBARS) in complex biological tissues—were commonly used. The early studies reported that the predominant source for formation of free radicals during exercise is from leakage from the electron-transport chain in the mitochondria (as much as 3% to 5% of the total oxygen consumed by mitochondria was suggested to undergo one electron reduction with the generation of superoxide). It was assumed that this source of ROS production was directly related to the rate of oxygen uptake by muscle tissue, which can increase up to 100-fold during exercise compared with rest. This assumption, of course, implies that potentially a 100-fold increase in superoxide generation by skeletal muscle could occur during aerobic exercise. These assumptions became firmly rooted and extensively quoted in the subsequent literature, but more recent research in this area has not supported them (Jackson 2007; Powers and Jackson 2008).

Since 2000, the development of improved techniques has established that the primary ROS generated by skeletal muscle are nitric oxide and superoxide. Mitochondria are cited as the major site of superoxide generation in tissues, but some recent findings have argued against the previously high estimates of rates of formation of superoxide within mitochondria. The most recent estimates of the rate of production of ROS by mitochondria indicate that no more than about 0.15% of the electron flow gives rise to ROS (i.e., less than 10% of the original minimum estimate), and it is becoming increasingly clear that even this low rate of production may be further reduced by intrinsic control mechanisms. As for exercise, the most recent data indicate that muscle intracellular ROS production increases by only a modest two- to fourfold during contractions (Jackson 2007), which seems to support the suggestion that there is considerable internal control of mitochondrial ROS generation.

Studies have identified the reduced nicotinamide adenine dinucleotide phosphate (NADPH) oxidase enzymes associated with the sarcoplasmic reticulum (SR) of cardiac and skeletal muscle as additional sources of ROS. The superoxide generated by these enzymes seems to influence calcium release by the SR through oxidation of the ryanodyne receptor. An NADPH oxidase somewhat similar to that found in phagocytic cells of the immune system has also been described; this is located in the plasma membrane, triads, and transverse tubules of skeletal muscle and is activated by membrane depolarization. Many studies have indicated that skeletal muscle cells release superoxide into the extracellular space and that nonmuscle cells contain other plasma membrane redox systems capable of undertaking electron transfer across the plasma membrane to effect transfer of electrons from intracellular reductants to appropriate extracellular electron acceptors (Jackson 2007). Other enzyme systems that can generate ROS in skeletal muscle tissue include phospholipases and xanthine oxidase. Skeletal muscle fibers themselves have been reported not to contain significant amounts of xanthine oxidase, although this enzyme will inevitably be present in associated endothelial cells of the blood vessels in muscle tissue.

Thus, skeletal muscle has multiple potential sites for generation of ROS, and data are increasingly casting doubt about whether mitochondria are the major dominant site for ROS generation in skeletal muscle during contractile activity. In particular, the inability to detect an increase in intracellular ROS activity at the levels predicted by the original studies of mitochondrial ROS generation and the increasing debate about the degree of internal regulation of mitochondrial ROS generation contrast sharply with the observations that superoxide is specifically generated by nonmitochondrial systems (such as the transverse tubule-localized NAD(P)H oxidase enzymes) in response to physiological stimuli. These nonmitochondrial ROS generation systems are clearly stimulated by physiological processes and seem to be linked to signaling processes acting to modify muscle gene expression and adaptations to exercise. The various potential pathways of ROS generation within muscle are illustrated in figure 10.6. The old view that ROS are by-products of metabolism and have only a deleterious effect on muscle function is now replaced by the concept that specific ROS are generated in a controlled manner by skeletal muscle fibers in response to physiological stimuli and play important roles in the physiological adaptations of muscle to contractions. These roles include optimization of contractile performance and initiation of key changes in gene expression that result in muscle training adaptations.

Antioxidant Mechanisms

An antioxidant is a compound that protects biological systems against the harmful effects or reactions that create excessive oxidants. Dietary antioxidants significantly decrease the adverse effects of ROS. Enzymatic and nonenzymatic antioxidants prevent oxidation initiated by ROS by

- preventing ROS formation;
- intercepting ROS attack by scavenging the reactive metabolites and converting them to less-reactive molecules;
- binding transition metal ion catalysts, such as copper and iron, to prevent initiation of free-radical reactions;
- reacting with chain-propagating radicals, such as the peroxyl and alkoyl species, to prevent continued hydrogen abstraction from FA side chains; and
- providing a favorable environment for the effective functioning of other antioxidants or acting to regenerate the nonenzymatic antioxidant molecules.

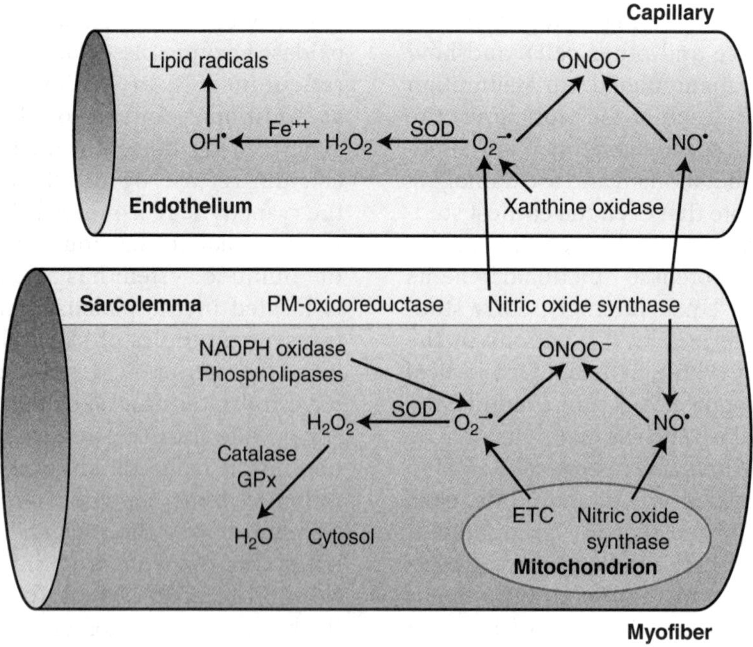

Figure 10.6 Simplified diagram of the processes that contribute to ROS generation in exercising muscle.

Antioxidant enzymes can affect free-radical generation at the initiation and propagation stages. The antioxidant enzymes superoxide dismutase (SOD) and catalase can inhibit the initial phase by inactivating precursor molecules of ROS production (see figure 10.7). At the propagation stage, glutathione peroxidase, another antioxidant enzyme, can scavenge $\cdot OH$ and lipid peroxides as described earlier. The trace elements copper and manganese are required as cofactors of SOD, and selenium is also a component of antioxidant defense because it is a cofactor of glutathione peroxidase–reductase and thus influences the quenching of ROS. The effects of exercise on manganese and selenium status are presently unknown, but training is associated with increased levels of antioxidant enzymes, which suggests there may be an increased requirement for these trace elements during periods of increased training. As with other minerals, losses of manganese and selenium in urine and sweat are likely higher in athletes than in nonathletes. Any supplements, however, should be taken with caution. Selenium supplements of amounts up to the RDA appear nontoxic, but the safety of larger doses has not been confirmed, and intakes of 25 mg (approximately 40 times the RDA) have been associated with vomiting, abdominal pain, hair loss, and fatigue.

Besides the enzyme defense system, some low-molecular-weight substances act as scavengers of radicals. These substances include vitamins A, C, and E; carotenoids such as beta-carotene; and compounds such as plant **polyphenols**. Fat-soluble vitamin E is a chain-breaking free-radical scavenger and is particularly effective at preventing initiation and propagation of lipid peroxidation in cellular membranes and thus maintaining membrane stability. Water-soluble vitamin C is capable of regenerating vitamin E in the antioxidant cascade as illustrated in figure 10.7.

Polyphenol compounds scavenge peroxyl, superoxide, and nitric oxide radicals. Rich sources of polyphenols include tea, wine (particularly red wine), fruits, and vegetables. Flavonoids, a subclass of polyphenols that includes the flavonols, flavanones, and anthocyanidins, contain a number of phenolic hydroxyl (-OH) groups attached to ring structures that confer their antioxidant activity. Differences in the antioxidant power of individual flavonoids result from the variation in the number and arrangement of the hydroxyl groups and the extent and nature of the glycolation of these groups. Flavonoids are reported to inhibit the enzyme lipoxygenase and to inhibit oxidant generation by neutrophils in a manner similar to vitamin E. As with vitamin E, the antioxidant power of the flavonoids results from donating a hydrogen atom from a hydroxyl moiety. But studies in chemical systems show flavonoids to be 3 to 10 times more effective than vitamin E in their

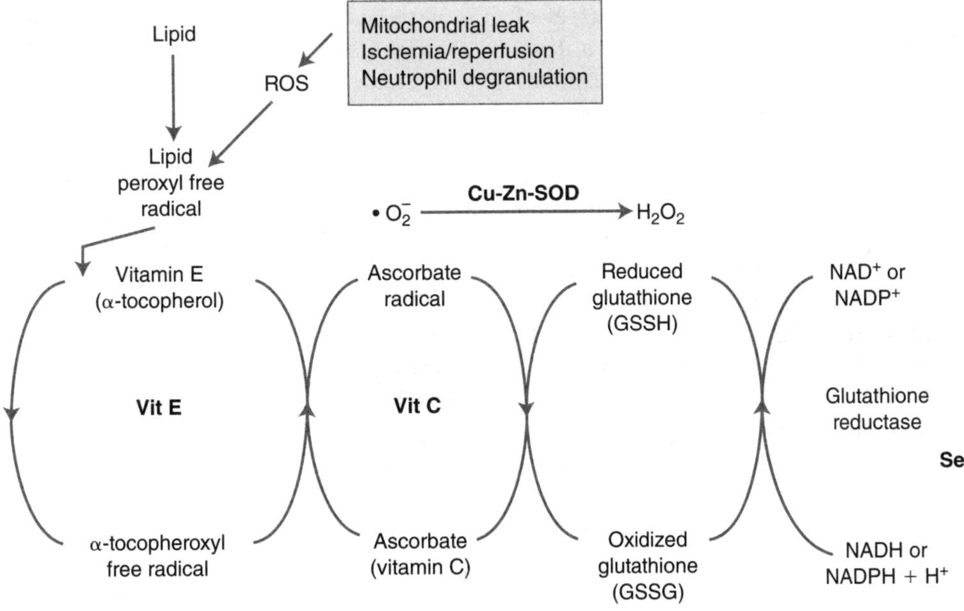

Figure 10.7 The antioxidant action cascade.

scavenging abilities. In addition, they may have anti-inflammatory effects. Flavonoids are used clinically to decrease inflammation and endothelial damage in diseases in which free radicals play a major role.

Flavonoids and Free Radicals

Some flavonoids are excellent scavengers of free radicals such as $\cdot O_{2^-}$ and $\cdot OH$. All subgroups of flavonoids decrease oxidant-induced lipid peroxidation and membrane permeability to potassium ions in isolated human erythrocytes (Meydani et al. 1993). Therefore, the ability of these compounds to chelate metal ions and prevent free-radical formation suggests that they may play an important protective role. In addition, flavonoids are also scavengers of the $\cdot NO$ radical. The $\cdot NO$ radical generated by inflammatory cells is reported to be toxic after reaction with the $\cdot O_2$- radical. Scavenging $\cdot NO$ radicals could therefore contribute to the proposed beneficial effect of the flavonoids.

Arteriosclerosis begins in a process in which $\cdot NO$ radicals play an unfavorable role, which adds additional weight to the possibility that flavonoids reduce the risk of CHD (Acker et al. 1995). Further support for this possibility was provided by the Dutch Zutphen elderly study, which showed an inverse correlation between intakes of flavonoids and incidence of CHD (Hertog et al. 1993). Moreover, a higher flavonoid intake from red wine may explain why the French have a lower mortality from CHD compared with the British, despite the fact that the consumption of saturated fat in France is greater than that in the United Kingdom.

The in vivo evidence for a protective effect of increased flavonoid intake is limited. The antioxidant capacity of plasma is increased in response to the oral ingestion of phenol-rich beverages, such as red wine and teas, or phenol-rich foods, such as dark chocolate. Polyphenols are rapidly absorbed, and peak plasma concentrations are reached within 1 hour of consuming nonalcoholic red wine. In vitro studies have demonstrated that alcohol-free red wine displays a stronger antioxidant activity than does alcohol-free white wine, and the only consistent chemical difference between the two wines is the phenol content, which is 20 times higher in red wine than in white wine. The higher phenol content results from the incorporation of the grape skins into the fermented grape juice during production of red wine. White wine production uses the fermented grape juice and not the grape skins. The biological actions of phenols may add significantly to the suggested protective effects of increased consumption of fruits and vegetables, such as the reduced risk of various cancers and CHD. Indeed, red wine inhibits LDL oxidation in vitro and reduces the susceptibility of plasma components to lipid peroxidation.

Possible Risks of High-Dose Antioxidant Supplementation

Antioxidants obviously provide some defense against the damaging effects of free radicals, and the media commonly extols the potential health benefits of a high antioxidant intake. This publicity has prompted many people to take large doses of antioxidant vitamins. Excessive antioxidant ingestion, however, may not be uniformly helpful. For example, in heavy smokers, increased intake of vitamin E and beta-carotene actually increases the incidence of lung cancer (Blot 1997; De Luca and Ross 1996). One possible reason for this effect is that antioxidants may interfere with important processes needed to kill cancer cells. Administration of antioxidants inhibits apoptosis (cell death), which is an important defense mechanism that inhibits tumor development by eliminating new mutated cells. ROS are intermediate messengers in several apoptosis signaling pathways. Therefore, excess antioxidants may effectively "shoot the messengers." Thus, in situations in which people have damaged their DNA (e.g., through heavy smoking, through exercise), the administration of antioxidants may prevent the effective removal of damaged cells.

Some side effects are associated with consuming excessive amounts of individual antioxidant vitamins. Very large doses of vitamin C are associated with urinary stone formation, impaired copper absorption, and diarrhea. Excess intakes of vitamin A by pregnant women can cause birth defects, and recent evidence suggests that high doses of vitamin A may be associated with reduced bone density and increased risk of hip fractures in postmenopausal women. Large intakes of vitamin E can impair absorption of vitamins A and K. Thus, more is not always better.

The controversy continues about whether physically active people should consume large amounts of antioxidant compounds. At present, the data are insufficient to recommend antioxidant supplements for athletes. In the last few decades, the role of ROS in exercise physiology has received considerable attention. Acute exercise has been shown to induce elevated generation of ROS in skeletal muscle through various mechanisms, and clear evidence shows that ROS formation in response to vigorous physical exertion can result in oxidative stress (Jackson 2007). Research has revealed the important role of ROS as signaling molecules that modulate contractile function and adaptive processes in skeletal muscle (Powers, Kavazis, and McClung 2007; Steensberg et al. 2007). In particular, ROS seem to be involved in the modulation of gene expression through redox-sensitive transcription pathways (Ji 2007). This potentially represents an important regulatory mechanism that has been suggested to be involved in the process of training adaptation. In this context, the adaptation of endogenous antioxidant systems in response to regular training reflects a potential mechanism responsible for augmented tolerance of skeletal muscle to exercise-induced stress. If so, it is likely that recommendations to athletes on antioxidant supplements may soon change. Consumption of high-dose supplements could impair the athlete's ability to adapt to the training stimulus, and considerable evidence for this has emerged from animal and human studies. In fact, there have now been more than 20 published studies reporting that antioxidant supplementation interferes with exercise training-induced adaptations. The main findings of these studies (reviewed by Peternelj and Coombes 2011) are that, in many situations, loading the tissues with high doses of antioxidants leads to a blunting of the effects of exercise training. The expected increases in mitochondrial biogenesis, GLUT4 expression, and antioxidant enzyme expression are smaller when athletes ingest daily high doses of antioxidant vitamins or other compounds with high antioxidant capacity. High-dose antioxidant supplementation can also interfere with ROS-mediated physiological processes such as vasodilation and insulin signaling. Therefore, more research needs to be done to produce evidence-based guidelines regarding the use of antioxidant supplementation during periods of exercise training. The best approach that can be currently recommended to athletes is to avoid the use of high-dose antioxidant supplements but aim to achieve an adequate intake of vitamins and minerals through a varied and balanced diet to maintain optimal antioxidant status. The following facts may help athletes determine whether to supplement with antioxidants:

- Numerous studies indicate that the body's natural antioxidant defense system is upregulated as an adaptation to exercise training.
- Antioxidant supplementation does not improve exercise performance, and some studies indicate that antioxidant supplementation may impair the adaptive response to exercise training.
- People who exercise regularly have a lower incidence of CHD, obesity, diabetes, and some (though not all) types of cancer compared with sedentary people, which suggests that the benefits of regular physical exercise outweigh the risks of free-radical-mediated damage.
- **Megadoses** of antioxidant vitamins can have undesirable side effects in some individuals.
- Athletes can obtain sufficient intakes of natural antioxidants by consuming well-balanced diets that are rich in a variety of fruits and vegetables.

Oxygen Transport

It is well recognized that optimal endurance exercise performance is dependent on the effective delivery and use of oxygen by the contracting muscles. Iron, as a component of hemoglobin, myoglobin, and cytochromes, is essential for both processes. Hemoglobin is the protein in red blood cells that transports oxygen. Myoglobin is the respiratory pigment found inside the muscle fibers. The cytochromes are components of the electron-transport chain located on the inner mitochondrial membrane that are involved in oxidative phosphorylation (ATP resynthesis from the oxidation of carbohydrates and fat).

Thus, iron is essential for oxygen transport and use. Besides the iron in the "functional compartment," mainly in hemoglobin and myoglobin, about one-fourth, or 1,000 mg, of the total body iron content in adult men is in storage. In contrast, iron stores are typically lower in adult women (300-500 mg), even lower in 18- to 21-year-old women (< 200 mg), and virtually absent in adolescents and young children. Unlike most adult male athletes, female and adolescent athletes need a regular supply of dietary iron to maintain iron balance and avoid anemia.

The gradual depletion of iron from the body when dietary intake is inadequate is commonly referred to as iron drain. This condition is thought to progress through a number of stages with different functional and diagnostic criteria as described in table 10.12. Iron is stored in the body complexed with **ferritin**, which is a protein found mostly in the liver, spleen, and bone marrow. Soluble ferritin is released from cells into the blood plasma in direct proportion to cellular ferritin content. Hence, the plasma, or serum, ferritin concentration can be used to indicate the status of the body's iron stores.

FREE RADICALS AND ANTIOXIDANTS: STUDIES IN EXERCISE-INDUCED MUSCLE DAMAGE

After eccentric exercise-induced damage to muscle, the phase of greatest loss of muscle force generation (sometimes referred to as the secondary injury because it follows an immediate mechanical damage to the muscle) is associated with considerable infiltration of phagocytic cells (blood neutrophils and monocytes) into the damaged fibers. This secondary damage has been mostly attributed to ROS released by these activated phagocytic invaders, and neutrophils in particular have been identified as the major contributors to the oxidative damage in muscle (Pizza et al. 2005).

Several studies have attempted to determine whether pretreatment with antioxidants can reduce or alter the time course of eccentric exercise-induced muscle damage. In an animal study, mice treated with SOD, the antioxidant enzyme involved in the elimination of the superoxide radical, showed smaller reductions in muscle force output 3 days after eccentric exercise (Zerba, Komorowski, and Faulkner 1990). The finding that SOD reduced loss of muscle function supports the role of free radicals in damage induced by eccentric contraction. But muscle levels of SOD and free-radical activity were not measured in this study. Furthermore, force reduction in mice given SOD supplements was found only in older mice. Endogenous levels of protective antioxidant enzymes decline with age (Meydani et al. 1993). These studies suggest that humans and animals have increased susceptibility to muscle damage with increasing age. Similarly, Cannon et al. (1990) compared the effect of an antioxidant supplement with a placebo treatment in two age groups (younger than 30 years and older than 55 years) using downhill running as the muscle-damaging exercise protocol. The authors found that vitamin E supplementation eliminated the differences between the two age groups.

Maughan et al. (1989) measured serum lipid peroxide concentration as total TBARS and found that subjects with the greatest increase in serum CK showed the highest TBARS concentrations, suggesting that free-radical reactions and subsequent loss of membrane integrity could be responsible for the release of muscle-derived enzymes into the circulation. Although TBARS may be a useful indicator of free-radical damage, methodological difficulties mean that care should be taken when interpreting results of such studies. One of the problems of free-radical research has been the difficulty in directly measuring free-radical activity, particularly in vivo (see Duthie 1999 for a review). But these indirect measures of free-radical activity suggest that free radicals are formed during exercise.

Although free radicals are difficult to detect directly, electron spin resonance (ESR) has been used to try to measure increased free-radical production. Davies et al. (1982) observed a two- to threefold increase in ROS concentration in the muscles and liver after exercise to exhaustion in rats. More recent studies support these findings. Fielding et al. (1993) demonstrated a relationship between neutrophil infiltration, ultrastructural damage, and increased muscle membrane permeability after downhill running in humans. Postexercise muscle infiltration and in vitro neutrophil superoxide generation were closely related to the time course of release of CK into the circulation and muscle ultrastructural damage. These events may be causally related to other symptoms of muscle damage, such as loss of muscle strength and muscle soreness.

A study by Jackson (2000) reported that dietary vitamin E deficiency in rats increased the susceptibility of skeletal muscles to contractile damage as indicated by CK release, but rats supplemented with 240 mg $\cdot$ kg^{-1} $\cdot$ day^{-1} of vitamin E exhibited lower CK release after a downhill run. Moreover, the peak CK activity in serum was significantly correlated to neutrophil superoxide release. In contrast, van der Meulen et al. (1997) found that 5 to 8 days of intravenous injections in mice increased vitamin E content threefold but did not alter the extent of eccentric-exercise-induced muscle damage in situ. Moreover, vitamin E did not alter the force deficit or change the percentage of muscle fibers damaged. In the same study, however, postexercise CK levels were significantly reduced with vitamin E injections, which suggests that vitamin E may help reduce membrane damage related to enzyme efflux but may not alter other indices of muscle damage induced by eccentric contractions. Neither antioxidant capacity nor ROS production was measured in these studies.

Warren et al. (1992) investigated rat muscle susceptibility to oxidative stress and observed lower CK release in a group given vitamin E supplements compared with a control group. Although force loss was similar in both groups, the susceptibility of the muscles to oxidant stress decreased after supplementation. The authors concluded that vitamin E supplementation may be useful in reducing free-radical damage but does not appear to alter muscle-fiber damage caused by eccentric exercise.

Several human studies have also shown contrasting findings. Cannon et al. (1990) reported that vitamin E supplementation (400 IU/day) for 48 days increased the amount of CK in the plasma of subjects older than 55 years. Moreover, plasma CK activity correlated with superoxide release from neutrophils at the time of peak CK levels; however, significant increases in plasma lipid peroxides were not observed. The authors concluded that free radicals are involved with the delayed increase in muscle-membrane permeability after damaging exercise but are not involved in the initial injury.

Meydani et al. (1993) studied the effects of a 45-minute run at 75% of maximal heart rate. The subjects were given either a placebo or vitamin E (800 IU) for 48 days before the exercise. Those given the vitamin E supplement decreased production of urinary TBARS after eccentric exercise, which suggested that vitamin E reduced free-radical-mediated damage. But the reliability of TBARS as a measure of lipid peroxidation has been questioned. Kaminiski and Boal (1992) studied the effect of vitamin C supplementation for 7 days after exercise in a double-blind crossover trial. Although this study noted that vitamin C treatment reduced muscle damage as indicated by muscle soreness, it did not measure any biochemical markers of muscle damage, and a carryover effect from the previous bout of exercise was likely.

Studies using a well-characterized model of lengthening contractions in rodents in which a single discrete muscle (in this case the extensor digitorum longus [EDL]) is damaged in a highly reproducible manner have investigated in more detail the effects of vitamin E supplementation on exercise-induced muscle damage. The findings from these studies have provided evidence that the EDL muscle was under considerable oxidative stress after lengthening contractions and that vitamin E had differential effects on individual measures of damage to muscle (van der Meulen et al. 1997). Animals subjected to a protocol of repeated lengthening contractions had a significant force deficit and morphological damage to the EDL fibers on histological examination at 3 days postexercise. This was associated with a significant elevation of serum CK activity at 3 hours and 3 days postexercise. Prior vitamin E supplementation of the rats had no effect on the loss of force generation by the EDL or on the percentage of damaged fibers but, surprisingly, prevented the rise in circulating CK activity that occurred postexercise. This apparent selective effect of vitamin E on the release of CK (a cytosolic enzyme) from the damaged muscle is consistent with previous in vitro data suggesting that vitamin E can stabilize muscle membranes by interaction with phospholipids (Phoenix, Edwards, and Jackson 1991) and may provide an explanation for at least some of the apparently discrepant data in this area. Other sources of antioxidants have also been examined in relation to reducing the effect of exercise-induced muscle damage. For example, tart cherries and their constituents have received growing attention for application in sport as a means of enhancing recovery from damaging exercise regimens, and the evidence for these effects has recently been reviewed by Bell et al. (2014). The food science, animal, and human literature currently available clearly demonstrate the anti-inflammatory and antioxidative effects of cherries (Bell et al. 2014). The research suggests that there are some limited benefits of tart cherry juice consumption in enhancing recovery and reducing muscle soreness following damaging exercise. There is also controversy regarding the manipulation of the stress responses to exercise (inflammation and oxidative stress) with antioxidant supplements, with a suggestion that adaptation may be blunted as a result of downregulating the stress response (Gomez-Cabrera et al. 2005, 2008). However, it should be noted that such negative adaptive effects have not been reported in cherry studies or any other functional foods and perhaps warrant further investigation. The specific compounds responsible for any beneficial effects of cherry juice have not been identified but could include quercetin and anthocyanins and their metabolites.

Because of the inconsistent and often contradictory findings, whether antioxidant vitamins are helpful in reducing free-radical-mediated damage is not clear. These conflicts may be the result of different indices of muscle damage being measured, variations in mode and intensity of exercise, previous training, the dose and the length of time of supplementation, and

(continued)

FREE RADICALS AND ANTIOXIDANTS *(continued)*

the ages of the subjects. Antioxidants react with free radicals and deactivate them, which lowers the amount of ROS produced and therefore may reduce or prevent secondary muscle damage. In addition, any effects that they may have in reducing the initial damage will likely result in a reduction in the later infiltration of neutrophils and macrophages with consequent attenuation of secondary damage. Caution must be exercised, however, because some studies have even reported deleterious effects on muscle function with antioxidant supplementation following exercise-induced muscle damage (e.g., Close et al. 2006).

TABLE 10.12 Stages of Iron Drain From Normal Iron Status to Iron Deficiency Anemia

Stage	Characteristics	Blood hemoglobin (g/L)	Serum ferritin (µg/L)	Serum transferrin saturation (%)
Normal iron status	Normal iron status measurements and normal appearance of RBCs	>120 (F) >140 (M)	>30 (F) >110 (M)	20-40 (M, F)
Iron depletion	Normal hematocrit and hemoglobin but low serum ferritin with normal to high transferrin saturation	>120 (F) >140 (M)	<30 (M, F)	20-40 (M, F)
Iron deficiency	Normal hemoglobin but low serum ferritin, iron, and transferrin; low transferrin saturation	>120 (F) >140 (M)	<12 (M, F)	<16 (M, F)
Iron deficiency anemia	Low hematocrit and hemoglobin; low serum ferritin, iron, and transferrin saturation; small and pale RBCs	<120 (F) <140 (M)	<10 (M, F)	<16 (M, F)

M = male; F = female; RBCs = red blood cells (erythrocytes). Hematocrit is packed cell volume (normal is 38%-45% for women and 42%-48% for men). Serum iron concentration is normally 0.4-1.4 mg/L. Characteristics of each stage and the associated diagnostic criteria are based on blood measures.

Adapted from Deakin (2000)

Iron depletion (low iron stores as evidenced by a serum ferritin concentration of < 12 µg/L) is common in female athletes (with a lesser incidence in male athletes), but whether this deficiency affects athletic performance in the absence of anemia remains controversial. Researchers have reported that depletion of the body's iron stores without anemia can be associated with increased lactate production during maximal exercise, which is indicative of reduced oxygen use by working muscle, and it can also be associated with an increased subjective feeling of exercise overload in elite athletes. A few studies indicate that some performance benefits may result from iron supplementation in iron-depleted female athletes who are not anemic (Brownlie et al. 2002; Brutsaert et al. 2003). Furthermore, adaptations to endurance training, including improvements in maximal oxygen uptake and endurance performance, are enhanced by iron supplementation in iron-depleted, nonanemic women (Brownlie et al. 2002; Hinton et al. 2000).

Other studies have shown that $\dot{V}O_2$max, endurance performance, and muscle oxidative enzyme activity can be maintained even when body iron stores are severely depleted. What seems certain is that if the condition should progress to a state of iron deficiency that results in anemia (low blood hemoglobin concentration [see table 10.12]), athletic performance is negatively affected. At this stage, not enough iron is available in the bone marrow to manufacture normal amounts of hemoglobin and red blood cells, which leads to the production of small, pale red blood cells.

Anemia lowers the oxygen-carrying capacity of the blood and reduces exercise performance. In severe cases of anemia, affected people report sensations of breathlessness on mild exertion and generally feel so lethargic that they can no longer carry out everyday activities. Impaired functioning of several enzymes that require iron as a cofactor may result in mental dysfunction, impaired temperature control, and weakened immunity, which exacerbate the symptoms of reduced exercise tolerance.

Iron deficiency is reported to be the most widespread micronutrient deficiency in the world, and field studies consistently associate iron deficiency with increased morbidity from infectious disease. The incidence of iron-deficiency anemia is rare and is similar among athletes and the general population. The cause of anemia in athletes may be low energy intake, insufficient iron intake to maintain iron stores (see figure 10.8), or low meat intake (which provides the most readily available dietary source of iron). The routine testing of iron status in athletes is recommended.

Exercise may cause some destruction (hemolysis) of red blood cells (possibly due to footstrike hemolysis during running), alterations of iron metabolism, and increased losses of iron in sweat and urine. In some susceptible individuals, additional losses caused by gastrointestinal bleeding may occur during prolonged strenuous exercise. Research has shown that the liver-derived hormone hepcidin is elevated for 3 to 6 hours after endurance exercise, which may negatively affect the ability to absorb dietary iron and to recycle iron taken up by macrophages subsequent to any exercise-induced hemolysis (Peeling and Goodman 2015). The body adapts to endurance training by increasing the red blood cell mass and the myoglobin content of skeletal muscle. Altitude exposure causes an additional increase in red blood cell production. Hence, regular exercise increases the dietary requirement for iron. Furthermore, female athletes are at a greater risk of iron deficiency than their male counterparts due to menstrual blood loss and suboptimal dietary iron intake.

The periodic screening of serum ferritin levels in athletes is recommended because changes in the storage and transport of iron typically precede decreases in functional iron (hemoglobin) levels. During training, some athletes experience a transient fall in hemoglobin concentration and hematocrit, which is probably caused mostly by the increase in plasma volume that is commonly associated with the initiation of training or a sudden increase in the training load. This form of hemodilutional iron deficiency, sometimes called sports anemia, has no apparent effect on exercise performance.

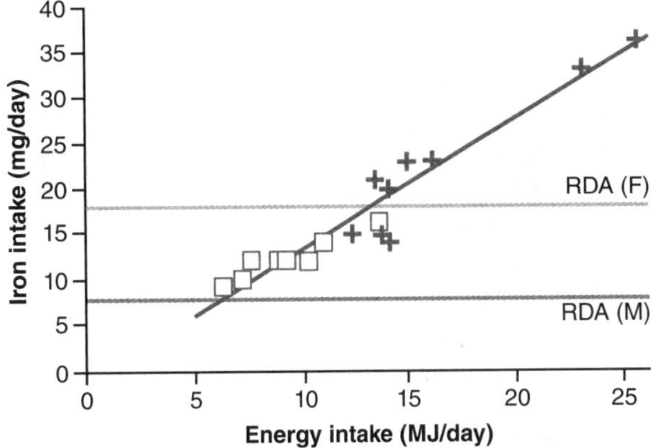

Figure 10.8 The relationship between mean intake of dietary energy and iron intake in male (crosses) and female (squares) athletes. Each point represents a mean value for a group.

Adapted from van Erp-Baart (1989b).

About 60% of iron in animal tissues is in the heme form; that is, it is associated with hemoglobin and myoglobin and thus found only in animal foods. Nonheme iron is found in animal and plant foods. Heme iron is absorbed better than nonheme iron. About 10% to 30% of ingested heme iron is absorbed in the gut, whereas only about 2% to 10% of nonheme iron is absorbed. The form in which it is consumed influences the bioavailability of iron (and many other minerals).

Some substances found in foods may promote or inhibit absorption of minerals. For example, vitamin C prevents the oxidation of Fe^{2+} to Fe^{3+}. Because ferrous iron is more readily absorbed, vitamin C facilitates nonheme iron absorption but has no effect on heme iron absorption. Thus, drinking a glass of fresh orange juice improves the absorption of iron from bread or cereals. Some natural substances found in foods such as tannins (e.g., in tea), phosphates, phytates, oxalates, and excessive fiber may decrease the bioavailability of nonheme iron. Iron absorption is also a function of storage: The larger the stores are, the poorer the absorption is, and vice versa. Thus, people with inadequate stores have better absorption regardless of diet.

The low bioavailability of iron in vegetarian diets possibly contributes to lower serum ferritin levels in athletes who consume a modified vegetarian diet, and iron may also be lacking in a lactovegetarian diet because of the absence of heme iron. A number of studies have failed to find that exercise per se decreased iron status, although this failurc may be attributed to the relatively low training volumes employed. The consensus is that all athletes should include foods rich in heme iron, such as lean red meat, poultry, and fish, in their daily diets.

Because prolonged bouts of exercise increase the losses of iron in feces, urine, and sweat, most athletes need more iron in their diets than sedentary people. Weaver and Rajaram (1992) noted that iron losses may be around 70% higher in athletes compared with the reference value for sedentary people. Men can achieve an iron intake equivalent to twice the RDA through consumption of a well-balanced diet sufficient to meet daily energy requirements. Studies of various groups of athletes have shown that iron intake is proportional to energy intake (see figure 10.8) such that male athletes who consume more than 10 MJ/day (2,390 kcal/day) from a varied food base will obtain the RDA of iron. Thus, male endurance athletes who match their energy intake (from varied food sources) to their energy expenditure are likely to obtain more than enough iron. The same cannot be said for women. Without consuming iron-fortified cereals or other iron-fortified foods, it is challenging for 16- to 40-year-old women, even those who consume energy-balanced diets, to consume the RDA for iron. Those at particularly high risk for poor iron status are those athletes who consume a low-energy diet or avoid food sources rich in heme iron. Vegetarian athletes should ensure that plant food choices are iron dense (e.g., green leafy vegetables, legumes), and they should include iron-fortified products (breads, cereals, breakfast bars), whole-grain breads, and pasta in their diets.

To maintain sufficient iron stores, dietary intakes of iron of 8 mg/day for adult men and 18 mg/day for adult women are recommended (Peeling and Goodman 2015). This can be achieved through the consumption of both heme iron sources, such as meat (which typically provides about 20% of dietary iron intake), and the less efficiently absorbed nonheme iron from plant foods such as green leafy vegetables, beans, and pulses. Because the absorption of dietary iron can be impaired by postexercise elevations of circulating hepcidin, it may be best to ingest foods high in dietary iron outside the first few hours following an exercise session. Daily oral iron supplements, usually in the form of 100 mg iron sulfate, can elevate the serum ferritin concentration by 30% to 50% over a 6- to 8-week period. The absorption of iron from supplements is thought to be more efficient when taken together with vitamin C (a convenient dietary source is orange juice) and less efficient when taken with caffeinated products such as coffee and tea. If a faster increase in iron status is required (e.g., due to diagnosis of anemia or chronic fatigue or in the lead-up to impending competition), then the use of intramuscular or intravenous injection of iron may be considered by the sports physician (Garvican et al. 2011, 2014).

Megadoses of iron are not advised, and routine oral iron supplements should not be taken without medical supervision following the diagnosis of iron deficiency by a physician. Only after laboratory confirmation of very low iron status or iron deficiency anemia should iron supplements be used. Oral iron supplementation can result in gastrointestinal distress, constipation, and dark-colored stools. Prolonged consumption of large amounts of iron can cause a disturbance in iron metabolism in susceptible individuals. Iron may accumulate in the liver, and the risk of developing hemochromatosis will increase. Hepatic iron accumulates as a compound called hemosiderin, which in excess can cause cell damage in the 0.3% of the population who are genetically predisposed. This condition causes cirrhosis and can be fatal. Excess intake of iron may also reduce absorption of other divalent cations, particularly zinc and copper. Groups at risk for insufficient iron intake who may be suitable candidates for iron supplementation include female endurance athletes, gymnasts, vegetarians, and those who have restricted energy intakes.

Anemia can also arise from deficiencies of vitamin B_6, vitamin B_{12}, folic acid, and copper. Vitamin B_6 is required for the synthesis of the porphyrin ring component of hemoglobin and myoglobin. Vitamin B_{12}, which contains the trace element cobalt, is required for the synthesis of nucleic acids, which are essential for the proliferation of stem cells that develop into red and white blood cells in the bone marrow. For the same reason, folic acid is also required for normal blood cell production. Deficiencies of these micronutrients are associated with megaloblastic or pernicious anemia, reduced blood leukocyte count, and impaired lymphocyte proliferation. Major food sources of vitamin B_{12} are meat, liver, and milk. Hence, athletes who avoid animal foods are at risk for cobalt and vitamin B_{12} deficiency. Some food products, notably breakfast cereals and milk, are fortified with vitamin B_{12}. For example, 120 g (4 oz) of cornflakes, or 40 g (1 oz) of cornflakes with 150 ml (5 fl oz) of pasteurized whole milk, provides 1 mg of vitamin B_{12} (67% of the RNI). Copper is a cofactor of many enzymes and plays an important role in the formation of red blood cells.

Phosphorus, besides being a constituent of bones, teeth, and cell membranes, is a component of 2,3-diphosphoglycerate (2,3-DPG), which is found predominantly in red blood cells. It alters the affinity of hemoglobin for oxygen and promotes more effective unloading of oxygen from the erythrocytes in the tissue capillaries, where the partial pressure of oxygen is lower than it is in the arteries. In response to altitude exposure, the erythrocyte concentration of 2,3-DPG increases.

Cofactors in Enzyme Catalyzed Reactions

Many of the B vitamins are reusable coenzymes in energy metabolism. Some of their roles can be seen in figure 10.9. Vitamins B_3, B_6, and B_1 are involved in carbohydrate metabolism; vitamin B_2, thiamin, pantothenic acid, and biotin are involved in fat metabolism; and vitamins B_6 and K are involved in protein metabolism. Niacin is the precursor of the important coenzymes nicotinamide adenine dinucleotide (NAD^+) and nicotinamide adenine dinucleotide phosphate (NADP); riboflavin is the precursor of flavin adenine dinucleotide ($FADH_2$) and flavin mononucleotide (FMN). These nicotinamide and flavin nucleotides are involved in oxidation and reduction reactions in energy metabolism, including some of the reactions of glycolysis, the TCA cycle, and the electron-transport chain (see figure 10.9). Pantothenic acid is the precursor of CoA, which is essential for the processes involved in both carbohydrate and fat oxidation (see chapter 3). A deficiency of these vitamins can result in premature fatigue and inability to maintain a heavy training program.

Zinc serves either a structural or a catalytic role in more than 200 human enzymes. It is a cofactor of several enzymes involved in energy metabolism and is required for normal cell replication, immune function, and wound healing. Some zinc-containing enzymes, such as carbonic anhydrase and lactate dehydrogenase, are involved in intermediary metabolism during exercise.

Studies have indicated that the intake of zinc among some groups of athletes (wrestlers, female endurance runners, and gymnasts) is considerably less than the RDA (11 mg/day and 8 mg/day for men and women, respectively). Prolonged exercise may cause significant losses of zinc and

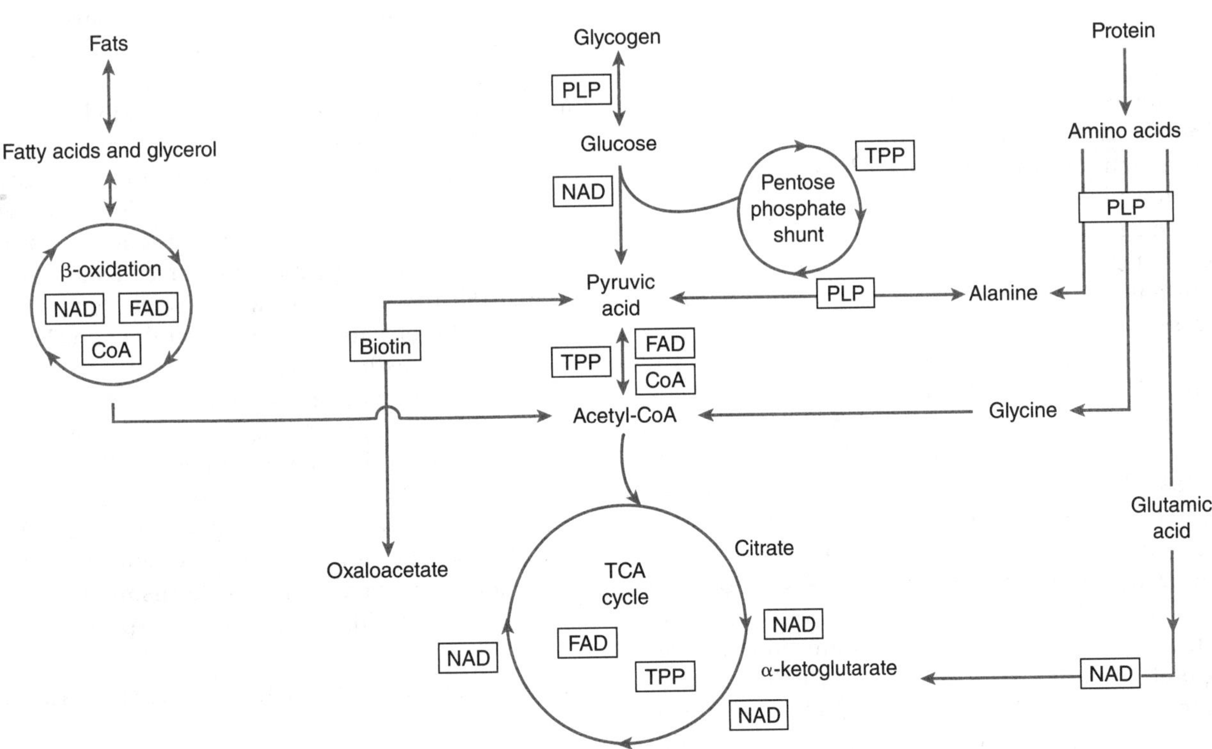

Figure 10.9 B vitamins as precursors of coenzymes in energy metabolism. CoA = coenzyme A; FAD = flavin adenine dinucleotide; NAD = nicotinamide adenine dinucleotide; PLP = pyridoxal phosphate; TPP = thiamin pyrophosphate.

magnesium in sweat. Losses of these minerals in urine also increase as a result of intensive training. The total amount of zinc in the human body is about 2 g, and most of it is in muscle (60%) and bone (30%). Hence, measurements of zinc concentrations in blood may not be meaningful. Although losses of zinc in sweat and urine increase in physically active people, no evidence indicates that these losses are sufficient to cause concern. Small amounts of zinc are present in many foods of both animal and plant origin, and no benefit of additional zinc supplements for health or performance has been established.

Magnesium is an essential cofactor for more than 300 enzymes involved in biosynthetic processes and energy metabolism. It is essential for the normal functioning of ATPases, including myosin ATPase involved in muscle contraction, and it is involved in glycogen breakdown, protein synthesis, and fat oxidation. Magnesium is also required for the maintenance of electrical potentials in muscles and nerves, so it is important for normal neuromuscular coordination. The total body content of magnesium is about 25 g (see table 10.5). The RDA for magnesium is 420 mg/day for men and 320 mg/day for women; hence, magnesium is a macromineral rather than a trace element. The main dietary sources of magnesium are listed in table 10.8. Several studies have reported low serum magnesium concentrations in athletes, and prolonged strenuous exercise is associated with increased losses of magnesium in urine and sweat. Although, as with zinc and iron, a single bout of exercise is extremely unlikely to induce substantial magnesium losses. A period of heavy training could induce a state of mild magnesium deficiency, particularly in a warm environment where sweat losses are high.

Magnesium deficiency in both humans and animals is associated with neuromuscular abnormalities, including muscle weakness, cramps, and structural damage of muscle fibers and organelles. The abnormalities may be caused by an impairment of calcium homeostasis secondary to an oxygen free-radical-induced alteration in the integrity of the membrane of the sarcoplasmic reticulum. Lack of magnesium may also be associated with depletion of selenium and reduced glutathione peroxidase activity, which would be expected to increase the susceptibility to damage by free radicals. Hence, magnesium deficiency possibly potentiates exercise-induced muscle damage and stress responses, but direct evidence for these is lacking. Magnesium deficiency exacerbates the inflammatory state after ischemic insult to the myocardium, which may be caused by a substance P–mediated increase in the secretion of proinflammatory cytokines in the magnesium-deficient state (substance P is a peptide that acts as a neurotransmitter).

Copper is a cofactor of many enzymes, including several oxidases, and appears to be needed for the proper use of iron. Copper plays an important role in energy metabolism and the synthesis of hemoglobin, catecholamines, and some peptide hormones. Copper is also required for the normal formation of erythrocytes and the development of connective tissue. The RDA for copper for adult men and women is 0.9 mg/day. Intakes up to 10 mg/day are safe, and toxicity from dietary copper ingestion is extremely rare. The main dietary sources of copper are shown in table 10.9. Even though copper deficiency is rare in humans, athletes who take zinc supplements may compromise the gastrointestinal absorption of copper because of the similar physicochemical properties of these two minerals. Athletes should also be aware that large doses of vitamin C can limit copper absorption.

The results of changes in copper status caused by exercise and training are controversial and perhaps reflect the inadequacy of measuring techniques or redistribution of copper between body compartments, although athletes have been reported to lose copper in sweat. Compared with sedentary control subjects, several groups of athletes have similar or higher resting blood levels of copper. Thus, the copper status of athletes seems to be normal. After an acute bout of prolonged exercise, the plasma copper concentration may rise or remain unchanged. One study reported a substantial increase in plasma copper concentration during the first 8 days of a 20-day running road race, and this elevation persisted for the remainder of the race. This increase was attributed to a rise in the production of ceruloplasmin by the liver as part of the acute-phase response. Ceruloplasmin is a glycoprotein that binds copper and is thought to exert a protective effect against cellular damage caused by free radicals. As explained previously, manganese and selenium are cofactors of the antioxidant enzymes superoxide dismutase and glutathione peroxidase–reductase, respectively.

Immune Function and Resistance to Infection

Heavy exercise and nutrition exert separate influences on immune function; these influences appear to be greater when exercise stress and poor nutrition act synergistically. The poor nutritional status of some athletes very likely predisposes them to immunodepression and increased risk of infection. Several vitamins, including vitamin B_{12} and folic acid, are needed for the normal production of white blood cells that defend the body against invading pathogens. Other vitamins, including A, C, D, and E, are needed for normal functioning of these cells. Several minerals, including zinc, iron, copper, and selenium, are also essential for optimal immune function. Deficiencies of these vitamins and minerals can result not only in increased risk of infections but also in more severe and longer lasting symptoms when illness does occur. Another negative outcome is that wound healing and recovery from injury can be impaired. The role of micronutrients and macronutrients in immune function and resistance to infection is discussed in detail in chapter 13.

Electrolytes in Body Fluids

An electrolyte conducts an electric current when dissolved in water. Electrolytes, which include acids, bases, and salts, usually dissociate into ions carrying either a positive charge (cation) or a negative charge (anion). The major electrolytes in the body fluids are sodium, potassium, chloride, bicarbonate, phosphate, sulfate, magnesium, and calcium. Of these, sodium, potassium, and chloride are found in the highest concentrations, although their distribution differs between the intracellular and extracellular fluids.

Sodium and chloride are found in higher concentrations in the extracellular fluid, whereas potassium is found in higher concentration inside cells. These concentration differences arise because of active transport mechanisms in cell membranes. The sodium–potassium ATPase actively pumps three sodium ions out of the cell for every two potassium ions pumped into the cell, which sets up an electrical potential (charge) difference across the cell membrane; the interior of the cell is slightly negative compared with the outside. This electrical potential difference can be measured as a voltage difference. Amounts in most cells are about 70 millivolts (mV). This resting membrane potential can be reversed by a sudden influx of positive ions into the cell, which is the basis of the action potential generated in nerve and muscle fibers when sodium channels in the membranes of these cells are temporarily opened.

Sodium, as the principal cation in the extracellular fluids (see table 10.5), serves primarily to maintain normal body fluid balance, osmotic pressure, and blood pressure. The role of excess sodium intake in the etiology of high blood pressure (hypertension) is discussed in chapter 2. Normal body fluid levels of sodium are critical for nerve impulse transmission and muscle contraction. The body has effective hormonal control mechanisms for dealing with wide variations in dietary sodium intake.

If the plasma concentration of sodium falls, aldosterone secretion from the adrenal glands increases, and this steroid hormone stimulates the kidney to reabsorb more sodium so that less is excreted in the urine. When the plasma concentration of sodium rises, aldosterone production falls, allowing increased urinary excretion of sodium. Other hormones, notably vasopressin or ADH, through their effects on water reabsorption by the kidney, help to maintain normal sodium concentration in the body fluids. During prolonged moderate exercise or short durations of high-intensity exercise, the plasma sodium concentration increases, which helps maintain blood volume. Exercise also leads to increased secretion of aldosterone and ADH, which results in the conservation of body sodium and water.

The estimated minimum daily requirement for sodium in adults is 0.5 g (the amount in 1.25 g of table salt), the adequate intake of sodium is 1.5 g, and the upper recommended intake of sodium is 2.4 g. Sodium occurs in small amounts in most natural foods, but many processed foods have substantial amounts of salt added. For example, a 180 g (5 oz) serving of cooked fresh beans contains 25 mg of sodium, whereas an equal portion of canned beans contains 750 mg of sodium. Because of health concerns, in recent years food manufacturers have reduced the salt content of processed foods. Even so, the average consumption of sodium by people in the United States is reported to be about 4.5 g/day. About one-third of this amount is from natural foods, one-half is from processed foods, and the rest is from table salt.

The typical sodium content of several foods is shown in table 10.13. Fresh meats, fruits, and vegetables generally contain relatively small amounts of sodium, whereas several processed foods, such as sauces, pickles, chips, ready meals, and processed meats (e.g., sausages and burgers), contain much larger amounts of sodium.

Deficiency of sodium is rare, partly because of the widespread availability of sodium in many food products and partly because humans have a natural appetite for salt. Nevertheless, substantial losses of sodium and chloride from the body can result from prolonged sweating. Although sweat composition is quite variable, the average amounts

TABLE 10.13 Sodium Content of Common Food Items

Food item	Amount	Sodium content (mg)
Meat		
Luncheon meat	28 g (1 oz)	450
Beef	28 g (1 oz)	25
Chicken	28 g (1 oz)	13
White fish	28 g (1 oz)	33
Tuna (in oil)	28 g (1 oz)	270
Salmon (canned)	28 g (1 oz)	140
Pork sausage	28 g (1 oz)	70
Cereal and starch products		
Bread	1 slice	130
Cornflakes	28 g (1 oz)	280
Pretzels	28 g (1 oz)	890
Chips or crisps (plain, salted)	28 g (1 oz)	195
Chips or crisps (salt and vinegar)	28 g (1 oz)	335
Vegetables and fruit		
Beans (fresh, cooked)	28 g (1 oz)	5
Baked beans (canned)	28 g (1 oz)	150
Red kidney beans (canned)	28 g (1 oz)	85
Peas (canned)	28 g (1 oz)	55
Pickled onions	28 g (1 oz)	225
Potatoes (baked)	1 medium	6
Bananas	1 medium	1
Oranges	1 medium	1
Dairy products		
Milk (semi-skimmed)	100 ml (3 fl oz)	120
Butter	5 g (1 teaspoon)	50
Cheese	28 g (1 oz)	445
Cottage cheese	28 g (1 oz)	20
Other common products		
Margarine	5 g (1 teaspoon)	50
Spaghetti sauce	28 g (1 oz)	340
Soup	100 ml (3 fl oz)	500
Tomato ketchup	15 g (1 tablespoon)	100
Soy sauce	15 g (1 tablespoon)	1,020
Bolognese sauce	28 g (1 oz)	140
Gravy powder	28 g (1 oz)	1,620
Cakes and tarts	28 g (1 oz)	85
Isotonic sports drinks	100 ml (3 fl oz)	46
Table salt	5 g (1 teaspoon)	2,000

of sodium and chloride lost in sweat are about 1.2 g/L and 1.4 g/L, respectively. Because most people sweat at a rate of 1 to 2 L/h (0.3-0.5 gal/h) during strenuous exercise, even in ambient temperatures around 20 °C (68 °F), salt losses can be considerable. Thus, for the athlete exercising in the heat, short-term deficiencies of sodium and chloride may be incurred, which, if not corrected in the recovery period, can have debilitating effects on subsequent exercise performance.

Low blood sodium levels (hyponatremia) can also occur with excessive consumption of water over a period of several hours, which can lead to potentially fatal water intoxication (see chapter 9). Chloride is the major anion in the extracellular fluids (see table 10.5), and, like sodium, it is involved in the regulation of body fluid balance and electrical potentials across cell membranes. Chloride ions are also a component in the formation of hydrochloric acid in the stomach, which promotes the denaturation and digestion of dietary proteins. The estimated minimum daily requirement for chloride in adults is 0.75 g, and the adequate intake is currently set at 2.30 g. The dietary intake of chloride, as might be expected, parallels that of sodium.

Potassium is the major cation found inside cells. The intracellular concentration is about 150 mmol/L compared with around 4 mmol/L in the extracellular fluids. Potassium is also involved in body fluid homeostasis and in the generation of electrical impulses in nerves, skeletal muscle, and the heart. Excretion of potassium in the urine is, like that of sodium, regulated by aldosterone. A rise in the plasma potassium concentration stimulates the secretion of aldosterone, which leads to increased urinary excretion of potassium. Conversely, a fall in the plasma potassium concentration causes a reduction in aldosterone secretion from the adrenal cortex and hence greater potassium retention by the kidneys. The estimated minimum daily requirement for potassium in adults is 2 g, and the adequate intake is set at 4.7 g. Potassium is found in most foods and is particularly abundant in bananas, citrus fruits, vegetables, and milk (see table 10.14). Because potassium balance is tightly regulated in the body, long-term deficiencies or excesses are extremely rare. Short-term imbalances, however, may occur in certain circumstances. For example, low blood potassium levels (hypokalemia) have been reported in people with diarrhea, during prolonged fasting, and after diuretic drug administration.

Low plasma potassium concentrations can lead to muscle weakness and fatal cardiac arrest. A higher than normal blood level of potassium (hyperkalemia) is also potentially dangerous because this condition, too, can cause cardiac arrhythmias and result in death. For this reason, people should not take large doses of potassium supplements. During high-intensity exercise, active skeletal muscle releases potassium ions that enter the circulation and cause a temporary rise in the plasma potassium concentration. Under normal

TABLE 10.14 Potassium Content of Common Food Items

Food item	Amount	Potassium content (mg)
Meat		
Beef	28 g (1 oz)	100
Chicken	28 g (1 oz)	70
White fish	28 g (1 oz)	160
Cereal and starch products		
Bread	1 slice	65
Cornflakes	28 g (1 oz)	100
Vegetables and fruit		
Potatoes (baked)	1 medium	780
Carrots	1 medium	275
Broccoli	1 medium stalk	270
Bananas	1 medium	460
Oranges	1 medium	260
Apples	1 medium	35
Dairy products		
Milk (semi-skimmed)	100 ml (3 fl oz)	180
Butter	5 g (1 teaspoon)	10
Cheddar cheese	28 g (1 oz)	28
Yogurt	100 g (4 oz)	450

circumstances, however, normal potassium levels are rapidly restored during the recovery period. Some potassium is excreted in sweat, but these losses are relatively small (160-320 mg/L) compared with the losses of sodium and chloride, so potassium status can easily be restored with ingestion of a postexercise meal.

Other Tissue Functions

Calcium, besides being an important structural component of bone, is involved in nerve conduction and muscle excitation and contraction. In the sarcoplasm (cytosol) of resting muscle, the concentration of free calcium ions (Ca^{2+}) is low (about 10 nM), whereas in the extracellular fluid and SR, the concentration is much higher; the blood plasma concentration of free calcium, for example, is about 1 mM (100,000 times higher than in the muscle sarcoplasm). Release of calcium from the SR in response to membrane depolarization after the arrival of an action potential allows the myosin and actin filaments to interact, bringing about muscle contraction (see chapter 3). Calcium is then pumped back into the SR by an active transport mechanism, which restores the low cytosolic calcium ion concentration and allows relaxation of the muscle.

Calcium is also required for the activation of numerous enzymes involved in energy metabolism. For example, the activity of phosphorylase, the key enzyme involved in muscle glycogen breakdown, is stimulated by increased cytosolic calcium ion concentration. Several enzymes of glycolysis are also activated by increased levels of intracellular calcium, which neatly links the provision of energy to the same process that allows the muscle to perform work.

It is now recognized that vitamin D is important for optimal functioning of skeletal muscle. Vitamin D can modulate skeletal muscle function by both genomic and nongenomic events. The biologically active form of vitamin D, 1, $25(OH)_2D$ induces muscle gene transcription and protein synthesis to influence muscle cell proliferation and differentiation, calcium uptake, and phosphate transport across the sarcolemma (Hamilton 2010). The nongenomic responses include modulation of calcium uptake across the sarcolemma and the activation of mitogen-activated protein kinase signaling pathways in muscle fibers. Vitamin D also upregulates expression of insulin-like growth factor 1 (IGF-1) (Ameri et al. 2013), which has a well-recognized role in muscle remodeling, hypertrophy, and strength gains. IGF-1, which is mostly produced by the liver and bound by insulin-like growth factor binding protein 3 (IGFBP-3) in the serum, is a key component in muscle regeneration and could induce proliferation, differentiation, and hypertrophy of skeletal muscle. IGFBP-3 expression could be regulated by vitamin D because there are vitamin D response elements in the promoter region of the human IGFBP-3 gene, which might lead to higher circulating amounts of IGFBP-3 and therefore delay the normally rapid clearance of IGF-1 in the bloodstream. The obvious implication of these findings is that vitamin D status and vitamin D supplementation might affect muscle strength, endurance, and athletic performance. This has received considerable attention over the past decade, and the results of these studies have been the main focus of numerous recent reviews about vitamin D and the athlete (Angeline et al. 2013; Moran et al. 2013; Owens, Fraser, and Close 2015; Todd et al. 2015). The general consensus at present is that vitamin D deficiency could negatively affect athletic performance due to the influence of vitamin D on muscle function. However, there is insufficient evidence from a limited number of cross-sectional vitamin D status studies and longitudinal, randomized, placebo-controlled vitamin D_3 supplementation studies in athletes to conclude that vitamin D is a direct performance enhancer (Girgis et al. 2014).

Calcium and vitamin K are required for normal blood clotting. Vitamin K is required for the synthesis of blood-clotting factors. This vitamin is a coenzyme in the posttranslational modification of protein structure, specifically the addition of sugar moieties to form glycoproteins.

Iodine functions as a component of the thyroid hormones triiodothyronine and tetraiodothyronine, which act as important regulators of metabolism and cardiovascular function. Although compromised iodine intake is not typically considered to be a concern for athletes, emerging research suggests that deficiency is prevalent among certain subpopulations. Athletes at risk for compromised iodine status include those who do not consume iodized salt, those who consume little seafood and live in regions with iodine poor soils (Dean 2017; Krajcovicova-Kudlackova et al. 2003), or those who have heavy sweat rates (Smyth and Duntas 2005).

Zinc plays a role in appetite regulation. Oral zinc supplementation has been shown to be effective in restoring normal eating behavior and body weight in patients suffering from the eating disorder anorexia nervosa (see chapter 16). Zinc has been suggested to be involved in the pathogenesis of this eating disorder. Among female athletes, gymnasts and dancers have a particularly high incidence of eating disorders, and several dietary surveys indicate that these groups consume inadequate amounts of zinc. Indeed, in a study of female adolescent dancers and gymnasts, 75% were found to consume less than two-thirds of the RDA for zinc. Thus, athletes who attempt to maintain a low body weight should be sure to consume adequate amounts of zinc.

Besides being coenzymes in energy metabolism, several of the B-complex vitamins are also required for normal neuromuscular function. For example, vitamin B_6 is needed for the synthesis and metabolism of many neurotransmitters, including norepinephrine and dopamine. Vitamin A forms the visual pigments of the eye and is therefore important for normal vision, particularly in fading light.

Assessing Micronutrient Status

Vitamin (and mineral) status can be estimated directly from biopsy samples of body tissues (e.g., skeletal muscle), from blood cells or plasma, or indirectly from analysis of the diet. The vitamin status of an individual, however, is difficult to determine accurately. A diagnosis of vitamin deficiency is best made by considering a variety of sources of information, including blood analysis, an assessment of dietary intake, and clinical symptoms. Most studies that have used blood analysis (either by direct measurement of the plasma concentration of the vitamin or by indirect measurement of vitamin-requiring enzyme activities) have not revealed any distinct differences between athletic people and sedentary people. Furthermore, little evidence suggests that the vitamin intakes of athletes in general are inadequate, based on the RDAs, except in athletes with extremely low dietary energy intakes or in athletes who fail to consume well-balanced diets.

As for mineral status, assessment using blood markers is possible for some (e.g., iron, magnesium, zinc) but not for others (e.g., calcium, potassium, selenium), and the only alternative is to assess dietary intake using the methods described in chapter 1.

Dietary Surveys of Vitamin Intakes in Elite Athletes

Ideally, athletes should obtain all their nutrients from food. A well-balanced diet, including foods from each of the five food groups (meat, dairy, whole grains, fruit, and vegetables) should provide adequate amounts of all 13 essential vitamins, with the possible exception of vitamin D, which is mostly produced inside the body by the action of sunlight on the skin. Arguably, because total energy intake of most athletes exceeds that of sedentary nonathletes, a greater amount and variety of vitamins should be available to athletes through their dietary intakes. Unfortunately, surveys of the dietary habits of elite athletes indicate that they do not always consume well-balanced diets. Elite athletes are at risk for nutrient deficiencies because of the fatiguing and time-consuming demands of training. A combination of increased vitamin turnover, additional loss of some nutrients, poor food selection, and limited time for food preparation are contributing factors.

The first two comprehensive reports on the actual dietary intakes of athletes, published in 1981, revealed inappropriate macronutrient composition of the diets with fat and protein components being too high. In one study (Barry et al. 1981), this inadequate diet was coupled with suboptimal intakes of thiamin, niacin, and folic acid. Intakes of these vitamins among female athletes were well below the recommended daily requirements. Some dietary surveys performed on elite endurance athletes have reported low (<85% of the RDA) or excessively high (>200% of the RDA) intakes of vitamins. But apart from reports of low vitamin D intake in South African runners (Peters and Goetzsche 1997) and low vitamin A intake in Dutch elite strength athletes (van Erp-Baart et al. 1989b), deficient as well as excess intakes are reported consistently only for the water-soluble vitamins. Low intakes of vitamins A and D are likely attributable to the restriction of dietary fat intake in weight-conscious athletes. In a national dietary survey of Dutch athletes (van Erp-Baart et al. 1989b) who participated in endurance, strength, or team sports, intakes of vitamins B_2, B_6, and C appeared to be more than adequate in endurance athletes but were marginal in some strength athletes and team games players (see figure 10.10). This difference was attributed to the higher total dietary energy intakes in the endurance athletes. Several groups of athletes in this study consumed vitamin supplements well in excess of the RDA.

In contrast, the groups most at risk for inadequate intake of vitamins (B vitamins in particular) are female adolescent athletes and athletes who are attempting to maintain low body weight (e.g., wrestlers, gymnasts, ballet dancers) by restricting their total energy intake. Clearly, these athletes need to choose foods carefully or take vitamin supplements.

The daily ingestion of a multivitamin tablet that provides the RDA of all 13 vitamins is common-

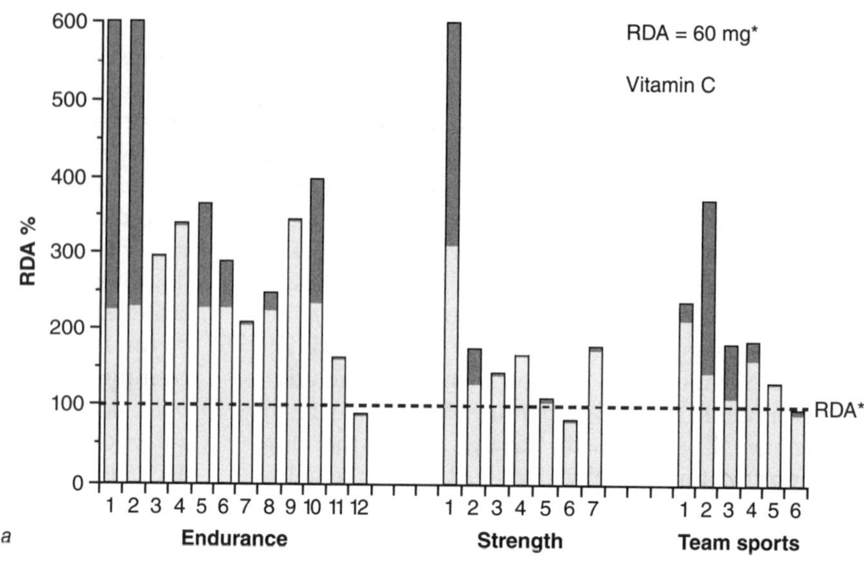

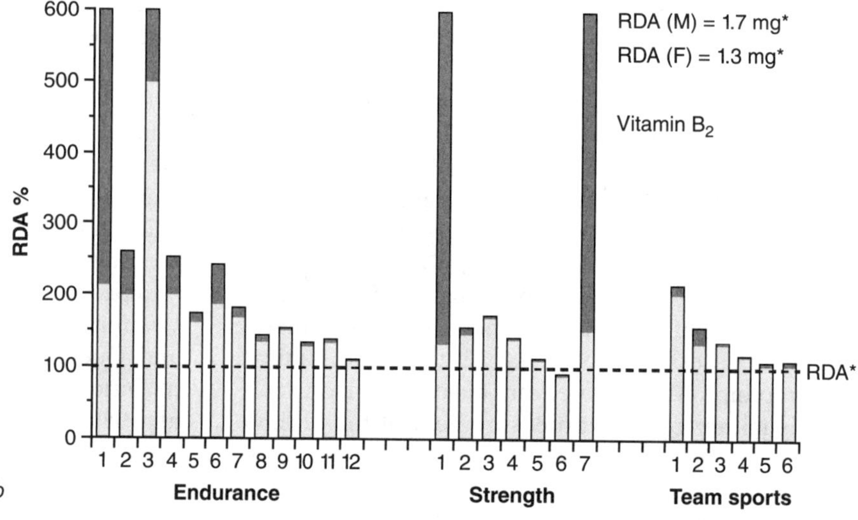

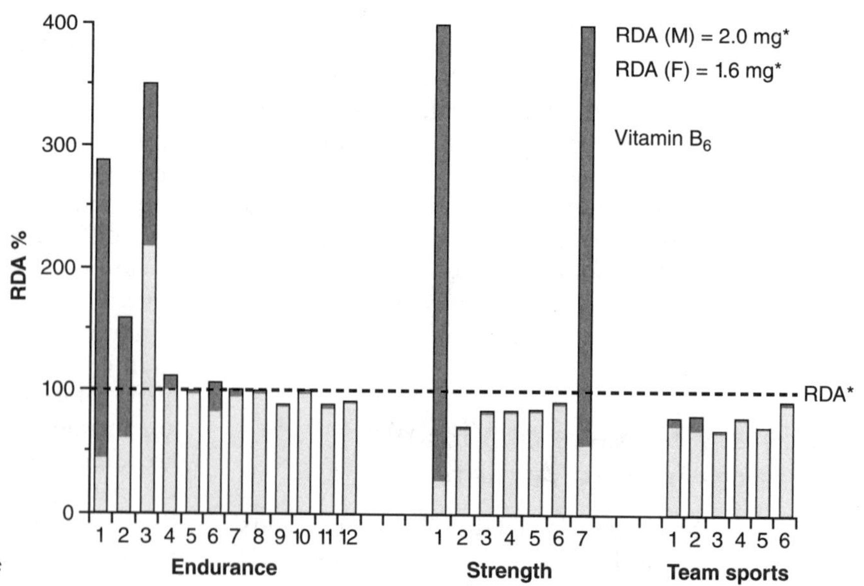

Figure 10.10 Daily intakes of *(a)* vitamin C, *(b)* vitamin B_2, and *(c)* vitamin B_6 in athletes from various sports. Open columns represent intake from food sources; filled columns indicate intake from supplements. M = male; F = female.

Endurance: 1 = Tour de France M; 2 = Tour de l'Avenir M; 3 = triathlon M; 4 = cycling M; 5 = marathon speed skating M; 6 = swimming M; 7 = rowing M; 8 = running M; 9 = rowing F; 10 = cycling F; 11 = running F; 12 = subtop swimming F.

Strength: 1 = bodybuilding M; 2 = judo M; 3 = weightlifting M; 4 = judo M; 5 = top gymnastics F; 6 = subtop gymnastics F; 7 = bodybuilding F.

Team sports: 1 = water polo M; 2 = soccer M; 3 = field hockey M; 4 = volleyball F; 5 = field hockey F; 6 = handball F.

*These are based on RDAs in 1989, which have since changed (see appendix C).

International Journal of Sports Medicine: From A.M.J. van Erp-Baart et al., "Nationwide Survey on Nutritional Habits in Elite Athletes. Part II: Mineral and Vitamin Intake," 1989; 10, suppl 1: S11-S16. Adapted by permission.

place among educated athletes and is the simplest and probably most effective means of correcting any vitamin deficiencies that arise from eating an unbalanced diet. Surveys of athletes on vitamin supplement use confirm the high prevalence of vitamin supplement use among elite athletes. For example, using questionnaires, Heikkinen et al. (2011) reported that 77% of Finnish Olympic athletes used vitamin supplements from 2002 to 2009. The main reason given by the athletes for taking supplements was to prevent nutritional deficiencies.

Dietary Surveys of Mineral Intakes in Elite Athletes

The interpretation of dietary records for adequacy of mineral (particularly trace element) intake should be done with some caution. This assessment is difficult because of the differences in the bioavailability of trace elements in various foods and because not all foods have been analyzed for their mineral composition. Furthermore, assessment of a person's mineral status based on a chemical analysis of blood or biopsy samples is not always possible. In many cases, the plasma concentration of a particular mineral does not accurately reflect the body stores of the mineral. Given those limitations, information based on dietary surveys of athletes and their blood chemistry suggest that iron, zinc, calcium, and magnesium status may be of some concern, especially for young athletes and female athletes of all ages.

Several groups of athletes may have low iron stores, including middle-distance and long-distance runners, female endurance athletes, and adolescent athletes. Nevertheless, the proportion of athletes with low iron stores is no greater than that found in the general U.S. population, in which the incidence of iron depletion (a serum ferritin level of less than 12 mg/L) is 21% of women and 25% of adolescent girls. The incidence of iron depletion in male athletes may be higher than it is for sedentary men, in whom iron deficiency is low (less than 2% of the male population in the United States). Men generally meet the RDA for calcium, but women, especially adolescents, do not. Young female athletes concerned with maintaining low body weight and low body fat, such as gymnasts, dancers, and runners, have low calcium intakes (Aulin 2000). The story is similar for zinc and magnesium; most male athletes appear to meet the RDA for these minerals, but many groups of female athletes do not. Limited information is available for other minerals, but reports of isolated trace element deficiencies in athletes, apart from iron and zinc, are extremely rare.

In a recent systematic review and meta-analysis of supplement use in elite and nonelite athletes, Knapik et al. (2016) reported that about 37% of male and female athletes regularly took a multivitamin and mineral supplement. The prevalence of taking an iron supplement was higher among women (23%) than men (11%), and the prevalence of taking a vitamin E supplement was higher among men (14%) than women (8%). The prevalence of taking calcium and zinc supplements was similar: 18% for men and 6% for women. Elite athletes (57%) were more likely to take a multivitamin and mineral supplement than nonelite athletes (36%).

Exercise and Micronutrient Requirements

Various experimental vitamin depletion studies have determined that inadequate vitamin status is associated with impaired exercise performance, particularly when more than one vitamin is deficient in the diet. Athletes are generally assumed to need increased vitamin intake because exercise increases vitamin requirements. Theoretically, exercise can induce a marginal vitamin status (deficiency) by causing decreased absorption from the digestive tract; increased excretion in sweat, urine, and feces; increased turnover (degradation); and increased requirement (retention) because of biochemical adaptation to training (e.g., increased mitochondrial density in skeletal muscle with endurance training and muscle hypertrophy with strength training).

A temporary depression of the free (unbound) plasma concentration of some trace elements (e.g., iron, magnesium, zinc, copper) may occur after prolonged exercise mainly because of a redistribution of the mineral to other tissue compartments (e.g., erythrocytes, leukocytes, muscle or adipose tissue) or because of the release of proteins from liver and neutrophils that chelate (bind) the mineral as part of the acute-phase response to inflammation (see figure 10.11). Regular exercise, particularly in a hot environment, incurs increased losses of several minerals in sweat and urine, which means that the daily requirement for most minerals increases in athletes engaged in heavy training. But with the exception of iron and zinc, isolated mineral deficiencies are rare.

Iron losses in sweat may be as high as 0.3 mg of iron per liter of sweat (see table 10.10). When an athlete exercises hard in a hot environment,

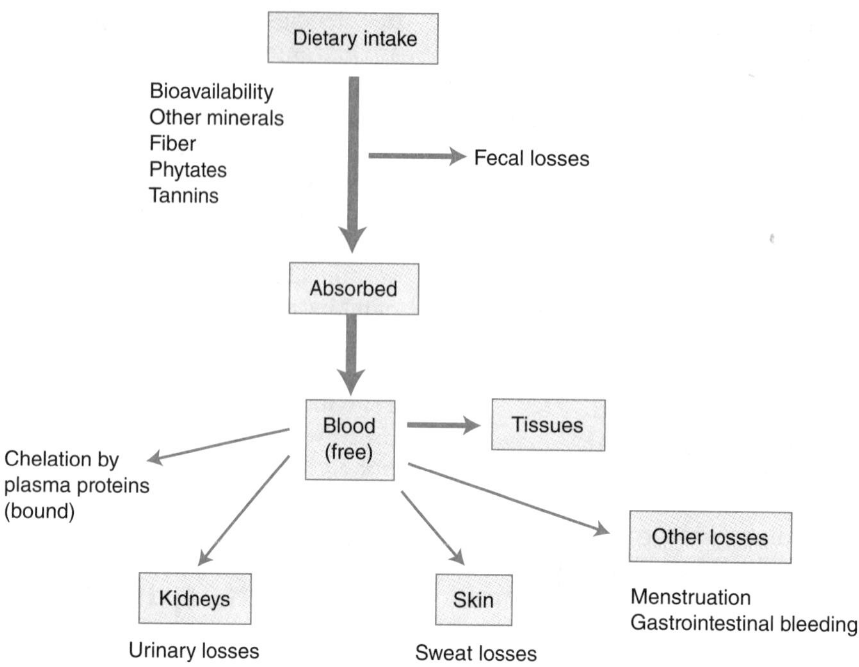

Figure 10.11 Factors that affect absorption and tissue distribution of minerals. Exercise may increase losses of minerals in urine and sweat, and several other components of the diet may interfere with mineral absorption.

sweat production can be about 2 L/h (0.5 gal/h). If the athlete exercises for 2 h/day in such conditions, the additional daily sweat loss is 4 L (1 gal), which incurs a loss of 1.2 mg of iron. Because, on average, only about 10% of dietary iron can be absorbed in the gut, the person must consume about 12 mg of extra iron in food to replace this loss of iron. The RDA for iron for men is 8 mg (18 mg for women), so the sweat losses approximately double the dietary requirement.

Controversy exists regarding iron losses in sweat and whether athletes can lose enough iron in sweat to cause iron deficiency. In a careful study that minimized iron loss in shed skin cells and iron contamination of skin, a much lower iron concentration in sweat (averaging only 23 mg/L) was reported (Brune et al. 1986). A subsequent study of exercising athletes (Waller and Haymes 1996) also suggested that losses of iron in sweat are modest and, furthermore, that the concentration of iron in sweat declines over time (at least during the first hour of exercise). These authors estimated that about 6% to 11% of the iron typically absorbed each day is lost in sweat during an hour of exercise and that losses for men are approximately twice those for women because of the higher sweat rate in men.

Exercise may further increase the requirement for iron because of the adaptive increase in muscle myoglobin concentration and red cell mass in response to endurance training (Eichner 2000). Some athletes are susceptible to gastrointestinal bleeding during prolonged strenuous exercise. About 20% of recreational runners are estimated to experience occult fecal blood after distance races. Bleeding may arise because of irritation of the stomach lining or superficial hemorrhage of the colon caused by ischemic insult (i.e., restricted blood supply because of constriction of blood vessels supplying the tissue). During strenuous exercise, blood is diverted to the working muscles, and when exercise is prolonged (particularly when accompanied by dehydration and hyperthermia), the restriction of blood flow to the colon may cause inflammation and blood vessel damage, which is called segmental hemorrhagic colitis (Eichner 2000). Measurement of fecal iron loss in elite male distance runners showed that during training and racing, gastrointestinal blood loss amounted to about 6 ml/day (Nachtigall et al. 1996).

Substantial amounts of magnesium are lost in sweat (see table 10.5), and increased urinary losses of both magnesium and zinc have been reported in athletes engaged in high-intensity exercise. These additional losses could cause magnesium and zinc deficiency with chronic training if they are not matched by increased dietary intakes. Several studies report lower resting serum concentrations of magnesium and zinc in athletes compared with sedentary control subjects, but serum levels of these minerals for athletes were still within the accepted normal ranges.

Ergogenic Effect of Micronutrient Supplementation

Many papers have been written about the effects of vitamin supplementation on exercise performance. Older studies suggested a potential ergogenic role of vitamins based on the argument that the RDAs may not represent optimal intake. But many of the early studies that claimed to show beneficial effects of vitamin supplementation on exercise performance were poorly designed and often had no control (placebo) group against which to compare the effects of supplementation or had no information about current vitamin status in the test subjects. More recent double-blind placebo-controlled studies have discredited the notion that excess vitamin intake improves exercise performance. Even so, many athletes consume relatively large amounts of vitamin and mineral supplements to prevent vitamin deficiency.

Severe or prolonged vitamin deficiencies are, of course, deleterious to health and would be expected to impair athletic performance. Vitamin and mineral supplementation may improve the nutritional status of people who consume marginal amounts of nutrients from food and may improve performance in those with deficiencies. Athletes should not rely on tablets to supply them with the necessary micronutrients. Besides the established vitamins, many other compounds present in small quantities in fresh fruit and vegetables are needed for optimal health.

Short-term inadequacy of vitamin intake is characterized by lowered vitamin concentrations in body tissues and fluids and decreased activities of certain enzymes. But functional disturbances, including decreased $\dot{V}O_2max$ or physical performance capacity, may not appear until weeks or months later. In the opposite scenario, large intakes of vitamins increase the body's vitamin stores (particularly fat-soluble vitamins) and the activity of some enzymes but will not necessarily improve physical work capacity. Furthermore, excessive intakes of the fat-soluble vitamins (A, D, E, and K) for prolonged periods can be harmful.

It is a similar story for most minerals. Correcting deficiencies (e.g., of iron, magnesium, zinc) may improve exercise performance, but supplements are unlikely to have any ergogenic effect for people who have adequate mineral status. Several studies indicate that magnesium supplementation may improve exercise economy during prolonged submaximal exercise due to lower oxygen uptake and better lactate clearance, and an association between magnesium intake and strength performance has been reported in athletes and older adults (Mooren 2015). Therefore, magnesium supplementation should be considered for athletes with magnesium deficiency.

Some minerals are specifically promoted as potential ergogenic aids to performance. These supplements, often consumed in bulk quantities a few hours before competition, include phosphates and sodium bicarbonate. Phosphate salts are suggested as a potential ergogenic aid because these ions are an important intracellular buffer. Phosphate groups are a component of the body's energy currency, namely ATP. Therefore, phosphate loading might increase the resynthesis rate of ATP from ADP and phosphate. Another possible ergogenic mechanism could be improving oxygen extraction from the blood by muscle fibers through an elevated erythrocyte 2,3-DPG concentration. At present, however, experimental evidence for these claims is lacking. Bicarbonate is an important extracellular buffer. Reliable evidence indicates that bicarbonate ingestion (most commonly consumed as sodium bicarbonate, although sodium itself has no independent effects in acid–base regulation) can improve performance in events in which lactic acid accumulation in the muscle is a major cause of fatigue, such as 400 to 1,500 m running (see chapter 11). But consumption of the amount of sodium bicarbonate necessary to sufficiently alter blood acid–base balance to influence performance (approximately 20 g) can cause gastrointestinal discomfort and diarrhea. Because of these unpleasant side effects, bicarbonate loading can temporarily result in inadequate absorption of essential micronutrients and carbohydrate and can delay the restoration of muscle glycogen stores after exercise. The side effects and their consequences are important factors to consider for sports events that involve competitions on successive days. Further details of phosphate and bicarbonate loading are found in chapter 11.

Summary of Recommendations for Micronutrient Intake in Athletes

In general, supplementation with individual vitamins, including the consumption of large doses of simple antioxidant mixtures, is not recommended. Consuming megadoses of individual vitamins (which is common among athletes) is likely to do more harm than good. Because most vitamins function mainly as coenzymes in the body, after these enzyme systems are saturated, the vitamin in free form can become toxic (as discussed earlier). Athletes should obtain complex mixtures of antioxidant compounds from increased consumption of fruits and vegetables.

Vitamin supplements are not necessary for athletes who eat well-balanced diets. Athletes who are concerned about adequate intakes of vitamins, especially during periods of intensive training and carbohydrate loading before competition, and want to avoid the risks of oversupplementation can take an over-the-counter multivitamin that provides an adequate and safe level of vitamin intake.

Most athletes do not require mineral supplements because their diets are already more than adequate to meet any increased requirements that result from the effects of regular intensive exercise. Some groups of athletes, notably those who compete in sports events in which low body weight is essential for success (e.g., gymnasts and dancers) or compete within certain body-weight categories (e.g., boxers, wrestlers, and weightlifters), are at risk for marginal mineral intake. Participants in such sports often train frequently and intensively but consume low-energy diets or undergo drastic weight-loss regimens to maintain or lose body weight before competition. Low energy intakes (< 8 MJ/day [< 1,912 kcal/day]) can lead to inadequate essential mineral and vitamin intakes. Because many athletes are young and still in a period of body growth and development, they can be detrimentally affected by micronutrient deficiencies.

The following specific recommendations can be given to athletes to ensure adequate calcium intake during an energy-restricted diet:

- Consume three servings per day of low-fat dairy foods.
- Include these dairy foods in high-carbohydrate meals (e.g., skim milk on cereal).
- Eat fish with bones (e.g., sardines).
- Include calcium-enriched soy products in the diet.
- Eat leafy green vegetables (e.g., cabbage, broccoli, spinach).

The following recommendations can be given to athletes to increase available iron intake in a high-carbohydrate diet:

- Eat foods rich in heme iron at least four times per week (e.g., liver or lean red meat).
- Eat iron-fortified foods (e.g., breakfast cereal).
- Include nonheme iron food sources (e.g., dried fruit, legumes, green leafy vegetables) in the diet.
- Combine nonheme iron foods with meat or foods rich in vitamin C (e.g., orange juice) to increase iron absorption.
- Avoid drinking tea or coffee at meals.

Other athletes who are at risk for marginal mineral intake are those who abstain from normal diets (i.e., consume extremely unbalanced diets with a low micronutrient density) and vegetarians. Micronutrient supplementation is recommended for such athletes.

Amenorrheic female athletes should certainly take calcium supplements, and other female athletes should consider taking calcium supplements to ensure adequate calcium status and maintain healthy bones. Moderately elevated intakes of calcium do not appear to be harmful, possibly because the blood calcium concentration is under tight hormonal regulation and moderate excesses can be excreted in the urine.

Athletes who train and compete in hot environments should also consider increasing their intake of minerals (particularly iron, zinc, and magnesium) because mineral losses in sweat can be considerable. Even so, daily supplements of these minerals should not exceed one to two times the RDA. As with vitamins, excessive intake of minerals can be toxic and can impair the absorption of other essential trace elements.

Poor diets are the main reason for micronutrient deficiencies in athletes, but in certain cases, regular strenuous exercise contributes to the deficiency. Eating a well-balanced diet can easily correct micronutrient deficiencies with the possible exceptions of iron, calcium, and vitamin D shortfalls. Inadequate knowledge of proper dietary practices, lack of time for food preparation, misleading advertisements for micronutrient supplements, and lack of qualified dietary advice are possible reasons for suboptimal micronutrient intakes in athletes. Few studies have definitively documented beneficial effects of mineral or vitamin supplementation on exercise performance except when supplementation was needed to correct an existing deficiency. Athletes who take micronutrient supplements are for the most part taking them to ensure good health, not to enhance sports performance. An unhealthy athlete is unlikely to perform to the best of his or her potential.

Key Points

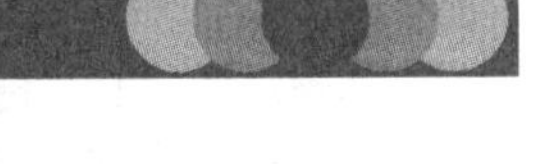

- Although vitamin and mineral supplementation may improve nutrition in athletes who consume marginal amounts of micronutrients from food and may improve performance in athletes with deficiencies, no convincing evidence indicates that doses in excess of the RDA improve performance.
- Vitamins and minerals are needed in the body for several important processes, including the growth and repair of body tissues, as cofactors in enzyme-catalyzed metabolic reactions, for oxygen transport and oxidative metabolism, for immune function, and as antioxidants. Any sustained deficiency of an essential vitamin or mineral will cause ill health, and an unhealthy athlete is extremely unlikely to perform to the best of his or her potential.
- Vitamins are organic compounds that are needed in small quantities in the diet. They are essential for specific metabolic reactions in the body and for normal growth and development. With the exception of vitamin D, which can be synthesized from sunlight, and vitamin K and some B vitamins, which can be produced by the bacterial microflora of the gastrointestinal tract, vitamins are not produced by the human body and must be consumed in the diet.
- Although vitamins do not directly contribute to energy supply, they play an important role in regulating metabolism by acting as reusable coenzymes in intermediary metabolism. A deficiency of some of the B-group vitamins, which act as cofactors of enzymes in carbohydrate (e.g., B_3, B_6, and B_1), fat (e.g., B_2, B_1, pantothenic acid, and biotin), and protein (B_6) metabolism, results in premature fatigue and inability to maintain a heavy training program. Other vitamins play a role in red and white blood cell production (folic acid and B_{12}) or assist in the formation of bones, connective tissue, and cartilage (e.g., vitamins C and D).
- The water-soluble vitamins—vitamins C, B_1, B_2, B_3, B_6, thiamin, riboflavin, pyridoxine, niacin, pantothenic acid, and biotin—are involved in mitochondrial energy metabolism. Folic acid and vitamin B_{12} are mainly involved in nucleic acid synthesis and hence are important for maintaining healthy populations of rapidly dividing cells in the body (e.g., red blood cells, immune cells, and the gut mucosa). Vitamin C is also an antioxidant.
- The fat-soluble vitamins are A, D, E, and K. Of these vitamins, only vitamin E has a probable role in energy metabolism. In addition, beta-carotene (provitamin A) and vitamin E have antioxidant properties. Vitamin K is required for the addition of sugar residues to proteins to form glycoproteins.
- Although physical activity may increase the requirement for some vitamins (e.g., vitamin C, riboflavin, and possibly pyridoxine, vitamin A, and vitamin E), this increased requirement typically is met by consuming a balanced high-carbohydrate, moderate-protein, low-fat diet. Vitamin and mineral intakes in athletes are correlated with energy intakes up to 20 MJ/day (4,780 kcal/day), so if energy intake matches the energy requirement, athletes get all the micronutrients that they need from food without any need for supplements (with the possible exception of vitamin D if sunlight exposure is insufficient).

- Evidence suggests that antioxidants provide an important defense mechanism in the body against the damaging effects of free radicals. Many athletes consume large doses of antioxidant vitamins (beta-carotene and vitamins C and E), but excessive antioxidant ingestion may not be uniformly helpful and may impair adaptation to training. The controversy continues about whether physically active people should consume antioxidant compounds in amounts above RDA values. At present, the data are insufficient to recommend antioxidant supplements for athletes.
- Most athletes do not require micronutrient supplements (with the possible exception of vitamin D) because their diets are already more than adequate to meet any increased requirements from the effects of regular intensive exercise. Particular groups of athletes, however, are at risk for marginal mineral and vitamin intake. These athletes compete in sports events in which low body weight is essential for success (e.g., gymnasts and dancers) or compete within certain body-weight categories (e.g., boxers, wrestlers, and weightlifters). Participants in these sports often train frequently and intensively but consume low-energy diets or undergo drastic weight-loss regimens to maintain or lose body weight before competition.
- Amenorrheic female athletes should certainly take calcium supplements, and other female athletes should consider taking them, to ensure adequate calcium status and maintain healthy bones. Athletes who train and compete in hot environments should also consider increasing their mineral intake (particularly iron, zinc, and magnesium) because mineral losses in sweat can be considerable. Even so, daily supplements of these minerals should not exceed one to two times the RDA. As with vitamins, excessive intakes of minerals can be toxic and can impair the absorption of other essential trace elements.
- Although poor diets are the main reason for micronutrient deficiencies among athletes, regular strenuous exercise can contribute to deficiency. Eating a well-balanced diet can easily correct these deficiencies, with the possible exceptions of shortfalls in iron, calcium, and vitamin D. Inadequate knowledge of proper dietary practices, lack of time for food preparation, misleading advertisements for micronutrient supplements, and lack of qualified dietary advice are possible reasons for suboptimal micronutrient intakes by athletes.

Recommended Readings

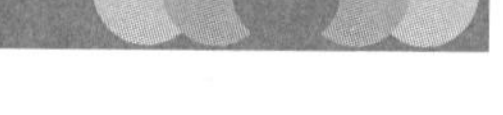

Chen, J. 2000. Vitamins: Effects of exercise on requirements. In *Nutrition in sport,* edited by R.J. Maughan, 282-291. Oxford: Blackwell Science.

Clarkson, P.M. 1991. Minerals: Exercise performance and supplementation in athletes. *Journal of Sports Sciences* 9:91-116.

Haymes, E.M. 1991. Vitamin and mineral supplementation to athletes. *International Journal of Sport Nutrition* 1:146-169.

Niess, A.M., and P. Simon. 2007. Response and adaptation of skeletal muscle to exercise—the role of reactive oxygen species. *Frontiers in Bioscience* 12:4826-4838.

Owens, D.J., W.D. Fraser, and G.L. Close. 2015. Vitamin D and the athlete: Emerging insights. *European Journal of Sport Science* 15:73-84.

Powers, S.K., K.C. DeRuisseau, J. Quindry, and K.L. Hamilton. 2004. Dietary antioxidants and exercise. *Journal of Sports Sciences* 22 (1): 81-94.

Quindry, J.C., A. Kavazis, and S.K. Powers. 2014. Exercise-induced oxidative stress: Are supplemental antioxidants warranted? In *Sport nutrition,* edited by R.J. Maughan, 263-276. Oxford: Blackwell Science.

van der Beek, E.J. 1991. Vitamin supplementation and physical exercise performance. *Journal of Sports Sciences* 9:77-89.

Volpe, S.L., and H.A. Nguyen. 2014. Vitamins, minerals and sport performance. In *Sport nutrition,* edited by R. J. Maughan, 217-228. Oxford: Blackwell Science.

Nutrition Supplements

Objectives

After studying this chapter, you should be able to do the following:

- Describe various categories of nutrition supplements
- Discuss the nutrition supplements that have ergogenic properties
- Discuss the potential hazards and risks of nutrition supplements
- Understand critical analyses of research findings and reports and the importance of them

The use of nutrition supplements is a widespread and legitimate part of the strategy employed by many athletes in the pursuit of sporting success. The use of **ergogenic aids** or nutrition supplements is not new. As long ago as 500 to 400 BC, dietary fads were being used to enhance performance (Applegate and Grivetti 1997). Many athletes today are still hopeful of finding a special beverage or pill that will improve performance.

Looking beyond genetic endowment and training, many athletes turn to ergogenic aids (Applegate 1999). Nutrition supplements, as the name implies, should be used to supplement the current diet rather than substitute for it. For many modern athletes, however, sport nutrition has become synonymous with nutrition supplements. The ideas and expectations that athletes have about nutrition supplements are heavily influenced by the manufacturers and sellers of those supplements, who claim that their products increase muscle mass, improve stamina, and so on.

Weight loss and muscle gain are important goals for many athletes and for people not involved in athletic training. Because achieving those goals is difficult with conventional methods (reducing energy intake and increasing energy expenditure through physical activity), supplements sound attractive to many. Nutritional supplements are used by 40% to 100% of athletes in one form or another (Burke, Collier, and Hargreaves 1993), and evidence suggests that athletes use several nutrition supplements at the same time and in extremely high doses. In this chapter, we review the claims and the experimental evidence for a selection of common supplements. We focus mainly on those supplements that are claimed to improve exercise performance, boost recovery, or promote fat loss. Thousands of nutrition supplements are now on the market. The global dietary supplement market was valued at $132.8 billion (USD) in 2016 and is expected to reach $220.3 billion in 2022 (Global News Wire 2017), and many of these supplements are targeted to athletes. Of course, we cannot review them all, but we will focus on some of the most popular ones where there is at least some reasonable scientific evidence to make an informed judgment on their efficacy. A fairly extensive list of common supplements is shown in the sidebar. For most there is little, if any, evidence to indicate that they are effective. For some supplements (e.g., beetroot juice, caffeine, ß-alanine, creatine, sodium bicarbonate) there is strong evidence that they

POPULAR NUTRITIONAL SUPPLEMENTS

- Acetylcholine
- Androstenedione
- Arginine
- Bee pollen
- Beetroot juice
- ß-alanine
- ß-hydroxy ß-methylbutyrate (HMB)
- Boron
- Branched-chain amino acids
- Caffeine
- Carnitine
- Carnosine
- Cherry juice
- Choline
- Chondroitin
- Citrulline
- Chromium picolinate
- Coenzyme Q10
- Conjugated linoleic acids
- Creatine
- Dehydroepiandrosterone (DHEA)
- Desiccated liver
- Dihydroxyacetone (DHA)
- Ephedra
- Fish oil
- Gamma oryzanol
- Ginseng
- Glandulars
- Glucosamine
- Glucose polymers
- Glutamine
- Glycerol
- Green tea
- Inosine
- Ketone salts
- Lactate salts and polylactate
- Lecithin
- Medium-chain triacylglycerol (MCT)
- Octacosanol
- Omega-3 fatty acids
- Pangamic acid (not available for sale)
- Phosphate salts
- Phosphatidylserine
- Phosphorus
- Polyphenols
- Pyruvate and dihydroxyacetone
- Quercetin
- Resveratrol
- Royal jelly
- Smilax
- Sodium bicarbonate
- Sodium citrate
- Sodium nitrate
- Sodium phosphate
- Spirulina
- Succinate
- Yohimbine
- Vanadium
- Wheat germ oil

are effective in improving exercise performance (Peeling et al. 2018) under certain conditions. The latter can include the supplement dose, timing of its ingestion in relation to exercise, and the intensity and duration of exercise. The impact of ingestion of carbohydrate, fat, fluid, protein, amino acids, and micronutrients on exercise performance was covered in previous chapters and will not be repeated here. Supplements that may modify training adaptations are mentioned in chapter 12, and supplements that may boost immunity and reduce susceptibility to infection are discussed in chapter 13.

Relative Importance of Supplements to a Normal Diet

When it comes to nutrition advice, many athletes appear to be more interested in supplements than in achieving a healthy balanced diet. This happens at all levels of sport from recreational weekend warriors to seasoned and professional athletes. Some beliefs about supplement use include the following:

- Supplements are more effective than a healthy diet.
- Supplements can provide a quick fix, whereas the positive effects of a balanced healthy diet take a long time.
- The diet is already balanced and healthy and the next thing to address is the use of supplements.
- The diet is unbalanced anyway and supplements are needed to compensate for this and help prevent deficiencies, or supplements are there as an insurance policy.
- Other athletes are using supplements, so not using them puts one at a disadvantage.

As mentioned previously, nutrition supplements should supplement the diet rather than replace it, and supplements should not be the main focus. One general lesson that can be learned from sport is that there are no quick fixes; success demands dedication and effort. This applies to sport nutrition as well.

Several sport nutrition conferences and review articles in the past two decades (e.g., Maughan and Shirreffs 2011) have emphasized that the amount, composition, and timing of food intake can profoundly affect sports performance. Evidence-based good nutritional practices that predominantly use natural foods and beverages have been established to help athletes perform and train more effectively, recover quickly, and adapt more effectively with less risk of illness and injury. Expert sport nutritionists repeatedly remind athletes that they should avoid the indiscriminate use of dietary supplements. Supplements that provide essential nutrients may be of help where food intake or food choices are restricted, but this approach to achieving adequate nutrient intake is normally only a short-term option. The use of supplements will not compensate for poor food choices and an inadequate diet. Athletes contemplating the use of supplements and foods or beverages developed for use by athletes should consider their efficacy, their cost, the risk to health and performance, and the potential for a positive doping test (see the last section of this chapter). Athletes can also benefit from the guidance of qualified sport nutrition professionals who can provide advice on individual energy, nutrient, and fluid needs and help develop sport-specific nutritional strategies for training, competition, and recovery (Maughan and Shirreffs 2011).

Serious athletes should ask themselves the following questions: How can I improve my nutrition intake to support my goals? Are there any sport nutrition products that can further support my goals on days of hard training or competition? Once those questions are adequately addressed, preferably following advice from a sport nutrition professional, it is sensible to ask a third question: Are there any supplements that, in addition to a balanced diet, can help improve my performance, training adaptation, or recovery? Supplements should be the last component rather than the foundation of a balanced diet.

Nonregulation of Nutrition Supplements

An abundance of information can be found in advertising and on the Internet about nutritional supplements. Most claims are not backed up by scientific studies, and many of them are unrealistic or even impossible. Claims are often based on studies in non-peer-reviewed journals or results from studies that are inappropriately extrapolated. The claims that manufacturers make about nutrition supplements are apparently difficult to regulate.

In contrast to prescription drugs, which are carefully regulated, nutrition supplements receive little governmental oversight, and retailers have enormous freedom in making marketing claims. For instance, the FDA strictly regulates the clinical testing, advertising, and promotion of prescription drugs, which prevents retailers from making unproved claims. Nutrition supplements are under no such regulation. Drugs are extensively tested for safety before they can be sold, but nutrition supplements are not tested. The Dietary Supplement Health and Education Act of 1994 created a new category of product called dietary supplements. These dietary supplements are considered to be part of nutrition (not medication) and are defined as "vitamins, minerals, herbs and botanicals, amino acids, and other dietary substances intended to supplement the diet by increasing the total dietary intake." The ingredients in the supplements may be in their natural form "or as any concentrate, metabolite, constituent or combination of these ingredients" (Federal Food, Drug, and Cosmetic Act 1938). Although manufacturers must submit information about new products (including the claims) to the FDA, this information is for notification rather than authorization (Ross 2000). Nevertheless, the

FDA is responsible for acting against any adulterated or misbranded dietary supplement product after it reaches the market. Under existing law, including the Dietary Supplement Health and Education Act of 1994, the FDA can take action to remove products from the market if the agency can establish that such products are adulterated (e.g., that the product is unsafe) or misbranded (e.g., that the labeling is false or misleading). The FDA keeps a list of tainted supplements on their website (www.fda.gov).

Critical Evaluation of Nutrition Supplement Studies

Athletes and others must critically examine claims made by the dietary supplement industry and the "scientific evidence" that supports the claims. The following are some factors that should be considered when evaluating reports of scientific studies:

- *Does the study have a clear hypothesis?* A well-designed study has a clear hypothesis and a strong theoretical basis for the expected outcome. Some studies, however, are designed with a shotgun approach. A supplement is given, and many variables are measured. The more variables that are examined, the greater the chance that some of them will change. The application of study results should have a sound, scientific rationale. For example, sodium bicarbonate may improve buffering capacity, which could result in improved 800 m running performance, but it cannot be expected to improve Ironman triathlon performance (an event that lasts 8-14 hours).
- *Was the study on cells, muscle, animals, or humans?* Results are often extrapolated from findings in cell cultures. These in vitro experiments greatly help our understanding of metabolism and molecular interactions. In vivo situations, however, may be quite different. For instance, test tube samples are not exposed to hormonal changes that exist in living organisms. Also, muscle cells in the body may behave differently from isolated muscle cell preparations. Even if living animals are tested, animal metabolism can be significantly different from human metabolism. Rats have relatively large stores of muscle glycogen and extremely small stores of intramuscular triacylglycerol compared with humans. High-fat diets in rats clearly improve exercise capacity (see chapter 7), but no evidence indicates that high-fat diets improve performance in humans. Some study results cannot simply be extrapolated to human athletes.
- *Was the population for which claims were made comparable to the population in the study?* Coenzyme Q10 supplementation improves $\dot{V}O_2$max and exercise capacity in cardiac patients but has no effect on $\dot{V}O_2$max or exercise capacity in healthy individuals. Vanadium supplementation increases insulin sensitivity (reduces insulin resistance) in patients with type 2 diabetes but does not seem to be effective in healthy people with normal insulin sensitivity. These examples show how outcomes can differ in a target group that has different ages, sexes, body compositions, or fitness levels than the study group.
- *Were external variables controlled?* In an ideal study, all variables and conditions are identical so the only difference between the trials is the treatment that each group receives. Then, all observed changes can be attributed with great certainty to the treatment. For example, if in examining the effect of caffeine on exercise performance the environmental conditions were different in the caffeine and control trials, the observed effects might be related to environmental conditions as much as they are to caffeine.
- *Was the study placebo controlled?* If subjects have prior knowledge or expectations with respect to a treatment or supplement, their performance could be affected. The proper choice of a placebo avoids this kind of performance bias. With some nutrition interventions, however, matching placebos are difficult to find. For example, BCAAs have an extremely bitter taste, and finding a placebo with a similar (horrible) taste is difficult. In this case, subjects may be aware of what they receive, which can influence the outcome.
- *Were adequate techniques used?* Endurance capacity (time to exhaustion) has large day-to-day variability (Jeukendrup et al. 1996). Methods used to measure this variability may not detect small differences in performance. Similarly, some measures of body composition have a relatively large error and thus will not be able to detect small changes in fat or fat-free mass. If a treatment (supplement) is said to have no effect, perhaps the particular method used in the study was not sensitive enough to pick up small differences (Currell and Jeukendrup 2008b). A small change in performance (<3%) that is undetectable in a laboratory setting may determine success or failure in a sports event (Currell and Jeukendrup 2008b; Hopkins 2000).
- *Were the trials randomized?* Randomization reduces the confounding effects of variables that were not controlled or could not be controlled. When a small number of subjects are tested, a counterbalanced design is preferred. If trials are

randomized, eight of ten subjects could be in the treatment group in the first trial (leaving only two subjects in the control group). A counterbalanced design prevents this imbalance by appointing equal numbers to the control and treatment groups in the first trial (i.e., half of the subjects will take the supplement first and the other half will take the placebo first). Failure to randomize treatments in a study may confound the outcome and hence make any conclusions untrustworthy.

- *Was a crossover design used?* In a crossover study design, the same subjects perform the treatment trial and the placebo trial, which allows comparisons to be made within the same person. Although this type of study design can cause complications, particularly if a test substance that exerts effects in the body for a long time is given before the placebo, it is considered the ideal study design. Failure to use a crossover design may not necessarily affect the trustworthiness of the conclusions, but it is likely that variation between subjects in the measured variables will be greater than that within the same subjects. Hence, if a crossover design is not used, many more subjects will have to be studied to obtain the same degree of confidence that the conclusions are valid.
- *Was the assignment random or was self-selection used?* If subjects are allowed to self-select their trial group, a significant bias may be introduced. For example, in a study of the effects of chromium on weight loss, subjects most motivated to lose weight would likely choose to be in the chromium group and not the placebo group.
- *Do other studies confirm the findings?* If one study reports an ergogenic effect of a supplement, the claim might be true. But if several studies come to the same conclusion, the supplement most likely does have an ergogenic effect. The more studies that have been conducted, the larger the variety of subjects tested, and the more varied the dosages of the supplement used, the more generalizable the conclusion is.
- *Was the study peer reviewed?* Papers sent for publication to peer-reviewed journals undergo a rigorous process whereby usually two or three referees, who are experts in the area, evaluate the paper based on specific criteria. Quality research withstands critical review and evaluation by colleagues. Articles published in popular magazines or on consumer-oriented websites do not undergo this extensive review process and are therefore often filled with errors and untruthful claims.

The most important supplements that are claimed to improve performance, boost recovery, or promote fat loss or muscle gain are discussed in the following sections. Table 11.1 contains a list of selected supplements that are discussed in this chapter, along with claims and scientific evidence for those claims. Supplements discussed in previous chapters, such as carbohydrate–electrolyte drinks (see chapter 6) and individual amino acids (see chapter 8) are not discussed.

Androstenedione

Androstenedione is one of the most popular nutrition supplements in the United States. It is believed to stimulate the endogenous synthesis of testosterone and thereby increase protein synthesis, build muscle mass, and improve recovery. Androstenedione was first developed in the former East Germany to enhance the performance of athletes. The regulations in the Dietary Supplement Health and Education Act of 1994 allow it to be sold as a food supplement, and it is available over the counter in almost any drugstore or pharmacy in the United States.

If androstenedione functions as an anabolic steroid, it also has the side effects of an anabolic steroid, including acne, growth of facial and body hair, growth of the prostate, and impaired testicular function. The evidence that androstenedione has anabolic properties, however, is far from convincing. Although only a few studies have investigated the effects of androstenedione on serum testosterone concentrations and muscle strength, some conclusions can be drawn from them.

A study determined effects of short-term (2 weeks) and long-term (8 weeks) oral androstenedione supplementation (300 mg/day) on serum testosterone and estrogen concentrations and skeletal muscle fiber size and strength in a group of people in a strength-training program (King et al. 1999). The group of 20 was randomly divided into a placebo group and an androstenedione group. No changes were observed in serum testosterone concentrations, but serum estradiol concentrations increased after androstenedione administration. Strength training resulted in increased strength, increased lean body mass, and increased cross-sectional area of type II muscle fibers after 8 weeks, but the androstenedione group and the placebo group showed no differences. A lack of effect on serum testosterone concentrations was also reported by three other studies in which 100 to 200 mg/day were ingested for 2 days to 12 weeks (Ballantyne et al. 2000; Rasmussen, Volpi, et al. 2000; Wallace et al. 1999). Rasmussen, Volpi, et al. (2000) did not find effects on protein synthesis and

TABLE 11.1 Selected Nutrition Supplements, Product Claims, and Supporting Scientific Evidence

Nutrition supplement	Description	Claim	Scientific evidence
Androstenedione	Synthetic product to stimulate testosterone synthesis	Increases testosterone, increases muscle mass, and improves recovery	Does not increase testosterone and has no effect on strength
Bee pollen	Mixture of bee saliva, plant nectar, and pollen	Increases energy levels, enhances physical fitness, improves endurance, and boosts immune function	No supporting evidence
Beetroot juice	A good source of dietary nitrate (NO_3^-)	Decreases the oxygen cost of exercise and improves endurance exercise performance	Decreases the oxygen cost of exercise and improves endurance exercise performance
ß-alanine	Amino acid that in combination with histidine forms the dipeptide carnosine, which is an important intracellular buffer	Buffers hydrogen ions in muscle and improves high-intensity exercise performance	Positive effects in high-intensity exercise capacity tests but evidence for improvements in performance tests is lacking
ß-hydroxy ß-methylbutyrate (HMB)	Metabolite of the essential amino acid leucine	Decreases protein breakdown, improves muscle mass, and increases strength	Possible small effects on lean body mass and strength
Boron	Trace element present in vegetables and noncitrus fruits	Improves bone density, muscle mass, and strength	Improves bone mineral density in postmenopausal women but no effect on bone density, muscle mass, or strength in men
Caffeine	Substance in coffee and chocolate	Increases performance and alertness	Improves performance in most events except short high-intensity exercise and increases cognitive functioning during exercise
Carnitine	Vitamin-like substance important for FA transport	Improves fat oxidation and endurance exercise performance, helps weight loss, and improves $\dot{V}O_2$max	Taken up by muscle; if coingested with carbohydrate, improves performance in endurance exercise
Choline	Precursor of the neurotransmitter acetylcholine	Improves performance and decreases fatigue	No supporting evidence
Chromium	Trace element that potentiates insulin action	Builds muscle and helps weight loss	No supporting evidence
Coenzyme Q10	Part of the electron-transport chain in the mitochondria	Improves $\dot{V}O_2$max, improves performance, and reduces fatigue	No supporting evidence
Creatine	High-energy phosphate carrier important for direct energy	Improves strength, reduces fatigue, and increases protein synthesis	Improves performance in single and repeated sprint bouts and improves recovery between bouts; anabolic properties unclear
Dehydroepiandrosterone (DHEA)	A precursor of testosterone and estradiol	Improves immune function, increases lifespan, protects against cardiovascular diseases, increases lean body mass, and increases well-being	Some evidence in humans for improved well-being
Dihydroxyacetone (DHA) and pyruvate	Intermediates of carbohydrate metabolism usually used in combination	Facilitate carbohydrate and fat metabolism and improve endurance performance, insulin sensitivity, and recovery and increases glycogen storage	Limited supporting evidence

Nutrition supplement	Description	Claim	Scientific evidence
Fish oil and omega-3 fatty acids	Polyunsaturated fatty acids	Increase $\dot{V}O_2$max and muscle protein synthesis, enhance recovery from damaging exercise, and improve cognitive function	No supporting evidence for increased $\dot{V}O_2$max but some evidence for the other effects with combinations of DHE and EHA
Ginseng	Root of the Araliaceous plant	Improves strength, performance, stamina, and cognitive functioning and reduces fatigue	No supporting evidence, but studies were poorly designed
Glandulars	Extracts of animal glands	Improves strength, performance, and stamina	No supporting evidence
Green tea	Plant leaf extract containing polyphenol catechins and caffeine	Increases fat oxidation at rest and during exercise	Limited supporting evidence
Glycerol	Backbone of a triacylglycerol molecule	Induces hyperhydration, decreases heat stress, and improves performance	Induces hyperhydration and decreases heat stress during exercise; effects on performance unclear
Inosine	Nucleoside	Increases ATP stores and improves strength, training quality, and performance	No supporting evidence
Ketone salts Lecithin	Sodium or potassium salts of ketone bodies (ß-hydroxy butyrate or acetoacetate)	Alternative fuel for muscle, is glycogen sparing, and increases endurance performance	No supporting evidence
Lecithin	Phosphatidylcholine	Increases $\dot{V}O_2$max and performance	No supporting evidence
Medium-chain triacylglycerol (MCT)	Synthesized from coconut oil	Supplies energy, reduces muscle glycogen breakdown, and improves performance	No supporting evidence
Pangamic acid	Varied composition depending on supplier	Increases oxygen delivery	No supporting evidence
Phosphate salts	Mineral	Increases ATP, provides energy, and buffers lactic acid	Possible ergogenic effects; improves performance in events 1 hour or shorter
Phosphatidylserine	Structural component of cell membranes	Reduces stress responses and improves recovery	Little supporting evidence
Polylactate and lactate salts	Polymers of lactate	Provide energy	No effect on performance
Pyruvate	Intermediate of carbohydrate metabolism	Facilitates carbohydrate metabolism and improves endurance performance and recovery	Limited supporting evidence
Polyphenols	Plant polyphenols such as flavonoids (e.g., quercetin)	Improves endurance performance	Limited evidence of improved performance in sufficient doses
Sodium bicarbonate	Buffer present in blood	Buffers lactic acid and improves high-intensity exercise performance	Improves high-intensity exercise performance
Sodium citrate	Buffer	Buffers lactic acid and improves high-intensity exercise performance	Can improve performance with larger doses
Sodium nitrate	Mineral source of nitrate	Decreases the oxygen cost of exercise and improves endurance exercise performance	Decreases the oxygen cost of exercise and improves endurance exercise performance
Vanadium	Trace element	Helps weight loss and improves insulin sensitivity and recovery	Increases insulin sensitivity in patients with insulin resistance; studies in healthy individuals lacking
Wheat germ oil	Extracted from embryo of wheat	Improves endurance	No supporting evidence

breakdown or phenylalanine balance across the leg. Therefore, the conclusions that androstenedione has no effect on the plasma testosterone concentration, does not change protein metabolism, has no anabolic effect, and does not alter the adaptations to resistance training seem appropriate.

Androstenedione may have negative health effects. A study reported a decrease in serum HDL cholesterol (Granados et al. 2014), a lack of which has been associated with increased risk of cardiovascular disease. Two reviews of the literature on prohormones concluded that, contrary to marketing claims, research to date indicates that the use of prohormone nutritional supplements (DHEA, androstenedione, androstenediol, and other steroid hormone supplements) does not produce either anabolic or ergogenic effects in men but may raise the risk for negative health consequences (Brown, Vukovich, and King 2006; Ziegenfuss, Berardi, and Lowery 2002). Ethical issues are also involved. Androstenedione is banned by the International Olympic Committee (IOC), and athletes have been disqualified and banned from their sport for using it.

Bee Pollen

Pollen is a fine, powdery substance produced by the anthers of seed-bearing plants. Bees collect it from the plants and store it in their hives. It has a rich mixture of vitamins, minerals, and amino acids and is therefore believed to be healthy and especially because it is a natural product as opposed to some of the multivitamin and mineral supplements. Pollen is often referred to as the perfect food or complete food, and manufacturers claim that it improves endurance, reduces free-radical damage, aids in weight control, increases longevity, and prevents asthma. But no reliable information exists to prove its effectiveness as an ergogenic aid. Based on the available information on supplementation with amino acids, vitamins, and minerals that are found in bee pollen (see chapters 8 and 10), ergogenic effects would not be expected. One study (Chandler and Hawkins 1984) in which the effect of bee pollen supplementation was investigated showed no influence on maximal oxygen uptake, exercise performance, or metabolism. Bee pollen can be harmful for people who are allergic to specific pollens.

Beetroot Juice

Studies suggest that beetroot juice, which is a good source of dietary nitrate, may improve endurance performance in some circumstances. Studies have examined the effect of ingesting nitrate in the form of sodium nitrate ($NaNO_3$) or vegetable sources of nitrate (usually beetroot juice) containing about 6 mmol of nitrate a few hours prior to performing prolonged exhaustive exercise. Bacteria in the mouth convert nitrate into nitrite, and dietary nitrate supplementation has been shown to increase plasma nitrite concentration, reduce the oxygen cost of submaximal exercise (Bailey et al. 2009; Lansley, Winyard, Bailey, et al. 2011; Lansley, Winyard, Fulford, et al. 2011; Larsen et al. 2007), improve high-intensity exercise tolerance, improve cycling economy (i.e., a higher power output for the same rate of oxygen uptake), and enhance 4 and 16 km (2.5 and 10 mi) cycling time-trial performance (Lansley, Winyard, Bailey, et al. 2011). Furthermore, daily consumption of 0.5 L (0.1 gal) of beetroot juice for 6 days can reduce resting blood pressure, lower the oxygen cost of high-intensity treadmill running by about 7%, and increase time to exhaustion by 15%. There is also some evidence that intermittent high-intensity exercise performance can be enhanced by nitrate ingestion (Bond, Morton, and Braakhuis 2012; Wylie, Mohr, et al. 2013), but so far, no studies have convincingly demonstrated any performance benefits during prolonged endurance exercise. Vegetables that have a high nitrate content (other than beetroot) include celery, cress, lettuce, rhubarb, and spinach. The effects of dietary nitrate are thought to be mediated by increased formation of nitrite and nitric oxide.

Dietary nitrate is absorbed through the intestine and is concentrated into the salivary glands and secreted into the oral cavity where some of it is converted to nitrite by commensal bacteria. When swallowed, it enters the systemic circulation where it is bioactive as nitrite or is further reduced to NO. There are several theoretical mechanisms of action: NO is known to be a factor in the regulation of local blood flow that causes vasodilation when a muscle is receiving less or using more oxygen. This does not explain the reduction in oxygen cost during exercise. Rather, nitrite and NO may act more directly because NO is able to inhibit cytochrome oxidase activity which slows conversion of oxygen to water. Also, NO may increase mitochondrial oxidative phosphorylation efficiency by increasing the phosphate/oxygen (P/O) ratio (i.e., more ATP is formed per amount of oxygen consumed). Skeletal muscle mitochondria harvested from muscle biopsies after nitrate supplementation display an increased P/O ratio, and the improved mitochondrial P/O ratio correlates with the reduction in oxygen cost during exercise (Larsen et al. 2011).

> Mechanistically, nitrate reduces the expression of ATP/ADP translocase, a protein involved in proton conductance. Thus, it appears that dietary nitrate has profound effects on basal mitochondrial function. (Gleeson 2014)

There is also the possibility that NO could reduce the ATP cost of exercise by lowering sarcoplasmic reticulum calcium ion (Ca^{2+}) release by protecting channels from Ca^{2+} release induced by reactive oxygen species since Ca^{2+} is energetically expensive to resequester via the Ca^{2+} ATPase (Bailey et al. 2010; Ferreira and Behnke 2011). NO also promotes mitochondrial biogenesis, thereby possibly enhancing adaptation to subsequent exercise. Since these discoveries there has been a great deal of research examining the acute and chronic effects of dietary nitrate supplementation on exercise performance in a variety of activities in subjects that range from sedentary people to elite athletes. The results of these studies suggest that nitrate may be less effective as an ergogenic aid in very highly trained or elite subjects compared with those who are sedentary or recreationally active (Boorsma, Whitfield, and Spriet 2014; Christensen, Nyberg, and Bangsbo 2013). No doubt more research on this supplement will emerge in the coming years. The fact that something as simple as this can change the oxygen cost of exercise seems remarkable and will surely prompt the search for other agents that might have similar effects.

Beetroot juice is currently the most popular and convenient means of ingesting sufficient quantities of dietary nitrate to affect oxygen uptake and exercise performance. A recent dose–response study (Wylie, Kelly, et al. 2013) found that exercise tolerance was improved with 8 mmol but not 4 mmol of nitrate, but there was no further improvement in performance when 16 mmol of nitrate was ingested. Thus, the effective dose is 6 to 8 mmol of nitrate, which is contained in about 500 ml of natural beetroot juice or 70 ml of a more concentrated beverage (e.g., Beet-It). This should be ingested 2 to 3 hours before exercise. Chronic ingestion of 6 to 8 mmol of nitrate per day for several days may be slightly more effective than a single acute preexercise dose.

ß-Alanine and Carnosine

For sports in which glycolysis is simulated and lactic acid production is high (e.g., middle-distance running), ß-alanine has been suggested to be an effective supplement. During intense exercise, the increased H^+ concentration is buffered by intra- and extramuscular buffering mechanisms. Sodium bicarbonate ($NaHCO_3$) is an extracellular buffer that will be discussed later in this chapter. The dipeptide carnosine or ß-alanyl-L-histidine is one of the most important intracellular buffers. Carnosine is synthesized from its precursors L-histidine and ß-alanine. It is present in relatively high concentrations in the cytoplasm of skeletal muscle (5-10 mM) and is thought to be responsible for approximately 10% of the total buffering capacity of the vastus lateralis muscle. Carnosine ingestion is not effective in increasing intramuscular carnosine concentration because it is broken down in the GI tract and absorption is poor. Also, carnosine is not taken up by muscle but is synthesized in muscle from its constituent amino acids by the enzyme carnosine synthase. ß-alanine is synthesized in the liver from uracil, a pyrimidine base that is used in the synthesis of RNA, and evidence suggests that ß-alanine supplementation can lead to an increase in muscle carnosine content of up to about 80%, which can result in enhanced intramuscular H^+ buffering. This has been shown to result in an increase in high-intensity exercise performance in untrained and trained individuals.

Dosing protocols include taking a single daily dose of 3.2 g of ß-alanine or up to eight daily doses of 0.4 to 1.6 g ß-alanine per dose to reach a total daily ingestion of 3.2 to 6.4 g/day over a range of 4 to 10 weeks, which results in a 60% to 80% increase in muscle carnosine contents (Harris et al. 2006; Hill et al. 2007). It has been documented that large acute doses of ß-alanine induce paresthesia (mild flushing and tingling sensations on the skin) that appears to dissipate within about 2 hours; this is why smaller doses are recommended. It can also be taken as a slow-release tablet (i.e., CarnoSyn). Despite the relatively consistent findings that ß-alanine supplementation leads to an increase in muscle carnosine, evidence for subsequent performance effects has been less clear. A study demonstrated that 4.8 g of ß-alanine per day for 4 weeks in trained 400 m runners improved fatigue resistance in repeated bouts of exhaustive dynamic contractions. But isometric endurance at about 25% of maximal voluntary contraction (MVC) force and 400 m race time were not affected (Derave et al. 2007). In another study, sprint performance was enhanced at the end of a simulated cycling race (Van Thienen et al. 2009). Other studies have demonstrated performance benefits in moderate-intensity (45% MVC) isometric exercise (Sale et al. 2012) and several dynamic high-intensity exercise capacity tests lasting between 1 and 4 minutes (Hobson et al. 2012; Sale and Harris 2014).

Most studies that have used an exercise protocol of longer than 1 minute in which acidosis was the primary cause of fatigue have demonstrated significant positive performance effects. Carnosine may limit acidosis by acting as a hydrogen ion buffer, but improved contractile performance may also be obtained by improved excitation-contraction coupling and defense against ROS because carnosine is also an antioxidant. High carnosine concentrations are found in people with a high proportion of fast-twitch fibers, because these fibers are enriched with the dipeptide. Muscle carnosine content is lower in women, declines with age, and is lower in vegetarians whose diets do not contain ß-alanine. Sprint-trained athletes display markedly high muscular carnosine, but the effect of several weeks of high-intensity training on muscle carnosine is rather small. High carnosine levels in elite sprinters are therefore either genetically determined or a result of slow adaptation to years of training. In light of the positive effects on performance, it is not surprising that ß-alanine is rapidly developing as a popular ergogenic nutritional supplement for athletes, though potential side effects and the mechanism of action require additional research. In summary, most of the studies that have found significant ergogenic effects to date have been carried out on untrained or recreationally active individuals performing exercise bouts under laboratory conditions. The studies on highly trained athletes performing single competition-like exercise tasks indicate that these athletes receive modest but potentially worthwhile performance benefits from ß-alanine supplementation. Some studies also provide evidence supporting the use of ß-alanine as a training aid to augment bouts of high-intensity training (Trexler et al. 2015). ß-alanine supplementation has also been shown to increase resistance training performance and training volume in team-sport athletes, which may allow for greater overload and superior adaptations compared with training alone (Trexler et al. 2015). The ergogenic potential of ß-alanine supplementation for elite athletes who perform repeated high-intensity exercise bouts during training or competition in sports that require repeated maximal efforts (e.g., football, rugby, hockey) needs further investigation. The effects of ß-alanine have been discussed in detail in a couple of reviews (Lancha et al. 2015; Saunders et al. 2017).

ß-Hydroxy ß-Methylbutyrate

ß-hydroxy ß-methylbutyrate (HMB) is a metabolite of the essential amino acid leucine (see figure 11.1), and it is synthesized in the body at an estimated rate of about 0.2 to 0.4 g/day (Nissen et al. 1996). Its use as a supplement has increased dramatically in the past few years, especially among bodybuilders, and it has become one of the most popular supplements. HMB is claimed to increase lean body mass and strength, improve recovery, improve immune function, reduce blood cholesterol, protect against stress, and reduce body fat.

The first studies of HMB were performed in rats, and the studies demonstrated that supplementing leucine can be anticatabolic, possibly through the actions of its metabolite HMB. Later studies investigated HMB as a potential anticatabolic agent in farm animals. No effect of HMB supplementation on protein metabolism was observed in growing lambs (Papet et al. 1997). Subsequently, HMB was hypothesized to reduce protein breakdown in humans, resulting in increased muscle mass and strength. In addition, subjects given HMB supplements were believed to have a decreased stress-induced muscle glycogen breakdown. HMB thus was claimed to benefit strength and endurance athletes.

Nissen et al. (1996) studied 41 untrained male volunteers who participated in a resistance-training program for 3 weeks. The program consisted of three 90-minute weightlifting sessions per week. Participants were divided into three groups, and each group received a different dose of HMB. The first group received placebo, the second group received 1.5 g of HMB per day, and the third group received 3 g/day. Lean tissue (determined by total-body electrical conductance, a technique with a similar principle as bioelectrical impedance analysis [BIA]) tended to increase more in the HMB groups, and this occurred in a dose-dependent manner (see figure 11.2). Lower-body strength also increased in a significant linear manner with HMB dosage (see figure 11.3).

The group that had the largest increase in lean body mass (3 g of HMB per day) was also the group with the lowest lean body mass and muscle strength to begin with. Therefore, this group would be expected to gain more than the placebo group, who already had a larger lean body mass. Also, this study had no diet control, so the leucine intake is not known.

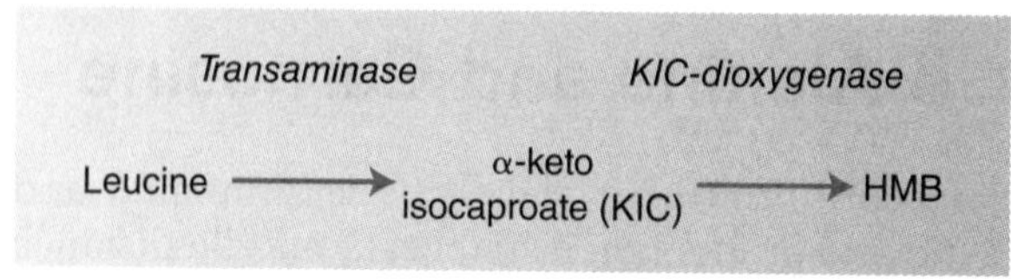

Figure 11.1 Synthesis of HMB from the amino acid leucine.

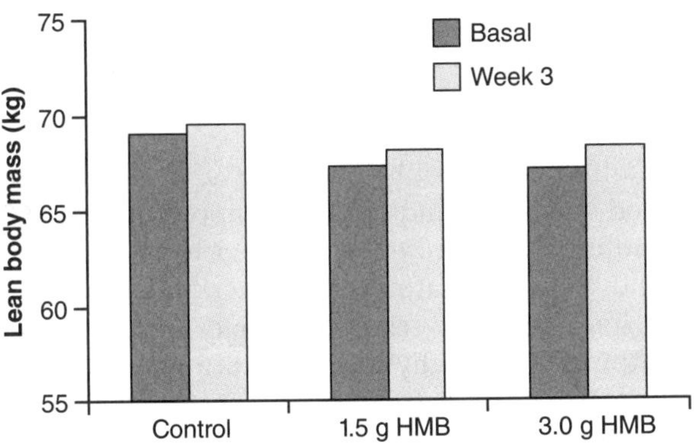

Figure 11.2 The effect of HMB supplementation on body composition.
Data from Nissen et al. (1996).

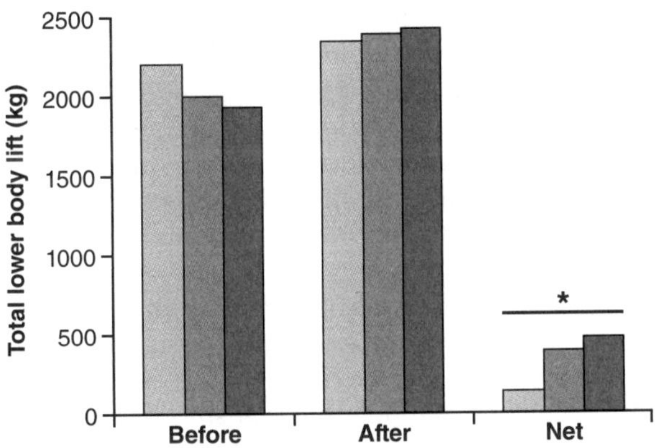

Figure 11.3 Change in total lower-body strength with placebo or HMB. The asterisk indicates significant linear effect of HMB supplementation for net increase in strength only. Gray columns: placebo; Light blue columns: 1.5 g HMB/day; Dark blue columns: 3.0 g HMB/day.

In the second part of the study by Nissen et al. (1996), subjects trained 6 days per week for 7 weeks and were given 3 g of HMB per day or placebo. This study showed an increase in fat-free mass in the HMB group after 14 days, but after 39 days, no differences were observed. Strength was also measured in this study, but no differences were found in the strength measurements except for bench press. A small improvement in bench press strength occurred with HMB supplementation (2.6 kg [5.7 lb] after 7 weeks of training with HMB versus 1.1 kg [2.4 lb] with placebo). Again, a point of criticism is that the diet was not controlled. Since then, other studies have provided mixed results. Some have found an increase in lean body mass or muscle strength (Jówko et al. 2001; Nissen et al. 2000; Panton et al. 2000), whereas others have found no effect on body composition and strength (Slater et al. 2001) or signs of muscle damage after eccentric exercise (Paddon-Jones, Keech, and Jenkins 2001). In a meta-analysis, HMB was found to increase net lean mass gains by 0.28% per week and strength gains by 1.4% per week (Nissen and Sharp 2003). More recently, it has also been suggested that HMB can increase aerobic exercise performance, although not all studies have found such improvements.

Nissen et al. (2000) collected data in nine studies that ranged from 3 to 8 weeks in duration. No negative effects of 3 g of HMB per day were noted on organ and tissue function, emotional perception, or GI tolerance. The authors concluded that 3 g/day is a safe dose. Some evidence suggests that HMB can result in increased lean body mass and muscle strength. A number of studies show that HMB has several positive effects, but an equal number show no effect of HMB. There is now compelling evidence in clinical muscle wasting conditions that HMB can be beneficial, and some evidence for a potential mechanism is also starting to emerge. HMB seems to reduce the breakdown of protein through inhibiting proteolytic pathways and to stimulate protein synthesis through stimulation of the transcription factor mammalian target of rapamycin (mTOR) (see chapter 12). Even though some of the research that has been performed with HMB in nonathletes has reported generally positive outcomes (Molfino et al. 2013), the results in athletes are still not very convincing. In older adults, there appears to be some protection against muscle wasting with HMB (Hickson 2015; Phillips 2015), but larger well-controlled studies are required that measure outcomes relevant to sarcopenia and outcomes relevant to athletic populations.

For more complete reviews of the effects of HMB on performance and body composition and a discussion of potential mechanisms, see Wilson, Wilson, and Manninen (2008) and Phillips et al. (2017). From a practical point of view, potential users should keep in mind that most of the studies have used 3 g of HMB per day, but most recovery products currently on the market contain extremely small amounts of HMB.

Boron

The trace element boron influences calcium and magnesium metabolism (Volpe, Taper, and Meacham 1993), steroid hormone metabolism, and membrane function. It is present in noncitrus fruits, leafy vegetables, nuts, and legumes. Although no RDA has been established for boron, the recommended daily intake is often 1 mg/day (Nielsen 1996). For humans, boron is not an essential trace element.

Boron has been studied in relation to osteoporosis. One of these studies found that boron supplementation for 48 days increased the serum estrogen and testosterone levels of postmenopausal women. It also reduced calcium, phosphorus, and magnesium excretion in urine and is therefore suggested to contribute to improved bone mineral density (Nielsen et al. 1987).

The finding that boron increased testosterone levels in postmenopausal women has been extrapolated to the claim that it may improve muscle growth and strength in strength athletes. The women in this study, however, had been deprived of boron for 4 months. Continued supplementation did not further elevate testosterone levels, and boron supplementation in men did not affect testosterone levels at all. Another placebo-controlled study investigated the effects of boron supplementation (2.5 mg of boron per day for 7 weeks) on serum testosterone, lean body mass, and strength in bodybuilders. Besides elevated plasma boron levels, no effect was found (Green and Ferrando 1994). Therefore, although interactions are shown between boron and calcium and magnesium metabolism (Volpe, Taper, and Meacham 1993), boron does not appear to be an ergogenic aid.

Caffeine

The use of **caffeine** dates back to Paleolithic times. The raw fruit of the coffee plant (Coffea arabica) was used to brew a drink with stimulant properties. This strongly caffeinated beverage was later replaced by a beverage prepared from roasted coffee beans. Other natural sources of caffeine include tea and chocolate. Over the past decade, the introduction and popularity of new caffeine-containing food products (especially synthetic caffeine-containing energy drinks) and changes in consumption patterns of the more traditional sources of caffeine have increased caffeine intake in the general population. Caffeine is by far the most widely consumed psychoactive drug in the world. The change in consumption patterns has also increased scrutiny by health authorities and regulatory bodies about the overall consumption of caffeine and its potential cumulative effects on behavior and physiology.

Caffeine originates naturally in 63 species of plants as several types of methylated xanthines. Caffeine and caffeine-like substances can be found in a variety of foods and drinks, but the main sources for these substances are coffee beans, tea leaves, cocoa beans, and cola nuts (see figure 11.4. and table 11.2). Coffee accounts for 75% of all caffeine consumption.

Caffeine is readily absorbed after ingestion. Blood levels rise and peak after approximately 60 minutes. The half-life is reported to be between 2 and 10 hours. Caffeine is primarily degraded in the liver, and the resulting single methyl group xanthines and methyluric acids are eliminated in urine. About 0.5% to 3.5% of ingested caffeine is excreted unchanged in urine. A study showed that significant amounts of caffeine are also excreted through sweat (Kovacs, Stegen, and Brouns 1998). Caffeine remains the most widely consumed drug in Europe and the United States (Curatolo and Robertson 1983), and athletes have long used it in the belief that it improves performance. On January 1, 2004, the IOC took caffeine off its list of banned substances. Before this, caffeine was one of the few compounds for which the IOC had set a tolerance limit. This limit was defined at a caffeine concentration in urine of 12 mg/ml. Because caffeine is a substance that can influence exercise performance, whether it should be used in sports is a question of ethics.

Here we will briefly summarize the evidence that caffeine is an ergogenic aid and explain some of the proposed mechanisms. For further readings and details on caffeine metabolism and the ergogenic effects of caffeine, see Armstrong (2002), Graham, Rush, and van Soeren (1994), Spriet (1995), and Doherty and Smith (2004, 2005).

Endurance Exercise

In the late 1970s it was observed that caffeine ingested 1 hour before the start of an exercise bout increased plasma FA concentration and improved

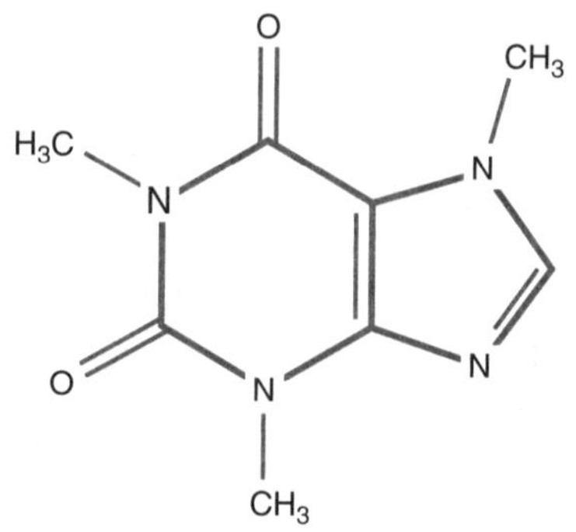

O
CH3
H3C
N
N
N
O
N
CH3

Figure 11.4 Chemical structure of caffeine and caffeine-like compounds.

TABLE 11.2 Caffeine Content in Foods, Beverages, and Medications

Item	Caffeine content (mg)	Item	Caffeine content (mg)
Coffee		**Pain relievers (per tablet)**	
Drip method (150 ml [5 oz])	110-150	Anacin	32
Percolated (150 ml [5 oz])	64-124	Excedrin	65
Instant (150 ml [5 oz])	40-108	Midol	32
Decaffeinated (150 ml [5 oz])	2-5	Aspirin	0
Starbucks grande (480 ml [16 oz])	550	Vanquish	33
Starbucks tall (360 ml [12 oz])	375	**Diuretics (per tablet)**	
Starbucks short (240 ml [8 oz])	250	Aqua Ban	200
Starbucks tall latte (360 ml [12 oz])	70	Pre-Mens Forte	100
Tea		**Cold Remedies (per tablet)**	
1 min brew (150 ml [5 oz])	9-33	Coryban-D	30
3 min brew (150 ml [5 oz])	20-46	Dristan	0
5 min brew (150 ml [5 oz])	20-50	Triaminicin	30
Instant tea (150 ml [5 oz])	12-28	**Weight-control aids (per tablet)**	
Iced tea (360 ml [12 oz])	22-36	Dexatrim	200
Chocolate		Prolamine	140
Made from mix	6	**Stimulants (per tablet)**	
Milk chocolate (30 g [1 oz])	6	Pro Plus	50
Baking chocolate	35	NoDoz	100
Chocolate bar (100 g [4 oz])	12-15	**Prescription pain relievers (per tablet)**	
Soft drinks		Cafergot	100
Mountain Dew (355 ml [12 fl oz])	55	Davron compound	32
Mello Yello (355 ml [12 fl oz])	52	Fiorinal	40
Coca-Cola (355 ml [12 fl oz])	46	Migramal	1
Diet Coke (355 ml [12 fl oz])	46		
Pepsi (355 ml [12 fl oz])	38		
Diet Pepsi (355 ml [12 fl oz])	36		
Dr. Pepper (355 ml [12 fl oz])	40		
Red Bull (250 ml [8 oz])	80		

performance (Costill et al. 1977; Essig, Costill, and Van Handel 1980; Ivy et al. 1979). Although not all studies show effects of caffeine on endurance performance, many well-conducted studies have shown improved endurance capacity after ingesting caffeine at a dose of 3 to 9 mg per kilogram of body weight (Costill, Dalsky, and Fink 1978; Graham and Spriet 1991; Pasman et al. 1995; Spriet et al. 1992). More recently, studies have used smaller doses of caffeine (as little as 1–3.2 mg per kilogram of body weight) and still observed positive effects on performance (Cox et al. 2002; Kovacs, Stegen, and Brouns 1998) (see the Dosage section).

At exercise intensities of about 85% of $\dot{V}O_2$max, improvements of 10% to 20% in time to exhaustion are typically found. A meta-analysis of published studies on caffeine and exercise performance (Doherty and Smith 2005) suggested that the magnitude of the performance-enhancing effect increases as the duration of exercise increases. In most of these studies, caffeine also decreased perceived ratings of exertion.

The improvement in performance was originally explained by the increased availability of plasma FAs, which supposedly resulted in a suppression of carbohydrate metabolism and consequently to a decrease in glycogen use. However, a number of studies did see performance improvements without changes in the rate of fat oxidation, and it is highly unlikely that this mechanism is behind the observed effects.

It has become clear in recent years that the effects of caffeine are due to its stimulant properties; a given exercise feels easier with caffeine. The fact that not all studies found that caffeine has a performance-enhancing effect might be related to various factors, including the dose of caffeine, the fitness level of the subjects, habitual caffeine consumption, and, perhaps most important, the type and duration of exercise.

Maximal Exercise

A few studies investigated the effects of caffeine ingestion on high-intensity exercise (about 100% of $\dot{V}O_2max$ lasting 3-8 minutes). Some, but not all, studies (Falk et al. 1989; Sasaki et al. 1987) demonstrated a positive effect of caffeine on exercise performance at these high intensities. Jackman et al. (1996) found that ingestion of 6 mg of caffeine per kilogram of body weight increased time to exhaustion at 100% of $\dot{V}O_2max$. Muscle glycogen concentrations, however, were still relatively high at exhaustion. Therefore, the authors concluded that the mechanism was not through glycogen sparing. Caffeine (150-200 mg) also improved 1,500 m (1 mi) time in well-trained runners (4:46.0 versus 4:50.2) (Wiles et al. 1992).

Generally, caffeine seems to improve performance during exercise near 100% of $\dot{V}O_2max$ that lasts approximately 5 minutes. The mechanism for this improvement is unknown but has been suggested to be an effect of caffeine on the neuromuscular pathways that facilitate recruitment of muscle fibers or increase the number of fibers recruited. In addition, caffeine possibly has direct effects on muscle ion handling or enhanced anaerobic energy production or an effect on the brain that decreases sensations of effort (Spriet 1995b).

Ball Sports and Team Sports

Ball sports and team sports are characterized by a more intermittent exercise pattern, and typically a lot of skill is involved. Cognitive functioning in these sports is very important, so it could be expected that caffeine should have profound effects. A review by Chia et al. (2017) did not find consistent performance outcomes with caffeine and concluded that the efficacy of caffeine varies depending on various factors, including the nature of the game, physical status, and caffeine habituation. Overall, however, it seems that the ingestion of 5 to 6 mg of caffeine per kilogram of body weight consumed before or during training or competition can improve motor skill and cognitive performance (Baker, Nuccio, and Jeukendrup 2014).

Supramaximal Exercise

The effects of caffeine on short-term supramaximal exercise performance are uncertain. Williams et al. (1988) reported no effect on power output or muscular endurance during 15-second sprints after caffeine ingestion. Similar findings were reported by Collomp et al. (1991), who found that ingestion of 5 mg of caffeine per kilogram of body weight did not affect 30-second Wingate test performance. A study investigated the effects of caffeine ingestion on repeated Wingate exercise tests (Greer, McLean, and Graham 1998) and found that caffeine had no effect on the first two Wingate tests but that it decreased power output during the third and fourth tests. Caffeine, therefore, seems to have no positive effect on sprint performance. Given the limited number of studies, however, this conclusion is not definitive.

Cognitive Functioning

Caffeine has an effect on cognitive functioning. In a study by Hogervorst et al. (1999), caffeine was added to a carbohydrate–electrolyte drink that was consumed before and during exercise. Cognitive functioning (attention, psychomotor skills, and memory) was measured immediately after a time trial (approximately 1 hour of all-out exercise). Caffeine improved all measures of cognitive functioning, and these effects were evident for the ingestion of 2 and 3 mg of caffeine per kilogram of body weight. More recently, the effects of caffeine (100 mg) in an energy bar (45 g of carbohydrate) were investigated. The energy bar was ingested immediately before exercise and twice during exercise (after 55 and 115 minutes), which was a total of 2.5 hours of cycling at 60% of $\dot{V}O_2max$ followed by a time to exhaustion test at 75% of $\dot{V}O_2max$. The researchers found that time to exhaustion was extended and that concentration, response speed and detection, and performance of complex cognitive tasks improved during and after exercise when an energy bar with caffeine was ingested. The energy bar with caffeine resulted in better cognitive function compared with an energy bar without caffeine and a control trial in which no carbohydrate or caffeine was ingested (Hogervorst et al. 2008).

Dosage

A few studies have investigated the effects of various doses of caffeine on exercise performance (or endurance capacity). In a study by Pasman et al. (1995), cyclists received three different doses of caffeine or placebo 1 hour before a ride to exhaustion at about 80% of $\dot{V}O_2$max. The dosages were 0, 5, 9, and 13 mg per kilogram of body weight. With the lowest dose (5 mg per kilogram of body weight), endurance capacity improved by 20%, but an increase in dosage had no further effect on performance (see figure 11.5). In another study, ingestion of 3 mg and 6 mg of caffeine per kilogram of body weight had positive effects on runners, whereas the improvement in time to exhaustion with 9 mg of caffeine per kilogram of body weight did not reach statistical significance (Graham and Spriet 1995).

In a study by Cox et al. (2002), small amounts of caffeine (1-2 mg per kilogram of body weight) resulted in significant performance improvements in a time trial at the end of 2 hours of cycling. Kovacs, Stegen, and Brouns (1998) studied the effect of adding relatively small amounts of caffeine (2, 3, or 4.5 mg per kilogram of body weight) to a carbohydrate-electrolyte solution during prolonged exercise. Time-trial cycling performance improved with the lowest dosage of 2 mg per kilogram of body weight and improved more with 3 mg per kilogram of body weight, but a higher dose did not further affect performance. These results suggest that a caffeine intake of 3 mg per kilogram of body weight exerts an ergogenic effect but that higher intakes will not produce increased benefit.

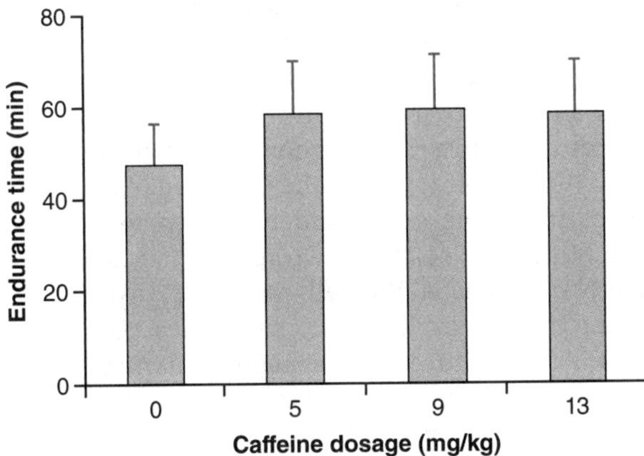

Figure 11.5 Effect of ingesting various amounts of caffeine 1 hour preexercise on time to exhaustion at about 80% of $\dot{V}O_2$max.

Data from Pasman, van Baak, Jeukendrup, and deHaan (1995).

Habitual Users

Studies have tried to address the question of whether habitual consumers of caffeine have an altered response during exercise. Although habitual caffeine users may have markedly different metabolic responses to caffeine (e.g., blunted FA response and blunted catecholamine excretion) (Dodd et al. 1991; Van Soeren et al. 1993), performance improvements with caffeine are similar (Gonçalves et al. 2017). There is only one study (Beaumont et al. 2017) that suggests that repeated daily caffeine supplementation (1.5-3.0 mg per kilogram of body weight for 4 weeks) diminished performance benefits of acute caffeine supplementation in low habitual caffeine consumers (<45 mg/day). However, giving caffeine to low habitual users for 4 weeks may be quite different from a habitual high intake. The study can also not exclude the possibility that high habitual users can still benefit from caffeine.

In one study, withdrawal from caffeine for 2 to 4 days had no effect on the observed performance effect of caffeine (Van Soeren and Graham 1998). Although caffeine (6 mg per kilogram of body weight) improved performance compared with placebo, performance did not change after 2 or 4 days of withdrawal. This study also suggested that the mechanisms by which caffeine works are not related to availability of substrate or catecholamines. Another study found performance benefits with acute caffeine supplementation during a 30-minute cycling time trial, but there were no differences between the groups with low, medium, or high habitual caffeine intake (Gonçalves et al. 2017). This also does not mean that refraining from caffeine products will increase the effects of caffeine. A study by Irwin et al. (2011) showed similar improvements in exercise with caffeine in habitual consumers regardless of a 4-day withdrawal period. Thus, it seems fair to conclude that the balance of evidence suggests that practicing caffeine withdrawal to get a better effect from caffeine is not required.

Carbohydrate Absorption

It was suggested that caffeine may also improve the absorption of carbohydrate. Van Nieuwenhoven, Brummer, and Brouns (2000) reported that caffeine (1.4 mg per kilogram of body weight) coingested with glucose (0.5 g/min) during 90 minutes of cycling produced higher rates of intestinal glucose absorption compared with glucose alone. Because absorption appears to be the rate-limiting step for exogenous carbohydrate delivery to the muscle, it was suggested that caffeine may increase exogenous carbohydrate oxidation (Yeo et al. 2005). In another study, it was shown that combined ingestion of caffeine (10 mg per kilogram of body weight, which is a very high dose) and glucose (0.8 g/min) resulted in 26% higher rates of exogenous carbohydrate oxidation compared with glucose (0.8 g/min). It is possible, however, this effect may be present only when a high dose of caffeine is given or when carbohydrate intake is relatively high. In a follow-up study with a lower dose of caffeine, the coingestion of caffeine (5.3 mg per kilogram of body weight) with carbohydrate (0.7 g/min) during exercise enhanced time-trial performance by 4.6% compared with carbohydrate and 9% compared with a water placebo. In this study, however, caffeine did not influence exogenous carbohydrate oxidation during exercise. So, although some evidence indicates that caffeine may help carbohydrate absorption and exogenous carbohydrate oxidation, the optimal carbohydrate and caffeine intakes needed to achieve this effect are uncertain.

Mechanisms of Action

Several theories of how caffeine could exert its effects have been proposed. The precise mechanisms behind the ergogenic effect of caffeine are still unclear but are unlikely to be related to changes in metabolism (increased fat metabolism and decreased muscle glycogen breakdown). The most likely explanations seem to be changes in central drive, muscle fiber recruitment, and perceived exertion caused by central nervous system effects of caffeine. The following are some of the mechanisms that have been suggested.

The traditional hypothesis for the ergogenic effect of caffeine is that caffeine stimulates lipolysis, increases fat oxidation, and thereby spares muscle glycogen, which is generally believed to improve endurance performance. Caffeine indeed stimulates lipolysis and the mobilization of FAs. These actions might occur indirectly by increasing the circulating epinephrine levels or directly by antagonizing adenosine receptors that normally inhibit hormone-sensitive lipase and FA oxidation.

Another possible mechanism is a direct effect of caffeine or one of its metabolites on skeletal muscle. Possibilities include the handling of ions, inhibition of phosphodiesterase leading to an increased concentration of 3′,5′-cyclic adenosine monophosphate (cAMP), and the direct effect on key regulatory enzymes such as phosphorylase. Most of these hypotheses are derived from in vitro studies in which unphysiologically high concentrations of caffeine were used, and whether similar effects would have been found with realistic physiological concentrations is unclear.

A third possibility, which is used to explain some of the suggested influences of caffeine on high-intensity exercise, is an increased influx of calcium from the extracellular space, increased release of calcium from the sarcoplasmic reticulum, and increased sensitivity of the myofilament to calcium. All of these result in increased excitability of the muscle fibers.

A fourth possible mechanism is the stimulating effect of caffeine on the central nervous system, which affects the perception of effort or affects the signal transduction from the brain to the neuromuscular junction. The cellular actions responsible for this central nervous system activation are not clear but may be related to catecholamine release and, more likely, to the release of neurotransmitters.

Caffeine Supplements Versus Coffee

As mentioned previously, coffee accounts for 75% of all caffeine consumption. The quantity of caffeine in coffee is highly variable and depends not only on the type of bean (e.g., Robusta coffee contains about 40%-50% more caffeine than Arabica coffee) but also on the method of preparation (see table 11.2) as well as other factors. Whatever the type of coffee, we would expect it to have the same effect as another source of comparable caffeine content. Studies suggest, however, that this may not be the case. Graham, Hibbert, and Sathasivam (1998) found that caffeine in coffee was less potent than caffeine given in a capsule. The differences in performance occurred despite similar plasma caffeine concentrations, and the authors concluded that another component in coffee may reduce the effect of caffeine. But when McLellan and Bell (2004) gave coffee before the ingestion of a capsule of caffeine, the coffee did not seem to dampen the effect of a relatively large caffeine dose. In a study by Hodgson, Randell, and Jeukendrup (2013), eight trained cyclists and triathletes performed time trials with caffeine taken as a supplement or consumed as coffee. Time trial performance was significantly faster and average power was significantly higher when caffeine or coffee was consumed compared with decaffeinated coffee or placebo. There was, however, no difference in performance between coffee and a caffeine supplement. Because the use of coffee seems to be less controversial than the use of a caffeine supplement, this may be the preferred caffeination option for many. Many will also enjoy the taste and smell of a cup of fresh espresso more than a supplement.

Side Effects

Caffeine use has side effects. People who normally avoid caffeine may experience GI distress, headaches, tachycardia, restlessness, irritability, tremor, elevated blood pressure, psychomotor agitations, and premature left ventricular contractions with intake of caffeine, all of which are caused by the effect of caffeine on the central nervous system. It is often stated that caffeine is a diuretic and should not be consumed in the hours before exercise when hydration is required. Studies have demonstrated, however, that moderate intake of caffeine does not affect urine loss or hydration status (Armstrong 2002; Armstrong et al. 2005). Furthermore, during exercise, the potential diuretic effect of caffeine is counteracted by catecholamines (Wemple, Lamb, and McKeever 1997), causing constriction of renal arterioles and reducing glomerular filtration rates. The catecholamines possibly increase sodium and chloride reabsorption rates in the proximal and distal tubules by affecting aldosterone, an antidiuretic hormone, resulting in greater water retention. Caffeine has no effect on sweat rates. Thus, caffeine taken in moderate amounts may not have a diuretic effect. Extremely high intakes of caffeine have been associated with peptic ulcer, seizure, coma, and even death. A review summarized the health effects of caffeine and concluded that for healthy adults, caffeine consumption is relatively safe, but for some vulnerable populations, caffeine consumption could be harmful and impair cardiovascular function and sleep (Temple et al. 2017). Although this conclusion relates to the general population, the same is probably true for athletes, and each athlete will have to establish his or her side effects from caffeine through trial and error.

Role of Genetics in Determining Responses

The effects of caffeine are highly individual due to genetics. Perhaps the most studied gene related to caffeine is CYP1A2, which regulates the breakdown of caffeine. This gene determines the rate at which a person metabolizes caffeine, but it does not actually affect the sensitivity to caffeine. Sensitivity to caffeine is mostly determined by the gene ADORA2A. Other genes that have been identified are AHR, which switches on gene CYP1A2 and indirectly regulates breakdown of caffeine, and COMT, which regulates the concentration of catecholamines. The combination of these genes will determine how a person responds to caffeine. It is possible to find out how someone will respond to caffeine by performing a genetic test.

Carnitine

Carnitine (also known as L-carnitine), a substance present in relatively high quantities in meat (the Latin word *carnis* means meat or muscle), has received much attention over the past 20 years. As a supplement, it has been popular among athletes, and it has been the focus of many studies. Carnitine became especially popular after rumors circulated that it helped the Italian national soccer team to become world champions in 1982.

Carnitine supplementation is said to increase $\dot{V}O_2max$ and reduce lactate production during maximal and supramaximal exercise and is also claimed to improve endurance exercise performance by increasing fat oxidation and sparing muscle glycogen. But the most important claims are that carnitine improves fat metabolism, reduces fat mass, and increases muscle mass. It is generally advertised as a fat burner. Therefore, carnitine is often used to lose weight, reduce body fat, and improve muscle definition (popular with body builders). Endurance athletes use carnitine to increase the oxidation of fat and spare muscle glycogen.

In the Body

Carnitine is derived from red meats and dairy products in the diet (see table 11.3) and from endogenous production in the body. Even when dietary sources are insufficient, healthy humans produce enough from methionine and lysine to maintain functional body stores. For this reason, carnitine is not regarded as a vitamin but as a vitamin-like substance.

Carnitine is synthesized in the liver and kidneys, which together contain only 1.6% of the whole-body carnitine store (about 27 g). About 98% of the carnitine in the human body is present in skeletal and heart muscle. Skeletal muscle and the heart depend on transport of carnitine through the circulation, which contains about 0.5 % of whole-body carnitine.

Muscle takes up carnitine against a very large (about 1,000-fold) concentration gradient (plasma carnitine is 40-60 µmol/L and muscle carnitine is 4-5 mmol/L) by a saturable active transport process

TABLE 11.3 Sources of Dietary Carnitine

Source	Total carnitine content (mg/100g)
Sheep	210
Lamb	78
Beef	64
Pork	30
Rabbit	21
Chicken	7.5
Milk	2.0
Eggs	0.8
Peanuts	0.1

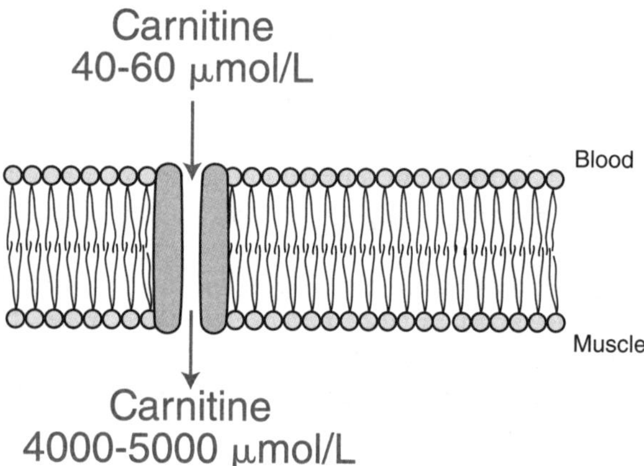

Figure 11.6 Transport of carnitine into the muscle sarcoplasm occurs against a large concentration gradient.

(see figure 11.6). Carnitine is an end product of human metabolism and is only lost from the body by excretion in urine and feces. Daily losses are minimal (<60 mg/day) and are reduced to less than 20 mg/day on meat-free and carnitine-free diets (Bremer 1983). These minimal losses imply that the rate of endogenous biosynthesis, which is needed to maintain functional body stores, is also only about 20 mg/day. The amounts lost in feces can usually be ignored except after ingestion of oral supplements.

Fat Metabolism

Carnitine plays an important role in fat metabolism. In the overnight fasted state and during exercise of low to moderate intensity, LCFAs are the main energy sources used by most tissues, including skeletal muscle. The primary function of carnitine is to transport LCFAs across the mitochondrial inner membrane because the inner membrane is impermeable to both LCFAs and fatty acyl-CoA esters (Bremer 1983) (see figure 7.6 in chapter 7). Once inside the mitochondria, FAs can be degraded to acetyl-CoA through ß-oxidation. The acetyl-CoA units will then be available for the TCA cycle to provide energy.

Carnitine plays an important role in maintaining the acetyl-CoA to CoA ratio in the cell. During high-intensity exercise, a large production of acetyl-CoA occurs, resulting in an increased acetyl-CoA to CoA ratio. This increased ratio, in turn, inhibits the pyruvate dehydrogenase (PDH) complex and reduces flux through the PDH complex and hence acetyl-CoA formation, resulting in increased lactate formation. Therefore, the acetyl-CoA to CoA ratio should be maintained. Acetyl-CoA reacts with free carnitine to form acetyl-carnitine and CoA:

$$\text{acetyl-CoA} + \text{carnitine} \leftrightarrows \text{acetyl-carnitine} + \text{CoA}$$

In theory, carnitine therefore acts as a sink for excess acetyl-CoA and blunts the accumulation of lactic acid, thereby enhancing high-intensity exercise performance. By increasing fat oxidation during exercise, it could also spare muscle glycogen and thereby enhance endurance exercise performance.

Slimming Agent

The belief that carnitine is a slimming agent is based on the assumption that regular oral ingestion of carnitine increases the muscle carnitine concentration. Another assumption is that if carnitine concentration in the muscle increases, fat oxidation also increases, thus leading to a gradual loss of body fat stores. Several carefully conducted studies (Barnett et al. 1994; Vukovich, Costill, and Fink 1994; Wachter et al. 2002), however, showed that oral carnitine ingestion (daily ingestion for up to 3 months) does not change the muscle carnitine concentration. Even infusion of carnitine for 5 hours did not increase muscle carnitine concentration. It seems that the reason carnitine was unable to increase muscle carnitine concentration in these studies was partly because of poor **bioavailability** (20% for a 2-6 g dose) and partly because the transport of carnitine into the muscle was limited. Any claims regarding effects of carnitine on fat oxidation or weight loss are, of course, unfounded if carnitine supplementation is unable to increase the carnitine concentration in muscle. In addition, enzyme kinetics indicate that human muscle in resting conditions has more than enough free carnitine to allow the enzyme CPT I to function at maximal activity. Other studies, however, indicate that if carnitine is coingested with carbohydrate, more substantial increases in the muscle carnitine concentration can be observed. While this might not necessarily be beneficial for losing weight, it could improve exercise performance.

In a series of studies, it was observed that it is possible to increase muscle carnitine concentration if carnitine is given when plasma insulin concentrations are elevated. Carnitine is transported into the muscle cell by a sodium-dependent active transport process. The transport protein involved is called the organic cation transporter OCTN2, and it was hypothesized that insulin may increase the sodium-dependent transport of carnitine. Initial studies used simultaneous infusion of insulin and carnitine and observed a 15% increase in muscle carnitine (Stephens et al. 2006). Further studies revealed that a certain (fairly high) level of insulin is necessary to achieve this effect (Stephens, Evans, et al. 2007). It has also been demonstrated that the insulin response resulting from carbohydrate feeding can be sufficient to increase the uptake of carnitine into the muscle (Stephens, Evans, et al. 2007). In this study, 3 g of carnitine was ingested each day followed by four 500 ml (17 fl oz) beverages that each contained 94 g of carbohydrate. It was observed that carnitine retention improved (less carnitine excretion in urine), which suggests increased muscle carnitine. Of course, whether this strategy is practical or meaningful is questionable, especially in a weight-loss situation. If four lots of 94 g of carbohydrate (372 g in total, which is equivalent to 6,000 kJ [1,434 kcal]) has to be ingested to increase muscle carnitine concentration, one might think that weight gain is more likely to result than weight loss! Also, the high carbohydrate intake will suppress fat oxidation. This suppression will be greater than the possible effect of carnitine. Nevertheless, the observations are interesting and have been subsequently followed up by a study that showed 12 weeks of daily carnitine and carbohydrate feeding in humans increases skeletal muscle total carnitine content and prevents body mass accrual associated with carbohydrate feeding alone (Stephens et al. 2013). No changes in fat oxidation were reported. It remains to be seen how practical and cost effective this daily supplementation of carnitine with carbohydrates is.

Endurance Exercise

The belief that carnitine is an ergogenic aid for endurance exercise is based on assumptions similar to the weight-loss assumptions (Wagenmakers 1991): that carnitine concentration in muscle becomes too low to allow CPT I to function at a high velocity and to support the increased rate of fat oxidation during exercise; that oral ingestion of carnitine increases the total carnitine concentration in muscle; and that the increase in muscle carnitine increases the oxidation rate of plasma FAs and intramuscular triacylglycerols during exercise, thereby reducing muscle glycogen breakdown and postponing fatigue.

During high-intensity exercise, the free carnitine concentration in muscle falls because it reacts with acetyl-CoA. During very high-intensity exercise, the free carnitine concentration falls to extremely low levels. Studies report values as low as 0.5 mmol/kg w.w. after 3 to 4 minutes at 90% of $\dot{V}O_2max$ (Constantin-Teodosiu et al. 1991). These values approach the K_m of CPT I for carnitine (250-450 μM) measured in vitro (Bremer 1983). K_m is the substrate concentration that results in an enzyme-catalyzed reaction proceeding at 50% of the maximum rate. At the typical muscle carnitine concentrations of 250 to 450 μM, the reaction catalyzed by CPT I is proceeding at about 50% of its maximum rate. (For further explanation of K_m, see appendix A.) This decrease in free carnitine has been suggested as one of the mechanisms by which plasma FA and intramuscular triacylglycerol oxidation are reduced during high-intensity exercise (Constantin-Teodosiu et al. 1991; Timmons et al. 1996).

As previously mentioned, early studies using direct measurements in muscle after 14 days on 4 to 6 g of carnitine per day failed to show increases in the muscle carnitine concentration (Barnett et al. 1994; Vukovich, Costill, and Fink 1994). This finding implies that carnitine supplementation cannot increase fat oxidation and improve exercise performance by the proposed mechanism. Indeed, many original investigations, which are summarized in numerous reviews (Heinonen 1996; Wagenmakers 1991), confirmed that carnitine supplementation on its own does not increase fat oxidation and reduce glycogen breakdown and does not improve performance during prolonged cycling and running exercise. However, a placebo-controlled study (Wall et al. 2011) has shown that substantial elevations (~20%) of muscle carnitine content do occur in humans following prolonged daily supplementation with carnitine tartrate when carbohydrate is ingested at the same time. Importantly, this study also showed that this results in muscle glycogen sparing during low-intensity exercise (consistent with an increase in fat oxidation) and lower lactate accumulation during high-intensity exercise. Furthermore, these changes were associated with an 11% improvement in a 30-minute work output exercise performance trial (Wall et al. 2011). Despite this important finding, there has been very little work to follow it up.

High-Intensity Exercise

As previously indicated, carnitine may increase the availability of free CoA and maintain the acetyl-CoA to CoA ratio (see figure 11.7). This function of carnitine is especially important during maximal and supramaximal exercise, such as competitive sprint and middle-distance running and 50 to 400 m swimming. If carnitine supplementation increases muscle carnitine concentration and, therefore, CoA availability in these conditions, the flux through the pyruvate dehydrogenase complex could increase and less lactic acid would be produced (see figure 11.7). Theoretically, this process could delay fatigue and improve exercise performance, but this now requires investigation using chronic supplementation of carnitine coingested with carbohydrate. One study compared the effects of a commercially available carbohydrate–protein supplement enriched with L-glutamine and carnitine tartrate to carbohydrate alone or placebo on sprint performance, muscle damage markers, and recovery from a 90-minute intermittent repeated sprint test (Naclerio et al. 2014). No significant effects of the supplement on performance and fatigue were found, but the accumulation of some biomarkers of muscle damage was attenuated.

Cherry Juice

Cherries and their constituents have received growing attention for application in sport as a means of enhancing recovery from damaging exercise regimens. The evidence for these effects has been

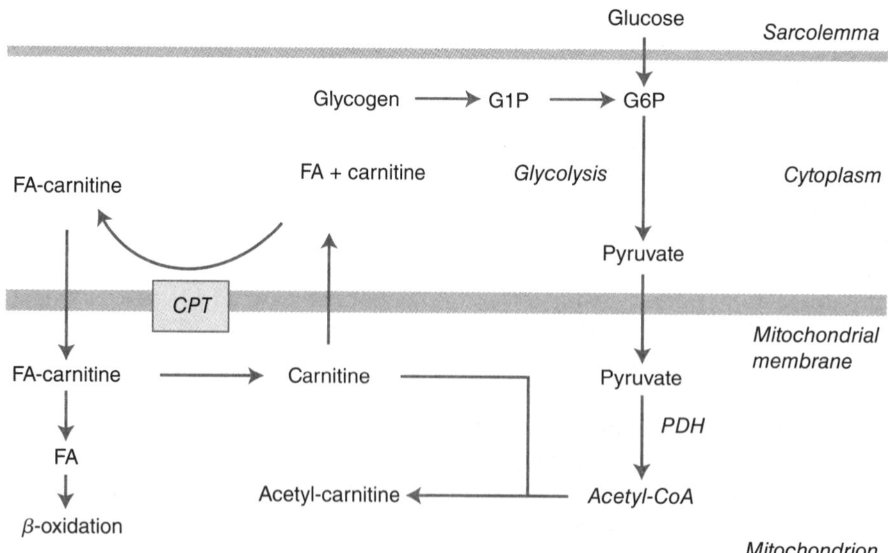

Figure 11.7 A potential link between FA uptake, carnitine, and glucose metabolism. Carnitine acts as a buffer for acetyl-CoA, thereby preventing a buildup of pyruvate and preventing lactate accumulation. This activity may, however, reduce free carnitine availability and, at least in theory, FA transport into the mitochondria. FA = fatty acid; PDH = pyruvate dehydrogenase; CPT = carnitine palmitoyl transferase.

reviewed by Bell et al. (2014). The food science, animal, and human literature currently available clearly demonstrate the anti-inflammatory and antioxidative effects of cherries. The research suggests that there are some limited benefits of tart cherry juice consumption in enhancing recovery from exercise and improving sleep quality, but the mechanisms of action are somewhat speculative with regard to recovery from exercise. As a result, confident prescription of the optimal supplementation strategy is troublesome, although efficacy for a loading phase has been established. There is also controversy regarding the manipulation of the stress responses to exercise (inflammation and oxidative stress) with antioxidant supplements, with a suggestion that adaptation may be blunted as a result of downregulating the stress response (Gomez-Cabrera etal. 2005, 2008). It should be noted, however, that such negative adaptive effects have not been reported in cherry studies or any other functional foods and perhaps warrant further investigation. The specific compounds responsible for any beneficial effects of cherry juice have not been identified but could include quercetin, anthocyanins, and their metabolites.

Choline

Acetylcholine transmits the electrical potential from the neuron to the muscle cell, which leads to calcium release from the sarcoplasmic reticulum and muscle contraction. Experimental studies in animals suggest that depletion of the neuromuscular transmitter acetylcholine contributes to fatigue during sustained electrical stimulation or exercise (Pagala, Namba, and Grob 1984). Whether this transmission defect is at the presynaptic or postsynaptic membrane or across the synapse has not been elucidated.

The precursor of acetylcholine, **choline**, is a normal component of the human diet. It is most abundant in meat and dairy products. It is also an integral part of several phospholipids incorporated into cell membranes, including phosphatidylcholine (**lecithin**), lysophatidylcholine, and sphingomyelin (Zeisel 1998). Peak serum concentrations of choline occur several hours after ingestion of lecithin (Zeisel et al. 1991). Ingestion of choline or lecithin raises plasma choline levels in a dose-dependent manner. Based on these functions, choline supplements have been hypothesized to affect nerve transmission, increase strength, or facilitate the loss of body fat.

Strenuous exercise decreases plasma choline levels. They were reduced by 40% in participants of the 1985 Boston Marathon (Conlay et al. 1986), and similar findings were reported after the 1986 Boston Marathon (Wurtman and Lewis 1991). Von Allworden et al. (1993) reported a 16.9% average decline in plasma choline concentration after 2 hours of strenuous cycling (35 km/h [22 mph]). Neuromuscular transmission can be impaired before the end of marathons or during the late stages of other forms of prolonged strenuous exercise unless choline is supplied by neuronal or muscular membrane phospholipids or ingestion. Low acetylcholine concentrations have been associated with impaired neuromuscular transmission and fatigue. The acetylcholine concentration in the brain is directly related to the plasma choline concentration. Several studies of choline uptake and distribution after intravenous administration of choline show that plasma choline and acetylcholine in kidney, liver, lung, and heart are directly proportional to the amounts administered. Haubrich et al. (1975) reported that intravenous infusion of choline in guinea pigs led to incorporation of choline into acetylcholine within minutes in a variety of tissues.

Whether this reaction is also the case for skeletal muscle in vivo is still unknown. Some evidence from in vitro studies, however, indicates that newly synthesized acetylcholine is released during neuromuscular stimulation when choline is added to the perfusion medium (Bierkamper and Goldberg 1980). Gardiner and Gwee (1974) infused choline in rabbits and measured an elevated choline concentration in all tissues, including muscle. Unfortunately, acetylcholine was not measured. Thus, prolonged neuromuscular efforts could result in depletion of plasma choline, which might lead to fatigue because of insufficient availability of acetylcholine. Increasing plasma choline levels by ingesting choline might increase acetylcholine availability and thereby reduce fatigue.

One preliminary report showed that ingestion of choline citrate during a 32 km (20 mi) run prevented the fall of plasma choline concentration, and performance improved compared with a placebo-treated group (Sandage et al. 1992). Spector et al. (1995) reported no effect on either brief supramaximal or prolonged submaximal cycling performance after the ingestion of 2.43 g of choline bitartrate. During the placebo trial, however, no fall in choline was observed and none of the subjects displayed choline depletion. In the absence of any choline depletion, choline ingestion is unlikely to improve performance. Interestingly, these authors reported a significant negative correlation between the decrease in choline concentration and time to exhaustion, which suggests that choline may play a role in the development of fatigue.

Von Allworden et al. (1993) gave subjects 0.2 g of lecithin per kilogram of body weight 1 hour before they cycled for 2 hours at 35 km/h (22 mph). Lecithin ingestion increased plasma choline concentrations by 26.9%, whereas placebo ingestion decreased choline concentrations by 16.9%. Unfortunately, exercise performance was not evaluated in this study. The claims of choline as a supplement are based largely on theory and findings of in vitro studies. Although some interesting observations have been made in humans, the grounds for recommending choline as an ergogenic aid are insufficient.

Chromium

Chromium is a popular supplement because it is said to be a muscle builder and fat burner, and enormous marketing hype has surrounded this supplement over the past few years. **Chromium** is a trace element that is present in foods such as brewer's yeast, American cheese, mushrooms, and wheat germ, and it is considered an essential nutrient. Because of insufficient methods to assess chromium status, the U.S. Food and Nutrition Board could not establish an RDA for chromium. Instead, an AI value of 20 to 45 mg/day is recommended. Anderson and Kozlovsky (1985) suggested that many people in the United States are not ingesting even 50 picograms (pg) per day (a picogram is 10^{-12} g) of chromium. The AI was established using less sophisticated equipment than is available today, so the recommended values may be too high (Stoecker 1996).

Chromium potentiates insulin action, and insulin stimulates glucose and amino acid uptake by muscle cells. The increase in amino acid uptake is thought to increase protein synthesis and muscle mass. Chromium supplements increase muscle mass and growth in animals (Stoecker 1996), but the effect of chromium on muscle mass in humans is less clear. Chromium is marketed predominantly in the form of chromium picolinate, although chromium nicotinate and chromium chloride supplements also exist. Picolinic acid is an organic compound that binds to chromium and is thought to enhance the absorption and transport of chromium (Evans 1989).

Evans (1989) was the first to report that ingesting chromium increased lean tissue in exercising humans. In those studies, untrained college students and trained football players were given 200 mg of chromium picolinate or a placebo each day for 40 to 42 days while they were on a resistance-training program. Those subjects who took chromium supplements gained significantly more lean body mass compared with the placebo group. But lean body mass was only estimated from circumference measures and the changes observed were small, so measurement error could have influenced the results.

Subsequent studies (Clancy et al. 1994; Hallmark et al. 1996; Hasten et al. 1992; Lukaski et al. 1996) have not confirmed Evans' results. In these carefully controlled studies that used more sophisticated techniques to measure body composition, no effects on lean body mass were found.

A study investigated the effects of chromium on muscle glycogen synthesis after exercise (Volek et al. 2006). Because it has been reported that chromium may affect insulin sensitivity, it was hypothesized that it may also enhance insulin sensitivity postexercise, thereby increasing glucose uptake and glycogen synthesis. Chromium supplementation for 4 weeks, however, did not augment glycogen synthesis during recovery from high-intensity exercise and high-carbohydrate feeding, although there was a trend for lower phosphoinositide-3-kinase activity (which is indicative of improved insulin sensitivity).

Thus, most of the studies show that chromium supplements are not effective in increasing lean body mass. Based on laboratory studies of cultured cells, chromium picolinate was suggested to accumulate in cells and cause chromosome damage (Stearns, Wise, et al. 1995). Although this finding has not been confirmed in human studies (McCarty 1996), caution must be exercised in the use of chromium supplements.

Coenzyme Q10

Coenzyme Q10 (CoQ10), or ubiquinone, is an integral part of the electron-transport chain of the mitochondria. Therefore, it plays an important role in oxidative phosphorylation. In heart muscle it has been used therapeutically to treat cardiovascular disease and promote recovery from cardiac surgery. CoQ10 supplementation in patients with those conditions improves oxidative metabolism and exercise capacity (Khatta et al. 2000), and it functions as an antioxidant, which promotes the scavenging of free radicals. Manufacturers extrapolated the results of improved $\dot{V}O_2$max in cardiac patients to healthy and trained athletes. CoQ10 is claimed to increase $\dot{V}O_2$max and increase stamina and energy.

A few studies have investigated the effects of CoQ10 supplementation in athletes. Although most of these studies report elevated plasma CoQ10 levels, no changes were observed in $\dot{V}O_2max$, performance, or blood lactate at submaximal workloads. Ingestion of 120 mg/day of CoQ10 for 20 days was reported to result in marked increases in plasma CoQ10 concentrations, but the muscle CoQ10 concentration was unaltered (Svensson et al. 1999). Of course, if CoQ10 supplementation does not alter muscle CoQ10 concentration, it cannot be expected to have any effects on any of the performance-related variables.

CoQ10 may have some negative effects. It possibly augments free-radical production during high-intensity exercise when an abundance of hydrogen ions are present in the cells (Malm et al. 1997). Ironically, this effect is the opposite of what CoQ10 is claimed to do.

Creatine

Creatine became a popular supplement after the 1992 Olympics in Barcelona. Gold medal winners Linford Christie (men's 100 m dash) and Sally Gunnell (women's 400 m hurdles) supposedly used creatine supplements. At the Olympic Games in Atlanta in 1996, approximately 80% of all athletes used creatine (Williams, Kreider, and Branch 1999). The worldwide creatine consumption by athletes is now estimated to be around 3,000,000 kg/year. This section discusses the efficacy of creatine in different sports and the supposed mechanisms of action. For more information on the role of creatine in metabolism and performance, see Casey and Greenhaff (2000), Greenhaff (1998), and Terjung et al. (2000). The book by Williams, Kreider, and Branch (1999) is also a complete source of information.

In the Body

Creatine, or methylguanidine-acetic acid, is a naturally occurring compound present mostly in muscle tissue. It is not an essential nutrient because it can be synthesized in the human body. In normal, healthy people, diet and oral ingestion provide approximately 2 g of creatine per day. Creatine is broken down to creatinine and excreted in the urine at approximately the same rate (2 g/day).

The primary dietary sources of creatine are fish and red meat (see table 11.4). Strict vegetarians and vegans have negligible creatine intake because plants contain only trace amounts. They are, therefore, dependent on endogenous synthesis of creatine. Oral ingestion of creatine suppresses the biosynthesis. When a creatine-deficient diet is consumed, the urinary excretion of creatine and creatinine decreases.

TABLE 11.4 Sources of Dietary Creatine

Food	Creatine content (g/100 g)
Fish	
Shrimp	Trace
Cod	0.30
Herring	0.65-1.10
Plaice	0.20
Salmon	0.45
Tuna	0.40
Meat	
Beef	0.45
Pork	0.40
Other	
Milk	0.01
Cranberries	0.0002

Creatine synthesis in the human body is a two-step reaction. First, the guanidino group of arginine is transferred to glycine, thereby forming guanidinoacetate. Second, creatine is formed by transfer of a methyl group from S-adenosylmethionine to guanidinoacetate. Most creatine synthesis in humans occurs in the liver and kidneys (see figure 11.8).

In a 70 kg (154 lb) man, the total-body creatine pool is approximately 120 g, 95% of which is in skeletal, heart, and smooth muscle. The remaining 5% is in the brain, liver, kidneys, and testes. Creatine synthesized in the liver and kidneys and absorbed from the diet is transported by blood to the muscle. Muscle takes up creatine against a concentration gradient by a sodium-dependent saturable active transport process. In the muscle cell, creatine is phosphorylated and then trapped within the muscle. This process helps create a high total-creatine gradient (30-40 mmol/kg w.w. or 120-160 mmol/kg dry matter (d.m.) in skeletal muscle, with 60%-70% in the form of phosphocreatine) (Wyss and Kaddurah-Daouk 2000). Type I and type II muscle fibers have differing creatine contents; type II fibers have about 30% more creatine than type I fibers.

Metabolic Process

The role of creatine and phosphocreatine is discussed in chapter 3 but will be briefly summarized here. As muscle contracts, ATP is degraded to ADP and Pi to provide energy:

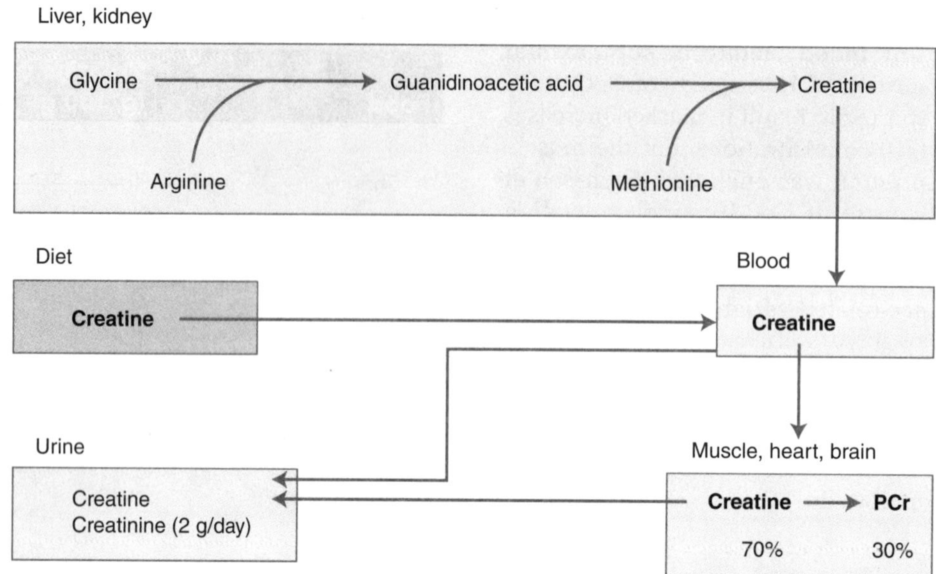

Figure 11.8 Creatine synthesis and transport in the body.

$$\text{ATP} \rightarrow \text{ADP} + \text{Pi} + \text{energy}$$

During intense maximal exercise, ATP stores can provide energy for only 1 to 2 seconds. When the whole-muscle ATP concentration falls by about 30%, the muscle fatigues (Hultman et al. 1991; Karlsson and Saltin 1970). To prevent fatigue, regeneration of ATP must occur at a rate similar to that of ATP hydrolysis to maintain ATP concentration close to resting levels. An important function of phosphocreatine in muscle is to provide the high-energy phosphate group for ATP regeneration during the first seconds of high-intensity exercise, thus allowing time for glycogen breakdown and glycolysis (the other main process generating cytosolic ATP during high-intensity exercise) to speed up to the required rate. Transfer of the phosphate group from phosphocreatine to ADP is catalyzed by the enzyme creatine kinase, which results in regeneration of ATP and release of free creatine:

$$\text{PCr} + \text{ADP} + \text{H}^+ \rightarrow \text{creatine (Cr)} + \text{ATP}$$

PCr is present in resting muscle in a concentration that is three to four times that of ATP (see appendix A). During the 100 m sprint, 22 g of ATP is estimated to be broken down per second, or about 50% of the ATP content per kilogram of active muscle. Because fatigue occurs in human muscle when the whole-muscle ATP concentration falls below 70% of its normal resting value, the need for rephosphorylation of the ADP formed during contraction is obvious.

Anaerobic degradation of PCr and glycogen is responsible for the extremely high rate of ATP resynthesis during the first seconds of high-intensity exercise (Hultman et al. 1991; Karlsson and B. Saltin 1970). The PCr store in muscle is limited and is depleted within 5 seconds of supramaximal exercise. The rapid breakdown of PCr after the onset of intense exercise allows the concentration of skeletal muscle ATP to be maintained to some degree during single bouts or repeated bouts of supramaximal exercise. Anaerobic ATP resynthesis, however, cannot be maintained at the same rate as during the first few seconds of supramaximal exercise. Consequently, over the course of 30 seconds, ATP turnover rates fall by about 20%. High PCr stores possibly reduce the need for anaerobic glycolysis and lactic acid formation during intense exercise, which might be another potential benefit of creatine supplementation.

Another important function of creatine is its potential buffering capacity for hydrogen ions because those ions are used during ATP regeneration, as shown in the previous equation. A higher creatine concentration in the muscle also implies increased flux through the creatine kinase reaction, which results in increased PCr synthesis during recovery from high-intensity exercise. The roles of creatine listed previously suggest that elevating muscle creatine and PCr stores will benefit high-intensity exercise performance.

Supplementation

Harris, Soderlund, and Hultman (1992) were the first to state that ingesting creatine monohydrate could increase total muscle creatine stores (creatine and phosphocreatine). In that study, ingesting 5 g of creatine four to six times per day for several days increased the total creatine concentration by an average of 25 mmol/kg d.m., and 30% of the increase in total creatine content was in the form of phosphocreatine. The authors suggested that these increases could improve exercise performance but did not test this suggestion in their study. The first performance study was conducted by Greenhaff, Casey, et al. (1993). Subjects ingested 20 g of creatine per day for 5 days, and creatine improved performance by about 6% during repeated bouts of maximal knee extensor exercise. After that study, more studies were performed that investigated different modes of exercise (Balsom, Ekblom, et al. 1993; Balsom, Harridge, et al. 1993; Birch, Noble, and Greenhaff 1994; Harris, Soderlund, and Hultman 1992; Volek et al. 1997). In 1999, of the 62 laboratory-based studies performed on creatine supplementation and high-intensity exercise performance, 42 reported positive effects, and the remainder showed no effects (Williams, Kreider, and Branch 1999). Since then, the number of positive studies has accumulated.

Loading Regimens

Most studies used a creatine loading regimen of 20 g/day in four portions of 5 g each given at different times of the day for a 6-day period. This regimen has been shown to increase muscle creatine concentration by about 25 mmol/kg d.m. on average. This increase corresponds to about 20% of the basal total muscle creatine concentration of about 125 mmol/kg d.m. Hultman et al. (1996) found that after an initial loading phase of 20 g/day for 6 days, a subsequent dose of 2 g/day was enough to maintain the high total creatine concentration for 35 days, whereas stopping creatine supplementation after 6 days caused a slow, gradual decline of the creatine concentration in muscle.

When creatine was ingested at a dose of 3 g/day, the rate of increase in muscle creatine was correspondingly lower, but after 28 days on 3 g/day, the total creatine concentration was similar to the rapid-loading regimen (see figure 11.9). Therefore, a loading dose of 20 g/day for 6 days followed by a maintenance dose of 2 to 3 g/day is advised if athletes want to increase muscle creatine to maximal levels quickly, whereas a continuous dose of 3 g/day leads to the same maximal level in about 1 month. The increase in muscle PCr concentration was about 40% of the increase in total creatine concentration with both procedures.

Considerable variation exists among subjects in the initial total muscle creatine concentration. The reasons for variation are largely unknown, but they may be at least partly related to the habitual diet. The largest increase in muscle creatine concentration is observed in people with the lowest initial concentrations, whereas those who already have high creatine concentrations benefit only marginally (Harris, Soderlund, and Hultman 1992) (see figure 11.10). A concentration of 160 mmol/kg d.m. appears to be the maximal creatine concentration achievable by creatine supplementation, but only about 20% of subjects reached this level after creatine supplementation.

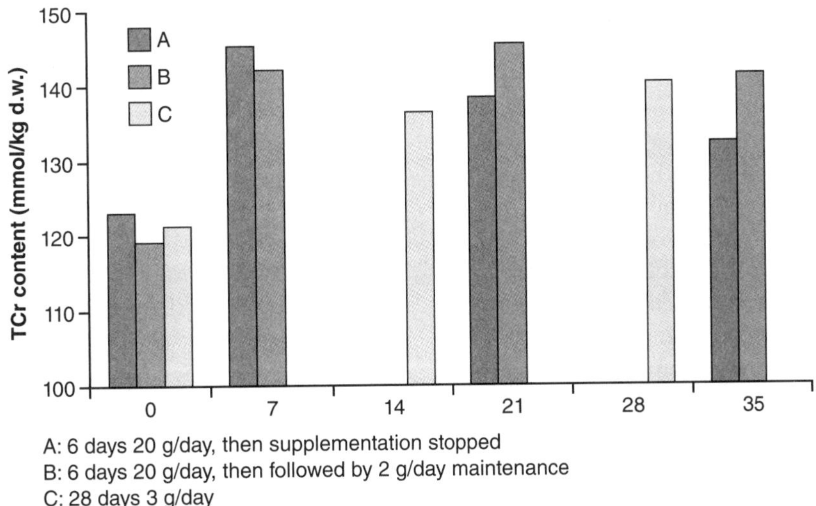

Figure 11.9 Different protocols of creatine loading. TCr = total creatine.

Data from Hultman et al. (1996).

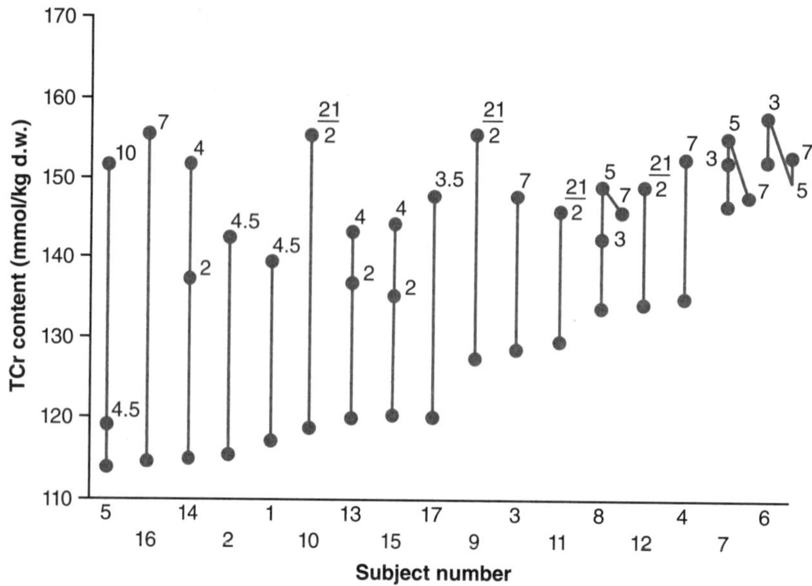

Figure 11.10 Individual responses to creatine loading. People with low creatine stores benefit most, whereas those who already have high creatine stores have minimal increases in muscle creatine. Numbers in the graph are days of supplementation at a rate of 20 to 30 g/day. 21/2 indicates subjects who ingested creatine on alternate days for 21 days.

Data from Hultman et al. (1996).

Total muscle creatine can be increased more (mean increase 30-40 mmol/kg d.m.) when creatine (20 g/day for 5 days) is ingested in solution with simple carbohydrate (Green et al. 1995, 1996). In a study, the total muscle creatine concentration increased in most subjects close to the upper limit of 160 mmol/kg d.m. Carbohydrate ingestion is thought to stimulate muscle creatine uptake through an insulin-dependent mechanism. Insulin may stimulate the sodium-potassium pump activity and thereby the sodium-dependent muscle creatine transport.

In a study by Casey et al. (1996) the changes in performance were related to the changes in total muscle creatine content (see figure 11.11). A strong correlation was observed in that people who displayed the largest increases in total muscle creatine concentration also exhibited the largest performance benefits. A change in muscle creatine content of about 20 mmol/kg d.m. (or 5 mmol/kg w.w.) is said to be necessary before significant changes in performance are observed. About 30% of all individuals do not display such large increases in muscle creatine and therefore do not benefit. They are often referred to as nonresponders.

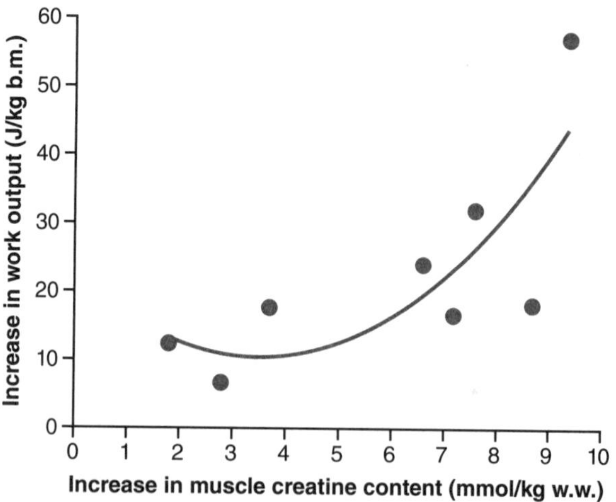

Figure 11.11 Relationship between individual changes in mixed muscle creatine concentration and changes in total work production after creatine loading (4-5 g/day for 5 days). Work production was measured during two bouts of 30 seconds of maximal isokinetic cycling exercises. The polynomial trend line indicates a significant correlation ($r = 0.78$).

Weight Gain

Creatine supplementation (20 g/day for 5-6 days) is generally accompanied by increases in body weight of 0.5 to 3.5 kg (1.1-7.7 lb). (For a complete overview, see Williams, Kreider, and Branch 1999.) The average increase in body mass is about 1 kg (2 lb). Theoretically, this increase in body mass and possible change in body composition results from increases in intracellular water, stimulation of protein synthesis, or a decrease in protein breakdown. Because the decrease in urine production exactly paralleled the time course of the increase in muscle creatine concentration (see figure 11.11), creatine likely causes water retention in skeletal muscle cells because of an increase of the intracellular osmolarity of the muscle fibers. Evidence suggests that some of the weight gain may be attributable to the anabolic effect of creatine (Kreider et al. 1998), although in the short term (5-6 days) this effect is not likely to be an important factor.

The increase in body mass may be beneficial or have no effect in some disciplines. But in sports that involve weight-bearing activities, such as running or gymnastics, the weight gain caused by creatine supplementation could have a negative effect on performance.

High-Intensity Exercise

The findings of Greenhaff, Casey, et al. (1993), who used high-intensity intermittent exercise, have been repeated in other studies using cycle ergometry, bench press, or running as the mode of exercise. About 70% of these studies found improvements in strength, force production, or torque.

Balsom, Ekblom, et al. (1993) randomly assigned 16 trained subjects to a creatine group (25 g/day for 6 days) and a placebo group. One test that these subjects performed was a repeated sprint test in which they sprinted 10 times for 6 seconds with 30 seconds of recovery between bouts. Although subjects fatigued with both creatine and placebo, after 7 sprints, fatigue was significantly greater in the placebo group. Casey et al. (1996) investigated the effect of acute creatine supplementation (20 g/day for 5 days) on isokinetic cycle performance (2 × 30 seconds with 4 minutes of recovery between bouts). Increases in peak power and total work were already observed in the first of the two bouts after creatine supplementation. The improvements in total work production were positively correlated with the increased concentration of PCr in type II muscle fibers after supplementation (see figure 11.12).

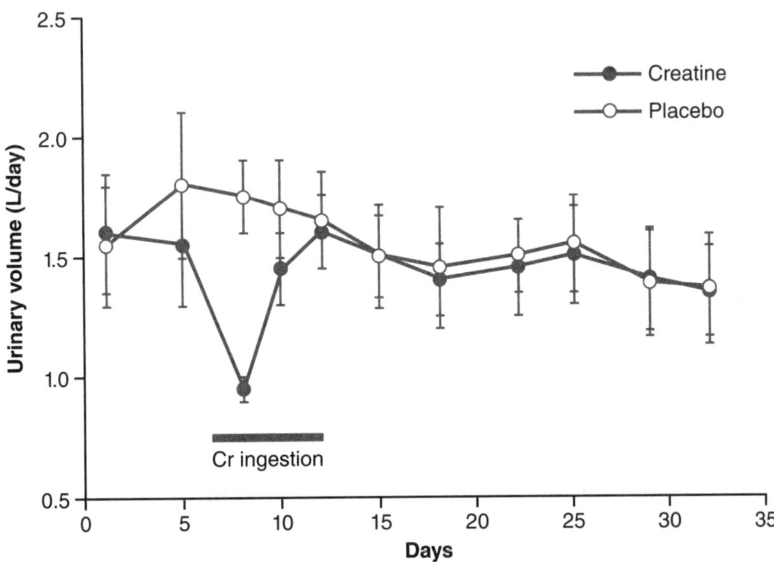

Figure 11.12 Urinary volume before and after placebo or creatine ingestion. Creatine was administered in 5 g increments four times per day for 5 days. A clear relationship was found between the decreased urinary output and the increase in body mass after creatine ingestion.

Reprinted from E. Hultman et al., "Muscle Creatine Loading in Men," *Journal of Applied Physiology* 81, no. 1 (1996): 232-237. Used with permission.

Several studies investigated the effect of creatine supplementation versus placebo on 25 m, 50 m, and 100 m performance in elite swimmers performing their best stroke (Burke, Pyne, and Telford 1996; Mujika et al. 1996; Peyrebrune et al. 1998). These studies failed to show an ergogenic effect of creatine supplementation. Two studies, however, showed improvements in 10 × 50 m or 8 × 45 m swimming velocity (Leenders, Lamb, and Nelson 1999; Peyrebrune et al. 1998). Rossiter, Cannell, and Jakeman (1996) observed an ergogenic effect of creatine versus placebo supplementation on the 1,000 m performance of competitive rowers. When two groups of rugby union players received creatine or placebo, no differences were observed in body composition between the groups (Chilibeck, Magnus, and Anderson 2007). The group receiving creatine supplementation had a greater increase in the number of repetitions for combined bench press and leg press tests compared with the placebo group.

Findings suggest that creatine also improves high-intensity exercise performance in competitive squash players (Romer, Barrington, and Jeukendrup 2001). The players fatigued less toward the end of a game when supplemented with creatine. Thus, creatine supplementation may have a positive effect on performance in competitive situations in some sports. Whether creatine has an effect may depend on the initial muscle creatine concentrations, the type of exercise, and the level of the athlete.

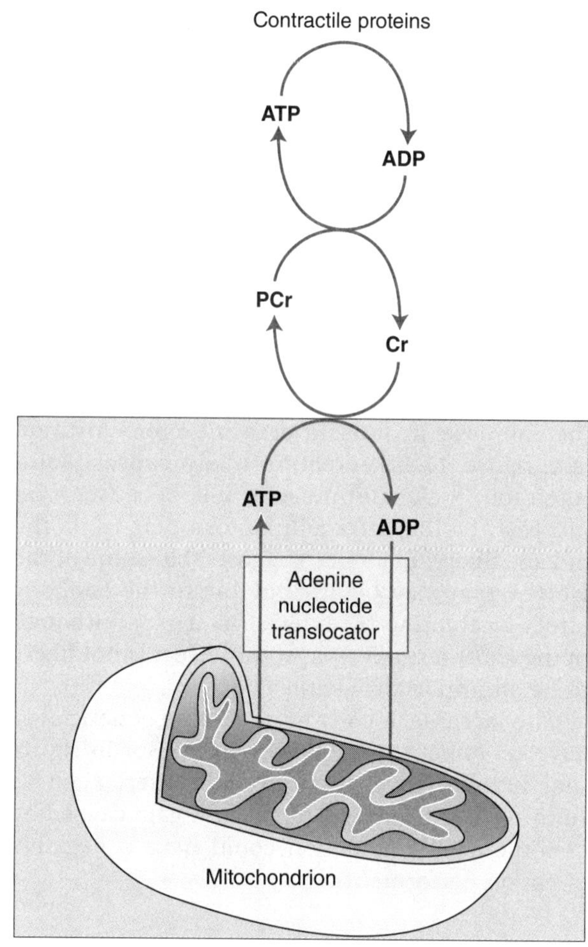

Figure 11.13 Transfer of ATP from the site of synthesis (mitochondria) to the site of usage (contractile proteins). Creatine and PCr play important roles in this process.

Data from Wagenmakers (1999b).

Endurance Exercise

In endurance exercise, most ATP is resynthesized by oxidative phosphorylation in the mitochondria. Net PCr breakdown and the net contribution of PCr to energy production are minimal. But creatine and PCr provide a shuttle system for the transfer of high-energy phosphate groups from the ATP production site (the mitochondria) to the ATP consumption site (the contracting myofibrils) (see figure 11.13). A phosphate group of ATP produced in the mitochondria is donated to creatine to form PCr. From PCr, the phosphate group is donated to ADP, and ATP is formed and can be used for muscle contraction. Theoretically, creatine could, therefore, facilitate aerobic energy production and enhance performance in prolonged exercise.

Balsom, Harridge, et al. (1993) investigated the effect of creatine supplementation for 6 days on endurance exercise performance in well-trained runners. No effect occurred during a supramaximal treadmill run to exhaustion in the laboratory, but a significant decrease in performance occurred during a 6 km (4 mi) terrain run. Subjects showed an increase in body weight of 0.5 to 1 kg (1-2 lb), which possibly explains the negative result during the terrain run. In another study, 5 days of creatine supplementation (20 g/day) had no influence on oxygen uptake, respiratory gas exchange, and blood-lactate concentration during submaximal incremental treadmill exercise and recovery. These data seem to suggest that the availability of creatine and PCr is not rate limiting for the diffusion of energy-rich phosphate groups through the cytosol and that creatine supplementation, therefore, does not affect muscle metabolism in endurance exercise. The studies that have investigated the effects of creatine supplementation on endurance performance generally have not reported an ergogenic effect.

Resistance Training

Vandenberghe et al. (1997) investigated the effect of creatine loading on muscle PCr phosphate concentration, muscle strength, and body composition after a 10-week resistance-training program. Compared with placebo, maximal strength of the trained muscle groups increased 20% to 25% more, maximal intermittent exercise capacity of the arm flexors increased 10% to 25% more, and fat-free mass increased 60% more with creatine supplementation. This study and others suggest that the combination of creatine ingestion and strength training is more effective than strength training alone. In addition, Wagenmakers (1999b) suggested that creatine supplementation allows more repetitions and thus better quality of training and also may have an anabolic effect.

Creatine causes fluid retention, which may result in muscle cell swelling. Cell swelling acts as a universal anabolic signal, causing an increase of protein synthesis and net protein deposition (Lang et al. 1998). Although several animal and clinical studies suggest that creatine ingestion has anabolic effects, no evidence in healthy individuals indicates that creatine affects protein metabolism.

Mechanisms of Action

Several mechanisms by which creatine exerts its effects have been proposed.

- The most obvious explanation is increased PCr availability, particularly in type II muscle fibers (Casey et al. 1996). Evidence indicates that increased PCr stores in the muscle improve contractile function by maintaining ATP turnover.
- Another possible mechanism is the increased rate of PCr resynthesis (Greenhaff et al. 1994), which is particularly important in short recovery periods during repeated bouts of maximal exercise.
- The increased use of PCr as an energy source could reduce anaerobic glycolysis and lactic acid formation. This activity could theoretically reduce hydrogen ion formation in the muscle and delay fatigue caused by increased muscle acidity.
- Creatine could buffer some of the hydrogen ions produced during high-intensity exercise. This process would delay fatigue in high-intensity exercise that is limited by lactic acid formation.
- As indicated in figure 11.13, creatine plays an important role in shuttling high-energy phosphates from the site of ATP production (mitochondria) to the site of ATP breakdown (myofibrils). This role of creatine was suggested as a potential mechanism for improved performance in endurance activities, but these types of activities are not affected by creatine supplementation, which suggests that this mechanism may not be important.
- Creatine may have anabolic properties.

Safety

No studies have reported detrimental health effects of creatine. According to numerous anecdotal reports, however, creatine supplementation causes ailments; GI, cardiovascular, and muscular problems; nausea, vomiting, and diarrhea; alterations in kidney and liver function; muscle cramps; and elevated blood pressure. As pointed out in a roundtable discussion by the American College of Sports Medicine,

> the evidence is not definitive and/or it is incomplete to indict the practice of creatine supplementation as a health risk; at the same time, our lack of information cannot be taken as an assurance that creatine supplementation is free from health risks. Ignorance provides little comfort of untoward effects yet to be discovered. (Terjung et al. 2000)

Dehydroepiandrosterone

Dehydroepiandrosterone (DHEA) and its sulfated ester dehydroepiandrosterone sulfate (DHEAS) are relatively weak androgen steroid hormones synthesized primarily in early adulthood (20-25 years of age) by the adrenal cortex. DHEA is not present in large quantities in the diet, but when taken as a supplement it becomes a precursor for at least two hormones: testosterone and estradiol. Because DHEA is a precursor for testosterone, it is thought to increase testosterone concentration and thereby increase protein synthesis and muscle mass. DHEA is, therefore, one of the most popular supplements, especially in the United States. Synthetic DHEA is categorized as a nutrition supplement because the substance also occurs naturally. Because of its classification, the FDA has no control over what manufacturers say about the product. They call DHEA a superhormone that increases lean body mass, slows the aging process, boosts immune function, and protects against heart disease. Because the plasma DHEA concentration decreases with age, many studies have focused on the effects of the supplement in older people. Manufacturers abuse the results of this research and claim that restoring blood DHEA concentrations to youth levels slows the aging process. Little is known about the physiological role of DHEA or the cellular and molecular mechanisms of its action, but it is known to interact with the receptors of the neurotransmitter γ-aminobutyric acid (GABA) in the brain.

Early support for DHEA as a supplement came from animal studies in which animals were given this hormone. The test animals showed improved immune function and resistance to arteriosclerosis, cancer, viral infections, obesity, and diabetes. Some studies even reported an extended life span. Rats, however, normally have extremely low DHEA levels and may respond very differently than humans. Human studies showed a decreased risk of cardiovascular diseases in men with high DHEA levels but an increased risk in women. Subsequent studies reported minimal protective effects of DHEA in men and no effects or negative effects in women (Johannes et al. 1999). In one study, DHEA supplementation resulted in enhanced protection against cardiovascular diseases (Jakubowicz, Beer, and Rengifo 1995). In general, though, the results of various studies are not consistent, and whether DHEA really protects against cardiovascular disease is difficult to determine (Sirrs and Bebb 1999).

Studies that investigated the effects of DHEA on body composition showed a rise in blood androgen levels after supplementation (100-1,600 mg of DHEA per day), but no effects on body weight or lean body mass were observed. In addition, Welle, Jozefowicz, and Statt (1990) did not observe effects on energy or protein metabolism. Nestler et al. (1988) reported a small decrease in fat mass without a change in total body mass, which suggests that DHEA resulted in an increase in lean body mass. In a study by Mortola and Yen (1990), 100 mg of DHEA per day for 3 months resulted in a 1% increase in lean body mass. In that study, fat mass decreased in men but increased in women. A study of obese subjects who received 1,600 mg of DHEA per day for 28 days did not report any changes in body composition. These results, although varied and not convincing, seem to indicate that DHEA has a small effect on muscle mass and immune function. Most of these studies were performed in 40- to 75-year-old subjects, and little is known about the effects in young adults.

Because so little is known about the possible side effects of DHEA, various researchers and institutions have expressed concerns. DHEA is an uncontrolled substance and is readily available in pharmacies, in drugstores, and over the Internet. Clinicians fear that elevated plasma DHEA through supplementation might stimulate dormant prostate tumors or cause hypertrophy of the prostate gland itself. Ethical questions also arise about the use of hormones as ergogenic substances. Both the IOC and the U.S. Olympic Committee have placed DHEA on the list of banned substances with zero tolerance. In March 2007, a bill introduced in the U.S. Senate attempted to classify DHEA as a controlled substance under the category of anabolic steroids.

Fish Oil and Omega-3 Fatty Acids

Fish oil is a natural source of long-chain omega-3 FAs, including DHA and EPA. An omega-3 fatty acid is a polyunsaturated FA (PUFA), meaning it contains two or more double bonds with one of the double bonds at the third carbon from the methyl end (see chapter 7). PUFAs are considered essential nutrients because the human body cannot manufacture them in appreciable amounts. The essential fatty acid α-linolenic acid (ALA) can be converted to EPA and DHA within the body, but only in small amounts. Omega-3 fats have been the focus of a great deal of exercise and cognitive performance research since they are known to be incorporated into the membranes of cells, improve muscle protein synthesis, decrease inflammation, and improve cognitive function, which all have performance and health implications for athletes. Studies have either provided omega-3 fatty acids as fish oil or as purified isolated extracts of EPA and DHA.

Guezennec et al. (1989) suggested that increasing the fraction of PUFAs in the phospholipids of erythrocyte (red blood cell) membranes improves membrane fluidity and increases red blood cell deformability (flexibility), which results in improved peripheral oxygen supply. They conducted a study in which 14 male subjects were divided into two groups; for 6 weeks, one group received a normal diet and the other received a diet rich in fish oil. The fraction of omega-3 FAs increased in erythrocyte membranes, but no change in red blood cell deformability was seen under resting conditions. During hypobaric exercise, red blood cell deformability decreased less with consumption of fish oil.

Brilla and Landerholm (1990) studied the effects of fish oil intake and exercise training in 32 sedentary men and found that exercise training resulted in an increased $\dot{V}O_2max$, whereas fish oil supplementation had no effect. Oostenbrug et al. (1997) supplemented trained cyclists for 3 weeks with placebo or fish oil (6 g/day). Fish oil did not alter red blood cell characteristics in this study and had no effect on $\dot{V}O_2$max, maximal power output, or time-trial performance.

Physical training improves red blood cell deformability and changes the FA composition of membranes toward a higher percentage of unsaturated FAs, so the enhanced fluidity under resting conditions could be masked by physical training (Kamada et al. 1993). The enhanced membrane fluidity may be especially important when the uptake of oxygen becomes limiting, such as during exercise under hypoxic conditions. The physiologic consequences of PUFAs derived from fish oils are still hypothetical, however, and further studies are necessary to evaluate the possible effects on hemorheological changes during exercise.

To date, most studies examining the effects of omega-3 fatty acids on muscle protein synthesis have been conducted in older populations (>60 years of age) or animals. In one study, omega-3 fatty acid intake appeared to result in greater activation of the protein complex known as the molecular/mammalian target of rapamycin complex 1 (mTORC1) during periods of high insulin and amino acid infusions in elderly adults (Smith et al. 2011a). mTORC1 activity is necessary for resistance exercise, increased amino acid availability, and leucine to increase muscle protein synthesis. It is also required for muscle regeneration after injury (Baar and Heaton 2015). In a follow-up study, Smith et al. (2011b) found that the anabolic response to insulin and amino acid infusion was greater after daily supplementation with 4 g of long chain omega-3s (including 1.86 g EPA and 1.50 g DHA) for 8 weeks. These findings suggest that when insulin and amino acid levels are high, such as following a large carbohydrate and protein-containing meal, adequate amounts of omega-3 fatty acids may improve muscle protein synthesis through the activation of mTORC1. Further research is needed to determine whether these findings extend to elite athletes.

Several forms of exercise (e.g., resistance training and games such as soccer, rugby, and American football) result in significant amounts of damage to muscle, and this damage accumulates as the season progresses. One of the natural responses to damage is inflammation within the muscle that promotes adaptations that strengthen the muscle and make it more resistant to injury. Although some inflammation may be essential for normal training adaptation, too much inflammation can impair or delay the muscle's ability to recover postexercise. Omega-3 FAs are known to have anti-inflammatory properties. DHA and EPA decrease the expression of inflammatory cytokines by leukocytes and also give rise to a family of anti-inflammatory mediators called resolvins (Calder 2006). DHA also alters the activity of phagocytic cells such as neutrophils and macrophages (see chapter 13 for further details about these immune cells), which are the initiators of inflammation following exercise-induced muscle damage (Peake et al. 2017).

Several studies have shown that ingestion of EPA and DHA can decrease DOMS following eccentric exercise. One such study (Tartibian, Maleki, and Abbasi 2009) had untrained subjects consume 1.8 g of an omega-3 supplement (0.32 g EPA and 0.22 g DHA) per day for 30 days before completing a knee extensor eccentric exercise protocol. Subjects who took the omega-3 supplement reported reductions in perceived muscle soreness and displayed improved knee range of motion 48 hours postexercise even at this low dose. A similar study using a higher daily dose of omega-3 oils (2 g EPA and 1 g DHA) also showed a decrease in DOMS 48 hours after an eccentric exercise session (Jouris, McDaniel, and Weiss 2011). Further research is required to confirm similar effects in more highly trained individuals, but there appears to be potential for omega-3 supplements to improve recovery of muscle from damaging exercise. Several studies (e.g., Fontani et al. 2005) also suggest that improvements in cognitive function, reaction time, and attention span result from supplementation with omega-3 fatty acids, and these effects could be important for many team games and racquet sports.

Dietary sources of omega-3 fatty acids for ALA include flaxseed, flaxseed oil, nuts, nut butters, algae, seeds, soybean oil, and rapeseed oil, and EPA and DHA are found in fish (e.g., cod, mackerel, salmon, tuna), fish oils, and krill oil. The U.S. Institute of Medicine recommends that men consume 1.6 g of ALA per day. Although there are currently no established recommendations for EPA and DHA intake, the ingestion of about 1 g daily of these fatty acids seems appropriate to obtain the benefits described.

One potential disadvantage of omega-3 consumption could be that the anti-inflammatory effects may add to the anti-inflammatory and immunosuppressive effects of intensive endurance training and hence worsen the infection risk for athletes, but as of yet there is no direct evidence for this. The evidence on omega-3 fatty acid supplementation for athletes is ambiguous, but it is recommended that good sources of EPA and DHA be included in the diet.

Ginseng

Ginseng, which is most commonly used in the form of *Panax ginseng* derived from the root of the Araliaceous plant family, is a popular supplement among athletes. It is commonly described as an *adaptogen*, which is a substance that helps the body adapt to stress situations. Ginseng has been used for several thousand years in Asia. Its effects are said to include improved sleep, improved memory, reduced fatigue, and relief of heart pain, headache, and nausea. The known varieties of ginseng are American, Chinese, Korean, Japanese, and Siberian, and the three main medicinal species are *Panax ginseng* (Chinese or Korean ginseng), *Panax japonicum* (Japanese ginseng from India, southern China, and Japan), and *Panax quinquefolium* (American ginseng). Siberian, or Russian, ginseng, although claimed to have a similar stimulant effect, is an entirely different plant, *Eleutherococcus senticosus*. It is used as a cheaper substitute for *Panax ginseng*.

The main active constituents of the *Panax ginseng* species are triterpenoid glycosides, or saponins (also referred to as ginsenosides or panaxosides). The structure and distribution of saponins may vary with species and variety. At least 13 different saponins exist. *Panax ginseng* is believed to be the most potent form of ginseng and has become the standard.

Animal studies support some of the claims about ginseng. Running performance in rats improved 132% after acute administration of ginseng and 179% after 7 days of administration. The ingestion of ginseng was accompanied by an increase in the basal ACTH and cortisol levels in rats. In humans, the effects are not clear, and several studies show inconsistent results. Most of the human studies did not have an appropriate design and were not placebo controlled or were not randomized. Some of these uncontrolled studies reported improvements in $\dot{V}O_2max$ and exercise performance. In one study, five subjects ingested 2 g of *Panax ginseng* per day for 4 weeks, and six subjects acted as a control group. Measurements included substrate use, plasma hormone concentrations, ratings of perceived effort, and endurance capacity. No differences were found in any of these variables between the group given ginseng and the control group. Other researchers reported similar findings (Allen et al. 1998; Engels and Wirth 1997). At present, little or no evidence in the literature supports the claim that ginseng is an ergogenic aid.

Glandulars

Glandulars are extracts from animal glands such as the adrenals, the thymus, the pituitary, and the testes. They are claimed to enhance the function of the equivalent gland in the human body. For example, orchic extract from the testes supposedly enhances testosterone levels (Williams 1993). Glandular extracts are degraded during the digestive process and are inactive when absorbed; therefore, they cannot exert a pharmacological effect.

Glycerol

Glycerol is a three-carbon molecule that normally serves as the backbone of a triacylglycerol molecule. We ingest a fairly large amount of glycerol as part of triacylglycerol on a daily basis. Glycerol is also released into the bloodstream after lipolysis. Thus, during exercise, when lipolysis is stimulated, plasma glycerol concentrations become elevated.

Fuel Source

Studies have investigated the efficacy of glycerol as a fuel, but they found the contribution of glycerol to the overall energy expenditure to be relatively small. Glycerol cannot be directly oxidized in large amounts in the muscle; therefore, it must be converted into a glucose molecule in gluconeogenesis in the liver before being used as a fuel. This process is relatively slow, so the contribution of glycerol to fuel supply during exercise is negligible.

Hyperhydrating Agent

When ingested with a relatively large volume of water (1 to 2 L [0.3-0.5 gal]), glycerol improves water absorption (Wapnir, Sia, and Fisher 1996) and increases water retention in the extracellular space, especially in plasma (Gleeson, Maughan, and Greenhaff 1986; Koenigsberg et al. 1995). This action can occur through either of two mechanisms: (1) Glycerol may move to the extracellular space and, through osmosis, draw water into this compartment (in other words, glycerol acts like a sponge); or (2) a small increase in the plasma osmolarity may increase ADH secretion from the posterior pituitary gland, thus decreasing urine production. Hyperhydration with glycerol before exercise decreases overall heat stress during exercise as indicated by a lower heart rate and body temperature (Lyons et al. 1990). The recommended protocol for the intake of glycerol and water before exercise is given in table 11.5.

TABLE 11.5 Recommended Protocol for Glycerol and Water Intake to Optimize Preexercise Hydration

Timing of ingestion	Dosage
150 min preexercise	5 ml/kg (0.2 fl oz/kg) glycerol in a 20% solution
120 min preexercise	5 ml/kg water
105 min preexercise	5 ml/kg water
90 min preexercise	5 ml/kg glycerol in a 20% solution + 5 ml/kg water
60 min preexercise	5 ml/kg water
0 min	Start exercise

Stated doses are in milliliters per kilogram of body weight.

Although these studies look promising, several other studies found no effect of glycerol on thermoregulation (Inder et al. 1998; Latzka et al. 1997, 1998). In these studies, the volume of water consumed (500 ml [17 fl oz]) may have been too small. In a study by Murray et al. (1991), no indications of hyperhydration were found. Generally, however, the ingestion of 1 g of glycerol per kilogram of body weight with 1 to 2 L of water seems to protect against heat stress and thus may have some health benefits for those who exercise in extreme conditions. Some studies showed that reduced cardiovascular stress and decreased body temperature resulted in improved exercise performance. This finding could not be confirmed, even though those studies reported indications of improved thermoregulation. Whether glycerol improves endurance performance remains unclear. Glycerol has significant side effects, including nausea, heartburn, blurred vision, headaches, GI problems, dizziness, and light-headedness. Also, the large volume of fluid that needs to be consumed with the glycerol causes many users to feel bloated. Glycerol was prohibited as an ergogenic aid by the World Anti-Doping Agency (WADA) in 2010 due to its plasma expansion properties and consequent potential use as a masking agent. However, in 2018, glycerol was removed from the WADA prohibited list as research since 2012 indicated that these effects were minimal.

Green Tea

Green tea is made from the leaves of the *Camellia sinensis* plant, which is rich in polyphenol catechins and caffeine. There is increasing interest in the potential role of green tea extract (GTE) in oxidative stress and fat metabolism and its influence on health and exercise performance. Several studies report that GTE increases fat oxidation at rest and during exercise while attenuating levels of oxidative stress markers after exercise (Hodgson, Randell, and Jeukendrup 2013). Overall, however, the literature on GTE and exercise performance and recovery from damaging exercise is inconclusive. The fact that not all studies observed effects may be related to differences in study designs, GTE bioavailability, and variation of the measurement (fat oxidation). In addition, the precise mechanisms of GTE in the human body that increase fat oxidation are unclear. The often-cited in vitro catechol-O-methyltransferase mechanism is used to explain the changes in substrate metabolism with little in vivo evidence to support it. Also, changes in expression of fat metabolism genes with longer term GTE intake have been implicated at rest and with exercise training, including the upregulation of fat metabolism enzyme gene expression in the skeletal muscle and downregulation of adipogenic genes in the liver. The exact molecular signaling that activates changes to fat metabolism gene expression is unclear but may be driven by PPAR gamma coactivator 1α and PPARs. To date, however, evidence from human studies to support these adaptations is lacking. Clearly, more studies must be performed to elucidate the effects of GTE on fat metabolism as well as to improve our understanding of the underlying mechanisms. A couple of studies have provided some evidence of the ergogenic potential of GTE and have shown that its antioxidant effects do not impair exercise training adaptations in recreationally active subjects (Roberts et al. 2015) and male sprinters (Jówko et al. 2015).

Inosine

Inosine is a nucleoside, a purine base comparable to adenine, which is one of the structural components of ATP. Inosine is obtained through the diet or synthesized endogenously in the body. Manufacturers claim that inosine increases ATP stores, thereby improving muscle strength, training quality, and performance. In addition, inosine is thought to improve oxygen delivery to the cells and to improve endurance. The latter belief is based on the role that inosine plays in the formation of 2,3-diphosphoglycerate, a substance in erythrocytes that facilitates the release of oxygen to the tissues. Other suggested mechanisms for ergogenic effects of inosine include augmenting cardiac contractility, vasodilating activity, and stimulation of insulin release, increasing glucose delivery to the myocardium. The studies that have investigated the effects of inosine on strength and endurance performance do not provide support for the claims and theories.

In one carefully conducted study, trained men ($n = 4$) and women ($n = 5$) were administered 6 g of inosine or placebo per day for 2 days (Williams et al. 1990). No change occurred in 5 km (3 mi) treadmill run time, $\dot{V}O_2max$, or perceived exertion, and blood lactate levels were also similar. After a 30-minute break, subjects performed another run in which speed was kept constant but the gradient gradually increased. Time to fatigue in this run decreased with inosine (i.e., it had an **ergolytic** effect).

Another study investigated the effects of 5 g of inosine or placebo per day for 5 days (Starling et al. 1996). No effects were found on performance in a 30-second Wingate test or a 30-minute self-paced time trial. In addition, a supramaximal constant-load sprint test was performed, and fatigue occurred 10% earlier with inosine compared with placebo, again indicating that inosine can be detrimental to performance. No effects were observed in heart rate or ratings of perceived exertion.

A study investigated the effects of 10 g of inosine supplementation per day over periods of 5 days and 10 days (McNaughton, Dalton, and Tarr 1999). Seven trained volunteers performed tests—a 5 × 6-second sprint, a 30-second sprint, and a 20-minute time trial. Inosine supplementation did not affect performance. In addition, no changes in erythrocyte 2,3-DPG concentrations were observed.

Inosine has adverse effects in that it increases serum uric acid levels. The levels observed by Starling et al. (1996) are often associated with gouty arthritis, particularly pain in the knee and foot joints. Because inosine has no ergogenic effects, supplements should be avoided.

Ketone Salts

Ketone salts are among the most recent popular supplements, and ketone esters are talked about a lot in the media. The ketone bodies ß-hydroxybutyrate and acetoacetate are produced in the body as by-products of fat metabolism. Essentially, ketone bodies are formed in the body when there is an excess of FAs available, such as during periods of starvation. During prolonged starvation, ketone bodies become a fuel for the brain. This is believed to be their most important function. Ketone bodies are also a readily used substrate for oxidation in the muscle. Dietary strategies to increase blood concentrations of ketone bodies require a high-fat, extremely low carbohydrate diet (ketogenic diet) for at least 3 to 4 days. Reducing carbohydrate availability may impair performance, because carbohydrate forms a key fuel source for intense exercise; therefore, adding ketone bodies to carbohydrate has been suggested as a strategy to add a substrate for oxidation while maintaining carbohydrate stores (Pinckaers et al. 2017). It has also been suggested that ketone bodies can help promote training adaptations, but there are no human studies to show this. Although some ketone body supplements (ketone salts and esters) may be used to rapidly increase ketone body availability without first adapting to a ketogenic diet, the extent to which ketone bodies can contribute as fuel for skeletal muscle metabolism during prolonged exercise remains unknown. At present, there are no data available to suggest that ingestion of ketone bodies during exercise improves performance when other established nutritional strategies are applied appropriately.

One of the limitations is that most products on the market contain ketone salts, and typically these deliver ketone bodies in small amounts that are unlikely to affect metabolism or performance. Ingesting larger amounts has implications for taste because large amounts of sodium or potassium are ingested at the same time, and this also affects the tolerance. Ingesting these ketone salts in large amounts will likely result in gastrointestinal problems.

Under the leadership of Professor Kieran Clarke at the University of Oxford, a ketone ester was developed that seemed to prevent some of these issues (a ketone ester will deliver less salt for the same amount of energy). However, so far this has mostly been used in animal studies and very little information on performance is available. This ketone ester is prohibitively expensive, still has a poor taste profile, and may still cause gastrointestinal problems. Time will tell whether ketone esters can become a practical solution to fueling for endurance athletes.

Lactate Salts and Polylactate

Lactate is a good fuel for the human heart, and in several studies the rate of lactate clearance and oxidation exceeded the rates achieved by glucose. Most of the lactate that appears in the blood during moderate-intensity exercise is oxidized by the active muscle fibers with a high oxidative capacity. The lactate molecule possibly serves as a shuttle for transport of glucose-derived carbon moieties between various organs and cells (e.g., from the exercising muscle to the heart, from type II fibers in an active muscle to the neighboring type I fibers in the same muscle or to the type I fibers of another active muscle) (Brooks 1986). Lactate ingestion during exercise may provide a good fuel for the muscle.

Lactate Salts

Lactate can be provided as sodium or potassium lactate. A solution containing these salts, however, has extremely high osmolarity when significant amounts of lactate must be ingested. The amounts of sodium or potassium that would also have to be ingested are large and are likely to produce severe GI problems. Solutions of lactate salts can be taken in maximal bolus amounts of about 10 g without causing GI problems. The performance effects of these amounts have not been investigated but are expected to be nonexistent given the amount of endogenous lactate formed.

Polylactate

The problem of too much lactate salt could theoretically be solved by using polylactate, a lactate polymer:

CH_3-CH(OH)-COOH CH_3-CH(OH)-COO^- CH_3-CH(OH)-CO[O-CH(CH_3)-CO]n-OCH(CH_3)-COOH (polylactate)

This would reduce the osmolarity yet provide relatively large amounts of lactate.

Polylactate is used as a supplement and is included in some sports drinks. It can be produced through controlled chemical synthesis. If polylactate dissolved in water and could be quickly hydrolyzed in the GI tract of humans, similarly to glucose polymers, it could be the ideal chemical form to ingest carbohydrate. But polylactate does not normally occur in food products and does not dissolve well in water. The human body does not contain enzymes to degrade polylactate. Thus, the bioavailablity and intestinal absorption are extremely low or even zero (Wagenmakers 1999b). Because of its slow biodegradability, polylactate is used by orthopedic and dental surgeons to replace steel plates in the repair of broken bones. Polylactate, in the true chemical sense, cannot function to generate lactate at a high rate and cannot function as a nutritional ergogenic aid during exercise.

Nevertheless, two studies (Fahey et al. 1991; Swensen et al. 1994) claim to have investigated the performance effects of polylactate. A careful reading of the published papers reveals that the authors appear to have investigated the effects of a commercial product called Poly-L-lactate. This supplement contains molecules of lactate bound to amino acids. Because of the much larger molecular mass of the amino acids, the lactate content of this supplement is relatively low (< 50% lactate). One of the amino acids is arginine, which is known to cause GI problems when ingested in large amounts. Swensen et al. (1994) indeed observed severe GI distress (abdominal cramping, diarrhea, and in some cases vomiting) when Poly-L-lactate was administered in concentrations of 5% (w/v) (~2.5% w/v lactate). To prevent gastric distress, Swensen et al. (1994) added only 0.75% Poly-L-lactate to a 6.25% glucose polymer solution and compared that with a 7% glucose polymer solution. As expected, given the fact that the energy content of the drinks was almost identical, no difference occurred in time to exhaustion during exercise at 70% of $\dot{V}O_2max$. Polylactate can therefore not be considered an ergogenic aid. The main problem with lactate supplements (in all available forms) is that performance effects occur only at ingestion rates that are not tolerated by the GI tract.

Lecithin

Lecithin, or phosphatidyl choline, is a phospholipid that occurs naturally in a variety of food items, including beans, eggs, and wheat germ. It contains choline and phosphorus and is theorized to be an ergogenic aid. It is claimed to improve strength and reduce fatigue. A study investigated the effect of lecithin on 15-minute, all-out cycling performance after a 105-minute ride at 70% of $\dot{V}O_2max$ (Burns et al. 1988). No effects of two dosages of lecithin that contained 1.1 g and 1.8 g of choline were observed. The only observed change was a rise in plasma choline concentration. Lecithin, therefore, does not appear to be an ergogenic aid. (See also the sections on choline and phosphorus.)

Medium-Chain Triacylglycerol

MCT is sold as a supplement to replace normal fat because MCT is said not to be stored in the body and is suggested to help athletes to lose body fat. For a while, this was a popular supplement among bodybuilders. It was also used as an extra energy source in various energy bars. MCT is normally present in our diet in small quantities, and a few natural sources are available. MCT is usually synthesized from coconut oil. After hydrolysis of the oil, the medium-chain and long-chain FAs are separated, and the fraction of MCFAs is subsequently esterified to form an MCT. MCFAs are used in enteral and parenteral nutrition to provide patients with a rapidly available energy source. Because of this clinical use, a possible role for MCFAs in sport nutrition became the subject of investigation.

MCFAs contain 8 to 10 carbons, whereas LCFAs contain 12 or more carbons. Unlike most LCTs, MCTs are liquid at room temperature partly because of the small molecular size of MCTs. MCTs are more polar and therefore more soluble in water. Greater water solubility and smaller molecular size have consequences at all levels of metabolism. MCTs are more rapidly digested and absorbed in the intestine than LCTs are. Furthermore, MCFAs follow the portal venous system and enter the liver directly, whereas LCFAs pass into the lacteals and follow the slow lymphatic system (Bach and Babayan 1982; Isselbacher 1968).

MCT may therefore be a valuable exogenous energy source during exercise in addition to carbohydrates (Jeukendrup et al. 1995). In addition, MCT ingestion may improve exercise performance by elevating plasma FA levels and sparing muscle glycogen (Van Zeyl et al. 1996) because it increases the availability of plasma FAs, reduces the rate of muscle glycogen breakdown, and delays the onset of exhaustion.

In one study, MCT added to carbohydrate drinks did not inhibit gastric emptying (Beckers et al. 1992). In fact, the drinks with MCT emptied faster from the stomach than isoenergetic carbohydrate drinks. In a subsequent study, the oxidation rates of orally ingested MCT were investigated (Jeukendrup et al. 1995). In a randomized crossover design, eight well-trained athletes cycled 180 minutes at 57% of $\dot{V}O_2max$. Subjects ingested carbohydrate, carbohydrate plus MCT, or MCT. During the 60- to 120-minute period, the amount of MCT oxidized was 72% of the amount ingested with carbohydrate plus MCT, whereas during the MCT trial, only 33% was oxidized. It was concluded that more MCT is oxidized when ingested in combination with carbohydrate. Data confirmed that oral MCT might serve as an energy source in addition to glucose during exercise. The metabolic availability of MCT was high during the last hour of exercise, and oxidation was as high as 70% of the ingestion rate. The maximal amount of oral MCT tolerated in the GI tract is about 30 g, and this small amount limited the contribution of oral MCT to between 3% and 7% of total energy expenditure (see figure 11.14).

Horowitz et al. (2000) argued that MCT ingestion might be particularly effective in reducing muscle glycogen breakdown in conditions where FA availability may be limiting fat oxidation, such as during high-intensity exercise. During exercise at 85% of $\dot{V}O_2max$, plasma FAs are reduced to

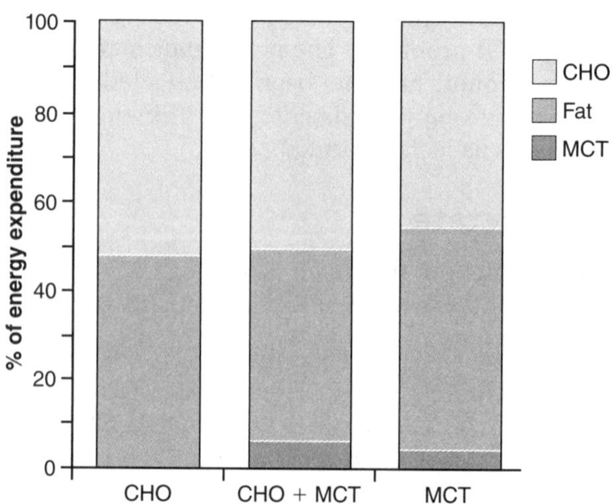

Figure 11.14 Small contribution of MCT to total energy expenditure.

extremely low levels, which reduces fat oxidation (Romijn et al. 1995). Therefore, Horowitz et al. (2000) fed their subjects 25 g of MCT 1 hour before 30 minutes of exercise at 84% $\dot{V}O_2$max. Plasma ß-hydroxybutyrate levels were elevated after MCT ingestion, but plasma FA concentrations remained low during exercise. Thus, the MCT feedings did not affect glycogen breakdown. Van Zeyl et al. (1996) reported a reduction in the rate of muscle glycogen oxidation when a larger amount of MCT was ingested (86 g in 2 hours). They also claimed that MCT added to a 10% (w/v) carbohydrate solution improved time-trial performance in trained cyclists compared with a 10% carbohydrate solution alone. The authors did not report GI disturbances. The same research group repeated the study with a low dose and a high dose of MCT (27 g and 54 g, respectively, in 2 hours) (Goedecke et al. 1999) but could not reproduce the previous findings. In fact, although MCT ingestion did not affect GI symptoms in this study and plasma FA and ß-hydroxybutyrate levels were elevated, fuel oxidation and exercise performance were unchanged. When a large amount of MCT was ingested in a study by Jeukendrup et al. (1998) (86 g in 2 hours), subjects experienced GI problems, and their performance did not improve. In fact, MCT ingestion caused deterioration in performance compared with the placebo (water) treatment. Angus et al. (2000) studied the effects of carbohydrate plus MCT ingestion on 100 km (62 mi) cycling time-trial performance. Subjects ingested 42 g of MCT per hour in combination with carbohydrate during their time trials, but performance was not affected. MCT ingestion can increase the concentrations of ketone bodies in the blood and could therefore be an alternative to ketone salts or ketone esters (although the evidence does not currently support the use of either ketone salts or MCT).

In conclusion, MCT is rapidly emptied from the stomach, absorbed, and oxidized, and the oxidation of exogenous MCT is enhanced when coingested with carbohydrate. Ingestion of 30 g MCT does not affect muscle glycogen breakdown, and the contribution of MCT to energy expenditure is small. Ingestion of larger amounts of MCT results in GI distress. Therefore, MCT does not appear to have the positive effects on performance that are often claimed.

Pangamic Acid

Pangamic acid, often referred to as vitamin B_{15}, has many unfounded claims. Most of these claims are based on anecdotal reports of athletes (or manufacturers), and they include increased maximal oxygen uptake, reduced lactate formation, and improved performance. Two studies have found no effect of pangamic acid on lactate concentration in the blood or on performance (Girandola, Wiswell, and Bulbulian 1980; Gray and Titlow 1982). Pangamic acid is not a vitamin, it is not essential, and it has no known function in the human body. Synthetic pangamic acid has been shown to be harmful (Herbert 1979), and FDA guidelines forbid the sale of pangamic acid as a dietary supplement or as a drug.

Phosphatidylserine

The supplement phosphatidylserine is usually a natural, soy-derived glycerophospholipid. It is a typical structural component of cell membranes, and it has been hypothesized to alter the cell membrane phospholipid composition and hence the properties of the membrane. Theoretically, when phosphatidylserine is incorporated in cell membranes, it can alter the number and the affinity of various receptors. Phosphatidylserine has been suggested to alter the neuroendocrine response to stress (including exercise stress).

In one study, subjects received 800 mg/day of phosphatidylserine for 10 days (Monteleone et al. 1992). The stress response (as measured by plasma ACTH and cortisol concentration) after three 6-minute intervals of strenuous exercise was smaller than with placebo. These results agreed with earlier observations by the same researchers that phosphatidylserine injection reduced hypothalamic–pituitary–adrenal axis activation in humans (Monteleone et al. 1990). Phosphatidylserine potentially affects cognitive functioning. It reversed a memory decline that occurred in 25- to 65-year-old healthy humans (Crook et al. 1991). The authors of the study argued that phosphatidylserine is rapidly absorbed by the gut into the bloodstream and transported across the blood–brain barrier. It may also be rapidly incorporated into membranes of the central nervous system, which have naturally high phosphatidylserine content. This action could help to activate and regulate proteins involved in generation, storage, and reception of nerve impulses. Before definite conclusions can be drawn, however, more studies are needed.

Phosphatidylserine supplements that are for sale are derived from soybeans, whereas the phosphatidylserine in the previously mentioned studies was bovine derived (cerebral cortex). The possibility cannot be excluded that soy-derived phosphatidylserine has no effects or different effects than those reported in the studies. Also, whether the observed decreases in serum ACTH and cortisol concentrations are a desirable effect is not clear. Although cortisol is generally known as a catabolic hormone and decreasing cortisol is hypothesized to decrease catabolism, no evidence supports this conclusion.

Phosphorus and Phosphate Salts

The body contains about 850 g of phosphorus (phosphate salts), 80% of which is found in bone. Besides having a structural function in bone and teeth, phosphorus is a component of nucleic acids and cell membranes. Phosphorus is a component of the high-energy phosphates (ATP and PCr) and thus plays an important role in energy metabolism. It is also a cofactor or component for many B vitamins and 2,3-DPG in erythrocytes. Phosphate salts also serve as an important intracellular buffer.

Phosphorus is an essential nutrient. The RDA for men and women 11 to 24 years of age is 1,200 mg. Persons older than 25 years have lower requirements (800 mg). Diets usually contain sufficient phosphorus because it is present in relatively large quantities in many foods.

Ingestion of larger amounts of phosphorus, or phosphate loading, has been suggested to result in improved performance. The proposed mechanisms include increased ATP synthesis (Chasiotis 1983) and improved oxygen extraction in muscle cells because of elevations of 2,3-DPG in erythrocytes. For these purposes, phosphate salts are usually ingested in relatively large quantities of 4 g/day. One study observed an increased $\dot{V}O_2max$ and decreased lactate concentration at submaximal workload when eight cyclists ingested 4 g of sodium phosphate per day for 3 days (Cade et al. 1984). The study did not have a crossover design, but the control group, who received a placebo, did not show improvements. Three other studies reported similar findings after subjects ingested 3.6 to 4 g of sodium phosphate or tribasic sodium phosphate (Kreider et al. 1992, 1990; Stewart et al. 1990). In addition, improvements in 8 km (5 mi) run and 40 km (25 mi) time-trial performance were reported. Other studies did not find differences in $\dot{V}O_2max$, performance, or lactate concentrations (Bredle et al. 1988; Duffy and Conlee 1986; Galloway et al. 1996; Mannix et al. 1990).

The inconsistencies in these findings may be related to the differences in the experimental protocols (the amount of phosphate ingested, the timing of the ingestion, the type of subjects, the exercise mode, and so on). In addition, most of these studies used small numbers of subjects, which can make relatively small changes in exercise performance difficult to detect. At present, little scientific evidence indicates that phosphate loading improves exercise performance, and more studies are needed before we can confidently recommend phosphate as an ergogenic aid (Tremblay, Galloway, and Sexsmith 1994).

Polyphenols

Polyphenols are compounds found in many plants, including edible fruits and vegetables, as well as other plant-derived products, including chocolate, fruit juices, wines, and teas. There are thousands of different plant polyphenols, and the type and quantity present differ substantially between different fruits, vegetables, leaves, and seeds. Based on their chemical structure, polyphenols can be grouped into at least 10 classes, but the four major classes are the phenolic acids, flavonoids, stilbenes, and lignans. Individual polyphenols are generally not found in abundant amounts in normal foods, so their intake from the diet is generally low. There also issues with bioavailability. This has led to the popularity of isolated polyphenols as dietary supplements, and an increasing number of supplements are available. Several polyphenols in supplement form, including curcumin, **quercetin**, **epigallocatechin gallate (EGCG)**, and **resveratrol**, have been suggested to act as antioxidants, anti-infectives, and anti-inflammatories in humans that may modify immune function (see chapter 13), promote recovery from damaging exercise, increase training adaptations (see chapter 12), and improve exercise performance with chronic use in doses of a few grams per day.

Although there is evidence that antioxidants dampen training adaptations, it is thought that polyphenols can influence other mechanisms, such as stimulating stress-related cell signaling pathways that promote mitochondrial biogenesis and improving blood flow by increasing endothelial nitric oxide synthesis, and that these effects could potentially lead to improvements in exercise performance. In addition, quercetin also acts as an adenosine receptor antagonist, so that could improve performance in a similar manner to caffeine. Potential mechanisms of polyphenol action and the evidence that they are effective in increasing endurance exercise performance, reducing oxidative stress, and improving recovery from muscle-damaging exercise have been reviewed by Myburgh (2014). The author concluded the current evidence is insufficient to make recommendations for or against the use of polyphenol supplementation (neither specific polyphenols nor specific doses) for either the recreationally active or elite athlete populations. Here we will concentrate on possible performance enhancement by polyphenols.

A meta-analysis of the overall effects of polyphenols on human exercise performance (Somerville, Bringans, and Braakhuis 2017) examined results from 14 randomized controlled trials that were either single or double blind. The polyphenol intervention was either dietary (i.e., food-based polyphenol combinations), a polyphenol mixture, or individual polyphenol supplements (quercetin, resveratrol, catechins, or anthocyanins). On average, the polyphenol intake was 0.7 g/day for an intervention period of 31 days. The pooled results demonstrated a performance improvement of 1.9% with most trials using exercise performance or capacity tests of high intensity lasting between 30 seconds and 80 minutes. Subset analysis of the seven trials that used quercetin identified a performance increase of 2.8%. If performance improvements were mostly due to improved training adaptation, one would imagine that larger gains could be obtained with longer periods of supplementation. However, of the three studies that used quercetin and reported significant performance improvements, only one used elite athletes in continuous training (MacRae and Mefferd 2006). Another used recreationally active people who were not highly trained (Davis et al. 2010), and the third used men who had been sedentary for the previous 6 months (Nieman et al. 2010). Therefore, the results should be viewed with some caution. Overall, there is insufficient evidence of performance improvements with mixed or isolated polyphenol supplements to recommend their use as an ergogenic aid.

Pyruvate and Dihydroxyacetone

Pyruvate and **dihydroxyacetone (DHA)** are three-carbon intermediates of carbohydrate metabolism. They are formed in the glycolytic pathway. Some evidence suggests that supplementation or infusion of these metabolites can influence metabolism. Pyruvate and dihydroxyacetone are claimed to increase fat oxidation during exercise. They are also claimed to increase muscle glycogen storage, improve endurance capacity, and alter body composition (decrease fat mass).

Suggestions from the literature regarding the efficacy of pyruvate are based on long-term supplementation of pyruvate (7 days or more). Although only one study investigated the acute effects of pyruvate and lactate infusion, the results suggest a negative effect on running performance in rats compared with saline or glucose infusion (Bagby et al. 1978). Pyruvate infusion seemed to accelerate carbohydrate metabolism and increase muscle and liver glycogen breakdown.

When pyruvate was given as a supplement to human subjects for 7 days, improved endurance capacity was observed in two studies from the same research group (Stanko, Robertson, Galbreath, et al. 1990; Stanko, Robertson, Spina, et al. 1990). In the first study, subjects received 100 g/day of a mixture of dihydroxyacetone and pyruvate (3:1) or placebo (maltodextrins) for 7 days and performed arm ergometry to exhaustion before and after the supplementation period (Stanko, Robertson, Galbreath, et al. 1990). Muscle biopsies taken from the triceps showed that muscle glycogen concentrations at rest were significantly elevated by the dihydroxyacetone–pyruvate supplementation (88 versus 130 mmol/kg w.w.). Endurance times increased from 133 minutes after the control diet to 160 minutes after dihydroxyacetone–pyruvate supplementation. In the second study, subjects consumed a high-carbohydrate diet for 7 days or a high-carbohydrate diet supplemented with 75 g of dihydroxyacetone and 25 g of pyruvate (Stanko, Robertson, Spina, et al. 1990). Subjects performed cycling exercise to exhaustion at 70% of $\dot{V}O_2$max. Again, the supplement increased endurance time (79 minutes versus 66 minutes).

Morrison, Spriet, and Dyck (2000) administered a much smaller dose of pyruvate (7 g/day for 7 days) or placebo to seven trained cyclists in a randomized crossover trial. Subjects cycled to exhaustion at 74% to 80% of $\dot{V}O_2$max. Time to exhaustion did not increase with pyruvate, and with this smaller dose, no changes in blood pyruvate concentration were found.

No explanation is apparent for the improved endurance times reported by Stanko and colleagues (Stanko, Robertson, Galbreath, et al. 1990). They measured fractional extraction of glucose across one leg at rest and during exercise and found that glucose uptake increased after dihydroxyacetone–pyruvate supplementation. They also observed that carbohydrate oxidation was unaffected, which suggests that subjects used less muscle glycogen when supplemented with dihydroxyacetone–

pyruvate. In the first study, muscle glycogen was not measured, so this question could not be answered. In the second study, muscle biopsies were taken from the vastus lateralis, but no differences were found between the control diet and the dihydroxyacetone–pyruvate supplemented diet. Inconsistencies between the studies by Stanko, Robertson, Galbreath, et al. (1990) and Morrison, Spriet, and Dyck (2000) may be related to the different dosages of pyruvate, the different training statuses of the subjects, or the coingestion of dihydroxyacetone in the studies. More studies are needed before definitive conclusions can be drawn about the ergogenic effect of pyruvate.

Sodium Bicarbonate

When maximal exercise is performed for more than 30 seconds, most of the energy is derived from anaerobic glycolysis (see chapter 3). Lactic acid is formed at high rates, and the increased acidity of the muscle is an important limiting factor for performance in events lasting 1 to 10 minutes. Reducing the muscle acidity and increasing the buffering capacity are theoretical ways of improving performance in such events, and bicarbonate ingestion has been proposed as one of the ways to achieve these effects. A group of substances with this buffering function is the **alkalinizers** (e.g., sodium bicarbonate, sodium citrate). This section summarizes only the research findings on bicarbonate, but a number of detailed reviews have been published the past few years that are well worth studying (Horswill 1995; Linderman and Gosselink 1994).

Anaerobic Glycolysis

Events of 60 seconds to 10 minutes (e.g., 400 m, 800 m, and 1,500 m running; track cycling events; speed skating) rely heavily on anaerobic glycolysis for ATP regeneration. In this process, lactic acid is produced, which results in decreased pH in the muscle cell. This increased acidity interferes with the contraction process and causes fatigue. From the moment this high-intensity exercise starts, lactic acid (hydrogen ions and lactate) builds up in the muscle and is transported into the blood. The decrease in muscle pH is, with some delay, reflected by the blood pH.

The pH of blood is normally 7.4 and may decrease to 7.1 or slightly lower after high-intensity exercise. The pH of muscle is normally around 7.0 and may decrease to about 6.5. The body has several systems to adjust and regulate the acid–base balance. Chemical buffers provide an effective and rapid way of normalizing the H^+ concentration. Other systems include excretion of carbon dioxide by pulmonary ventilation and H^+ excretion by the kidneys.

The primary buffers in the muscle are phosphates and tissue proteins. The most important buffers in the blood are proteins, hemoglobin, and bicarbonate. During intense exercise, the intracellular buffers are insufficient to buffer all the hydrogen ions formed. The efflux of H^+ into the circulation increases, and bicarbonate has a role in buffering them:

$$H^+ + HCO_3^- \rightarrow H_2CO_3 \rightarrow H_2O + CO_2$$

The mechanism by which bicarbonate supposedly exerts its action is through this buffering of H^+ in the blood (not in the muscle as is often claimed). The buffering of H+ in the blood, however, increases the H^+ gradient and increases efflux of H^+ from the muscle. Numerous studies on the effects of bicarbonate ingestion and exercise performance have yielded equivocal results.

Various studies suggest that a minimal dose of bicarbonate ingestion is needed to improve performance. Meta-analyses from the available literature suggest a dose–response relationship between the amount of bicarbonate ingested and the observed performance effect (Horswill 1995; Matson and Vu Tran 1993) (see figure 11.15). A dose of 200 mg per kilogram of body weight ingested 1 to 2 hours before exercise seems to improve performance in most studies (Sale and Harris 2014), whereas 300 mg per kilogram of body weight seems to be the

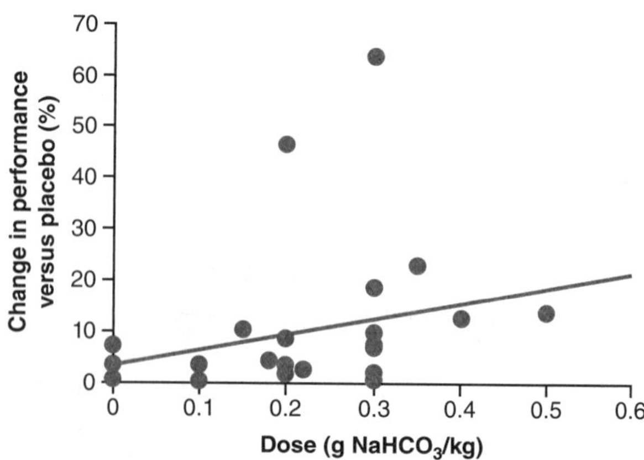

Figure 11.15 Effect of different dosages on exercise performance.

International Journal of Sports Nutrition: From C.A. Horswill, "Effects of Bicarbonate, Citrate, and Phosphate Loading on Performance," 1995, 5: S111-S119. Adapted by permission.

optimum dose (with tolerable side effects for most athletes). Doses of less than 100 mg per kilogram of body weight do not affect performance. This finding seems to make sense because a minimal amount of bicarbonate is needed to cause a significant increase in the buffering capacity of the blood. Intakes greater than 300 mg per kilogram of body weight tend to result in GI problems (bloating, abdominal discomfort, and diarrhea). No studies show an effect on exercise performance in high-intensity exercise that lasts less than 1 minute (Sale and Harris 2014). Exercises such as squat, bench press, and jumping are unaffected. Also, exercise of long duration is generally unaffected. Therefore, a window for efficacy of bicarbonate has been identified between approximately 1 and 7 minutes. A study by McNaughton, Dalton, and Palmer (1999), however, showed improved performance in a 1-hour time trial, and this was accompanied by higher blood pH throughout the exercise.

Side Effects

The side effects of sodium bicarbonate intake in such large doses can be severe. At doses of 300 mg per kilogram of body weight, many athletes experience diarrhea, GI discomfort, bloating, and cramps 1 hour after loading. The effects are dose dependent. The main causes of these problems are the large amount of sodium that is ingested with the bicarbonate and the reaction of bicarbonate with the hydrochloric acid in the stomach, which generates a large volume of carbon dioxide that distends the stomach wall. Drinking large amounts of water during the loading is likely to alleviate some of the problems.

Sodium Citrate

Sodium citrate works similarly to bicarbonate. It increases the buffering capacity of the extracellular space to increase the efflux of hydrogen ions from the intracellular space. Sodium citrate is effective in limiting the decrease in blood pH and improving high-intensity exercise performance of 2- to 4-minute durations (McNaughton 1990; McNaughton and Cedaro 1992). One study also showed improved performance in a 30 km (19 mi) cycling time trial (Potteiger et al. 1996). The typical doses for sodium citrate are 300 to 500 mg per kilogram of body weight. Like sodium bicarbonate, sodium citrate is likely to cause GI problems such as diarrhea, cramping, and bloating. Sodium citrate may act as a buffering agent and improve exercise performance in events up to about 10 minutes (Lancha et al. 2015; Sale and Harris 2014). It is said to improve high-intensity (~80% $\dot{V}O_2max$) endurance performance, but this claim has not been proved.

Sodium Nitrate

Sodium nitrate is a chemical source of nitrate that has been used in some experimental studies to confirm that acute preexercise nitrate ingestion can reduce the oxygen cost of exercise and improve endurance performance. However, natural sources of dietary nitrate, such as beetroot juice (discussed earlier), are preferred as ergogenic supplements for endurance athletes and game players because there is far less risk of harmful overdosing.

Vanadium

Vanadium, a trace element that is widely distributed in nature and normally present in human tissues, has insulin-like properties. Foods that contain vanadium include cereal and grain products, dietary oils, meat, fish, and poultry. In supplements, vanadium is usually ingested as vanadyl sulfate or bis(maltolato)oxovanadium (BMOV). One of the reasons to ingest vanadium in these compounds is that less-toxic effects have been shown in rats.

The insulin-like effects of vanadium compounds are well documented in vitro and in vivo (Verma, Cam, and McNeill 1998). In humans with type 2 diabetes mellitus, an increase in insulin-mediated glucose uptake (Halberstam et al. 1996), glycogen synthase activity, and glycogen synthesis has been demonstrated after vanadium administration (Cohen et al. 1995). These observations in insulin-resistant populations lead to suggestions that vanadium can help weight loss, improve insulin sensitivity, and increase muscle glycogen storage.

No studies in healthy humans without insulin resistance are available that demonstrate insulin-like effects after acute or chronic administration of vanadium compounds. In fact, one study did not show changes in insulin sensitivity measured with an oral glucose tolerance test in non-insulin-resistant subjects after acute or chronic (7 days) vanadyl sulfate administration (Jentjens and Jeukendrup 2002). The amounts required for biological effects of vanadium in humans (1 to 2 $mg \cdot kg^{-1} \cdot day^{-1}$) obviously greatly exceed the amounts that can be consumed in the diet (< 30 mg/day) (Verma, Cam, and McNeill 1998).

Neither the short- or long-term toxicities of the agents have been systematically studied in humans. Currently, no human studies are available that describe toxic effects after 2 to 10 weeks of vanadyl sulfate administration at dosages between 100 and 125 mg/day (Boden et al. 1996; Cohen et al. 1995; Halberstam et al. 1996). Some people may experience diarrhea, cramps, and nausea after intake of vanadium compounds. In rats, vanadium in excess amounts is toxic. Although some evidence indicates that vanadium can influence insulin sensitivity in patients with type 2 diabetes, such does not seem to be the case in healthy people. Thus, no evidence supports an ergogenic role of vanadium.

Wheat Germ Oil

Wheat germ oil is extracted from the embryo of wheat. It is high in linoleic acid, vitamin E, and octacosanol, a solid white alcohol that is theorized to have ergogenic effects. Wheat germ oil is advertised to increase endurance, stamina, and vigor. Several theories have been developed about the possible physiological effects of wheat germ oil, including enhanced glycogen metabolism and increased maximal oxygen uptake. Although many studies have focused on the metabolic effects of wheat germ oil, no evidence supports the contention that it is an effective ergogenic aid.

Additive Effects of Combining Different Supplements

Considering that acute preexercise ingestion of supplements such as bicarbonate, carbohydrate, caffeine, and nitrate-rich beetroot juice has been found to enhance exercise performance via different mechanisms, their combined effects on performance could potentially be additive. In other words, the preexercise ingestion of beetroot juice and caffeine, for example, could theoretically improve performance more than intake of either beetroot juice or caffeine alone. Furthermore, supplements that have been shown to be effective in improving performance by different mechanisms with chronic supplementation, such as creatine, ß-alanine, and carnitine, might also be more effective in combination than alone. This is of obvious interest to athletes. To date, there are relatively few studies on the effects of combining different dietary ergogenic aids either chronically or as acute preexercise supplements.

The combined ingestion of caffeine and carbohydrate during exercise has been shown to be more effective in improving endurance exercise performance than either caffeine or carbohydrate alone. For example, the inclusion of caffeine in a cereal bar consumed during prolonged exercise was found to enhance cycling time to exhaustion at 75% $\dot{V}O_2max$ compared with placebo or the cereal bar alone (Hogervorst et al. 2008). In another study, 10 endurance-trained cyclists performed three experimental trials consisting of 105 minute steady-state cycling at 62% $\dot{V}O_2max$ followed by a time trial that lasted approximately 45 minutes (Hulston and Jeukendrup 2008). During exercise, subjects ingested one of the following: a 6.4% glucose solution, a 6.4% glucose plus caffeine solution (5.3 mg of caffeine per kilogram of body weight), or a placebo. Performance times were 43.5 ± 0.9 minutes, 45.5 ± 1.1 minutes, and 47.4 ± 1.3 minutes for glucose plus caffeine, glucose, and placebo, respectively. Therefore, the combined ingestion of carbohydrate and caffeine enhanced time-trial performance by 4.6% ($P < 0.05$) compared with carbohydrate alone and 9% ($P < 0.05$) compared with placebo. In a study that examined simulated soccer performance, the addition of caffeine to a carbohydrate–electrolyte beverage during 90 minutes of intermittent shuttle running improved sprint and countermovement jump performance compared with the carbohydrate–electrolyte beverage alone (Gant, Ali, and Foskett 2010). In a meta-analysis of similar studies, Conger et al. (2011) concluded that combined caffeine and carbohydrate ingestion provides a significant but small effect to improve endurance performance compared with carbohydrate alone.

To date, only two studies have been published on the single and combined effects of beetroot juice and caffeine supplementation on endurance exercise performance. One study found that caffeine (3 mg per kilogram of body weight) administered in the form of a caffeinated gum increased cycling time-trial performance lasting 50 to 60 minutes by 3% to 4% in men and women, but the addition of beetroot juice (supplying 8 mmol of nitrate) supplementation did not further enhance performance (Lane et al. 2014). Another study that examined the effect of combined preexercise beetroot-caffeine ingestion prior to a time to exhaustion cycle ride at 80% $\dot{V}O_2max$ reported a likely additive effect on exercise capacity of combining these supplements compared with either supplement alone (Handzlik and Gleeson 2013).

There have been a few studies on the effects of combining creatine and ß-alanine supplementation for several weeks on subsequent performance in incremental cycling (Stout et al. 2006; Zoeller et al. 2007) and repeated 30-second sprint cycling (Okudan et al. 2015), but only the latter study reported significant performance improvements with combined ß-alanine and creatine compared with ß-alanine or creatine alone. There is certainly scope for more research to be done on the effects of combinations of established nutritional ergogenic aids on exercise performance. In theory at least, if two different ergogenic aids have different modes of action that do not interfere with each other, there is a good chance that their combined effects will be greater than with the individual supplements alone.

Contamination of Nutrition Supplements

It is now well-known that supplements can be contaminated with doping substances and their use can result in positive doping tests. The available data indicate that between 40% to 70% of athletes use supplements, and that between 10% to 15% of supplements may contain prohibited substances. These data indicate that there is a considerable risk of accidental doping through the use of supplements (Maughan et al. 2018; Outram and Stewart 2015). Although some forms of estimation can be made, it is suggested that it is currently not possible to quantify the scale of the problem.

The steroid nandrolone has been especially prominent. Some competitive athletes are afraid to take supplements because of uncertainty over which supplements are contaminated and which are clean. The IOC-accredited laboratory in Cologne, Germany, reported that various steroids—including nandrolone and testosterone, as well as their precursor compounds—were found in various dietary supplements. In fact, of the 634 supplements tested, 94 (nearly 15%) contained enough anabolics to cause a positive result on a drug test. None of these products gave any indication on the label that they contained steroid compounds. Of the supplements made in the United States, almost 20% of the 240 tested products contained **prohormones**.

The substances in the following list have been identified in supplements and are either directly banned by the IOC or cause a positive doping outcome in some people:

- Ephedrine
- Strychnine
- Androstenedione, androstenediol, DHEA (may lead to an elevated testosterone to epitestosterone ratio)
- 19-Norandrostenedione, 19-norandrostenediol, and related compounds (may lead to a positive test for metabolites of the steroid nandrolone)

Because athletes sign codes of conduct, they are responsible for what they take, including supplements. Caffeine and pseudoephedrine were on this list as well, but because they have been taken off the list of banned substances and placed on a monitoring program, they will no longer cause positive doping tests.

Unfortunately, current legislation does little to protect athletes and other consumers from insufficiently labeled, mislabeled, contaminated, or even unsafe ingredients in dietary supplements. Although regulations vary widely from country to country, food supplements are never subject to the standards of manufacture and quality control that are required of foods and drugs. In addition, legislation regarding product claims is less strict. Many manufacturers make claims that have never been proved scientifically. With clever marketing techniques and numerous retail outlets, supplement sellers make their products attractive and easy to obtain by athletes who do not know about the source or purity of the ingredients. Thus, if an athlete decides that the benefits of taking a supplement outweigh the risks, a product from a large, respectable company is probably the best choice. Reputable brands of vitamins, minerals, and other common supplements manufactured by major food and drug companies are normally manufactured to high standards and should be safe. Contamination is a problem especially in some smaller and more exotic companies. Companies that do not sell steroids and prohormones are less likely to have their products contaminated by those substances.

Given the overall possibility of supplement contamination, the risk of taking a mislabeled supplement is a threat to elite athletes who have to undergo drugs tests and a threat to the health of all consumers. Some products can be unintentionally adulterated with substances (including heavy metals, pesticides, or other unwanted substances), and others may be inadvertently contaminated with sport-prohibited substances. There are examples of cases in which supplements were purposely contaminated with doping substances. Many supplements are safe and pure, but always keep in mind that one batch of a supplement could be contaminated with a dangerous or sport-prohibited substance. This could happen when manufacturing equipment isn't cleaned to the required standards and contains remnants of ingredients from other products. This is similar to what can happen in a factory that manufactures nut products with other products such as cereals and breads. If the machines aren't cleaned correctly or if particles or dust permeate manufacturing areas, the breads or cereals can contain remnants or traces of nuts, which can be potentially dangerous to those with nut allergies.

There are a number of certificates that supplement companies can get to show that they have done everything to reduce these risks. Programs such as Informed Sport and Trusted Sport provide labels that indicate drug tests have been performed on certain batches. You can check their websites to see which batches were tested and whether a particular supplement was part of that batch. Although this may not guarantee that there is no contamination, it is probably as much a guarantee as you can get. It is highly recommended that anyone who is drug tested use products that have been batch tested.

In addition, the U.S. Anti-Doping Agency (USADA) recommends the following four steps to minimize risk for the athlete:

1. Seek advice from a health professional, dietitian, or sport nutritionist to make sure there is a clear nutritional benefit of using a supplement and that there are no food alternatives.
2. Look for third-party certification, but also recognize that certification is not a guarantee that the product is safe or free from prohibited substances. If the supplement you are thinking of using is not certified by a third-party agency, find an equivalent product that is certified or a real food alternative that you can use.
3. If this is not possible, look for specific warnings on your product by visiting the Supplement 411 High Risk List (www.usada.org/substances/supplement-411), where you must first create an account (it is free to do so) and then login to access the list. You can also check out supplements on the FDA Health Fraud page (www.fda.gov/ForConsumers/ProtectYourself/HealthFraud/default.htm).
4. Evaluate your product by looking for red flags. If you find any, it may mean the product is too risky to use. The following are examples of red flags:
    - There are substances that you know are prohibited listed on the label.
    - The product is in a bodybuilding, weight loss, preworkout or energy, or sexual enhancement category.
    - There is a health warning or a warning that the product may be banned in some sports.
    - The product claims to treat or cure a disease (e.g., the common cold, diabetes, arthritis).
    - The product claims to be all natural but to have similar effects to those of a prohibited substance (e.g., amphetamines, erythropoeitin, growth hormone, IGF-1, or testosterone or other steroids).
    - The product claims to be approved by USADA or the World Anti-Doping Agency (these organizations do not approve or endorse products).
    - The product lists a proprietary blend or contains trademarked ingredients, but you can't find good information about the ingredients.

Adapted from USDA n.d.

In the end, each athlete must do a cost–benefit analysis. On one side of the equation is the potential benefit of taking a product, which necessitates a thorough evaluation of the evidence to determine whether the benefit is real. On the other side is the risk that the supplement has a negative effect on performance and the possibility that a seemingly innocent product may result in a positive doping test and all the consequences that follow. Figure 11.16 can be used to decide whether a supplement is worth the risk.

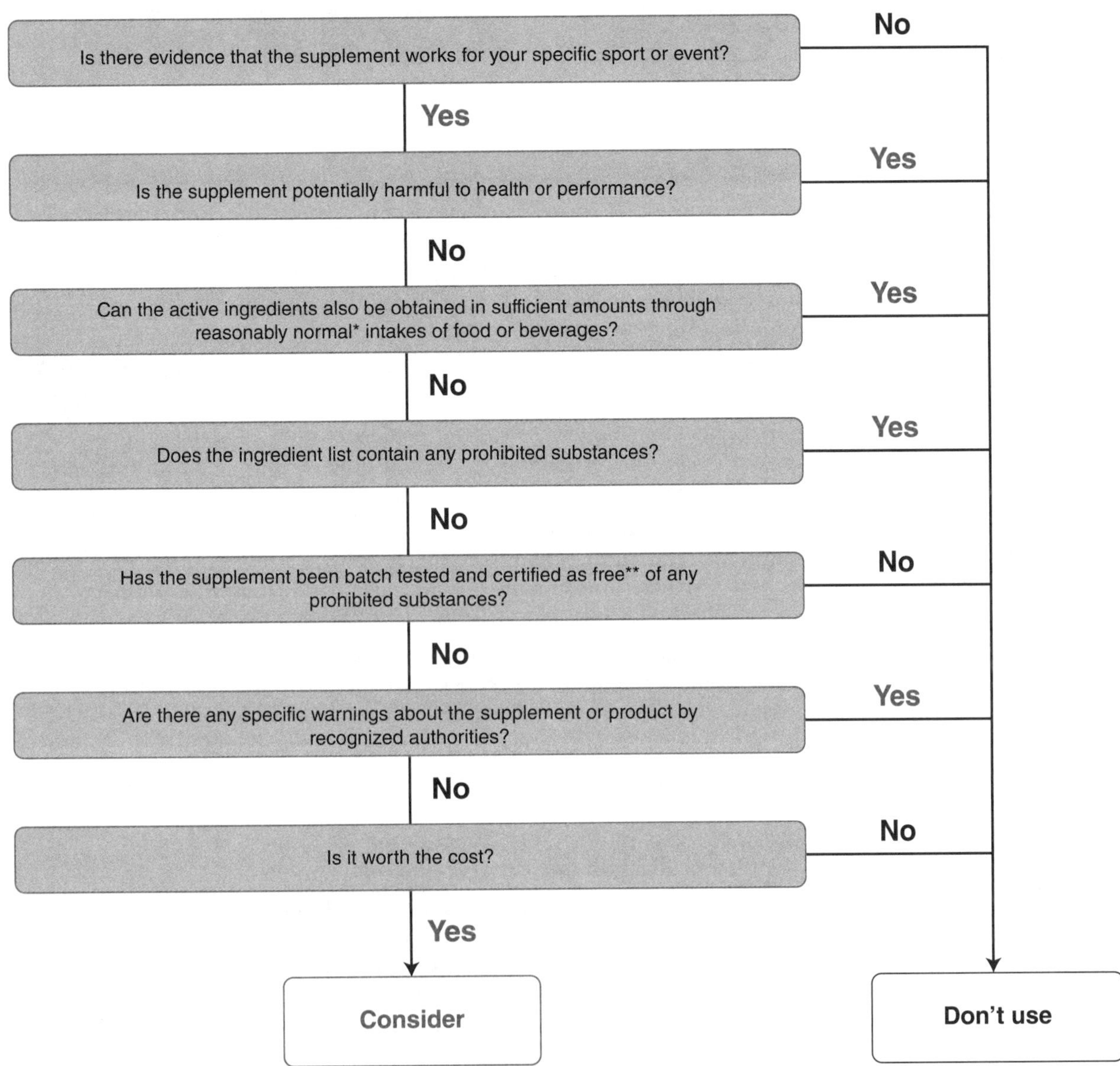

Figure 11.16 Supplement decision chart. *Some ingredients can be obtained from normal foods but normal intakes would not have performance-enhancing effects (e.g., creatine can be obtained from meat, but to obtain 20 g/day of creatine you would have to eat 10 kg [22 lb] of meat per day). **Manufacturers can batch test for several prohibited substances, including the more common banned stimulants and steroids, but no test addresses all prohibited substances; therefore, there is no guarantee that the supplement is free of all prohibited substances.

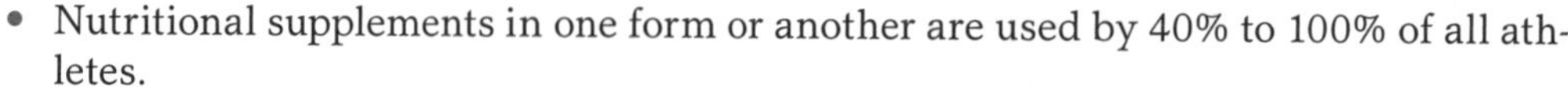

Key Points

- Nutritional supplements in one form or another are used by 40% to 100% of all athletes.
- From a regulatory point of view, dietary supplements are treated as nutritional products rather than medicine and are defined as vitamins, minerals, herbs and botanicals, amino acids, and other dietary substances intended to supplement the diet by increasing the total dietary intake, or as any concentrate, metabolite, constituent, or combination of these ingredients. No strict regulations apply to testing, advertising, and promoting nutrition supplements.
- Few nutrition supplements have proven benefits in terms of performance, recovery, or effects on body weight or body composition.
- There are some supplements for which there is good evidence of efficacy in certain conditions or situations. These supplements include caffeine, ß-alanine, creatine, sodium bicarbonate, and dietary nitrate (beetroot juice).
- Ingesting nitrate in the form of sodium nitrate ($NaNO_3$) or vegetable sources of nitrate (usually beetroot juice) containing about 6 mmol of nitrate a few hours prior to exercise improves performance in prolonged continuous or intermittent high-intensity exercise.
- For sports in which glycolysis is simulated and lactic acid production is high (e.g., middle-distance running), ß-alanine, a precursor of the intramuscular buffer carnosine, is an effective supplement. A daily dose of 3.2 to 6.4 g ß-alanine over 4 to 10 weeks results in a 60% to 80% increase in muscle carnosine content.
- Caffeine (3-9 mg per kilogram of body weight) has an ergogenic effect in endurance exercise (1-2 hours) and exercise around 100% of $\dot{V}O_2max$ that lasts approximately 1 to 5 minutes as well as effects on cognitive functioning. Caffeine also has side effects, such as GI distress, headaches, tachycardia, and restlessness.
- Oral creatine supplementation of 20 g/day for 5 days increases total muscle creatine content in men by about 20% (30% to 40% of the increase is phosphocreatine). A subsequent daily dose of 2 g is enough to maintain this concentration. This quantity allows an increase in the amount of work performed during single and repeated bouts of short-term, high-intensity exercise but may also result in some weight gain.
- A dose of 200 mg of sodium bicarbonate per kilogram of body weight ingested 1 to 2 hours before exercise seems to improve performance in most studies, but 300 mg per kilogram of body weight seems to be the optimum dose. Side effects of use include diarrhea, GI discomfort, bloating, and cramps 1 hour after loading.
- Supplements can be contaminated with doping substances and their use can result in positive doping tests. Between 40% to 100% of athletes are reported to use supplements, and between 10% to 15% of supplements may contain prohibited substances. These data indicate that there is a considerable risk of accidental doping through the use of supplements.

Recommended Readings

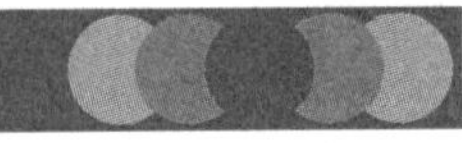

Bahrke, M.S., and C.E. Yesalis. 2002. *Performance enhancing substances in sport and exercise.* Champaign, IL: Human Kinetics.

Castell, L.M., S.J. Stear, and L.M. Burke, eds. 2015. *Nutritional supplements in sport, exercise and health: An A-Z guide.* London: Routledge.

Maughan, R.J., ed. 2014. *Sports nutrition.* Chichester: Wiley, Blackwell.

Maughan, R.J., L.M. Burke, J. Dvorak, D.E. Larson-Meyer, P. Peeling, S.M. Phillips, E.S. Rawson, N.P. Walsh, I. Garthe, H. Geyer, R. Meeusen, L.J.C. van Loon, S.M. Shirreffs, L.L. Spriet, M. Stuart, A. Vernec, K. Currell, V.M. Ali, R.G. Budgett, A. Ljungqvist, M. Mountjoy, Y.P. Pitsiladis, T. Soligard, U. Erdener, and L. Engebretsen. 2018. IOC consensus statement: Dietary supplements and the high-performance athlete. *British Journal of Sports Medicine* 52 (7): 439-455.

Peeling, P., M.J. Binnie, P.S.R. Goods, M. Sim, and L.M. Burke. 2018. Evidence-based supplements for the enhancement of athletic performance. *International Journal of Sport Nutrition and Exercise Metabolism* 28 (2): 178-187.

Wagenmakers, A.J. 1999. Amino acid supplements to improve athletic performance. *Current Opinion in Clinical Nutrition and Metabolic Care* 2 (6): 539-544.

Williams, M.H. 1998. *The ergogenic edge.* Champaign, IL: Human Kinetics.

Williams, M.H., R.B. Kreider, and J.D. Branch. 1999. *Creatine: The power supplement.* Champaign, IL: Human Kintics.

12

Nutrition and Training Adaptations

Objectives

After studying this chapter, you should be able to do the following:

- Describe the main adaptations to resistance and endurance training
- Discuss the mechanisms behind these changes and the molecular mechanisms underlying such changes
- Discuss the timeline of changes that may occur at molecular, cellular, and organ levels during the training process
- Discuss how carbohydrate intake can influence signaling, protein synthesis, and training adaptations
- Discuss how antioxidants can influence signaling, protein synthesis, and training adaptations
- Discuss how carbohydrate intake can reduce symptoms of overreaching
- Discuss the effects of nutrition on sleep quality and rehabilitation from injury

Regular physical activity results in adaptations that eventually result in improved physiological function. Exercise training makes use of this principle by planning and systematically applying exercise activities with the goal of optimizing those adaptations and thus improving performance. Many adaptations occur at all levels and in different organs in the body, including increased capillarization, fast-to-slow muscle fiber type conversion, increased heart size, increased mitochondrial mass, increased muscle mass, and so on. Table 12.1 lists several adaptations to resistance or endurance exercise. Adaptations to exercise or exercise training are specific to the exercise performed. High-intensity (predominantly anaerobic) exercise will result in adaptations that are different from those for moderate-intensity, longer-duration (aerobic) exercise. Resistance exercise typically results in a different phenotype than endurance training. With resistance exercise, hypertrophy is one of the main adaptations, whereas endurance training will not increase muscle mass and may even decrease it. Endurance training, however, will result in greater oxidative capacity and increase the fatigue resistance of the muscle. This chapter will answer the following questions: How does exercise result in training adaptations? Which signals and mechanisms are involved? How is it possible that different types of exercise training result in very different training adaptations? How can nutrition modify these adaptations?

Initially, we will look at the signals responsible for the changes. Then, we will study the effects of exercise on a variety of proteins in the body, and we will look at ways nutritional manipulation can improve the training adaptations. Finally, we will consider how nutritional interventions can promote sleep and recovery from injury.

TABLE 12.1 Training Adaptations

	Endurance training	Strength training
Capillary density	++	=
Muscle glycogen	++	++
Number of mitochondria	++	+
Mitochondrial density	++	+
Resting ATP	-	+
Resting PCr	-	+
Glycolytic enzymes	-	+
Phosphofructokinase	-	+
Oxidative enzymes	++	-/+
Succinate dehydrogenase	++	+
Citrate synthase	++	+
ß-hydroxyacyl dehydrogenase	++	+
Maximum cardiac output	++	+
Maximum oxygen uptake ($\dot{V}O_2max$)	++	+
Maximum heart rate	-	-
Plasma volume	++	=
Muscle fiber size	-	++
Fat oxidation	++	+

++ large increase; + increase; = no change; - decrease

Training Adaptations

Resistance training results in a number of adaptations in the muscle, including an increase in the muscle cross-sectional area (hypertrophy) and altered neural recruitment patterns. For hypertrophy to occur, the rate of myofibrillar protein synthesis must exceed the rate of myofibrillar protein breakdown over a certain period. Myofibrillar hypertrophy can occur through two processes: an increase in the number of nuclei within each muscle fiber or an increase in the amount of contractile material supported by each nucleus. Generally, resistance training does not increase the oxidative capacity of the muscle much, although some studies have observed improvements in oxidative enzyme activity (citrate synthase). The type and intensity of resistance training and the length of the recovery intervals may determine whether such adaptations take place.

Endurance exercise training is characterized by the development of improved fatigue resistance partly because of increased skeletal muscle mitochondrial density and thus mitochondrial protein. In addition, alterations occur in neural recruitment patterns, substrate use, and acid–base balance. Intramuscular glycogen stores as well as triacylglycerol stores increase after endurance training, although the amounts of both these fuel stores depend on the time since the last exercise session and the adequacy of nutrition in the postexercise period. Reliance on carbohydrate (glycogen) as a fuel decreases, and the ability to oxidize fat increases. These changes result in sparing of muscle glycogen during exercise. Endurance training does not greatly alter muscle fiber size, although an increase of around 20% in the cross-sectional area of type I fibers has been observed in some studies. Endurance training can increase the mitochondrial protein content of the muscle by 50% to 100% in 6 weeks (Hoppeler and Fluck 2003). The training adaptation is only temporary, and if the training stimulus is not maintained, mitochondrial proteins will be broken down again. Their half-life is only about 1 week. The best predictors of performance improvements are mitochondrial density and mitochondrial enzyme activity. The increase in size and number of mitochondria is usually referred to as **mitochondrial biogenesis.**

Another important adaptation to training is the improvement in blood supply to the muscles involved in the exercise. This is caused by increased numbers of capillaries in the muscle, and this process is referred to as **angiogenesis.** These increases are greatest in type I and type IIA muscle fibers. It turns out that angiogenesis is tightly coupled to the mitochondrial content of the muscle fibers. If one increases, the other seems to increase in parallel. It is believed that shear stress on endothelial cells resulting from an increased blood flow and stretch of the muscle are the main triggers of angiogenesis. It is thought that shear stress results in formation of nitric oxide by nitric oxide synthases in the endothelial cells and that, in response to muscle stretching (active or passive), vascular endothelial growth factor (VEGF) is secreted. These signals are important for the promotion of angiogenesis. Angiogenesis is also mediated by the actions of **peroxisome proliferator-activated receptor γ coactivators (PGCs),** which are the responsible for the transcriptional activation of hundreds of genes as described later in this chapter.

Exercise will increase net muscle protein synthesis after resistance and endurance exercise (see chapter 8) if dietary protein and energy intakes are adequate. Studies have typically looked at mixed muscle protein synthesis without specifically looking at which proteins are synthesized. It is likely that with resistance exercise there is synthesis of predominantly actin and myosin, whereas endurance exercise results mostly in mitochondrial biogenesis with little or no change in the synthesis of myofibrillar proteins. A study confirmed this in humans: Resistance exercise increased protein synthesis specifically in the myofibrillar fraction, and endurance exercise increased protein synthesis predominantly in the mitochondrial fraction (Wilkinson et al. 2008). The increase in protein synthesis after resistance or endurance exercise may last for up to 2 to 3 days after the last training session.

Ultimately, all adaptations, whether an increase in muscle mass or an increase in mitochondrial mass, result from increases in certain proteins. The complex process of exercise-induced adaptation in skeletal muscle starts with a blend of stresses that trigger specific molecular events. These stresses are different for endurance and for strength training; with strength training, stresses are mostly mechanical, while during endurance exercise, stresses are mainly metabolic. There are generally four categories of stresses:

1. Mechanical load
2. Neuronal activation
3. Hormonal adjustments
4. Metabolic disturbances

A blend of these stresses triggers specific molecular events, which in turn trigger an increase in protein synthesis. More specifically, signaling mechanisms activated by exercise stress initiate replication of deoxyribonucleic acid (DNA) genetic sequences (**genes**) that enable subsequent translation of the genetic code into a series of amino acids to synthesize new proteins (see appendix A for a basic description of the processes involved). The synthesis of these specific proteins ultimately results in adaptations. As discussed earlier, adaptations to training are highly specific to the type of training, which suggests that different signaling events may be involved. The signaling events and the resulting increases in messenger ribonucleic acid (mRNA), as well as the synthesis of proteins, depend on the intensity and duration of exercise, the type of exercise performed, and the intake of specific nutrients. The following section examines the molecular signaling events that underlie the training adaptations and the effects that different modes of exercise and nutrition can have on these events as well as on the outcomes.

Signal Transduction Pathways

Protein synthesis is regulated by **signal transduction pathways** that sense and compute local and systemic signals and regulate various cellular functions. The main signaling mechanisms are the phosphorylation of serine, threonine, and tyrosine residues by **kinases** and their dephosphorylation by phosphatases. The growth, metabolism, and proliferation of muscle fibers and most other functions depend on signals such as nutrient availability, pH, partial pressure of oxygen, ROS, and mechanical stimuli. The nervous and endocrine systems provide further inputs. Cells detect this ever-changing mix of signals through specific sensor proteins. Examples of sensor proteins are cell membrane receptors and amino acid-, calcium-, or AMP-sensing proteins. Activation of a sensor protein will trigger a cascade of reactions. These cascades of reactions form the link between the signals and the change in cellular function.

Protein kinases are typically part of a cascade of reactions that generally follows the sequence of events depicted in figure 12.1. This model is oversimplified because many signals converge or branch off.

These signal transduction pathways can then influence a number of cellular events (see the sidebar Control by Signal Transduction Pathways and figure 12.2) and will ultimately result in altered function. The preceding general description of signaling pathways probably applies to most cells in most situations. The details of these signaling cascades and the triggers, proteins, and kinases involved are different in different tissues and different situations. To understand adaptations in muscle cells in response to exercise training, the signaling pathways in muscle have to be studied in more detail.

During exercise, cellular homeostasis is disturbed and initiates a cascade of events that ultimately result in an adaptation that will cause less disturbance of homeostasis the next time that

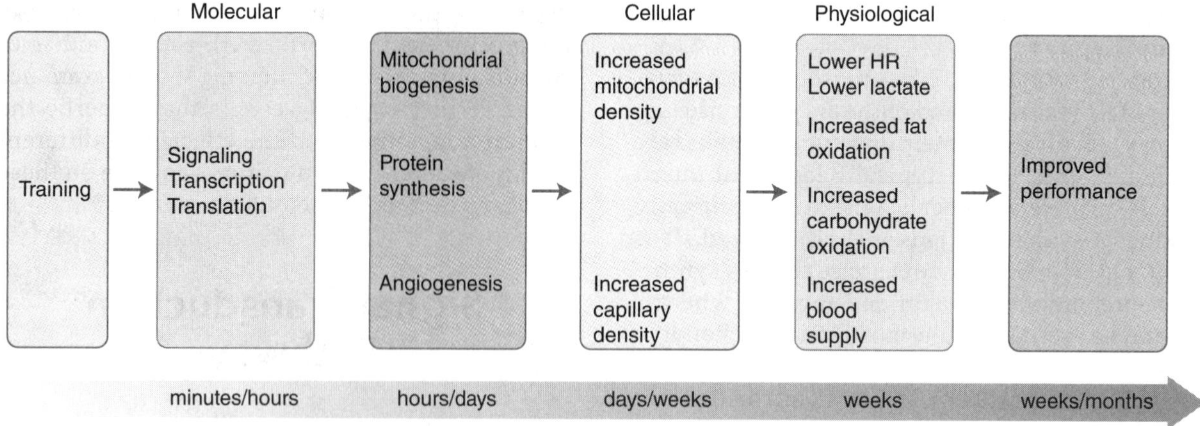

Figure 12.1 Simplified model of a typical kinase signaling pathway. HR = heart rate.

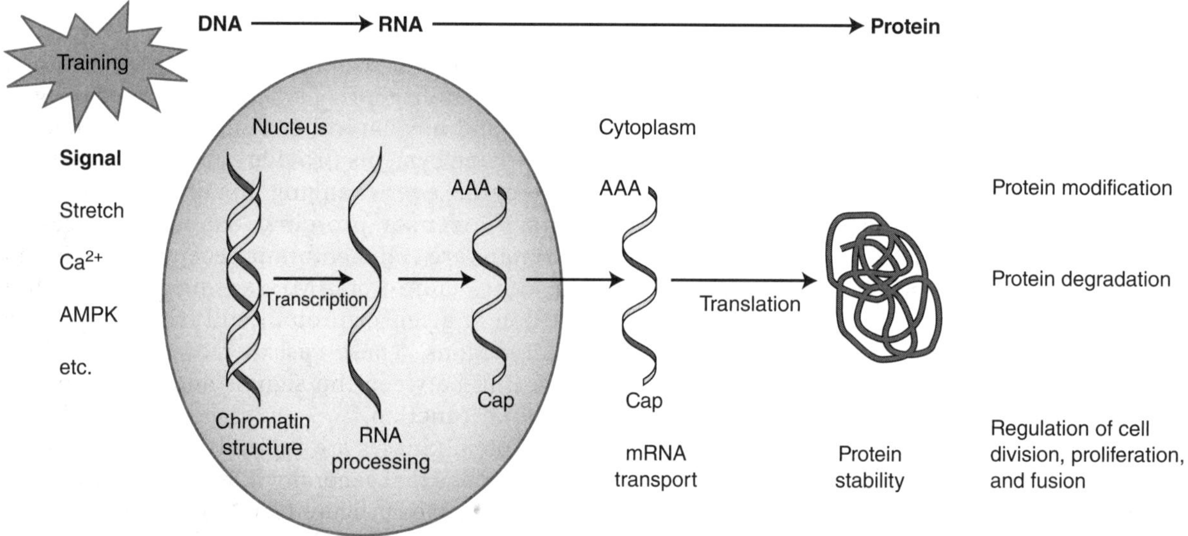

Figure 12.2 Training adaptations result from an increase in protein synthesis in response to repeated exercise sessions. It is believed that an exercise session causes a signal to transcribe DNA in the nucleus into RNA, which is then transported out of the nucleus and translated into protein. The signal caused by the exercise stimulus determines which proteins are synthesized. The amount of protein formed is determined not only by the signal, the transcription, and translation but also by the RNA processing and the stability of proteins. AAA indicates a triplet codon (in this case it is composed of 3 adenine bases which codes for the amino acid lysine).

the same exercise is performed. During exercise, these signals include changes in muscle stretch or tension, changes in intracellular Ca^{2+} concentrations, changes in the energy charge of the cell, and changes of the redox potential. Certain hormones and other ligands that can bind to receptors on the cell surface can alter these signals. These primary messengers may then trigger a series of secondary molecular events that increase or decrease transcription or translation as described in figure 12.3. The following section looks at the primary signals in detail.

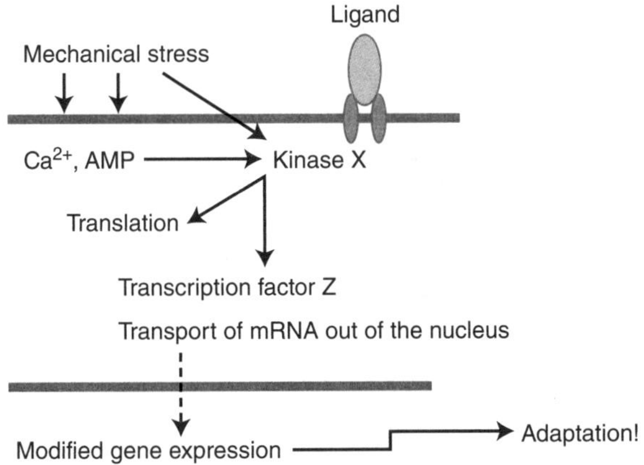

Figure 12.3 Simplified model of signal transduction in relation to exercise. Muscle contraction may result in a disturbance of homeostasis. Mechanical stress (stretch, tension), Ca^{2+}, and the accumulation of AMP or metabolites are primary signals that affect the phosphorylation state of various kinases. These kinases can influence the transcription process, the transport of mRNA out of the cell, and translation. Hormones and other ligands can influence these signals. The changes in gene expression can result in different adaptations.

Starting a Signaling Cascade

The basis for any training adaptation is a disturbance of homeostasis. Metabolic or mechanical changes in the muscle start a signaling cascade that results in the relevant proteins being broken down and synthesized. These initial signals are discussed next.

Muscle Stretch and Tension

Mechanical perturbations of skeletal muscle cells cause activation of a number of signaling pathways. More specifically, muscle stretch or altered tension can induce activation of calcineurin, mitogen-activated protein kinase (MAPK), and insulin-like growth factor (IGF) signaling cascades.

Calcium Ions

Neural activation of skeletal muscle generates an action potential that results in Ca^{2+} release from the T-tubules of the sarcoplasmic reticulum. When the exercise is stopped, the Ca^{2+} returns back from the cytoplasm to the sarcoplasmic reticulum. The fluctuations in Ca^{2+} concentration or the release and reuptake of Ca^{2+} in the sarcoplasmic reticulum are different for different types of activities, which could at least partly explain the differences in the adaptive response to exercise. Endurance exercise, for example, results in more prolonged and moderately elevated concentrations, whereas high-intensity exercise causes shorter periods of very high Ca^{2+} concentrations. Elevations of Ca^{2+} concentration in the muscle cytoplasm activate calmodulin kinase (CaMK) and calcineurin (CaN).

CONTROL BY SIGNAL TRANSDUCTION PATHWAYS

Signal transduction pathways control the following processes:

- Transcription of genes (specific sequences of DNA) into mRNA
- Translation of mRNA into protein
- Protein modification altering catalytic activity
- Regulation of protein degradation
- Regulation of cell division, proliferation, and fusion

Perturbations in Cellular Energy Balance

During muscle contraction, ATP is broken down to provide energy. In this process, ADP and Pi are formed. ADP is then resynthesized to ATP by glycolysis or oxidative phosphorylation. Some ADP is further broken down to AMP. The ratio of metabolites ADP, AMP, and Pi relative to that of ATP is often referred to as the energy charge. If there is a lot of ATP present but few metabolites, the energy charge is high. If the concentration of metabolites rises, the energy charge is low. These metabolites are important regulators of metabolism, but they also serve as signaling molecules. AMP, in particular, can activate **AMPK**, a potent secondary messenger. AMPK seems to play a role in the regulation of a variety of processes, including glucose uptake, fatty acid oxidation, hypertrophy, and gene expression. The redox potential is another indicator of the energy status of the cell. If the ratio of the oxidized form of the coenzyme NAD^+ to its reduced form (NADH) is high, poor energy status is indicated. The maintenance of redox potential produces volatile free-radical oxygen molecules (ROS). These ROS are also thought to play a role in the exercise-induced signaling that will ultimately be responsible for training adaptations. This signaling may work by ROS acting on transcription factors such as nuclear factor kappa B (NFKB) and activator protein 1 (AP1).

Hormones can affect the activation of kinases as well. The hormone or other ligand binds to a receptor, which then changes the phosphorylation state of a kinase. For example, when thyroid hormone (triiodothyronine or T_3) binds to its receptor, the process induces phosphorylation of AMPK in skeletal muscle.

The primary messengers activate a series of secondary messengers. These secondary messengers are often kinases and phosphatases, which are activated to pass on the exercise-induced signal. The secondary messengers often involve a complex series of reactions (cascades), which are highly regulated. Next, we will discuss some of the most studied messengers.

Secondary Signals

The initial signals almost immediately trigger a secondary response. This response usually involves the phosphorylation of certain kinases (or dephosphorylation of phosphatases). These kinases will then activate or deactivate another kinase or have a direct effect on a specific protein that alters the function. Only the most relevant and most investigated signals will be discussed here.

AMPK

AMPK plays a crucial role in energy metabolism and acts as a metabolic master switch that regulates several intracellular systems, including the cellular uptake of glucose, the ß-oxidation of fatty acids, and the biogenesis of GLUT4 and mitochondria (figure 12.4). The energy-sensing capability of AMPK can be attributed to its ability to detect and react to fluctuations in the AMP to ATP ratio that take place during rest and exercise. Muscle contraction is associated with an increase in the demand for cellular ATP, which subsequently increases the AMP to ATP ratio. AMPK is activated by an increase in the AMP to ATP ratio. Acute activation of AMPK results in a response that aims to conserve energy (limit ATP use) and generate more ATP. For example, AMPK activation results in an increase in glucose uptake and an increase in fat oxidation so that ATP can be generated. When AMP is high and ATP is low, AMP activates AMPK by dislodging ATP from the α-subunit of AMPK and makes it more sensitive to phosphorylation by AMPK kinases (Scott et al. 2007). In skeletal muscle, the major AMPK kinase appears to be liver kinase B1 (LKB1), also known as serine/threonine kinase 11, although the Ca^{2+}/calmodulin-dependent kinases (CaMK) and the transforming growth factor (TGF)-ß-activating kinase may also activate AMPK (figure 12.4).

Winder and Hardie (1996) were the first to demonstrate that AMPK could be activated by exercise. They demonstrated that when rats ran at a high intensity, AMPK activity increased two-and-a-half times within the first 5 minutes and did not increase any further after 30 minutes (Winder and Hardie 1996). In humans, 20 minutes of cycling at 70% of $\dot{V}O_2$max increased the activity of the α2 AMPK isoform without altering α1 AMPK activity (Fujii et al. 2000). Cycling at a lower intensity (50% of $\dot{V}O_2$max) for 20 minutes did not activate either α1 or α2 AMPK. Together these data suggest that intense endurance exercise activates α2 AMPK. It has been suggested that resistance exercise may be different. In a study in which muscles were electrically stimulated, Atherton et al. (2005) showed

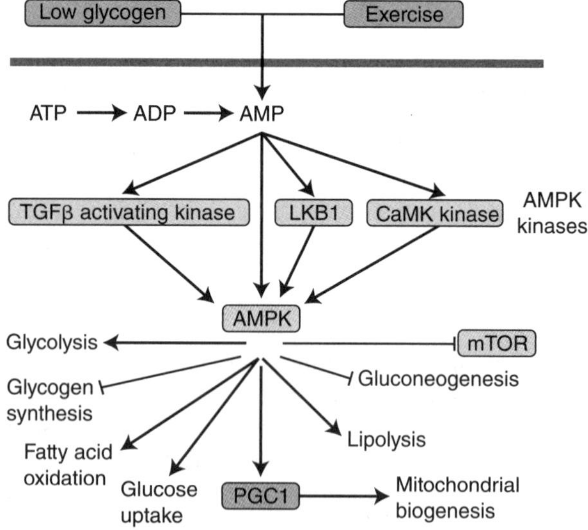

Figure 12.4 A change in the AMP to ATP ratio activates AMPK by activating AMPK kinases (LKB1, CaMK, and the TGF-ß-activating kinase). AMPK then acts as a metabolic master switch by turning on processes that generate ATP and turning off processes that use ATP. It also causes an adaptation so that the next time the same stress is applied, the cell will be better adapted.

that after endurance exercise, AMPK was activated, but with resistance exercise no change in AMPK activation occurred. However, it has also been demonstrated that humans who are unaccustomed to resistance exercise can also show increased activation of AMPK (Coffey et al. 2006). It was also shown that endurance-trained athletes have a blunted AMPK response after endurance exercise.

CaMK is a family of various kinases that can detect and respond to changes in calcium concentrations. It has been shown that certain isoforms of CaMK (CaMKII) can also respond to muscle stretch. After CaMK is activated, a number of other signaling molecules are activated, including nuclear factor of activated T-cells (NFAT) and histone deacetylase (HDAC). Calcineurin is another molecule that is activated by Ca^{2+}. Calcineurin is known to act as a coregulator of **muscle hypertrophy** in combination with **insulin-like growth factor (IGF)**, but it also has a role in fiber-type transformation (fast twitch to slow twitch) and the expression of the genes of oxidative enzymes.

The insulin and insulin-like growth factor pathways play an important role in muscle hypertrophy. Contractile activity stimulates the release of IGF-1, which binds to its receptor and initiates a cascade of molecular events (figure 12.5).

After IGF binds to its receptor, insulin receptor substrate 1 (IRS-1) is activated, and this in turn activates phosphatidylinositide 3-kinase (PI3K). The latter activates phosphoinoisitide-dependent kinase 1 (PDK1), which in turn phosphorylates

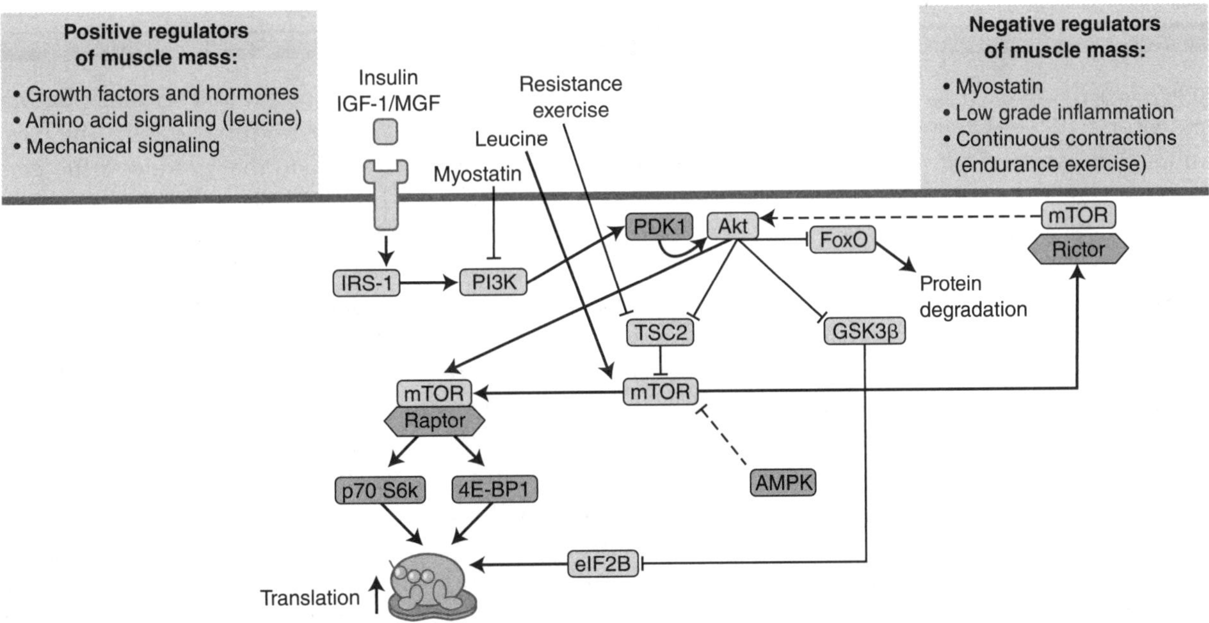

Figure 12.5 The insulin and insulin-like growth factor pathways play an important role in muscle hypertrophy through the Akt-mammalian target of rapamycin (Akt-mTor) signaling cascade. The lines ending in arrows indicate positive influences and the dashed lines ending in bars indicate negative (inhibitory) influences. eIF2B = eukaryotic translation initiation factor 2B.

INCREASED SIGNALING DOES NOT NECESSARILY MEAN INCREASED PROTEIN SYNTHESIS

Several studies have investigated the signaling pathways that are activated by exercise, but few studies have linked these changes with actual changes in protein synthesis. Note that although these signals can increase the synthesis of mRNA, protein synthesis may not necessarily increase. The rate of protein synthesis depends on mRNA degradation, additional translational control mechanisms, transport of mRNA out of the nucleus, and the translation process.

Akt (also known as protein kinase B). Akt has numerous targets, including those involved in protein synthesis (mTOR and tuberous sclerosis complex 2 [TSC2]), glycogen synthesis (glycogen synthase kinase 3 [GSK3ß]), protein degradation (forkhead Box proteinO, FoxO), and glucose transport (Akt substrate of 160 kilodaltons, AS160). There is strong evidence that the **Akt-mTOR pathway** is involved in hypertrophy through activating translation initiation as well as increasing the ribosomal protein content. The response of Akt to exercise is unclear at the moment, and studies have found either increases or no change in response to exercise. This is likely because of the central role of Akt in regulating muscle hypertrophy as well as glucose transport. The Akt response may therefore be highly specific to the type of exercise and is probably influenced by many other factors. mTOR responds to a number of different stimuli and can have effects on mRNA translation, the synthesis of ribosomes, and metabolism.

Two mTOR protein complexes exist where mTOR binds with a G-ß-L protein (one of a family of guanosine nucleotide-binding proteins) and either a rapamycin-sensitive raptor or a rictor protein. mTOR-raptor complex is a positive regulator of cell growth, and mTOR-rictor appears to have a key role in Akt activation and actin cytoskeleton regulation. Primary downstream targets of mTOR-raptor include p70 S6 kinase (p70 S6K), eIF4E-binding protein (4E-BP1), and eukaryotic translation initiation factor 4B (eIF4B; not shown in figure 12.5). These downstream targets increase

EFFECT OF TRAINING TYPE

In an elegant study, Wilkinson et al. (2008) investigated changes in signaling and protein synthesis before and after a 10-week training program consisting of endurance or resistance (strength) exercise. They distinguished between mitochondrial and myofibrillar protein synthesis. They found that untrained subjects increased both mitochondrial and myofibrillar protein synthesis after a bout of resistance exercise (when fed). Endurance exercise resulted in an increase only in mitochondrial protein synthesis. After 10 weeks of training, however, the response was more specific. Resistance exercise resulted in an increase only in myofibrillar protein synthesis and endurance training only in mitochondrial biosynthesis. Differences in translation initiation explained few of these observed differences in protein synthesis, so the mechanism for the distinctly different adaptations to resistance and endurance exercise lies in the different signaling pathways that are activated or inhibited by endurance and resistance exercise.

It is very clear that exercise training regimens designed to promote strength or endurance result in distinctly different adaptations and phenotypes. Endurance capacity, which is closely related to the capacity of the muscle to use oxygen for the regeneration of ATP, is primarily controlled at the level of gene transcription. In this process, PGC-1α is the central regulator of mitochondrial biogenesis and also plays a role in the regulation of angiogenesis. Resistance exercise is predominantly controlled by mTOR, and this is considered the key governor of protein synthesis. Several pathways can activate mTOR; the most important ones are mechanical signaling, growth factors, and amino acid availability. There is also cross talk between the pathways involved with endurance exercise and strength exercise, and generally, they seem to inhibit each other's adaptations at least to some degree. For example, it has been suggested that AMPK inhibits the mTOR pathway, as illustrated in figure 12.5. Contraction-induced changes in mechanical strain, calcium flux, and mechanosensation as well as substrate metabolism influences, including altered redox balance, ATP turnover, and increased ROS production, have all been implicated in the activation of signal transduction cascades that regulate skeletal muscle gene expression and altered protein synthesis that lead to exercise training adaptations. A summary of these trigger mechanisms and the various cellular sensors and signal transduction pathways that convert these homeostatic perturbations to induce training adaptation is illustrated in figure 12.6. The nature of the exercise challenge (strength or endurance) determines the acute metabolic and molecular responses, which result in the phenotypic changes associated with long-term physiological adaptation to exercise training.

mRNA translation and increased protein synthesis. It is generally thought that mTOR plays a central role in the adaptation to resistance exercise.

PGCs

One family of transcriptional regulators in particular, the PGCs family—PGC-1α, PGC-1ß, and the PGC-1 related coactivator (PRC)—is important in driving mitochondrial biogenesis and angiogenesis. The PGCs are coactivators of the peroxisome proliferator-activated receptor-γ (PPAR-γ). A transcription coactivator is defined as a protein or protein complex that increases the probability of a gene being transcribed by interacting with transcription factors but does not itself bind to DNA in a sequence-specific manner. The activity and the expression of PGCs rapidly increase following a single bout of endurance exercise. PGC mRNA increases 1.5 to 10 times following a single bout of exercise (Pilegaard, Saltin, and Neufer 2003; Baar et al. 2002; Wright et al. 2007). PGCs increase oxidative capacity and endurance performance. Therefore, the goal of endurance athletes and coaches should be to maximize the activation of PGC signaling pathways in skeletal muscle.

Consequently, it has been hypothesized that AMPK might mediate the increase in PGCs in response to training. Indeed, in humans, moderate to high-intensity endurance exercise increases the amount of AMPK in muscle cells (McGee et al. 2003). These findings put AMPK directly upstream of PGCs, potentially governing the level of PGCs and therefore the metabolic state of the muscle.

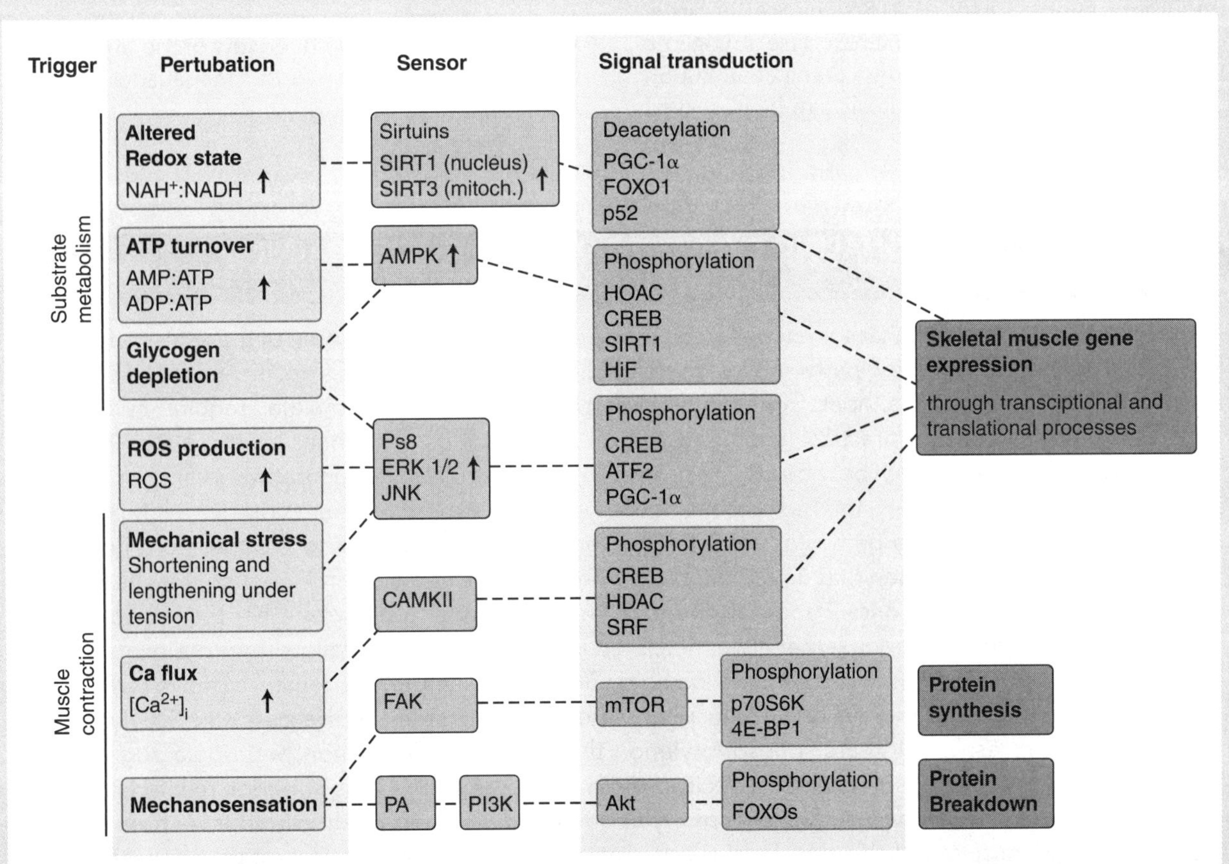

Figure 12.6 The initiation of mechanical and metabolic perturbations by skeletal muscle contraction during exercise that are detected by intracellular sensor mechanisms leads to the activation of networks of signaling molecules, including protein kinases, phosphatases, and deacetylases, which in turn alter the states of transcription factors and transcriptional coregulators that result in altered gene expression and altered rates of protein synthesis and breakdown.

Adapted from Egan and Zierath (2013).

As a result, training that increases AMPK activity should be beneficial for endurance performance. It has also been suggested that central nervous system activity through ß-adrenergic receptors may play a significant role in the activation of PGCs and the subsequent increase in mitochondria.

Time Course of Events

Typically, the initial response to exercise occurs within seconds or minutes. For example, changes in intracellular calcium are instant. Then, a cascade of reaction follows. The activation of various kinases can take a bit longer, and some kinases may not reach their maximal activity until several hours after exercise. Gene expression seems to peak between 4 and 12 hours after exercise, possibly depending on the gene and the type of exercise performed. In one study, myogenic and metabolic genes peaked at 4 to 8 hours after resistance exercise. After endurance exercise, myogenic genes peaked after 8 to 12 hours (Yang et al. 2005). The changes in protein synthesis can be observed within hours after exercise but may peak many hours later. In fact, studies have demonstrated increased protein synthesis up to 48 hours after exercise. An overview of the changes is depicted in figure 12.7.

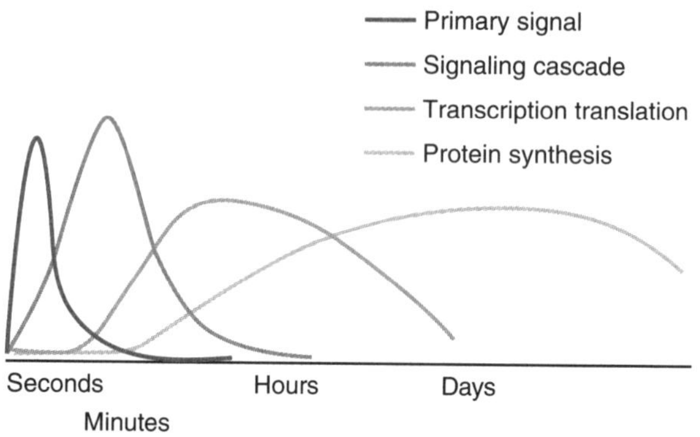

Figure 12.7 A rough overview of the time course of changes in various events that cause an adaptation to exercise training.

CAN SIGNALING EVENTS BE USED TO GUIDE TRAINING OR NUTRITION INTAKE?

The practical question that sometimes arises is whether we can measure some of these responses, such as anabolic signaling pathways, to guide training. The short answer is no, it cannot be solely based on these markers. Apart from the fact that it is an invasive procedure (i.e., requires cutting the skin) and not very practical (you need to take muscle biopsies to measure these markers), there often is a mismatch between the responses of the anabolic signaling pathways and muscle protein synthesis. In part, this has to do with the way these experiments are conducted. Muscle biopsies are taken at a particular point in time (and often only once) and are therefore just a snapshot. Thus, if we see that a particular intervention, say whey protein ingestion, results in a greater molecular response 2 hours after intake, there is no way to know whether the molecular response would have been larger if we measured it at a different time following protein intake.

Another issue relates to a potential threshold effect. For example, the activity of the mTORC1 pathway is assessed by measuring phosphorylation of the proteins in the pathway. So, if one intervention results in greater phosphorylation than another intervention, we would suggest that the former results in greater muscle protein synthesis and is thus superior to the latter. There is evidence, however, that phosphorylation has to hit a certain threshold level before a reaction is triggered. If this threshold is not met, the response of muscle protein synthesis to the two interventions will be no different.

The final issue to highlight is the fact that the methods to quantify anabolic signaling pathways are semi-quantitative and, in many cases, not accurate enough to use at an individual level. In conclusion, nutrition or exercise interventions cannot be based solely on information about anabolic signaling pathways. These methods can be used in research and will help us understand how training adaptations occur, but in sport they are not practical and not predictive enough.

Nutrition and Effects on Training Adaptations

Nutrients can affect signaling and thus have the potential to regulate or alter the training adaptation. In chapter 8, for example, we discussed that the amino acid leucine not only serves as a building block for protein synthesis but also can function as a signaling molecule. This function of leucine can result in greater rates of protein synthesis. Similar functions have been suggested for muscle glycogen, ROS, cytokines, and various inflammatory markers. Nutrition can play an important role in modulating the levels of these molecules. Here we will discuss some of these effects starting with muscle glycogen, which has received the most attention.

Glycogen and the Signaling Response

A single bout of endurance exercise will increase transcription or mRNA content for various metabolic and stress-related genes. Typically, transcriptional activity peaks within the first few hours of recovery and returns to baseline within 24 hours. These findings have led to the overall hypothesis that training adaptations in skeletal muscle may be generated by the cumulative effects of transient increases in **gene transcription** during recovery from repeated bouts of exercise.

A number of studies have reported that altering substrate availability during exercise (e.g., by increasing dietary fat intake or commencing exercise with low muscle glycogen) can influence metabolic gene transcription, suggesting that modification of the training response may be possible through specific diet interventions. It has been shown that commencing endurance exercise with low muscle glycogen increases the activity of several metabolic genes and signaling proteins. In a study by Pilegaard et al. (2002), six untrained male volunteers performed 2.5 hours of cycling at 45% of $\dot{V}O_2$max. One day before the experiment, subjects performed 90 minutes of one-legged cycling to reduce the muscle glycogen content in that leg. On the day of the experiment, muscle biopsies were taken from both legs at rest before exercise, immediately postexercise, and 2 and 5 hours postexercise. Compared with the control leg, the leg that exercised the previous day had 45% lower resting preexercise muscle glycogen content. Following 2.5 hours of cycling at 45% of $\dot{V}O_2$max, it was found that transcriptional activity of pyruvate dehydrogenase kinase 4 (PDK4), uncoupling protein 3 (UCP3), and hexokinase II (HKII) was significantly higher in the leg that exercised with low muscle glycogen. Because the control leg and the low-glycogen leg were exposed to the same systemic concentrations of metabolites, hormones, catecholamines, and cytokines, it is reasonable to assume that increased transcriptional activity was in some way directly related to low muscle glycogen content.

The role of muscle glycogen could be explained by the fact that some signaling proteins (e.g., AMPK) possess glycogen-binding domains and that when glycogen is low, these proteins are more active toward their specific targets. In support of this, Wojtaszewski et al. (2003) reported that AMPK activity was elevated when a standardized bout of exercise (1 hour of cycling at 70% $\dot{V}O_2$max) was undertaken with low muscle glycogen (160 compared with 900 mmol/kg d.w.). Elevated AMPK activity with low muscle glycogen may be beneficial to individuals undertaking exercise training because AMPK is believed to play a critical role in regulating the adaptive response. Commencing endurance exercise with low muscle glycogen has also been shown to increase the activity of p38 MAPK, and like AMPK, p38 MAPK is thought to be a regulator of mitochondrial biogenesis and endurance-training adaptations.

The aforementioned studies provide early evidence to suggest that training with low muscle glycogen might be a useful strategy to promote endurance-training adaptations. Further studies are clearly needed before this proposition can be confirmed or dismissed. Because glycogen plays such an important role, it is logical to speculate that manipulating it could enhance training adaptations. Indeed, studies have tried to train athletes with low glycogen to see if this could enhance the signaling response and the adaptations in the muscle. Generally, the available studies support this idea, as discussed in the following sections.

Train Low, Compete High

Only one study has determined whether long-term training with low muscle glycogen can enhance the adaptive response to endurance training. Hansen et al. (2005) recruited seven untrained men to undertake a 10-week program of knee extensor exercise. Each of the subjects' legs was trained according to a different schedule, but the total amount of work performed by each leg was kept the same. One leg was trained twice a day every second day, whereas the other leg was trained once daily. This protocol meant that the leg that trained twice every second day commenced half of the sessions with low muscle glycogen. Compared with the leg that trained with normal glycogen levels, the leg that commenced half of the training sessions with low muscle glycogen had more pronounced increases in resting muscle glycogen content and citrate synthase activity. Time to fatigue at 90% of maximal power output increased in both legs after training (figure 12.8). Performance times, however, were nearly twice as long in the leg that trained with low muscle glycogen (19.7 ± 2.4 vs. 11.9 ± 1.3 min). These remarkable findings demonstrate that, under the specific conditions of the study, training with low muscle glycogen enhanced adaptations in skeletal muscle and improved exercise performance. However, a number of details make it difficult to extrapolate these findings. First, the subjects recruited were untrained, so it is not yet known whether training with low muscle glycogen will translate into improved adaptations in well-trained athletes. Second, subjects performed a fixed amount of work even though higher glycogen stores would normally allow exercise to be performed at higher intensities or longer durations. Third, it is difficult to translate the results from a single-leg kicking exercise to that of real-life sporting situations that involve activities such as running, cycling, or swimming.

To take these findings to a more realistic sporting situation, researchers in Melbourne (Australia) and Birmingham (United Kingdom) investigated the effects of a 3-week training program in which all the training was performed in the glycogen-loaded state or in which half of the training was performed in a glycogen-depleted state (Yeo et al. 2008). The performance during the self-paced training sessions in the glycogen-depleted state was significantly impaired. The subjects who always trained when glycogen loaded trained at higher absolute intensities. Despite this, however, at the end of the training period, performance improved equally in the low-glycogen group and the high-glycogen group. The metabolic adaptations in the two groups were very different though. The low-glycogen group had a greater oxidative capacity as evidenced by greater citrate synthase (TCA cycle enzyme) and ß-hydroxyacyl dehydrogenase (rate-limiting enzyme of FA ß-oxidation) activities as well as greater cytochrome c oxidase subunit IV (COX IV) content. Fat oxidation was also enhanced in the low-glycogen group. These findings partly confirm the findings of the single-leg study by Hansen et al. (2005). The difference is that although adaptations were observed in metabolism, no differences in performance occurred after 3 weeks. Of course, it may be that 3 weeks is sufficient to see differences in metabolism but not long enough to see improvements in performance. Future studies should investigate longer-term training protocols.

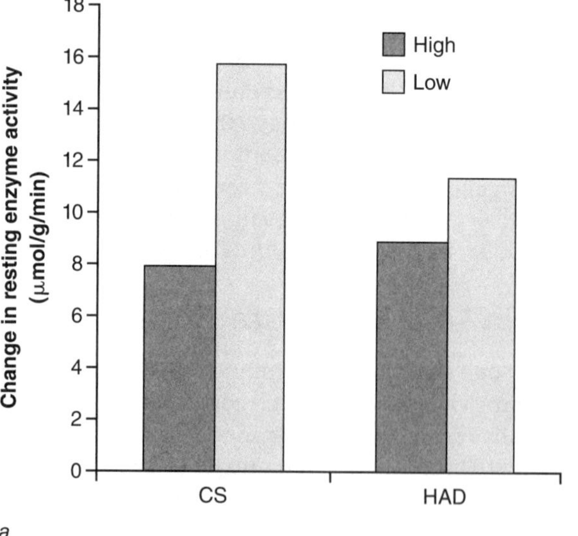

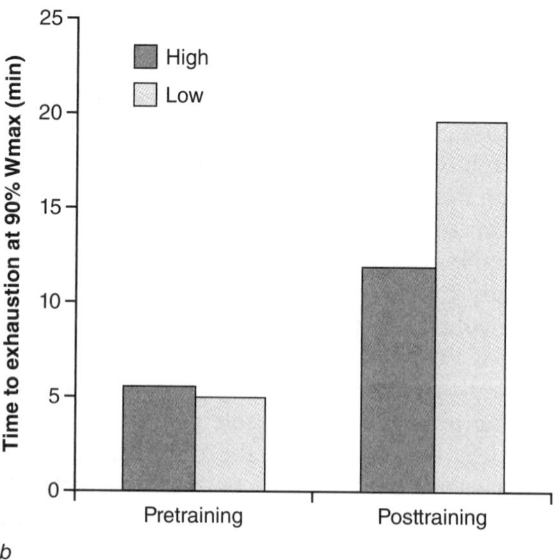

Figure 12.8 Single-leg training study in which one leg trained with low glycogen 50% of the time (low) and the other leg always trained with high glycogen (high). Training with low glycogen resulted in *(a)* an increase in oxidative enzymes (citrate synthase and ß-hydroxyacyl-CoA dehydrogenase) and *(b)* improved endurance capacity after 10 weeks of knee extensor training.

Data from Hansen (2005).

It seems fair to conclude that endurance training in a glycogen-depleted state results in improved capacity to use fat to fuel exercise. The mechanisms behind this adaptation are unclear but may involve activation of the PPARs. The PPARs are a group of nuclear receptor proteins that function as transcription factors that regulate the expression of genes. PPARs play an essential role in the regulation of metabolism and many other processes.

Narkar et al. (2008) showed that training rats on a treadmill while at the same time giving them a drug that activated a transcription factor called PPAR-δ resulted in the same change that occurs when training in the glycogen-depleted state: increased capacity to use fat as a fuel. PPAR-δ increases the concentration of the enzymes that are required for oxidizing fatty acids. The result in this study was that the rats that got the drug and trained on the treadmill increased their ability to run at about 50% of $\dot{V}O_2max$ by 70% over those that only ran on the treadmill. It is possible that exercising in a glycogen-depleted state activates PPAR-δ to a greater extent than training in the glycogen-loaded state does. PPAR-δ seems to be activated by a by-product of the breakdown of fat in muscle. As discussed earlier, exercising in the glycogen-depleted state increases circulating FA concentration and oxidation of fat during exercise, which results in more of the by-product and more PPAR-δ activation.

Few studies have investigated the effects of high- and low-carbohydrate diets on longer-term training adaptations. Simonsen et al. (1991) determined the effect of 4 weeks of moderate or high carbohydrate intake (5 or 10 g per kilogram of body weight per day) on muscle glycogen concentration, training capacity, and exercise performance in 22 collegiate rowers (12 men and 10 women). Rowers trained twice daily throughout the 4-week period. Morning training sessions consisted of 40 minutes at 70% of $\dot{V}O_2max$, whereas evening training sessions consisted of 2,500 m time trials or high-intensity interval training (~90% of $\dot{V}O_2max$). Consuming the moderate-carbohydrate diet maintained muscle glycogen concentrations throughout the 4-week period, but consuming the high-carbohydrate diet resulted in a progressive increase in muscle glycogen concentrations, which were 65% higher by the end of the fourth week of training. Power output during 2,500 m time trials increased by 1.6% and 10.7% after 4 weeks of training with moderate- and high-carbohydrate diets, respectively. These were the first findings to demonstrate that consuming a high-carbohydrate diet can improve training adaptation and enhance performance following training. Subsequent studies have shown that high carbohydrate intake during periods of intensified training can delay or reduce the magnitude of overreaching symptoms such as decreased performance, reduced endocrine responsiveness to exercise, and disturbed mood state (Achten et al. 2004; Halson et al. 2004), as discussed later in this chapter. Much earlier studies established the importance of high carbohydrate intake to maximize glycogen stores for optimal competition performance in endurance events (see chapter 6), so there is never any question that athletes should "compete high."

Although the results of studies suggest that training with low glycogen could have some metabolic advantages, whether this results in improvements in performance is not clear. Studies may show enhanced adaptations in muscle, but there is little evidence that exercise performance is also improved. In addition, this type of training is harder and recovery may take longer, the risk of overreaching or overtraining is greater, and immunodepression may be more profound. Therefore, training with low carbohydrate availability is promising, but it needs to be applied with caution. If it is used as part of periodized nutrition program (see chapter 17), training low might be a useful approach, at least in endurance sports.

Athletes and coaches have started to incorporate training low into their weekly training practice. In chapter 17, we will mention how this type of training can fit into a weekly or yearly schedule (often referred to as periodized training) and how it can be used in conjunction with training high. It is also important to remember that training low is different from being on a low-carbohydrate diet. Training low could result in some positive adaptations but always training low, such as on a low-carbohydrate diet, is not recommended (as discussed in previous chapters).

Fasted Training

For many years, endurance athletes (mainly runners and cyclists) have used exercise without breakfast as a way to increase the oxidative capacity of the muscle. This protocol has often been termed *fat-burning training.* Ingesting carbohydrate in the hours before exercise will raise plasma insulin and subsequently suppress fat oxidation by up to about 35% (Achten and Jeukendrup 2003). This effect of insulin on fat oxidation may last as long as 6 to 8 hours after a meal, so the highest fat oxidation rates can be achieved after an overnight fast. A study was performed at the University of Leuven in Belgium in which the effect of an endurance-training program (6 weeks, 3 days/week, 1-2 hours) in the fasted or carbohydrate-fed state was investigated (DeBock et al. 2008). The investigators observed a decrease in muscle glycogen use, and the activity of various proteins involved in fat metabolism increased after training in the fasted state. Fat oxidation during exercise was the same in the two groups. It is possible, however, that small but significant changes in fat metabolism occur after fasted training, but in this study, changes in fat oxidation might have been masked by the fact that these subjects received carbohydrate during their experimental trials. Note that training after an overnight fast may reduce exercise capacity and may therefore be suitable only for low- to moderate-intensity exercise sessions. More research is needed to find out whether training in the fasted state has any advantages over training in the fed state. Note that training in the fed or fasted state is a different concept from training with low muscle glycogen. After an overnight fast, liver glycogen may be low, but muscle glycogen would be unaffected.

Carbohydrate Intake During Exercise

It has been suggested that carbohydrate intake during exercise may interfere with training adaptations. This notion is based on the observation that carbohydrate intake during exercise can reduce the expression of the mRNA of certain proteins after exercise. For example, carbohydrate ingestion has been shown to reduce CPT I mRNA, mitochondrial UCP3, and the FA transporter FAT/CD36 as well as the activation of AMPK (Akerstrom et al. 2006; Civitarese et al. 2005). This finding could indicate that training adaptations could be compromised when carbohydrate is ingested during training. Another study did not show any difference in the activation of AMPK (Lee-Young et al. 2006). Although it was shown that glucose ingestion during moderate-intensity exercise reduced the expression of PDK4 and UCP3, the expression of the gene for PGC-1, the PPAR-γ transcription coactivator responsible for longer-term adaptations, was not altered (Cluberton et al. 2005). From these studies that investigated the acute effects of one exercise bout, it is difficult to predict the long-term effects on protein synthesis and training adaptation.

A training study was performed in which subjects trained with or without carbohydrate ingestion in each training session for a period of 10 weeks (using a single-leg kicking model). It was found that citrate synthase and ß-hydroxyacyl dehydrogenase activity and muscle glycogen increased but that there were no differences between the carbohydrate-fed and placebo-fed groups. Performance also improved after training, but the improvement was identical for the carbohydrate and placebo groups (Akerstrom et al. 2009). The authors concluded that glucose ingestion during exercise does not alter training adaptation related to substrate metabolism, mitochondrial enzyme activity, glycogen content, or performance.

At present drawing any firm conclusions is impossible, but it seems unlikely that carbohydrate ingestion negatively influences training adaptations. Differences in the findings between acute studies and the training study described earlier may be explained by differences in the exercise protocol, including the exercise model used (one-legged kicking versus two-legged cycling exercise) and the training status of the subjects. Note that carbohydrate feeding may allow the athlete to train harder or longer; therefore, metabolic perturbations and changes in gene expression may be greater in those situations.

Leucine and the Signaling Response

Exercise increases muscle protein synthesis by stimulation of signaling pathways inside the contracting muscle cells. However, when no source of protein or amino acids is provided and there is no increased availability of amino acids, a net gain of tissue protein will not occur (see chapter 8). In chapter 8, we also mentioned that increased amino acid intake is necessary for two reasons: to stimulate the signaling pathways and to provide building blocks for the new proteins being synthesized. The BCAAs, particularly leucine, stimulate the muscles' signaling pathways.

One study is often cited to demonstrate the importance of BCAA for increasing muscle protein synthesis and ultimately the training adaptation. Anthony et al. (1999) studied protein synthesis in rats that ran for two hours on a treadmill. They observed that muscle protein synthesis was decreased significantly following the exercise. When leucine was given to these animals, the signaling pathways were stimulated and protein synthesis increased. However, it is important to note that protein synthesis only increased to preexercise levels. In humans, exercise does not decrease muscle protein synthesis like it did in these rats. The leucine did not increase protein synthesis in these rats above preexercise levels; it merely returned muscle protein synthesis to the levels observed before the exercise. In other words, if there is a catabolic state, leucine may be effective, but whether leucine would be effective in humans where such a catabolic state cannot be observed postexercise remains unclear.

Several studies have demonstrated that signaling is increased postexercise with the ingestion of BCAA. However, no studies in humans have measured protein synthesis in combination with these measurements. It is not unlikely, however, that, although BCAAs alone can stimulate the signaling cascades, this would not result in increased protein synthesis if the amino acid building blocks are not supplied at the same time. Protein synthesis not only depends on the activation of the protein synthetic machinery but also on its substrate.

This line of thought led some researchers to theorize that a protein source that provides all amino acids and has a slightly higher leucine content could optimize protein balance postexercise. Koopman et al. (2004, 2005, 2007) demonstrated that the addition of protein to carbohydrates following resistance exercise increases muscle protein synthesis. However, when they added extra leucine to the carbohydrate–protein mixture, this did not result in further improvement in protein balance (Koopman et al. 2005). It seems likely that by giving a source of protein postexercise, muscle protein synthesis is already stimulated to maximum (by the combination of exercise and protein) and leucine cannot stimulate it any further.

Although BCAAs (particularly leucine) have a role in signaling that enhances protein synthesis, it is unlikely that leucine alone will stimulate protein synthesis postexercise because the other amino acids have to be supplied as well to serve as building blocks. In some situations, muscle protein synthesis may be compromised, and in these situations BCAAs are more likely to have an effect. At this stage, however, the role of BCAAs and the possible effects on protein balance are not entirely clear.

Antioxidants and Training Adaptations

Skeletal muscle is repeatedly subjected to bouts of oxidative stress during exercise. Considerable evidence now indicates that aerobic contractile activity is associated with an increase in free-radical production in skeletal muscle (see chapter 10 for further details). This increased production arises because a proportion of the molecular oxygen used in normal respiration undergoes one-electron reduction to produce superoxide radicals, the production of which increases with the large increase in oxygen flux in muscle mitochondria during exercise. This process leads to release of superoxide ($\cdot O_2^-$) and hydrogen peroxide by the muscle cell and the local formation of hydroxyl radicals ($\cdot OH$); collectively, these are known as ROS. Other mechanisms also contribute to free radical production by exercising muscle, including the release of ROS from activated leukocytes that infiltrate and accumulate in the damaged muscle fibers after damaging eccentric exercise. Much work has been undertaken to examine the possibility that this free-radical production is the cause of exercise-induced muscle damage, and much research has focused on the detrimental effects of free radicals. But considerable evidence indicates that muscle cells adapt to this increased free-radical activity to reduce the risk of free-radical damage to the tissue. Thus, exercise training has been shown to increase the activity of several antioxidant enzymes, such as superoxide dismutase and catalase in muscle, and to increase muscle heat-shock protein content following exercise. It is now recognized that these adaptations can protect skeletal muscle against further bouts of (normally) damaging contractile activity.

In the past decade, it has become clear that physiological concentrations of free radicals may have advantageous effects. ROS and reactive nitrogen species (RNS) are involved in modulation of cell signaling pathways and the control of several (redox-sensitive) transcription factors (see figure 12.6). Although high levels of ROS may interfere with muscle function, moderate levels of ROS are essential in the development of optimal force production in muscle (Powers and Jackson 2008).

These findings also raise a number of important questions concerning the possible role of free-radical species as signals for wider adaptive responses in these and other tissues; they question the approach to protection of tissues that involves the use of widespread supplementation with antioxidant nutrients. It is entirely feasible that the adaptations to stress mediated by free radicals play an important role in maintaining cell viability in tissues routinely subjected to repeated stresses (e.g., muscle following exercise) and that increased consumption of some antioxidant nutrients might interfere with these necessary adaptive processes (Slattery, Bentley, and Coutts 2015).

In one study, 14 men were trained for eight weeks (Gomez-Cabrera et al. 2008). Five of the men were supplemented daily with an oral dose of 1 g of vitamin C. The administration of vitamin C significantly hampered endurance capacity. The adverse effects of vitamin C may result from its capacity to reduce the exercise-induced expression of key transcription factors involved in mitochondrial biogenesis: peroxisome proliferator-activated receptor co-activator 1 (PGC-1α), nuclear respiratory factor 1 (NRF1), and mitochondrial transcription factor A (Tfam). Vitamin C also prevented the exercise-induced expression of cytochrome C (a marker of mitochondrial content) and of the antioxidant enzymes superoxide dismutase and glutathione peroxidase. The authors concluded that vitamin C supplementation decreased training efficiency because it prevented some cellular adaptations to exercise.

Subsequently, more than 20 published studies have reported that antioxidant supplementation interferes with exercise training-induced adaptations. The main findings of these studies (reviewed by Peternelj and Coombes 2011) are that, in many situations, loading the tissues with high doses of antioxidants leads to a blunting of the effects of exercise training (e.g., mitochondrial biogenesis, increased GLUT4 expression, increased antioxidant enzyme expression) and interferes with ROS-mediated physiological processes such as vasodilation and insulin signaling. Much more research needs to be done to produce evidence-based guidelines regarding the use of antioxidant supplementation during periods of exercise training. The best approach that can be currently recommended to athletes is to avoid the use of high-dose antioxidant supplements and to aim for an adequate intake of vitamins and minerals through a varied and balanced diet to maintain optimal antioxidant status. For an in-depth discussion of the potential effects of antioxidant supplementation on training adaptation and changes in exercise performance, see the book edited by Lamprecht (2015).

Nonsteroidal Anti-Inflammatory Drugs and Training Adaptations

Nonsteroidal anti-inflammatory drugs (NSAIDs), such as ibuprofen, aspirin (acetylsalicylic acid), naproxen, diclofenac, flurbiprofen, and ketoprofen, are perhaps the most widely known therapy in the treatment of muscle damage. Athletes often take these drugs to relieve pain or soreness following strenuous exercise. Some studies show a reduction in muscle pain with the use of these drugs, and some studies show no change. Studies have, however, consistently shown a reduction in the CK response after damaging exercise. The appearance of elevated levels of CK in plasma is often used as a marker of muscle damage, although it does not always correlate well with delayed-onset muscle soreness and other markers of muscle damage, such as loss of strength. NSAIDs inhibit the synthesis of certain prostaglandins, which are potential mediators of edema and pain during acute inflammation. NSAIDs may therefore interfere with the normal inflammatory response after damaging exercise, and it is possible that this inflammatory response plays a role in the adaptation that occurs postexercise. Some evidence indicates that tissue protein synthesis is suppressed following high-intensity eccentric exercise as a result of over-the-counter doses of ibuprofen and paracetamol (1,200 mg and 4,000 mg/day, respectively) (Trappe et al. 2002). Animal studies also provide evidence that NSAIDs can interfere with muscle regeneration and hypertrophy. Given the equivocal acute effects of NSAIDs and their likely negative effect on training adaptation, NSAIDs should not be recommended as a strategy to treat symptoms of muscle damage. These findings provide more evidence that strategies that interfere with the normal signaling pathways have the potential to reduce training adaptations and cause training to be less effective.

Overreaching and the Overtraining Syndrome

We discussed in previous sections the role of nutrition in the development of training adaptations. Athletes often train extremely hard (and even several times a day) to push their bodies to new levels. Often they push their bodies so hard that their performance deteriorates and may be substandard even after several days, weeks, or even months of rest. If recovery takes days, we generally think of this circumstance as normal; if it takes a week or more, we may call this condition overreaching, which could be regarded as an early stage of what is called the overtraining syndrome. Athletes with the overtraining syndrome (also called the unexplained underperformance syndrome by some scientists) have reduced performance and display a number of symptoms, including disturbed eating and sleeping and mood changes (Meeusen et al. 2013). The cardinal symptom of overreaching and the overtraining syndrome is reduced performance. Because reduced performance could also be the result of fatigue, overreaching is diagnosed based on reduced performance in combination with

DEFINITIONS OF OVERREACHING AND OVERTRAINING

Overreaching

An accumulation of training or nontraining stress that results in a short-term decrement in performance capacity with or without related physiological and psychological signs and symptoms of overtraining. Restoration of performance capacity may take from several days to several weeks.

Overtraining

An accumulation of training or nontraining stress that results in a long-term decrement in performance capacity with or without related physiological and psychological signs and symptoms of overtraining. Restoration of performance capacity may take several weeks or months.

sustained disturbances in mood state, consistent inability to perform normal training, and a prolonged recovery period.

Overreaching and the overtraining syndrome can occur when the total of all life stresses (and exercise training is only one of them) exceeds the ability of the body to cope with them. Managing overreaching means that the stresses have to be managed. Because poor nutrition is one of these stresses, we will discuss how nutrition can reduce the symptoms of overreaching and reduce the risk of developing overtraining syndrome.

Overreaching and Muscle Glycogen

Because overreaching is believed to be brought about by high-intensity training with limited recovery, it is thought that the fatigue and underperformance associated with overtraining are at least partly attributable to a decrease in muscle glycogen levels. Therefore, two studies have attempted to elucidate the role of carbohydrate and dietary intake on performance after intensified training.

SYMPTOMS OF OVERTRAINING AND OVERREACHING

Symptoms may be different during overreaching and overtraining and can be highly individual. Not everyone will have all symptoms, and not everyone will have the same symptoms. The following are possible symptoms:

- Drop in performance (note that without a decrease in performance, there is no overtraining or overreaching)
- Feeling washed-out, tired, or drained; lacking energy
- Mild leg soreness, general aches and pains
- Pain in muscles and joints
- Sleeping problems, insomnia
- Headaches
- Decreased immunity (increased number of colds, sore throats)
- Decreased training capacity or intensity, inability to complete training sessions
- Moodiness and irritability
- Depression
- Loss of enthusiasm for the sport
- Decreased appetite, eating problems
- Increased incidence of injuries
- Reduced maximal lactate
- Reduced maximal heart rate
- Elevated resting heart rate, elevated sleeping heart rate
- No increase in cortisol in response to a stressful bout of exercise

Costill et al. (1988) investigated this possibility by examining the effects of 10 days of increased training volume on performance and muscle glycogen levels. Of the 12 swimmers participating in the investigation, four were unable to tolerate the increase from 4,000 to 9,000 m/day and were consequently classified as nonresponders. The group of nonresponders consumed approximately 4.2 MJ (1,000 kcal) per day less than their estimated energy requirement and consumed less carbohydrate than the responders (5.3 vs. 8.2 g per kilogram of body weight per day). Notably, however, muscular power, sprint swimming ability, and swimming endurance ability were not affected in either the responders or the nonresponders. Costill et al. (1988) concluded that the glycogen levels of the nonresponders were sufficient to maintain performance but inadequate for the energy required during training and thus fatigue resulted. Because overreaching and overtraining are primarily defined by a reduction in performance, the ability to ascertain whether the nonresponders were overreached is limited.

These findings directed Snyder et al. (1995) to examine performance responses to intensified training with the addition of sufficient dietary carbohydrate in a bid to determine whether overreaching could still occur in the presence of normal muscle glycogen levels. To ensure sufficient carbohydrate intake, subjects consumed drinks that contained 160 g of carbohydrate in the 2 hours following exercise. Subjects completed 7 days of normal training, 15 days of intensified training, and 6 days of minimal training. Resting muscle glycogen was not significantly different when compared between normal training (531 mmol/kg dry matter) and intensified training (571 mmol/kg dry matter) as determined by needle biopsy of the vastus lateralis muscle. Subjects were reported to be overreached, although maximal power output during an incremental cycle test was not statistically different after intensified training. Only four of the eight subjects demonstrated both a decline in maximal power output and an increase in responses to questionnaires about mood disturbance. Therefore, it appears that in this study, only half of the subjects could be classified as overreached. From the two studies cited earlier, the role of carbohydrate intake and glycogen depletion in overreaching is unclear. Again, this is partly due to inappropriate analysis of performance.

One of the most important performance-determining factors is the resynthesis of muscle glycogen after training or competition. In a study by Costill et al., well-trained runners ran 16 km (10 mi) on three consecutive days (Costill, 1971). Muscle glycogen levels decreased from 141 mmol/kg w.w. after the first run to 73 mmol/kg w.w. after the third run when a 40% to 50% carbohydrate diet was consumed (see figure 6.4). This decrease was much smaller (in fact, muscle glycogen levels were well maintained) when the runners received a high-carbohydrate diet.

Decreased glycogen levels can result in disturbances of the endocrine milieu. Glycogen depletion is related to high levels of catecholamines (epinephrine and norepinephrine), cortisol, and glucagon while insulin levels are very low. Such hormonal responses will result in changes in substrate mobilization and use (e.g., high epinephrine levels in combination with low insulin will increase lipolysis and stimulate the release of fatty acids).

Although insufficient carbohydrate intake (or energy intake) can contribute to the development of overtraining syndrome, overtraining may also develop when carbohydrate intake is adequate. In a study at the University of Maastricht in the Netherlands, the training intensity and volume of well-trained cyclists were increased for two weeks. All cyclists showed signs of overtraining and were classified as overreached. The decrease in performance was accompanied by lower heart rates during exercise (time trial) and lower submaximal and maximal plasma lactate levels (Jeukendrup et al. 1992). Three factors can theoretically explain lower lactate levels. First, lactate clearance may have increased. This occurrence is unlikely because normal training does not induce such an effect. A second explanation could be decreased glycogen concentration. When glycogen levels are low, rates of glycolysis will decrease, and, therefore, lactate formation will be reduced. But when the same research group repeated the study and provided carbohydrate supplements to avoid a decrease in muscle glycogen breakdown, the cyclists still showed signs of overreaching (Snyder et al. 1995). Submaximal and maximal lactate levels again decreased, and muscle glycogen levels remained constant. A third explanation for the lower lactate levels, therefore, could be a decreased sympathetic drive or a reduced sensitivity of adrenoceptors. This view was put forward by Barron et al. (1985) and can be the result of an increased stress level and increased levels of circulating catecholamines. After a while, a downregulation of receptors will occur, which results in decreased sensitivity of the target tissues (e.g., liver, muscles, heart) to catecholamines and a decreased rate of glycolysis and, hence, lower lactate levels.

Because repeated days of hard training and carbohydrate depletion seem to be linked to the development of overreaching, it is tempting to think that carbohydrate supplementation can reverse the symptoms. In a group of runners who ran 16 to 21 km (10-13 mi) daily for 7 days and treated all those runs as races, performance dropped significantly when a moderate carbohydrate intake of 5.5 g per kilogram of body weight per day was maintained (Achten et al. 2004). The runners also displayed a range of symptoms that indicated they were overreached. But when the daily carbohydrate was increased to 8.5 g per kilogram of body weight per day, the drops in performance were much smaller and symptoms were reduced. Recovery from this week of hard training was more complete with the high-carbohydrate treatment. In this study, the dietary intake was strictly controlled and the subjects were fed to maintain energy balance. In a follow-up study, subjects received a carbohydrate supplement, but their dietary intake the rest of the day was recorded but not controlled (Halson et al. 2004). A group of well-trained cyclists were required to perform 8 days of intensive endurance training (normal training volume was doubled). This training was performed on two occasions separated by a washout, or recovery, period of at least 2 weeks. On one occasion, subjects consumed a 2% carbohydrate solution before, during, and after training (moderate carbohydrate), and on the other occasion, subjects consumed a 6.4% carbohydrate solution before and during training and a 20% carbohydrate solution after training (high carbohydrate). Total carbohydrate intake was 6.4 g per kilogram of body weight per day with moderate carbohydrate and 9.4 g per kilogram of body weight per day with high carbohydrate. The intensified training protocol induced overreaching as indicated by a decrease in performance (time to fatigue at ~74% of $\dot{V}O_2max$), although the decrease in performance was significantly less with high carbohydrate intake, suggesting that high-carbohydrate diets can reduce the severity of overreaching. By forcing the subjects to consume supplements that contained a larger amount of carbohydrate, the total energy intake increased as well (13 vs. 16.5 MJ/day [3,107 vs. 3,944 kcal/day] for moderate and high carbohydrate intakes, respectively). Athletes in hard training seem to reduce their spontaneous food intake, and unless they supplement with carbohydrate, they may be in negative energy balance during periods of intensified training. It also appeared that the amount of carbohydrate ingested during training influenced the length of time needed for recovery. After 2 weeks of recovery (reduced volume and intensity) from intensified training with moderate carbohydrate intake, performance remained below that of the baseline, whereas performance improved compared with the baseline after 2 weeks of recovery from intensified training with high carbohydrate intake. Besides carbohydrate depletion, dehydration and negative energy balance can increase the stress response (increased catecholamines, cortisol, and glucagon and reduced insulin levels), which increases the risk of overtraining.

Branched-Chain Amino Acids and Overtraining

In the 1990s, Newsholme et al. (1991) launched a hypothesis in which the amino acid tryptophan was associated with central fatigue. Trp is the precursor of 5-hydroxytryptamine (5-HT; serotonin). During exercise, the plasma concentrations of the BCAAs leucine, isoleucine, and valine decline, and the concentration of free Trp increases. This is caused by an increased concentration of plasma fatty acids during exercise, which forces Trp to be released from its binding sites on albumin. As a result, the ratio of free Trp to BCAA in the plasma increases.

Because BCAA and free Trp use the same transport mechanism (the large neutral amino acid [LNAA] transporter) across the blood–brain barrier, they compete for transport. An increased plasma free Trp to BCAA ratio allows more Trp to enter the brain, which could lead to increased synthesis of 5-HT. An increased concentration of this neurotransmitter in certain areas of the brain could result in fatigue. A situation such as overtraining could result in chronic elevation of the free Trp to BCAA ratio. This circumstance may explain some of the symptoms of the overtraining syndrome. Supplementation of BCAA would reduce the free Trp to BCAA ratio and thereby reduce fatigue. As discussed in chapter 8, however, it seems that BCAA supplementation has no effect on performance. Although the effect on overtraining has not been directly studied, the efficacy of BCAA feedings should be questioned.

Nutrition and Effects on Sleep

Sleep quantity and quality are important for athletes. Sleep has many important physiological and cognitive functions that may be particularly important for physical and mental performance. Recent evidence and anecdotal information suggest that athletes may experience reduced quality or quantity of sleep particularly during periods of intensified training. Lack of sufficient sleep can have significant effects on athletic performance especially for prolonged, submaximal exercise. Compromised sleep may also influence learning, memory, cognition, pain perception, immunity, and inflammation. Furthermore, changes in glucose metabolism and neuroendocrine function due to chronic partial sleep deprivation may result in alterations in carbohydrate metabolism, protein synthesis, appetite, and food intake. These factors can ultimately have a negative influence on an athlete's nutritional, metabolic, and hormonal status and could therefore potentially reduce athletic performance. Research has identified a number of neurotransmitters (e.g., 5-HT, γ-aminobutyric acid, orexin, melanin-concentrating hormone, norepinephrine, histamine) that are associated with the sleep–wake cycle. There are some nutritional interventions that can influence these neurotransmitters in the brain and may also influence sleep. For example, carbohydrate, Trp, valerian, melatonin, and others have been investigated as possible sleep inducers and represent promising potential interventions to improve sleep quantity and quality. Here we examine a few of the factors that influence sleep quality and quantity in athletic populations and consider the potential benefits of nutritional interventions to promote good sleep.

Sleep has important biological functions regarding physiological processes, learning, memory, and cognition. Sleep allows recovery from previous wakefulness and prepares the body for functioning in the subsequent wake period. A person's recent sleep history therefore has an effect on daytime functioning, including exercise and mental performance. Restricting sleep to less than 6 hours per night for 4 or more consecutive nights has been shown to impair cognitive performance, mood, glucose metabolism, appetite regulation, and immune function (Halson 2014). It is generally recommended that adults obtain 8 hours of sleep per night to prevent neurobehavioral deficits. Although there has been considerable scientific research on the amount and quality of sleep needed for optimal function by adults in general, there are few published studies on the sleep habits and requirements of athletes. One common measure of sleep quality is the percentage of time spent sleeping in relation to total time in bed after lights out. This is termed *sleep efficiency*, and in the general adult population it is typically about 90% to 95%. Taking more time to get to sleep and frequent awakenings during the night result in lower sleep efficiency. Sleep quantity and quality can be measured noninvasively by actigraphy, whereby movements and heart rate are continuously monitored by a monitor worn on the wrist. Some actigraphy studies in athletes indicate that sleep efficiency during normal training in cyclists is about 85% to 90%, which is somewhat lower that in the general population (Killer et al. 2015). Furthermore, during periods of intensified training (Killer et al. 2015) or overreaching (Hausswirth et al. 2014), sleep efficiency drops by a further 2% to 6%. Thus, interventions (nutritional or otherwise) that could improve sleep quality during intensified training could allow high-intensity training to be maintained for longer periods or delay the onset of overreaching symptoms such as depressed mood and chronic fatigue, which ultimately promotes better training adaptation.

Dietary precursors can influence the rate of synthesis and function of a small number of neurotransmitters in the brain, including 5-HT and melatonin. Synthesis of 5-HT in the brain is dependent on the availability of its precursor, Trp. As mentioned previously, Trp is transported across the blood–brain barrier by a transport system that is shared by LNAA, including the BCAAs leucine, isoleucine, and valine. Thus, the ratio of Trp to LNAA in the blood is crucial to the rate of transport of Trp into the brain. Ingestion of protein generally decreases the uptake of Trp into the brain because Trp is the least abundant amino acid; therefore, other LNAA are preferentially transported into the brain. The ingestion of carbohydrate, however, increases brain Trp because the rise in circulating insulin (as a result of the increase in blood glucose concentration) stimulates the uptake of LNAA into skeletal muscle; this results in an increase in free Trp in the circulation, which promotes its uptake into the brain. There have been numerous investigations of the effects of Trp supplementation on sleep (for review see Silber and Schmitt 2010), and it appears that Trp doses as low as 1 g can improve sleep latency and subjective sleep quality.

Melatonin is a hormone released from the pineal gland at the base of the brain that transmits information regarding the light–dark cycle and influences the sleep–wake cycle by inducing a sleep-promoting effect. Light exposure of the retinas results in a suppression of melatonin secretion. Some nutritional interventions that increase Trp availability or reduce the plasma concentration of LNAA can increase melatonin production and promote sleep. This can be achieved by several means, including a high protein diet that contains more Trp than LNAA; ingestion of carbohydrate, which may increase the ratio of free Trp to LNAA and facilitate the release of insulin, which promotes the uptake of BCAA into the muscle; ingestion of a high-fat meal, which may increase free fatty acids and result in increased free Trp; and submaximal exercise, which can also increase the circulating concentration of free fatty acids. Research investigating the use of melatonin for primary insomnia has demonstrated inconclusive results. A meta-analysis reported a reduction in sleep-onset latency of 7 minutes and concluded that while melatonin appeared safe for short-term use, there was no evidence that melatonin was effective for most primary sleep disorders (Buscemi et al. 2005). Another nutritional supplement that has received attention and has become particularly popular with game players is tart cherry juice, which contains relatively large amounts of phytochemicals, including melatonin. The ingestion of tart cherry juice has been shown to increase urinary melatonin. When consumed for a 1-week period, it was shown to result in modest improvements in sleep time and quality (Howatson et al. 2012) compared with placebo.

Studies on the effects of carbohydrate ingestion on indices of sleep quality and quantity (reviewed by Halson 2013) indicate that high carbohydrate meals consumed in the hour before bedtime improve sleep quality and reduce wakefulness. Solid compared with liquid meals tend to reduce sleep onset latency (time to fall asleep) up to 3 hours after ingestion, and a high glycemic index meal significantly improves sleep-onset latency compared to a low glycemic index meal if it is consumed 4 hours (but not 1 hour) before bedtime. A few studies have investigated more chronic manipulations of habitual dietary intake on sleep, and these suggested that diets higher in carbohydrate result in shorter sleep-onset latencies, diets higher in protein result in fewer wake episodes, and diets high in fat may negatively influence total sleep time.

Valerian is an herb that binds to γ-aminobutyric acid type A receptors and is thought to induce a calming effect by regulation of the nervous system. Results of a meta-analysis investigating the efficacy of valerian showed a subjective improvement in sleep quality (Fernandez-San-Martin et al. 2010). Although valerian is one of the more common ingredients found in supplements that claim to promote sleep, side effects such as daytime drowsiness, dizziness, and allergic reactions have been observed.

There are numerous other traditional sleep aids, including passionflower, kava, St. John's wort, lysine, glycine, magnesium, lavender, skullcap, lemon balm, magnolia bark, and nucleotides. Although most of these have not been adequately investigated in the scientific literature, many can be found in supplements that are claimed to improve sleep quantity and quality.

The following are some practical recommendations to improve sleep via nutritional interventions:

- High glycemic index foods, such as white rice, pasta, bread, and potatoes, may promote sleep, but they should be consumed more than 1 hour before bedtime.
- High-carbohydrate diets may result in shorter sleep latencies.
- High-protein diets may result in improved sleep quality.
- High-fat diets may negatively influence total sleep time.
- When total caloric intake is decreased, sleep quality may be disturbed.
- Small doses of tryptophan (1 g) may improve sleep latency and sleep quality. This can be achieved by consuming a supplement or approximately 300 g of turkey.
- The hormone melatonin and foods that have a high melatonin concentration (e.g., tart cherries) may decrease sleep onset time.
- Subjective sleep quality may be improved with the ingestion of the herb valerian.

Nutrition and Effects on Rehabilitation

Injuries are an unavoidable aspect of participation in sport and high levels of physical activity. Nutrition is important for optimal wound healing and recovery, but little information about nutritional support for injuries exists. After skeletal muscle injury, a regeneration process takes place to repair muscle. Immediately following injury, wound healing begins with an inflammatory response. Excessive anti-inflammatory measures during this early period after injury may impair recovery. Many injuries result in prolonged periods of limb immobilization to reduce further potential damage and allow repair of bone and skeletal muscle and connective tissue. Immobilization results in muscle disuse and consequently a loss of muscle mass due to increased periods of negative muscle protein balance that results from decreased basal muscle protein synthesis and resistance to anabolic stimuli, including protein ingestion. The extent of muscle loss during injury strongly influences the level and duration of rehabilitation required. Therefore, consideration should be given to nutritional strategies to reduce muscle loss. During rehabilitation and recovery, nutritional needs are very much like those for any athlete who desires muscle hypertrophy to increase strength and power (Tipton 2013). Reduced physical activity during recovery from injury will result in a decrease of muscle oxidative capacity and loss of aerobic fitness. Therefore, physical training programs will need to be designed to restore endurance and muscle strength to preinjury levels during the rehabilitation period.

Skeletal muscle recovery is a highly coordinated process that involves cross talk between immune and muscle cells. Studies have demonstrated that nutrients such as amino acids, n-3 polyunsaturated fatty acids, polyphenols, and vitamin D can improve skeletal muscle regeneration by targeting key functions of immune cells, muscle cells, or both. For a detailed review, see Wall, Morton, and van Loon (2015). Intake of supplemental vitamin D_3 (1,000-4,000 IU/ day), additional protein, and adequate energy in combination with treatment and resistance training promotes recovery after injury and improved capacity to exercise. The most important consideration is to avoid malnutrition; nutrient and energy deficiencies should be avoided. Energy expenditure may be reduced during immobilization, but inflammation, wound healing, and the energy cost of ambulation limit the reduction of energy expenditure. Neuromuscular electrical stimulation may be applied to evoke involuntary muscle contractions and support muscle mass maintenance in the injured athlete. During rehabilitation and recovery from immobilization, increased activity (especially resistance exercise) will increase muscle protein synthesis and restore sensitivity to anabolic stimuli. Ample, but not excessive, protein and energy must be consumed to support muscle growth. Dietary protein consumption is of critical importance for stimulating muscle protein synthesis rates throughout the day. Given that the injured athlete greatly reduces physical activity levels, maintaining muscle mass while avoiding gains in fat mass can be challenging. Nevertheless, evidence suggests that maintaining or increasing daily protein intake by focusing on the amount, type, and timing of dietary protein ingestion throughout the day (see chapter 8 for an in-depth discussion of these issues) can restrict the loss of muscle mass and strength during recovery from injury. There is also a theoretical rationale for leucine and omega-3 fatty acid supplementation to help reduce muscle atrophy (Tipton 2013). Although more applied work is required to translate laboratory findings directly to the injured athlete, current recommendations for those who want to limit the loss of muscle mass and strength following injury can be summarized as follows:

- Avoid nutrient and energy deficiencies.
- Ingest 1,000 to 4,000 IU of supplemental vitamin D_3 daily and ingest 1 to 2 g of omega-3 fatty acid supplements daily.
- Ingest sufficient dietary energy to maintain energy balance.
- During rehabilitation, when resistance training is possible, ingest protein in the postexercise period in sufficient doses ($\sim$0.4 g per kilogram of body weight per meal) and in up to three other meals distributed throughout; the total daily dietary protein intake should be 1.4 to 1.6 g per kilogram of body weight.
- Choose rapidly digested proteins with a high leucine content for the postexercise meal (e.g., whey, skim milk).
- For other meals, choose mostly lean, high-quality proteins that contain all the essential amino acids in approximately equal proportions (e.g., beef, ham, lamb, poultry, fish).

Key Points

- Exercise leads to adaptations that eventually result in improved physiological function. Exercise training makes use of this principle by planning and systematically applying exercise activities with the goal of optimizing these adaptations and thus improving performance.
- Adaptations to exercise or exercise training are specific to the exercise performed. Resistance exercise results in muscle hypertrophy, which makes the muscle stronger, and endurance training, which results in increased oxidative capacity and makes the muscle more fatigue resistant.
- Training adaptations in skeletal muscle may be generated by the cumulative effects of transient increases in gene transcription during recovery from repeated bouts of exercise.
- The complex process of exercise-induced adaptation in skeletal muscle starts with specific molecular events that trigger an increase in protein synthesis. Signaling mechanisms triggered by exercise stress initiate replication of DNA genetic sequences that enable subsequent translation of the genetic code into a series of amino acids to synthesize new proteins.
- Signal transduction pathways control the transcription of genes (specific sequences of DNA) into mRNA, the translation of mRNA into protein, the protein modification that alters catalytic activity, the regulation of protein degradation, and the regulation of cell division, proliferation, and fusion.
- During exercise, changes in muscle stretch or tension, intracellular calcium ion concentrations, the energy charge of the cell, and the redox potential are primary signals that may then trigger a series of secondary molecular events that can increase protein synthesis.
- AMPK is activated by a high AMP to ATP ratio and plays a crucial role in energy metabolism by acting as a metabolic master switch that regulates several intracellular systems, including the cellular uptake of glucose, the ß-oxidation of fatty acids, and the synthesis of GLUT4 and biogenesis of mitochondria.
- Insulin and insulin-like growth factor pathways play an important role in muscle hypertrophy through the Akt-mTOR signaling cascade.
- PGCs are important in driving mitochondrial biogenesis.
- The rate of protein synthesis depends on mRNA degradation, additional translational control mechanisms, transport of mRNA out of the nucleus, and the translation process.
- A single bout of endurance exercise will increase transcription or mRNA content for various metabolic and stress-related genes.
- Substrate availability during exercise (e.g., low muscle glycogen) can increase metabolic gene transcription, which suggests that modification of the training response may be possible with specific dietary interventions.
- Although results of some studies suggest that training with low glycogen could have some metabolic advantages, whether this can also result in improvements in performance is not clear.
- BCAAs, particularly leucine, are signaling molecules and building blocks for protein synthesis. Although the BCAAs alone can stimulate signals in the muscle, this increased signaling will not result in increased synthesis if other amino acids in the blood are not available.
- Antioxidant supplementation may decrease training efficiency by preventing some cellular adaptations to exercise.

- Although a high-carbohydrate diet can maintain muscle glycogen stores and reduce or delay symptoms of overreaching during prolonged periods of intensified training, overreaching cannot be prevented by high carbohydrate intake.
- Modest improvements in sleep quality can be achieved through nutritional interventions. High-carbohydrate diets result in shorter sleep-onset latencies, high-protein diets result in fewer wake episodes, and high-fat diets may negatively influence total sleep time.
- During rehabilitation and recovery, nutritional needs are very much like those for any athlete who desires muscle hypertrophy to increase strength and power. Maintaining or increasing daily protein intake by focusing on the amount, type, and timing of dietary protein ingestion throughout the day can restrict the loss of muscle mass and strength during recovery from injury. Nutrients such as amino acids, n-3 polyunsaturated fatty acids, polyphenols, and vitamin D can improve skeletal muscle regeneration by targeting key functions of immune cells, muscle cells, or both.

Recommended Readings

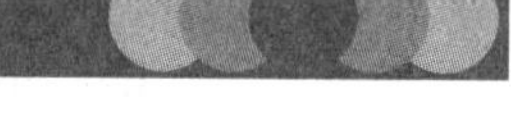

Egan, B., J.A. Hawley, and J.R. Zierath. 2016. Snapshot: Exercise metabolism. *Cell Metabolism* 24 (2): 342-342.

Egan, B., and J.R. Zierath. 2013. Exercise metabolism and the molecular regulation of skeletal muscle adaptation. *Cell Metabolism* 17 (2): 162-184.

Hargreaves, M., and D. Cameron-Smith. 2002. Exercise, diet, and skeletal muscle gene expression. *Medicine and Science in Sports and Exercise* 34:1505-1508.

Hawley, J.A., M. Hargreaves, M.J. Joyner, and J.R. Zierath. 2014. Integrative biology of exercise. *Cell* 159 (4): 738-749.

Hawley, J.A., and J.P. Morton. 2014. Ramping up the signal: Promoting endurance training adaptation in skeletal muscle by nutritional manipulation. *Clinical and Experimental Pharmacology and Physiology* 41 (8): 608-613.

Hawley, J.A., K.D. Tipton, and M.L. Millard-Stafford. 2006. Promoting training adaptations through nutritional interventions. *Journal of Sports Sciences* 24 (7): 709-721.

Hoppeler, H. 2016. Molecular networks in skeletal muscle plasticity. *Journal of Experimental Biology* 219 (Pt 2): 205-213.

Hoppeler, H., and M. Fluck. 2003. Plasticity of skeletal muscle mitochondria: Structure and function. *Medicine and Science in Sports and Exercise* 35:95-104.

Lamprecht, M., ed. 2015. *Antioxidants in sport nutrition.* Boca Raton, FL: CRC Press/Taylor & Francis.

Peternelj, T.T., and J.S. Coombes. 2011. Antioxidant supplementation during exercise training: Beneficial or detrimental? *Sports Medicine* 41 (12): 1043-1069.

Slattery K., D. Bentley, and A.J. Coutts. 2015. The role of oxidative, inflammatory and neuroendocrinological systems during exercise stress in athletes: Implications of antioxidant supplementation on physiological adaptation during intensified physical training. *Sports Medicine* 45 (4): 453-471.

Spriet, L.L., and M.J. Gibala. 2004. Nutritional strategies to influence adaptations to training. *Journal of Sports Sciences* 22:127-141.

Wall, B.T., J.P. Morton, and L.J.C. van Loon. 2015. Strategies to maintain skeletal muscle mass in the injured athlete: Nutritional considerations and exercise mimetics. *European Journal of Sport Science* 15(1): 53-62.

Nutrition and Immune Function in Athletes

Objectives

After studying this chapter, you should be able to do the following:

- Describe the main components and functional mechanisms of the immune system
- Describe the common illnesses and allergies that are experienced by athletes
- Distinguish between infection, allergy, and intolerance
- Describe the effects of exercise and training on immune function and susceptibility to infection
- Describe the mechanisms by which nutrition may influence immune function
- Describe the roles of several vitamins and minerals that are required to maintain immune function
- Discuss nutritional strategies that may be effective in improving immune function or reducing exercise-induced immunodepression
- Comment on studies that have investigated the effects of nutritional supplements on exercise-induced immunodepression
- Describe groups of athletes who may be at increased risk for immunodepression and susceptibility to infection

The **immune system** is involved in tissue repair after injury and in the protection of the body against potentially damaging (pathogenic) microorganisms such as bacteria, viruses, and fungi. In some circumstances, the immune system can become functionally depressed (known as **immunodepression**), which may result in an increased susceptibility to infection. Several forms of stress, including a heavy schedule of training and competition, can lead to immunodepression in athletes, which places them at greater risk for opportunistic infections and particularly upper respiratory tract infections (URTIs). An abundance of epidemiological evidence and clinical data suggest that nutritional deficiencies impair immune function and increase the risk of infection and that even medically harmless infections may significantly impair athletic performance.

Although many factors influence exercise-induced immunodepression (e.g., physical, environmental, and psychological stresses), nutrition plays a critical role. This chapter examines the role of

---

nutrition in exercise-induced immunodepression and the effects of excessive and insufficient nutrient intakes on immune function. Because much of the present literature concerning nutrition and immune function is based on studies with sedentary subjects, the need for research that directly investigates the interrelationship between exercise immunology and nutrition is emphasized. Some important questions that must be answered include the following:

- Which aspects of nutrition are crucial to normal immune function? Are the reported dietary practices of athletes optimal for immune function?
- Do any specific nutritional practices impair immune function or exacerbate the temporary immunodepression that follows an acute bout of prolonged strenuous exercise?
- Does feeding of supplements (e.g., carbohydrate, amino acids, vitamins) during and after prolonged exercise reduce the stress on the immune system?
- Can nutrient supplements reduce the risk of infection after heavy exertion?
- What practical guidelines can be given to athletes to help them reduce their risk of infection?

Because readers of this book are unlikely to have detailed knowledge of the physiology of the immune system, the following section provides a summary of the main components of the immune system and their role in defending the body against pathogenic microorganisms.

Functions of the Immune System and Its Cellular Components

Simply put, the immune system recognizes, attacks, and destroys things that are foreign to the body. The functions of this homeostatic system are actually far more complex and involve the precise coordination of many cell types and molecular messengers. Like any other homeostatic system, the immune system is composed of redundant mechanisms to ensure that essential processes are carried out.

The immune system has two broad functions, innate (natural, or nonspecific) immunity and adaptive (acquired, or specific) immunity, which work synergistically. The attempt of an infectious agent to enter the body immediately activates the innate system. This first line of defense comprises three general mechanisms (see figure 13.1) that have the common goal of restricting microorganism entry into the body:

1. Physical or structural barriers (skin, epithelial linings, and mucosal secretions)
2. Chemical barriers (pH of bodily fluids and soluble factors)
3. Phagocytic cells (e.g., **neutrophils** and **macrophages** or **monocytes**)

Failure of the innate system and the resulting infection activates the adaptive system, which aids recovery from infection. Adaptive immunity is helped greatly by T-lymphocyte and B-lymphocyte acquisition of receptors that recognize the foreign molecules (called antigens) and engender specificity and memory that enable the immune system to mount an augmented response when the host is reinfected by the same **pathogen.**

The components of the immune system comprise cellular and soluble elements, which are listed in table 13.1. The white blood cells (**leukocytes**) have diverse functions despite their common origin from the stem cells of the bone marrow. Leukocytes consist of the granulocytes (60%-70%), monocytes (10%-15%), and **lymphocytes** (20%-25%). Various subsets of the latter can be identified through use of monoclonal antibodies, which are used to identify specific proteins (clusters of differentiation or cluster designators [CD]) that are expressed on the cell surface of a particular cell type. For example, all T-lymphocytes express the protein CD3 on the cell surface and so are designated as CD3+. B-lymphocytes do not express CD3 but express CD19, CD20, and CD22. A subset of T-lymphocytes called helper T-cells specifically express the CD4 protein, whereas the cytotoxic T-cells express CD8. T-cells recognize short peptide sequences from antigens only if they are held on the surface of the cell and complexed with a major histocompatibility complex (MHC) molecule. The characteristics of the various cells of the immune system are summarized in tables 13.2 and 13.3, and the relative distribution of these cells in the blood compartment is illustrated in figure 13.2. The ability of the immune system to distinguish self from nonself depends largely on the MHC, a group of protein markers that is present on the surface of every cell and is slightly different in each person.

Soluble factors of the immune system activate leukocytes, neutralize (kill) foreign agents, and

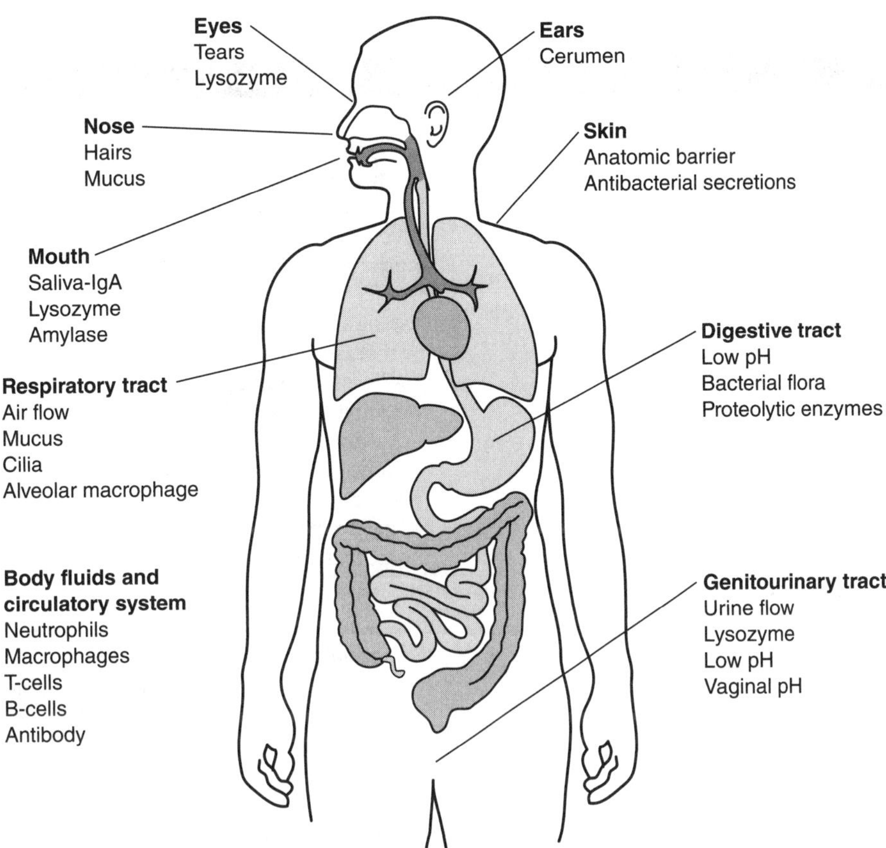

Figure 13.1 The body's barriers and innate defenses against invading microorganisms.

TABLE 13.1 Main Components of the Immune System

Innate components	Adaptive components
Cellular	**Cellular**
Natural killer cells (CD16+ and CD56+) Phagocytes (neutrophils, eosinophils, basophils, monocytes, and macrophages)	T-cells (CD3+, CD4+, and CD8+) B-cells (CD19+, CD20+, and CD22+)
Soluble	**Soluble**
Acute-phase proteins Complement Lysozymes Cytokines (interleukins [IL], interferons [IFN], colony-stimulating factors [CSF], tumor necrosis factors [TNF])	Immunoglobulins (IgA, IgD, IgE, IgG, and IgM)

regulate the immune system. The factors include the **cytokines**, which are proteins that act as chemical messenger substances (like hormones) to stimulate the growth, differentiation, and functional development of immune system cells through specific receptor sites on secretory cells (autocrine function) or on immediately adjacent cells (paracrine function). Cytokine action is not confined to the immune system; cytokines also influence the central nervous system and the neuroendocrine system.

Other soluble factors include **complement**, lysozyme, and the specific antibodies formed by the reaction of B-cell-derived **immunoglobulins (Ig)**

TABLE 13.2 Characteristics of Leukocytes

Leukocyte	Main characteristics
Granulocytes	60%-70% of leukocytes
Neutrophils	>90% of granulocytes Phagocytose (i.e., ingest and destroy) bacteria and other foreign material (antigens) Have a receptor for antibody: phagocytose antibody–antigen complexes
Eosinophils	2%-5% of granulocytes Display little or no capacity to recharge their killing mechanisms once activated
Basophils	0%-2% of granulocytes Phagocytose parasites Triggered by IgG to release toxic lysosomal products Produce chemotactic factors The basophils found in tissues other than blood are called mast cells, which release an eosinophil chemotactic factor
Monocytes or macrophages	10%-15% of leukocytes Egress into tissues (e.g., liver and spleen) and differentiate into the mature form: the macrophage Phagocytose bacteria and viruses enabling antigen presentation Secrete immunomodulatory cytokines Retain their capacity to divide after leaving the bone marrow
Lymphocytes	20%-25% of leukocytes Activate other lymphocyte subsets Produce lymphokines Recognize antigens Produce antibodies Exhibit memory Exhibit cytotoxicity

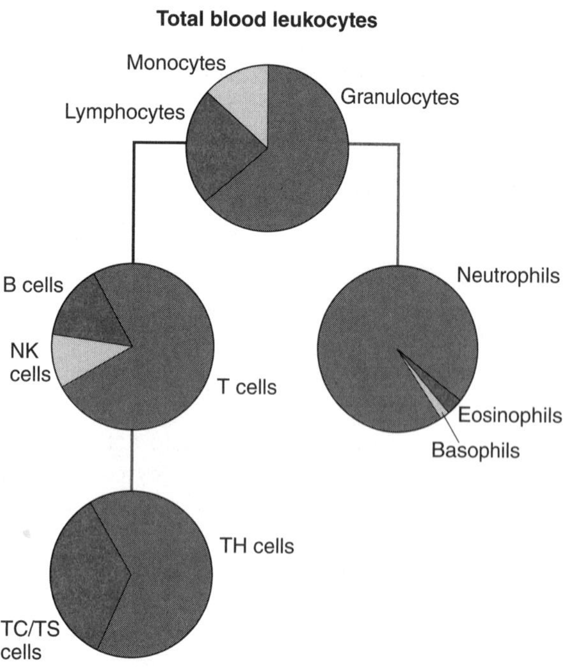

Figure 13.2 The average distribution of the different leukocyte subsets in the blood compartment at rest in a healthy adult. B = bursa- or bone-marrow derived; NK = natural killer; T = thymus derived; TH = T helper; TC/TS= T cytotoxic/suppressor.

with specific antigens. The actions of the innate soluble factors are summarized in table 13.4. The immunoglobulins are defined by the structure of the constant region of their heavy chains, which are associated with differences in biological activity and function.

General Mechanisms of the Immune Response

The introduction of an infectious agent to the body initiates an inflammatory response that augments the response of the immune system. Acute **inflam-**

TABLE 13.3 Lymphocyte Functions and Characteristics

Lymphocyte subset	Main functions and characteristic
T-cells (CD3+) TH (CD4+)	60%-75% of lymphocytes 60%-70% of T-cells Helper T-cells Recognize antigen to coordinate the acquired response Secrete cytokines that stimulate T-cell and B-cell proliferation and differentiation
TC/TS (CD8+)	30%-40% of T-cells TS (suppressor T-cells) involved in the regulation of B-cell and other T-cell proliferation by suppressing certain functions TS may be important in switching off the immune response TC (cytotoxic T-cells) kill a variety of targets, including some tumor cells
B-cells (CD19+, CD20+, and CD22+)	5%-15% of lymphocytes Produce and secrete Ig specific to the activating antigen Exhibit memory
Natural killer (NK) cells (CD16+ and CD56+)	10%-20% of lymphocytes Large, granular lymphocytes Express spontaneous cytolytic activity against a variety of tumor-infected and virus-infected cells MHC independent Do not express the CD3 cell-surface antigen Triggered by IgG Control foreign materials until the antigen-specific immune system responds

TABLE 13.4 Producers and Actions of the Innate Soluble Factors

Soluble factor	Producers and immune actions
Cytokines IL-1	Produced mainly from activated macrophages IL-1α tends to remain cell associated IL-1ß acts as a soluble mediator Stimulates IL-2 production from CD3+ and CD4+ cells Increases IL-1 and IL-2 receptor expression Increases B-cell proliferation Increases TNF-α, IL-6, and CSF levels Stimulates secretion of prostaglandins
IL-2	Produced mainly by CD4+ cells Stimulates T-cell and B-cell proliferation and expression of IL-2 receptors on their surfaces Stimulates release of IFN Stimulates NK cell proliferation and killing
IL-6	Produced by activated helper T-cells, fibroblasts, and macrophages; also released from exercising muscle Stimulates the differentiation of B-cells, inflammation, and the acute-phase response Endogenous pyrogen (induces fever)
TNF-α	Produced from monocytes, T-cells, B-cells, and NK cells Enhances tumor cell killing and antiviral activity
Acute-phase proteins (APP)	Made in the liver and secreted into the blood Encourage cell migration to sites of injury and infection Activate complement Stimulate phagocytosis
Complement	Found in the serum Consists of 20 or more proteins Stimulates phagocytosis, antigen presentation, and neutralization of infected cells Amplifies the response

CSF = colony stimulating factor; IFN = interferon; IL = interleukin; NK = natural killer; TNF = tumor necrosis factor.

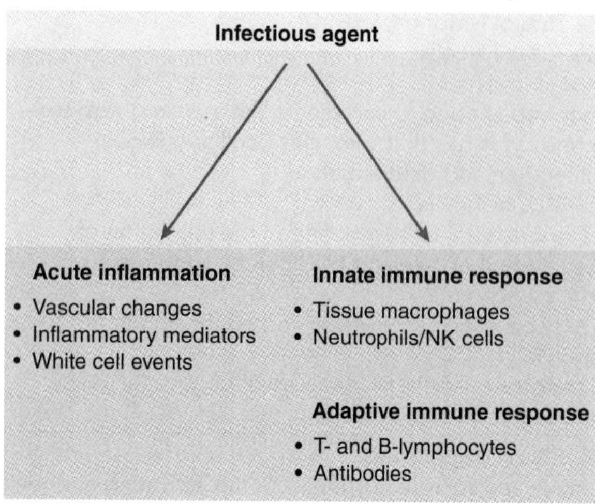

Figure 13.3 The relationship between the inflammatory and the immune response.

mation increases local blood flow in the infected area, which, coupled with increased permeability of blood capillaries, facilitates the entry of leukocytes and plasma proteins into the infected tissue (see figure 13.3). The immune response itself varies according to the nature of the infectious agent (parasitic, bacterial, fungal, and viral), but a general response pattern is evident, as illustrated in figure 13.4. The key player is the macrophage, which expresses toll-like receptors (TLRs) on its cell surface that detect the presence of certain molecules on the surface of microorganisms and subsequently initiates an immune response to destroy potentially harmful invaders. The macrophage ingests foreign material and presents antigens on its cell surface that, in turn, activate T-lymphocytes and B-lymphocytes specific for the antigen. Infectious agents also activate nonspecific (innate) host defense mechanisms, including complement, phagocytic cells (e.g., neutrophils), and NK cells.

The action of the macrophage on the invading microorganism initiates a chain of events. The macrophage first ingests the foreign organism and isolates it within a membranous vesicle (vacuole) inside the cell (phagocytosis). Digestive enzymes (e.g., lysozyme and elastase) and oxidizing agents (e.g., hydrogen peroxide) are secreted by the macrophage. The foreign proteins

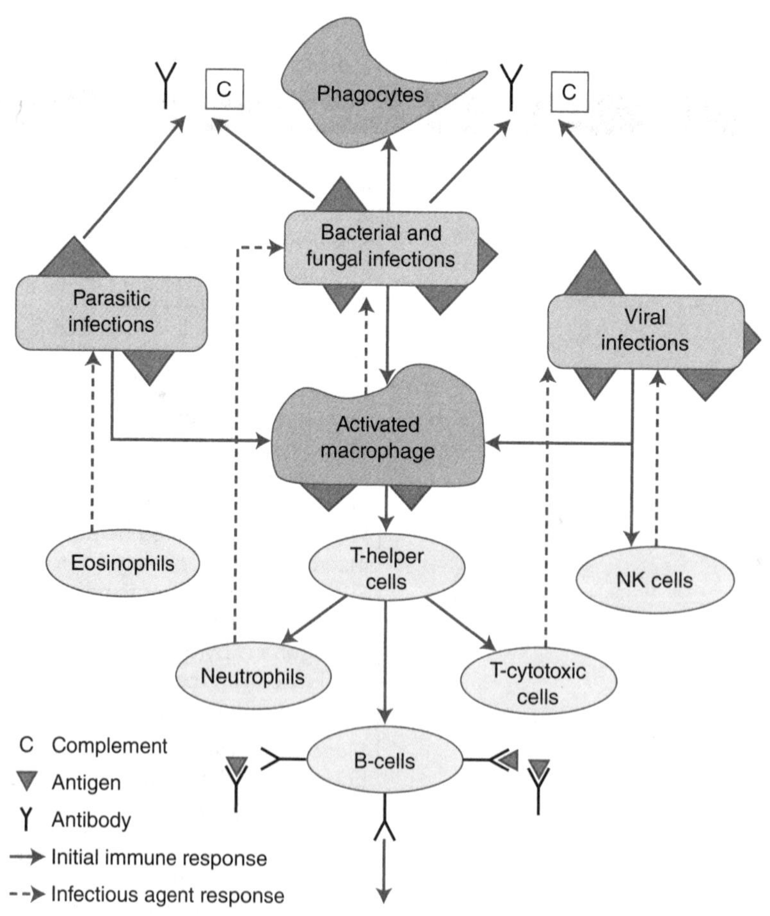

Figure 13.4 The general scheme of the immune response to various infectious agents.

(antigens) normally found on the surface of the microorganism are digested and processed by the macrophage and incorporated into its own cell surface. The antigen can now be presented to the other cellular immune components. Helper T-cells (CD4+) coordinate the response through cytokine release to activate other immune cells. Mature B-cell stimulation results in proliferation and differentiation into immunoglobulin-secreting (**antibody**-secreting) plasma cells. Reaction of the immunoglobulin with a specific antigen forms an antibody–antigen complex. Antibodies are essential to antigen recognition and memory of earlier exposure to specific antigens.

Clonal Selection and Immunological Memory

An antigen that enters the body selectively activates only a tiny fraction of the quiescent lymphocytes, which then grow and divide to form a clone of identical effector cells (clonal selection). Each antigen (usually a foreign protein or lipopolysaccharide) carries several antigenic determinants that each activate a different clone, and an invading bacterium carries a number of antigens. So, a particular species of bacterium invading the body activates a number of clones of lymphocytes.

The first encounter with any antigen causes the primary immune response to that antigen. After several days, clones of lymphocytes selected by the antigen multiply and differentiate to become effector B-cells and T-cells. After several more days, specific antibodies from B-cells appear in the blood, as illustrated in figure 13.5. During the lag time, pathogenic organisms may enter the body and multiply in sufficient numbers to cause illness.

A second exposure to the same antigen (even years later) produces a much quicker, stronger, and longer-lasting secondary response. This response depends on memory cells, which are produced at the same time as effector cells during the primary response. Effector cells usually last for only a few days, but memory cells may last for decades. When a second exposure to an antigen occurs, memory cells rapidly multiply and differentiate to create a large number of effector cells and a large quantity of antibodies dedicated to attacking the antigen. This enhanced antibody response usually prevents symptoms of infection from developing (i.e., immunity to the antigen has been acquired).

Cellular Immune Response

Many pathogens, including all viruses, are parasites that can reproduce only within host body cells. The

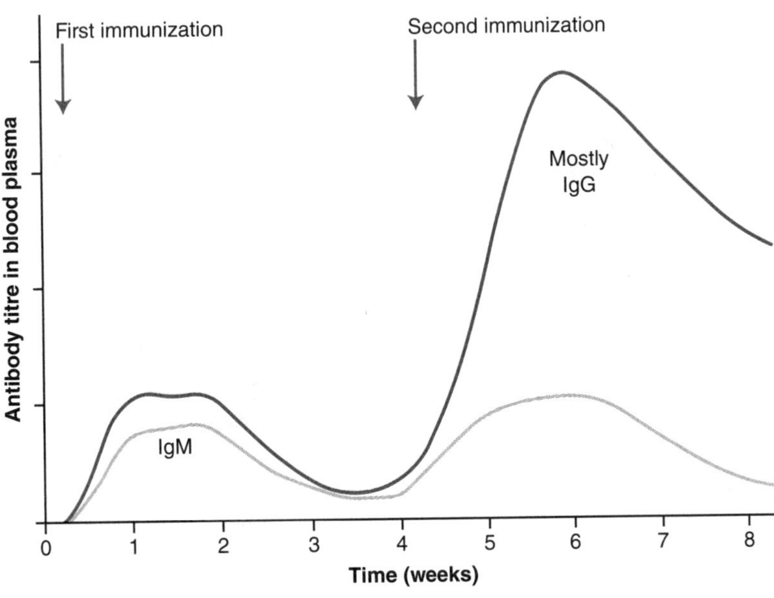

Figure 13.5 Specific antibody production (IgM and IgG subclasses) after first exposure to an antigen (at 0 weeks) and on subsequent exposure to the same antigen (at 4 weeks). Note the markedly larger and more rapid IgG response after the second exposure.

cellular immune response fights pathogens that have already entered cells. Activated T-lymphocytes include memory cells and cytotoxic T-cells (killer cells) that attack infected host cells or foreign cells. Helper T-cells and suppressor T-cells are also important in mobilizing and regulating the whole immune response.

When helper T-cells bind to specific antigenic determinants displayed with MHC proteins on the cell surface of macrophages, the macrophage is stimulated to release a cytokine called **interleukin**-1 (IL-1), which causes the T-cells to grow and divide. The activated T-cells release another cytokine, IL-2, which further stimulates proliferation and growth of helper T-cells and cytotoxic T-cells (see figure 13.6). IL-2 and other cytokines from helper T-cells also stimulate B-cells to respond to specific antigens by differentiating into antibody-forming plasma cells. Cytotoxic T-cells recognize and attach to cells that have on their surface appropriate antigenic determinants coupled with the MHC complex. Cytotoxic T-cells then release perforin, a protein that causes puncture of the cell membrane so that a lethal cocktail of digestive enzymes can be passed from the T-cell into the infected cell, causing cell necrosis (death) and lysis (breakup) of the infected host cell. NK cells exert cytotoxic activity in a similar way. The fragments of the lysed cell are then ingested and digested by **phagocytes**.

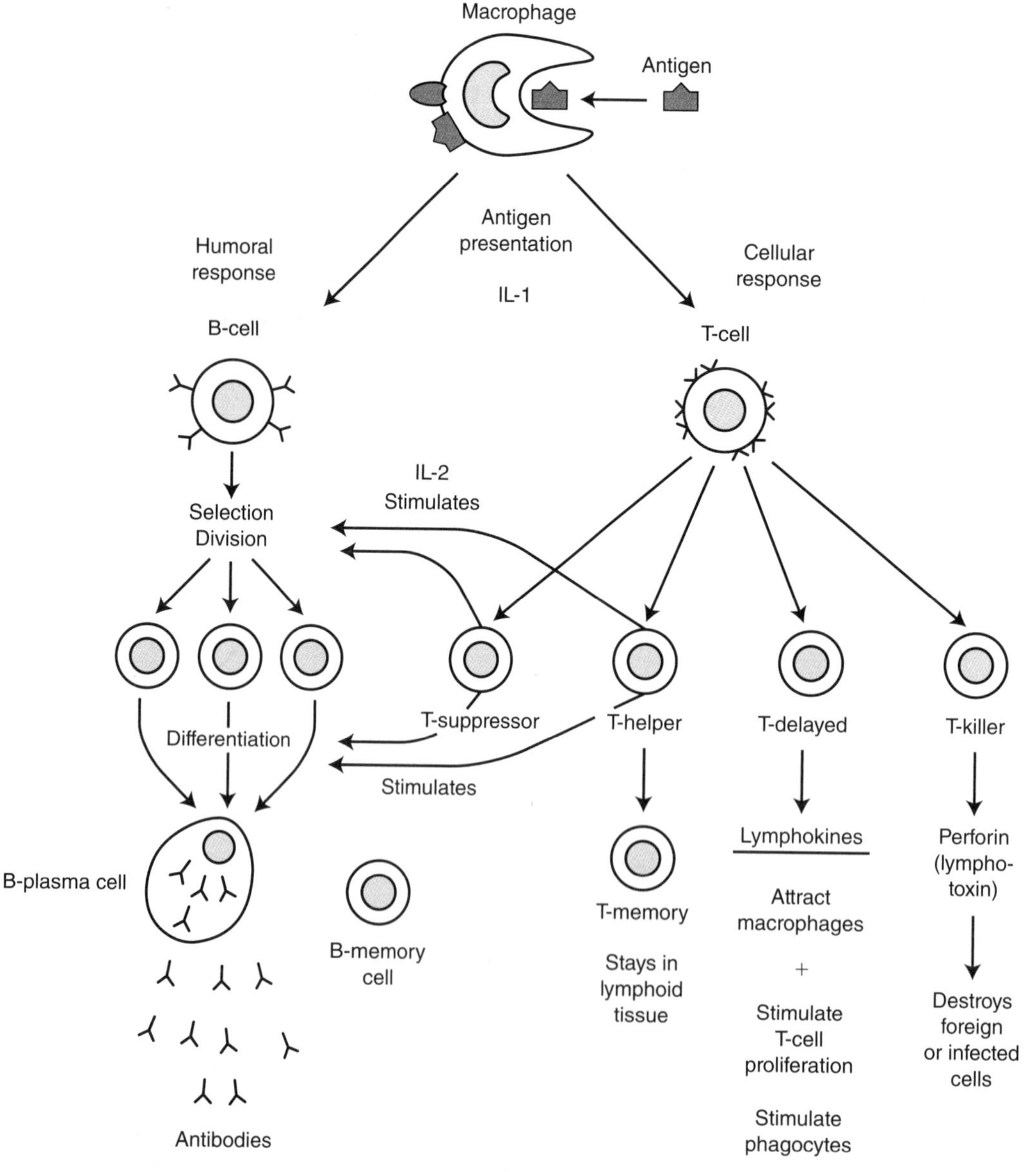

Figure 13.6 The cellular immune response (showing interaction with humoral response).

Humoral (Fluid) Immune Response

B-lymphocytes are also coated with receptors that are specific for particular antigenic determinants. Most antigens activate B-cells only when the B-cells are stimulated by cytokines from helper T-cells; they are T-cell-dependent antigens. Some antigens are T-cell independent. They usually have a repetitive structure and bind with several receptors on the B-cell surface at once (capping). As shown in figure 13.7, the antigen is taken into the cell and activates it. Exposure to an antigen causes appropriate clones of B-cells to proliferate and differentiate into memory cells and plasma cells. The latter are the effector cells of **humoral** immunity and can secrete a large amount of antibody during their brief life of 4 to 5 days.

The antibodies circulate in the blood and lymph and bind to antigen and contribute to the destruction of the organism bearing it. Antibodies belong to a class of proteins called immunoglobulins. Each antibody molecule can bind to a specific antigen and assist with the destruction of the antigen. Every antibody has separate regions for each of these two functions. The regions that bind the antigen differ from molecule to molecule and are called variable regions. Only a few humoral

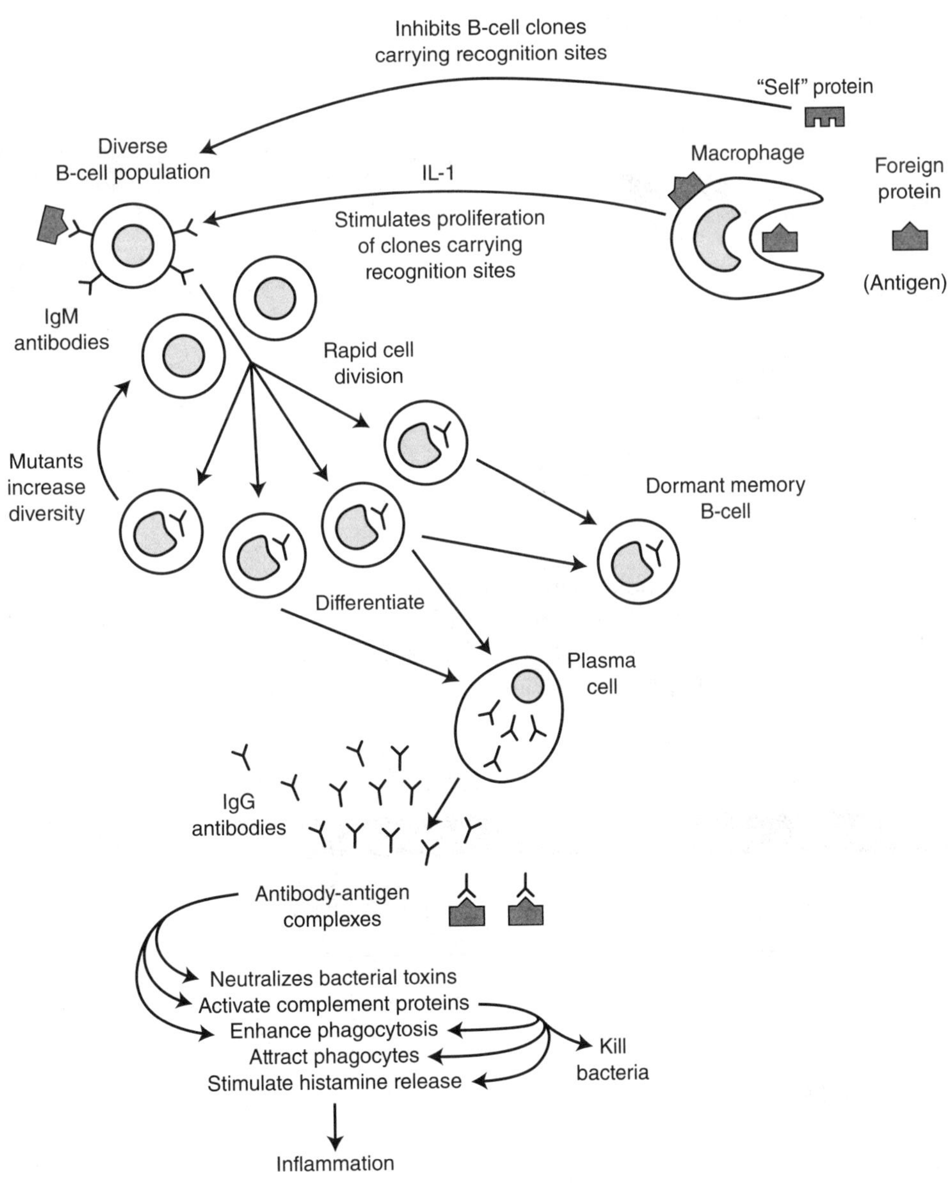

Figure 13.7 The humoral immune response.

effector mechanisms exist to destroy antigens, so only a few kinds of regions—the constant regions—are involved. An antibody molecule consists of two pairs of polypeptide chains: two short, identical light (L) chains and two longer, identical heavy (H) chains. The chains are joined together to form a Y-shaped molecule (see figure 13.8). The variable regions of H chains and L chains are located at the ends of the arms of the Y, where they form the antigen-binding sites. Thus, each antibody molecule has two antigen-binding sites, one at each tip of the antibody's two arms. The rest of the antibody molecule, which consists of the constant regions of the H and L chains, determines the effector function of the antibody. Along with the five types of constant region are five major classes of antibodies called IgM, IgG, IgA, IgD, and IgE. Their different roles in the immune response are described in table 13.5. Within each class is a multitude of subpopulations of antibodies, each specific to a particular antigen.

Antibodies cannot destroy antigen-bearing invaders directly. Instead, they tag foreign molecules and cells for destruction by various effector mechanisms. Each mechanism is triggered by the selective binding of antigens to antibodies to form antigen–antibody complexes. The antibodies may simply block the potential toxic actions of some antigens (neutralization), or they may cause antigens or foreign cells to clump together (agglutination); these can then be ingested by phagocytes (see figure 13.9). Precipitation is a similar mechanism in which soluble antigen molecules are cross-linked to form inactive and immobile precipitates that are captured by phagocytes. Antibody–antigen complexes on the surfaces of invading microor-

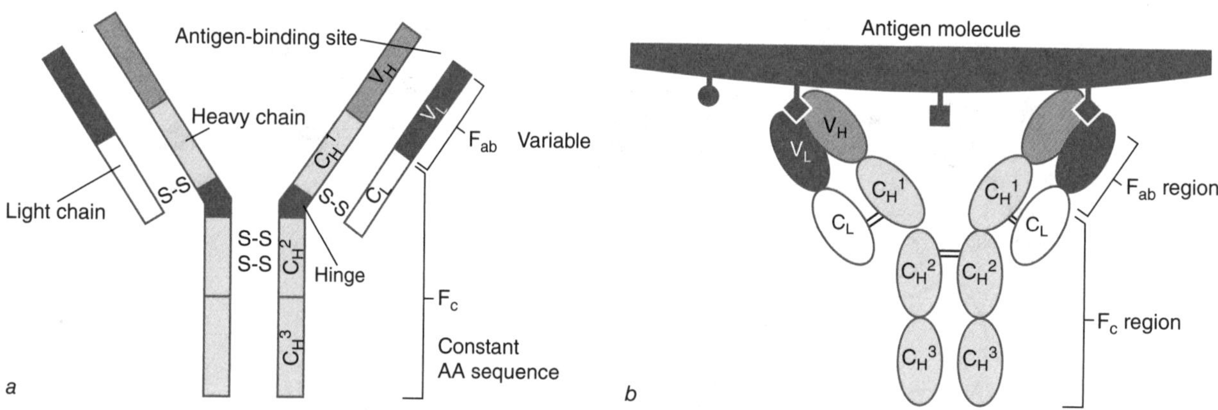

Figure 13.8 The structure of immunoglobulins or antibodies. *(a)* Antibodies are composed of two heavy polypeptide chains (H) and two light polypeptide chains (L). *(b)* Variable (V) and constant (C) regions within the heavy and light chains. Antigens combine with the variable regions as shown in *(b)*. Each antibody molecule is divided into an F_{ab} (antigen-binding) fragment and an F_c (constant) fragment.

TABLE 13.5 Physiological Properties of the Five Classes of Ig in Extracellular Fluid

Class	Mean adult serum level (g/L)	Serum half-life (days)	Physiological function
IgM	1.0	5	Complement fixation Early immune response Stimulation of ingestion by macrophages
IgG	12	25	Complement fixation Placental transfer Stimulation of ingestion by macrophages
IgA	1.8	6	Localized protection in external secretions (e.g., saliva)
IgD	0.03	3	Function unknown
IgE	0.0003	2	Stimulation of mast cells Parasite expulsion

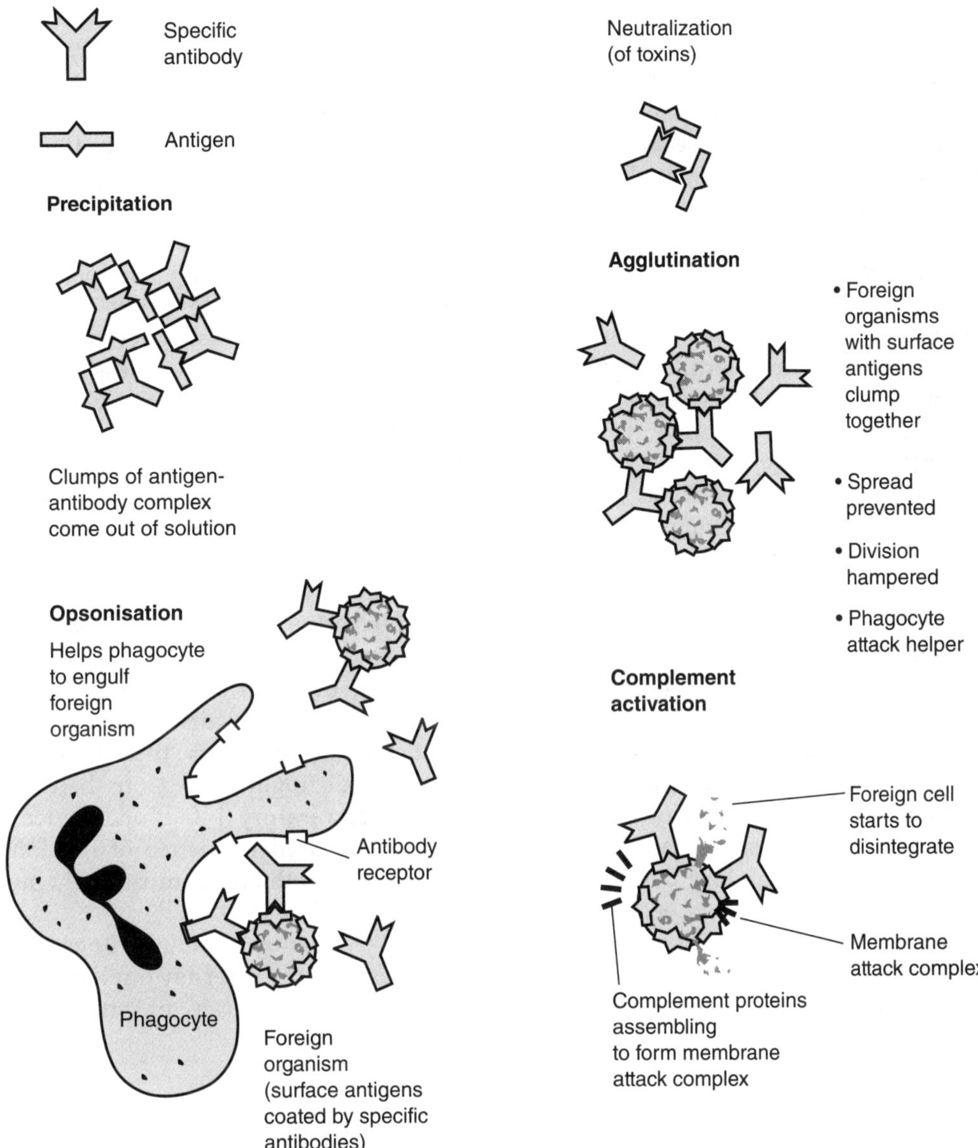

Figure 13.9 Types of antibody–antigen reactions.

ganisms usually cause complement activation. Complement proteins then attack the membrane of the invader or, by coating the surface of foreign material, make it attractive to phagocytes (opsonization).

Causes of Illness in Athletes

Infections of the upper respiratory tract caused by viruses (i.e., the common cold and influenza) are the most common illnesses in athletes and in the general population. Adults typically experience between two and four episodes of respiratory illness per year, and these infectious illnesses occur most frequently during the winter. Similar symptoms (e.g., sore throat, runny nose, dry cough) can develop due to an **allergy** or inflammation affecting the mucosal lining of the upper respiratory tract. This noninfectious airway inflammation can be brought on by the inhalation of cold, dry, or polluted air (Bermon 2007). The symptoms are generally not severe, but no matter whether the symptoms and inflammation are caused by an infection, allergy, or adverse reaction, they can cause an athlete to miss training, underperform, or be unable to participate in an important competition. Studies that have examined the incidence of reported illnesses among athletes competing in major games, such as the Olympics and World Athletics Championships, indicate that typically illnesses affecting the upper respiratory tract account for 40% to 50% of all reported illnesses with confirmed infection in about 20% of respiratory illness cases (Alonso et al. 2012). The other most frequently reported causes of sickness are associated with exercise-induced dehydration and gastroenteritis or diarrhea.

The performance of prolonged bouts of strenuous exercise (usually longer than 90 minutes and of a continuous rather than intermittent nature) have been shown to result in transient depression of white blood cell (leukocyte) functions, which can consequently impair defense against infectious pathogens, including viruses and bacteria. It has been suggested that such changes create an open window of decreased host protection during which time pathogens can gain a foothold, thereby increasing the risk of developing an infection (Walsh, Gleeson, Shephard, et al. 2011). Other factors, such as inadequate nutrition (particularly deficiencies of protein and essential micronutrients), psychological stress, and lack of sleep, can also depress immunity (Walsh, Gleeson, Pyne, et al. 2011) and lead to increased risk of infection. There are also some situations, such as proximity to large crowds, coming into close contact with people who are suffering from infections, and being exposed to environments with poor hygiene, in which an athlete's exposure to infectious agents may be increased. Thus, the degree of exposure to pathogens in the athlete's environment and the status of the athlete's immune system are the two important determinants of infection risk. Various strategies, including behavioral and nutritional ones, can be employed to reduce these risk factors. Of course, in many professional sports that attract large numbers of spectators, the competitors' exposure to large crowds is unavoidable. Air travel to foreign countries may also increase the risk of picking up infections. Recently, international travel was shown to be associated with significantly more upper respiratory illness symptoms (URS) in professional rugby players who traveled across multiple time zones (Fowler, Duffield, and Lu 2016; Schwellnus et al. 2012). International travel was an independent risk factor for illness in another prospective study among elite cross-country skiers (Svendsen et al. 2016).

During dynamic exercise, exposure of the lungs to airborne bacteria and viruses increases because of the higher rate and depth of breathing. However, URS can also arise due to allergy and inflammation of the airways caused by breathing cold, dry, or polluted air; the URS that result from this are indistinguishable from the URS that result from a respiratory infection. Hence, the cause of the increased incidence of respiratory illness symptoms in athletes is most likely multifactorial (figure 13.10).

The frequency of acute illness in elite-level athletes during international competition has been studied in a variety of settings, including the

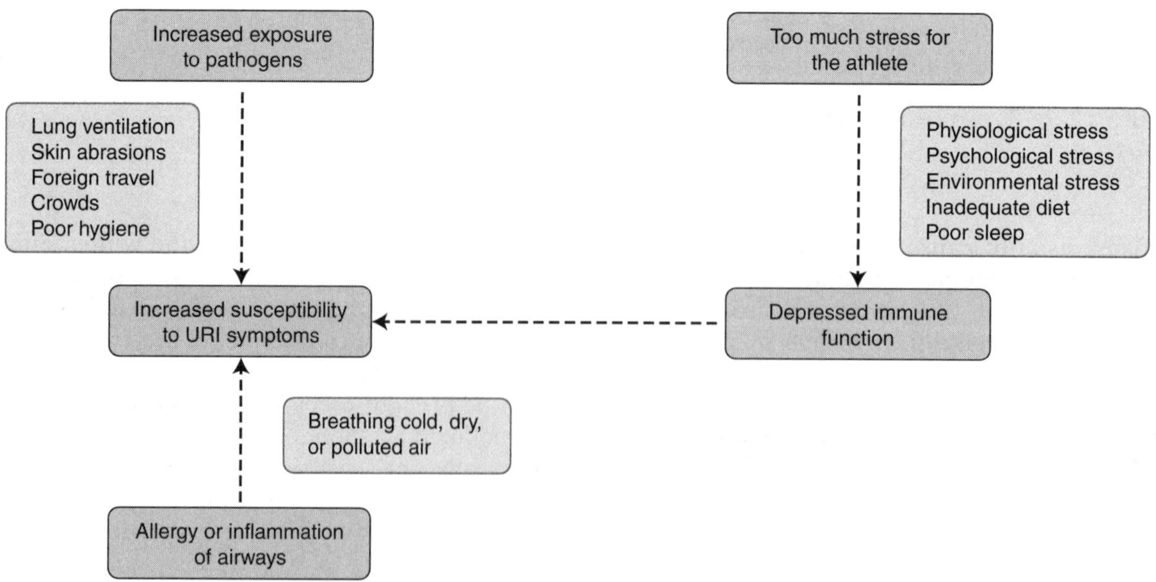

Figure 13.10 Factors that contribute to respiratory illness symptom incidence in athletes.

Summer and Winter Olympic Games, the Winter Youth Olympic Games, the Summer and Winter Paralympic Games, and other international athletic and aquatic sport competitions (Schwellnus et al. 2016). These data indicate that in major international games that last 9 to 18 days, 6% to 17% of registered athletes are likely to suffer an illness episode. Interestingly, illness appears to be consistently more common in female athletes compared with their male counterparts, which is the opposite of what is found for the general adult population. Furthermore, the incidence of illness appears to be higher in Winter Olympic Games compared with the Summer Olympic Games, and data from one study indicate that athletes who participate in the Paralympic Games appear to have a higher incidence of illness than those who compete in the Olympic Games (Derman et al. 2016).

Several of the body's organ systems can be detrimentally affected by infections, and this can result in impaired exercise performance through a variety of mechanisms, including impaired motor coordination, decreased muscle strength, decreased aerobic capacity, and alterations in metabolic function (Schwellnus et al. 2016). Furthermore, the presence of an infection-associated elevated resting core body temperature (commonly known as a fever) impairs the body's ability to regulate body temperature and increases fluid losses, thereby impairing endurance performance. It can typically take 2 to 4 days for exercise performance to be fully restored following the cessation of respiratory illness symptoms, and it has been reported that runners who start a distance running race with systemic illness symptoms are two to three times less likely to complete the race (Van Tonder et al. 2016). It has also been reported that in 33% of cases, an infection (most commonly of the respiratory tract) was the reason that elite Great Britain athletes from 30 different Olympic sports missed training sessions. Perhaps more importantly, some forms of infective illness can also increase the risk of developing serious medical complications during prolonged intensive exercise and may even increase the risk of sudden death.

Other common illnesses in athletes are those that affect the skin, digestive tract, and genitourinary system. Ear infections are more common in aquatic sports. In contact sports, skin abrasions may occur, thereby increasing the risk of transdermal infections. In some situations, food hygiene can be a problem, which increases the risk of gastrointestinal infections.

Forms of illness that are quite common in athletes but are noninfectious include dehydration and heat illness. An increase in gut permeability may allow entry of gut bacterial endotoxins into the circulation, particularly during prolonged exercise in the heat, which can increase the risk of heat illness. Other forms of noninfectious illness include allergies that involve the respiratory tract, skin, or digestive system and are caused by a hypersensitivity of the immune system to certain molecules (often proteins) that are inhaled (e.g., pollen), come into contact with the skin (e.g., latex), or are eaten (e.g., wheat gluten). All of these involve the inappropriate activation of the immune system against a compound that is normally tolerated well by most people. The inflammation caused by this hypersensitivity is the major cause of the illness symptoms. Similar symptoms may arise with intolerance to certain food items, although this does not directly involve immune system activation, as explained in the following section.

Allergies and Intolerance

When the term *allergy* was first introduced in 1906, it referred to an adverse reaction to a food or other substance not typically regarded as harmful or bothersome. For most people this is still what allergy means, although doctors use the word rather differently, and this can be misleading and confusing. Doctors use the word allergy to mean an adverse reaction of the immune system to a substance not recognized as harmful by most people's immune systems. True allergies (e.g., to pollens, dust mites, fish, shellfish, nuts) are typically associated with the formation of antibodies. Some people (doctors refer to these people as *atopic*) have an inherited tendency to this type of allergy and they tend also to be prone to asthma, eczema, and hay fever; this condition is known as atopy. In certain circumstances, and especially during the first few years of life, atopic people may develop IgE antibodies when exposed to an allergy-inducing protein in a process called sensitization. When sensitization has occurred, the allergy-inducing protein is referred to as an allergen and the resulting antibody (also a protein) as allergen-specific IgE. Although doctors use the term allergy when referring to an adverse reaction that involves the immune system, the term *intolerance* is preferred when an adverse reaction shows no evidence of immune system involvement. The scientific term for an intolerance is *nonallergic hypersensitivity*.

Food Allergy

A true gluten allergy—not to be confused with gluten sensitivity or celiac disease—is caused by gliadin, a glycoprotein that, along with another protein called glutenin, helps form the gluten protein. Gluten is found in wheat and other similar cereal grains such as barley, oats, and rye. The symptoms of gluten allergy are similar to those of gluten intolerance but can be more severe. Gliadin is also one of the major allergens associated with wheat allergies and a known trigger for celiac disease, which is a serious autoimmune disorder of the small intestine. In a person with a gluten allergy, small amounts of gluten may be tolerated, but a person with celiac disease cannot tolerate any gluten at all. When a person with celiac disease eats gluten, the immune system initiates an unnecessary inflammatory response, and this eventually damages the lining of the small intestine. Celiac disease restricts absorption of nutrients and may lead to malnutrition and weight loss. Because celiac disease shares symptoms with a number of other disorders, including a gluten allergy, it is important that a test is conducted to confirm the condition. Gluten allergies and celiac disease are major public health concerns. It is estimated that 0.6% of children and 0.9% of adults in the United States have a gluten allergy and another 1% suffer from celiac disease.

A less common but dangerous allergy is to proteins in nuts. Each year there are several reported cases of fatalities due to a rapid, severe anaphylactic shock following ingestion of nuts or, usually, to inadvertently eating foods (e.g., curries, cakes, pastries, cookies) that contain nuts or nut extracts by people with nut allergies.

Food Intolerance

Food intolerance can occur when the body fails to produce a sufficient amount of a particular enzyme needed to digest a food component before it can be absorbed. For example, if a person suffers abdominal discomfort with flatulence and bloating or diarrhea every time he or she consumes milk or milk-derived products (e.g., cream, yogurt, cheese), the person may be suffering from lactose intolerance, which is a condition caused by lack of lactase (the enzyme that digests the main sugar in milk, which is a disaccharide called lactose). This is caused by the lactose not being absorbed but instead being fermented by the microbes in the intestine. Food intolerances are normally dose related, meaning the more you eat the worse the reaction is likely to be. There may also be a threshold amount required to be consumed before experiencing any symptoms, which can make it difficult to determine the specific cause.

If a person suffers nervous system symptoms because of an amount of caffeine in a mug of strong coffee (which would be tolerated by most people), this person would be suffering from a drug-like or pharmacological food intolerance. This can occur because of an intolerance to chemicals naturally present in foods (such as theobromine in chocolate or tyramine in aged cheeses) or an intolerance to food additives such as sulphites or benzoates.

Although enzymatic and pharmacological food intolerance reactions only affect some people, toxic food reactions can affect anyone when an excessive amount of a food constituent is ingested. A good example is the reaction that can occur when sufficient amounts of histamine accumulate in the flesh of spoiled tuna (known as the scombroid reaction). Because histamine is also the natural agent in the human body involved in allergic reactions, scombroid food poisoning is often misidentified as a food allergy. This condition is named after the Scombridae family of fish, which includes tunas, mackerels, and bonitos, because early descriptions of the illness noted an association with those species; however, other nonscombroid fish, including mahi-mahi and amberjack, are also known to cause this problem. Cooking the fish does not prevent illness, because histamine is not destroyed at normal cooking temperatures.

As noted previously, some people have gluten sensitivity (also known as gluten intolerance) and symptoms such as bloating, abdominal pain, or diarrhea. However, because immune and autoimmune symptoms are not involved, it is not considered as serious as celiac disease or gluten allergy. As many as 6% of people in the United States have gluten sensitivity.

Note that these examples of food intolerance involve the immune system. For this reason, none can result in life-threatening allergy or anaphylaxis, but they can result in severe abdominal discomfort.

With the exception of lactose intolerance, no reliable forms of testing exist for food intolerance. However, recent scientific studies point to a delayed-type food allergy in which the immune system is involved even though allergen-specific IgE is not present. For this reason, the controversial view that certain medically unexplained symptoms might be related to a delayed form of food allergy rather than to an unexplained or psychosomatic mechanism may prove to have some scientific worth. Studies that have used food exclusion followed by blind and placebo-controlled food challenges have suggested that this kind of mechanism may apply in some cases of migraine,

HOW DO YOU KNOW IF YOU HAVE AN ALLERGY?

The only way to find out if you have a gluten allergy is to be tested. One of the most common tests is an elimination diet. In an elimination diet, a person removes all gluten-containing foods from the diet for a period of time to see if symptoms resolve. However, an elimination diet will not rule out celiac disease or gluten sensitivity.

The conventional allergy tests used by doctors to detect other allergies depend on the presence of allergen-specific IgE antibodies. The two most used are the skin prick test and the specific IgE blood test (previously called a RAST test). However, it is very important to realize that although allergy is unlikely when allergen-specific IgE is absent, the presence of allergen-specific IgE only indicates that sensitization has occurred; it does not diagnose the allergy. When completely healthy and symptom-free people are tested for allergies, positive results are often found. These results are called false positives. For this reason, reliable allergy diagnosis is dependent on an allergy-focused history. A good allergy clinician can usually identify the likely allergen(s) from the history alone, and allergy tests may not be needed. However, because a negative allergy test may point to a different, unrecognized allergy or a different explanation altogether, allergy tests are very useful to confirm the diagnosis. This is especially important in the case of suspected food allergy when an inaccurate diagnosis might commit the patient to lifelong, but unnecessary, food avoidance. Allergy tests are also useful if there is any confusion as to whether symptoms are being caused by true allergy or whether some other condition is involved. This is why allergy tests need to be interpreted by a health-care professional who is qualified in allergy and who will interpret the results in light of an allergy-focused history. This also explains why it is important not to test everybody for every known allergen, which would inevitably lead to erroneous diagnosis.

Occasionally, clinicians may be faced with situations in which the allergy history points strongly in one direction but an allergy test points strongly in another. This is when a provocation challenge test may be useful. The test is only undertaken under specialist supervision in a hospital. The patient is exposed to tiny, but gradually increasing, amounts of the suspected allergen source (typically a food such as peanut or cereal) until there is the tiniest hint of a rash, swelling, breathing difficulty, or drop in blood pressure (the initial signs of an anaphylactic reaction). This is the gold standard among allergy tests.

Another available allergy test is the skin contact (or patch) test that is used by skin specialists in cases of contact dermatitis. The test diagnoses a delayed, or cell-mediated (as opposed to antibody-mediated), type of allergy that mainly affects the skin. Unconventional allergy tests that are considered to be of no value include skin end-point titration tests (in which increasing amounts of a diluted allergen solution are injected under the skin until a reaction occurs), applied kinesiology (based on measurements of muscle strength, the idea being that muscle weakness may become evident when the individual is exposed to the suspected allergen), auricular cardiac reflex (based on measurements of the pulse at the wrist), hair analysis (based on a pseudoscientific concept called bioresonance), blood cytotoxic tests (based on an examination of the white blood cells when exposed to a suspected allergen) and the Vega test (based on acupuncture theory and electromagnetism).

Another common test that has become popular among athletes and others is the IgG blood test. In IgG testing, the blood is tested for IgG antibodies instead of being tested for IgE antibodies (i.e., the antibodies typically associated with food allergies). Some practitioners (particularly unconventional ones) claim that the existence of serum IgG antibodies toward specific foods is an effective tool to diagnose food allergy or intolerance. The problem with this is that IgG is a memory antibody, which means that IgG signifies previous exposure to a food rather than an actual allergy to a food. Because a normally functioning immune system should make IgG antibodies to foreign proteins, a positive IgG test to a food is a sign of a properly working immune system. In fact, a positive result can indicate tolerance for the food rather than intolerance. Thus, there is no good scientific evidence to support IgG testing for the diagnosis of food allergies.

arthritis, and irritable bowel syndrome. With the exception of dietitian-supervised food exclusion and food challenges, no validated test for this type of food allergy has so far emerged.

Allergies in Athletes

There are some claims that athletes may be more susceptible to symptoms of food sensitivities because the stress of constant training taxes the immune system. In other words, a stressed body will be less able to handle foods that cause inflammation. However, there is currently no convincing scientific evidence to back this up. Although there is some belief among athletes that gluten intolerance is higher in those who are highly physically active, much of this may arise from the recent trend to have food intolerance tests performed using nonvalidated methods, such as the IgG blood test or hair analysis mentioned previously. Unrecognized intolerance to foods or supplements consumed during exercise could lead to increased risk of gastrointestinal problems and could be a potential cause of impaired performance in certain sports and particularly endurance events.

It has been established that high-level athletes—especially those who take part in endurance sports, such as swimming or running, and in winter sports—present an increased risk for asthma and allergies that affect the respiratory tract (Sliva and Moreira 2015). Classical postulated mechanisms behind exercise-induced asthma or bronchoconstriction include the osmotic, or airway-drying, hypothesis. Hyperventilation leads to evaporation of water and the airway mucosal surface liquid becomes hyperosmolar, which provides a stimulus for water to move by osmosis from any cell nearby. This results in the shrinkage of cells and the consequent release of inflammatory mediators that cause airway smooth muscle contraction. The exercise-induced asthma or bronchoconstriction explanatory model in athletes probably also involves the interaction between environmental training factors, such as increased lung exposure to airborne pollutants and allergens; ambient conditions, such as temperature, humidity, and air quality; and the athlete's personal risk factors, such as genetic and neuroimmune-endocrine determinants.

Effects of Exercise on the Immune System

Athletes who engage in heavy training programs, particularly endurance events, appear to be more susceptible to infection than the general population. For example, sore throats and flulike symptoms are more common in these athletes (Gleeson et al. 2013). The modern-day athlete who participates in elite sports is exposed to high training loads and an increasingly saturated competition calendar. Emerging evidence (Schwellnus et al. 2016) indicates that inappropriate load management is a significant risk factor for acute illness and the overtraining syndrome. The IOC recently convened an expert group to review the scientific evidence for the relationship of load (e.g., rapid changes in training and competition load, competition calendar congestion, psychological load, travel) and health outcomes in sport. They concluded that there is some evidence that changes in external training load (increased volume and intensity of training) and internal training load (the physiological and psychological responses to external load in each individual) are associated with an increased risk of illness and that participation in competitions (single or multiple) is associated with an increased risk of illness (Schwellnus et al. 2016). They stated, however, that it is not yet possible to quantify which amount of training load increase is related to increased risk of a specific illness or to identify which sports are related to increased risk of illness. They also said the factors responsible for increased illness risk as a result of intensive training and competition are likely to be multifactorial and also need to be explored in future studies. Some convincing evidence suggests that this increased susceptibility to infection arises due to a depression of immune system function (for detailed reviews, see Gleeson, Bishop, and Walsh 2013 and Walsh, Gleeson, Pyne, et al. 2011).

The main component of the immune system is the white blood cells or leukocytes. The circulating numbers and functional capacities of leukocytes may be decreased by repeated bouts of intense, prolonged exercise. The cause may be increased levels of stress hormones (e.g., epinephrine and cortisol) and anti-inflammatory cytokines (e.g., IL-6, IL-10) during exercise and the entry of less mature leukocytes from the bone marrow into the circulation. Increased free radical production during exercise is another potential inhibitor of several immune cell functions. Drops in the blood concentration of glutamine have also been suggested as a possible cause of the immunodepression associated with heavy training, although the evidence for this is less compelling. Inflammation caused by muscle damage may be another factor.

The relationship between exercise and susceptibility to infection has been modeled as a J-curve (Nieman 1994). This model suggests that although engaging in moderate activity may enhance immune function above sedentary levels, excessive amounts of prolonged, high-intensity exercise may induce detrimental effects on immune function. Although the literature provides strong evidence in support of the latter point, relatively little evidence is available to suggest any clinically significant difference in immune function between sedentary and moderately active people. Thus, the portion of the J-curve that represents this part of the relationship should perhaps be flattened out, as shown in figure 13.11. Matthews et al. (2002) reported that regular performance of about 2 hours of moderate exercise per day was associated with a 29% reduction in the risk of URTI compared with a sedentary lifestyle. Similarly, in a study of more than 1,000 participants, Nieman et al. (2011) observed that doing moderate exercise 5 or more days per week was associated with a 30% lower risk of URTI than doing 1 or fewer days of exercise per week. This finding emphasizes that the benefit of regular, moderate exercise in improving resistance to infection is quite small; a more active lifestyle, however, does have substantial cardiovascular and metabolic health benefits.

Acute Effects of Exercise on Immune Function

Prolonged strenuous exercise has a temporary depressive effect on immune function, and this effect has been associated with increased incidence of infection. For example, Peters and Bateman (1983) and Nieman et al. (1990) described a substantially higher (two- to sixfold) frequency of self-reported symptoms of URTI in athletes who completed long-distance foot races compared with control runners who did not compete in the events.

Prolonged intensive exercise has a transient negative effect on immune function. The extent of the depression in immune function following exercise is most pronounced when the exercise is prolonged (> 1.5 h), of moderate to high intensity (55%-75% of aerobic capacity), continuous rather than intermittent, and performed without any carbohydrate intake (Gleeson 2013). Numerous aspects of innate immunity, including neutrophil chemotaxis, phagocytosis, oxidative burst activity, and degranulation (figure 13.12), together with monocyte TLR expression and natural killer cell cytotoxic activity are depressed by prolonged

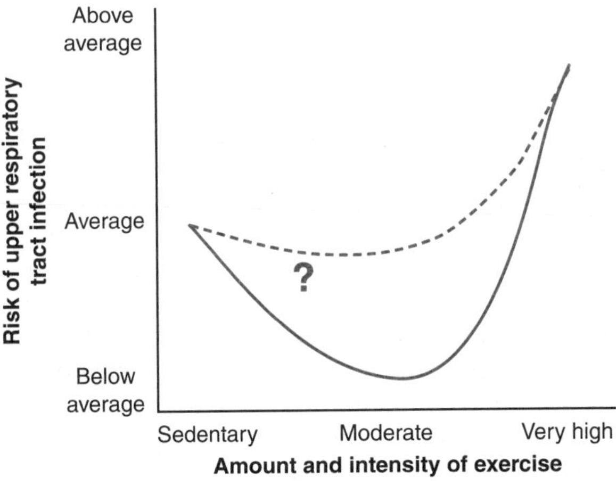

Figure 13.11 The J-curve model implies that risk of URTI is reduced by moderate activity but is progressively elevated by heavier training loads. The dashed line between the two levels of exercise may be a more appropriate representation of the relationship between training load and URTI risk.

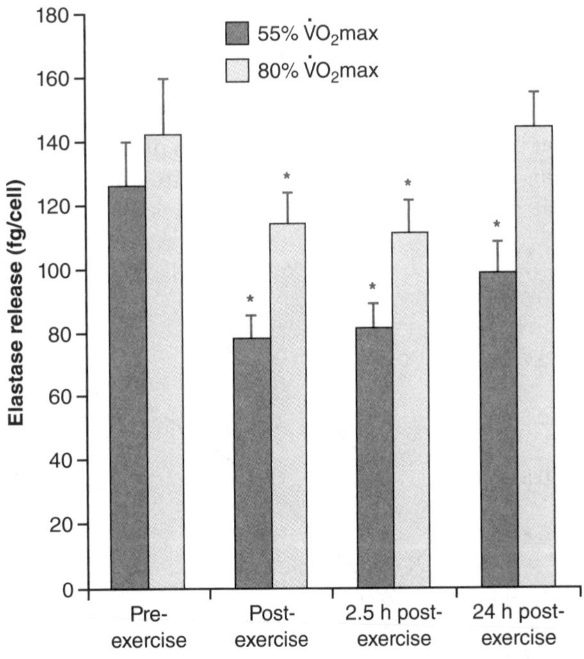

Figure 13.12 Changes in the in vitro lipopolysaccharide-stimulated neutrophil degranulation response (elastase release per cell) after 3 hours of cycling at 55% of $\dot{V}O_2$max and after cycling to fatigue at 80% of $\dot{V}O_2$max (mean exercise duration 38 minutes) in 10 well-trained cyclists. Data are means and SEM. $*P < 0.05$ compared with pre-exercise. $P < 0.05$: 55% of $\dot{V}O_2$max versus 80% of $\dot{V}O_2$max.

International Journal of Sports Medicine: From P.J. Robson et al., "Effects of Exercise Intensity, Duration, and Recovery on in Vitro Neutrophil Function in Male Athletes," 1999; 20: 128-135. Reprinted by permission.

strenuous exercise. Furthermore, after a prolonged bout of moderate- to high-intensity exercise, many important acquired (specific) immune cell functions, including antigen presentation by monocytes and macrophages, immunoglobulin production by B-lymphocytes, T-lymphocyte cytokine (e.g. interferon-gamma) production, and T-lymphocyte proliferation (figure 13.13), are reduced. Mucosal immune protection may also be temporarily impaired; many studies on endurance athletes have reported falls in the concentration and secretion rates of salivary secretory immunoglobulin A (SIgA) following very prolonged bouts of exercise such as running a marathon (Walsh et al. 2011b). The increase in circulating stress hormones (e.g., epinephrine and cortisol) is a likely causal factor for immune depression after prolonged exercise. Another important contributing factor is thought to be an alteration in the pro-/anti-inflammatory cytokine balance mostly due to elevated circulating levels of IL-6, IL-10, IL-1 receptor antagonist (IL-1ra), and soluble tumor necrosis factor receptors (sTNFr) that have inhibitory actions on proinflammatory cytokine actions and immune activation.

Studies examining the alteration of leukocyte gene expression after prolonged exercise indicate that there is an increased expression of many genes that code for proteins involved in anti-inflammatory actions. Furthermore, genes of the TLR receptor signaling pathway that leads to proinflammatory cytokine production and activation of the immune system are downregulated following prolonged exercise (Abbasi et al. 2013, 2014). The factors responsible for this altered pattern of gene expression after exercise may include cortisol, epinephrine, growth hormone, heat shock proteins, and muscle-derived IL-6 (Gleeson et al. 2011). Cortisol and IL-6 are probably the two key players in orchestrating this broad anti-inflammatory reaction. During prolonged exercise, IL-6 is released from contracting muscle fibers and causes release of other anti-inflammatory mediators, including IL-10, IL-1ra, sTNFr, adrenocorticotrophic hormone, and cortisol, as well as acute phase reactants of hepatocytes (e.g., α1 acid glycoprotein and C-reactive protein). The anti-inflammatory cytokine response to exercise is rather different from that involved with sepsis because there appears to be no initial proinflammatory response with exercise. In contrast, with sepsis the primary cytokine response is a large increase in the circulating concentration of several proinflammatory cytokines, such as TNF-α and IFN-γ, which is later followed by a counter-regulatory secretion of anti-inflammatory cytokines, such as IL-6 and IL-10.

With exercise, in addition to the anti-inflammatory effects induced by IL-6, there may be additional mechanisms at work in promoting anti-inflammatory reactions. One such mechanism has been suggested to be the rapid induction of microRNAs (Tonevitsky et al. 2013) during and following exercise. Some microRNAs are capable of interfering with TLRs and downstream signaling, and this would be an effective means of inducing the anti-inflammatory response to exercise (Abbasi et al. 2014). The various events that contribute to the anti-inflammatory effects of exercise and the associated immunodepression are summarized in figure 13.14.

During recovery from exercise, NK cell numbers and activity fall below preexercise levels (see figure 13.15), and if the exercise bout was of high intensity or was prolonged, the number of circulating lymphocytes may decrease below preexercise levels for several hours and the T-lymphocyte CD4+ to CD8+ (helper to suppressor) ratio decreases. After prolonged strenuous exercise, the production of immunoglobulins by B-lymphocytes is inhibited. The plasma concentration of glutamine falls by about 20% and may remain depressed for some time. These changes during early recovery from exercise appear to weaken the potential immune response to pathogens and possibly provide an open window for infection (Pedersen and Bruunsgard 1995). A temporary reduction in

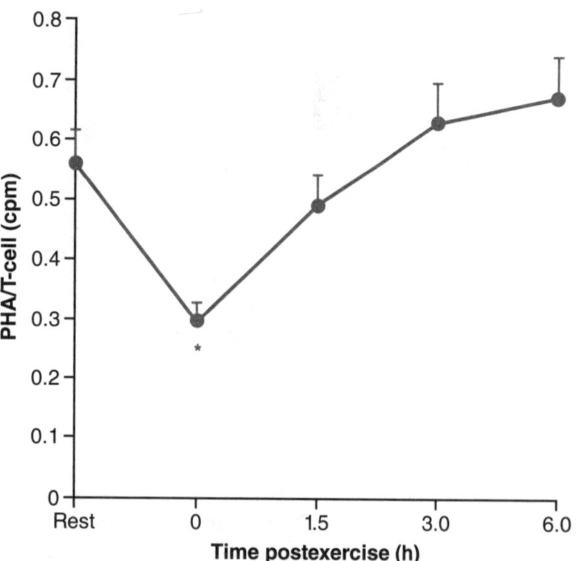

Figure 13.13 Change in phytohemagglutinin-stimulated (PHA) lymphocyte proliferation after 2.5 hours of running.

International Journal of Sports Medicine: From P.J. Robson et al., "Effects of Exercise Intensity, Duration, and Recovery on in Vitro Neutrophil Function in Male Athletes," 1999; 20: 128-135. Reprinted by permission.

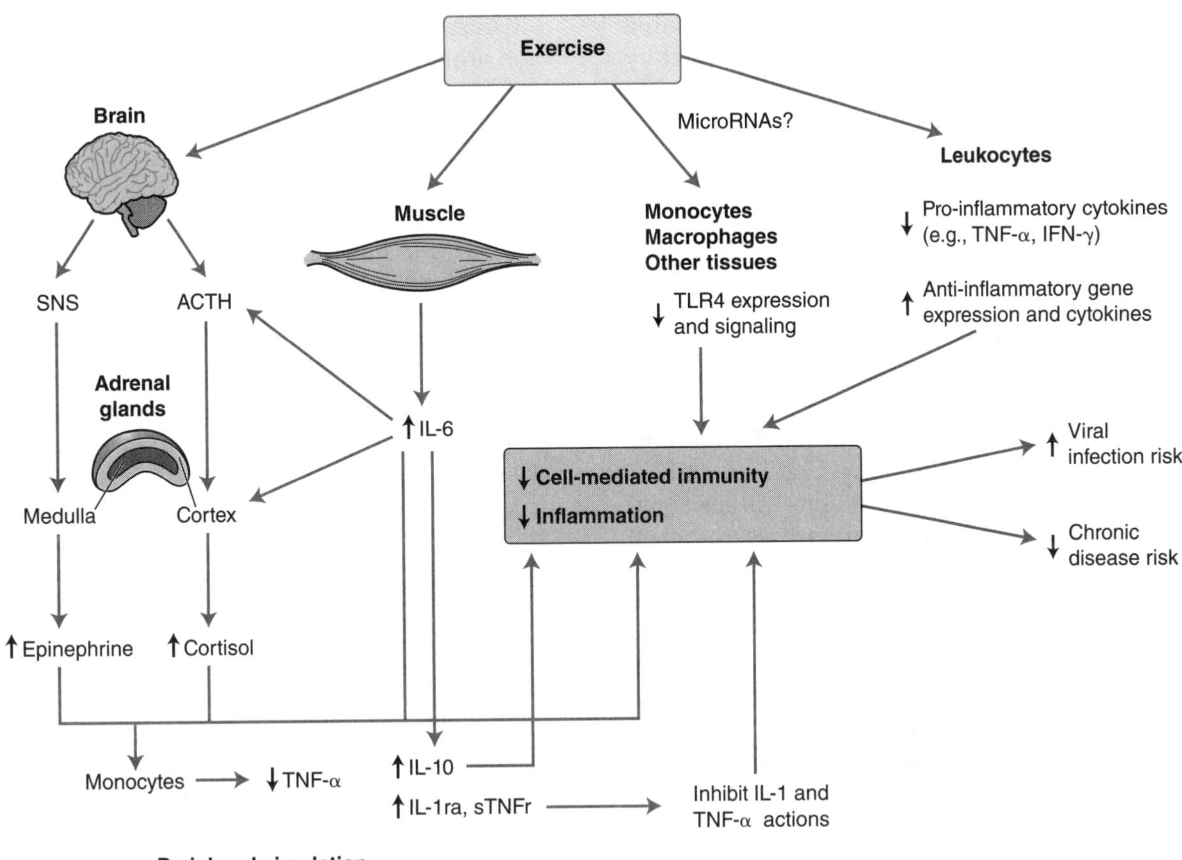

Figure 13.14 The potential mechanisms by which prolonged exercise causes anti-inflammatory and immunodepressive effects.

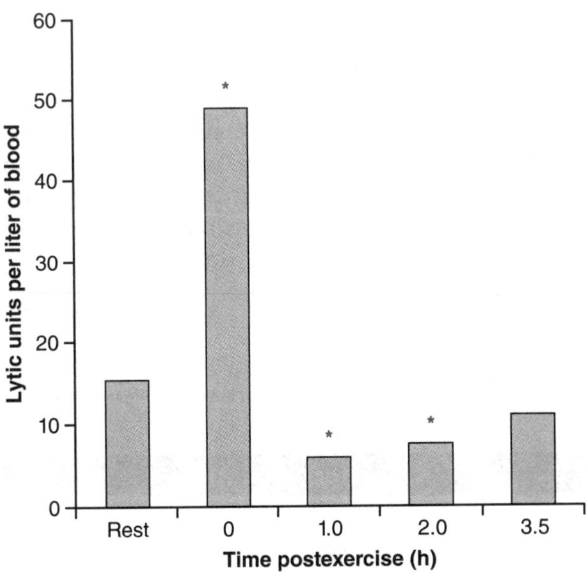

Figure 13.15 Change in natural killer cell cytotoxic activity (NKCA, expressed as lytic units per liter of blood) after 2.5 hours of running. *Significantly different from rest, $P<0.05$.

Based on Nieman et al. (1993).

several aspects of innate immune function occurs at this time, and athletes should be encouraged to adopt practices that can minimize the risk of infection as described later in this chapter.

Chronic Effects of Exercise Training on Immune Function

Circulating numbers of leukocytes are generally lower in athletes at rest compared with sedentary people (see table 13.6). A low blood leukocyte count may arise from the hemodilution (expansion of the plasma volume) associated with training, or it may represent altered leukocyte kinetics, including diminished release from the bone marrow. Indeed, the large increase in circulating neutrophil numbers that accompanies a bout of prolonged exercise could, over periods of months or years of heavy training, deplete the bone marrow reserve of these important cells. The blood population of these cells seems to be less mature than in sedentary individuals, and the phagocytic activity of blood neutrophils has been reported to be markedly lower in well-trained cyclists compared with age-matched and weight-matched sedentary control subjects. However, most indices of immune function that have been measured in athletes in the true resting state (i.e., at least 24 hours after the last exercise bout) are generally not very different from their sedentary counterparts. One exception to this general rule is when athletes are engaged in periods of intensified training. In this situation, immune function may not fully recover from the last training session and a more chronic depression of immunity may develop within 1 to 2 weeks (Gleeson, Bishop, and Walsh 2013). For example, when well-trained athletes undertake a period of intensified training, there are falls in stimulated B-cell immunoglobulin synthesis and SIgA levels. Furthermore, there are decreases in circulating numbers of type 1 T-cells, reduced T-cell proliferative responses to mitogens, and inhibition of type 1 T-cell cytokine production. However, the only immune variable that has been consistently associated with increased infection incidence is SIgA; low concentrations of SIgA and substantial transient falls in SIgA are associated with increased risk of URS episodes (Neville et al. 2008). In contrast, following a few weeks of regular, moderate exercise training in previously sedentary individuals, SIgA levels have been reported to rise and could, at least in part, contribute to the apparent reduced susceptibility to URS associated with regular, moderate exercise compared with a sedentary lifestyle (Walsh et al. 2011).

Low SIgA secretion rate and higher IL-10 production in whole blood cultures exposed to an antigen challenge in vitro (Gleeson and Bishop 2013) have been reported in illness-prone athletes. Other factors that are associated with increased susceptibility to URS in athletes include low vitamin D status, high training loads, and no prior infection with cytomegalovirus and Epstein-Barr virus (He et al. 2013).

Recurrent infections can be debilitating for some athletes and catastrophic when they occur just before or during major competitions. A study by Neville et al. (2008) provides some encouragement for using SIgA measures as a monitoring tool and predictor of impending infection risk. On retrospective analyses of the salivary samples of 38 America's Cup athletes taken once every week over a period of 50 weeks, this study showed that when relative SIgA values fell by 40% or more, the athletes had a one in two chance of contracting an upper respiratory infection within the next 3 weeks. In the near future, the development of new handheld devices will likely will allow rapid salivary analysis in the field that provides useful data for sport science support personnel and coaches that may inform them when their athletes are most vulnerable to infection so problems associated with increased training loads might be avoided.

It is generally assumed that getting cold and wet increases the probability of picking up a respiratory infection such as the common cold, but the available scientific evidence does not indicate that this is the case for either athletes or the general population. Although the inhalation of cold, dry air can reduce upper airway ciliary movement and decrease mucous flow, it appears that when athletes train and compete in cold conditions, they do not experience a greater reduction in immune function compared with thermoneutral conditions (Walsh et al. 2011). Indeed, there is no data supporting more frequent, more severe, or longer-lasting infections in athletes who regularly train and compete in cold conditions. Other environmental extremes, such as high altitude and hot weather, do not seem to have a marked effect on immune responses to exercise (Walsh et al. 2011). Moreover, moderate levels of dehydration do not have an obvious influence on immune defenses apart from a transient lowering of the saliva secretion rate, which is quickly restored by fluid intake.

TABLE 13.6 Numbers of Circulating Leukocytes in Endurance-Trained Men and Sedentary Men

Blood cell count (×10^9/L)	Sedentary (n = 8)	Trained* (n = 8)
Total leukocytes	6.62 (0.87)	4.36 (1.15)
Neutrophils	3.83 (0.86)	2.46 (0.87)
Lymphocytes	2.02 (0.27)	1.36 (0.20)

*$P < 0.01$, trained versus sedentary subjects.

Subjects were matched for age and body mass.

Data from Blannin et al. (1996).

Nutritional Manipulations to Decrease Immunodepression in Athletes

Poor nutritional practices may contribute to impaired immunity in athletes. Some athletes adopt diets that are extremely high in carbohydrate content at the expense of protein and fat. By avoiding foods that are high in animal fat, athletes are reducing their intake of fat-soluble vitamins and essential FAs. Many sports have strict weight categories that lead some competitors to follow energy-restricted diets that are often unbalanced and place them at risk of several nutrient deficiencies.

Anecdotal and media reports promote the supposed performance benefits of certain vitamins and minerals, but most athletes do not realize that micronutrient supplementation is only beneficial when it corrects a deficiency and that excessive intake of individual micronutrients can be toxic or can limit the absorption of other essential trace elements. Deficiencies or excesses of various dietary components have a substantial effect on immune function and may exacerbate the immunodepression associated with heavy training loads.

Mechanisms of Nutritional Influences on Immune Function in Athletes

Nutrient availability potentially affects almost all aspects of the immune system because many nutrients are involved in energy metabolism and protein synthesis. Most immune responses involve cell replication and the production of proteins with specific functions (e.g., cytokines, antibodies, acute phase proteins). Immune system functions that may be compromised include the humoral and secretory antibody production, cell-mediated immunity, bactericidal capacity of phagocytes, complement formation, and T-lymphocyte proliferative response to mitogens.

A nutritional deficiency is said to have a direct effect when the nutritional factor has primary activity within the lymphoid system and an indirect effect when the primary activity affects all cellular material or an organ system that functions as an immune regulator. For example, carbohydrate availability directly affects a number of leukocyte functions but also indirectly affects the lymphoid system through its influence on circulating levels of the catecholamines, ACTH, and cortisol. Changes in plasma levels of these stress hormones are probably mostly responsible for the observed changes in immune function after an acute bout of exercise (see figure 13.16).

The effect of a nutrient deficiency on the immune system depends on the duration of the deficiency as well as on the athlete's nutritional status as a whole. The severity of the deficiency is also a factor, although even a mild deficiency of a single nutrient can alter the immune response. Because the availability of one nutrient may enhance or impair the action of another and nutrient deficiencies often occur together, nutrient–nutrient interactions on immune function are also an important consideration. Athletes who are training hard eat to satisfy their energy demands and consume more macronutrients (carbohydrate,

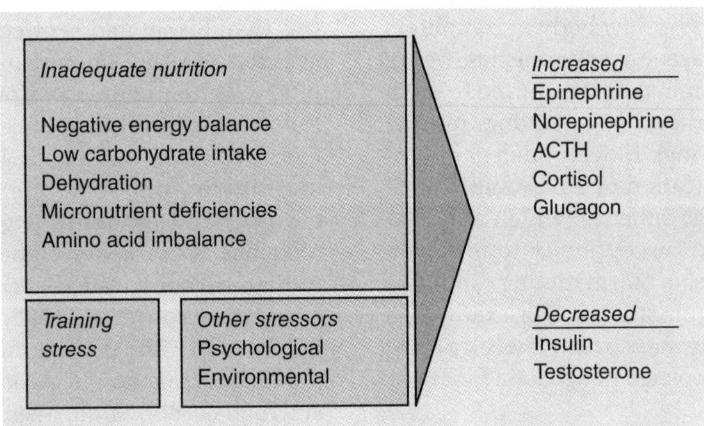

Figure 13.16 Various factors that can influence the stress hormone response to exercise.

Reprinted by permission from M. Gleeson and N.C. Bishop, "Modification of Immune Responses to Exercise by Carbohydrate, Glutamine and Anti-oxidant Supplements" *Immunology and Cell Biology* 78, (2000): 554-561.

protein, and fat) and micronutrients (vitamins and minerals) than their sedentary counterparts. Therefore, they may ingest excessive amounts of some nutrients. Excessive amounts of specific nutrients (e.g., omega-3 polyunsaturated FAs, iron, zinc) can have detrimental effects on immune function.

The 1991 Consensus Conference on Foods, Nutrition, and Sports Performance (Williams and Devlin 1992) gave the following dietary advice: "In the optimum diet for most sports, carbohydrate is likely to contribute about 60% to 70% of the total energy intake and protein about 12%, with the remainder coming from fat."

Athletes are generally advised to eat well-balanced diets that consist of a variety of foods in sufficient quantity to cover their energy expenditures. Many athletes, however, follow high-protein, high-carbohydrate, or high-fat diets or very low-energy diets; fast; or consume megadoses of vitamins and minerals. Such dietary extremes may compromise immune function. For example, diets that are excessively high in carbohydrate, which are favored by many athletes to keep glycogen stores high, are generally low in meat products and thus are low in protein (an important nutrient for immune function) and vitamin B_{12} (essential for DNA and RNA synthesis). Many athletes avoid dairy products to minimize intake of saturated fat, but this omits major sources of vitamin D, B-group vitamins, and calcium, all of which play roles of varying importance in maintaining immune function. If fat intake is a concern, athletes should select nonfat or low-fat dairy products that provide the same (or higher) levels of calcium, vitamin D, and vitamin B_{12} as full-fat dairy products. Only milk (regardless of fat content) is likely to be fortified with vitamin D.

Energy-restricted diets are not uncommon in sports in which leanness or low body mass confers a performance advantage (e.g., gymnastics, figure skating, endurance running) or is required to meet certain body-weight criteria (e.g., boxing, martial arts, weightlifting, rowing). Indeed, such demands have led to the identification of a new subclinical eating disorder, *anorexia athletica,* which is associated with an increased susceptibility to infection (see chapter 16). Even short-term dieting can influence immune function in athletes. For example, a loss of 2 kg (4 lb) of body mass over a 2-week period adversely affects macrophage phagocytic function.

Carbohydrate

The importance of adequate carbohydrate availability for maintenance of heavy training schedules and successful athletic performance is unquestionable (see chapter 6). During periods of heavy training, athletes should consume sufficient carbohydrate to cover about 60% of their energy costs. The recommended daily intake is 8 to 10 g of carbohydrate per kilogram of body weight for athletes who train more than 2 hours per day (see chapter 6). These recommendations are principally aimed at restoring muscle and liver glycogen stores to ensure sufficient carbohydrate availability for skeletal muscle contraction for training on successive days.

Glucose is also an important fuel for cells of the immune system, including lymphocytes, neutrophils, and macrophages. Phagocytes use glucose at a rate that is 10 times higher than the rate at which they use glutamine when both substrates are present in a culture medium at normal physiological concentrations. The importance of glucose for the proper functioning of lymphocytes and macrophages is further emphasized in a study that found mitogen-stimulated proliferation of these cells in vitro depends on a glucose concentration over the physiological range. Cells of the immune system have extremely high metabolic rates, and this finding highlights the importance of adequate nutrition for the provision of fuels to maintain immunocompetence.

Because elevated levels of stress hormones seem to cause many aspects of exercise-induced immune function impairment, nutritional strategies that effectively reduce the stress hormone response to exercise would be expected to limit the degree of exercise-induced immune dysfunction. The size of the glycogen stores in muscle and liver at the onset of exercise influences the hormonal and immune response to exercise. The amount of glycogen stored in the body is limited (usually less than 500 g) and is affected by recent physical activity and the amount of dietary carbohydrate intake. When people perform prolonged exercise following several days on very low-carbohydrate diets (typically < 50 g of carbohydrate per day), the magnitude of the stress hormone (e.g., adrenaline, cortisol) and cytokine (e.g., IL-6, IL-1ra, IL-10) response is markedly higher than it is on normal or high-carbohydrate diets, as illustrated in figure 13.17 (Gleeson et al. 1998; Mitchell et al. 1998). Furthermore, the postexercise fall in plasma glutamine concentration is greater than it is on normal and high-carbohydrate diets. It has been speculated that athletes deficient in carbohydrate are placing themselves at risk from the immunosuppressive effects of cortisol and reduced glutamine availability, including the suppression of antibody

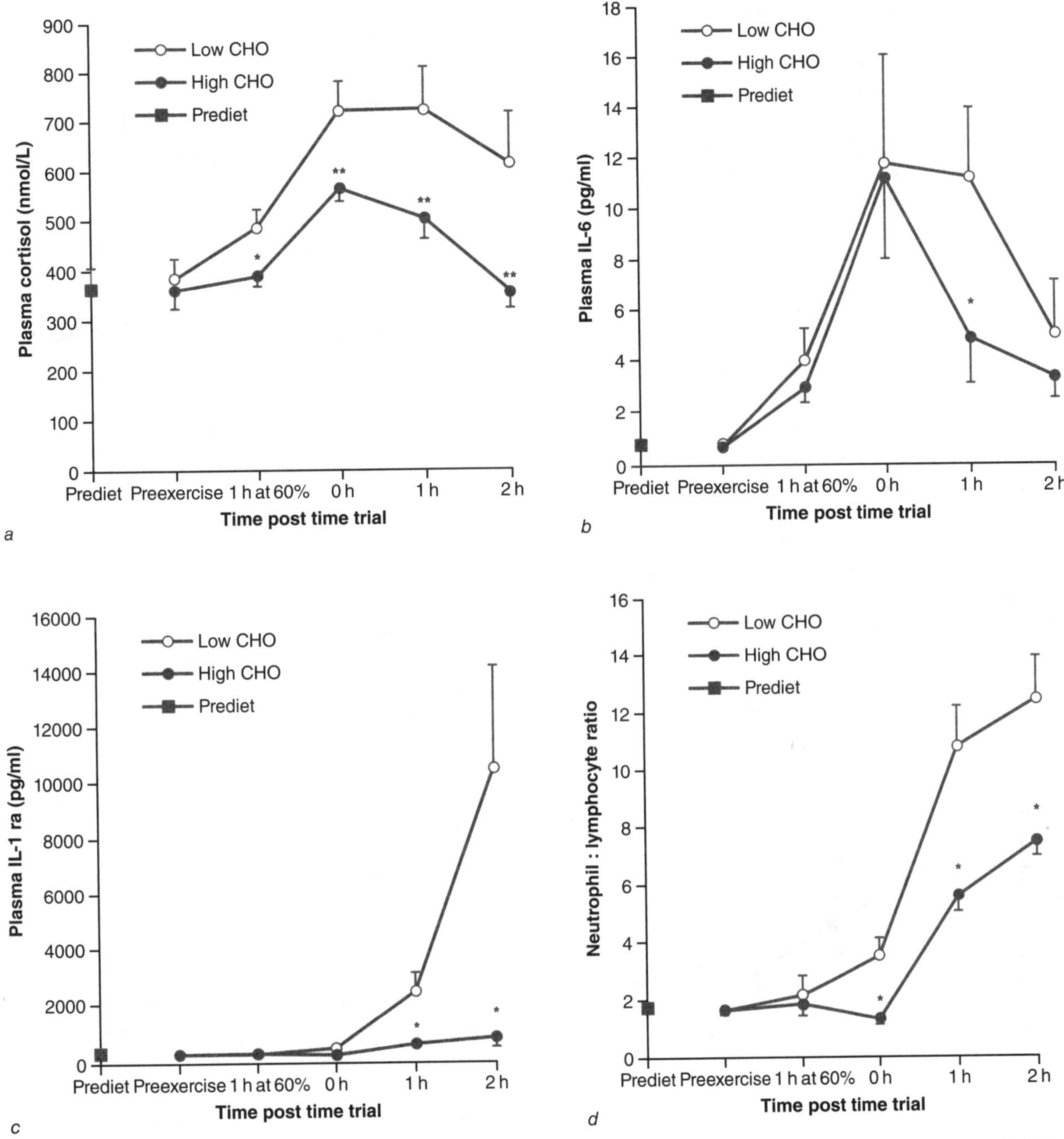

Figure 13.17 Changes in the concentrations of *(a)* plasma cortisol, *(b)* plasma interleukin-6 (IL-6), *(c)* plasma IL-1ra, and *(d)* the blood neutrophil-to-lymphocyte ratio after 1 hour of cycling at 60% of $\dot{V}O_2max$ immediately followed by a half-hour time trial (work rate around 80% of $\dot{V}O_2max$). For the 3 days before the exercise trial, subjects (n = 12) consumed either a high-carbohydrate (CHO) diet or a low-carbohydrate diet. Data are presented as mean and SEM. *Significantly different from low carbohydrate, $P < 0.05$. **Significantly different from low carbohydrate, $P < 0.01$.

Reprinted by permission from M. Gleeson and N.C. Bishop, "Modification of Immune Responses to Exercise by Carbohydrate, Glutamine and Anti-oxidant Supplements," *Immunology and Cell Biology* 78, (2000): 554-561.

production, lymphocyte proliferation, and NK cell cytotoxic activity. In the study by Mitchell et al. (1998), it was observed that exercising (for 1 hour at 75% of $\dot{V}O_2max$) in a glycogen-depleted state (induced by prior exercise and 2 days on a low-carbohydrate diet) resulted in a greater fall in circulating lymphocyte numbers at 2 hours postexercise compared with the same exercise performed after 2 days on a high-carbohydrate diet. In this study, the manipulation of carbohydrate status did not affect the decrease in mitogen-stimulated lymphocyte proliferation that occurred after exercise. But a study by Bishop, Walker, et al. (2005) showed that lymphocyte proliferation responses to mitogen and influenza were lower 24 hours following a 90-minute intermittent high-intensity exercise bout when subjects consumed a placebo beverage compared with a carbohydrate beverage before, during, and after the exercise bout (figure 13.18). These differences were independent of changes in the plasma cortisol concentration, which implies that these carbohydrate effects were mediated by a different mechanism.

Consumption of carbohydrate during prolonged exercise attenuates rises in plasma epinephrine, cortisol, and cytokines (Nehlsen-Cannarella et al. 1997); attenuates the trafficking of most leukocyte and lymphocyte subsets, including the rise in the neutrophil-to-lymphocyte ratio (see figure 13.19); prevents the exercise-induced fall in neutrophil function (see figure 13.20); and reduces the extent of the diminution of mitogen-stimulated T-lymphocyte proliferation (on a per-cell basis) after prolonged exercise (Henson et al. 1998) (see figure 13.21). It was shown that consuming 30 to 60 g of carbohydrate per hour during 2.5 hours of strenuous cycling prevented both the decrease in the number and percentage of interferon-gamma (IFN-γ) positive T-lymphocytes and the suppression of IFN-γ production from stimulated T-lymphocytes (figure 13.22) observed on the placebo control trial (Lancaster et al. 2005). IFN-γ production is critical to antiviral defense, and it has been suggested that the suppression of IFN-γ production may be an important mechanism that leads to increased risk of infection after prolonged exercise bouts (Konig et al. 1997).

The consumption of carbohydrate in beverages during exercise may have the additional benefit of helping maintain saliva flow rate during exercise. Saliva contains several proteins with antimicrobial properties, including IgA, lysozyme, and ß-amylase. During periods of heavy training, athletes

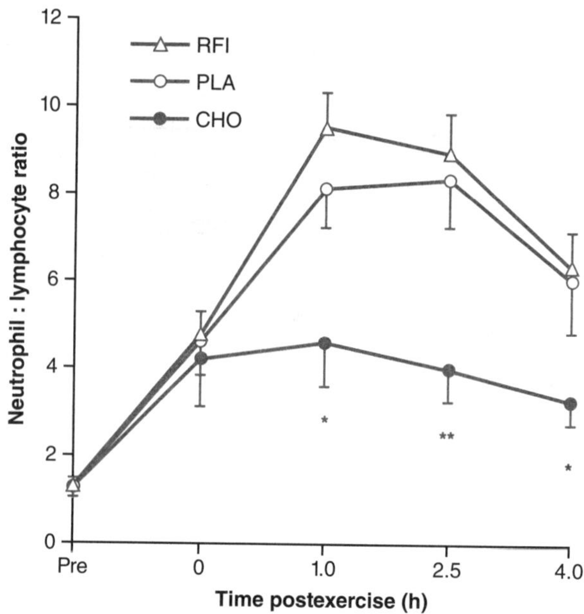

Figure 13.19 Changes in the neutrophil to lymphocyte ratio after 2 hours of cycling at 60% of $\dot{V}O_2$max when fed a 6% w/v carbohydrate solution (CHO), the same volume of an artificially sweetened placebo solution (PLA), or a restricted fluid intake (RFI). *Significantly different from placebo trial, $P < 0.05$. **Significantly different from placebo trial, $P < 0.01$.

Reprinted by permission from M. Gleeson and N.C. Bishop, "Modification of Immune Responses to Exercise by Carbohydrate, Glutamine and Anti-oxidant Supplements" *Immunology and Cell Biology* 78, (2000): 554-561; Data from Bishop, Blannin, Rand, Johnson, and Gleeson. (1999).

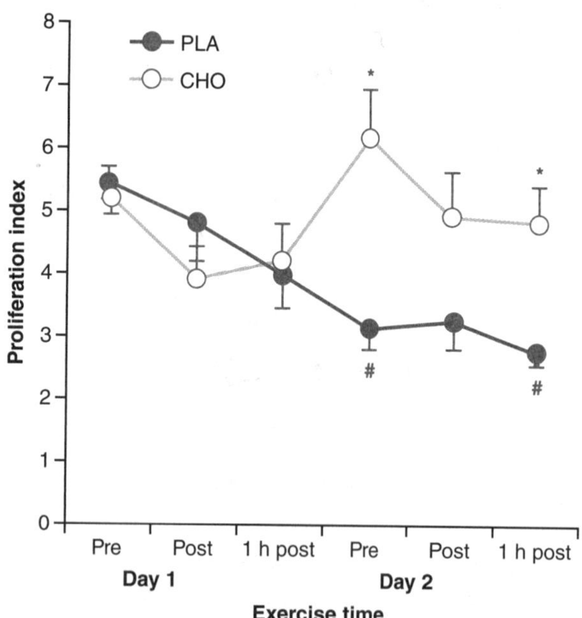

Figure 13.18 Mitogen (phytohemagglutinin)-stimulated T-lymphocyte proliferative response (fold increase relative to unstimulated cells) before and after two bouts of high-intensity intermittent exercise performed on consecutive days with either carbohydrate (CHO, 6.4% w/v) or placebo (PLA) beverage ingestion before, during, and after exercise bout. *Significantly higher than PLA, $P < 0.05$. **Significantly lower than preexercise on day 1 (PLA only), $P < 0.05$.

Based on Bishop et al. (1999b).

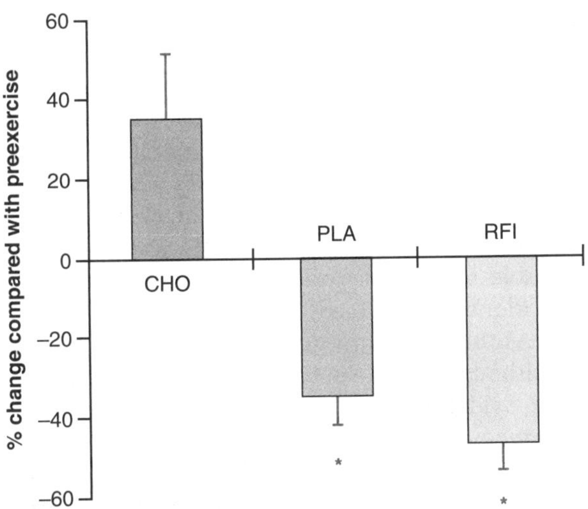

Figure 13.20 Percentage change (compared with preexercise) in the lipopolysaccharide-stimulated neutrophil degranulation response immediately after 2 hours of cycling at 60% of $\dot{V}O_2$max when fed a 6% w/v carbohydrate solution (CHO), the same volume of an artificially sweetened placebo solution (PLA), or a restricted fluid intake (RFI). *Significant change from preexercise, $P < 0.05$.

Reprinted by permission from M. Gleeson and N.C. Bishop, "Modification of Immune Responses to Exercise by Carbohydrate, Glutamine and Anti-oxidant Supplements" *Immunology and Cell Biology* 78, (2000): 554-561; Data from Bishop, Blannin, Rand, Johnson, and Gleeson. (1999).

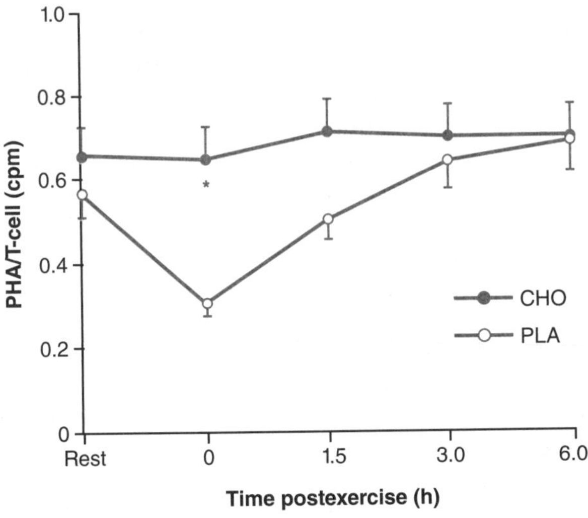

Figure 13.21 Change in phytohemagglutinin-stimulated (PHA) lymphocyte proliferation after 2.5 hours of running when fed a 6% w/v carbohydrate (CHO) solution or the same volume of an artificially sweetened placebo (PLA) solution. *Significantly different from PLA, $P < 0.05$.

Reprinted by permission from M. Gleeson and N.C. Bishop, "Modification of Immune Responses to Exercise by Carbohydrate, Glutamine and Anti-oxidant Supplements" *Immunology and Cell Biology* 78, (2000): 554-561; Data from Heson et al. (1998).

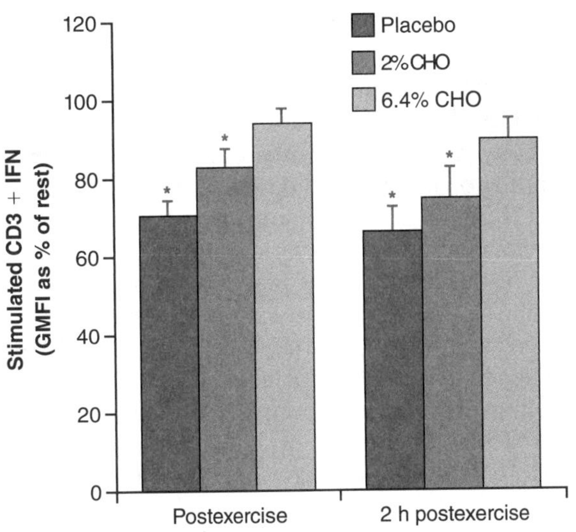

Figure 13.22 Consumption of 30 to 60 g of carbohydrate per hour as a 6.4% w/v beverage during 2.5 hours of strenuous cycling exercise prevents the suppression of IFN-γ production from stimulated T-lymphocytes observed on the placebo control trial. Note that ingesting a small amount of carbohydrate as a 2% w/v beverage is not as effective. The volume of drinks consumed was 500 ml immediately preexercise and 200 ml every 20 minutes during exercise. *Significantly lower than preexercise, $P < 0.05$.

Data from Lancaster et al. (2005).

have lower levels of IgA in their saliva, and this condition may contribute to their increased incidence of URTI (Mackinnon 1999; Neville, Gleeson, and Folland 2008). Saliva secretion is under neural control. The sympathetic nervous system stimulation that occurs during exercise causes vasoconstriction of the blood vessels to the salivary glands and results in a reduction in saliva secretion. Regular fluid intake during exercise prevents this effect, and a study (Bishop, Blannin, and Gleeson 2000) has confirmed that regular consumption of carbohydrate-containing drinks helps maintain saliva flow rate and, hence, saliva IgA secretion rate during prolonged exercise.

Although carbohydrate feeding during exercise appears to be effective in minimizing some of the immune perturbations associated with prolonged strenuous exercise, it does not prevent the fall in the plasma glutamine concentration and seems less effective for less-demanding exercise such as football (Bishop et al. 1999) or rowing training (Nieman et al. 1999). Carbohydrate feeding is not as effective in reducing immune-cell trafficking and functional depression when exercise is performed to the point of fatigue (Bishop et al. 2001).

Preexercise feeding of carbohydrate is not effective in limiting exercise-induced changes in leukocyte trafficking or depression of neutrophil function. In a study that investigated the effect of carbohydrate ingestion during 2 hours of treadmill running on cell-mediated in vivo immunity (using experimental skin contact hypersensitivity with the novel antigen diphenylcyclopropenone), there was no difference from placebo (both treatments exhibited a 46% drop in skin fold response compared with resting controls) (Davison et al. 2016). Evidence that any beneficial effect of carbohydrate feeding on immune responses to exercise translates to reduced incidence of URTI after prolonged exercise (e.g., marathon races) is currently lacking. Although a trend for a beneficial effect of carbohydrate ingestion on postrace URTI was reported in a study of 98 marathon runners (Nieman, Henson, Fagoaga, et al. 2002), this finding did not achieve statistical significance. Larger-scale studies are needed to investigate this possibility.

Fat

The International Consensus Conference on Foods, Nutrition, and Sports Performance advised athletes that 20% of energy intake should come from fat, whereas the *Dietary Guidelines for Americans* (U.S. Department of Agriculture 2005) recommended that total fat intake should be between 20% and 35% of total energy intake. More recently, for athletes at least, it is recognized that recommendations for macronutrient intake, specifically carbohydrate and protein, should be given as amounts needed in grams per day or grams per kilogram of body mass per day (as described in chapters 6 and 8) and that fat makes up the rest to meet the overall total daily energy need. Thus, fat intake is commonly 20% to 35% of dietary energy, but this is not actually a recommendation. The type of dietary fat consumed, however, is important. In 1994, the UK Department of Health recommended that saturated fats contribute no more than 10% of daily energy intake, and the *Dietary Guidelines for Americans* (U.S. Department of Agriculture 2005) made an identical recommendation and advises that the remainder of fat intake be provided by MUFAs (15%), PUFAs (6%), linoleic acid (1%), linolenic acid (0.2%), and *trans* FAs (<2%). Two groups of PUFAs are essential to the body: the omega-6 (*n*-6) series derived from linoleic acid and the omega-3 (*n*-3) series derived from linolenic acid. Adequate intakes of omega-6 FAs for adult men and women are 17 and 12 g/day, and AIs for omega-3 FAs are 1.6 and 1.1 g/day (U.S. Department of Agriculture 2005). These FAs cannot be synthesized in the body and therefore must be derived from the diet. Diets rich in either of these PUFAs improve the conditions of patients suffering from diseases characterized by an overactive immune system, such as rheumatoid arthritis, and there is also evidence that fish oil omega-3 FA supplements can help minimize respiratory symptoms in individuals who are susceptible to exercise-induced bronchoconstriction (Mickleborough, Head, and Lindley 2011). These PUFAs thus have immunomodulatory functions.

Although FAs are used as fuels by lymphocytes, their oxidation does not appear to be crucial for lymphocyte function, because the inhibition of FA oxidation does not affect the ability of lymphocytes to proliferate in response to mitogens. FAs exert either direct effects (by altering cell membrane fluidity) or indirect effects (as precursors of cell-signaling molecules called eicosanoids) on immune function, which generally result in reduced IL-2 production and suppressed mitogen-induced lymphocyte proliferation. But supplementation with vitamin E or vitamin C appears to provide partial protection against some of these immunosuppressive effects.

Relatively little is known about the potential contribution of FAs to the regulation of exercise-induced modification of immune function. Although no study has been done in athletes, excessive intake of PUFA could possibly further potentiate the exercise-induced suppression of IL-2 production and lymphocyte proliferation. High intakes of arachidonic acid relative to intakes of omega-3 FAs may also exert an undesirable influence on inflammation and immune function during and after exercise. Alteration of essential FA distribution through dietary changes or nutritional supplementation is already being applied in the treatment of chronic inflammatory diseases. More research is needed on the effects of altering essential FA intake on immune function after exercise and during periods of heavy training. A study that investigated the effects of endurance training for 7 weeks on carbohydrate-rich (65% of dietary energy) or fat-rich (62% of dietary energy) diets concluded that diet during training may influence natural immunity because NK cell activity increased on the carbohydrate-rich diet compared with the fat-rich diet (Pedersen et al. 2000). The results of this study suggest that a fat-rich diet is detrimental to immune function compared with a carbohydrate-rich diet but do not clarify whether this effect is the result of a lack of dietary carbohydrate or an excess of a specific dietary fat component.

Protein and Amino Acids

The daily protein requirement of athletes is approximately twice that of the sedentary population. An intake of less than 1.6 g of protein per kilogram of body weight per day is likely to be associated with a negative nitrogen balance in athletes who are training hard (particularly endurance athletes). If athletes consume well-balanced diets that meet their requirements for energy, the increased requirement for protein will be met. Those at greatest risk for protein deficiency are athletes who are undertaking a program of food restriction to lose weight, vegetarian athletes, and athletes who are consuming unbalanced diets (e.g., with an excessive amount of carbohydrate at the expense of protein).

Inadequate intake of protein impairs host immunity and has particularly detrimental effects on the T-cell system, which results in increased incidence of opportunistic infections. One of the most dramatic manifestations of this development is widespread atrophy of lymphoid tissue. In humans, protein-energy malnutrition (PEM) depresses the number of mature, fully differentiated T-lymphocytes and the in vitro response to T-lymphocyte mitogens, although the latter is reversible with nutritional repletion. In addition, the T-lymphocyte CD4+ to CD8+ ratio is markedly decreased in PEM. Essentially all forms of immunity are affected by PEM in humans, depending on the severity of the protein deficiency relative to energy intake. These effects include impaired phagocytic cell function, decreased cytokine production, and reduced complement formation. Although athletes are unlikely to reach a state of extreme malnutrition unless they are dieting very severely, some impairment of host-defense mechanisms is observed even in moderate protein deficiency.

Excessive dietary protein could also be harmful to immune function. A diet rich in protein (24% protein, 72% fat, and 3% carbohydrate) consumed for 4 days caused a 25% lowering of muscle and plasma glutamine levels. This decline was attributed to increased renal uptake of glutamine to reestablish normal acid–base balance because a high intake of protein combined with a low intake of carbohydrate induces chronic metabolic acidosis. Furthermore, falls in the plasma glutamine concentration after prolonged strenuous exercise are greater when consuming a low-carbohydrate diet compared with a normal diet. Ingesting carbohydrate during exercise, however, does not prevent the postexercise fall in plasma glutamine.

The ingestion of protein stimulates protein synthesis, and this may be particularly important in the postexercise period to promote muscle repair and adaptation to training (see chapter 8). It has also been shown that postexercise ingestion of about 20 g protein (0.3 g per kilogram of body weight) can help to restore some aspects of immune function during the recovery period (Papacosta et al. 2015, Witard et al. 2013) and reduce respiratory infection incidence in overreaching athletes, which emphasizes the importance of encouraging athletes to develop feeding strategies that focus on the postexercise period as part of their overall nutritional plans.

Glutamine is the most abundant free amino acid in human muscle and plasma, and it is used at extremely high rates by leukocytes to provide energy and optimal conditions for nucleotide biosynthesis. Indeed, glutamine is important, if not essential, to lymphocytes and other rapidly dividing cells, including the gut **mucosa** and bone marrow stem cells. Glutamine is also required for optimal macrophage phagocytic activity. Prolonged exercise is associated with a fall in the plasma concentration of glutamine, and such a decrease has been hypothesized to impair immune function. The overtraining syndrome is associated with a chronic reduction in plasma glutamine levels, which may be partly responsible for the immunodepression apparent in this condition. Interestingly, evidence indicates that an additional intake of 20 to 30 g of protein per day can restore depressed plasma glutamine levels in overtrained athletes.

Several scientists have suggested that exogenous provision of glutamine supplements may be beneficial by preventing the impairment of immune function after prolonged exercise. The evidence that oral glutamine supplements reduce the incidence of URTI after endurance events is limited (Castell and Newsholme 1996). Several studies that have investigated the effect of glutamine supplementation during and after exercise on various indices of immune function have failed to find any beneficial effect. A glutamine solution (0.1 g per kilogram of body weight) given at 0 minutes, 30 minutes, 60 minutes, and 90 minutes after a marathon race prevented the fall in the plasma glutamine concentration but did not prevent the fall in mitogen-induced lymphocyte proliferation and lymphocyte-activated NK cell activity (Rohde et al. 1998). Similarly, maintaining the plasma glutamine concentration by consuming glutamine in drinks taken during and after 2 hours of cycling at 60% of $\dot{V}O_2$max did not affect leukocyte subset trafficking or prevent the exercise-induced fall in neutrophil function (Walsh et al. 2000). Unlike carbohydrate consumed during exercise, glutamine supplements do not seem to affect immune function perturbations, and a review article (Hiscock and Pedersen 2002) concluded that falls in plasma glutamine are not responsible for exercise-induced immunodepression. However, two studies have provided some evidence that glutamine may help reduce exercise-induced immunodepression following exercise. Caris et al. (2014) observed a positive effect of glutamine and carbohydrate in modulating the Th1–Th2 (helper cells) balance after exercise and the postexercise ratio of CD4+ helper to CD8+ cytotoxic/suppressor cells was reported to be higher in athletes provided with glutamine rather than placebo after heavy load training (Song et al. 2015).

Bassit and colleagues (2002) reported that supplementation of BCAAs (6 g/day for 15 days) before a triathlon or 30 km (19 mi) run prevented the approximately 40% decline in mitogen-stimulated lymphocyte proliferation observed in the placebo control group after exercise. BCAAs are precursors for glutamine, and BCAA supplementation prevented the postexercise fall in plasma glutamine concentration and was associated with increased IL-2 and interferon production. More research is needed to resolve these conflicting findings of BCAA and glutamine supplementation on immune responses to exercise.

Alcohol and Caffeine

Increasing evidence suggests that consumption of light to moderate amounts of polyphenol-rich alcoholic beverages, such as wine or beer, could have health benefits. Scientists have long debated the effects of alcohol on immune function. On the one hand, high doses of alcohol consumption can directly suppress a wide range of immune responses, and alcohol abuse is associated with an increased incidence of a number of infectious diseases. On the other hand, moderate alcohol consumption seems to have a beneficial effect on the immune system compared with alcohol abuse or abstinence, and epidemiological studies have indicated that moderate alcohol consumption is associated with lower morbidity (Romeo et al. 2007). This may be because the ethanol in alcoholic beverages has largely detrimental effects, whereas some of the polyphenol compounds in wine and beer may have antioxidant, anti-inflammatory, or beneficial immunomodulatory effects. At present, the link between alcohol consumption, immune response, and infectious and inflammatory processes is not completely understood. Of course, other factors that are unrelated or are indirectly related to immune function, such as drinking patterns, beverage type, amount of alcohol, or gender differences, may well affect the influence that alcohol consumption has on the immune system. It is clear, however, that binge drinking of alcohol depresses immune function for several hours (Afshar et al. 2015) and athletes should avoid this, particularly after heavy training sessions or competition. With alcoholic beverage consumption more is not better, and all people should be aware of the serious health risks of consuming more than two drinks per day.

Caffeine is the most widely consumed drug in Europe and the United States (Curatolo and Robertson 1983), and athletes have long used it in the belief that it improves performance (see chapter 11). Caffeine is an adenosine receptor antagonist, and several immune cell types, including neutrophils and lymphocytes, express adenosine receptors. Furthermore, caffeine ingestion results in elevated circulating epinephrine (adrenaline) concentration at rest and during exercise, so it could affect immune cell functions indirectly through actions on adrenoreceptors. At present, little information is available about the effects of caffeine on immune function at rest. Addition of pharmacological doses of caffeine to cell culture media has been associated with dose-dependent suppression of in vitro mitogen-stimulated lymphocyte proliferative responses in humans (Rosenthal et al. 1992). But in vivo administration of 18 mg of caffeine per kilogram of body weight per day in rats was associated with a significant increase in mitogen-stimulated T-cell proliferation (Kantamala, Vongsakul, and Satayavivad 1990). In the same study, B-cell proliferative responses to mitogen significantly decreased following administration of 6 mg of caffeine per kilogram of body weight per day.

Several exercise studies have demonstrated that caffeine compared with placebo ingestion 1 hour before a bout of intensive endurance exercise was associated with greater perturbations in numbers of circulating lymphocytes, CD4+ cells, and CD8+ cells. Moreover, caffeine ingestion was associated with an increased percentage of T-helper (CD4+) and T-cytotoxic (CD8+) lymphocytes expressing the early activation marker CD69 in vivo before and after exercise (Bishop, Fitzgerald, et al. 2005). Furthermore, the postexercise fall in stimulated neutrophil oxidative burst responses was attenuated by caffeine ingestion (Walker et al. 2006). It is thought that these effects may be largely mediated through the action of caffeine as an adenosine receptor antagonist.

Vitamins

Vitamins are essential organic molecules that cannot be synthesized in the body and therefore must be obtained from food (see chapter 10). Several vitamins are essential for normal immune function: fat-soluble vitamins A and E and water-soluble vitamins B_{12} and C. Other vitamins (e.g., B_6 and folic acid) also play important roles in immune function, but dietary deficiencies of these vitamins in humans are extremely rare.

No indications in the literature suggest that vitamin intake among athletes in general is insufficient with the exception of vitamin D. Athletes tend to ingest above-average quantities of most micronutrients, and this may satisfy any increase in need. Vitamin D is an exception because it is mostly derived from endogenous synthesis, which requires the action of sunlight on the skin; only a small amount comes from dietary sources. The requirement for most vitamins is not thought to be increased in athletes compared with the general population. For example, vitamin loss through sweat during exercise is negligible, and vitamin metabolism is largely unaffected by exercise.

Antioxidant Vitamins

Vitamins with antioxidant properties, including vitamins C, E, and beta-carotene (provitamin A), may be required in increased quantities in athletes to inactivate the products of exercise-induced lipid peroxidation (Packer 1997). Oxygen free-radical formation that accompanies the dramatic increase in oxidative metabolism during exercise (see chapter 10) could potentially inhibit immune responses.

ROS inhibit locomotory and bactericidal activity of neutrophils, reduce the proliferation of T-lymphocytes and B-lymphocytes, and inhibit NKCA. Sustained endurance training appears to be associated with an adaptive upregulation of the antioxidant defense system. Such adaptations, however, may be insufficient to protect athletes who train extensively, and these individuals should consider increasing their intakes of nutritional antioxidants, such as vitamins C, E, and beta-carotene, to reduce free-radical damage.

Vitamin C (ascorbic acid) occurs in high concentration in leukocytes and is implicated in a variety of anti-infective functions, including promotion of T-lymphocyte proliferation, prevention of corticosteroid-induced suppression of neutrophil activity, production of interferon, and inhibition of virus replication. It is also a major water-soluble antioxidant that is effective as a scavenger of ROS in intracellular and extracellular fluids. It can act as an antioxidant directly (e.g., in the prevention of auto-oxidative dysfunction of neutrophil bactericidal activity) and indirectly through its regeneration of reduced vitamin E (α-tocopherol). Vitamin C occurs in high concentration in the adrenal glands and is necessary for the production of several hormones that are secreted in response to stress, such as epinephrine, norepinephrine, and cortisol.

Studies report that daily supplementation of large doses of vitamin C reduced the incidence of symptoms of URTI in athletes after they participated in ultramarathon races (Peters et al. 1993, 1996). The results of one of these studies are illustrated in figure 13.23, which also shows that the supplementation of additional dietary antioxidants (vitamin E and beta-carotene) does not confer any additional beneficial effects. The doses of vitamin C used in these studies (600-1,000 mg/day) are considerably higher than the daily dosage of 200 mg that is associated with accelerated clinical improvement in elderly patients hospitalized with acute respiratory infection after 4 weeks of daily supplementation (Hunt et al. 1994). In a more recent randomized, double-blind, placebo-controlled study, intake of 1,500 mg of vitamin C per day for 7 days before an ultramarathon race and consumption of vitamin C in a carbohydrate beverage during the race (subjects in the placebo group consumed the same carbohydrate beverage without added vitamin C) did not affect oxidative stress, cytokine, or immune function measures during and after the race (Nieman, Henson, McAnulty, et. al 2002). In contrast, it has been reported (Fischer et al. 2004) that 4 weeks of combined supplementation of vitamin C (500 mg/day) and vitamin E (400 IU/day) before a 3-hour knee extension exercise protocol reduced muscle IL-6 release and reduced the systemic rise in circulating IL-6 and cortisol (figure 13.24). Some degree of blunting of the plasma cortisol response to exercise and better-maintained neutrophil function after exercise were reported in a placebo-controlled study that used the same daily dose of vitamin C and E supplements and examined immunoendocrine responses to 2.5 hours of cycling after 4 weeks of supplementation (Davison, Gleeson, and Phillips 2007). Furthermore, administration of the antioxidant N-acetyl-L-cysteine (a precursor of glutathione) to mice prevented the exercise-induced reduction in intracellular glutathione concentration and markedly reduced postexercise apoptosis in intestinal lymphocytes (Quadrilatero and Hoffman-Goetz 2004). Thus,

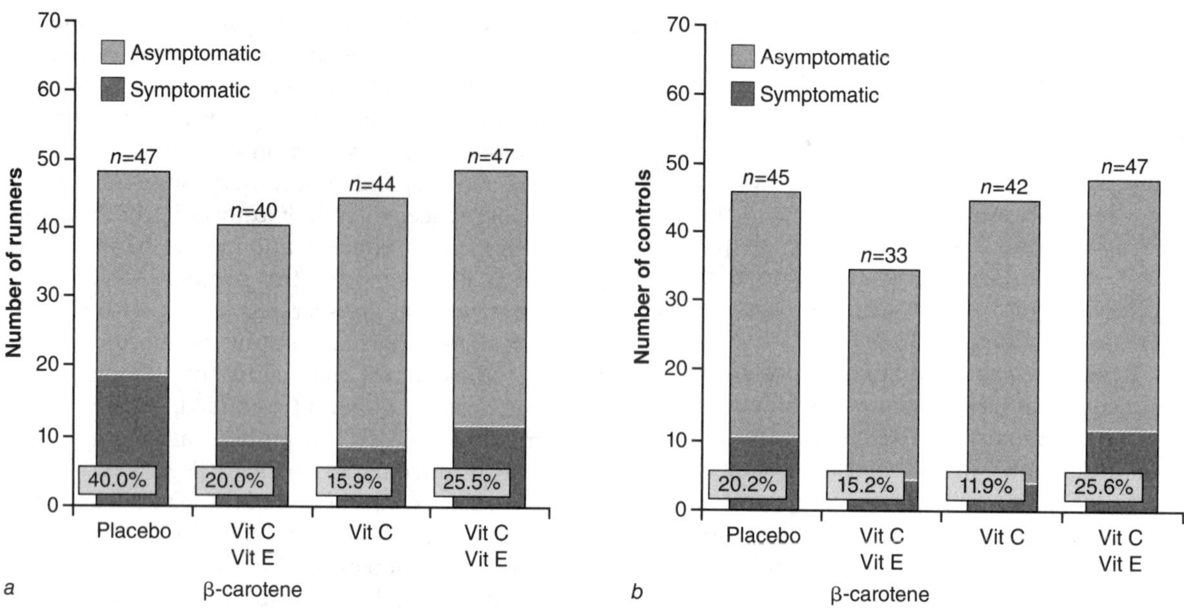

Figure 13.23 The incidence of URTI in the week after the 1993 Comrades Ultramarathon (90 km [56 mi]) in South Africa. Different groups of runners *(a)* or control subjects *(b)* received different combinations of antioxidant supplements or placebo for 3 weeks before the ultramarathon.

Adapted from E.M. Peters et al., "Vitamin C as Effective As Combinations of Anti-Oxidant Nutrients In Reducing Symptoms of Upper Respiratory Tract Infections in Ultramarathon Runners," *South African Journal of Sports Medicine* 11, (1996): 23-27.

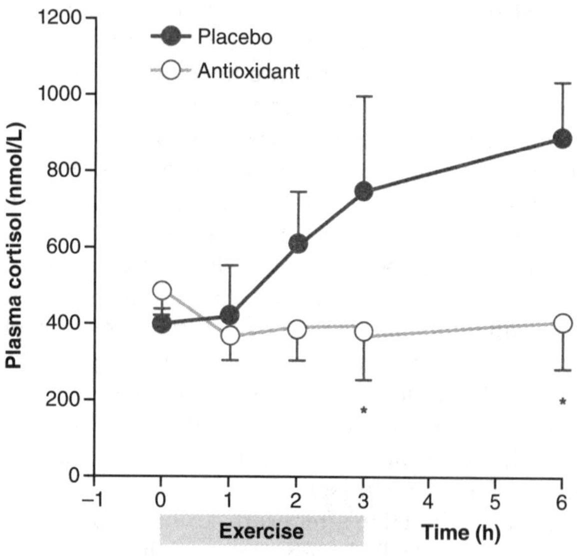

Figure 13.24 The effect of 4 weeks of antioxidant supplementation (500 mg/day of vitamin C and 400 IU/day of vitamin E) compared with placebo on plasma cortisol responses to 3 hours of dynamic knee extensor exercise. *Significantly different from placebo, P<0.05.

Based on Fischer et al. (2004).

although some inconsistencies are seen in the literature regarding antioxidant supplementation and immune responses to exercise, some basis is present for believing that such supplementation could have beneficial effects in alleviating exercise-induced immunodepression through the mechanisms summarized in figure 13.25.

The most recent Cochrane meta-analysis examined the evidence that daily doses of more than 200 mg vitamin C were more effective than placebo in preventing or treating the common cold (Douglas et al. 2007). Twenty-nine trial comparisons involving 11,077 study participants contributed to this meta-analysis on the relative risk (RR) of developing a cold while taking prophylactic vitamin C. The pooled RR was 0.96 (95% CI: 0.92-1.00). A subgroup of six trials that involved physically active subjects (a total of 642 marathon runners, skiers, and soldiers on subarctic exercises) reported a pooled RR of 0.50 (95% CI: 0.38-0.66). Thirty comparisons that involved 9,676 respiratory episodes contributed to the meta-analysis on common cold duration during vitamin C or placebo supplementation. A consistent benefit of vitamin C was observed, representing a reduction in cold duration of 8% (95%: CI 0.03-0.13) for adult participants and 13.5% (95% CI: 0.0-0.21) for child participants. Fifteen trial comparisons that involved

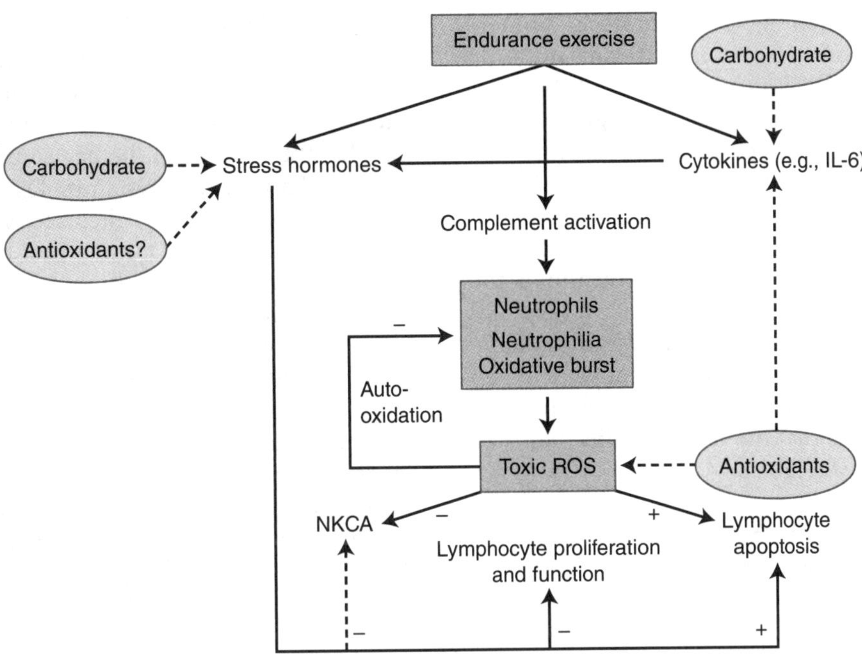

Figure 13.25 The possible mechanisms by which dietary antioxidant supplementation reduces stress-induced or exercise-induced immunodepression.

7,045 respiratory episodes contributed to the meta-analysis of severity of episodes experienced while on prophylaxis, and the results revealed a benefit of vitamin C when days confined to home and off work or school were taken as a measure of severity. A limited number of trials had examined cold duration and severity during therapy with vitamin C that was initiated after the onset of cold symptoms, and no significant differences from placebo were found. The authors concluded that the failure of vitamin C supplementation to reduce the incidence of colds in the normal population indicates that routine mega-dose prophylaxis is not generally justified but that individuals subjected to brief periods of severe physical exercise or cold environments may gain some benefit.

Even if high-dose antioxidant supplementation offers some protective effect on infection risk, athletes need to consider the risks, which may include the blunting of some of the adaptations to training. Chapter 12 discusses this issue in detail.

Animal studies show an increased oxidation of vitamin E during exercise that could result in reduced antioxidant protection. Dietary vitamin E stimulates mononuclear cell production of IL-Iß through its influence on the arachidonic acid metabolic pathways, and cytokine production is further facilitated by a vitamin E–influenced inhibition of prostaglandin E2 (PGE2) production. Severe vitamin E deficiency results in impaired cell-mediated immunity and decreased antibody synthesis.

Vitamin A is also essential for immunocompetence. Vitamin A deficiency in animals and humans results in atrophy of the thymus, decreased lymphocyte proliferation in response to mitogens, increased bacterial binding to respiratory tract epithelial cells, and impaired secretory IgA production. Consequently, vitamin A–deficient humans have a higher incidence of spontaneous infection. Vitamin A–deficient experimental animals also demonstrate reduced NKCA, lower production of interferon and antibodies, impaired delayed cutaneous hypersensitivity, and less-effective macrophage activity.

Beta-carotene acts as an immunostimulant; it increased the number of CD4+ helper T-cells in healthy human volunteers and stimulated NKCA when added in vitro to human lymphatic cultures. Furthermore, elderly men who had been taking beta-carotene supplements (50 mg on alternate days) for 10 to 12 years were reported to have significantly higher NKCA than did elderly men on placebo. Beta-carotene also functions as an antioxidant; thus, the requirement may increase in athletes who are involved in heavy training schedules that stimulate increased production of ROS.

However, supplementing ultramarathon runners with beta-carotene had an insignificant effect on the incidence of URTI after the 90 km Comrades Ultramarathon in South Africa (see figure 13.23).

Because there is little evidence of any immune benefit from excessive supplementation with antioxidant vitamins (with the possible exception of vitamin C), this practice cannot be recommended. Indeed, oversupplementation can diminish the body's natural antioxidant defense system and may attenuate some endurance training adaptations such as mitochondrial biogenesis (Ristow et al. 2009; Yfanti et al. 2010). The best option is probably to ensure that the diet contains plenty of fresh fruits and vegetables.

Vitamin B_{12} and Folic Acid

Vitamin B_{12} and folic-acid deficiencies have profound effects on immune function. Both of these vitamins are essential for the synthesis of nucleic acids and hence are required for the normal production of red and white blood cells in the bone marrow. Vitamin B_{12} can be absorbed from the gut only in the presence of the glycoprotein intrinsic factor. Lack of this factor or deficiency of vitamin B_{12} causes pernicious anemia, which has detrimental effects on immune function. For example, impaired lymphocyte proliferative responses to mitogens and a modest reduction in the phagocytic and bactericidal capacity of neutrophils have been reported in people with primary pernicious anemia. The only natural sources of vitamin B_{12} are of animal origin. As such, vegetarian athletes and athletes who avoid dairy products to minimize saturated fat intake are at high risk for deficiency of this vitamin. If fat intake is a concern, then athletes should select nonfat or low-fat dairy products that provide the same (or higher) levels of B_{12} as full-fat dairy products.

Vitamin D

As mentioned, most athletes who consume a varied diet sufficient to meet their energy needs should meet their micronutrient requirements; vitamin D is an exception (He et al. 2013; Owens et al. 2015). It has been established that vitamin D is not only important for calcium homeostasis and bone health but also for the optimal function of skeletal muscle and immune function as well as some other health outcomes (Bendik et al. 2014; Bischoff-Ferrari 2014; Owens et al. 2015; Prietl et al. 2013; Shuler et al. 2012). These aspects are covered in chapter 10; here we focus on the importance of vitamin D for immune function.

Vitamin D is not actually a vitamin but a secosteroid hormone that is mostly produced in the skin from 7-dehydrocholesterol after exposure to sunlight UVB radiation. Two forms of vitamin D can be obtained from dietary sources: vitamin D_3 (cholecalciferol) and vitamin D_2 (ergocalciferol). The endogenously synthesized vitamin D_3 and diet-derived D_2 and D_3 must first be hydroxylated in the liver into 25-hydroxy vitamin D (25(OH) D), the main storage form. In the second hydroxylation, 25(OH)D is converted to the biologically active form, 1,25-dihydroxy vitamin D (1, $25(OH)_2D$), by 1-α-hydroxylase in the kidney or some cells in nonrenal compartments, such as cells of the immune system, including T-cells, B-cells, macrophages, and dendritic cells (Aranow 2011).

New insights indicate that sufficient vitamin D is required for the production of antimicrobial proteins, such as cathelicidin and defensins, following toll-like receptor stimulation; as such, vitamin D is purported to play a central role in the antibacterial defenses that characterize the innate immune response (Laaksi 2012). These vitamin D–responsive antimicrobial proteins are produced by monocytes, macrophages, and epithelial cells. In the lungs, they are secreted into the thin layer of fluid that covers the inner surface of the airways, thereby creating a barrier that is chemically lethal to microbes. In addition to its effects on antimicrobial proteins, the biologically active form of vitamin D (1, $25(OH)_2D$) strengthens epithelial barrier functions by upregulating genes for the proteins required in tight junctions (e.g., occludin), gap junctions (e.g., connexin 43), and adherens junctions (e.g., E-cadherin) in epithelial cells, fibroblasts, and keratinocytes (Clairmont et al., 1996; Gniadecki et al., 1997; Palmer et al., 2001). Furthermore, 1, $25(OH)_2D$ enhances the effectiveness of monocytes and macrophages in killing microbes by enhancing the generation of ROS and the expression of inducible nitric oxide synthase in these phagocytic cells (Sly et al. 2001) as well as augmenting IL-1ß secretion and upregulating the expression of CD14, the lipopolysaccharide (LPS) receptor. Recent studies on natural killer cell function indicate that 1, $25(OH)_2D$ upregulates the expression of NK cell surface cytotoxicity receptors, downregulates the expression of the killer inhibitory receptor CD158, and enhances NK cell cytolytic activity (Al-Jaderi & Maghazachi, 2013). It is also recognized that vitamin D is essential in activating and controlling the T-cell antigen receptor and thus enhancing the recognition of antigens by T-lymphocytes (Kongsbak et al., 2013; von Essen et al., 2010), which leads to an activation of the cellular immune response in response to pathogen exposure. These findings indicate that vitamin D is crucial for the activation of the acquired immune system and is therefore very important for the effective clearance of viral infections. Vitamin D may also modulate cytokine secretion by lymphocytes and monocytes, which increases proinflammatory cytokine production following antigen exposure (He et al. 2013) and promotes anti-inflammatory IL-10 production in order to resolve inflammation and speed recovery from illness or injury. Although the actions of vitamin D do not alter numbers of circulating leukocytes, neutrophils, monocytes, or lymphocytes, the proportions of lymphocyte subsets, particularly within the T-cell compartment, can be modified as can the functions of various immune cells associated with innate and acquired immunity. The actions of 1, 25(OH)$_2$D on the human immune system are summarized in table 13.7.

It is generally accepted that the best measure of vitamin D status is the serum concentration of 25-hydroxy vitamin D (25(OH)D) which is formed in the liver. Vitamin D deficiency (serum 25(OH)D < 40 nmol/L) is not uncommon among athletes and the general population, particularly when sunlight exposure is limited in the winter months. Because of severe concern about vitamin D deficiency in Finland, the Ministry of Social Affairs and Health instigated the fortification of milk (0.5 µg or 20 IU per 100 ml) and margarines (10 µg or 400 IU per 100 g) with vitamin D from 2003 onward, and the vitamin D status of the general population has since substantially improved in Finland (Laaksi 2012).

TABLE 13.7 Main Effects of 1, 25-Dihydroxy Vitamin D on the Immune System

Tissue site of action and function	Actions of 1, 25(OH)$_2$D
Antigen-presenting cells (monocytes, macrophages, and dendritic cells, which are initiators of immune responses to pathogens)	Increases the production of antimicrobial proteins and peptides (e.g., cathelicidin, ß-defensins) and the generation of ROS and NO synthase activity Increases macrophage phagocytosis and upregulates CD14 expression Downregulates CD40 (required for B-cell activation), CD80/86 (required for T-cell activation), and major histocompatibility complex II (MHCII) expression Increases IL-10 production and inhibits production of proinflammatory cytokines
Salivary glands (produce saliva which has antimicrobial properties)	Increases saliva flow and antimicrobial protein secretion
Epithelial cells (protective mucosal linings of airways, gut, and so on)	Upregulates genes for gap, adherens, and tight junction proteins, which strengthens barrier function
Natural killer cells (important in innate immunity; kill cells infected with viruses)	Downregulates production of IFN Upregulates expression of NK cytotoxicity receptors and promotes IL-2-activated cytolysis
T-cells (coordinate immune responses; responsible for cell-mediated immunity)	Increases vitamin D receptor expression Inhibits production of proinflammatory cytokines IL-2 and IFN-γ by Th1 cells and increases IL-4 production by Th2 cells Suppresses the development of Th17 cells and inhibits their cytokine production Induces Treg cells and increases their IL-10 production Generally increases antigen-specific T-cell activation and proliferation
B-cells (responsible for humoral immunity)	Increases vitamin D receptor expression Suppresses B-cell proliferation and immunoglobulin production Inhibits the differentiation of B-cells into plasma cells

A study in university athletes reported a higher level of plasma cathelicidin and salivary SIgA secretion in those who had plasma 25(OH)D greater than 120 nmol/L compared with those who had lower vitamin D status (He et al. 2013). Furthermore, low vitamin D status (25(OH)D < 30 nmol/L) was associated with substantially lower in vitro antigen-stimulated production of the proinflammatory cytokines (IL-6, IFN-γ and TNF-α) by whole blood culture than in athletes with high vitamin D status (25(OH)D > 90 nmol/L). A higher proinflammatory cytokine production in response to an antigen challenge with better vitamin D status could be seen as being beneficial to host defense against pathogenic microorganisms, and in the He et al. (2013) study, those athletes with relatively high vitamin D status had fewer URTI episodes during 4 winter months than those with inadequate levels of vitamin D. Moreover, in those who experienced at least one URTI episode, the severity and duration of symptoms were negatively associated with vitamin D status.

Most of the vitamin D present in the adult human body (~80%-90%) comes from skin sunlight exposure; dietary vitamin D typically accounts for about 10% to 20%. The main dietary sources of vitamin D_3 are found in food of animal origin, such as egg yolk, cod-liver oil, and salmon, and vitamin D_2 is present in some plants and fungi. Some breakfast cereals, dairy products, and margarines may also be fortified with vitamin D. Because of the limited sunlight and weak strength of the UVB rays during the winter months in northern latitudes, vitamin D from the diet or supplements becomes increasingly important in maintaining vitamin D status (Laaksi et al. 2010). The amount of sunlight exposure needed to avoid vitamin D deficiency is about 15 minutes in the middle of the day several times each week (Powers et al. 2011). The recommended dietary intake of vitamin D in the United States is currently 15 µg/day (600 IU/day) for bone health, but it seems likely that this amount should be higher to maintain or optimize immune function; but more research on this is needed (Ross et al. 2011; He et al. 2016).

Vitamin D insufficiency has been reported to be common in athletes in the United Kingdom especially during training in the winter months (Close et al. 2013; He et al. 2013; Morton et al. 2012). A study that assessed the vitamin D status of UK-based professional athletes (latitude 53° north) reported that 62% of athletes (n = 61), including professional rugby players, soccer players, and jockeys, had inadequate serum total 25(OH)D concentrations (< 50 nmol/L) in the winter months (Close et al. 2013). In a study of elite soccer players in the English Premier League, 65% (n = 20) of players presented with serum total 25(OH)D concentrations of less than 50 nmol/L in December (Morton et al. 2012). Another study on a large university student cohort of endurance athletes and game players reported that 55% (n = 181) had serum total 25(OH)D concentrations of less than 50 nmol /L at the end of the 4-month winter training period (He et al. 2013). Therefore, it seems probable that vitamin D supplementation could be desirable to increase vitamin D concentrations to levels that are normally seen in the summer months. In theory, this should upregulate the expression of antimicrobial proteins and possibly reduce the risk of respiratory infections, but additional large-scale, placebo-controlled supplementation studies are needed to confirm this. Athletes who are particularly susceptible to vitamin D deficiency are those who live at latitudes above 35° north during the winter months, train indoors, or wear clothing that covers most of their skin. Another risk factor for having low vitamin D status is having darker skin due to the relationship of skin pigmentation to vitamin D synthesis (Powers et al. 2011).

In summary, the overwhelming evidence points to the benefits of avoiding vitamin D deficiency to maintain immunity and prevent respiratory infection in athletes (see review by He et al. 2016). Although the Institute of Medicine describes vitamin D sufficiency (for bone health) as a circulating 25(OH)D level greater than 50 nmol/L recent evidence tentatively supports a level of 75 nmol/L to prevent upper respiratory infections (He et al. 2016).The practical recommendation is to get adequate but safe summer sunlight exposure. During the winter months, a daily 25 µg or 1,000 IU vitamin D_3 supplement can maintain vitamin D sufficiency. In people who are deficient, a daily supplement of 100 µg or 4,000 IU of vitamin D_3 can bring them to optimal vitamin D status within 2 months (He et al. 2016). Further studies are required in athletes to determine the effects of these recommendations on immune function and respiratory infection risk.

Vitamin Supplements and Megadoses

In general, supplementation with individual vitamins or consumption of large doses of simple antioxidant mixtures is not recommended. Athletes should obtain complex mixtures of antioxidant compounds from consumption of fruits and vegetables. A suitable alternative is commercially available capsules of dried fruit and vegetable juice.

Consuming megadoses of individual vitamins is likely to do more harm than good. Because most vitamins function mainly as coenzymes in the body, after the enzyme systems are saturated, the vitamins in free form can have toxic effects. For example, 300 mg of vitamin E (as α-tocopherol acetate) given daily to 18 men for 3 weeks produced a significant depression in the bactericidal activity of peripheral blood leukocytes and mitogen-induced lymphocyte proliferation. Some people suffer from diarrhea following ingestion of large doses of vitamin C, and prolonged intake of very large doses (>1,000 mg/day) of vitamin C is associated with kidney oxalate stone formation, impaired absorption of copper, and, in susceptible individuals, excessive absorption of iron and predisposition to gout. These side effects, however, seem to be rare. Consuming megadoses of vitamin A may impair the inflammatory response and complement formation and have other pathological effects (e.g., causing fetal abnormalities when consumed by pregnant women, reducing bone mineral density). Vitamin D_3 in doses of up to 100 µg or 4,000 IU/day is known to be safe, but toxicity becomes a risk (e.g., hypercalcemia, kidney stones) at daily doses that exceed 250 µg or 10,000 IU/day.

Minerals

Minerals are classified as macrominerals or microminerals (trace elements), based on the extent of their occurrence in the body (see chapter 10). The trace elements constitute less than 0.01% of total body mass, and 14 are known to be essential for maintenance of health. Some of these, including zinc, iron, selenium, and copper, are known to exert modulatory effects on immune function (see table 13.8), but with the exception of zinc and iron, isolated deficiencies are rare. Iron deficiency is reported to be the most widespread nutrient deficiency in the world and is consistently associated with increased morbidity from infectious disease.

Zinc

Zinc plays an essential role as a cofactor of more than 100 metalloenzymes and is required for development of the immune system and for normal immune cell functions. Zinc is needed by rapidly dividing cells, such as bone marrow stem cells and lymphocytes, because it is a cofactor for several enzymes involved in the transcription of DNA and protein synthesis. For example, zinc is a cofactor for the enzyme terminal deoxynucleotidyl

TABLE 13.8 Roles of Minerals in Immune Function and the Effects of Dietary Deficiency or Excess

Mineral	Role in immune function	Effect of deficiency	Effect of excess
Iron	Oxygen transport and cofactor of metalloenzymes	Anemia and increased infections	Hemochromatosis, liver cirrhosis, heart disease, and increased infections
Zinc	Cofactor of metalloenzymes, protein synthesis, and antioxidant enzymes such as superoxide dismutase	Impaired growth, impaired healing, increased infections, and anorexia	Impaired absorption of iron and copper, increased HDL to LDL cholesterol ratio, anemia, nausea, vomiting, and immune system impairment
Selenium	Cofactor of glutathione peroxidase (antioxidant)	Cardiomyopathy, cancer, heart disease, impaired immune function, and erythrocyte fragility	Nausea, vomiting, fatigue, and hair loss
Copper	Promotes normal iron absorption and cofactor of superoxide dismutase (antioxidant)	Anemia and impaired immune function	Nausea and vomiting
Magnesium	Protein synthesis and cofactor of metalloenzymes	Muscle weakness, fatigue, apathy, muscle tremor, and cramp	Nausea, vomiting, and diarrhea

From M. Gleeson, "Minerals and Exercise Immunology," in *Nutrition and Exercise Immunology*, edited by D.C. Nieman and B. Klarlund Pedersen (Danver, MA: CRC Press, 2000), 137-154.

transferase, which is required by immature T-cells for their proliferation, differentiation, and functioning. Dietary zinc deficiency in humans results in lymphoid atrophy, decreased delayed-hypersensitivity cutaneous responses, decreased IL-2 production, impaired mitogen-stimulated lymphocyte proliferative responses, and decreased NKCA. Zinc is also a cofactor for superoxide dismutase, which is an important enzyme in antioxidant defense. The consequences of sustained zinc deficiency include impaired growth, delayed wound healing, and increased infections.

Vegetarian athletes and those who eat very low-energy diets to lose weight are at risk for zinc deficiency because meat and seafood are the richest dietary sources (see table 10.9). Although whole grains, wheat germ, asparagus, spinach, nuts, and legumes (beans, lentils, peanuts, and peas) are potentially good sources of zinc, the high levels of fiber normally found in these foods can decrease zinc absorption. For these reasons, zinc deficiency is more common in athletes who compete in sports in which a low body mass confers a performance advantage. Zinc is lost from the body mainly in sweat and urine (see table 10.10), so heavy training in hot weather could induce a zinc deficiency in athletes. Urinary zinc excretion is increased by exercise and is another significant route of zinc loss for athletes. Research on urinary zinc loss in athletes has shown that highly trained women have significantly higher urinary zinc excretion compared with untrained control subjects. In well-trained male game players, an acute bout of high-intensity exercise increases daily urinary zinc excretion by 34% compared with a day of rest.

Although male and female athletes have lower plasma zinc concentrations than untrained people, there have been very few studies on the relationship between immune function, exercise, and zinc status in athletes. One study of male runners found that 6 days of zinc supplementation (25 mg of zinc and 1.5 mg of copper twice per day) inhibited the exercise-associated increase in superoxide free-radical formation by activated neutrophils (as shown in figure 13.26) and exaggerated the exercise-induced suppression of T-lymphocyte proliferation in response to mitogens. Such effects might temporarily predispose athletes to opportunistic infection. Although zinc supplementation may be warranted for some athletes, it is important to be aware that megadoses of zinc have detrimental effects on immune function. For example, healthy men who ingested a large zinc supplement (150 mg twice per day) for 6 weeks exhibited reduced T-lymphocyte proliferative responses to mitogen

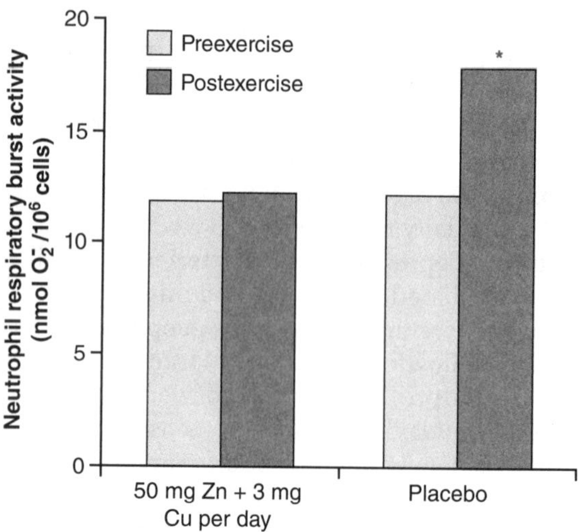

Figure 13.26 The effect of zinc and copper supplementation versus placebo on the exercise-induced change in neutrophil respiratory burst activity. *Significant difference between placebo and zinc-copper supplement after exercise, $P<0.05$.
Data from Singh, Failla, and Deuster (1994).

stimulation and impaired neutrophil phagocytic activity. Hence, megadoses of zinc should be avoided unless advised otherwise by an expert physician. Athletes should be encouraged to consume zinc-rich foods (e.g., poultry, meat, fish, dairy products) that can form part of a well-balanced, healthy diet. Vegetarians are advised to take a 10 to 20 mg supplement of zinc daily (the RDA is 10 mg and 12 mg for women and men, respectively), but in view of the findings just discussed, supplements at the lower end of this range may be more suitable.

The efficacy of zinc supplementation as a treatment for the common cold has been investigated in over a dozen studies published since 1984. The findings have been equivocal, and several reviews of this topic conclude that further research is necessary before the use of zinc supplements to treat the common cold can be recommended (Macknin 1999; Marshall 2000). Although only limited evidence suggests that taking zinc supplements reduces the incidence of URTI (McElroy and Miller 2002; Veverka et al. 2009), in the studies that have reported a beneficial effect of zinc in treating the common cold (i.e., reduction of symptom duration, severity, or both) zinc lozenges with high ionic zinc content (>75 mg/day) had to be taken within 24 hours of the onset of symptoms to be of any benefit (Hemila 2011). Potential problems with zinc supplements include nausea, bad taste reactions, lowering of HDL cholesterol, depression of some immune cell functions (e.g., neutrophil oxidative burst), and interference with the absorption of copper (Gleeson 2000).

Iron

Iron deficiency is prevalent throughout the world. By some estimates, as much as 25% of the world's population is iron deficient. Endurance athletes risk potential iron deficiency because of increased iron losses in sweat, urine, and feces. The incidence of iron depletion among athletes, however, is no greater than that in the general population as the dietary iron intakes of athletes tend to be higher because of their higher energy intakes. Nevertheless, exercise may contribute to an iron-depleted state. The acute-phase host response to stress (including exercise) involves the depression of circulating free iron levels. Stress-induced elevation of IL-1 causes granulocyte release of the iron-binding protein lactoferrin within the circulation. Lactoferrin is then thought to bind (chelate) iron from transferrin and form lactoferrin-iron complexes, which leads to a depression of plasma iron concentration that is independent of plasma volume changes.

The immune system appears to be particularly sensitive to the availability of iron, although iron deficiency has neither completely harmful nor enhancing effects on immune function. On the one hand, free iron is necessary for bacterial growth. Removal of iron with the help of chelating agents, such as lactoferrin, reduces bacterial multiplication, particularly in the presence of a specific antibody. A study reported that iron-deficient mice had a lower mortality after infection with *salmonella* compared with iron-replete mice. Thus, iron deficiency may protect a person from infection, and supplementation may predispose a person to an infectious disease because iron catalyzes the production of hydroxyl free radicals and high intake of iron can impair gastrointestinal zinc absorption. On the other hand, iron deficiency depresses various aspects of immune function, including macrophage IL-1 production, the lymphocyte proliferative response to mitogens, NKCA, neutrophil phagocytic activity, and delayed cutaneous hypersensitivity (an index of cell-mediated immune function).

A number of causes of iron deficiency in endurance athletes involved in heavy training have been suggested. Exercise may cause reductions in gastrointestinal iron absorption, and iron is lost in sweat, which contains 0.3 mg/L of iron (see table 10.10). This process can cause losses of up to 1 mg of iron per day in athletes who are training extensively. Because only about 10% of dietary iron is absorbed, such losses increase the dietary requirement by about 10 mg/day, which is approximately double the normal daily iron requirement (the RDA is 15 mg for women and 10 mg for men). In addition, because some damage to red blood cells (hemolysis) may occur in runners and game players (because of foot strike) and in swimmers (because of body friction from moving through the water), loss of hemoglobin in the urine will occur; however, this loss is thought to be a negligible drain on iron stores. Some athletes are also susceptible to gastrointestinal bleeding during exercise, which may increase fecal iron losses.

The bioavailability of iron is lower in vegetarian diets because of the lack of heme iron, which is more easily absorbed. All athletes should include foods that are rich in heme iron, such as lean red meat, poultry, and fish, in the daily diet. Increased iron requirements for endurance athletes can be met through the diet (see table 10.9) without the need for artificial supplements. Vegetarian athletes should ensure that plant food choices are iron dense (e.g., green leafy vegetables, legumes, whole-grain breads and pasta, iron-fortified products). Some breakfast cereals, bars, and breads are fortified with iron, but usually in amounts that are lower than the RDA. Megadoses of iron are not advised, and routine oral supplements of iron should not be taken without medical advice.

Selenium

Selenium deficiency can affect all components of the immune system. Selenium is a cofactor of glutathione peroxidase and reductase and thus influences the quenching of ROS. As such, the requirement for selenium may increase in athletes who are involved in regular intensive training programs. Selenium supplements should not exceed the RDA for the reasons explained in chapter 10. .

Copper

The effects of copper deficiency on immune function include impaired antibody formation, inflammatory response, neutrophil phagocytosis, NKCA, and lymphocyte stimulation responses. The results of changes in copper status because of exercise and training are controversial and perhaps reflect the inadequacy of techniques used to measure copper status. Some redistribution of copper between body compartments may occur with exercise, and athletes have been reported to lose copper in sweat collected after exercise. Although copper deficiency is rare in humans, athletes who take zinc supplements may compromise the gastrointestinal absorption of copper because of the similar physicochemical properties of these two minerals.

Magnesium

Magnesium is an essential cofactor for many enzymes involved in biosynthetic processes, including protein synthesis. It is therefore needed particularly by lymphocytes for rapid cell proliferation and antibody production. Details of magnesium requirements, food sources, and effects of deficiency can be found in chapter 10.

Other Trace Elements

Manganese is important as a cofactor of the enzyme superoxide dismutase, which aids in protection against free radicals and can impair some immune cell functions. Cobalt is important as a component of vitamin $B_{12,}$ and is needed for normal production of leukocytes in the bone marrow. Deficiencies are associated with pernicious anemia, reduced blood leukocyte counts, impaired lymphocyte proliferation, and impaired bactericidal capacity of neutrophils. Fluorine, although not directly required for normal immune function, is needed for the normal formation of healthy bones and teeth, and it protects against dental caries (tooth decay by oral bacteria). Details of manganese, cobalt, and fluorine requirements, food sources, and effects of deficiency can be found in chapter 10.

Dietary Immunostimulants

Certain supplements may boost immune function and reduce infection risk in immunocompromised people, including athletes who are engaged in heavy training and competition. There are many nutritional supplements on the market (besides those already mentioned) that claim to boost immunity. These include ß-glucans, bovine colostrum, probiotics, and herbals such as echinacea, Kaloba (the brand name of an extract of the geranium plant *Pelargonium sidoides*), ginseng, and curcumin. The claims for many of these supplements are often based on selective evidence of efficacy in animals, in vitro experiments, children, the elderly, or clinical patients in severe catabolic states. Direct evidence for their efficacy for preventing exercise-induced immune depression or improving immune system status in athletes is usually lacking. In recent years, however, the effects of some of these supplements on immune function or infection incidence have been evaluated in physically active populations. Some of the ones that show the most promise are discussed in the sections that follow. Table 13.9 provides a summary of some of the more commonly used supplements, and their efficacy in enhancing immunity and reducing infection risk in athletes is rated based on the available scientific evidence.

Echinacea and Other Herbals

Several herbal preparations are reputed to have immunostimulatory effects, and consumption of products containing *Echinacea purpurea* is widespread among athletes. In a double-blind, placebo-controlled study, the effect of a daily oral pretreatment for 28 days with pressed juice of *Echinacea purpurea* was investigated in 42 triathletes before and after a sprint triathlon (Berg, Northoff, and Konig 1998). A subgroup of athletes was also treated with magnesium as a reference for supplementation with a micronutrient that is important for optimal muscular function. During the 28-day pretreatment period, none of the athletes in the echinacea group became ill compared with three subjects in the magnesium group and four subjects in the placebo group. Pretreatment with echinacea appeared to reduce the release of soluble IL-2 receptor before and after the race and increased the exercise-induced rise in IL-6.

Numerous experiments have shown that *Echinacea purpurea* extracts exert significant immunomodulatory effects in vitro. The active ingredients of echinacea extracts are thought to include alkamides, chicoric acid, and polysaccharides. The immunomodulatory effects include the activation of macrophages, neutrophils, and natural killer cells (Barrett 2003), and there are a few reports of changes in the numbers and activities of T-cell and B-cell leukocytes. However, evidence of positive effects on leukocyte activities in vitro does not mean that these effects will also be observed in vivo. Several dozen human experiments, including a number of blind, randomized trials, report modest health benefits (particularly those that have examined the effects of *Echinacea purpurea* extracts in the treatment of acute URTI). Most of these trials, however, were limited in size and in methodological quality. In a randomized, double-blind, placebo-controlled trial, administering unrefined echinacea at the onset of symptoms of URTI in 148 college students did not provide any detectable benefit or harm compared with placebo (Barrett et al. 2002).

In a meta-analysis of 22 well-controlled trials (Linde et al. 2006), three trials investigated prevention of colds and 19 trials tested treatment of colds. A variety of different echinacea preparations were used. None of the comparisons in the

TABLE 13.9 Nutrition Supplements That Claim to Boost Immunity and Reduce URS Incidence in Athletes

Supplement	Type of compound	Proposed mode of action	Efficacy rating*
ß-glucans	Polysaccharides derived from the cell walls of yeast, fungi, and oats	Stimulate innate immunity	●●○○○
Bovine colostrum	First milk of the cow that contains antibodies, growth factors, and cytokines	Boosts mucosal immunity, which increases resistance to infection	●●●○○
Carbohydrate	Macronutrient	Maintains blood glucose during exercise, lowers stress hormone and anti-inflammatory cytokine responses, and thus counters immune dysfunction	●●●○○
Echinacea	Herbal extract	Has stimulatory effects on macrophages	●○○○○
Glutamine	Nonessential amino acid (but conditionally essential in some situations)	Is a precursor in the synthesis of nucleic acids and is important for rapidly dividing cells; also is an important fuel for immune cells	●○○○○
Kaloba	Herbal medicine	Has stimulatory effects on macrophages	●○○○○
Omega-3 polyunsaturated fatty acids	Fatty acids that contain more than one double bond	Have anti-inflammatory effects	○○○○○
Probiotics	Live bacteria administered orally	Increase the beneficial bacteria in the gut and modulate gut-associated and systemic immune functions	●●●○○
Quercetin	Plant flavonoid	Has anti-inflammatory, antioxidative, and antipathogenic effects	●●●○○
Quercetin with EGCG	Flavonoid mixture	Has anti-inflammatory and antioxidative effects and is claimed to improve immune function above that of quercetin alone	●●●○○
Vitamin C	Essential water-soluble antioxidant vitamin	Quenches reactive oxygen species and reduces interleukin-6 and cortisol responses to exercise	●●○○○
Vitamin D_3	Fat soluble vitamin that is mostly produced via the action of sunlight in the skin	Induces production of antimicrobial proteins, enhances natural killer cell cytolytic activity, increases the generation of ROS in phagocytes, and modifies leukocyte cytokine secretion	●●●●○
Vitamin E	Essential fat-soluble antioxidant vitamin	Quenches exercise-induced ROS and is known to boost immunity in the elderly	●○○○○
Zinc	Essential mineral	Is a cofactor of many enzymes and is required for normal immunity	●○○○○

*Items are rated based on scientific evidence; ●●●●● indicates very strong evidence and ○○○○○ indicates limited to no evidence of the supplement's efficacy in enhancing immunity or reducing infection risk in athletes.

Adapted from Gleeson (2013).

prevention trials showed any benefit of echinacea over placebo. In the trials that examined the effectiveness of echinacea versus placebo in the treatment of colds, there was a significant beneficial effect reported in nine comparisons, a trend in one, and no difference in six. The authors' main conclusions were that there is some evidence that preparations based on the aerial parts of the echinacea plant might be effective for the early treatment of colds in adults but that results have not been fully consistent. In the relatively few large-scale, well-controlled, randomized trials that have been performed, no beneficial effects of echinacea have been shown. Hence, there is still uncertainty regarding whether echinacea has any real value in preventing or treating URTI in the general population, and only a very few trials with small numbers of subjects have attempted to examine its effectiveness for reducing URS in athletes.

Other herbals are also claimed to have various antiviral, antibacterial, and immune-modulating actions, and many also act as antioxidants (for details see Roxas and Jurenka 2007). Some of the more common examples include extracts of elderberries (*Sambucus nigra*), Kaloba (the brand name for an extract of the roots of *Pelargonium sidoides*), ginseng (*Panax quinquefolium*), astragalus (*Astragalus membranaceus*), and leaves of the olive tree (*Olea europaea*). There have been very few well-controlled, large-scale studies of the clinical efficacy of these extracts, and most of the evidence for their use comes from in vitro studies that demonstrate immune cell stimulatory effects or direct antiviral actions (preventing viral entry into host cells or viral replication). Several preparations, such as Kaloba and echinacea, are classed as herbal medicines that are used to reduce the severity and duration of cold symptoms rather than to prevent infections. It is debatable whether these are any more effective than taking antiviral medications or nonprescription cold remedies for the alleviation of upper respiratory illness symptoms.

Curcumin

Curcumin (diferuloylmethane) is a component of turmeric (a spice commonly found in curry powders and sauces). Traditionally, curcumin has been known for its anti-inflammatory effects, and several studies have demonstrated that curcumin is a potent immunomodulatory agent that can modulate the activation of T-cells, B-cells, NK cells, neutrophils, macrophages, and dendritic cells (Jagetia and Aggarwal 2007). Curcumin can also downregulate the expression of various proinflammatory cytokines (including TNF, IL-1, and IL-2) most likely through inactivation of the transcription factor NFKB. At low doses, however, curcumin can also enhance antibody responses (Jagetia and Aggarwal 2007).

Polyphenols

The plant kingdom uses tens of thousands of secondary metabolites (generally referred to as phytonutrients), including terpenes, alkaloids, and phenolics for defense against fungal, bacterial, and viral infections, attraction of insects for pollination, and protection against oxidative stress and strong sunlight. The phenolic compounds or polyphenols play key roles in the growth, regulation, and structure of plants and are divided into four main classes: flavonoids (~50% of all polyphenols), phenolic acids, lignans, and stilbenes. Flavonoids are further classified into six simple (flavan-3-ols, flavanones, flavones, isoflavones, flavonols, and anthocyanins) and two complex (condensed and derived tannins) subgroups. In foods, flavonoids, lignans, and stilbenes are usually found as glycosides and phenolic acids are found as esters with various polyols, and structural variations influence their absorption and bioavailability. Most flavonoids are potent antioxidant compounds and many exert antiviral effects, modulate NK cell activities and regulatory T cell properties, and influence macrophage inflammatory responses (Kim et al. 2015). A recent systematic review and meta-analysis showed that flavonoid supplementation (0.2-1.2 g/day in 14 selected studies) decreased acute URS episode incidence by 33% compared with control or placebo treatments (Somerville, Braakhuis, and Hopkins 2016).

One flavonoid in particular, quercetin, has received a lot of attention in recent years in relation to its possible effects on exercise performance, training adaptation, and immune function. Quercetin is found in variety of fruits and vegetables, and there are relatively high amounts in apples, blueberries, broccoli, curly kale, hot peppers, onions, and tea. Quercetin generally provides about 75% of total daily flavonol intake (which ranges from 13-64 mg depending on the population studied). The bioavailability of quercetin from food or supplements is good, and elimination from the body is quite slow (reported half-life ranges from 11-28 hours).

Studies in mice indicate that 7 days of quercetin feeding improved survival following an influenza virus inoculation (Davis et al. 2008). Several small-scale human trials have now been conducted and a double-blind, placebo-controlled study with 40 cyclists showed that ingesting a daily dose of 1,000 mg of quercetin for 3 weeks significantly increased circulating quercetin concentration and reduced URTI incidence during the 2-week period following 3 successive days of exhaustive cycling exercise (Nieman et al. 2007). In this study, an unusually high proportion of subjects in the placebo group (9 out of 20) reported URTI symptoms in the 2-week post-training period, whereas only 1 out of 20 subjects in the quercetin group were similarly affected. Despite the apparent difference in susceptibility to stress-induced URTI, none of the measured markers of immune dysfunction, inflammation, and oxidative stress were different between the groups, and the authors suggested that quercetin may have exerted direct antiviral effects. A few studies support the notion that coingestion of quercetin with other flavonoids and food components can improve and extend quercetin's bioavailability and bioactive effects. The compounds examined in this context included the flavonoid epigallocatechin gallate (EGCG) from tea; isoquercetin, which is the glycosylated form of quercetin in onions and other foods; omega-3 PUFAs, such as EPA and DHA; vitamin C; and folic acid. In a study with 39 trained cyclists, a combination supplement incorporating quercetin, EGCG, isoquercetin, and omega-3 PUFAs was more effective than quercetin alone in partially countering exercise-induced oxidative stress (Nieman et al. 2009), but currently there is no data on relevant markers of immune function and URTI incidence in humans.

Other naturally occurring polyphenolic compounds are present in foods such as green leafy vegetables, onions, apples, pears, citrus fruits, and red grapes and in some plant-based beverages such as citrus juices, green tea, red wine, and beer. A large-scale study of more than 1,000 physically active men and women revealed that a high fruit intake was associated with reduced self-reported respiratory illness incidence (Nieman et al. 2011). Diets that contain large amounts of fruit and vegetables tend to be bulky, and this can be a problem for athletes who need to ingest relatively large amounts of carbohydrate (and protein) to meet their energy requirements. A suitable alternative to ensure a high polyphenol intake is to ingest commercially available fruit extract concentrates formulated as powders, tablets, or capsules.

In a study that investigated the effects of regular ingestion of nonalcoholic beer polyphenols before and after a marathon (Scherr et al. 2012) (see figure 13.27), it was found that male runners who drank 1 to 1.5 L (0.3-0.4 gal) per day of a nonalcoholic beer had reduced blood markers of inflammation immediately after the race and 24 hours later and had a 3.25 times lower incidence of URTI compared with the placebo beverage group during the 2-week postmarathon period. In contrast, another study that examined the effects of regular ingestion of cocoa polyphenols in the form of dark chocolate prior to an exhausting bout of cycling (Allgrove et

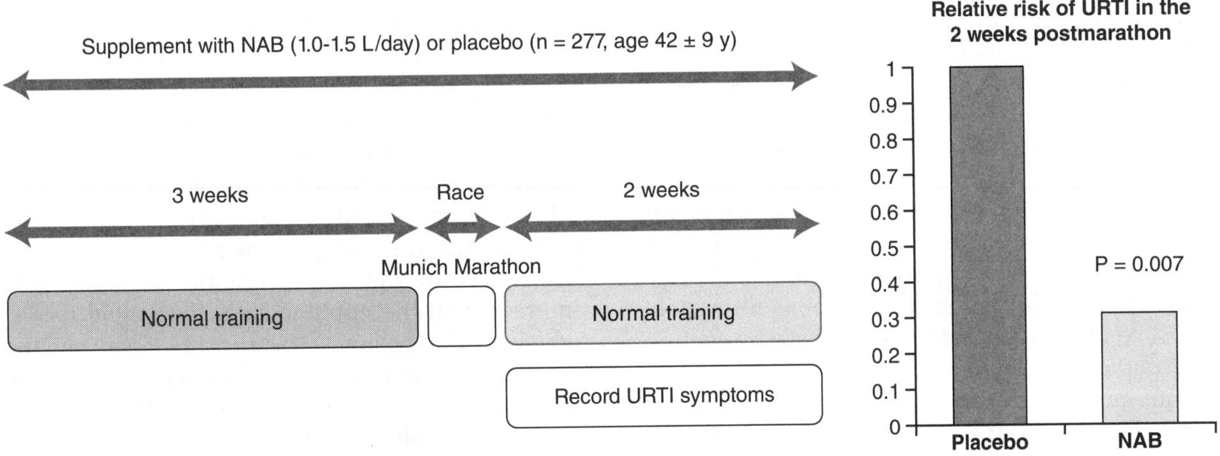

Figure 13.27 Reduction in proportion of runners reporting upper respiratory illness symptoms in the 2 weeks postmarathon with daily nonalcoholic beer consumption compared with a placebo beverage.
Data from Scherr et al. (2012).

al. 2011) reported that oxidative stress markers were lower but none of the measured hormonal or immune responses to the exercise were different compared with the placebo control (cocoa liquor-free chocolate).

β-Glucans

ß-Glucans are present as major structural components of the cell walls of yeast, fungi, and some bacteria and are present in the diet as part of the endosperm cell wall in cereals such as barley and oats. ß-Glucans are carbohydrates that consist of linked glucose molecules and differ in macromolecular structure depending on the source. ß-Glucans from bacteria are unbranched 1,3 ß-linked glycopyranosyl residues. The cell wall ß-glucans of yeast and fungi consists of 1,3 ß-linked glycopyranosyl residues with small numbers of 1,6 ß-linked branches, whereas oat and barley cell walls contain unbranched ß-glucans with 1,3 and 1,4 ß-linked glycopyranosyl residues. The specific characteristics of the various ß-glucans may influence their immune-modulating effects. For example, Brown and Gordon (2003) have suggested that high molecular weight or particulate ß-glucans from fungi directly activate leukocytes, whereas low molecular weight ß-glucans from fungi only modulate the response of immune cells when they are stimulated (e.g., with cytokines). This implies that the addition of ß-glucans to the diet may be used to modulate immune function and might improve the resistance against invading pathogens in humans.

To date, there is limited evidence for immune-promoting effects of orally administered oat ß-glucans in animals and humans. Intragastric administration of oat ß-glucans in mice enhanced resistance to bacterial and parasitic infections (reviewed by Volman, Ramakers, and Plat 2008). Furthermore, Davis et al. (2004) demonstrated that daily ingestion of oat ß-glucan counteracted the decrease in macrophage antiviral resistance induced by exercise stress in mice. Results both from in vitro studies from animals treated with ß-glucans suggest that ß-glucans enhance the immune response in leukocytes and epithelial cells. In the in vivo situation, there is now substantial evidence that these effects ultimately translate into an enhanced survival after infection with pathogens (Volman, Ramakers, and Plat 2008). In this respect, effects are observed irrespective of the ß-glucan source or route of administration. It has been suggested that the protective effects of orally administered 1,3 ß-glucans are mediated through receptor-mediated interactions with microfold cells (specialized epithelial cells for the transport of macromolecules in the Peyer's patches) that lead to increased cytokine production and enhanced resistance to infection. Therefore, it might be possible to modulate immune function by increasing the dietary ß-glucan intake by developing functional foods, for example. This may have benefits for specific target populations, such as the elderly or type 2 diabetic patients, and for athletes who are involved in heavy training; all of these are characterized by a suppressed (Th1) immune response (Gleeson 2006). One trial in humans found no effect of 3 weeks of oat ß-glucan supplementation on immune responses to exercise or infection incidence during the 2-week period following 3 successive days of exhaustive exercise (Nieman et al. 2008). More recently, however, another human study reported a 37% reduction in the number of URS days following a marathon with yeast ß-glucan supplementation versus placebo, which the authors attributed to a postexercise increase in salivary IgA (McFarlin et al. 2013).

Probiotics

Probiotics are food supplements that contain live microorganisms that, when administered in adequate amounts, confer a health benefit on the host. There is now a reasonable body of evidence that regular consumption of probiotics can modify the population of the gut-dwelling bacteria (microbiota) and influence immune function (Matsuzaki 1998; Mengheri 2008; Borchers et al. 2009; Minocha 2009), though it should be noted that such effects are strain specific. Probiotics survive transit through the acid conditions of the stomach into the intestine where they may modify the intestinal microbiota such that the numbers of beneficial bacteria increase and numbers of species that are considered harmful usually decrease. These effects have been associated with a range of potential benefits to the health and functioning of the digestive system and modulation of immune function. Probiotics have many mechanisms of action. By their growth and metabolism, they help inhibit the growth and reduce any harmful effects of other bacteria, antigens, toxins, and carcinogens in the gut. In addition, probiotics are known to interact with the gut-associated lymphoid tissue, which leads to positive effects on the innate and the acquired immune system. This is possible because the gut, as the largest surface area of the body, has a significant role to play in immunity; every day it has to deal with three different immune challenges. First, it must differentiate and tolerate the large commensal microbiota; otherwise, inflammation will occur. Second, it must tolerate the food antigens. Third, it must be able to mount a defense against any potential pathogens as required. This explains why 85% of the body's lymph nodes are located in the gut and why probiotics, as functional foods that target the gut, are able to affect the health of the whole body.

Studies have shown that probiotic intake can improve rates of recovery from rotavirus diarrhea, increase resistance to enteric pathogens, and promote antitumor activity (Kopp-Hoolihan 2001). Some evidence even suggests that probiotics may be effective in alleviating some allergic and respiratory disorders in young children (Kopp-Hoolihan 2001). Although to date there are few published studies of the effectiveness of probiotic use in athletes, interest is beginning to grow, mostly in examining their potential to help maintain overall general health, enhance immune function, or reduce URTI incidence and symptom severity or duration (Gleeson et al. 2012; West et al. 2009).

In a double-blind, placebo-controlled, crossover trial in which 20 healthy elite distance runners received the probiotic *Lactobacillus (L.) fermentum* or a placebo daily for 28 days with a 28-day washout period between the initial and the second treatment, the athletes suffered fewer days of respiratory illness and lower severity of respiratory illness symptoms when taking the daily probiotic (Cox et al. 2010; see figure 13.28). The probiotic treatment elicited a twofold greater change in whole-blood culture IFN-γ production compared with placebo, which may be one mechanism underpinning the positive clinical outcomes. In another study, a one-month course of daily probiotic (*L. acidophilus*) ingestion in athletes presenting with fatigue and impaired performance restored an apparent deficit in blood T-helper cell IFN-γ production (Clancy et al. 2006). Another small study found that consumption of an *L. casei* probiotic yogurt drink for one month limited the observed decrease in natural killer cell activity after an exercise stress test (Pujol et al. 2000).

In a somewhat larger-scale, randomized, double-blind intervention study, 141 marathon runners received *L. rhamnosus* GG (LGG) or placebo daily for a 3-month training period and then participated in a marathon race with a 2-week follow-up of illness symptoms (Kekkonen et al. 2007). Although there were no differences in the number of respiratory infections or GI-symptom episodes, the duration of GI-symptom episodes in the LGG group was shorter than in the placebo group during the training period (2.9 vs. 4.3 days) and during the 2 weeks after the marathon (1 vs. 2.3 days). In a study on soldiers participating in 3 weeks of commando training followed by a 5-day combat course, no difference in respiratory infection incidence was observed for those taking a daily *L. casei* probiotic supplement compared with placebo (Tiollier et al. 2007). However, there was a significant decrease in salivary IgA concentration after the combat course in the placebo group with no change over time in the probiotic group. A randomized, placebo-controlled trial in 64 university athletes reported a lower incidence of URTI episodes during a 4-month winter training period in subjects that received a twice-daily *L. casei* supplement compared with placebo, and this study also reported better maintenance of salivary IgA in the probiotic group (Gleeson et al. 2011). Others have also reported increased levels of salivary IgA (O'Connell et al. 2009) and natural killer cell function (Nagao et al. 2000) in healthy nonathletes after a few weeks of daily *L. casei* ingestion. Another study using *L. fermentum* reported reduced URTI incidence among

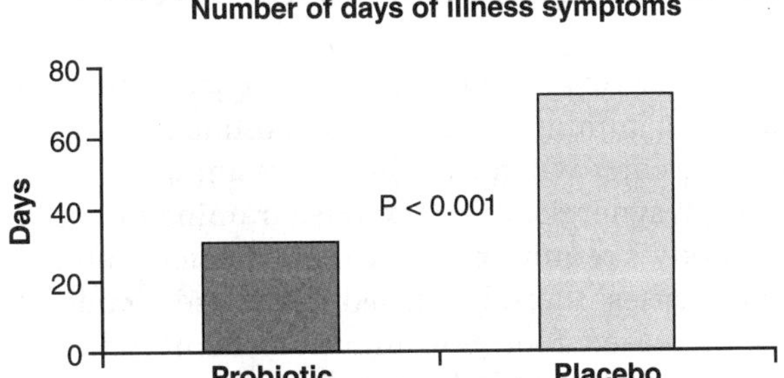

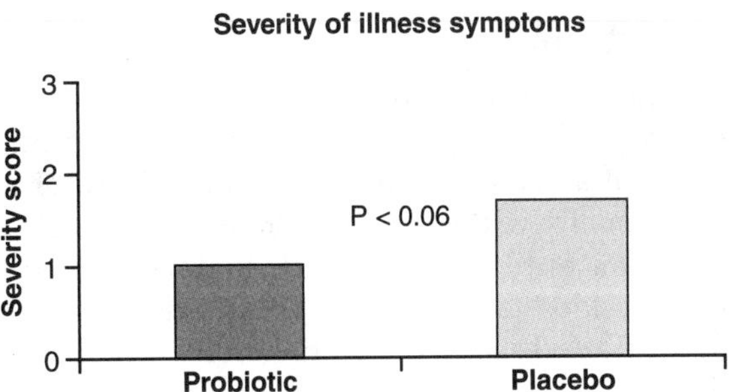

Figure 13.28 Reduction in number of URS symptom days and symptom severity with a daily probiotic supplement in male runners.
Data from Cox et al. (2010).

male but not female athletes during 11 weeks of training (West et al. 2011). A recent large-scale, randomized, placebo-controlled trial involving 465 physically active men and women reported fewer URTI episodes (relative risk ratio 0.73) in those who ingested daily a *Bifidobacterium animalis* subspecies *lactis* Bl-04 compared with placebo over a 150-day intervention period (West et al. 2014). Although most studies to date have examined probiotic effects in recreationally active individuals or endurance sport athletes, a recent study on elite rugby players provides evidence that beneficial effects of probiotics in reducing URTI incidence, but not severity, may extend to team game players (Haywood et al., 2014).

From the research reviewed here, one cannot be certain of a health benefit with regular probiotic ingestion for athletes, but there is sufficient understanding of the mechanism of action of certain probiotic strains and enough evidence from trials with athletes to signify that this is a promising area of research with mostly positive indications at present. A meta-analysis using data from athlete and nonathlete studies involving 3,451 participants concluded that there is a likely benefit in reducing URTI incidence (Hao et al. 2011). Another potential benefit of probiotics could be a reduced risk of gastrointestinal infections, which are a particular concern when traveling abroad. Further large-scale studies are needed to confirm that taking probiotics can reduce the number of training days lost to infection and to determine the most effective probiotics since their effects are strain specific. The studies to date that have shown reduced URS incidence in athletes have mostly used *Lactobacillus* and *Bifidobacterium* species in daily doses of about 10^{10} live bacteria. Given that some probiotics appear to provide some benefit with no evidence of harm and are low cost, there is no reason why athletes should not take probiotics, especially if they are traveling abroad or are illness prone.

Colostrum

Bovine colostrum is the first collection of a thick, creamy-yellow liquid produced by the mammary gland of a lactating cow shortly after birth of her calf (usually within the first 36 hours). Colostrum contains antibodies, growth factors, enzymes, gangliosides (acid glycosphingolipids), vitamins, and minerals and is commercially available in liquid and powder forms. Numerous health claims have been made for colostrum ranging from performance enhancement to preventing infections, but well-controlled studies in athletes are rare. The gangliosides in colostrum may modify the gut microbiota and act as decoy targets for bacterial adhesion as well as have some direct immunostimulatory properties (Rueda 2007). A few studies suggest that several weeks of bovine colostrum supplementation can elevate levels of antibodies in the circulation and saliva. In a study of 35 middle-aged distance runners who consumed a supplement of either bovine colostrum or placebo for 12 weeks, median levels of salivary IgA increased by 79% in the colostrum group after the 12-week intervention with no change in the placebo group (Crooks et al. 2006). While this result was statistically significant, its physiological interpretation must be viewed with caution due to the small numbers in this study and the large variability in salivary IgA levels. Davison and Diment (2010) reported that 4 weeks of daily bovine colostrum supplementation prevented exercise-induced falls in salivary lysozyme and speeded the recovery of neutrophil function after 2 hours of strenuous cycling in healthy men compared with placebo. Further studies are needed to confirm and extend these observations of effects on immune responses to exercise and to establish whether bovine colostrum can reduce the incidence of URTIs in athletes. Regular ingestion of bovine colostrum may also limit the increase in gut permeability caused by prolonged strenuous exercise and reduce the risk of developing heat stroke (Marchbank et al. 2011). Several studies have also reported that daily oral bovine colostrum supplementation reduces the total number of days with self-reported URS (Crooks et al. 2006, 2010, Jones et al. 2014, Shing et al. 2013), the incidence of URS episodes (Crooks et al. 2006, Jones et al. 2014, Shing et al. 2007, 2013), and the duration of self-reported URS episodes (Jones et al. 2014, Shing et al. 2013) in adults involved in exercise training.

Conclusions and Recommendations

Heavy exercise and nutrition exert separate influences on immune function; these influences appear to be greater when exercise stress and poor nutrition act synergistically. Exercise training increases the body's requirement for most nutrients and, in many cases, these increased needs are countered by increased food consumption. Some athletes, however, adopt unbalanced dietary regimens, and many surveys indicate that few athletes follow the best dietary patterns for optimal sport nutrition. Certainly, the poor nutritional statuses of some athletes can predispose them to immunodepression and increase their risk of infection. Despite an abundance of studies investigating the effects of nutrition on immune function and the effects of nutrition on physical performance, relatively few have investigated the interrelationships between nutrition, performance, and immune function concurrently. Therefore, some of the conclusions drawn in this chapter remain speculative because they rely on generalizations about sedentary populations that are applied to athletic populations. Although countering the effects of all of the factors that contribute to exercise-induced immunodepression is impossible, minimizing many of the effects is possible. Athletes can help themselves by eating well-balanced diets that include adequate carbohydrate, protein, and micronutrients.

Consumption of carbohydrate drinks during training and competition is recommended because this practice appears to attenuate some of the immunosuppressive effects of prolonged exercise. The ingestion of individual amino acids, echinacea, vitamin E, and zinc is unlikely to be of significant clinical benefit in preventing common infections, such as URTI. The dangers of oversupplementation of vitamins and minerals is emphasized because many micronutrients given in quantities beyond a certain threshold reduce immune responses and may also pose a risk to health.

The following are current recommendations for immunonutrition support in athletes (Bermon et al. 2017; Gleeson 2016), and they are likely to be of the most benefit to people who are particularly prone to illness:

- Overall daily energy intake should match energy needs, and more than 50% should come from carbohydrate.
- Ingest 30 to 60 g of carbohydrate per hour during strenuous training sessions.
- Ingest adequate amounts of protein (1.2-1.6 g per kilogram of body weight per day). Of this, 0.3 g per kilogram of body weight per day should be ingested in meals following training sessions.
- Ingest adequate amounts of micronutrients (a daily multivitamin supplement that meets the RDAs can ensure this).
- Take a daily oral vitamin D_3 supplement of 25 µg or 1,000 IU from early autumn until early spring.
- Take a daily probiotic supplement that contains at least 10 billion live bacteria.
- Include a variety of fruit and vegetables as part of the normal diet at least 5 days per week. This can be supplemented with plant polyphenol supplements or beverages (e.g., green tea, nonalcoholic beer) or concentrated fruit and vegetable extracts.
- Consider taking a daily 10 to 20 g bovine colostrum powder supplement.
- Consider taking zinc and Kaloba supplements in the days leading up to an important competition in case cold symptoms begin at that time.

It is important to remember that nutrition is only one factor with regard to infection risk. There are several other strategies that can minimize the risk of developing immune function depression or reduce the degree of exposure to pathogens and thus limit infection risk, such as reducing other life stresses, maintaining good oral and skin hygiene, obtaining adequate rest, and spacing prolonged training sessions and competitions as far apart as possible (Schwellnus et al. 2016). The practices listed in the sidebar are recommended.

PRACTICAL STRATEGIES TO MINIMIZE RISKS OF INFECTION

- Allow sufficient time between training sessions for recovery. Include 1 or 2 days of resting recovery in the weekly training program; more training is not always better.
- Avoid extremely long training sessions. Restrict continuous activity to less than 2 hours per session. For example, a 3-hour session might be better performed as two 1.5-hour sessions, one in the morning and one in the evening.
- Avoid training monotony by ensuring variation in the day-to-day training load. Follow a hard training day with a light training day.
- When increasing the training load, do so on the hard days. Do not eliminate recovery days.
- When recovering from overtraining or illness, begin with very light training and build gradually.
- Monitor and record mood, feelings of fatigue, and muscle soreness during training; decrease the training load if the normal session feels harder than usual.
- Keep other life, social, and psychological stresses to a minimum.
- Avoid rapid weight loss.
- Get at least 6 hours of good quality sleep per night.
- Avoid contact with people who have symptoms of infection, and wear a disposable mask when appropriate.
- Minimize contact with animals and young children, who are common carriers of infectious agents.
- Practice good personal and oral hygiene. Wash hands with soap and water effectively and regularly apply antimicrobial gels on hands. Brush teeth regularly and use an antibacterial mouth rinse.
- Never share drink bottles, cups, cutlery, towels, and so on with other people.
- Increase rest as needed after travel across time zones to allow circadian rhythms to adjust.
- Avoid touching surfaces that are frequently handled by the public, such as doorknobs, handrails, and telephone receivers.
- Avoid crowded areas and shaking hands.
- Quickly isolate a person with infection symptoms from others.
- Use disposable paper towels and limit hand-to-mouth, -nose, and -eye contact when suffering from URS or gastrointestinal illness (these are major routes of viral self-inoculation).
- Avoid getting a dry mouth during competition and at rest by drinking at regular intervals and maintaining hydration status.
- Use properly treated water for consumption and swimming.
- Avoid shared saunas, showers, and whirlpool tubs.
- Be aware of elevated vulnerability after training or competition.
- Discuss vaccination with your coach or doctor. Influenza vaccines require 5 to 7 weeks to take effect. Intramuscular vaccines may have a few small side effects, so receiving vaccinations out of season is best. Do not get a vaccination before a competition or if symptoms of illness are present.

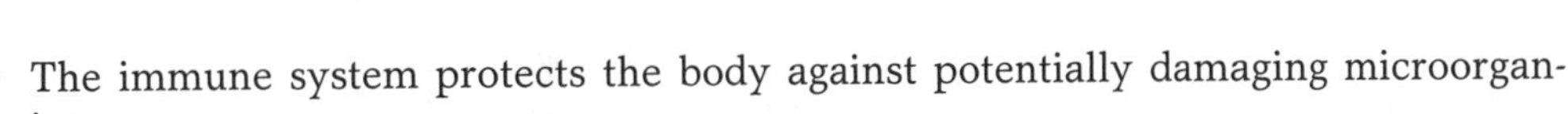

Key Points

- The immune system protects the body against potentially damaging microorganisms.
- Athletes engaged in heavy endurance training programs often have depressed immune function and suffer from an increased incidence of URTIs. Training and competitive surroundings may increase the athlete's exposure to pathogens and provide optimal conditions for pathogen transmission.
- Acute infective or allergic illness can cause a reduction in exercise performance through a number of mechanisms, including impaired motor coordination, decreased muscle strength, decreased aerobic capacity, and alterations in metabolic function. Furthermore, the presence of fever causes a decrease in the body's ability to regulate body temperature and increases fluid losses, thereby impairing endurance performance.
- Heavy, prolonged exertion is associated with numerous hormonal and biochemical changes, many of which can have detrimental effects on immune function. Improper nutrition can compound the negative influence of heavy exertion on immunocompetence.
- An athlete who exercises in a carbohydrate-depleted state experiences larger increases in circulating stress hormones and a greater perturbation of several immune-function indices.
- Consuming carbohydrate (but not glutamine) during exercise attenuates rises in stress hormones, such as cortisol, and appears to limit the degree of exercise-induced immunodepression.
- The poor nutritional status of some athletes may predispose them to immunodepression. For example, dietary deficiencies of protein and specific micronutrients are associated with immune dysfunction.
- Adequate intakes of iron, zinc, and B vitamins are particularly important, but the dangers of oversupplementation should also be considered. Many micronutrients given in quantities beyond a certain threshold reduce immune responses and may have other toxic effects.
- Sustained endurance training appears to be associated with an adaptive upregulation of the antioxidant defense system. Such adaptations may be insufficient to protect athletes who train extensively, and these individuals should consider increasing their intake of nutritional antioxidants.
- In general, supplementation of individual micronutrients or consumption of large doses of simple antioxidant mixtures is not recommended. Athletes should obtain complex mixtures of antioxidant compounds from consumption of fruits and vegetables.
- Consuming megadoses of individual vitamins is likely to do more harm than good. Vitamin D supplementation is an exception, because many athletes do not exhibit adequate vitamin D status during the winter months.
- Some supplements, including probiotics, plant polyphenols, and bovine colostrum, may benefit immunity and reduce risks of infection if taken regularly in sufficient doses.
- Countering the effects of all the factors that contribute to exercise-induced immunodepression is impossible, but minimizing many of them is possible. Athletes can help themselves by eating well-balanced diets that include sufficient protein and carbohydrate to meet their energy requirements. Such diets ensure adequate intakes of trace elements without special supplements.
- By adopting sound nutritional practices, reducing life stresses, maintaining good hygiene, obtaining adequate rest, and spacing prolonged training sessions and competitions as far apart as possible, athletes can reduce their risk of infection.

Recommended Readings

Bermon, S., L.M. Castell, P.C. Calder, N.C. Bishop, E. Blomstrand, F.C. Mooren, K. Krüger, A.N. Kavazis, J.C. Quindry, D.S. Senchina, D.C. Nieman, M. Gleeson, D.B. Pyne, C.M. Kitic, G.L. Close, D.E. Larson-Meyer, A. Marcos, S.N. Meydani, D. Wu, N.P. Walsh, and R. Nagatomi. 2017. Consensus statement: Immunonutrition and exercise. *Exercise Immunology Review* 23:8-50.

Calder, P.C., C.J. Field, and H.S. Gill. 2002. *Nutrition and immune function.* Oxford: CABI.

Chandra, R.K. 1997. Nutrition and the immune system: An introduction. *American Journal of Clinical Nutrition* 66:460S–463S.

Douglas R.M., H. Hemila, E. Chalker, and B. Treacy. 2007. Vitamin C for preventing and treating the common cold. *Cochrane Database of Systematic Reviews* 3:CD000980.

Gleeson, M. 2013. Exercise, nutrition and immunity. In *Diet, immunity and inflammation*, edited by P.C. Calder and P. Yaqoob, 652-685. Cambridge: Woodhead Publishing.

Gleeson, M. 2016. Immunological aspects of sport nutrition. *Immunology and Cell Biology* 94:117-123.

Gleeson, M., N.C. Bishop, and N.P. Walsh, eds. 2013. *Exercise immunology*. Abingdon: Routledge.

He, C.-S., X.H. Aw Yong, N.P. Walsh, and M. Gleeson. 2016. Is there an optimal vitamin D status for immunity in athletes and military personnel? *Exercise Immunology Review* 22:42-64.

Konig, D., A. Berg, C. Weinstock, J. Keul, and H. Northoff. 1997. Essential fatty acids, immune function and exercise. *Exercise and Immunology Review* 3:1-31.

Nieman, D.C., and B.K. Pedersen, eds. 2000. *Nutrition and exercise immunology.* Boca Raton, FL: CRC Press.

Pedersen B.K., K. Ostrowski, T. Rohde, and H. Bruunsgaard. 1998. Nutrition, exercise and the immune system. *Proceedings of the Nutrition Society* 57:43-47.

Peters, E.M. 1997. Exercise, immunology and upper respiratory tract infections. *International Journal of Sports Medicine* 18 (Suppl 1): S69-S77.

Pyne, D.B., N.P. West, A.J. Cox, and A.W. Cripps. 2015. Probiotics supplementation for athletes—clinical and physiological effects. *European Journal of Sport Science* 15:63-72.

Scrimshaw, N.S., and J.P. SanGiovanni. 1997. Synergism of nutrition, infection and immunity: An overview. *American Journal of Clinical Nutrition* 66:464S–477S.

Walsh, N.P., M. Gleeson, D.B. Pyne, D.C. Nieman, F.S. Dhabhar, R.J. Shephard, S.J. Oliver, S. Bermon, and A. Kajėnienė. 2011. Position statement part two: Maintaining immune health. *Exercise Immunology Review* 17:64-103.

Walsh, N.P., M. Gleeson, R.J. Shephard, M. Gleeson, J.A. Woods, N.C. Bishop, M. Fleshner, C. Green, B.K. Pedersen, L. Hoffman-Goetz, C.J. Rogers, H. Northoff, A. Abbasi, and P. Simon. 2011. Position statement part one: Immune function and exercise. *Exercise Immunology Review* 17:6-63.

Body Composition

Objectives

After studying this chapter, you should be able to do the following:

- Describe normal ranges of body weight and body fat for adults and various athlete populations
- Describe the principles of methods available to measure body composition
- Compare different techniques of measuring body composition and discuss their advantages and limitations

Body weight and body composition are important determinants of performance in many sports. Quantifying human body composition has played an important role in monitoring the efficacy of athlete training and dietary regimens especially in gravitational, weight class, and aesthetic sports in which the tissue composition of the body can have a profound effect on performance (Ackland et al. 2012). Some athletes try to gain weight and others try to lose weight. In some sports, reducing body fat is important, whereas in other sports, increasing lean body mass is important. In most weight-bearing activities, such as running and jumping, extra weight is a disadvantage, although in some contact sports, such as American football and rugby, extra weight may be an advantage. Every sport has an optimal physique, and in some sports, a specific discipline or position requires a specific body type. For dancing and gymnastics, leanness is important mainly for aesthetic reasons.

The desire to lose or gain weight is not limited to competitive athletes; it is also common among recreational athletes and sedentary people who wish to change their physical appearance. Although obesity is a growing problem, images in the media create continuous pressure to be lean and well proportioned. The stereotypical athlete is particularly lean and toned. Many athletes try to lose weight through diet or exercise or both. This chapter discusses how body composition can be assessed and how it relates to performance in various sports. In the next chapter, the problems associated with weight loss and weight gain and the applications in various categories of sports will be discussed.

Optimal Body Weight and Composition

Body size, structure, and composition are separate yet interrelated aspects of the body that make up the physique. Body size refers to the volume, mass, length, and surface area of the body; body structure refers to the distribution or arrangement of body parts such as the skeleton, muscle, and fat; and body composition refers to the amounts of constituents in the body. Size, structure, and composition all contribute to optimal sports performance. Evidence from sports participants in various age groups demonstrates an inverse relationship between fat mass and performance of physical activities that require translocation of body weight either vertically (e.g., jumping) or horizontally (e.g., running). Excess fat is detrimental to performance in these types of activities because it adds mass to the body without adding capacity to produce force. In addition, acceleration is directly proportional to force but inversely proportional to mass, so at a given level of force application, excess fat results in slower changes in velocity and direction. Excess fat also increases the metabolic cost of physical activities that require movement of the total body mass. Thus, in most performances that involve movement of body mass, a relatively low percentage body fat is advantageous mechanically and metabolically.

By studying the **anthropometry** of high-level athletes, we can gather ideas about optimum body size, structure, and composition for various sports. In some sports, a low percentage body fat is a requirement. Generally, body composition of athletes can be used in three ways:

1. To track changes in body composition to monitor the effectiveness of a training program or dietary regimen
2. To estimate optimal body weight or competition weight in weight-category sports such as boxing, lightweight rowing, and wrestling
3. To screen and monitor the health status of athletes to prevent disorders associated with extremely low levels of body fat

Male athletes with the lowest estimates of body fat (less than 6%) include middle-distance and long-distance runners and bodybuilders. Male basketball players, cyclists, gymnasts, sprinters, jumpers, triathletes, and wrestlers average between 6% and 15% body fat. Olympic marathon runners have 3% to 4% body fat, and Tour de France cyclists have between 4% and 6% body fat. Male athletes involved in power sports such as football, rugby, and ice and field hockey have slightly more variable levels of body fat (6% to 19%). Linebackers in American football have between 12% and 15% body fat, whereas defensive linemen have 16% body fat or more. Female athletes with the lowest estimates of body fat (6% to 15%) participate in bodybuilding, cycling, triathlons, and running events; higher fat levels (10% to 20%) are found in female athletes who participate in racquetball, skiing, soccer, swimming, tennis, and volleyball. The estimated minimal level of body fat compatible with health is 5% for men and 12% for women, but optimal body fat percentages for a particular athlete may be much higher than these minimums and should be determined on an individual basis.

Body mass may also be dramatically different in different sports. Female distance runners may weigh 50 to 55 kg (110-120 lb), whereas female shot putters may weigh 75 to 85 kg (165-185 lb). Ballet dancers may weigh no more than 45 kg (100 lb). These body composition assessments reveal that athletes generally have physique characteristics that are unique to their specific sports and disciplines.

Athletes who strive to maintain body weight or body-fat levels that are inappropriate or have body-fat percentages below the minimal levels may be at risk for an eating disorder or other health problems related to poor energy and nutrient intakes. This topic will be discussed in detail in chapter 16.

The human body is made up of various components. We can look at these components at different levels. In body composition research, five levels are usually distinguished: atomic, molecular, cellular, tissue or organ, and whole body. At the atomic level, for example, the body is mostly made up of four elements: carbon, hydrogen, oxygen, and nitrogen. Together these elements make up about 96% of the weight. The remaining 4% comes mostly from minerals (particularly calcium in bones).

Most available techniques for measuring body composition help quantify the most important structural components of the body: muscle, bone, and fat. Body composition measurements are usually performed at important time points in the athletic season. Often, athletes and coaches discuss the measurements with a sports dietitian, sports medic, or sports scientist. Regular measurements (once every 3 months) are important to note trends in body composition. Changes in body composition do not occur overnight, and sufficient time must pass between measurements to allow changes to become evident. Some techniques have more variation than others, and demonstrating changes with those measurements is even more difficult. A simple way of tracking changes in body composition is to look at body fat, lean body mass, or the fat-free mass (FFM) divided by fat mass (FM). This is often referred to as the FFM to FM ratio.

Body Composition Models

To understand the science of body composition assessment, it is important to understand the theoretical models that underlie these measurements of human body composition. Information about the composition of the human body has been obtained from the analysis of human cadavers, mostly in the 1950s, that quantified the total fat, protein, water, and mineral content of the body. These studies formed the basis of body composition models that divide the body into two or more components.

Two-Component Model

The two-component model partitions body mass into its lean (FFM) and fat (FM) compartments:

$$\text{body mass} = \text{FFM} + \text{FM}$$

The term *lean body mass* is occasionally used, but *fat-free mass* is probably more appropriate. Lean body mass is a more anatomic concept that includes some essential lipids, whereas FFM is a biochemical concept. This model has had the widest application in the study of body composition, including many studies of athletes. FM is the more labile of the two compartments; it is readily influenced by diet and training. A shortcoming of the two-component model is the heterogeneous composition of FFM; it includes water, protein, mineral (bone and soft-tissue mineral), and glycogen.

Three-Component Model

To account for interindividual differences in hydration, a three-component model was developed that includes FM and partitions FFM into total body water (TBW) and fat-free dry mass (FFDM):

$$\text{body mass} = \text{TBW} + \text{FFDM} + \text{FM}$$

Water is the largest component of body mass, and it is most located in lean tissues. FFDM includes protein, glycogen, and mineral in bone and soft tissues. The use of dual X-ray absorptiometry (DXA) is based on this three-component model (see the later section about DXA).

Four-Component Model

With the development of techniques to measure bone mineral, the four-component model is a logical extension of the preceding model. FFDM is partitioned into bone mineral (BM) and the residual:

$$\text{body mass} = \text{TBW} + \text{BM} + \text{FM} + \text{residual}$$

The four-component model is more accurate than the two-component model but also requires more measurements. All models measure FM, and this component is of particular interest in this chapter.

Normal Ranges of Body Weight and Body Fat

Body fat consists of essential body fat and storage fat. Essential body fat is present in the nerve tissues, bone marrow, and organs (all membranes), and we cannot lose this fat without compromising physiological function. Storage fat represents an energy reserve that accumulates when excess energy is ingested and decreases when more energy is expended than consumed. Essential body fat is approximately 3% of body mass for men and 12% of body mass for women. Women are believed to have more essential body fat than men because of childbearing and hormonal functions. In general, the total body-fat percentage (essential plus storage fat) is between 12% and 15% for young men and between 25% and 28% for young women (Lohman and Going 1993) (see also table 14.1). Average percentages of body fat for the general population and for various athletes are presented in tables 14.2 and 14.3.

Different sports have different body composition requirements. In some contact sports, such as American football and rugby, a higher body weight is generally seen as an advantage. In sports

TABLE 14.1 Body Fat Percentages for Men and Women and Their Classification

Men	Women	Rating
5-10	8-15	Athletic
11-14	16-23	Good
15-20	24-30	Acceptable
21-24	31-36	Overweight
>24	>36	Obese

These are rough estimates. The term *athletic* in this context refers to sports in which low body fat is an advantage.

TABLE 14.2 Body Fat Percentages for the Average Population

	<30 yr	30-50 yr	>50 yr
Women	14-21	15-23	16-25
Men	9-15	11-17	12-19

TABLE 14.3 Body-Fat Percentages for Athletes

Sport	Male	Female	Sport	Male	Female
Baseball	12-15	12-18	Rowing	6-14	12-18
Basketball	6-12	20-27	Shot putting	16-20	20-28
Bodybuilding	5-8	10-15	Skiing (cross-country)	7-12	16-22
Cycling	5-15	15-20	Sprinting	8-10	12-20
Football (backs)	9-12	No data	Soccer	10-18	13-18
Football (linemen)	15-19	No data	Swimming	9-12	14-24
Gymnastics	5-12	10-16	Tennis	12-16	16-24
High and long jumping	7-12	10-18	Triathlon	5-12	10-15
Ice and field hockey	8-15	12-18	Volleyball	11-14	16-25
Marathon running	5-11	10-15	Weightlifting	9-16	No data
Racquetball	8-13	15-22	Wrestling	5-16	No data

such as gymnastics, marathon running, and other weight-bearing activities, a lower body weight and a high power-to-weight ratio are extremely important. Therefore, in these sports low body fat and low body weight are necessary. In sports such as bodybuilding, increasing lean body mass and increasing body weight without increasing body fat are desirable. No accepted standards for percentage body fat exist for athletes. The ideal body composition depends largely on the sport or discipline, and athletes should discuss this topic with the coach, a physiologist, and a nutritionist or dietitian. Body weight and body composition should be discussed in relation to functional capacity and exercise performance.

Body Composition Measurement Techniques

Body composition measurement methods are continuously being developed and perfected. The methods range from simple manual anthropometry to ones that require complex or expensive equipment. The latter include multisegmental and multifrequency bioelectrical impedance analysis; quantitative magnetic resonance for total body water, fat, and lean tissue measurements; and imaging to further define ectopic fat depots (Lemos and Gallagher 2017). Available methods permit the measurement of FM, total adipose tissue and its subdepots (visceral, subcutaneous, and intermuscular), ectopic fat (i.e., fat that is tissues other than adipose tissue that normally contain only small amounts of fat, such as the liver, skeletal muscle, and heart), lean (fat-free) mass, bone mass and mineral content, total body water, extracellular water, and skeletal muscle.

A variety of techniques have been developed to measure body composition (see table 14.4). Such measurements are more meaningful than the traditional weight–height relationship. All methods, including the simple anthropometric measurements, will be discussed in detail in the following sections.

Anthropometry

Anthropometry involves the systematic measurement of the physical properties of the human body, primarily dimensional descriptors of body size and shape. The most obvious ones are body height and body weight and derived values such as the **body mass index (BMI)**. Anthropometric measures can also include body segment girths such as the circumference of the chest, waist, and hips. Height–weight charts, such as the one shown in figure 14.1, provide a normal range of body weights for any given height. These charts have limitations, however, especially when applied to an athletic population. For instance, a bodybuilder (180 cm, 100 kg [6 ft, 220 lb]) may have very low body fat but could be classified as overweight. Clearly the "extra" weight is muscle, not body fat, which would lead to erroneous classification and possibly mistaken advice.

Body Mass Index

A rough but better measure than the height–weight chart is body mass index (BMI), which is also shown in figure 14.1.The BMI, also known as the Quetelet index, is derived from body mass and height and is calculated as follows:

TABLE 14.4 Techniques to Measure Body Composition

Method	Description
Anthropometry	Measurements of body height, body weight, and body segment girths to predict body fat
Densitometry	Underwater weighing based on Archimedes' principle to estimate lean body mass and fat mass
Skinfold thickness	Measurement of subcutaneous fat with a caliper that gives an estimation of lean body mass and fat mass
Bioelectrical impedance analysis (BIA)	Measurement of resistance to an electrical current to estimate total-body water, lean body mass, and fat mass
Dual-energy X-ray absorptiometry (DXA or DEXA)	X-ray scan at two intensities to measure total-body water, lean body mass, fat mass, and bone-mineral density
Computed tomography (CT)	Computer-assisted X-ray scan to image body tissues and measure bone mass
Quantitative magnetic resonance imaging	Similar to CT but uses electromagnetic rather than ionizing radiation to image body tissues and organs
Air displacement plethysmography (Bod Pod)	Measurement of air displacement to estimate lean body mass and fat mass

Are you at a healthy weight?

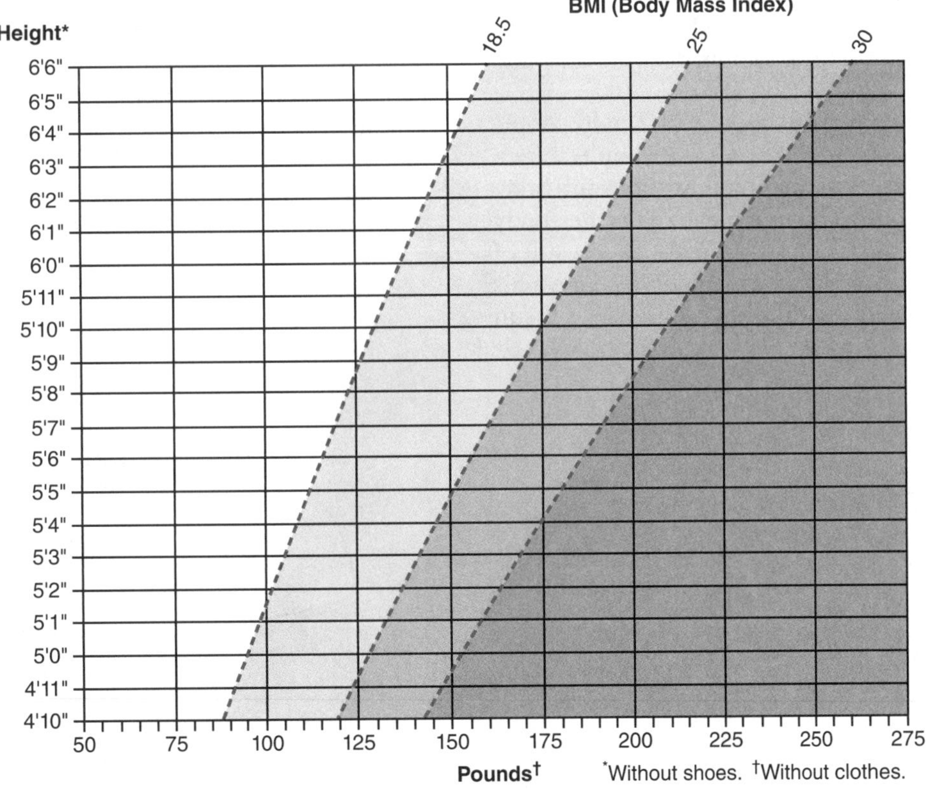

BMI measures weight in relation to height. The BMI ranges shown above are for adults. They are not exact ranges of healthy and unhealthy weights. However, they show that health risk increases at higher levels of overweight and obesity. Even within the healthy BMI range, weight gains can carry health risks for adults.

Directions: Find your weight on the bottom of the graph. Go straight up from that point until you come to the line that matches your height. Then look to find your weight group.

- Healthy Weight BMI from 18.5 up to 25 refers to healthy weight.
- Overweight BMI from 25 up to 30 refers to overweight.
- Obese BMI 30 or higher refers to obesity. Obese persons are also overweight.

Figure 14.1 Relationship between height, weight, and body mass index (BMI) and criteria for healthy BMI, overweight BMI, and obese BMI.

Adapted from U.S. Department of Agriculture (2000).

$$\text{BMI} = \text{body mass in kilograms} / (\text{height in meters})^2$$

A person who is 1.76 m (5 ft 9 in.) tall and weighs 72 kg (158 lb) has a BMI of $72 / (1.76)^2 = 23.2$. The normal range is between 18.5 kg/m^2 and 25 kg/m^2. People with a BMI higher than 25 kg/m^2 are classified as overweight, and people with a BMI higher than 30 kg/m^2 are classified as obese.

Body Mass Index Classifications

< 18.5 Underweight

18.5-24.9 Normal weight

25.0-29.9 Overweight

30.0-34.9 Obesity class I

35.0-39.9 Obesity class II

>40.0 Obesity class III (extreme obesity)

Even when using BMI, the previously mentioned bodybuilder would be classified as overweight or even obese because the equation does not take into account body composition ($\text{BMI} = 100 / (1.80)^2 = 30.9$). As illustrated in figure 14.2, two people might have the same BMI (in the example shown it is 28.0 kg/m^2) but completely different body compositions. One could achieve his or her body weight with primarily muscle mass as a result of hard training, whereas the other could achieve his or her body weight with fat deposition as a result of a sedentary lifestyle. Without information about body composition, they both might be classified as obese. In children and older people, BMI is difficult to interpret because muscle and bone weights are changing in relationship to height.

The BMI, however, does provide useful information about risks for various diseases and is used in many epidemiological and clinical studies. For example, BMI correlates with the incidence of cardiovascular complications (hypertension and stroke), certain cancers, type 2 diabetes, gallstones, osteoarthritis, and renal disease (Calle et al. 1999). The BMI, however, is best used for populations rather than individuals. When used for individual assessment, BMI needs to be used in coordination with other measurements, such as waist circumference, body composition, and so on.

Waist Circumference or Waist-to-Hip Ratio

The waist-to-hip ratio (WHR) measurement gives an index of body-fat distribution (figure 14.3) and can be used to help determine obesity. The distribution of fat is evaluated by dividing waist size by hip size. A person with a 75 cm (30 in.) waist and 100 cm (39 in.) hips would have a ratio of 0.75; one with an 82 cm (32 in.) waist and 78 cm (31 in.) hips

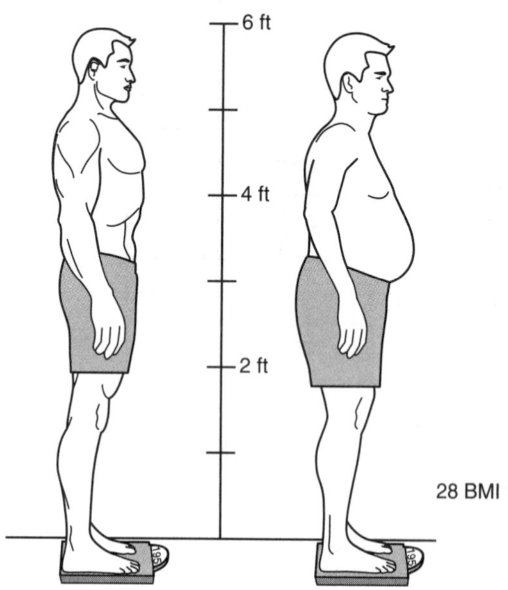

Figure 14.2 Two people with the same height and weight and the same BMI but very different body compositions.

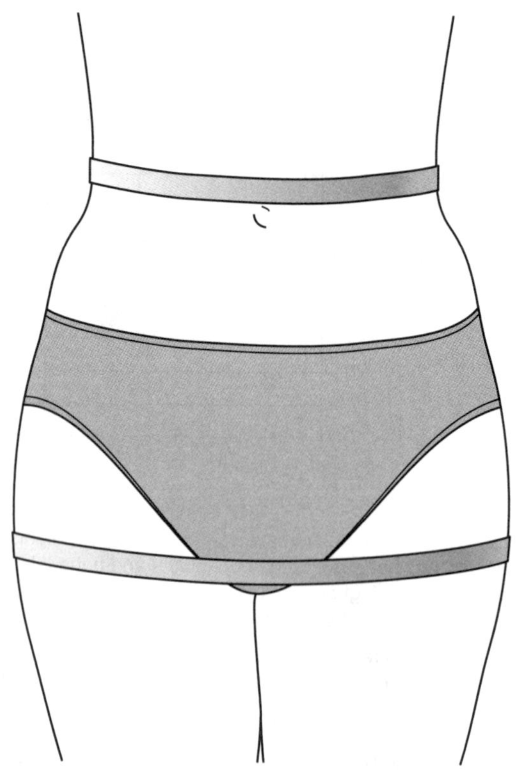

Figure 14.3 Waist-to-hip ratio.

would have a ratio of 1.05. The higher the ratio is, the higher the risk of heart disease and other obesity-related disorders is. Women and men with WHRs greater than 0.80 and 0.91, respectively, have a higher risk of developing cardiovascular disease, diabetes, hypertension, and certain cancers. WHRs smaller than 0.73 for women and 0.85 for men indicate a low risk. WHR is also a better predictor of mortality in older people than waist circumference or BMI. Other studies have found waist circumference, not WHR, to be a good indicator of cardiovascular risk factors, body fat distribution, and hypertension in type 2 diabetes. Although WHR and waist circumference are simple measures, they are of limited use to athletes.

Densitometry

Several techniques of **densitometry** have been developed to measure body composition and to distinguish the most important components: carbohydrate (typically < 1% of body mass), minerals (~4%), fat (~15%), protein (~20%), and water (~60%). Each of these components has a different density. Density is mass divided by volume and is usually expressed in grams per cubic centimeter (g/cm^3). The density of bone, for instance, is 1.3 to 1.4 g/cm^3, the density of fat is 0.9 g/cm^3, and the density of fat-free (lean) tissue is 1.1 g/cm^3. A lower total-body density value represents a higher FM.

The Greek inventor Archimedes (287 BC-212 BC) discovered a fundamental principle to assess human body composition. King Heron II of Syracuse had commissioned a goldsmith to make a crown of pure gold. When the goldsmith delivered the crown, the king noticed that the color of the gold was slightly lighter than usual. Suspecting that some of the gold had been replaced with silver, the king asked Archimedes to invent a way to measure the gold content of the crown without melting it down. Archimedes thought hard about this problem for several weeks. Then, stepping into a bath filled to the top with water and watching the overflow, he realized that he had found a way to measure the density of an object. Archimedes jumped from the bath and ran naked through the streets, shouting his famous words, "Eureka, eureka!" Archimedes had found a way to solve the mystery of the king's crown. He reasoned that a substance must have a volume proportional to its mass, and measuring the volume of an irregularly shaped object would require submersion in water and collecting the overflow. He found that pure gold with the same mass as the crown displaced less water than the crown and that silver displaced more water. He concluded that the crown was made of a mixture of gold and silver and thus confirmed the king's suspicions.

Assume that a 1,000 g crown is an alloy of 70% gold and 30% silver. Because its volume is 64.6 cm^3, it displaces 64.6 g of water (water has a density of 1.00 g/cm^3). The crown's apparent mass in water is thus 1,000 g - 64.6 g = 935.4 g. The 1,000 g of pure gold has a volume of 51.8 cm^3, so its apparent mass in water is 1,000 - 51.8 g = 948.2 g. If both crowns were suspended on opposite ends of a scale immersed in water, the apparent mass is 935.4 g at one end and 948.2 g at the other end—an imbalance of 12.8 g. Scales from Archimedes' time could easily detect such an imbalance in mass.

The same principle can be used to distinguish between FM and FFM in the human body (see figure 14.4). With underwater weighing or hydrostatic weighing, a person is submerged in water and the body weight is accurately measured before and after submersion. Assume that a 75 kg (165 lb) person is submerged in water and weighs 3 kg (6.6

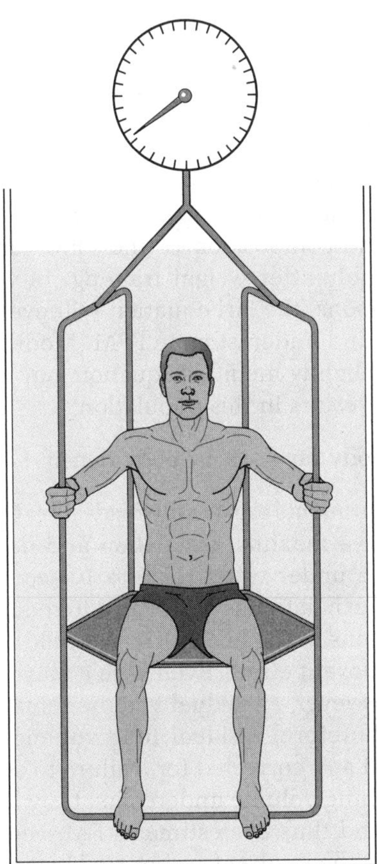

Figure 14.4 With the underwater or hydrostatic weighing technique, a person's body density is determined using Archimedes' principle.

lb) in water. According to Archimedes' principle, the loss of weight in water of 72 kg (158.4 lb) equals the weight of the displaced water.

The volume of the water displaced must be corrected for the temperature of the water at the time of weighing because water density changes with temperature. The density is 1.00 g/cm^3 at 4 °C (39.2 °F), but measurements are usually performed in warmer water. Without correction, the body density in our example would be 75,000 / 72,000 = 1.0417 g/cm^3.

Siri (1956) developed a method to estimate the percentage body fat from these measurements. The method assumes a density of 0.90 g/cm^3 for the density of fat and 1.10 g/cm^3 for the density of fat-free tissues. The equation for calculating the percentage body fat, often referred to as the Siri equation, is as follows:

$$\% \text{ body fat} = (495 / \text{body density}) - 450$$

Using the same example of a 75 kg (165 lb) person, the percentage body fat is (495 / 1.0417) - 450 = 25.2%. FM can then be calculated as 25.2% of 75 kg = 18.9 kg, and FFM is 75 kg - 18.9 kg = 56.1 kg.

Although this technique generally works well and is considered by some to be the best current method available for assessing percentage body fat, it has several limitations. The calculations are based on a two-compartment model (FM and FFM). The composition of the FFM can change considerably after weight training. In very muscular persons, the Siri equation will overestimate body fat and underestimate FFM (Modlesky et al. 1996). A slightly modified equation may give more accurate results in this population:

$$\% \text{ body fat} = (521 / \text{body density}) - 478$$

Measurements are usually made after the person has made a maximal exhalation and held her or his breath under water for 5 to 10 seconds. This maximal exhalation is performed to reduce the air that remains in the lungs, which would otherwise exert a buoyant effect. Even with a maximal exhalation, however, a residual volume remains in the lungs. Therefore, residual lung volume must be measured and corrected for. Failure to correct for residual lung volume underestimates whole-body density and thus overestimates FM. Food intake, especially the intake of carbonated beverages, can also affect the measurement and should be avoided in the hours before measurement.

Skinfold Thickness

The most frequently used technique to estimate body fat is measuring the thickness of skinfolds. These measurements are based on the interrelationships between the fat located underneath the skin (subcutaneous fat), internal fat, and whole-body density. Skinfolds can be measured using a caliper, which usually indicates the thickness in millimeters (see figure 14.5). The skinfold should be held between the operator's thumb and forefinger as illustrated in figure 14.5, placed between the two arms of the caliper, and the measurement read within 2 seconds to avoid skinfold compression. Considerable experience is necessary to produce accurate skinfold measurements. When comparing skinfold thickness, measurements should always be taken by the same person to guarantee consistency.

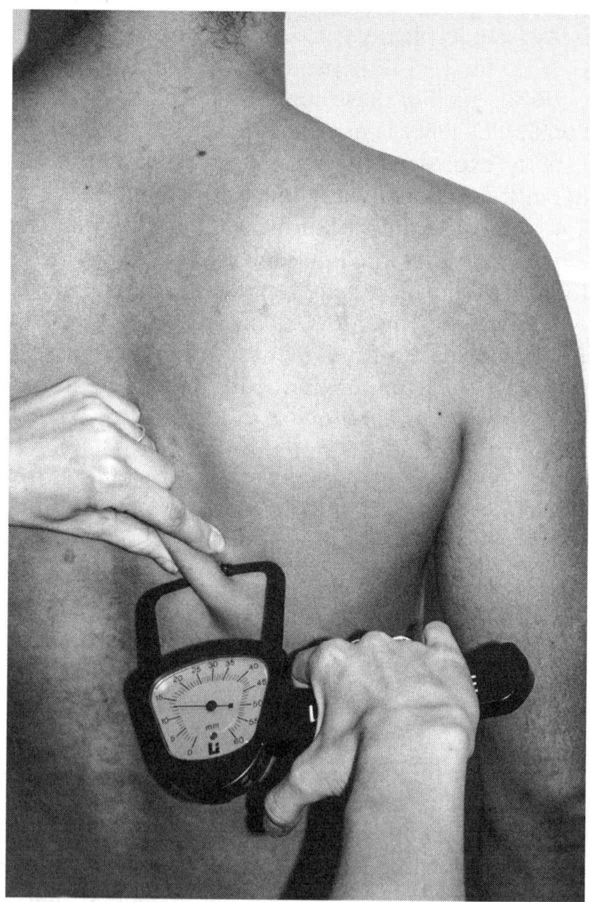

Figure 14.5 Skinfold measurement using calipers (subscapular site).

Several anatomical sites can be used for skinfold measurements. The four most common sites are the biceps, triceps, subscapularis, and abdominals. These sites are shown in figure 14.6. Sometimes other sites on the upper thigh and chest are used. Often the sum of four skinfolds is chosen, but other methods take the sum of seven or even 10 skinfolds.

The sum of skinfolds can then be used to predict body density and body-fat percentage. This prediction is usually based on previous research in which the skinfold measurements were compared with the results of underwater weighing. Various experimenters have put forward equations that are used either with skinfold thickness alone or in conjunction with other measurements, such as body circumference or limb lengths. Two of the most common sets of equations used are attributable to Durnin and Womersley (1974) (skinfolds alone) and to Jackson and Pollock (1978) (skinfolds and body measurements).

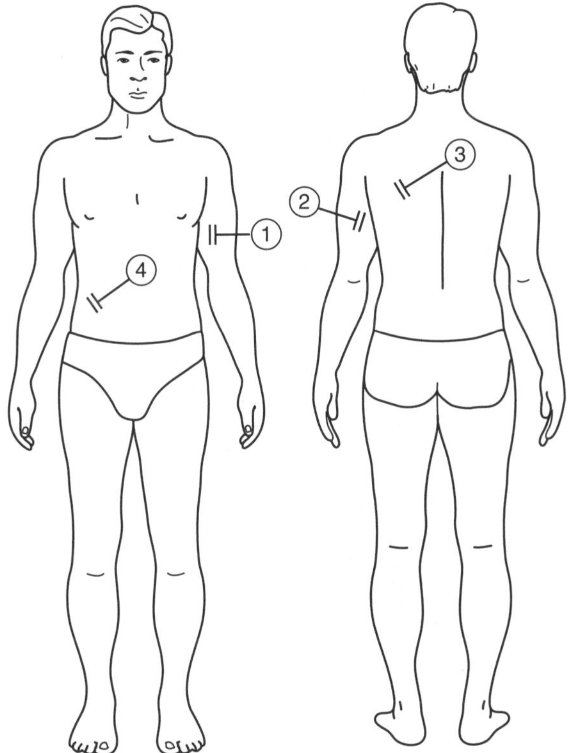

Figure 14.6 The four sites used for measuring skinfold thickness.

Based on Jackson and Pollock (1978).

After skinfold thickness has been measured using the sum of four skinfold measurements, body density can be calculated based on the equation and values shown in table 14.5 (Durnin and Womersley 1974). The appropriate values of C and M can be read from the table, and the equation can be solved to determine body density (g/cm^3) according to gender, age, and sum of the four skinfolds (in millimeters).

Percentage body fat is calculated using the Siri equation. For ease of reference, tables have been generated for percentage body fat values for men (table 14.6) and women (table 14.7) based on the sum of four skinfold measurements. Results are shown for each 2 mm increment of skinfold thickness.

Measurements at three skinfold sites (different ones for men and women as illustrated in figures 14.7 and 14.8, respectively) can also be used to estimate percentage body fat. When using three skinfold measurements, the body density equations of Jackson and Pollock are used:

$$\text{male body density} = 1.0990750 - 0.0008209\,(X2) + 0.0000026\,(X2)^2 - 0.0002017\,(X3) - 0.005675\,(X4) + 0.018586\,(X5)$$

where $X2$ = sum of the chest, abdomen, and thigh skinfolds in millimeters; $X3$ = age in years; $X4$ = waist circumference in centimeters; and $X5$ = forearm circumference in centimeters.

TABLE 14.5 Linear Regression Equations for the Calculation of Body Density

	17-19 yr	20-29 yr	30-39 yr	40-49 yr	≥50 yr
C	1.1620 (male) 1.1549 (female)	1.1631 (male) 1.1599 (female)	1.1422 (male) 1.1423 (female)	1.1620 (male) 1.1333 (female)	1.1715 (male) 1.1339 (female)
M	0.0630 (male) 0.0678 (female)	0.0632 (male) 0.0717 (female)	0.0544 (male) 0.0632 (female)	0.0700 (male) 0.0612 (female)	0.0779 (male) 0.0645 (female)

Body density = C - [M($\log_{10}$ sum of all four skinfolds)]

Based on Durnin and Womersley (1974).

TABLE 14.6 Percentage Body Fat for Male Subjects According to Age and Skinfold Thickness

	AGE (YR)				
Skinfold thickness*	**17-19**	**20-29**	**30-39**	**40-49**	**≥50**
10 mm	0.41	0.40	5.05	3.30	2.63
12 mm	2.46	2.10	6.86	5.61	5.20
14 mm	4.21	3.85	8.40	7.58	7.39
16 mm	5.74	5.38	9.74	9.31	9.31
18 mm	7.10	6.74	10.93	10.84	11.02
20 mm	8.32	7.96	12.00	12.22	12.55
22 mm	9.43	9.07	12.98	13.47	13.95
24 mm	10.45	10.09	13.87	14.62	15.23
26 mm	11.39	11.03	14.69	15.68	16.42
28 mm	12.26	11.91	15.46	16.67	17.53
30 mm	13.07	12.73	16.17	17.60	18.56
32 mm	13.84	13.49	16.84	18.47	19.53
34 mm	14.56	14.22	17.47	19.28	20.44
36 mm	15.25	14.90	18.07	20.06	21.31
38 mm	15.89	15.55	18.63	20.79	22.13
40 mm	16.51	16.17	19.17	21.49	22.92
42 mm	17.10	16.76	19.69	22.16	23.66
44 mm	17.66	17.32	20.18	22.80	24.38
46 mm	18.20	17.86	20.65	23.41	25.06
48 mm	18.71	18.37	21.10	24.00	25.72
50 mm	19.21	18.87	21.53	24.56	26.35
52 mm	19.69	19.35	21.95	25.10	26.96
54 mm	20.15	19.81	22.35	25.63	27.55
56 mm	20.59	20.26	20.73	26.13	28.11
58 mm	21.02	20.69	23.11	26.62	28.66
60 mm	21.44	21.11	23.47	27.09	29.20
62 mm	21.84	21.51	23.82	27.55	29.71
64 mm	22.23	21.90	24.16	28.00	30.21
66 mm	22.61	22.28	24.49	28.43	30.70
68 mm	22.98	22.65	24.81	28.85	31.17
70 mm	23.34	23.01	25.13	29.26	31.63
72 mm	23.69	23.36	25.43	29.66	32.07
74 mm	24.03	23.70	25.73	30.04	32.51
76 mm	24.36	24.03	26.01	30.42	32.93
78 mm	24.68	24.36	26.30	30.79	33.35
80 mm	25.00	24.67	26.57	31.15	33.75

*Sum of all four skinfolds.

TABLE 14.7 Percentage Body Fat for Female Subjects According to Age and Skinfold Thickness

	AGE (YR)				
Skinfold thickness*	**17-19**	**20-29**	**30-39**	**40-49**	**≥50**
10 mm	5.34	4.88	8.72	11.71	12.88
12 mm	7.60	7.27	10.85	13.81	15.10
14 mm	9.53	9.30	12.68	15.59	16.99
16 mm	11.21	11.08	14.27	17.15	18.65
18 mm	12.71	12.66	15.68	18.54	20.11
20 mm	14.05	14.08	16.95	19.78	21.44
22 mm	15.28	15.38	18.10	20.92	22.64
24 mm	16.40	16.57	19.16	21.95	23.74
26 mm	17.44	17.67	20.14	22.91	24.76
28 mm	18.40	18.69	21.05	23.80	25.71
30 mm	19.30	19.64	21.90	24.64	26.59
32 mm	20.15	20.54	22.70	25.42	27.42
34 mm	20.95	21.39	23.45	26.16	28.21
36 mm	21.71	22.19	24.16	26.85	28.95
38 mm	22.42	22.95	24.84	27.51	29.65
40 mm	23.10	23.67	25.48	28.14	30.32
42 mm	23.76	24.36	26.09	28.74	30.96
44 mm	24.38	25.02	26.68	29.32	31.57
46 mm	24.97	25.65	27.24	29.87	32.15
48 mm	25.54	26.26	27.78	30.39	32.71
50 mm	26.09	26.84	28.30	30.90	33.25
52 mm	26.62	27.40	28.79	31.39	33.77
54 mm	27.13	27.94	29.27	31.86	34.27
56 mm	27.63	28.47	29.74	32.31	34.75
58 mm	28.10	28.97	30.19	32.75	35.22
60 mm	28.57	29.46	30.62	33.17	35.67
62 mm	29.01	29.94	31.04	33.58	36.11
64 mm	29.45	30.40	31.45	33.98	36.53
66 mm	29.87	30.84	31.84	34.37	36.95
68 mm	30.28	31.28	32.23	34.75	37.35
70 mm	30.67	31.70	32.60	35.11	37.74
72 mm	31.06	32.11	32.97	35.47	38.12
74 mm	31.44	32.51	33.32	35.82	38.49
76 mm	31.81	32.91	33.67	36.15	38.85
78 mm	32.17	33.29	34.00	36.48	39.20
80 mm	32.52	33.66	34.33	36.81	39.54

*Sum of all four skinfolds.

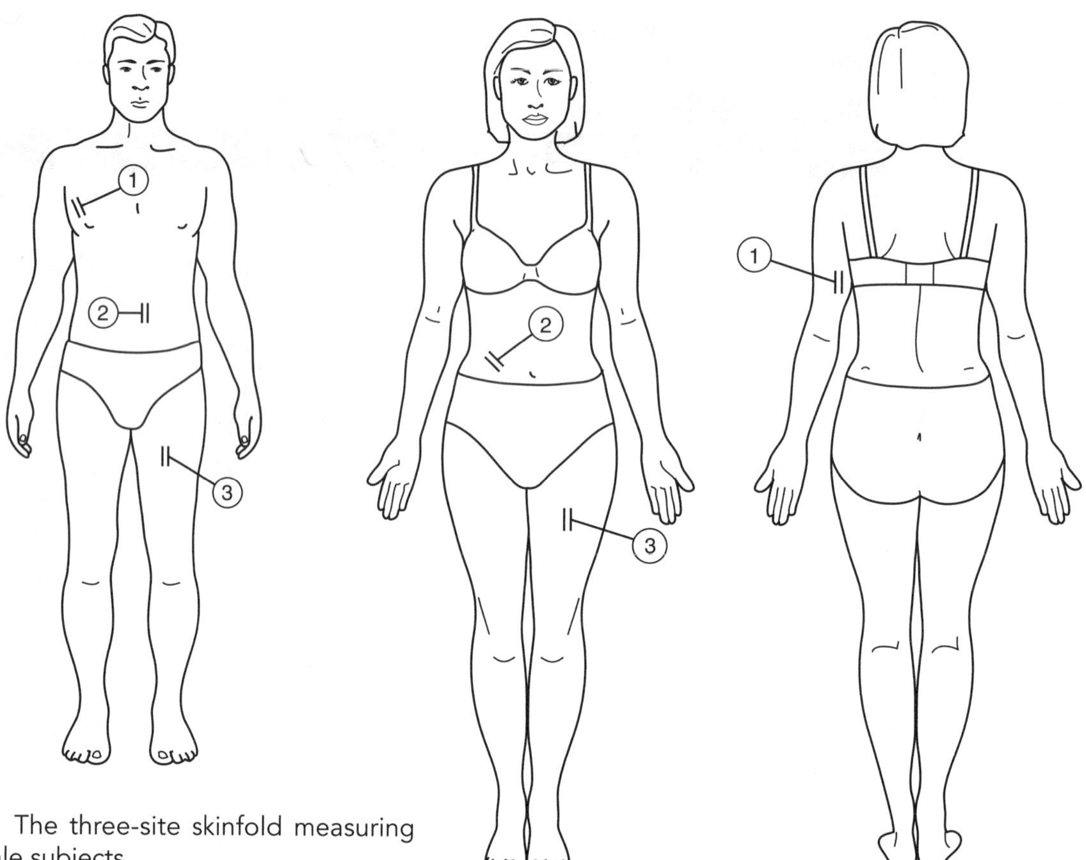

Figure 14.7 The three-site skinfold measuring system for male subjects.

Based on Jackson and Pollock (1978).

Figure 14.8 The three-site skinfold measuring system for female subjects.

Based on Jackson and Pollock (1978).

$$\text{female body density} = 1.1470292 - 0.0009376\,(X3) + 0.0000030\,(X3)2 - 0.0001156\,(X4) - 0.0005839\,(X5)$$

where $X3$ = sum of triceps, thigh, and suprailiac skinfolds in millimeters; $X4$ = age in years; and $X5$ = gluteal circumference in centimeters.

Again, percentage body fat is then calculated using the Siri equation. The correct tables must be used because the relationship between skinfold thickness and body fat may vary depending on the gender, age, and ethnicity of the individual. Estimating percentage body fat for populations other than the population the equations were based on may result in large errors. Skinfold measurements, when properly taken, correlate highly (r = 0.83-0.89) with hydrostatic weighing with a standard error of only about 3% or 4%. This error should always be kept in mind when using tables or equations to convert skinfold thickness to a percentage body fat. Sport scientists often stay with the skinfold thickness measurement and don't convert it to a body fat percentage. Skinfold measurement is especially useful when repeated and regular measurements are made of the same athlete.

Bioelectrical Impedance Analysis

Bioelectrical impedance analysis (BIA) is based on the principle that different tissues and substances have different impedance (resistance) to an electrical current. For example, impedance or conductivity is quite different for fat tissue and water (see figure 14.9).

Electrodes are placed on different parts of the body, often the hand and foot, and a current applied to one of those electrodes can be measured at the other electrode. The less the measured resistance is, the higher the body-water content is. Adipose tissue has high resistance, or impedance, whereas muscle (of which 75% is water) has low resistance. Based on these differential effects of applied electrical current, BIA can be

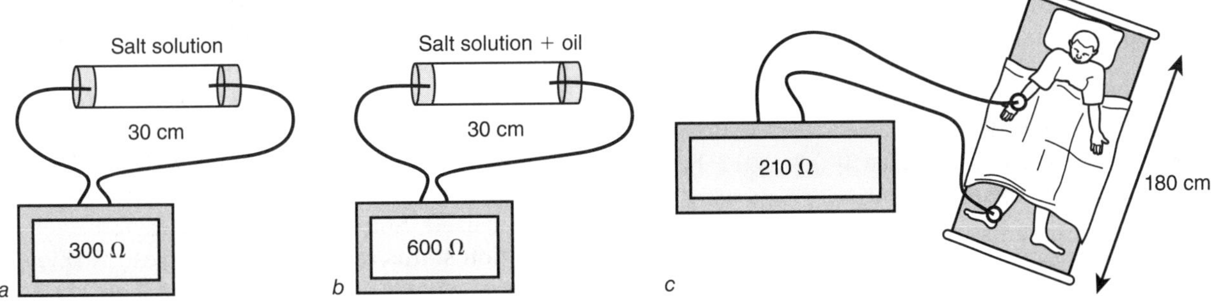

Figure 14.9 Bioelectrical impedance analysis. *(a)* If the resistance is measured to a known current in a tube with a salt solution and a known length (30 cm [12 in.]), the volume can be calculated. *(b)* If the same tube contains oil in addition to the salt solution, the resistance changes and a new calculation of volume is obtained. *(c)* The same principle can be applied to the human body, which can be viewed as five tubes (two arms, two legs, and one trunk).

used to estimate percentage body fat, percentage lean body mass, and percentage body water. BIA is often used to measure body composition, but it can also be used to estimate fluid levels in different body segments.

A simple example of a device for measuring impedance is a tube that contains a highly conductive salt solution with electrodes inserted at each end (see figure 14.9*a*). An electrical current is sent through one of the electrodes, and resistance (Z) is measured between the two electrodes. If the length of the tube (L) and the specific resistivity (ρ) of the salt solution are known, the volume (V) can be calculated:

$$V = \rho \times L^2 / Z$$

If some of the salt solution is replaced with oil, the measured resistance increases and the new volume of the salt solution is calculated. By deduction, the percentage of oil in the solution can be determined (see figure 14.9*b*). The principle is the same when measuring body impedance and calculating body composition. For this purpose, the measured body impedance and the subject's height are used.

Most BIA devices are tetrapolar, meaning that they have four electrodes: two that apply the current and two that receive a signal. The device applies a current of 500 μA to 800 μA at a single frequency of 50 kHz or more, which is too weak to be felt by the subject.

The subject lies on a nonconducting surface with arms at least 20 cm [8 in] apart and not touching the trunk and legs. Shoes, socks, and metal objects (jewelry) are removed. The contact surfaces on the hand and ankle should be cleaned with alcohol. The resistance measured can then be used in various formulas in a similar manner to the tube examples. The body can be viewed as five tubes: two arms, two legs, and one trunk (see figure 14.9*c*).

The example of the tubes is an oversimplification. In reality, several factors can affect impedance and invalidate the assumptions. A larger tube increases conductivity. Warming the tube also increases conductivity. Changes in the skin temperature alter whole-body conductivity and have a profound effect on the measurement. Higher skin temperature results in an underestimated body-fat content (Baumgartner, Chumlea, and Roche 1990). Often, when the measurements are performed, the subject may sweat more; a wet surface also reduces impedance and underestimates body-fat content.

Factors such as hydration status and distribution of water can also affect impedance. Even small changes in the hydration level can have a marked effect on the accuracy of the measurement and can influence the calculated body-fat content (Koulmann et al. 2000; Saunders, Blevins, and Broeder 1998). If a person is dehydrated, impedance decreases, whereas if a person drinks a lot of fluid before the measurement, impedance could increase. Thus, losing body water through prior exercise or voluntary fluid restriction will overestimate body-fat content. Hyperhydration has the opposite effect and will underestimate body-fat content.

Body position is important, and the fluid shifts that occur can affect impedance. The orientation of tissues can also affect impedance. For example, current is more easily transported along muscle fibers than against muscle fibers. The testing conditions under which BIA is run should be extremely well controlled. Usually subjects are advised as follows:

- Abstain from alcohol for 8 to 12 hours before the measurement.
- Avoid vigorous exercise for 8 to 12 hours before the measurement.
- Measurements are performed at least 2 hours after the last meal (or drink).
- Measurements are performed within 5 minutes of lying down.

BIA seems like a convenient technique, but it requires considerable experience, expertise, and control of the testing conditions. When BIA is performed in the best possible way, the results are extremely reliable, but they may not be as accurate as skinfold measurements (Broeder et al. 1997; Stolarczyk et al. 1997).

Dual-Energy X-Ray Absorptiometry

Dual-energy X-ray absorptiometry (DXA or DEXA) has become the clinical standard for measuring bone density. The principle is based on absorption of low-energy X-rays. The short duration of exposure gives only a minimal dose of radiation.

During the measurement, the subject lies supine on a table. A source and detector probe pass across the body at a relatively low speed (about 60 cm/min; a whole-body scan may take 6-15 minutes). The subject is exposed to these low-energy X-rays, and the loss of signal in various parts of the tissue is recorded. The measurement is performed at two intensities so the instrument's software can distinguish not only between soft tissues and bone-mineral content but also between FFM and FM. The derivation of fat and fat-free soft tissue from DXA scans is based on the ratio of soft-tissue attenuation of the low-energy and high-energy photon beams as they pass through the body. The attenuation of the low-energy and high-energy soft tissues is known based on scans of pure fat and fat-free soft tissues and theoretical calculations. The DXA instrument is linked with appropriate computer algorithms to derive estimates of bone mineral, fat-free soft tissue, and fat-tissue content of the total body. The algorithms also permit division of the body into anatomical segments—arms, legs, trunk, and head—to permit estimates of regional body composition.

DXA seems to be an accurate technique that shows excellent agreement with other independent techniques to measure bone-mineral content (Going et al. 1993; Heymsfield et al. 1990). In addition, small changes in body composition can be detected with this method (Going et al. 1993).

DXA may underestimate body-fat content somewhat compared with underwater weighing. In addition, with DXA, test conditions must be standardized (Kohrt 1995) because factors such as hydration status can influence the results (Elowsson et al. 1998). The software and hardware of the various commercially available DXA scanners are different, which is also a source of error (Van Loan et al. 1995). Although DXA has limitations, it appears to be one of the better ways to measure body composition, and it has advantages over other methods because it can distinguish FFM (i.e., lean body mass) and FM and also assess bone density. With this technique it is important to control for hydration status and standardize the measurements as much as possible.

Computed Tomography

Computed tomography (CT) uses ionizing radiation by an X-ray beam to create images of body segments. The CT scan produces qualitative and quantitative information about the total area of the tissue investigated and the thickness and volume of tissues within an organ. With this method, fat surrounding a tissue as well as fat within a tissue can be measured.

Quantitative Magnetic Resonance Imaging

With **magnetic resonance imaging (MRI)**, pictures can be obtained from body tissues and compartments. The results are somewhat similar to those obtained by CT scan, but with MRI, electromagnetic radiation is used rather than potentially damaging ionizing radiation. The MRI scanner itself is a cylinder-shaped, open-ended machine in which you lie on your back. MRI uses magnetic fields and radio waves to produce an image of the body. Passing these strong waves through the body affects the atoms within the body. The nucleus within each atom is forced into a different position, and when it returns to its normal position, this produces a second radio wave. The machine picks this up and translates the information into an image. All the tissues within our bodies contain water, and water contains hydrogen atoms that play a large part in how the image appears. Those structures with a high proportion of hydrogen atoms appear much brighter than those with a lower proportion. For this reason, fatty tissue appears much brighter than bone. Generally, for body-fat mass estimation, MRI shows good agreement with other methods. A study found excellent agreement between MRI and underwater-weighing estimates in overweight and nonoverweight women, which suggests that MRI may be a satisfactory substitute for the more-established methods of body-fat estimation in adult women. In fact, MRI showed the smallest day-to-day variation in measurement within an individual (see figure 14.10). Calculations of body fat from MRI scans are highly dependent on software, however, and this dependency can introduce error. MRI produces far more detailed pictures than X-rays or CT scans, so it is often used by clinicians for detecting conditions such as brain tumors, strokes, and heart defects. Sports injuries, such as meniscus tears and anterior cruciate ligament ruptures, are often scanned by MRI to confirm diagnosis prior to surgery.

Air Displacement Plethysmography

A relatively new and promising method for estimating whole-body volume is a small chamber in which air displacement is measured. The technique is called air displacement plethysmography, and it is marketed commercially as Bod Pod. The advantages of this technique are that it is convenient for the subject because it takes place while the subject is sitting in a small chamber, measurements take only 3 to 5 minutes, and the reproducibility is good.

The subject is first accurately weighed outside the Bod Pod. He or she then sits in the 750 L (198 gal) Bod Pod, which consists of a dual chamber made out of fiberglass (see figure 14.11). The person's volume is the original volume in the chamber minus the air that has been displaced with the subject inside. The subject breathes into an air circuit to assess pulmonary gas volume, which, when subtracted from measured body volume, yields true body volume. Body density can then be calculated from body mass and body volume. Although this technique has good reproducibility, it generally gives lower percentages of body fat compared with hydrostatic weighing and DXA (Collins et al. 1999; Wagner, Heyward, and Gibson 2000; Weyers et al. 2002).

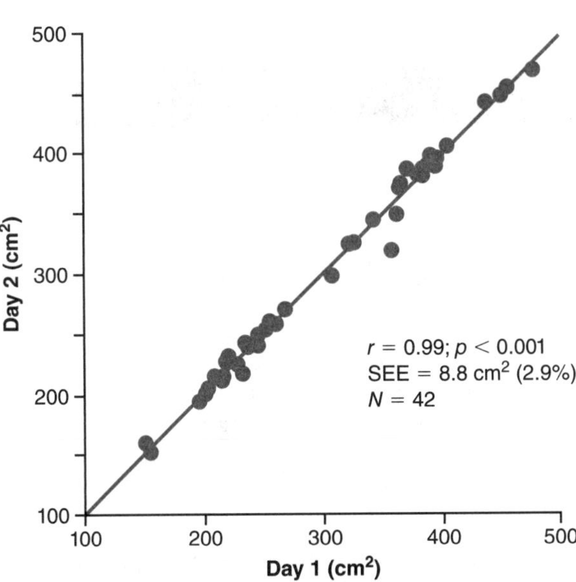

Figure 14.10 Comparison of typical in vivo magnetic resonance images obtained on two separate days from the same subject at the midthigh. Regression between cross-sectional adipose tissue–free skeletal muscle areas from 42 pairs of magnetic resonance images (six subjects and seven images each). SEE = SE of estimate; N = number of images. The solid line is the regression line.

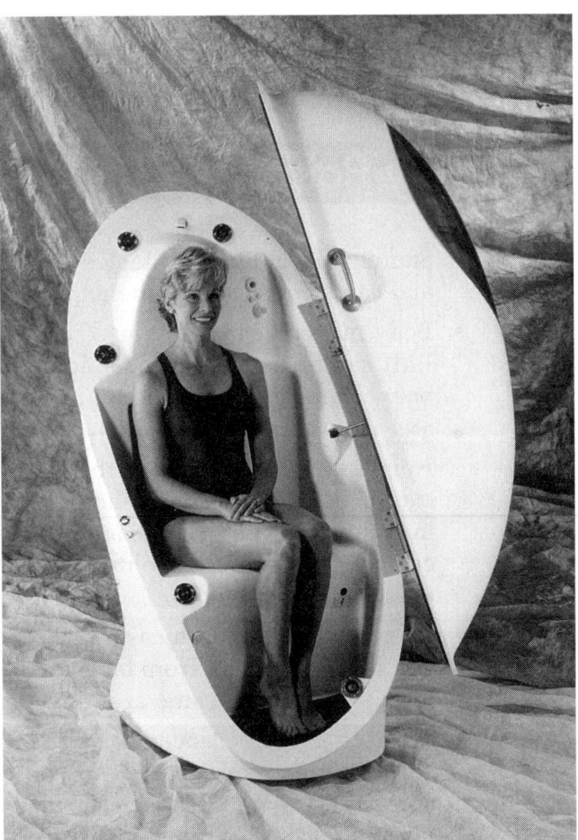

Figure 14.11 The Bod Pod.

From Life Measurement, Inc.

CONSIDERATIONS FOR BODY COMPOSITION ASSESSMENT OF ATHLETES

All methods of assessing body composition have some inherent problems whether in measurement methodology or in the assumptions they make. To date, there is no universally applicable criterion or gold standard methodology for body composition assessment of athletes (Ackland et al. 2012), although underwater weighing and DXA are probably the two methods that are often used as a gold standard. Generally, the more complex models are more accurate, but they are often unsuitable for conditions outside a laboratory or clinical setting. The best available methods for percentage body fat measurement are underwater weighing and DXA, but the most user-friendly method is probably skinfold measurement. Periodic measurement with the best available techniques is recommended to obtain accurate information about body composition. To track athletes in field conditions, the same person should collect the skinfold measurements, and the sum of skinfolds should be used as the outcome measure rather than a conversion to percentage body fat, which can be inaccurate and can cause unnecessary variation.

Multicomponent Models

Multicomponent models use a combination of methods, such as hydrostatic weighing, BIA, and DXA, to reduce the errors associated with using a single method (Wagner, Heyward, and Gibson 2000). Although the traditional two-component model is based on separating FM and FFM to determine body composition, these models assume that the density of FFM is 1.1 g/cm^3 and that the components of the FFM (water, protein, and minerals) are constant for all individuals. These assumptions may not always hold true, and accuracy can therefore be improved by measuring these components. Multicomponent models can combine measures of whole-body density with measures of body-water and bone-mineral density. This approach is generally believed to give the most accurate results.

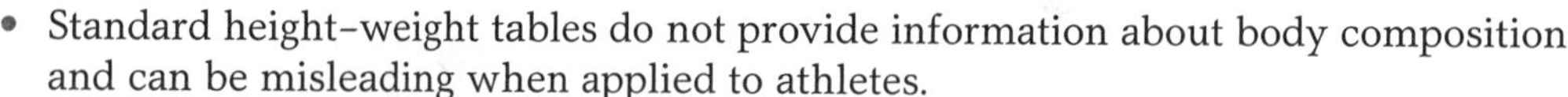

Key Points

- Standard height–weight tables do not provide information about body composition and can be misleading when applied to athletes.
- Body mass index is often used as a rough measure of body composition. Although BMI can be useful in epidemiological and clinical studies, it does not distinguish between muscle mass and fat mass.
- The technique of densitometry is based on Archimedes' principle that the loss of weight in water is equal to the volume of the displaced water. The same principle can be used to determine the density of the human body by submerging a person in water and measuring his or her body weight before and after submersion. After correcting for residual volume, the percentage of body fat can be calculated based on underwater weight.
- The sum of skinfold measurements can be used to estimate body fat percentage. For accuracy, values from tables that have been established for specific populations (e.g., same gender, same age range) must be used.
- Bioelectrical impedance analysis is a convenient technique that requires considerable experience, expertise, and control of environmental conditions to obtain reliable results. When BIA is performed in the best possible circumstances, the results may be reliable, but they may still be less accurate than skinfold measurements.
- Dual-energy X-ray absorptiometry is based on the principle that compartments with different densities absorb different amounts of low-energy X-rays. The advan-

tage of DXA is that it can distinguish FM and FFM and also assesses bone density. DXA has become the clinical standard to measure bone density.

- Imaging technologies, such as computed tomography (CT) and magnetic resonance imaging (MRI), can provide images of body fat in different parts of the body.

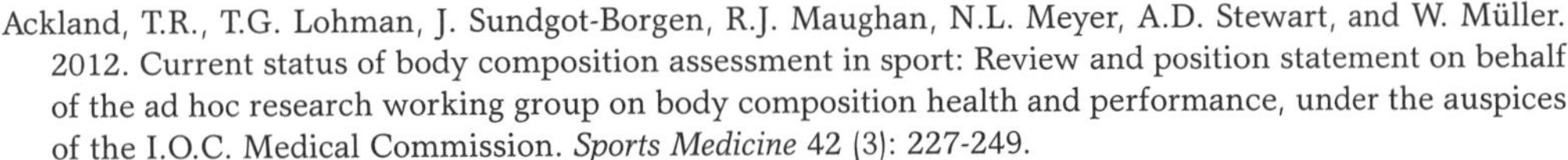

Recommended Readings

Ackland, T.R., T.G. Lohman, J. Sundgot-Borgen, R.J. Maughan, N.L. Meyer, A.D. Stewart, and W. Müller. 2012. Current status of body composition assessment in sport: Review and position statement on behalf of the ad hoc research working group on body composition health and performance, under the auspices of the I.O.C. Medical Commission. *Sports Medicine* 42 (3): 227-249.

Bouchard, C. 1994. Genetics of obesity: Overview and research directions. In *The genetics of obesity,* edited by C. Bouchard, 223-233. Boca Raton, FL: CRC Press.

Bouchard, C., A. Tremblay, J.P. Despres, A. Nadeau, P.J. Lupien, G. Theriault, J. Dussault, S. Flatt, J.-P. 1995. Use and storage of carbohydrate and fat. *American Journal of Clinical Nutrition* 61:952S-959S.

Heymsfield, S.B., T.G. Lohman, Z. Wang, and S.B. Going. 2005. *Human body composition.* Champaign, IL: Human Kinetics.

Heyward, V.H., and D.R. Wagner. 2004. *Applied body composition assessment.* Champaign, IL: Human Kinetics.

Lemos, T., and D. Gallagher. 2017. Current body composition measurement techniques. *Current Opinion in Endocrinology Diabetes and Obesity* 24 (5): 310-314.

Moorjani, S. Pinault, and G. Fournier. 1990. The response to long-term overfeeding in identical twins. *New England Journal of Medicine* 322:1477-1482.

Roche, A.F., S.B. Heymsfield, and T.G. Lohman. 1996. *Human body composition.* Champaign, IL: Human Kinetics.

Weight Management

Objectives

After studying this chapter, you should be able to do the following:

- Understand the factors that control appetite
- Describe ways of losing body fat and body weight by dieting
- Describe the role of exercise in losing body fat and body weight
- Describe the benefits and risks of making weight and discuss the ways of minimizing the risks

Maintaining an optimal body weight and composition is important for performance in many sports. Seasonal changes in body weight may occur in athletes such as games players where there is an off season. Usually any weight gained during the off season will have to be lost when the players return for preseason training before competitive matches begin. Many athletes try to lose body weight (particularly body fat) even if they are not overweight. For some, this weight loss offers an advantage because it increases the power-to-weight ratio (which is particularly important in jumping events). For others, weight loss means a reduction in energy expenditure when competing (such as when running). Weight reduction is also common in weight-category sports in which athletes often compete well below their normal weight. Another reason that athletes want to get rid of body fat is simply to enhance physical appearance and live up to the stereotype of the lean, toned, and strong athlete. Athletes can attempt to lose weight by reducing dietary energy intake, increasing energy expenditure by doing more exercise, or both.

Weight loss is not always a good idea, and it can sometimes be detrimental to performance. A reduction in body mass is usually accompanied by a reduction in muscle mass, and it may reduce muscle glycogen stores as well. Excessive weight loss has also been associated with chronic fatigue and increased risk of injuries. Too much emphasis on losing weight can lead to the development of eating disorders, which are discussed in chapter 16.

There are also situations in which an athlete may want to gain weight. This will usually be a desire to increase lean muscle mass in order to improve strength and power. This is commonplace in sports such as hammer throwing, discus throwing, shot put, weightlifting, American football, and rugby. There may also be a need for some athletes to restore muscle mass that may have been lost during a period of immobilization or bedrest caused by injury or illness. The key to putting on weight is to have energy intake exceed energy expenditure. To increase lean body mass rather than fat mass, the main focus will be to increase protein intake and perform some resistance training. This chapter discusses genetic factors in weight loss and weight gain, how **appetite** is controlled, and the various diet and exercise strategies that can be employed to modify body weight and composition, together with the associated problems of achieving desired weight changes while minimizing risks to health and performance.

Genetics

A significant portion of the variation in individual body-fat levels is genetically determined. Perhaps 25% to 40% of adiposity is the result of our genes (Bouchard 1994). Evidence from genetic epidemiology and molecular epidemiology studies suggests that genetic factors determine susceptibility to gaining or losing body fat in response to dietary energy intake (Perusse and Bouchard 2000). To study the influence of genetics on the effects of overfeeding, identical twins were investigated. In one study, monozygotic twins were subjected to an energy surplus of 4.2 kJ/day (1,000 kcal/day) on 6 days/week for 100 days (Bouchard et al. 1990). The excess energy intake over the entire period was 353 MJ (84,369 kcal). The average body mass gain was 8.1 kg (17.9 lb), but there was considerable variation among participants. The variation between pairs was more than three times greater than the variation within pairs, which suggests an important genetic component. The variation between pairs was even greater for changes in abdominal visceral fat, which indicates that the site of storage is also genetically determined.

Similarly, when identical twins completed a negative energy balance protocol by exercising over a period of 93 days without increasing energy intake, more variation occurred between pairs than within pairs (Bouchard et al. 1990). The energy deficit was estimated to be 244 MJ (58,317 kcal), and the mean body-weight loss was 5 kg (11 lb). The range of weight loss, however, was 1.0 to 8.0 kg (2.2-17.6 lb) (see figure 15.1).

These classic early studies demonstrate a genetic factor in the development of obesity. This link has been confirmed by molecular epidemiology studies, and now more than 250 genes are believed to have the potential to influence body fatness (Rankinen et al. 2002). Several risk factors associated with weight gain, such as a low resting metabolic rate, high reliance on carbohydrate metabolism, and a lower level of spontaneous activity, almost certainly have a genetic basis, but the relative contribution of genetic versus environmental factors is still a subject of debate.

Energy and Macronutrient Intake

A negative energy balance is necessary to lose weight, and it can be induced by reducing energy intake, increasing energy expenditure, or a combination of these two. These alterations in energy balance are just part of the picture. Macronutrient (carbohydrate, fat, and protein) intake and expenditure must also be considered. Excess intake of carbohydrate and protein can be converted to fat, although this process requires energy. For many years, it was believed that although de novo lipogenesis (the biochemical process of synthesizing

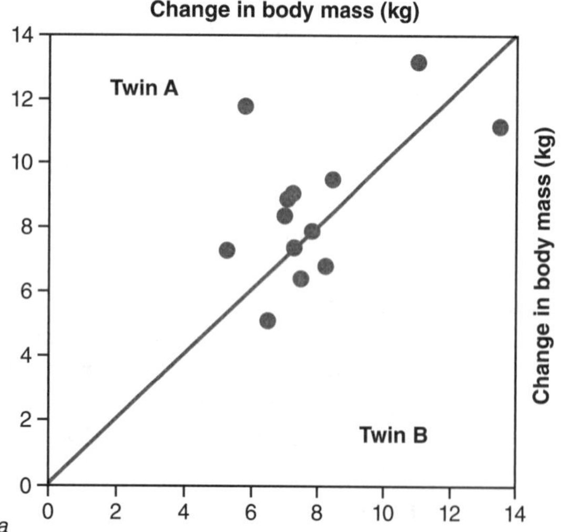

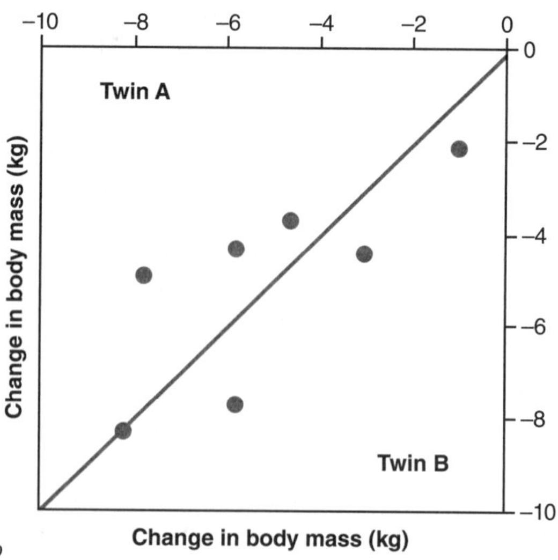

Figure 15.1 Changes in body mass in identical twins *(a)* after overfeeding and *(b)* after being subjected to a negative energy balance by exercise. Considerably more variation occurred between pairs than within pairs, which strongly suggests a genetic component in the regulation of body mass.

Based on Bouchard et al. (1990).

fatty acids from acetyl-CoA subunits that are produced from a number of different pathways within the cell, most commonly carbohydrate catabolism) did exist, it did not play an important role in human metabolism. Evidence now shows that overfeeding with carbohydrate can increase de novo lipogenesis (Aarsland, Chinkes, and Wolfe 1997). The liver plays only a minor role in this process, and the majority of de novo lipogenesis probably takes place in adipose tissue. The subjects in the study of Aarsland et al. (1997) were overfed and received a large amount of excess energy (2.5 times their requirements). Therefore, it could be questioned whether increased de novo lipogenesis could occur in athletes who are in energy balance. Jeukendrup and colleagues (unpublished) performed a study in which endurance-trained athletes exercised 2 h/day at moderate intensity while maintaining energy balance, thereby mimicking a normal training situation. Subjects stayed in a respiration chamber so energy intake and expenditure could be accurately monitored. Subjects received two diets. One was a normal diet, and the other was a low-fat, high-carbohydrate diet that contained virtually no fat and a large amount of carbohydrate. Subjects exercised daily for 10 days, and substrate use was measured during their exercise sessions and during the rest of the day. On the low-fat, high-carbohydrate diet, 24-hour fat oxidation exceeded fat intake; consequently, the subjects were in negative fast balance and in positive carbohydrate balance. Over a 10-day period, body composition would have to change or carbohydrate had to be turned into fat. No changes were observed in body composition after 10 days, which suggested that carbohydrate had been converted to fat. This notion was confirmed with stable isotopes; ^{13}C tracer ingested with carbohydrate was found in fatty acids in adipose tissue and plasma. It was found only in those fats that are the product of de novo lipogenesis. No such changes were observed with the control diet. These data show that even in a situation of energy balance, de novo lipogenesis can occur and that this pathway can become quantitatively important.

The body increases the oxidation rate of carbohydrate and protein immediately when excess amounts are ingested, but fat is different. Generally, fat is not converted into protein or carbohydrate. In addition, when excess amounts of fat are ingested, oxidation rates do not increase immediately, which makes it more likely that fat will be stored in adipose tissue (Abbott et al. 1988; Westerterp 1993).

The macronutrient composition of the diet, therefore, plays an important role in daily energy intake and expenditure (Westerterp et al. 1995). These substrate balances are influenced by a variety of genetic, environmental, cultural, and socioeconomic factors (Flatt 1995). For example, dietary intake is different in different socioeconomic classes. Lower socioeconomic classes typically have a higher fat intake and lower carbohydrate intake than higher socioeconomic classes. There are also cultural differences in diets and in acceptability of exercise. People in some African countries, for example, have a very high carbohydrate intake (>70%), but carbohydrate intake among people in the Western world is typically around 40% to 50%.

A simple example illustrates the importance of substrate balances together with the metabolic inefficiencies and adaptations that limit, to some degree, the consequences of consuming too much dietary energy. Someone who eats 50 g of sugar (e.g., by drinking half a liter of a soft drink) daily in addition to the normal diet is in positive energy balance by approximately 800 kJ/day (191 kcal/day). This level of intake is 292,000 kJ/year (69,789 kcal/year), which over the course of 30 years amounts to 8,760 MJ (2,093,690 kcal). Assuming an energy density of adipose tissue of 19.0 kJ/g (4.5 kcal/g), this person should gain 284 kg (626 lb) in those 30 years. Clearly, this amount of weight gain does not occur; this person would probably gain only a few kilograms. Increased body weight results in an increased metabolic rate and an increased oxidation of energy substrates. Also, some of the energy ingested as carbohydrate is lost in the conversion to fat. These effects limit the amount of fat accumulated and weight gained. The preceding example is a theoretical one; in real life the ingestion of additional foods or drinks will most likely also affect appetite.

Regulation of Appetite

It is well established that the hypothalamic region of the brain plays a key role in the central regulation of eating behavior in humans (figure 15.2). The hypothalamus, in particular the arcuate nucleus, constantly receives and processes neural, metabolic, and endocrine signals from the periphery. This enables it to maintain energy homoeostasis by adjusting energy intake as well as energy expenditure. Peripheral signals are generated mostly by the gastrointestinal tract but also by other organs such as the pancreas and the adipose tissue. In response to feeding, the gastrointestinal tract produces several appetite-regulating hormones, such as cholecystokinin (CCK), glucagon-like peptide-1 (GLP-1), and peptide YY (PYY). Ghrelin, which is produced mostly by the stomach, plays an important role by stimulating appetite. Ghrelin concentrations increase before meals and stimulate the conscious sensation of hunger that makes us want to eat food. After eating meals, ghrelin returns to baseline concentrations. Meal size and composition influence the secretion of these hormones and contribute to the sensation of satiety (feeling full) as the foods consumed are digested and absorbed (see chapter 5). Adiposity signals such as insulin and leptin act in the arcuate nuclei to provide a background tone, and this tone in turn determines the sensitivity of the brain to satiation signals that influence how much food is eaten at any one time. Note that these homeostatic mechanisms provide at most a background influence and only subtly influence intake during any given meal. Social factors, palatability, habits, stress, and many other factors are always at work and influence not only when meals occur but also how much food is consumed. Only when extraneous factors are tightly controlled in laboratory animal experiments or when ingestion is precisely monitored and quantified over periods of days or weeks in free-feeding humans do the effects of these homeostatic signals become apparent. The physiology of appetite will be discussed in the following section, but it is important to keep in mind that although physiological factors contribute to appetite and eating behavior, it is widely accepted that strong social and environmental influences can easily overcome normal physiology.

Feeding Control Circuits and Regulators

To protect the human species from extinction through periods of famine, protective mecha-

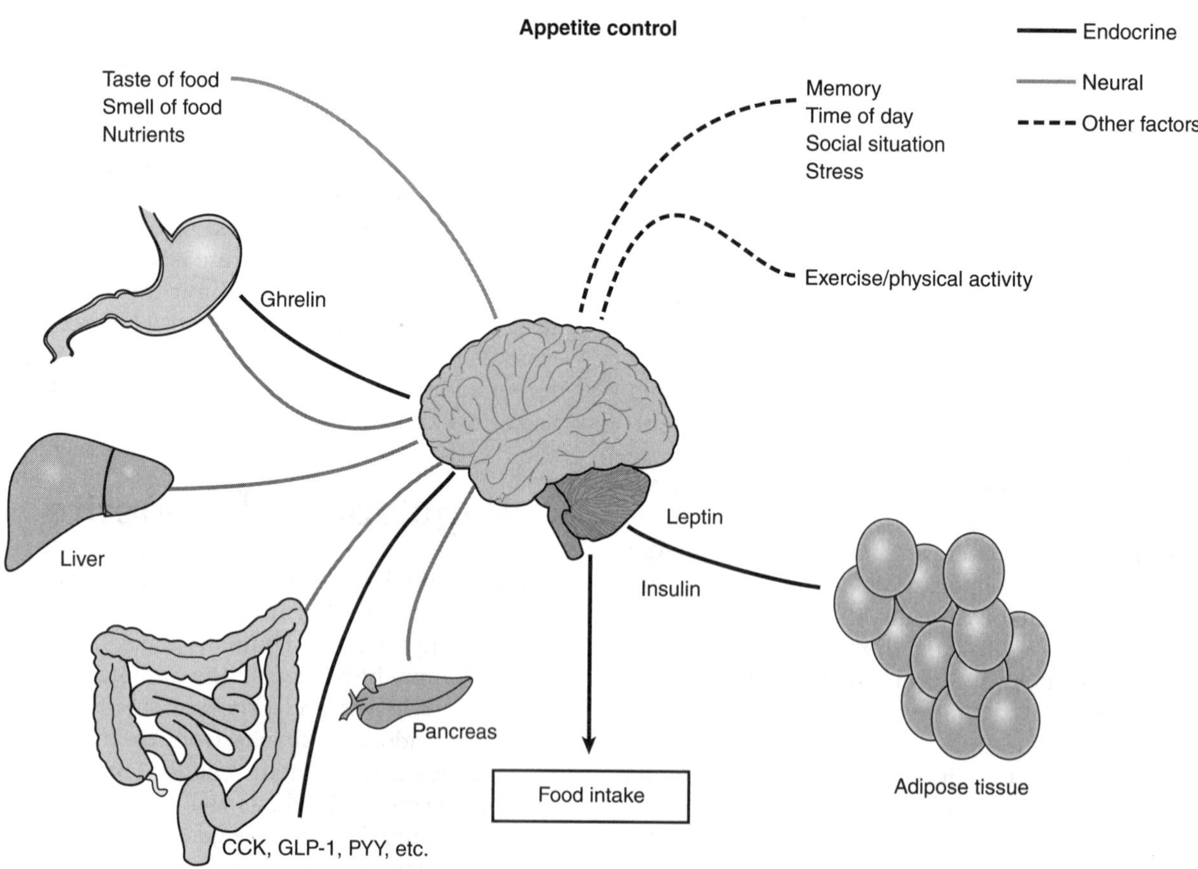

Figure 15.2 Appetite is sensed in the brain. The brain constantly receives and processes neural (gray lines), metabolic, and endocrine (black lines) signals from the periphery. In addition, many other factors (dashed lines) influence the eventual outcome (food intake).

nisms have evolved to resist fat loss and maintain body weight. According to metabolic needs, several homeostatic brain circuits, especially in the hypothalamus and brain stem, regulate feeding behavior by promoting food intake or suppressing appetite in response to peripheral hormonal and neural signals. A summary of these is described in the following sections; see reviews by Wynne et al. (2005) and Perry and Wang (2012) for further details. Feeding behavior is also influenced by the brain's reward systems. The hypothalamus plays a key role in monitoring, processing, and responding to peripheral signals. Ghrelin or appealing, high-calorie foods prompt people to eat. Satiety hormones such as leptin, insulin, and so-called brain–gut peptides can inhibit feeding behavior. Furthermore, cognitive structures involved in this process, such as emotions, can influence human eating behavior.

The main parts of the hypothalamus are the arcuate nucleus (ARC), the paraventricular nucleus, the ventromedial nucleus, the dorsomedial nucleus, and the lateral hypothalamic area, and all of them are involved in energy homeostasis regulation. Peripheral signals contact the brain to regulate energy homoeostasis. Gut hormones in the gastrointestinal tract communicate information and transfer it to regulatory appetite centers based in the brain via the so-called gut–brain axis. There are two means of communication: afferent nerve signaling and blood circulation. The ARC is adjacent to the third ventricle and the median eminence, where there is a thin blood–brain barrier that allows hormones and nutrient signals to directly diffuse into the extracellular fluid. This means that neural regulation and humoral regulation affect the ARC to give it a major role in feeding control circuits.

Vagal afferent fibers can sense the signals of nutrients and transfer them to the brain. Most of the vagal afferent fibers that innervate the viscera and gastrointestinal tract project to brain regions that control food intake through actions on dopamine signaling in motivation- and reward-related areas. The pleasantness of food and the emotional and cognitive aspects of eating behavior are determined in the reward system of the brain. This system is comprised of a number of limbic and cortical areas that communicate with each other and with the hypothalamus predominantly through dopamine, opioid, and endocannabinoid neurotransmission. Highly flavored, energy-dense comfort foods can override normal eating and weight-control mechanisms and generate paradoxically high but ineffective levels of appetite-suppressing hormones.

Brain–Gut Peptides as Feeding Control Regulators

The gastrointestinal tract is the largest endocrine organ in which many kinds of peptides are produced and released and have several distinct effects. External cues contact the central nervous system to control feed and coordinate with the brain's internal signals and transfer messages about the presence and composition of foods in the gut. These gastrointestinal peptides are either orexigenic (appetite promoting) or anorexigenic (appetite suppressing) related to food intake and are called brain–gut peptides. There are two types of brain–gut peptides: (1) short-term signals, which keep in step with each episode of eating; these include ghrelin, CCK, PYY, pancreatic polypeptide, neuropeptide Y, GLP-1, nesfatin-1, oxyntomodulin, glucagon, gastric inhibitory polypeptide (GIP), and amylin, to name a few; and (2) long-term signals, which reflect the metabolic state of adipose tissue, such as insulin and leptin. The short- and long-term signals interact with each other to determine eating behavior.

Short-Term Signals

Ghrelin is mostly secreted into the bloodstream by the stomach and exerts its orexigenic effect via the growth hormone secretagogue receptor, located in the hypothalamic ventromedial nucleus and ARC nucleus, to increase food intake. During fasting, the plasma concentration of ghrelin increases, and after eating, it falls to stimulate hunger. Currently, ghrelin is the only known gut hormone with orexigenic effects. The plasma level of ghrelin is mainly regulated by nutrients but not water. Ghrelin has been shown to stimulate appetite and promote food intake and may facilitate weight gain. Circulating levels of ghrelin follow a cyclical pattern, increasing before meals and decreasing shortly thereafter. The postprandial reduction is influenced by the relative proportion of macronutrients in a meal; there is a greater decrease after protein and carbohydrate ingestion than after fat ingestion. Ghrelin is also produced in the hypothalamus, where it acts as a neurotransmitter to adjust appetite. Ghrelin may also influence the reward system in the brain, in which the emotional wanting or reward value for highly desirable foods is increased.

CCK was the first gut hormone discovered to affect feeding and appetite. CCK is secreted from cells predominantly located in the wall of the proximal small intestine, mainly in response to fatty acids. Plasma CCK levels increase within 15 minutes after a meal, but its half-life in the circulation is only a few minutes. The vagal nerve and the hypothalamus express CCK receptors that can lead to early meal termination and reduce food intake when CCK binds to them.

Several pancreatic peptide (PP)-fold peptides, which share a PP-fold (hairpin-like fold) in their polypeptide chain structure, including neuropeptide Y, pancreatic polypeptide, and PYY, are secreted following feeding and act to inhibit appetite and eating. Pancreatic polypeptide is released from the pancreas in proportion to the number of ingested calories and acts via the brain stem and hypothalamus as an appetite suppressant. PYY is secreted in proportion to nutrients (particularly fat) ingested but is not affected by gastric distension. Parts of the hindbrain can produce GLP-1, and it is released in proportion to the number of calories ingested. Carbohydrate and fat stimulate GLP-1 secretion. GLP-1 activates neurons in the hypothalamus, which leads to satiety and reduced hunger.

Long-Term Signals

The long-term signals of feeding regulators are leptin and insulin. The release of leptin from adipose tissue is proportional to body-fat content. Leptin acts directly on the feeding control centers in the brain to reduce food intake and increase energy expenditure. It therefore plays a role in preventing obesity by inhibiting appetite. A lack of leptin or a leptin-receptor dysfunction may lead to overeating and obesity. Insulin, which is secreted from the pancreatic islets into the circulation in response to an increase in the blood glucose concentration also acts to inhibit appetite via its actions on the hypothalamic nuclei.

MACRONUTRIENTS AND SATIETY

The term *satiety* refers to the inhibition of eating following a meal, and it is measured by the interval between meals and by the amount consumed at the next meal. Different macronutrients have different effects on satiety. It has been demonstrated that protein has a much stronger effect on satiety than fat and carbohydrate do. The effects of very high-protein diets on satiety and weight loss will be discussed later in the chapter.

Nutrients as Feeding Control Regulators

Nutrients can also transfer satiating signals to the hypothalamus. Specific receptors or transporters sense the signals from macronutrients. These receptors are mostly located in the enteroendocrine cells in the intestinal epithelium and can trigger the release of gastrointestinal regulatory peptides, such as CCK, ghrelin, PYY, GLP-1, and others. Increased levels of blood glucose can also be detected by the brain and reduce sensations of hunger. Receptors in the small intestine can sense the presence of nonesterified fatty acids in a length-dependent manner. After digestion, proteins are degraded to amino acids and small peptides. The latter are detected by μ-opioid receptors in the neurons of the portal vein walls, which are known to influence food intake at the brain level through signals sent via vagal and ascending spinal nerves. The relatively larger increase in plasma amino acid concentrations after ingestion of specific proteins (e.g., whey versus casein) appears to have a greater stimulatory effect on gastrointestinal hormones, such as CCK and GLP-1, and these effects probably account for the greater satiety after ingesting protein compared with carbohydrate and fat. It is also worth remembering that eating food slowly will allow more time for nutrients to be digested and absorbed and for the satiety signals to kick in, which means that you may eat smaller portions or no longer want dessert after your main meal.

The products of macronutrient digestion and their circulating metabolites are known to act as signals to stimulate and initiate eating that thereby determine eating frequency, signals to stop eating and thereby control meal size, and signals that activate brain reward systems that may, to some degree, dysregulate healthy eating. Over time, various diets have been proposed to accentuate or minimize each macronutrient to achieve a desired effect on appetite or energy intake; however, none has been widely successful. This is likely due to their failure to adequately address effects on eating frequency and meal size concurrently and their failure to address that eating behavior is strongly influenced by many cognitive and environmental factors in addition to sensory appeal, appetite, metabolic, endocrine, and neural signals that arise as a result of food intake, digestion, and metabolism. There may be health, training adaptation, or sport performance reasons to emphasize one macronutrient over another in a diet, but from the perspective of energy balance, total energy intake, rather than its source, is the most important factor to address.

SOCIAL AND BEHAVIORAL INFLUENCES ON EATING BEHAVIOR

Eating behavior is crucial to the maintenance of body weight, and this behavior is easily influenced by an athlete's lifestyle. Many sports have a specific eating culture, and in some sports, athletes are often exposed to foods in a cafeteria setting where limited choices may be available (e.g., pizza, fried fish, burgers, and French fries may be offered but no salad or lean grilled meat). In some sports, alcohol consumption is part of the culture (as a team-bonding experience), and the often-excessive consumption of alcohol can have dramatic effects on body weight and composition. Some sports are characterized by pressure to achieve a particular low body weight or low body fat percentage, and striving to reach that goal can result in disordered eating (see chapter 16).

Effect of Exercise on Appetite

Appetite and postexercise energy intake depend on many factors, including the intensity, duration, and mode of exercise. Studies by King, Burley, and Blundell (1994) showed that high-intensity exercise suppressed appetite for a short period, but no difference in food intake occurred when measured over 2 days. Hunger is suppressed only when the exercise is long enough (60 minutes or more) and intense enough (more than 70% $\dot{V}O_2$max). Few studies have investigated the effects of mode of exercise on appetite. Blundell et al. (1995) compared treadmill exercise with cycling and did not observe a difference in appetite. Although anecdotal evidence indicates that swimming increases appetite more than other activities do, no scientific evidence backs this up. One study compared cycling submerged in cold (20 °C [68 °F]) water to cycling in neutral-temperature (33 °C [91 °F]) water and observed an increased appetite in the cold conditions, thereby suggesting an effect of water temperature and consequently skin or body temperature on feelings of hunger.

Evidence suggests that in the short to medium term (up to 16 days), exercise is able to produce a negative energy balance with no substantial compensatory responses in energy intake. In the long term (more than 16 days), however, an increase in energy intake is likely to be observed. This compensation is usually partial and incomplete and generally accounts for only 30% of the energy cost associated with exercise, therefore allowing the attainment of a negative energy balance and some degree of weight loss (Blundell et al. 2003). In the short term, exercise may in fact be more effective than dieting in producing a negative energy balance. This notion is supported by the finding that an acute energy deficit created by dietary restriction (low-energy versus high-energy breakfast) induced a significant increase in subjective hunger, subsequent energy intake, and food cravings during the day. On the other hand, a similar energy deficit created by exercise failed to induce any significant change in these variables, thereby allowing the attainment of a short-term negative energy balance (Hubert, King, and Blundell 1998). It is becoming recognized that the major influences on the expression of appetite arise not only from changes in the episodic secretion of gut peptides, including ghrelin, CCK, and GLP-1 and other hormones such as insulin, but also from long-term influences of peptides, such as leptin, and other factors, including FFM, FM, and RMR. It is also clear that exercise can influence all of these factors, which influences the drive to eat through the modulation of hunger and adjustments in postprandial satiety via an interaction with food composition (Blundell et al. 2015). The effect of exercise on each of the aforementioned factors will vary in strength from person to person and with the intensity and duration of exercise. Therefore, individual appetite responses to exercise will be highly variable and difficult to predict.

Physical Activity and Energy Expenditure

Resting metabolic rate is an important component of daily energy expenditure. It has been suggested that exercise can increase RMR and thereby increase energy expenditure during the rest of the day. The increase in RMR postexercise is often measured as postexercise oxygen consumption (EPOC) (Borsheim and Bahr. 2003). It is well established that immediately after exercise, EPOC may be elevated, although this may only occur if the exercise is long enough (at least 30 minutes) and vigorous enough (at least equivalent to 60% of aerobic capacity). The longer and more intense the exercise, the greater the total EPOC. Even if the exercise meets these criteria, the postexercise increase in RMR seems only temporary and relatively small. After several hours, RMR will return to baseline values. Suggestions that RMR is chronically increased have been refuted, and although some studies have reported an increased RMR, several other studies have even observed a decrease in RMR after training.

Exercise training, and especially aerobic exercise training, results in a shift from carbohydrate to fat metabolism Increased mitochondrial density and increased capillarization of the muscle ensure an increase in the supply of substrates and oxygen to the muscle and in the capacity to take up oxygen and substrates. Studies have consistently observed a decreased reliance on carbohydrate as a fuel and an increased capacity to oxidize fat in response to as little as 4 weeks of exercise training. This increased ability to oxidize fat may help to reduce fat mass in a situation of energy restriction.

Dietary Weight-Loss Methods

Methods for losing body weight include pharmacological and surgical procedures as well as diet and exercise methods (see the sidebar), but here we focus only on the weight-loss strategies that involve diet, exercise, or a combination of the two. Several different diets exist, some of which have been commercialized. Some diets are effective, whereas others are a list of erroneous assumptions and claims. For the athlete, distinguishing between the facts and the fallacies is often difficult. This section reviews some of the most common dietary regimens and weight-loss methods.

Energy Restriction and Reduced Fat Intake

It is important to appreciate that some food calories are not the same as others. Different food sources are metabolized via different pathways in the body and the energy cost of this metabolism is higher for some foods than for others. Further-

METHODS TO ACHIEVE WEIGHT LOSS

Dietary Methods

- Fasting
- Energy restriction
- Low-fat diet
- High-protein diet
- High-carbohydrate diet
- Low-carbohydrate diet (e.g., Atkins, Sugar Busters)
- Ketogenic diet
- Zone diet
- Food-combining diet
- Low glycemic index diet
- Low-energy density diet
- Consumption of calcium and dairy products

Exercise

- Increased physical activity
- Regular exercise
- Endurance exercise
- High-intensity interval exercise

Surgical Procedures

- Stomach stapling
- Removal of a section of the small intestine
- Liposuction

Pharmacological Methods

- Stimulants
- Appetite suppressants
- Drugs that reduce fat absorption

more, calories from different food sources can have markedly different effects on hunger, hormones, and the brain regions that control food intake. In this sense, not all calories from food are equal (see the sidebar). Even though calories are important, in many cases, simple changes in food selection can lead to the same (or better) results for weight loss than calorie restriction.

Debate continues over whether weight loss can be achieved by reducing energy intake or by reducing only fat intake. For reducing body weight, epidemiological evidence suggests that reducing the percentage of fat in the diet is more effective than reducing the absolute amount of fat (Sheppard, Kristal, and Kushi 1991). The most important factor, however, is the reduction in energy intake. Although energy restriction and low-fat eating result in weight loss, energy restriction usually results in a larger reduction in energy intake than ad libitum (as desired) low-fat eating does. Therefore, energy restriction may initially result in a larger weight loss, although studies show that both diets are effective over the long term (Jeffery et al. 1995; Schlundt et al. 1993).

The advantage of reduced fat intake is that relatively high carbohydrate content can be maintained, which results in reasonable glycogen stores and better recovery. Many athletes adopt low-fat diets with a small reduction in energy intake so they can still replenish their carbohydrate stores. This type of diet seems to be a sensible way of reducing weight, although suboptimal carbohydrate intake can still interfere with normal training. Thus, weight reduction should occur slowly and in the off-season.

Metabolic adaptation or adaptive thermogenesis occurs in response to reduced energy intake, which results in a decrease in resting metabolic rate (i.e., energy expenditure). Moreover, any lean body mass that is lost over time will further lower resting energy expenditure. The commonly observed failure to lose more weight as diets progress over time is explained by these adaptations (Weck, Bornstein, and Blüher 2012). However, the question of whether the magnitude of the reduced resting energy expenditure is actually sufficiently large to exceed the original calorie deficit prescribed for weight loss remains controversial (Westertep 2013). In summary, during periods of caloric restriction, the commonly quoted equivalency of a loss of 0.46 kg (1 lb) of fat from a 15 MJ (3,585 kcal) dietary deficit no longer holds to the extent that energy intake, expenditure, and body weight are interrelated. Nonetheless, this remains a useful approximation with the proviso that the discrepancy represents metabolic adaptation (Howell and Kones 2017).

Very Low-Energy Diets

Very low-energy diets (VLEDs) or very low-calorie diets (VLCDs) are used to achieve rapid weight loss in people who are obese. These diets tend to consist mostly of liquid meals that contain the recommended daily intakes of micronutrients but only 1,600 to 3,200 kJ/day (400-800 kcal/day). These liquid meals contain relatively large amounts of protein to reduce muscle wasting and relatively small amounts of carbohydrate (less than 100 g/day). Such diets are extremely effective in rapidly reducing body weight. In the first week, the weight loss is predominantly glycogen and water. Fat and protein are also lost during the initial phase, but those losses are a relatively small proportion of the total weight loss. After the initial rapid weight loss, the weight reduction is mainly from adipose tissue, although some loss of body protein occurs. The increased fat oxidation results in ketosis (formation of ketone bodies, acetoacetate, and β-hydroxybutyrate).

Because carbohydrate intake is low, blood glucose concentration is maintained by gluconeogenesis from various precursors (glycerol and alanine). Although increased physical activity is also encouraged when very low-energy diets are prescribed, the diets are effective without the exercise component. Because of the associated chronic glycogen depletion, exercise capacity is severely impaired. For this reason, such diets are not advised for athletes, who would likely be unable to complete their normal training sessions. Even in the off-season, such diets are not advised because the loss of body protein can be significant. Side effects of these diets include nausea, halitosis (bad breath), hunger (which may decrease after the initiation of ketosis), light-headedness, and hypotension. Dehydration is also common with such diets, and electrolyte imbalances may occur.

Intermittent-Fasting Diets

Intermittent-fasting diets (IFDs), of which there are several, have become popular in recent years partly due to media coverage and backing from celebrities. There is reasonable evidence that they can be effective because they reduce weekly energy intake to some degree. They may not be quite as beneficial for women as they are for men, and they may also be a poor choice for people who are prone to eating disorders. People should eat healthy foods while following these diets.

A CALORIE IS A CALORIE, BUT....

Strictly speaking, a calorie is, of course, a calorie. The first law of thermodynamics states that energy can neither be created nor destroyed but only transformed. Thus the human body is constantly transforming energy, in this case calories, by combusting foodstuff to produce heat and metabolic processes. Of course, no matter what the food source, one dietary kilocalorie (or Calorie with a capital C) contains 4,184 Joules of energy and represents the amount of energy needed to raise the temperature of one liter of water by 1 °C. While it is true that in absolute terms all calories have the same amount of energy, when it comes to your body, things are not that simple.

The human body is a highly complex biochemical system with elaborate processes that regulate energy balance. Different foods go through different biochemical pathways such as digestion, absorption, and metabolism, including the biosynthesis of macromolecules (e.g., glycogen from glucose, protein from amino acids), and these have different energy costs. Some are more inefficient than others and cause some of the energy from food to be lost as heat.

Furthermore, different foods and macronutrients have a major effect on the hormones and brain centers that control our hunger and eating behavior and can affect the biological processes that govern when, what, and how much we eat. The following are five evidence-based examples of why a calorie is not simply a calorie:

1. *The metabolic pathways for protein are less efficient than the metabolic pathways for carbohydrate and fat.* Protein contains 17 kJ/g (4 kcal/g), but a large portion of the protein calories are lost as heat when it is metabolized. The thermic effect of food (see chapter 4) is a measure of how much different foods increase energy expenditure due to the energy required to digest, absorb, and metabolize the nutrients. The thermic effect of fat is 1% to 3% and for carbohydrate it is 5% to 10%, but for protein it is 20% to 30% (Tappy 1996). The relatively strong thermic effect of protein may be mediated by the high ATP costs of postprandial protein synthesis. Protein thus requires more energy to metabolize than fat and carbohydrate. This means that 418 kJ (100 kcal) of dietary protein would end up as 293 to 335 kJ (70-80 kcal) of stored energy, but a 418 kJ (100 kcal) of fat would end up as 406 to 414 kJ (97 to 99 kcal) of stored energy. Therefore, calories from protein may be less fattening (i.e., they cause less weight gain) than calories from carbohydrate and fat because protein takes more energy to metabolize. Whole foods also require more energy to digest than processed foods.

2. *Protein reduces appetite more effectively, which results in reduced energy intake.* Studies show that protein is the most fulfilling macronutrient by far. Increasing dietary protein intake

One IFD involves fasting every other day. Some versions of this diet allow up to 500 calories on the fasting days. A full fast every other day seems rather extreme and could lead to insufficient protein intake with negative consequences for muscle mass, so it is not recommended for athletes. A less extreme version of this IFD diet is the 5:2 diet (also known as the Fast Diet), which was popularized by TV medic Dr. Michael Mosley (Mosley and Spencer 2014). This diet involves eating normally 5 days of the week and restricting calories to 500 for women or 600 for men on 2 days of the week (usually these are separated by 2 to 3 days; e.g., fasting on Mondays and Thursdays). On the restricted-calorie days, the suggestion is to eat two small, high-protein meals (for better satiety and to maintain muscle mass).

Another IFD involves 24-hour fasts (that begin with the evening meal) two days of the week. The evening meal before the fast should be the same size as usual; in addition, eating slowly and having a high-protein meal will help with satiety. Another simple IFD is to skip one meal (usually lunch) during the day. This is suitable for athletes who do morning and afternoon training sessions and want to do the second session of the day in a

as a percentage of the total daily energy intake (i.e., substitute some fat and carbohydrate for extra protein) results in weight loss without counting calories.

3. *Different simple sugars are metabolized differently and have different effects on appetite.* The two main simple sugars in the diet are glucose and fructose. Although they have the same chemical formula ($C_6H_{12}O_6$), glucose can be metabolized by all of the body's tissues, but fructose can only be metabolized by the liver in any significant amount. Following feeding, fructose does not reduce levels of the appetite-stimulating hormone ghrelin as much as glucose, which means there is a tendency to want to eat more calories with fructose. Furthermore, fructose does not stimulate the satiety centers in the brain the same way glucose does, which leads to reduced satiety.

4. *Studies show that refined carbohydrates lead to faster and bigger spikes in blood sugar, which lead to cravings and increased food intake.* Refined carbohydrates have a high glycemic index, tend to be low in fiber, and get digested and absorbed quickly, which leads to more rapid and larger spikes in blood glucose. Within 1 to 2 hours of eating a food that causes a rapid spike in blood sugar, blood sugar levels fall below normal (see chapter 6). When blood sugar levels drop, this stimulates the appetite center in the brain and results in cravings for additional high-carbohydrate snacks. Studies show that people eat up to 80% more calories when given ad libitum access to a high glycemic index meal compared with a low one.

5. *Different foods have different effects on satiety.* Some foods affect satiety more than others, and this affects how many calories are consumed in subsequent meals. The satiety index is a measure of the ability of foods to reduce hunger, increase feelings of fullness, and reduce energy intake in the hours after a meal. If you eat foods that are low on the satiety index, then you will be hungrier and end up eating more. If you choose foods that are high on the satiety index, you will end up eating less and losing weight. Some examples of foods with a high satiety index are meat, eggs, boiled potatoes, beans, and fruits, and foods that are low on the satiety index include doughnuts, cookies, and cake.

The takeaway message is that calories from different food sources can have markedly different effects on hunger, hormones, energy expenditure, and the brain regions that control food intake. Even though calories are important, in many cases simple changes in food selection can lead to the same (or slightly better) results for weight loss than limited calorie restriction. However, there is no escaping the fact that significant weight loss (i.e., more than a few kilograms) can only be achieved by more substantial reductions in energy intake and can be further improved with increased energy expenditure.

glycogen-depleted state to improve training adaptation (as discussed in chapter 12). Another IFD, the Warrior Diet, was popularized by ex-army fitness expert Ori Hofmekler and involves eating small amounts of raw fruits and vegetables during the day and then eating one large meal in the evening. The diet also emphasizes food choices (whole, unprocessed foods) that are quite similar to a Paleo diet, which encourages the consumption of anything that could be hunted or gathered in the Paleolithic era (also known as the Stone Age), including foods like meats, fish, nuts, leafy greens, regional vegetables, and seeds, and the avoidance of processed foods such as ready meals, pasta, bread, cereal, and candy.

The largest evidence base for the efficacy of IFDs comes from studies that have used some of the more extreme forms, such as alternate-day fasting (Johnstone 2007). According to one review (Barnosky et al. 2014), IFDs can lead to 3% to 8% body-weight loss over a period of 3 to 24 weeks. With alternate-day fasting, the rate of weight loss averages about 0.75 kg/week (1.65 lb/week); with other IFDs the rate of weight loss is less at about 0.25 kg/week (0.55 lb/week) (Johnstone 2007).Studies comparing intermittent fasting and continuous calorie restriction show no difference in weight loss if calories are matched between groups (Barnosky et al. 2014). It is difficult to combine these diets with quality training and thus they are not recommended for the majority of athletes.

Low-Fat Diets

Reducing dietary fat intake can be an effective way to reduce energy intake and promote weight loss for the following reasons:

- Fat is energy dense. It has more than twice the amount of energy as the same weight of carbohydrate or protein.
- High-fat foods generally taste good, which leads to a tendency to eat more. Studies show that increasing the fat content of the diet increases the spontaneous intake of food.
- A large body of evidence has shown that fat is less satiating than protein or carbohydrate (de Castro 1987; de Castro and Elmore 1988).
- Fat is stored efficiently and requires little energy for digestion.
- Fat intake does not immediately increase fat oxidation.

Reducing dietary fat is best achieved by cutting out foods with high fat contents, such as fatty meats, sauces, cheese, creams, pizza, cakes, and cookies and substituting some foods or beverages with lower-fat alternatives (e.g., skim milk, low-fat yogurt, reduced-fat coleslaw). Body-weight and body-fat losses on a low-fat diet will largely depend on by how much daily energy intake is reduced. See the section on low-carbohydrate diets for a comparison of the efficacy of these with low-fat diets for weight loss.

Food-Combining Diets

Food-combining diets are based on a philosophy that certain foods should not be combined. Although many types of food-combining diets exist, most warn against the combination of protein and carbohydrate foods. Such combinations supposedly cause a buildup of toxins that have negative side effects, such as weight gain. These diets are often tempting because they promise easy, rapid weight loss, and they have worked for many people. When these diets are strictly followed, energy and fat intake are likely to be reduced compared with the normal diet. These reductions in energy and fat, rather than the fact that certain foods were not combined, lead to weight loss. Because energy and carbohydrate intakes are lower, glycogen stores decrease and performance and recovery may be impaired.

High-Protein Diets

Protein provides about 10% to 15% of the calories in most diets; with a high-protein diet, however, this is increases to about 30%. Recommendations for increased protein consumption are among the most common approaches of popular or fad diets. Some have argued that high-protein diets suppress the appetite, which might be a mechanism for facilitated weight loss. Protein also has a larger thermic effect and a relatively low coefficient of digestibility compared with a mixed, equicaloric (isoenergetic) meal. Several studies have demonstrated that increased protein content of the diet, particularly in combination with exercise training, may improve weight loss and reduce the loss of lean body mass in overweight and obese people during low-energy dieting (for a review, see Layman and Walker 2006). Furthermore, less weight is regained after the energy-restricted period ends when protein intake is high compared with more normal dietary compositions (Paddon-Jones et al. 2008).

Part of the effect of protein is visible only in free-living conditions when energy intake is not controlled. This circumstance points to an effect of protein on satiety. On an isoenergetic, high-protein (30% protein, 20% fat, 50% carbohydrate) diet, satiety was increased compared with a normal weight-maintaining diet (15% protein, 35% fat, 50% carbohydrate). When subjects were on an ad libitum high-protein diet for 12 weeks, their mean spontaneous daily energy intake decreased by 1,845 kJ (441 kcal) and they lost, on average, 4.9 kg (10.8 lb) of body weight and had a mean decrease in fat mass of 3.7 kg (8.2 lb) (Weigle et al. 2005). As protein has a greater effect on satiety than the other macronutrients, it can be helpful in a weight-loss situation. Note that increasing the proportion of protein in the diet also permits a simultaneous reduction in the proportion of fat.

As mentioned previously, protein has a higher thermogenic effect than carbohydrate or fat. In one study, increasing the amount of dietary protein from 10% to 20% of total energy intake resulted in a 63% to 95% increase in protein oxidation depending on the protein source (Pannemans et al. 1998). For example, Mikkelsen, Toubro, and Astrup (2000) observed a higher diet-induced thermogenesis with pork meat than with soy protein.

Another possible mechanism through which protein may aid weight loss is maintaining muscle mass in an energy-restricted situation. Little evidence is available, but it seems that protein is able to prevent some of the muscle mass loss that is inevitable with energy restriction. This means that a larger muscle mass can be maintained, and because muscle is the most metabolically active tissue, RMR could increase, thus helping weight loss.

Most studies on the effectiveness of high protein diets for weight loss have been conducted in nonathletes and inactive populations, including elderly and obese subjects. The relevance of these findings for athletes in training is questionable. The few studies in athletes seem to provide conflicting data on the effect of increased protein intake during weight loss. One study using nitrogen balance supports the idea that increased protein intake preserves muscle during low-calorie dieting in bodybuilders (Walberg et al. 1988). A more recent study, however, found no effect of increased protein or BCAA intake on lean body mass loss during weight loss in athletes (Mourier et al. 1997). Overall, evidence is accumulating that the protein content of a diet can be an important tool in weight management.

PROTEIN IN WEIGHT LOSS AND MAINTENANCE

Protein may be an effective and healthy means of supporting weight loss and maintenance for the following reasons:

1. Protein has a greater effect on satiety than carbohydrate or fat does.
2. Protein has a greater thermogenic effect than carbohydrate or fat does.
3. Protein may have a role in maintaining muscle mass in a situation of energy restriction, thereby preserving metabolically active tissue.
4. High-protein diets are associated with lower levels of ghrelin (the hunger hormone).
5. Protein supports gluconeogenesis and reduces plasma triacylglycerol concentrations.

The Zone Diet

The Zone diet was proposed by Barry Sears in his book *The Zone: A Dietary Road Map* (Sears 1995). The diet opposes the traditional recommendations of a high-carbohydrate, low-fat diet for athletes. By reducing carbohydrate intake, insulin response decreases and a favorable insulin-to-glucagon ratio is established. The benefits are increased lipolysis and improved regulation of eicosanoids, which are hormone-like derivatives of FAs in the body that act as cell-to-cell signaling molecules. The diet increases the "good" eicosanoids and decreases the "bad" eicosanoids.

The good eicosanoids improve blood flow to the working muscle and enhance the delivery of oxygen and nutrients, which eventually results in improved performance. To enter the zone, the diet should consist of 40% carbohydrate, 30% fat, and 30% protein divided into a regimen of three meals and two snacks per day. The diet is also referred to as the 40:30:30 diet.

Although some arguments by Sears are scientifically sound, the book has problems, pitfalls, and errors in assumptions, and it contains some contradictory information. Many of the promised benefits of the Zone diet are based on selective information about hormonal influences on eicosanoid metabolism. Opposing evidence is conveniently left out.

Eicosanoid metabolism is extremely complex and highly unpredictable, and previous diet manipulation studies have been unsuccessful in stimulating the synthesis of good eicosanoids relative to bad eicosanoids. Very small changes in insulin concentration are sufficient to reduce lipolysis significantly, and such effects persist for up to 6 hours after a meal. To avoid reductions in lipolysis after a meal, carbohydrate intake must be extremely low (even less than that proposed by the Zone diet). Meals with the 40:30:30 combination are difficult to compose unless the dieter buys the energy bars marketed by Sears.

Nevertheless, the Zone diet seems to work for some people, and anecdotal evidence indicates weight loss with the diet. The successes are expected because the Zone diet is low in energy (4,200-8,400 kJ/day [1,000-2,000 kcal/day]). Even for athletes who train hard, the energy intake does not increase much and they are in a relatively large energy deficit.

The principle of vasodilating muscle arterioles by altering eicosanoid production is correct in theory, but the little evidence available from human studies does not support any significant contribution of eicosanoids to active muscle vasodilation. In fact, the key eicosanoid reportedly produced in the Zone diet and responsible for improved muscle oxygenation is not found in skeletal muscle. The best available scientific evidence suggests that the Zone diet is more ergolytic than ergogenic to performance.

Low-Carbohydrate Diets

Some of the best-known low-carbohydrate diets are the Atkins diet (Atkins 1992) and Sugar Busters (Andrews et al. 1998). These diets are based on the premise that reducing carbohydrate intake results in increased fat oxidation. When the more extreme forms of the diets are used, in which carbohydrate intake is restricted to less than 20 g/day, ketone body production will increase (just as it does with fasting), which may suppress appetite. Ketones may also be present in urine, which could result in loss of calories through urine. Although all of the preceding may be true, the losses achieved in this diet are extremely small. The excretion of ketone bodies in urine is small, at most 400 to 600 kJ/day (95 to 143 kcal/day). These diets can be effective, but they are no more effective than a well-balanced, energy-restricted diet. Although these diets may provide better satiety than high-carbohydrate diets, most of the effect can be attributed to the relatively high protein content. For athletes, these very low-carbohydrate or ketogenic diets are likely detrimental because of reduced glycogen stores and exercise capacity (as discussed in chapter 7).

The main premise of the Atkins diet is that severe restriction of carbohydrate confers a substantial metabolic advantage that allows large amounts of fat to be consumed without significant weight gain. The low carbohydrate intake reduces circulating insulin levels, which promote lipolysis and fat oxidation and increases energy expenditure (to claimed amounts in the range of 1,673-2,510 kJ/day [400-600 kcal/day]) and should therefore result in body-fat loss over time. This has become known as the carbohydrate–insulin hypothesis, and two well-controlled studies (Hall et al. 2015, 2016) have rigorously investigated it. The essential findings were that the premises of decreased insulin secretion and increased fat oxidation were verified, but the premise that increased energy expenditure and body-fat loss would result from this was not. In fact, both studies reported less body-fat loss with low-carbohydrate diets than with isocaloric diets when protein intake was equated.

Some scientists believe that low-carbohydrate, high-fat diets have some beneficial effects for health because studies show that these diets improve several markers of cardiovascular risk, including lowering elevated blood glucose, insulin, triglyceride, and LDL cholesterol concentrations, while increasing HDL cholesterol concentration and reducing blood pressure and body weight (Noakes and Windt 2017). A meta-analysis of the efficacy of currently popular diets (without specific energy intake targets) for reducing body weight in overweight adults concluded that the Atkins diet had been tested in the greatest number of clinical trials and had the most evidence in producing meaningful long-term weight loss (Anton et al. 2017); however, this review used only body-weight loss as the outcome measure and did not consider the effects of the diet on body composition. Another comprehensive systematic review and meta-analysis (Hall and Guo 2017) does not support the use of low-carbohydrate diets for body-fat loss. The meta-analysis included 32 controlled feeding studies ($n = 562$) with isocaloric substitution of dietary carbohydrate for fat but with equal dietary protein content. As the proportion of dietary carbohydrate to fat changed, daily energy expenditure and body-fat changes were recorded, which allowed a direct comparison of the efficacy of low-fat and low-carbohydrate diets across a wide range of study conditions. The main findings were that the pooled weighted mean difference in energy expenditure was 109 kJ/day (26 kcal/day) higher with the lower fat diets, and the rate of body-fat loss was 16 g/day greater with lower fat diets. In fact, only three of the studies showed an improvement in body-fat loss with the low-carbohydrate diet, and the overwhelming majority showed greater body-fat loss with the low-fat diet. These results do not support the carbohydrate–insulin hypothesis and refute any so-called metabolic advantage conferred by low-carbohydrate diets.

In their review of the effects of high-fat, low-carbohydrate or low-fat, high-carbohydrate diets on weight loss, Howell and Kones (2017) concluded that weight changes are not primarily determined by varying proportions of carbohydrate and fat in the diet but instead by the number of calories ingested. Changes in energy expenditure, which metabolic pathways are used, and other considerations are quite modest when compared with actual caloric intake. Table 15.1 provides a summary of expected body-fat losses on different diets.

TABLE 15.1 A Summary of The Efficacy of Different Diets for Body-Fat Loss in Slightly Overweight Adults

Diet	What it involves	Weekly energy deficit	Weekly body-fat loss
Very low energy	3.4 MJ (800 kcal) liquid meals high in protein	49.8 MJ (11,900 kcal)	1.3 kg (2.9 lb)
Alternate-day fast	Fast completely every other day	36.6 MJ (8,750 kcal)	1.0 kg (2.2 lb)
5:2	2.1 MJ (500 kcal) intake on 2 days/week	16.7 MJ (4,000 kcal)	0.4 kg (0.9 lb)
Skip lunch	No lunch (2.1 MJ [500 kcal]) 3 days/week	6.3 MJ (1,500 kcal)	0.15 kg (0.33 lb)
Low carbohydrate (Atkins)	8.4 MJ/day (2,000 kcal/day) with <20 g carbohydrate daily in first 2 weeks, up to 50 g/day thereafter	14.7 MJ (3,500 kcal)	0.4 kg (0.9 lb)
Zone	6.3 MJ/day (1,500 kcal/day) with 40% carbohydrate, 30% fat, and 30% protein	29.3 MJ (7,000 kcal)	0.7 kg (1.5 lb)
Low fat	8.4 MJ/day (2,000 kcal/day) with <10% fat	14.7 MJ (3,500 kcal)	0.4 kg (0.9 lb)
High protein	8.4 MJ/day (2,000 kcal/day) with 30% protein	17.6 MJ (4,200 kcal)	0.5 kg (1.1 lb)

Assumes (1) normal energy intake is 10.5 MJ/day (2,500 kcal/day) with 15% coming from protein, (2) some diets will reduce appetite compared with normal due to higher protein or lower energy density, (3) body-fat losses are average weekly losses over a 10-week period on each diet, and (4) approximately 0.46 kg (1.01 lb) of body fat is lost for each 14.7 MJ (3,500 kcal) energy intake deficit in first 5 weeks and 0.30 kg (0.66 lb) is lost for each 14.7 MJ (3,500 kcal) energy intake deficit thereafter (accounting for metabolic adaptation to energy restriction). Note that body-weight losses will be higher than the body-fat losses shown here because some diets will also cause some loss of body water, glycogen, and lean tissue.

Manipulation of Energy Density

The **energy density** of a diet may play an important role in weight maintenance. A small quantity of food that is rich in fat has a very high energy content; therefore, visual cues may not prevent a large intake of energy on a high-fat diet. A number of studies have shown that subjects tend to eat a similar weight of food regardless of the macronutrient composition (Stubbs et al. 1995a, 1995b, 1996). Because a 500 g (18 oz) meal that consists mainly of carbohydrate will contain significantly less energy than a 500 g high-fat meal, lower energy intake will automatically result.

In an elegant series of studies, Stubbs and colleagues (Stubbs, Habron, et al. 1995; Stubbs, Ritz, et al. 1995; Stubbs, Harbron, and Prentice 1996) demonstrated that when subjects received a diet that contained 20%, 40%, or 60% fat and could eat ad libitum, the weight of the food that they consumed was the same. Because of differences in energy density, however, the total amount of energy consumed with the higher-fat diets was greater and therefore weight gain was greater. This result happened in both controlled laboratory conditions and free-living conditions. When the fat content of the diet was altered but the energy density was kept the same, the subjects still consumed the same weight of food, but this time the energy intake was the same, independent of the fat content of the diet. Figure 15.3 summarizes the results of these studies. Figure 15.3*a* shows the effects of ad libitum energy intake and figure 15.3*b* shows the weight of food consumed in subjects who consumed diets that had 20%, 40%, and 60% of energy from fat. The left column in each panel represents the findings in carefully controlled conditions in which the subjects lived in a laboratory calorimeter, and the middle column represents free-living conditions. In these two projects, the energy density (ED) between diets was different. In the third study (right column), also in

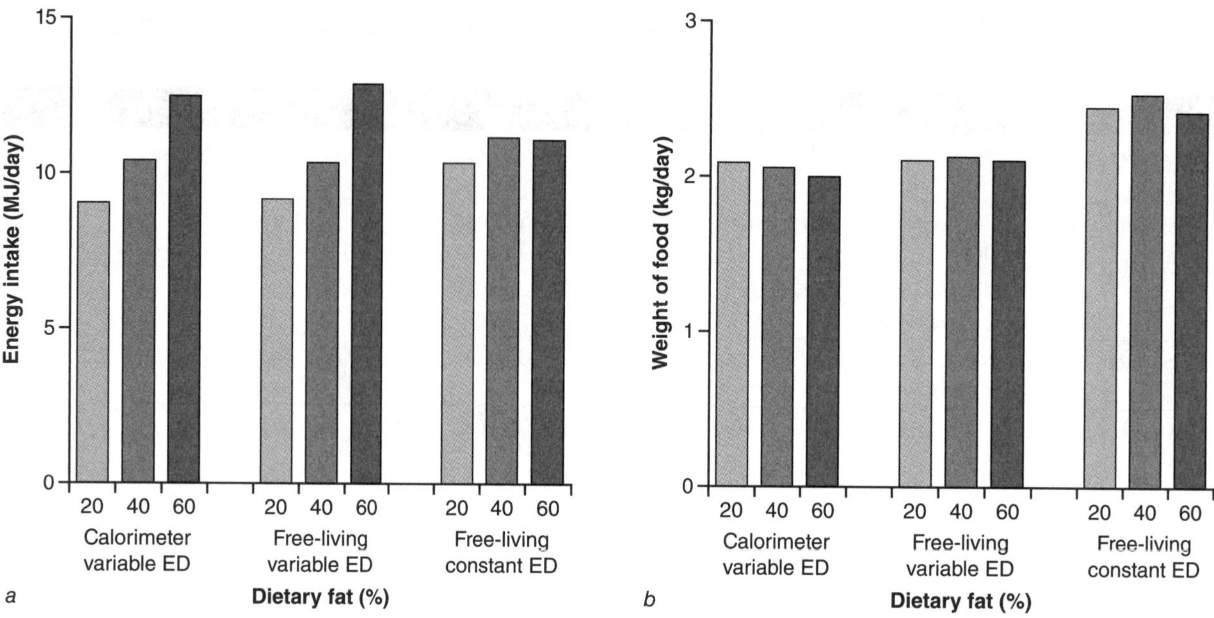

Figure 15.3 Ad libitum energy intake *(a)* and weight of food consumed *(b)* in subjects who consume diets that have 20%, 40%, and 60% of their energy as fat. ED is the energy content of the diets consumed.

Based on Stubbs et al. (1995a); Stubbs et al. (1996).

free-living conditions, the energy density was the same despite differences in composition. Note that subjects ate a constant weight of food in all three conditions, independent of energy, and that the energy density of the meals is a major determinant of energy intake.

Several large-scale longitudinal and cross-sectional studies involving thousands of participants and a number of review articles have clearly shown that an increase in energy density results in an increase in energy intake, whereas a decrease in energy density results in a decrease in intake (Poppitt and Prentice 1996; Ledikwe et al. 2006), as illustrated in figure 15.4. These studies also indicate that normal-weight people consume diets with a lower energy density than obese people and that people who have a high fruit and vegetable intakes have the lowest dietary energy density values and the lowest prevalence of obesity. This is not surprising, because fruits and vegetables generally have high water and fiber contents that provide bulk but less energy than most other food sources.

Only subtle changes to the diet are needed to alter its energy density. For example, the energy density of many popular foods, such as pies, pizzas, sandwiches, and stews, can be decreased without noticeably affecting palatability or portion size by reducing the fat content and adding vegetables and fruits. Furthermore, modifying food selection can lead to healthier eating patterns that are consistent with the most recent Dietary Guidelines for Americans (U.S. Department of Agriculture 2015) as explained in chapter 2. These studies clearly demonstrate the important role of the energy density of the diet and suggest that manipulation of energy density is a good tool in weight management.

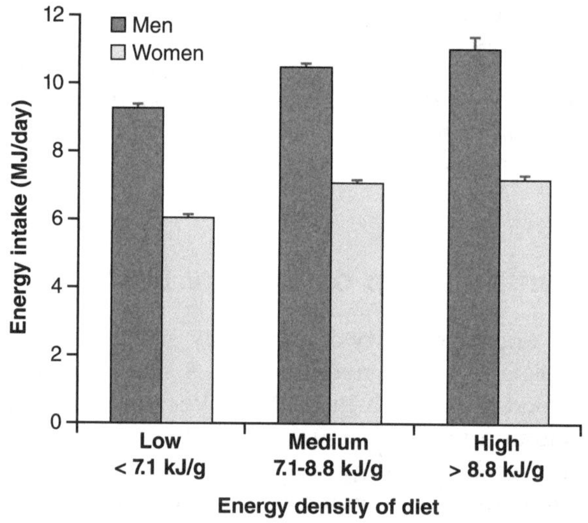

Figure 15.4 Energy intakes of men and women who consumed low-, medium-, or high-energy-density diets.

Data from Ledikwe et al. (2006).

Calcium and Dairy Products

The possible weight-reducing effect of dairy products was first observed by accident in a study in which the effects of dairy products on hypertension were investigated. As hypothesized, a higher dairy intake that provided 1,000 mg of calcium per day reduced hypertension compared with a control diet that provided 400 mg of calcium per day. But the authors were surprised to find that the subjects in the supplemented group lost 4.9 kg (10.8 lb) of body fat (Zemel et al. 2000). Similar trends were observed in several large population-based studies summarized by Zemel (2004). Furthermore, a meta-analysis of 37 randomized control trials involving 184,802 adult participants that investigated the impact of dairy consumption on body weight and body composition (Geng et al. 2018) concluded that high dairy intervention increased body weight and lean mass and decreased body fat and waist circumference overall. Among participants without dietary energy restriction, the consumption of dairy products increased body weight, but among participants with energy restriction, dairy consumption decreased body weight, body fat, and waist circumference. This meta-analysis suggests a beneficial lowering effect of dairy consumption on body weight and body fat but only for participants engaged in caloric restriction.

A suggested mechanism is that dietary calcium modulates circulating calcitriol 1,25-$(OH)_2$-D, which regulates intracellular calcium. This intracellular calcium plays a crucial role in fat metabolism in adipocytes. It has been suggested that reducing calcitriol by increasing dietary calcium intake results in a reduction of body fat in the absence of energy restriction. In combination with energy restriction, it may result in increased body fat and weight loss.

Dairy calcium appears to be more effective than just calcium, because the protein and amino acids in dairy products may have additional benefits. These could be related to the effects of protein on satiety and to the effects on angiotensin-converting enzyme (ACE), which has a role in adipose tissue fat metabolism.

Although several possible mechanisms have now been proposed and some studies provide evidence of a positive effect of dairy products on weight management, debate continues about the issue. In a comprehensive review, a large number of clinical trials were compared (Lanou and Barnard 2008). Of the 49 randomized trials that assessed the effect of dairy products or calcium supplementation on body weight, 41 showed no effect, two demonstrated weight gain, one showed a lower rate of gain, and five showed weight loss. Four of 24 trials reported differential fat loss. Another meta-analysis of randomized controlled trials assessed the effect of calcium on body weight and body composition through supplementation or increasing dairy food intake (Booth et al. 2015). Among 41 studies that met the inclusion criteria, calcium intake was approximately 900 mg/day higher in the supplement groups compared with control groups. In the increased dairy intake group, calcium intake was approximately 1,300 mg/day. The overall conclusion was that neither calcium supplementation nor increased dairy food intake significantly affected body weight or body fat compared with control. However, subanalyses revealed that in the presence of dietary energy restriction, dairy supplementation resulted in no change in body weight but resulted in about a 1 kg (2 lb) greater reduction in body fat over a mean of 4 months compared with control. This meta-analysis strongly suggests that increasing dietary calcium intake using supplements or increasing dairy intake is not an effective weight reduction strategy in adults but that approximately three servings of dairy may facilitate fat loss on weight reduction diets in the short term. Consequently, the majority of the current evidence from clinical trials does not support the hypothesis that calcium or dairy consumption aids in weight loss.

The debate about a role for dairy and calcium will continue. For a more detailed discussion, see several reviews (Lanou and Barnard 2008; Thorning et al. 2016; Zemel 2004; Zemel et al. 2005).

Nonnutritive Sweeteners

Nonnutritive sweeteners or artificial sweeteners are ecologically novel chemosensory signaling compounds that influence ingestive processes and behavior (see the sidebar). Five nonnutritive sweeteners with intense sweetening power have FDA approval (acesulfame-K, aspartame, neotame, saccharin, sucralose). These sweeteners, some of which contain hardly any energy, have the potential to moderate energy intakes while maintaining diet palatability. A critical review of the literature suggests that the addition of nonnutritive sweeteners to non-energy-yielding products may heighten appetite, but this result is not observed under the common condition in which nonnutritive sweeteners are ingested in conjunction with other energy sources. Substitution of a nonnutritive sweetener for a nutritive sweetener generally results in greater energy intake in the short term, but

NONNUTRITIVE SWEETENERS

Natural Sugar Substitutes

Brazzein—protein, 800 × sweetness of sucrose (by weight)
Curculin—protein, 550 × sweetness (by weight)
Erythritol—0.7 × sweetness (by weight), 14 × sweetness of sucrose (by food energy)
Fructose—1.7 × sweetness (by weight and food energy)
Glycyrrhizin—50 × sweetness (by weight)
Isomalt—0.45-0.65 × sweetness (by weight), 0.9-1.3 × sweetness (by food energy)
Lactitol—0.4 × sweetness (by weight), 0.8 × sweetness (by food energy)
Lo Han Guo—300 × sweetness (by weight)
Mabinlin—protein, 100 × sweetness (by weight)
Maltitol—0.9 × sweetness (by weight), 1.7 × sweetness (by food energy), E965*
Mannitol—0.5 × sweetness (by weight), 1.2 × sweetness (by food energy), E421
Monellin—protein, 3,000 × sweetness (by weight)
Pentadin—protein, 500 × sweetness (by weight)
Sorbitol—0.6 × sweetness (by weight), 0.9 × sweetness (by food energy), E420
Stevia—250 × sweetness (by weight)
Tagatose—0.92 × sweetness (by weight), 2.4 × sweetness (by food energy)
Thaumatin—protein, 2,000 × sweetness (by weight), E957
Xylitol—1.0 × sweetness (by weight), 1.7 × sweetness (by food energy), E967

Artificial Sugar Substitutes

Acesulfame potassium—200 × sweetness (by weight), Nutrinova, E950, FDA approved 1988
Aspartame—160-200 × sweetness (by weight), NutraSweet, E951, FDA approved 1981
Dulcin—250 × sweetness (by weight), FDA banned 1950
Neotame—8,000 × sweetness (by weight), NutraSweet, FDA approved 2002
P-4000—4,000 × sweetness (by weight), FDA banned 1950
Saccharin—300 × sweetness (by weight), E954, FDA approved 1958
Sucralose—600 × sweetness (by weight), Splenda, Tate & Lyle, E955, FDA approved 1998

*The E numbers of the sweeteners in packaged foods are commonly used to replace the chemical or common name of particular sweeteners. Other food additives that are used to enhance the color, flavor, and texture or prevent food from spoiling have also been assigned E numbers.

evidence of long-term efficacy for weight management is not available. The addition of nonnutritive sweeteners to the diet poses no benefit for weight loss or reduced weight gain without energy restriction. There are long-standing and recent concerns that inclusion of nonnutritive sweeteners in the diet promotes energy intake and has contributed to the obesity problem. More research is needed to understand the underlying mechanisms and the exact effects of nonnutritive sweeteners.

Exercise for Weight Loss

Exercise is another way to create a negative energy balance. In obese people, the effectiveness of exercise programs to achieve weight loss has been questioned because of problems with motivation, compliance, and impaired ability to exercise. In athletes, these factors are unlikely to be a problem. Most athletes can include exercise sessions with the specific aim of increasing energy expenditure, and they can exercise at an intensity high enough to cause a significant increase of energy expenditure. But athletes may have different problems. For example, coaches of athletes who compete in explosive events (e.g., sprints and jumps) are often reluctant to include aerobic exercise in their training programs. Athletes may have difficulty finding time to exercise in addition to performing their normal training without compromising recovery.

Generally, however, adding exercise to a weight-loss program results in weight loss that is fat loss (Ballor and Keesey 1991; Kraemer et al. 1995; McMurray et al. 1985). The combination of exercise and diet is the most effective way to maintain a lower body weight after weight reduction.

Exercise Intensity

Some argue that the optimal exercise intensity for weight and fat loss is related to fat oxidation and should be the intensity with the highest fat-oxidation rates. As discussed in chapter 7, fat oxidation increases as exercise increases from low to moderate intensity even though the percentage contribution of fat may decrease (see figure 7.8). Increased fat oxidation is a direct result of increased energy expenditure when going from light-intensity to moderate-intensity exercise. At high exercise intensities (>75% of $\dot{V}O_2max$), fat oxidation is inhibited, and the relative rate and the absolute rate of fat oxidation decrease to negligible values (Achten, Gleeson, and Jeukendrup 2002). The maximal rate of fat oxidation (typically around 0.5-1.0 g/min depending on aerobic capacity) generally occurs between 55% and 65% of $\dot{V}O_2max$ and has been referred to as the Fatmax intensity. In endurance trained people, Fatmax tends to be higher (62%-65% $\dot{V}O_2max$) than in less fit individuals (50%-55% $\dot{V}O_2max$). This is not surprising since we know that regular aerobic exercise training causes adaptations that allow the body to burn fat more effectively at higher exercise intensities. Whether regular exercise at this intensity is more effective than exercise at other intensities for body-weight and body-fat loss remains to be determined.

Mode of Exercise

The mode of exercise also affects maximal rates of fat oxidation. For example, fat oxidation is significantly higher during uphill walking and running compared with cycling (Achten, Venables, and Jeukendrup 2003; Arkinstall et al. 2001; Houmard et al. 1990; Nieman et al. 1998a, 1998b). No long-term studies have been conducted to compare different types of exercise and their effectiveness in achieving or maintaining weight loss. In addition, whether exercises that optimize fat oxidation are indeed an effective way to reduce body fat remains to be determined.

Comparisons of resistance training with endurance training have demonstrated favorable effects on body composition (Broeder et al. 1997; Van Etten, Verstappen, and Westerterp 1994) or similar effects in facilitating body-fat loss (Ballor and Keesey 1991). Resistance training seems more effective in preserving or increasing FFM. In turn, the amount of metabolically active tissue also increases, and the increase is suggested as one of the mechanisms by which exercise helps to maintain lower body weight after weight loss through energy restriction. The exercise preserves (or even increases) muscle mass, resulting in a smaller reduction of the RMR.

Current evidence indicates that resistance training is at least as effective as aerobic exercise in reducing body fat. One important factor, of course, is the duration of exercise, which largely determines the energy expended. Athletes who can spend more time exercising at relatively high intensities have greater opportunities to achieve negative energy balance and thus lose body weight.

High-Intensity Interval Training

Most exercise protocols designed to induce fat loss have focused on regular participation in relatively prolonged aerobic exercise, such as walking and jogging at a moderate intensity. For most people, in the absence of dietary caloric restriction, these kinds of protocols have led to rather slow and small losses of body fat and weight. This should not be surprising, as even exercising at an intensity that elicits maximal fat oxidation (i.e., 60%-65% $\dot{V}O_2max$ for a fit person) only results in fat oxidation of 0.5-1.0 g/min (30-60 g/h). Some scientists and fitness gurus have claimed that high-intensity intermittent exercise (HIIE) has the potential to be an economical and effective exercise protocol for reducing fat in overweight people (Boutcher 2011). HIIE protocols typically involve repeated bouts of brief sprinting at an all-out intensity (or at least at exercise intensities that exceed 90% $\dot{V}O_2max$) immediately followed by low-intensity exercise or rest. The lengths of the sprint and recovery periods have varied from 6 seconds to 4 minutes. A commonly used protocol has been the Wingate test, which consists of 30 seconds of all-out sprint with a hard resistance that is performed 4 to 6 times separated by 2 to 4 minutes of recovery. This protocol amounts to 3 to 4 minutes of actual exercise per session with each session typically performed 3 to 7 times a week. Other less-demanding HIIE protocols have also been used with shorter sprints or exercise intensities of 90%-150% of $\dot{V}O_2max$ but with shorter recovery periods. Thus, one of the characteristics of regular HIIE is that it involves markedly lower training volume, which makes it a time-efficient strategy to accrue training adaptations and possible health benefits compared with traditional aerobic exercise programs. These benefits have been shown to include increased aerobic and anaerobic fitness, lowering of insulin resistance, and increased skeletal muscle capacity for fatty acid oxidation and glycolytic enzyme content (Gibala and McGee 2008). Although this is good from the fitness and health perspective, there is limited evidence that regular HIIE results in significant body-fat and body-weight loss.

Studies that have carried out relatively short HIIE interventions (2-6 weeks) in young adults with normal body mass and BMI have reported negligible weight loss (Burgomaster et al. 2008; Perry et al. 2008). Research examining the effects of longer term HIIE on body-weight and body-fat loss in slightly overweight people has produced evidence to suggest that regular HIIE can result in modest reductions in subcutaneous and abdominal body fat (Trappe et al. 2008; Boutcher 2011). Studies using overweight (BMI $>29\,kg/m^2$), type 2 diabetic people have shown greater reductions in subcutaneous and abdominal fat (Boudou et al. 2003; Mourier et al. 1997). The mechanisms underlying the fat reduction induced by HIIE appear to include elevated fat oxidation in the postexercise period and suppressed appetite. However, the actual energy cost of HIIE is rather low; despite the intensity of the exercise being high, the duration is

WHAT SORT OF EXERCISE IS BEST FOR BODY-FAT LOSS?

Taken as a whole, the evidence suggests that for maximum fat burning during exercise, you should exercise aerobically at an intensity close to that which elicits your maximal fat oxidation rate. Depending on your aerobic fitness, this will be around 55%-65% of $\dot{V}O_2max$ (or 60%-80% of your maximum heart rate). As for duration and frequency of exercise sessions, the most important factor is your total energy expenditure over any given time period. So, for example, six dynamic exercise (e.g., cycling, running) 1-hour training sessions per week at 75% of your maximum heart rate (MHR) would be equivalent to three 2-hour sessions at the same relative exercise intensity. The goal is to increase your total volume (within reasonable limits) so you burn more fat. Fewer but longer sessions may be more advantageous because fat oxidation becomes an increasingly important fuel as the duration of exercise increases. An additional benefit of structuring sessions this way is that it allows longer periods of recovery in between each bout of exercise, and some of that recovery time could be used to do HIIE sessions that should increase your $\dot{V}O_2max$ and further increase your capacity for fat oxidation.

Furthermore, any fat loss program should ideally include some resistance training because this increases muscle mass and lean body mass. This is desirable because lean tissue is metabolically far more active than adipose tissue. Increasing your muscle mass by including some resistance training means that your resting metabolic rate can be increased to a small degree, which will help you to achieve your negative energy balance more easily. Two short (~30 min) sessions of resistance training per week comprised of 8 to 12 exercises designed to work all the major muscle groups (one to two sets of 10 to 15 repetitions per exercise with enough weight so the repetitions can just be completed) should produce good results in those who are not experienced resistance trainers.

These recommendations should be considered in light of the current training situation. In many team sports, such as soccer and rugby, body mass may increase during the off-season, and players return for preseason training carrying a little extra weight. Preseason training in these sports is usually harder than in-season training, and it may not be feasible to add extra exercise sessions in this situation because this will increase the risk of injury and illness (see chapter 13). Instead, the usual training plus a small degree of dietary energy restriction should be sufficient to allow normal training adaptation and simultaneous, but gradual, fat loss to occur.

so short that the actual energy expended usually does not exceed 418 kJ (100 kcal). Even taking into account the EPOC (say, in the extreme, a 10% increase in RMR over 12 hours), this only adds another 418 kJ at most, making the overall daily energy cost of an HIIE session no more than 837 kJ (200 kcal). If performed 5 times per week, this amounts to a 4,185 kJ (1,000 kcal) energy deficit. This amount of energy loss could be achieved by a single 10-mile run. Therefore, as previously mentioned, the athlete who wants to lose body weight relatively quickly (i.e., in a matter of weeks or months) would be best advised to exercise at relatively high but submaximal intensities for longer durations, incorporate some degree of dietary energy restriction, and maybe also increase the proportion of protein in the diet.

Decreased Resting Metabolic Rate With Weight Loss

It has been anecdotally reported that losing body weight becomes increasingly difficult as weight loss progresses, presumably because the body responds to weight loss by becoming more efficient. There are conflicting reports about whether RMR adapts or decreases beyond expected values based on changes in body composition in response to energy restriction and weight loss. If RMR exhibits metabolic adaptation, this would provide evidence that metabolic changes defend a certain body weight (set point), which could partly explain why people have difficulty maintaining weight loss. Several studies have reported that RMR decreases in response to weight loss (Dulloo and Jacquet 1998). Most studies have been performed in obese individuals. In a study, three groups of nonobese (although overweight) subjects were subjected to energy restriction for 6 months (Martin et al. 2007). One group was energy restricted by reducing food intake by 25%, one group was subjected to 12.5% energy restriction and a 12.5% increase in physical activity by structured exercise, and the third group served as the control group. Weight loss was similar in the two energy-restricted groups (loss of 10% of initial body weight). RMR adapted or decreased beyond values expected from changes in weight and body composition as a result of the energy deficit that was achieved through a food-based diet after 3 months and a food-based diet plus structured exercise after 6 months (Martin et al. 2007). The control group did not experience a decrease in RMR. At month 6, the combined data from the dieting groups demonstrated that RMR was lower than expected, resulting in 381 kJ/day (91 kcal/day) less energy expenditure compared with control participants even after differences in FFM were taken into consideration.

This decrease in resting metabolism is an autoregulatory feedback mechanism by which the body tries to preserve energy. This "food efficiency" may occur independently of a person's body mass or dieting history. It usually causes a plateau in weight loss and is a common source of frustration for dieters.

In a well-designed study by Leibel, Rosenbaum, and Hirsch (1995), maintenance of a 10% reduction in body weight was associated with a reduction in total energy expenditure of 25 kJ (6 kcal) per kilogram of FFM per day in nonobese subjects (see figure 15.5). Resting energy expenditure and nonresting energy expenditure each decreased 13-17 kJ (3-4 kcal) per kilogram of FFM per day. Maintenance of a 10% higher body weight was associated with an increase in total energy expenditure of 38 kJ (9 kcal) per kilogram of FFM per day. Maintenance of a reduced or elevated body weight is associated with compensatory changes in energy expenditure that oppose the maintenance of a body weight that is different from the usual weight. This study shows that the body has compensatory mechanisms that try to maintain a normal body weight.

Female athletes, especially runners, sometimes have extremely low energy intakes. Despite their training load (30-90 km [19-56 mi] of running per week), they may have energy intakes similar to their sedentary counterparts (Drinkwater et al. 1984; Myerson et al. 1991). Amenorrheic runners (those whose menstrual cycles are currently absent) had a significantly lower RMR than eumenorrheic runners (those with normal monthly menstrual cycles), and their energy intake was similar despite higher activity levels (Lebenstedt, Platte, and Pirke 1999; Myerson et al. 1991). These findings suggest that energy efficiency or food efficiency exists. Other reasons may account for the negative energy balance or low energy intake and expenditure in these female athletes. Not all studies of these athletes have found a reduced RMR (Beidleman, Puhl, and De Souza 1995; Wilmore et al. 1992). Alternative explanations include inaccuracies and underreporting of food intake by these athletes or reduced physical activity in the hours when they are not training.

The concept of food efficiency fits in with the theory that the body has a weight set point. Although interindividual differences in body

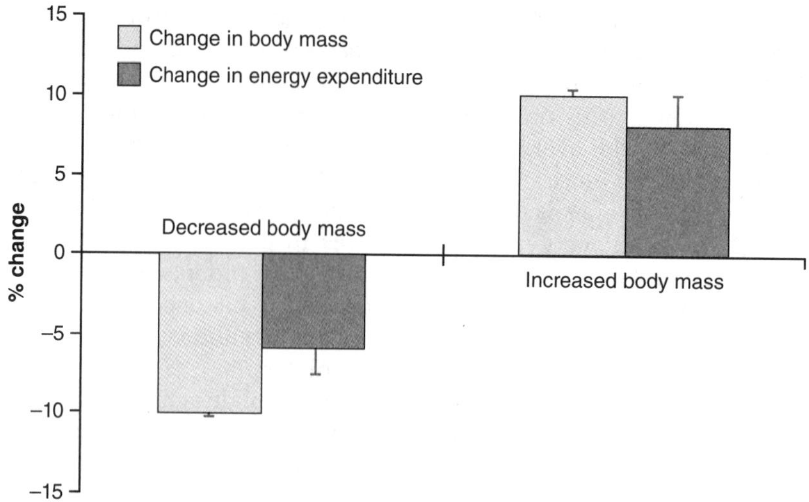

Figure 15.5 Changes in daily energy expenditure in response to weight loss or weight gain. A 10% reduction in body weight resulted in a 6% decrease in energy expenditure, and a 10% gain in body weight resulted in an 8% increase in energy expenditure. This finding shows that the body has compensatory mechanisms that try to maintain a normal body weight.

Based on Leibel, Rosenbaum, and Hirsch (1995).

weight are large, the body weight of an individual is usually fairly constant and typically varies only 0.5% over periods of 6 to 10 weeks (350 g [12 oz] for a person with a body mass of 70 kg [154 lb]). If rats are given an energy-restricted diet for several weeks, they lose body mass rapidly. When they are permitted to eat freely again, they restore this body mass within weeks and their weight becomes identical to their counterparts who had free access to food for the entire period. A similar change happens when rats are overfed. Evidence also exists for such a set point for body weight in humans (Keesey and Hirvonen 1997).

Weight Cycling

Often, the considerable effort applied to achieve weight loss is exceeded by the effort required to maintain the new lower body weight. After the weight is lost, it is regained in a relatively short period. This effect is usually referred to as the yo-yo effect. Studies in animals have documented this pattern of **weight cycling**. After a period of food restriction and weight reduction, animals tend to regain the weight quickly if they are allowed free access to food.

Several prospective studies have shown that weight fluctuation or weight variability is associated with increased mortality independent of the direction of weight change. When taking limited account of preexisting disease, however, studies show little evidence of negative side effects of weight cycling (Field et al. 1999; Wannamethee, Shaper, and Walker 2002). From a public health perspective, the risks from being overweight and obese far exceed the potential risks of weight cycling.

Gender Differences in Weight Loss

Meta-analyses of studies on weight loss after aerobic exercise training showed that weight loss, although modest, was greater for men (Ballor and Keesey 1991). These findings confirm earlier research in men concerning exercise-training effects on body mass and body composition and extend them to women and to a broader range of exercise types. These gender differences have been related to differences in body-fat distribution. Women store more fat in the gluteal–femoral region, whereas men store more fat in the visceral (abdominal) depot. Fat located in the upper body and abdominal regions (central fat) is more metabolically active and therefore has higher rates of lipolysis in response to adrenergic stimulation. During exercise, FAs are preferentially mobilized from these regions (Wahrenberg, Bolinder, and Arner 1991). In addition, postprandial fat storage may be higher in subcutaneous adipose tissue in women than in men. All these differences may play a role in the variation in net regional fat storage between men and women (Blaak 2001) and women's greater resistance to weight loss.

Practicalities of Weight Loss for Athletes

We have discussed the factors that influence body weight and body composition and the research and myths that surround weight loss, but we have not yet discussed how this information can be used to achieve weight loss in athletes. The studies discussed in the preceding section were predominantly performed on obese subjects, and little evidence has been obtained about athletes. These studies were concerned with longer term weight loss. Some information is available about athlete populations, but it generally concerns short-term weight loss programs for athletes in weight-category sports. This topic will be discussed in detail in a following section. Although the information on longer term weight loss obtained from obesity research can be informative, it is difficult to draw conclusions and come up with clear guidelines for athletes. The first step in the process should always be to define the goals: Is weight loss really required, and, if so, how much and over what period? With goals established, various strategies can be put in place to achieve the weight loss. Many mistakes can be made in weight management for athletes, and these will be discussed here as well.

Defining Goals

In conjunction with the coach and a nutritionist, weight-loss goals should be established. These goals should be carefully thought out and well defined. Whether the goal is a good idea depends primarily on the current body-fat percentage. Although individual differences exist, a body-fat percentage less than 5% for men and 12% for women is not recommended. As discussed earlier, some fat is essential, and people can lose only some of the storage fat without affecting physiological function.

Goals also have to be defined with a time schedule in mind. How much weight must be lost and how soon? A realistic weight loss is about a 1 kg (2 lb) every 2 weeks, so to lose 3 kg (7 lb) at least 6 weeks are needed. Achieving this goal means reducing energy intake by about 2,000 kJ/day (478 kcal/day). Faster weight loss will make training difficult or impossible.

Defining the Strategy

The next step is to establish a strategy that will help the athlete lose weight. Following are guidelines to help athletes achieve weight loss:

- Determine a realistic body-weight goal. The help of a sports dietitian is likely needed to identify a realistic target weight.
- Do not try to lose more than about 0.5 kg/week (about 1 lb/week), and do not restrict energy intake by more than 2-3 MJ (500-750 kcal/day).
- Eat more fruits and vegetables.
- Choose low-fat snacks.
- Study food labels and try to find substitutes for high-fat foods. Look not only at fat content but also at the energy content per serving.
- Limit fat add-ons such as sauces, sour cream, and high-fat salad dressings, or choose the low-fat versions of these products.
- Try to structure eating into five or six smaller meals.
- Avoid eating extremely large meals.
- Make sure carbohydrate intake is high, and consume carbohydrate immediately after training.
- A multivitamin and mineral supplement may be useful during periods of energy restriction. Seek the advice of a nutritionist or dietitian.
- Measure body weight daily and obtain measurements of body fat regularly (every 2 months). Keep a record of the changes.

Common Mistakes

When trying to lose weight, athletes make the following common mistakes:

- *Trying to lose weight too rapidly*. Like most people, athletes are impatient about weight loss. They want to see results within a couple of weeks, but unfortunately this expectation is not realistic. Although rapid weight loss is possible, this reduction is mostly dehydration, which reduces performance and the ability to train. Weight loss without performance loss has to occur slowly.
- *Trying to lose weight during the competitive season*. Athletes often try to lose weight during the competitive season, and this effort may result in underperformance. Because hard training is difficult when the energy intake is reduced, weight loss is best accomplished during the off-season.

- *Not eating breakfast or lunch.* Another weight-loss approach that athletes have tried is skipping breakfast and sometimes skipping lunch. Although this approach may work for some, it increases hunger feelings later in the day, and one large evening meal can easily compensate for the daytime reduction in food intake. In addition, exercise capacity and the ability to train may decrease without breakfast because glycogen stores may be low (see chapter 5).
- *Taking in too little carbohydrate.* When losing body weight (being in negative energy balance), athletes also risk losing muscle mass. This risk can be reduced by consuming relatively large amounts of carbohydrate. Carbohydrate intake has a protein-sparing effect.

Making Weight and Rapid Weight-Loss Strategies

Sports in which **making weight** is important are those with weight categories such as judo, wrestling, rowing, and boxing. In horse racing, jockeys are weighed before and after competition to ensure that each horse carries the precise assigned weight. In these sports, weight classes are clearly defined, and to compete in a particular weight class, body weight must be within the limits for that category at the weigh-in. Rowing, for instance, has a lightweight and a heavyweight division. In the lightweight division, male athletes are not permitted to exceed 72.5 kg (159.8 lb), and the crew must have an average weight of 70 kg (154 lb). For women, the maximum individual weight is 59 kg (130 lb), and the crew must have an average weight of 57 kg (126 lb). Weigh-ins can take place from 30 minutes to about 20 hours before competition, although sometimes the weigh-in is performed the day before the competition. Athletes commonly compete at a weight that is 2 to 6 kg (4-13 lb) below their normal weight, which implies that they must lose weight rapidly in the days or weeks before competition.

Most rapid weight loss is by dehydration, and athletes use various techniques to achieve it. The most common methods are energy or fluid restriction; dehydration by exercise, sauna, hotrooms, or steam rooms; and diuretics, stimulants, and laxatives. Exercise is often performed in a hotroom while wearing plastic or rubber garments. This rapid weight loss mainly affects body water, glycogen content, and lean body mass, and little or no loss of body fat occurs (Kelly, Gorney, and Kalm 1978; Oppliger et al. 1991).

Rapid weight loss by dehydration may result in reductions in plasma volume, central blood volume, and blood flow to active tissues and increased core temperature and heart rate. Cardiovascular changes can be observed with a weight loss of approximately 2% of body weight (see chapter 9). These rapid weight-loss strategies have also been reported to alter hormone status, impede normal growth and development, affect psychological state, impair academic performance, and affect immune function. Severe dehydration can result in heat illness and even death. Rapid weight loss strategies using dehydration in combination with food and fluid restriction are common practice among wrestlers who experience short periods of rapid weight loss about 7 to 15 times each year and approximately 100 times during a wrestling career (Tipton and Oppliger 1993).

In 1997, three previously healthy U.S. collegiate wrestlers died while engaged in rapid weight-loss programs to qualify for competition (Centers for Disease Control and Prevention 1998). In the hours preceding the official weigh-in, all three wrestlers engaged in a similar rapid weight-loss regimen that promoted dehydration through perspiration and resulted in hyperthermia. The wrestlers also restricted food and fluid intake and attempted to maximize sweat losses by wearing vapor-impermeable suits under cotton warm-up suits and exercising vigorously in hot environments. In response to these deaths, the National Collegiate Athletic Association (NCAA) rules were changed, and a wresting weight certification program was made mandatory to create a safer competitive environment (Davis et al. 2002). Other changes included establishing a weight-class system that better reflected the wrestling population, conducting weigh-ins close to competition (1 hour before) and for each day of a multiple-day tournament, and prohibiting use of tools that result in rapid dehydration (Davis et al. 2002). The current NCAA rules are now in line with the recommendations by the ACSM (Oppliger et al. 1996).

Another rapid weight loss technique that has been recently become popular is "water loading." This technique involves ingesting large amounts of water (7-10 L/day) for several days followed by fluid restriction. The idea is to target renal hormones and urine output. A recent study investigated the effects of ingesting 100 ml/kg b.m. of water for 3 days followed by 1 day of water restriction (Reale et al. 2017). It was demonstrated that indeed fluid losses were greater compared with fluid restriction alone. There was a small but potentially physiologically significant drop in plasma sodium that may have suppressed vasopressin release. This technique is thus effective but should not be performed without extensive medical supervision as drinking large amounts of water could result in life threatening hyponatremia (as discussed in chapter 9).

Weight Gain

Weight gain is a concern for athletes in sports in which higher body weight and increased muscle mass are advantages, such as hammer throwing, discus throwing, shot put, weightlifting, American football, and rugby. The key to gaining weight is to have energy intake exceed energy expenditure. To increase lean body mass rather than fat mass, a person must increase protein and carbohydrate intake and not fat intake. Whereas the body counteracts a decrease in body weight that occurs with energy restriction by decreasing resting energy expenditure, the body increases resting energy expenditure when energy intake increases in excess of expenditure. Just as expecting large weight losses in a short period is unrealistic, so is expecting large weight gains within days. Realistic weight gains are between 0.2 and 1.0 kg/week (0.4-2.2 lb/week) depending on the increase in energy intake. Protein synthesis is a slow process, and even with intake of excess protein, synthesis of muscle protein takes a long time and takes place only if combined with an adequate training program. For more information on protein synthesis and gaining muscle mass, see chapters 8 and 17.

Key Points

- An average body fat percentage for young adults is between 12% and 15% for men and between 25% and 28% for women. Approximately 3% of male body mass and 12% of female body mass is essential body fat.
- Appetite is sensed in the brain, which constantly receives and processes neural, metabolic, and endocrine signals from the periphery. In addition, a large number of external factors influence eventual food intake.
- Calories from different food sources can have markedly different effects on hunger, hormones, energy expenditure, and the brain regions that control food intake. Even though calories are important, in many cases simple changes in food selection can lead to the same (or better) results for weight loss than calorie restriction.
- Negative energy balance is required to lose weight. In addition, negative fat balance will promote fat loss. The resting metabolic rate, however, decreases in response to weight loss. This effect, referred to as food efficiency, makes losing weight more difficult. A common problem is the yo-yo effect, or weight cycling. After weight loss is achieved, the lost weight is often regained in a relatively short period.
- Studies clearly demonstrate the important role of energy density of the diet for voluntary food intake and suggest that manipulation of energy density is a useful tool in weight management.
- Common diet strategies to lose weight include very low-energy diets, intermittent-fasting diets, low-carbohydrate diets, food combination diets, and high-protein diets. For athletes seeking to lose weight, energy restriction and reduced fat intake while maintaining or increasing dietary protein are recommended. This strategy allows a reasonable carbohydrate intake, which enables athletes to perform high-intensity training without major reductions in lean body mass.
- Exercise can help create a negative energy balance, maintain muscle mass, and compensate for the reductions in RMR seen after weight loss.
- In weight-category sports such as judo, wrestling, rowing, and boxing, the need to make weight encourages athletes to try to lose weight in a relatively short time. Athletes should be aware of the risks of rapid weight loss. Rapid weight loss (mainly dehydration) can affect health and performance.

- The recommended method to gain weight is to maintain a positive energy balance without increasing fat intake. Most of the excess energy intake should come from carbohydrate.

Recommended Readings

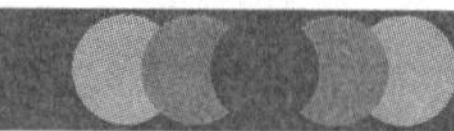

Barnosky, A.R., K.K. Hoddy, T.G. Unterman, and K.A. Varady. 2014. Intermittent fasting vs daily calorie restriction for type 2 diabetes prevention: A review of human findings. *Translational Research* 164 (4): 302-311.

Blundell, J.E., C. Gibbons, P. Caudwell, G. Finlayson, and M. Hopkins. 2015. Appetite control and energy balance: Impact of exercise. *Obesity Reviews* 16 (Suppl 1):67-76.

Blundell, J.E., R.J. Stubbs, D.A. Hughes, S. Whybrow, and N.A. King. 2003. Cross talk between physical activity and appetite control: Does physical activity stimulate appetite? *Proceedings of the Nutrition Society* 62:651-661.

Bouchard, C. 1994. Genetics of obesity: Overview and research directions. In *The genetics of obesity,* edited by C. Bouchard, 223-233. Boca Raton, FL: CRC Press.

Bouchard, C., A. Tremblay, J.P. Despres, A. Nadeau, P.J. Lupien, G. Theriault, J. Dussault, S. Moorjani, S. Pinault, and G. Fournier. 1990. The response to long-term overfeeding in identical twins. *New England Journal of Medicine* 322:1477-1482.

Flatt, J.-P. 1995. Use and storage of carbohydrate and fat. *American Journal of Clinical Nutrition* 61:952S-959S.

Hall, K.D., and J. Guo. 2017. Obesity energetics: Body weight regulation and the effects of diet composition. *Gastroenterology* 152 (7): 1718-1727.

Howell, S., and R. Kones. 2017. "Calories in, calories out" and macronutrient intake: The hope, hype, and science of calories. *American Journal of Physiology: Endocrinology and Metabolism.* 313(5):E608-E612.

Johnstone, A.M. 2007. Fasting: The ultimate diet? *Obesity Reveiws* 8:211-222.

Lanou, A.J., and N.D. Barnard. 2008. Dairy and weight loss hypothesis: An evaluation of the clinical trials. *Nutrition Reviews* 66:272-279.

Paddon-Jones, D., E. Westman, R.D. Mattes, R.R. Wolfe, A. Astrup, and M. Westerterp-Plantenga. 2008. Protein, weight management, and satiety. *American Journal of Clinical Nutrition* 87:1558S-1561S.

Poppitt, S.D., and A.M. Prentice. 1996. Energy density and its role in the control of food intake: Evidence from metabolic and community studies. *Appetite* 26:153-174.

Zemel, M.B. 2004. Role of calcium and dairy products in energy partitioning and weight management. *American Journal of Clinical Nutrition* 79:907S-912S.

Eating Disorders in Athletes

Objectives

After studying this chapter, you should be able to do the following:

- Describe the eating disorders that affect athletes
- Describe the characteristics of anorexia nervosa, bulimia nervosa, and eating disorders not otherwise specified
- Describe the prevalence of eating disorders in athletes
- Describe the risk factors for eating disorders
- Describe the effects of eating disorders on sports performance
- Describe the effects of eating disorders on the health of athletes
- Describe some effective strategies for the treatment and prevention of eating disorders

For people who consume 8 to 12 MJ (1,912-2,868 kcal) of dietary energy per day, a typical pattern of eating might be two or three main meals (e.g., breakfast, lunch, and dinner) with an occasional snack (e.g., biscuit or chocolate bar) between meals. For endurance athletes with higher energy intakes (typically 15-20 MJ/day [3,585-4,780 kcal/day]), a grazing pattern of eating is common with a substantial proportion of daily energy intake consumed between meals. In most cases, athletes are in energy balance, meaning that over the course of several days or weeks, energy intake generally matches energy expenditure. But some athletes (and nonathletes) experience **eating disorders** characterized by gross disturbances of eating behaviors. The major disorders are associated with abnormally low food intake or bouts of binge eating followed by purging the stomach contents, which results in low energy availability. If left undiagnosed and untreated, eating disorders can have detrimental effects on sports performance and damaging, long-lasting effects on health and can even be fatal. The potentially irreversible consequences of these conditions emphasize the critical need for prevention, early diagnosis, and treatment.

Evidence suggests that eating disorders are more common in certain athletic groups than in the general population, and the role of the sport nutritionist or dietitian working with athletes who are susceptible to eating disorders is crucial to prevention. Although these conditions were first identified in female athletes, research has shown that male athletes can also be susceptible to the same types of problems (Glazer 2008; Martinsen at al. 2010; Torstveit and Sundgot-Borgen 2014). Often, the best treatment is educating athletes about the health risks of eating disorders and counseling them about wise food choices and good eating habits. This chapter reviews the characteristics of various eating disorders, the prevalence of eating disorders in various sports, risk factors for eating disorders, and the effects of eating disorders on sports performance and health. Some practical guidelines on diagnosis, treatment, and prevention of eating disorders are also given.

Types of Eating Disorders

Among athletes there are several types of disordered eating behaviors, such as being obsessively preoccupied with body shape and body weight, restricting intake of particular foods, dieting, binge eating followed by vomiting, abusing of diuretic drugs, and using laxatives and so-called slimming pills. The main purpose of disordered eating behavior is usually to achieve a lower body weight and body-fat content to compensate for strong dissatisfaction with body image. What may begin with a moderate reduction of normal daily energy intake may escalate to more extreme behavior (e.g., strict dieting and increased volumes of exercise) to the degree that the athlete meets the criteria for a clinical eating disorder. Eating behavior can be considered as a spectrum ranging from healthy eating to overeating in one direction and clinical eating disorders in the other (figure 16.1). The major classified eating disorders include anorexia nervosa, bulimia nervosa, and **eating disorders not otherwise specified (EDNOS)** (American Psychiatric Association 1994). The characteristics of the three main clinical eating disorders are described in the following sections, and the current criteria for their diagnosis can be found in the 5th edition of the *Diagnostic and Statistical Manual of Mental Disorders* produced by the American Psychiatric Association (2013). For athletes who show significant symptoms of eating disorders but do not meet these criteria, a subclinical eating disorder separately classified as **anorexia athletica** has been proposed (Sundgot-Borgen 1994a).

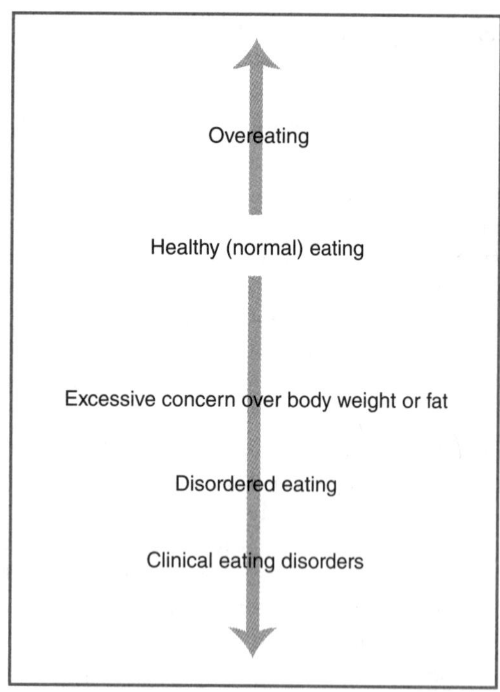

Figure 16.1 The spectrum of eating behavior.

Anorexia nervosa is characterized by an abnormally small food intake and an inability (intentional or not) to maintain normal body weight (according to what is expected for gender, age, and height). Sufferers have a distorted view of body image and an intense fear of being fat or overweight and of gaining weight. They often "feel fat" even when they are at least 15% below normal weight for age and height (this can be associated with low self-esteem), and they also often express denial of the seriousness of their current low body weight. The absence of at least three successive menstrual cycles (**amenorrhea**) is quite common in anorexic women and was one of the diagnostic criteria for anorexia nervosa; it was removed in 2013 because it cannot be applied to men or to women who are premenarcheal or post-menopausal or who are taking oral contraceptives. Anorexia nervosa primarily affects adolescent girls and young women. There are two main types of anorexia nervosa: the restricting type, in which the person does not regularly engage in binge eating and purging behavior (i.e., self-induced vomiting or the misuse of drugs to help lose weight, such as laxatives, diuretics, and enemas), and the binge eating and purging type, in which the person regularly engages in binge eating and purging behaviors.

The physical symptoms of people who suffer from anorexia nervosa or anorexia athletica are as follows (Thompson and Trattner-Sherman 1993; Sundgot-Borgen 1994b):

- Weight loss beyond that normally required for adequate sports performance
- Amenorrhea or some manifestation of menstrual dysfunction
- Dehydration
- High level of fatigue (beyond that normally expected after training or competition)
- Gastrointestinal problems (e.g., constipation, diarrhea, or distress after a meal)
- Hyperactivity
- **Hypothermia** (lower than normal body temperature)
- Low resting heart rate
- Muscle weakness
- Susceptibility to overuse injuries
- Reduced bone-mineral density and susceptibility to stress fractures

- Frequent infections, skin sores, and poor wound healing
- Low blood hemoglobin and **hematocrit** and low serum albumin, serum ferritin, glucose, HDL cholesterol, and estradiol levels

The psychological characteristics of those who suffer from anorexia nervosa or anorexia athletica are as follows (Thompson and Trattner-Sherman 1993):

- General anxiety
- Avoidance of eating and absence from meal situations
- Claims of being fat or feeling fat despite being thin and underweight
- Resistance to recommendations for weight gain
- Unusual weighing behaviors (e.g., excessive weighing, avoidance of weighing, negative reaction to being weighed, refusal to be weighed)
- Excessive training beyond that required for a sport or exercising while injured or when prohibited by coaching and medical staff
- Obsession with body image
- Compulsive behaviors regarding eating and physical activity
- Restlessness and inability or unwillingness to relax
- Social withdrawal
- Depression
- Tiredness and irritability
- **Insomnia** (difficulty with sleeping)

Most people who experience anorexia do not seem to realize they have a problem and therefore are unlikely to seek treatment. Hence, for the susceptible athlete, the coach, team doctor, physiologist, sport psychologist, or sport nutritionist or dietitian is crucial in identifying the problem and persuading the athlete to get medical attention. In many cases, anorexic athletes consider seeking help only when their sports performance declines.

Bulimia nervosa is an eating disorder in which affected individuals repeat cycles of binge eating (consumption of large amounts of usually energy-dense foods) followed soon after by purging the stomach contents (vomiting) before many of the nutrients from the heavy meal can be absorbed. The person often eats the food in secret and commonly disappears from view shortly after a meal to purge the stomach contents. Bulimic athletes do not usually volunteer information about their abnormal behavior until they think the situation is getting out of control or their habit is detrimentally affecting their sports performance. Besides purging, other compensatory behaviors, such as prolonged fasting or excessive exercise, may be used. Binge eating and inappropriate compensatory behaviors both occur at least once per week. People with bulimia may also use **laxatives** (drugs that promote defecation) and **diuretics** (drugs that promote urine formation) to achieve short-term weight loss. Some may also use enemas to lose weight; an enema involves the injection of liquid into the rectum through the anus to stimulate evacuation of the bowels.

These characteristics of bulimic people are quite similar to the purging type of anorexics. The main criterion difference involves weight, as an anorexic must be classified as underweight. For those with binge-purge anorexia, what they are doing results in a net energy intake lower than their energy expenditure for long enough to become, or maintain, a lower than normal body weight. For those with bulimia, their energy intake is enough to maintain or gain weight. People with bulimia may struggle just as much with weight-related thoughts as people with anorexia but the difference is the effect of their behavior on their bodies. Generally, the anorexic does not engage in regular bingeing and purging sessions but may do so occasionally. Characteristically, those with bulimia nervosa feel more shame and out of control of their behavior, whereas the anorexic meticulously controls intake, naive to the notion that it is, in fact, controlling her or him. For this reason, bulimics are more likely to admit to having a problem, as they do not feel they are in control of their behavior. Anorexics are more likely to believe they are in control of their eating and much less likely to admit that a problem even exists.

There are two main types of bulimia nervosa: the purging type, in which the person regularly engages in self-induced vomiting or misuses laxatives, diuretics, or enemas, and the nonpurging type, in which the person does not use vomiting or drugs to avoid weight gain but instead exhibits other inappropriate compensatory behaviors, such as fasting between binge eating episodes or engaging in excessive exercise. Unlike athletes with anorexia, many athletes with bulimia are at normal body weights. Therefore, the athlete's support team must be aware of the physical symptoms and psychological characteristics associated with bulimia nervosa. The physical symptoms are as follows (Thompson and Trattner-Sherman 1993):

- Calluses, sores, or abrasions on the fingers or the back of the hand used to induce vomiting
- Dehydration
- Dental or gum problems
- Edema, complaints of bloating, or both
- Serum electrolyte abnormalities
- Gastrointestinal problems
- Low weight despite apparent intake of large amounts of food
- Frequent and often extreme weight fluctuations
- Muscle cramps, muscle weakness, or both
- Swollen parotid salivary glands
- Menstrual irregularities

The psychological characteristics associated with bulimia nervosa are as follows (Thompson and Trattner-Sherman 1993):

- Binge eating
- Secretive eating and agitation when bingeing is interrupted
- Disappearing after eating meals
- Evidence of vomiting that is unrelated to illness
- Dieting
- Excessive exercise beyond that required for the sport
- Depression
- Self-criticism, especially concerning body image, body weight, and sports performance
- Substance abuse
- Use of laxatives, diuretics, or both that are unsanctioned by medical or coaching support staff

A person who does not meet all criteria for anorexia nervosa or bulimia nervosa is classified as having an EDNOS. For example, a person may meet all the criteria for anorexia nervosa except that, despite significant weight loss, the current body weight is within the normal range for sex, age, and height, or a person may meet all the criteria for bulimia nervosa except binge and purge behavior occurs less than once per week. Other examples of EDNOS are purging behavior that occurs after eating small amounts of food and repeatedly chewing large amounts of food but spitting it out rather than swallowing.

Binge eating disorder was included in the latest version of the *Diagnostic and Statistical Manual of Mental Disorders* (2013). A person who suffers from this disorder eats large amounts of food in a short period of time and then has feelings of anxiety, distress, guilt, or disgust. This behavior occurs, on average, at least once per week over a period of months, and it is associated with significant psychological problems. This is more extreme and far less common than overeating, which nowadays is commonplace in many developed countries. For athletes in most sports, this disorder would lead to rapid weight gain and deteriorating performance.

One increasingly common form of eating disorder is **orthorexia nervosa** (Michalska et al. 2016). Orthorexia is described as extreme concern about eating a healthy diet. It affects about 7% of the general population and is more frequent among men than women (Donini et al. 2004). The term was introduced by Bratman in 1997, and the condition is diagnosed when a person dedicates much of his or her daily activity to planning the diet and healthy lifestyle, often at the expense of a social life and job responsibilities. The relatively high prevalence of orthorexia is a direct consequence of Western tendencies to focus on appearance and increasing concern about health. Although concentration on one's health could be considered a positive trend, extreme dedication to researching healthy diets and restricting food choices to only those that are thought to be healthy or pure can result in health problems. For example, people who suffer from orthorexia will often avoid entire food groups (e.g., dairy products, meat, anything that contains fat), which can lead to nutritional deficits and social problems. Sometimes, people with orthorexia use a vegan diet to help justify or mask food restriction. In some cases orthorexia may develop in individuals who have adopted a vegan diet, but generally vegans are not more prone to orthorexia than other people. One of the main reasons for choosing to eat a vegan diet is compassion for animals rather than food restriction. A vegan diet does not demand an obsession with healthfulness or restrict foods beyond those of animal origin. Creating and following restrictive food rules that inhibit consumption of adequate nutrients is a form of disordered eating. Trying to eliminate all processed foods, avoid every gram of fat, or follow a strict "alkalizing" or "detox" diet and consuming too few calories are just a few of the characteristic traits of orthorexic behavior that may coincide with a vegan diet. Social problems commonly arise with orthorexia because often this lifestyle includes the majority of waking time dedicated to planning and research around foods that are acceptable. This can limit social gatherings and connections and lead to loss of relationships.. Diagnostic criteria of orthorexia are not well established, although new ones have been proposed (Dunn and Bratman 2016). The most important characteristics are obsessive-compulsive traits, health fanatic eating habits, an enduring pattern of abnormal behavior, and negative effects on a person's quality of life as a result of inappropriate eating patterns.

There are similarities between orthorexia and anorexia nervosa, such as rituals related to eating, concentration on food, strict dietary habits, and a very close relationship between eating and self-esteem. A major difference, though, is energy intake: Whereas people with anorexia severely restrict overall food intakes, people with orthorexia may have normal or only slightly subnormal intakes. This is exemplified by the much lower prevalence of orthorexic people who have very low BMIs. To date, there are very few published studies on orthorexia in athletes, but one study that compared 577 athletes with 217 matched controls reported higher positive results on an orthorexic tendency questionnaire and eating attitude test among athletes than among control subjects (Segura-García et al. 2012).

There are also some other, less common eating disorders within certain athlete groups. There are reports of athletes involved in bodybuilding, for example, who have an unhealthy preoccupation with increasing their muscle mass while decreasing their fat mass to look toned and lean. These people implement special dietary restrictions (selecting high protein, low-fat foods and whey protein supplements), have a dedication to sports (particularly bodybuilding ones), and use anabolic or fat-burning drugs to achieve adequate body mass. This problem is sometimes referred to as muscle dysmorphia, which is a variant of body dysmorphic disorder in which a person is preoccupied with the idea that his or her body is insufficiently muscular (Mosley 2009). It is also sometimes known as **bigorexia**. This problem is thought to affect approximately 10% of bodybuilders and is at least as common in men as it is in women (Pope et al. 2000).

Prevalence of Eating Disorders in Athletes

Currently, data on the prevalence of eating disorders in athletes are limited and equivocal, mainly because few studies have applied strict classification criteria (such as those in the *Diagnostic and Statistical Manual of Mental Disorders* [American Psychiatric Association 1994, 2013]) to athletes and nonathlete control subjects. Rather, most studies have looked at a limited number of symptoms of eating disorders, such as a preoccupation with body weight, body image, and food intake or the use of pathogenic means of weight control.

Some athlete populations exhibit a significantly greater preoccupation with body weight than nonathlete populations, particularly in sports that emphasize body shape, leanness, or body weight (Davis 1992). Some studies have relied exclusively on the use of questionnaires, which is likely to result in underreporting of eating disorders and underreporting of the use of purging methods, such as vomiting, laxatives, and diuretics (Sundgot-Borgen 1994a, 2000). Questionnaires also tend to result in overreporting of the incidence of binge eating compared with clinical evaluation by structured interviews (Sundgot-Borgen 1994a, 2000). Estimates of the prevalence of eating disorders among female athletes range from less than 1% to as high as 75% (Burckes-Miller and Black 1988; Gadpalle, Sandborn, and Wagner 1987; Sundgot-Borgen 1994a, 1994b; Warren, Stanton, and Blessing 1990), and among male athletes, estimates range from 0% to 57% (Burckes-Miller and Black 1988; Dummer, Rosen, and Heusner 1987; Rosen and Hough 1988; Rucinski 1989).

Studies generally indicate a substantially higher incidence of eating disorders among athletes compared with nonathletes and greater prevalence among women compared with men. Some studies report that eating disorders are at least 10 times more prevalent among women than men (Andersen 1995), although in recent years an increasing number of men have been diagnosed with anorexia and bulimia among distance runners, jockeys, and lightweight rowers. Classically defined anorexia nervosa does not seem to be much more prevalent (1.3%) in the female athletic population than in the general female population (Andersen 1990), whereas bulimia nervosa (8.2%) and subclinical eating disorders (8%) seem to be more prevalent among female athletes than female nonathletes. The prevalence of eating disorders appears to be higher among female athletes who compete in endurance and weight-category sports and, as can be seen in table 16.1, is especially high in those who participate in aesthetic sports (e.g., gymnastics and dance) compared with those who compete in team game sports, power sports, and technical sports. This is presumably the result of the relative importance of leanness to success in some sports or the perceived advantage to be gained by competing in a lower weight category.

TABLE 16.1 Prevalence of Eating Disorders Among Elite Female Athletes in Various Sports

Type of sport	*n*	Eating disorder present (%) and 95% CI
Aesthetic	64	34 (24-43)
Weight-dependent	41	27 (13-39)
Endurance	119	21 (14-28)
Technical	98	14 (8-20)
Ball games	183	11 (6-15)
Power	17	6 (5-11)
Nonathletes	522	5 (3-7)

Data are shown as mean percentage of individuals with an eating disorder in each sport type and the 95% CI.
Data from Sundgot-Borgen (2000).

Although the precise causes of eating disorders are unknown, several factors that increase the risk of eating disorders can be identified. These include gender, lifestyle, dieting, certain personality traits, and exercise dependence.

Gender and Athleticism

Women have a 10 times greater risk of experiencing eating disorders than men (Andersen 1995), but there is some evidence that the incidence of male eating disorders is on the rise (Byrne and McLean 2002). Athletes, particularly those at the elite level, seem to be more susceptible to eating disorders than the general population (Thompson and Sherman 2010), and this may be due to the additional stress associated with the elite athletic environment and encouragement by coaches to lose weight or body fat sometimes within a relatively short period of time, which requires a more extreme negative energy balance than gradual dieting. Male and female athletes who compete in sports that emphasize a lean body shape or low body weight have a significantly higher prevalence of eating disorders and eating-disorder symptoms than other athletes and nonathletes (Krentz and Warschburger 2011). Being an athlete, however, does not necessarily increase a person's risk for an eating disorder. The athletes who are particularly vulnerable are those who compete in sports in which being thin is considered essential or sports in which having a low body weight is necessary to be successful (Byrne and McLean 2002). This vulnerability may be a result of the additional physical, psychological, and social stresses associated with the athletic environment and lifestyle.

Studies suggest that a high training load may induce a negative energy balance in endurance athletes, which in turn may elicit physiological and social reinforcements that lead to eating disorders. Garner et al. (1987) reported a higher prevalence of eating disorders among top-level dancers compared with dancers in lower competitive levels. Heavy training loads, however, cannot be the prime cause of eating disorders because female cyclists, marathon runners, and triathletes expend more energy in their training than dancers and gymnasts. Nevertheless, there is no evidence to suggest that endurance athletes are more prone to developing eating disorders than dancers or gymnasts. Another possibility is that young athletes who take up serious sport at a prepubertal age may not select the sport that is most suitable for their adult body type and hence are subject to greater pressure to maintain a different (i.e., leaner, smaller) body type than is natural for them. Indeed, Sundgot-Borgen (1994b) found that athletes with eating disorders began sport-specific training at an earlier age than athletes who did not have eating disorders.

Dieting

A large, randomized, prospective study of 1,700 teenage boys and girls found that dieting and psychiatric morbidity were the most sensitive independent predictors of newly diagnosed clinical eating disorders (Patton et al. 1999). Girls who dieted at moderate and severe levels were 5 and 18 times more likely, respectively, to be diagnosed with clinical eating disorders 6 months later. Girls in the highest and second highest of four psychiatric morbidity categories were seven and three times more likely, respectively, to be diagnosed with clinical eating disorders 6 months later. Dieting is an established risk factor for eating disorders (Polivy and Herman 1995). Sudden periods of enforced inactivity (e.g., because of injury) or longer periods of positive energy balance (e.g., during the off-season) may result in weight gain, which the athlete is then told to lose. The athlete may begin to diet excessively or may develop an irrational fear of additional weight gain. Guidance to athletes about how best to lose weight is important at this point. In some cases, athletes may be asked to lose weight rapidly to remain on the team. As a result, they may undergo periods of restricted eating and weight cycling. This type of behavior has been suggested as an important factor in triggering eating disorders in athletes (Brownell, Steen, and Wilmore 1987; Sundgot-Borgen 1994b, 2000). Nutritional counseling is also essential for preventing inadvertent low energy availability, because energy deficits caused by too much exercise rather than by dietary restriction do not necessarily increase appetite for food (Hubert, King, and Blundell 1998). Thus, in some situations, low energy availability could occur inadvertently in the absence of clinical eating disorders, disordered eating behaviors, or even dietary restriction.

Personality Traits

Certain personality traits may predispose people to eating disorders. Most affected people are reported to have low self-esteem and to be excessively self-critical, particularly about body image (Sundgot-Borgen 2000). Those with bulimia consistently show high levels of impulsivity (DaCosta and Halmi 1992), and their addictiveness scores resemble those of drug addicts (DeSilva and Eysenck 1987). Athletes, at least the most successful ones, are by nature compulsive and focused. The same traits that encourage good sports performance in many athletes—perfectionism, dedication, and willingness to work hard and withstand discomfort—may lead to preoccupation with body image and body fat.

Exercise Dependence

Excessive exercising is widely reported to coexist with eating disorders and particularly among those who practice dietary restraint (Brewerton et al. 1995). Many of the reported characteristics of exercise dependence are evident in athletes with eating disorders (Touyz, Beumont, and Hook 1987). A study described 28% of female eating-disorder patients as "compulsive exercisers" (Brewerton et al. 1995), and another study reported that the prevalence of excessive exercising among such patients was as high as 78% (Davis et al. 1994).

Overactivity among those with eating disorders appears either as deliberate exercise to increase energy expenditure and promote fat loss or as involuntary and persistent restlessness often associated with sleep disturbance (Beumont 1995). Where the former is manifest, exercise is considered a secondary symptom of the disorder, and for athletes, distinguishing this motivation to exercise from the need to train for a sport may be impossible. Restless hyperactivity, on the other hand, may be a central feature of the eating disorder (Kron et al. 1978). This notion is supported by evidence of reduced food consumption in rats forced to exercise excessively and increased voluntary wheel running in food-deprived rats (Epling and Pierce 1988). Accordingly, a combination of excessive exercise and food restriction may be a self-perpetuating and mutually reinforcing cycle with potentially serious consequences. Currently, the precise role of exercise in the etiology of eating disorders remains unclear. Dieting is an established risk factor for eating disorders (Polivy and Herman 1995), but high levels of physical activity may play an important role in the perpetuation of an eating disorder. Davis et al. (1994) found that 75% of eating-disorder patients were most active during the period of lowest food intake and greatest weight loss.

Effects of Eating Disorders on Sports Performance

The effect of an eating disorder on exercise performance is determined by how long the disorder has been manifest and the severity of the disorder. Whether an eating disorder affects performance in a specific sport is also determined by the nature of the sport (i.e., whether the predominant requirement of the sport is power, strength, endurance, or motor skills). As in the early stages of dieting, the body adapts and uses up stored fat and certain minerals (e.g., iron) and vitamins. Decreased performance may not occur for some time, and the athlete may wrongly believe that the disordered eating behavior is harmless. In the early stages of weight loss, performance may transiently improve, but endurance performance is likely to deteriorate if liver and muscle glycogen levels are low or if the athlete becomes dehydrated or anemic (i.e., the blood hemoglobin concentration falls below normal).

Dehydration is common in anorexia nervosa and bulimia nervosa (Sundgot-Borgen 2000), and acute dehydration has other consequences for sports performance, such as loss of motor skills and coordination (Fogelholm 1994b). Reduced plasma volume in the dehydrated state impairs the ability to thermoregulate during exercise, which can also contribute to impaired exercise performance particularly in the heat (see chapter 9 for further details). Electrolyte disturbances are also likely to be detrimental to muscle function, and with time, a loss of lean body (muscle) mass will reduce strength and power. Short-term anaerobic performance and muscle strength are impaired after rapid weight loss, and restoration of performance requires 5 to 24 hours of rehydration (Fogelholm, Koskinen, and Lasko 1993). Possible performance consequences of eating disorders in athletes include the following:

- Decreased nerve conduction velocity
- Decreased reaction time
- Decreased concentration
- Light-headedness
- Decreased self-esteem and increased fear of failure
- Decreased speed of muscle contraction
- Muscle atrophy and loss of lean body mass
- Decreased strength and power
- Decreased endurance in static and dynamic exercise
- Decreased blood flow to skeletal muscle
- Decreased oxygen-carrying capacity of blood resulting in reduced delivery of oxygen to muscle
- Impaired oxidative metabolism in skeletal muscle
- Earlier onset of fatigue during exercise or development of chronic fatigue or overreaching symptoms
- Increased recovery time following exercise
- Increased number of training days missed due to musculoskeletal injuries or infections

Effects of Eating Disorders on Health

The health problems that can arise from chronic eating disorders are the effects of reduced energy availability and micronutrient deficiencies that are detrimental to the health of the athlete. A major problem with eating disorders is low energy availability, which is defined not simply as low dietary energy intake but rather as the dietary energy intake minus exercise energy expenditure. Energy availability is thus the amount of dietary energy available for other body functions after exercise training. When energy availability is too low, physiological mechanisms reduce the amount of energy used for cellular maintenance, thermoregulation, growth, bone development, and reproduction. Although the compensatory mechanisms tend to restore energy balance and promote survival, health becomes impaired. For female athletes in particular, inadequate intakes of calcium, iron, and B vitamins are a serious concern. Energy and macronutrient deficiencies may affect mood, growth and maturation, endocrine and reproductive function, bone health, and mortality.

Mood

Depression is a common symptom of eating disorders (Thompson and Trattner-Sherman 1993). Increased fatigue, anxiety, anger, and irritability are associated with low levels of energy and carbohydrate intake during periods of dieting to achieve rapid weight loss. Studies of the effects of eating disorders on mood state in athletes are currently lacking.

Growth and Maturation

Stunted growth in adolescent athletes may occur during prolonged periods of inadequate energy, protein, and micronutrient intake. The onset of puberty may be delayed in child athletes, and poor bone development can lead to increased susceptibility to fractures and problems in later life, particularly in girls.

Endocrine and Reproductive Function

Female reproductive function is affected by the negative energy balance that results from disordered eating coupled with intense training. Psychological stress and low body-fat content are other contributing factors that can lead to amenorrhea.

The pulsatile production of **gonadotrophic hormones** (follicle-stimulating hormone [FSH] and luteinizing hormone [LH]) from the anterior pituitary gland is inhibited during prolonged energy deficits, and the ovarian production of the sex steroid hormones estrogen and progesterone drops to extremely low levels (figure 16.2). Laboratory-based studies have shown that LH pulsatility is disrupted within 5 days when young women's energy availability is reduced by more than a third from 190 kJ (45 kcal) to 125 kJ (30 kcal) per kilogram of fat-free mass per day (Loucks and Thuma

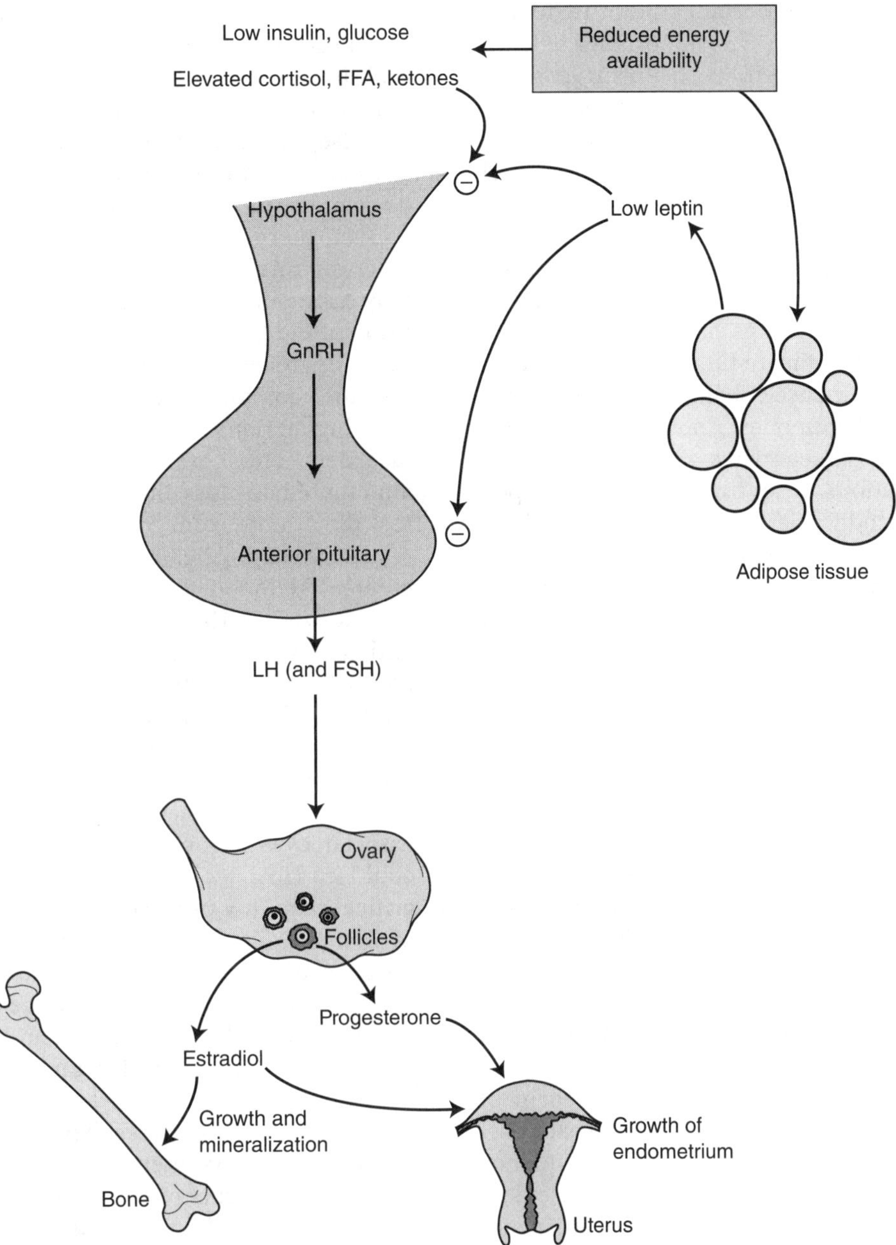

Figure 16.2 The role of hormonal disturbances in the development of amenorrhea and associated health problems, such as osteoporosis. The arrows indicate the effects of reduced energy availability that lead to inhibition (-) of GnRH and LH pulsatility.

2003). Menstrual irregularity ensues, which may be followed by amenorrhea and absence of **ovulation**. In this state, the person is infertile, and her endocrine status is akin to that of a postmenopausal woman. LH pulsatility reflects the pulsatile secretion of gonadotrophic-releasing hormone (GnRH) from the hypothalamus, and the GnRH pulse generator is influenced directly or indirectly by the levels of certain fuel substrates (glucose, free fatty acids, and ketones) and hormones (insulin, cortisol, growth hormone, and leptin). One or more of these is thought to constitute the signal to disrupt GnRH pulsatility in conditions of low energy availability. The most important of these may be **leptin**, which is an adipocyte-derived protein hormone that conveys a signal of the amount of energy stores in adipose tissue to the central nervous system. Recent advances in leptin physiology have established that the main role of this hormone is to signal energy availability in energy-deficient states.

Leptin also plays an important role in regulating neuroendocrine function. The importance of leptin in the reproductive system has been suggested by the reproductive dysfunction associated with leptin deficiency and resistance in both animal models and humans as well as the ability of leptin to accelerate the onset of reproductive function in animals Normal women have a pulsatile release pattern of leptin that is significantly associated with the variations in LH and estradiol levels. Studies in animals and human beings have shown that low concentrations of leptin are fully or partly responsible for starvation-induced changes in reproductive, thyroid, and IGF hormones. Anorexia nervosa and exercise-induced amenorrhea are associated with low concentrations of leptin and a similar spectrum of neuroendocrine abnormalities. It has been shown that leptin can restore ovulatory menstrual cycles and improve reproductive, thyroid, and IGF hormones and bone markers in hypothalamic amenorrhea (Chan and Mantzoros 2005).

The long-term effects of athletic amenorrhea on fertility are still unclear, although some evidence suggests that the reproductive deficiencies associated with amenorrhea are reversible when the problem is treated (Mishell 1993). Although low body-fat levels per se have not been implicated as the specific cause of menstrual dysfunction, evidence suggests that low energy availability is the major causal factor (Loucks 2006). Studies show that restricting energy intake below a critical threshold amount causes metabolic and hormonal adaptations. These changes may be mediated, at least in part, by the hormone leptin.

Athletic amenorrhea is an extreme form of menstrual dysfunction. Less-severe disturbances of the menstrual cycle, including reduced frequency of periods (oligomenorrhea) and luteal-phase deficiency, can result in depressed estrogen levels. Furthermore, in adolescent female athletes, the onset of puberty and **menarche** can be delayed (Manore 2002).

Bone Health

Ovarian steroid hormones, particularly estradiol, facilitate calcium uptake into bone (figure 16.2) and inhibit bone resorption; therefore, amenorrhea may predispose female athletes to osteoporosis, which is a premature loss of bone quality and quantity. This condition can occur despite the fact that load-bearing physical activity induces greater bone-mineral density (BMD). Weight-bearing, high-impact, fast movement exercise using a wide range of muscle groups and exceeding 70% of aerobic capacity or 70% of one-repetition maximum weightlifting appear to be most effective for bone building. This effect, however, is specific to the bones that receive the most impact stress during exercise, and even this degree of protection may not be enough to prevent net demineralization of bone in the face of inadequate estrogen secretion. In fact, there seems to be a threshold of dietary calcium intake below which physical activity may have minimal effect on increasing bone mass (Bloomfield 2001). Athletes with eating disorders have decreased spinal vertebral bone-mineral densities compared with normal values, but they have higher densities than nonathletes with eating disorders. Thus, exercise training may lessen the amount of bone loss, but exercise alone cannot protect the athlete from osteoporosis. Abnormal and restrictive eating behaviors seem to be related to a greater likelihood of fractures (Bennell, Matheson, and Heevwisse 1999; Golden 2002). Bone strength and the risk of fracture depend on the density and internal structure of bone mineral and on the quality of bone protein, which may explain why some people suffer fractures while others with the same BMD do not.

The withdrawal of estrogens at any age is associated with bone loss and reduced BMD that could lead to osteoporosis if prolonged and is more critical than low progesterone levels for the onset of bone demineralization (Cumming 1996). The absence of menstrual cycles and the associated low plasma estradiol levels may decrease BMD to such an extent that fractures occur under minimal impact loading (Snow-Harter 1994; Cumming 1996).

Peak bone mass is reached during the first 3 decades of life. Women attain 95% of maximum density by 18 years of age, and all women experience age-related bone loss after they reach their peak. Therefore, maximizing peak bone mass during the formative years is of utmost importance. Because the 2 to 3 years that constitute the pubertal growth spurt are accompanied by deposition of 60% of final bone mass, any dietary inadequacies and disruptions of the normal menstrual cycle may impair bone formation more severely at that time than at any other (Golden 2002; Sabatini 2001; Snow-Harter 1994). A female athlete's BMD reflects her cumulative history of energy availability and menstrual status as well as her genetic endowment and exposure to other nutritional, behavioral, and environmental factors. As is the case with sufferers of anorexia nervosa, athletes who experience estrogen deficiency because of low energy availability are usually chronically undernourished and have inadequate protein and micronutrient intakes, which further reduces the rate of bone formation. Low energy availability may also suppress bone formation through effects on other hormones, including cortisol and leptin.

As shown in figure 16.3, bone loss accelerates in women after the age of 40 to 50 years, when menopause occurs and when the ovaries stop producing estrogen. Child and adolescent female athletes who experience eating disorders are at high risk for osteoporosis because the premature cessation of estrogen production resulting from hormonal changes associated with reduced energy availability means that their peak bone mass will not be as high as it otherwise would have been. All physically active women who lose their periods because of heavy training or eating disorders are strong candidates for premature bone loss. Typically, they lose 2% to 6% of bone each year, which possibly results in the loss of 25% of total bone mass (Snow-Harter 1994). The result is that they reach the fracture threshold sooner than women who have normal menstruation up to menopause.

Studies report that the total number of years of regular menstrual cycles predicts lumbar spine BMD more accurately than any other training, dietary, or menstrual factor (Montagnani, Arena, and Maffulli 1992; Myburgh, Bachrach, and Lewis 1993). Over the past 15 years, numerous studies have reported that women with menstrual-cycle irregularities have BMD values that are significantly lower than those of normally menstruating female athletes and nonathletes (Kazis and Iglesias 2003). Consequently, the present concern is that many female athletes whose rigorous training schedules and restricted dietary practices have led to extended periods of amenorrhea may have suffered irreversible bone loss.

The development of osteoporosis is also accelerated by inadequate dietary intake of vitamin D or calcium (see chapter 10), which is an additional concern for athletes with eating disorders (Manore 2002). When amenorrhea is present, increasing the consumption of calcium to 120% of the RDA appears to help bones maintain density and develop properly. Such nutrition guidance should be given to low-body-weight women with amenorrhea.

The three conditions that are prevalent in female athletes—amenorrhea, disordered eating, and osteoporosis—are collectively known as the **female athlete triad syndrome** (see figure 16.4) (Nattiv et al. 2007). This has more recently been introduced as relative energy deficiency in sports (RED-S) (Mountjoy et al. 2014) with or without disordered eating or eating disorders. The underlying problem of RED-S is an inadequacy of energy to support the range of body functions involved in optimal health and performance (Mountjoy et al. 2014). Disordered eating underpins a large proportion of cases of low energy availability, but other situations, such as a mismanaged program to quickly reduce body mass or body fat, or an inability to match energy intake with high energy expenditure due to an

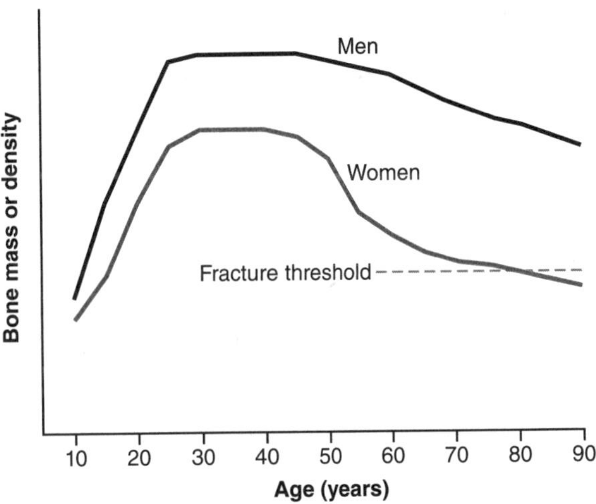

Figure 16.3 Changes in total bone mass or bone density with age in men and women. Peak bone mass is reached in the early 20s, and all women experience age-related bone loss after that. Note the drastic fall in bone mass following the age of the menopause (40-50 years). For men, bone mass is higher and relatively well maintained with only a gradual fall in later years. People (particularly women) with a lower than average peak bone mass reach the critical threshold for fractures at an earlier age.

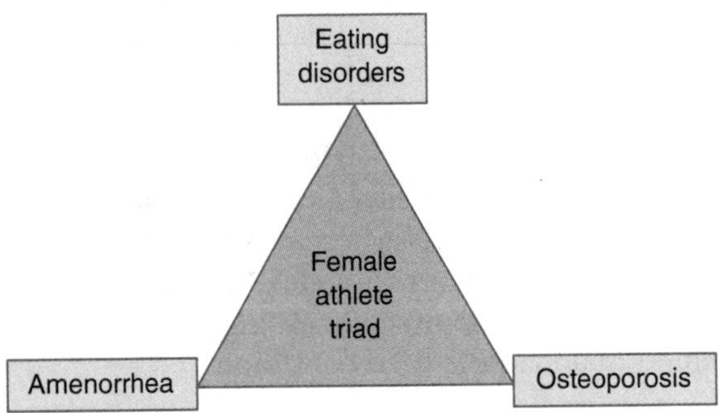

Figure 16.4 The female athlete triad syndrome (also known as relative energy deficiency in sports, RED-S).

extreme exercise commitment, may occur without the psychological problems that are associated with most eating disorders (Loucks 2004). Any female athlete is at risk, but women who participate in sports in which low body fat is advantageous (e.g., endurance running and gymnastics) or required (i.e., weight-category sports such as rowing and martial arts) are at the highest risk. Some studies indicate that the risk of musculoskeletal injuries is increased in those who suffer from the syndrome (Thein-Nissenbaum et al. 2011).

There has been some speculation that a male athlete triad exists, especially since two studies on male cyclists have found low bone-density values compared with controls (Rector et al. 2008; Smathers, Bemben, and Bemben 2009). Smathers, Bemben, and Bemben (2009) reported that 9% of male competitive cyclists compared with only 3% of age- and body mass-matched controls were classified as osteoporotic (i.e., had BMD >2.5 SD below normal), and as many as 25% of the cyclists compared with 10% of the controls were classified as osteopenic (i.e., had bone density between 1.0 and 2.5 SD lower than normal peak density but not low enough to be classified as osteoporotic). Rector et al. (2008) found that 63% of their cohort of recreational male cyclists had osteopenia of the spine or hip compared with 19% of a comparison group of runners. The authors concluded that, after controlling for age, body weight, and bone-loading history, cyclists were 7 times more likely to have osteopenia of the spine than runners. These effects may relate to the sport of cycling (which is a non-weight bearing form of exercise) and the low body fat content of professional male cyclists (see chapter 14) rather than the male athlete triad. However, a review of the literature by Tenforde et al. (2016) has presented evidence that an analogous process to the female athlete triad may occur in male athletes. The review indicated that some male athletes may experience adverse health issues that parallel those associated with the female athlete triad, including low energy availability (with or without disordered eating), low gonadotropic hormone secretion and associated hypogonadism, and low bone mineral density. As a result, male athletes experiencing these issues may be predisposed to developing bone stress injuries, and these injuries are likely to be the first presenting feature of associated male athlete triad conditions.

Mortality

Death rates from eating disorders among athletes are not known, but among patients with anorexia nervosa in the general population, increased mortality has been reported to range from less than 1% to as high as 18% (Thompson and Trattner-Sherman 1993). In patients with anorexia nervosa, death is usually caused by excessive fluid and electrolyte disturbance or is the result of suicide. Information on mortality in bulimia nervosa is not available, but clearly some deaths occur due to complications from vomiting behavior or suicide. The abuse of drugs, including diuretics, laxatives, **emetics** (which promote vomiting), and diet pills that commonly contain stimulants (e.g., amphetamines), is frequently reported among athletes with eating disorders (Sundgot-Borgen and Larsen 1993), and excessive or inappropriate use of some of these drugs may contribute to health problems and mortality in some cases. If dehydration or electrolyte disturbances are present because of an eating disorder, the athlete is at risk for cardiac arrest during exercise.

Treatment and Prevention of Eating Disorders

Perhaps the most effective means of preventing or treating eating disorders among athletes is education. Although educating athletes about the risks of eating disorders is only one element of a comprehensive program designed to prevent and treat disordered eating in athletes, many eating disorders may persist because of a lack of understanding of the effects they can have on health. Many people with eating disorders do not seem to know what constitutes a balanced meal or a normal pattern of eating. Because of misconceptions and poor understanding of nutritional principles, athletes may have an irrational fear of admitting (even to themselves) that they have a problem. Therefore, early diagnosis is vital because eating disorders are more difficult to treat the longer they progress. Eating disorders may also persist after appropriate education and counseling.

Eating disorders are extremely complex examples of psychological dysfunction. The coexistence of exercise dependence and depression is common among athletes with eating disorders. Some evidence suggests that a coincidence of an eating disorder with depression is most effectively treated by addressing the depressive illness first through a combination of therapy and antidepressant medication (Roth and Fonagy 1998). Managing depression is the immediate concern because it is the most life threatening. Treatment of the eating disorder would follow, generally in the form of cognitive-behavioral therapy for bulimia nervosa or interpersonal therapy for anorexia nervosa (Roth and Fonagy 1998). For athletes with long-term conditions, the readiness to listen and accept advice should be assessed with a mental health professional.

After the athlete's cooperation is gained, nutritional counseling can begin. The athlete's body weight and percent body fat should be measured to establish realistic goals, which also depend on the nature of the athlete's sport. An athlete who agrees to comply with all treatment regimens can continue to train and compete, but the athlete must be monitored closely. Effective treatment must always take precedence over sport.

Excessive exercising can aggravate medical complications of eating disorders (e.g., worsening electrolyte disturbances through sweating) (Pomeroy and Mitchell 1992). Exercise is employed in the treatment of depression and eating disorders in nonathletes (Beumont et al. 1994; Byrne and Byrne 1993), so a continued level of moderate exercise is preferable to stopping the athlete from exercising altogether. Nevertheless, the benefits of continued exercise should be weighed against the potential risks in each case. Furthermore, the exercise should be supervised, and signs of exercise dependence should be closely monitored.

The treatment of an athlete with an eating disorder should follow a team approach and incorporate a physician, dietitian, mental health practitioner, physiologist, and psychologist. These professionals all encourage the athlete to practice healthy eating habits and reinforce the message that the consequences of the condition are deterioration of health and sports performance. According to Thompson and Trattner-Sherman (1993), athletes should maintain a minimum body weight that is not less than 90% of "ideal" health-related body weight.

Athletes who have been amenorrheic for more than 6 months should be assessed for BMD and considered for hormone replacement therapy. Affected athletes should be referred to a dietitian for nutrition counseling and to have their energy availability estimated. Adequate amounts of bone-building nutrients such as calcium (1,000-1,300 mg/day), vitamin D (400-1,000 IU/day), and vitamin K (60-90 mg/day) are needed. Adequate protein intake is another concern. Increased energy availability should continue until menses resume and are maintained during training and competition.

Coaches should understand the influence that they can have on their athletes' eating and weight-control behaviors. Although the exact causes of eating disorders remain unknown, highly motivated but uninformed young athletes' pressure to succeed and satisfy the coach's demands can first result in dieting followed by unhealthy eating behaviors. If such behavior is reinforced by success and praise from the coach, it could lead to a full-blown eating disorder. Coaches should not comment on an athlete's body size, weight, or percentage of body fat. These comments should be left to the dietitian, who can advise the athlete on healthy eating and set up a structured, supervised weight-loss program when deemed necessary. For a more detailed discussion of the prevention, management, and treatment of eating disorders among athletes, see the comprehensive review by Torstveit and Sundgot-Borgen (2014).

Key Points

- Eating disorders are characterized by gross disturbances of eating behavior. The major disorders are associated with abnormally low food intake (anorexia nervosa) and bouts of binge eating followed by vomiting (bulimia nervosa). If left undiagnosed and untreated, eating disorders can have detrimental effects on sports performance and damaging, long-lasting effects on health.
- A higher incidence of eating disorders seems to occur among athletes compared with nonathletes, and female athletes have a much greater prevalence compared with male athletes. Classically defined anorexia nervosa does not seem to be much more prevalent in the female athlete population than it is in the general population, but bulimia nervosa and subclinical eating disorders seem to be more prevalent among female athletes than among female nonathletes.
- The prevalence of eating disorders appears to be higher among female athletes who compete in endurance and weight-category sports and is especially high in those

who participate in aesthetic sports, such as gymnastics and dance, compared with those who compete in team sports, power sports, and technical sports. Presumably, the higher prevalence is related to the importance of leanness in these sports or to the perceived advantage of competing in a lower weight category.

- Risk factors for eating disorders include gender, dieting, participation in an athletic lifestyle, and certain personality traits.
- Eating disorders are commonly associated with exercise dependence and depression.
- The precise causes of eating disorders are not known, and an eating disorder can progress from an initial desire or requirement to lose weight into a pathological fear of gaining weight. Highly motivated but uninformed, young, female athletes are probably most at risk.
- The major problem in eating disorders is low energy availability, which is defined as dietary energy intake minus exercise energy expenditure. When energy availability is too low, physiological mechanisms reduce the amount of energy used for cellular maintenance, thermoregulation, growth, bone development, and reproduction. Although the compensatory mechanisms tend to restore energy balance and promote survival, health becomes impaired.
- Eating disorders are likely to be detrimental to sports performance, although this consequence depends on the severity and duration of the disorder and the nature of the sport. Athletes who experience eating disorders may have low glycogen stores, be dehydrated, or exhibit electrolyte disturbances, so high-intensity and endurance exercise performance can be affected.
- Prolonged episodes of negative energy balance or of bingeing and purging are likely to result in micronutrient deficiencies that are detrimental to the health of the athlete. For female athletes in particular, inadequate intakes of calcium, iron, and B vitamins are a serious concern. Energy and macronutrient deficiencies are likely to affect mood, endocrine status, growth, reproductive function, and bone health.
- Athletic amenorrhea may predispose female athletes to premature osteoporosis because of the ovaries' failure to produce estrogen. This condition can occur despite the fact that load-bearing physical activity induces greater bone-mineral density.
- Amenorrhea, disordered eating, and osteoporosis are collectively known as the female athlete triad syndrome. Any female athlete is at risk, but women who participate in sports in which low body fat is advantageous or required have the highest risk.

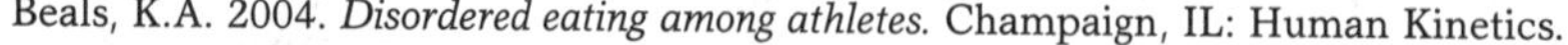

Recommended Readings

Beals, K.A. 2004. *Disordered eating among athletes.* Champaign, IL: Human Kinetics.

Beumont, P.J.V., J.D. Russell, and S.W. Touyz. 1993. Treatment of anorexia nervosa. *Lancet* 26:1635-1640.

Brownell, K.D., and J. Rodin. 1992. Prevalence of eating disorders in athletes. In *Eating, body weight and performance in athletes: Disorders of modern society,* edited by K.D. Brownell, J. Rodin, and J.H. Wilmore, 128-143. Philadelphia: Lea and Febiger.

Byrne, S., and N. McLean. 2001. Eating disorders in athletes: A review of the literature. *Journal of Science and Medicine in Sport* 4:145-159.

Clark, N. 1993. How to help the athlete with bulimia: Practical tips and case study. *International Journal of Sport Nutrition* 3:450-460.

Garner, D.M., L.W. Rosen, and D. Barry. 1998. Eating disorders among athletes: Research and recommendations. *Child and Adolescent Psychiatric Clinics of North America* 7:839-857.

Mountjoy, M., J. Sundgot-Borgen, L. Burke, S. Carter, N. Constantini, C. Lebrun, N. Meyer, R. Sherman, K. Steffen, R. Budgett, and A. Ljungqvist. 2014. The IOC consensus statement: beyond the Female Athlete Triad—Relative Energy Deficiency in Sport (RED-S). *British Journal of Sports Medicine* 48 (7): 491-497.

Nattiv, A., A.B. Loucks, M.M. Manore, C.F. Sanborn, J. Sundgot-Borgen, M.P. Warren, and American College of Sports Medicine. American College of Sports Medicine position stand: The female athlete triad. 2007. *Medicine and Science in Sports and Exercise* 39 (10): 1867-1882.

Redman, L.M, and A.B. Loucks. 2005. Menstrual disorders in athletes. *Sports Medicine* 35:747-755.

Sundgot-Borgen J. 1993. Prevalence of eating disorders in female elite athletes. *International Journal of Sport Nutrition* 3:29-40.

Tenforde, A.S., M.T. Barrack, A. Nattiv, and M. Fredericson. 2016. Parallels with the female athlete triad in male athletes. *Sports Medicine* 46 (2): 171-182.

Thompson, R.A., and R.T. Sherman. 2010. *Eating disorders in sport*. New York: Routledge.

Torstveit, M.K., and J. Sundgot-Borgen. 2014. Eating disorders in male and female athletes. In *Sports nutrition*, edited by R.J. Maughan, 513-525. Oxford: Blackwell Science.

Wilmore, J.H. 1991. Eating and weight disorders in female athletes. *International Journal of Sport Nutrition* 1:104-117.

Personalized Nutrition

Objectives

After studying this chapter, you should be able to do the following:

- Describe personalized nutrition
- Describe periodized nutrition
- Discuss the usefulness of nutrigenomics in sport
- Describe some differences in dietary guidelines for athletes in different age groups
- Describe some differences in dietary guidelines for female athletes
- Describe some nutrition guidelines for specific sports and situations

Products designed to meet specific personal needs are increasingly common. You can design your own shoes to your liking, get a shirt with your name on it, and so on. We also see this trend in medicine. *Precision medicine* was a term introduced in the United States to describe medical solutions that are personalized based on genetic tests. The argument is that having genetic information makes it possible to give better medication to patients. In nutrition and sport nutrition, we see a similar movement toward personalization.

There is no one-size-fits-all approach to sport nutrition, but there is still a question of how to develop a **personalized nutrition** plan. In this book, we mainly discuss the science of nutrition, but, with a few exceptions, we have not really discussed how the science should be translated to practical application. Much of the advice in this book is based on laboratory-based research studies and is expressed in units of dietary components (for example g/kg carbohydrate) rather than foods. Translating theoretical concepts to practical applications is usually the task of a practitioner (e.g., sport nutritionist, dietician, support staff, coach), but sometimes athletes have to figure this out for themselves. Extrapolating information from studies and applying it to real-life situations is not easy and is complicated by the fact that practitioners often need to make decisions quickly (minutes to hours) and science evolves slowly (months to years). The practitioner cannot usually ask athletes to wait until a more relevant research project is done. In previous chapters, we discussed carbohydrate, fat, protein, fluids, vitamins, and minerals in isolation. However, practitioners who work with athletes will have to use a more holistic approach that translates the individual athlete's needs for carbohydrates, fat, protein, fluids, and micronutrients into appropriate food choices and serving sizes. Athletes eat foods, not nutrients. This holistic approach is an important part of personalized nutrition. Many people, ourselves included, believe that personalized nutrition is the future of sport nutrition, but there is not yet a consensus about what personalized nutrition means.

Personalized nutrition plans provide advice on diet and supplements that is tailored to meet specific nutritional needs based on a person's phenotype, genotype, sex, age, and goals. The rules and restrictions regarding food availability will be different in different sports, and people have different preferences and tolerances. There are different physiological demands for different sports and positions. In general, however, differences in sport-specific factors (e.g., intensity, duration, goals) are far greater than the physiological differences. Thus, personalized nutrition in sport often focuses on these factors.

In this chapter, we focus on the practical applications of the information provided in previous chapters and the complications of converting science into meaningful advice. We will first discuss evidence that can inform personalized nutrition plans. Personalized nutrition must begin with the identification of factors that influence personal nutrition needs and the relative contributions of these factors and then identify the most important components of a diet plan that will meet the athlete's needs.. The following are the factors that should be considered when making a personalized nutrition plan:

Goals

Winning
Personal bests
Optimal performance
Finishing
Losing weight
Maintaining good health
Gaining muscle

Event

Duration of exercise
Intensity of exercise
Playing position (in team sports)
Sport type (e.g., track athletics)
Discipline (e.g., middle distance running)
Activity (e.g., competition)
Race distance (e.g., 1,500 m)
Training load

Individual

Genetics
Body mass
Fitness
Sweat rate
Metabolism
Preferences
Tolerances

Environment

Weather
Altitude

Genetic Influences

Undoubtedly, there is a significant genetic component to the impact of nutrition on health and the ability to adapt to training and exercise performance, and, not surprisingly, the media has a strong interest in this. Numerous companies offer genetic tests that provide information about your genome and various health-related outcomes. The Human Genome Project and advances in DNA sequencing technologies have revolutionized the identification of genetic disorders. Continually developing technological advances have radically changed genetic testing from an expensive and burdensome undertaking to one that is rapid, less costly, and serves many purposes. The utility of next-generation sequencing has established the diagnoses for hundreds of genetic disorders. The availability of genomic information has led to questions of whether there is a clinical benefit of sequencing the genomes of people who are not seeking diagnoses (i.e., generally healthy people) to provide anticipatory insights for their health care. These methods have also been criticized because there is little evidence on which to base conclusions and advice. We have seen these techniques offered to athletes to look at performance issues, but there are virtually no studies in this area, so it is difficult to draw conclusions with confidence. To provide an athlete with meaningful advice based on genetic tests, we need to understand gene–nutrient–exercise interactions (known as **nutrigenomics**, but studies in this area are very limited. Nutrigenomics is a demanding line of research because of the rigorous controls needed on all aspects of an intervention, the large sample sizes required (there is the expectation of a small effect size), and the high research costs. Progress in personalized sport nutrition can occur only if we are committed to carefully planned and well-executed human research in the future.

Let's look at an example. Current recommendations for carbohydrate intake are between 0 and 90 g per hour of exercise depending on the goals, the level of the athlete, and the duration of exercise. This is a very large range. From research studies, we know that there is a dose–response relationship during prolonged exercise (e.g., 60 g/h would result in better performance than 30 g/h). It is possible that genetic differences affect people's responses to carbohydrate feeding. Some people might benefit more than others, but this is pure speculation because we have no data to support this hypothesis. We could theorize which genes might be responsible for possible differences in response to the same carbohydrate feeding.

In studies, however, responses have been quite similar, and even if genetic differences exist they would be small. The differences in aerobic exercise performance with carbohydrate intakes of 30 g/h versus 90g/h would be several magnitudes larger than the genetic influences. Therefore, it is fair to conclude that, at least in this example, the other factors would probably far outweigh the influence of a genetic component. There is one exception, which is sensitivity to caffeine. It is clear that responses to caffeine differ between individuals, and it turns out that this relates to certain genes. In chapter 11 we discussed that CYP1A2 is a gene that regulates the breakdown of caffeine and determines the rate at which a person metabolizes caffeine, and sensitivity to caffeine is mostly determined by the gene ADORA2A. So measuring these genes will give some insight into how a person will respond to caffeine. This example, however, is unique, and we don't have many other single genes that predict relevant outcomes for athletes that are performance related.

Turning Science Into Practice

In previous chapters, we discussed science, mechanisms, physiology, and biochemistry in a bit of detail. We use studies as examples, and we give recommendations based on the evidence. Some translation is required, however, to turn these recommendations into practical advice. For example, we need to convert nutrient recommendations into foods or beverages that can be consumed by the athlete and we need to consider how relevant the conditions of a laboratory study might be to the athlete's actual sporting event and how nutrition can be used to support the athlete's particular goals on any given day.

Turning Nutrient Recommendations Into Foods

Recommendations for a specific nutrient may be given in grams per day or grams per meal, but this needs to be translated into how much of a certain food must be eaten to supply the recommended amount of the nutrient. For example, assume the recommendation is to consume 20 g of high-quality protein per meal. This may be meaningless to an athlete, who eats foods rather than protein. What does 20 g mean in food items? Dietitians are trained to make these conversions, but for an athlete, it is not always easy to do this. Table 17.1 gives examples of different foods in different amounts that contain 20 g of protein (the leucine and essential amino acid contents are also indicated in this table). In chapter 8 we discussed the importance of leucine and essential amino acids in driving optimal protein synthesis following resistance exercise training. Figure 17.1 gives examples of products

TABLE 17.1 Foods That Provide 20 g of Protein

Food	Typical portion size	Amount needed for 20 g protein	Energy content in the amount needed for 20 g protein	Total essential amino acids (EAA) (g)	Leucine in the amount needed for 20 g protein (g)
Bread (white)	75 g (2.6 oz)	238 g (8.4 oz)	2,385 kJ (570 kcal)	6.48	1.48
Spaghetti (boiled)	50 g (1.8 oz)	667 g (23.5 oz)	2,435 kJ (582 kcal)	10.11	2.20
Milk (semi-skimmed)	195 g (6.9 oz)	606 g (21.4 oz)	1,182 kJ (283 kcal)	10.27	2.03
Egg (raw)	60 g (2.1 oz)	160 g (5.6 oz)	979 kJ (234 kcal)	9.58	1.63
Steak, stewing (raw)	175 g (6.2 oz)	99 g (3.5 oz)	729 kJ (174 kcal)	9.16	1.60
Chicken (roasted)	85 g (3 oz)	75 g (2.6 oz)	449 kJ (107 kcal)	8.52	1.49
Lentils (boiled)	155 g (5.5 oz)	263 g (9.3 oz)	1,115 kJ (266 kcal)	7.91	1.55
Potato (new, boiled)	150 g (5.3 oz)	1,333 g (47 oz)	3,972 kJ (949 kcal)	7.58	1.27

Notice the very different amounts of food and the different energy contents for the same amount of total protein and for similar amounts of EAA.

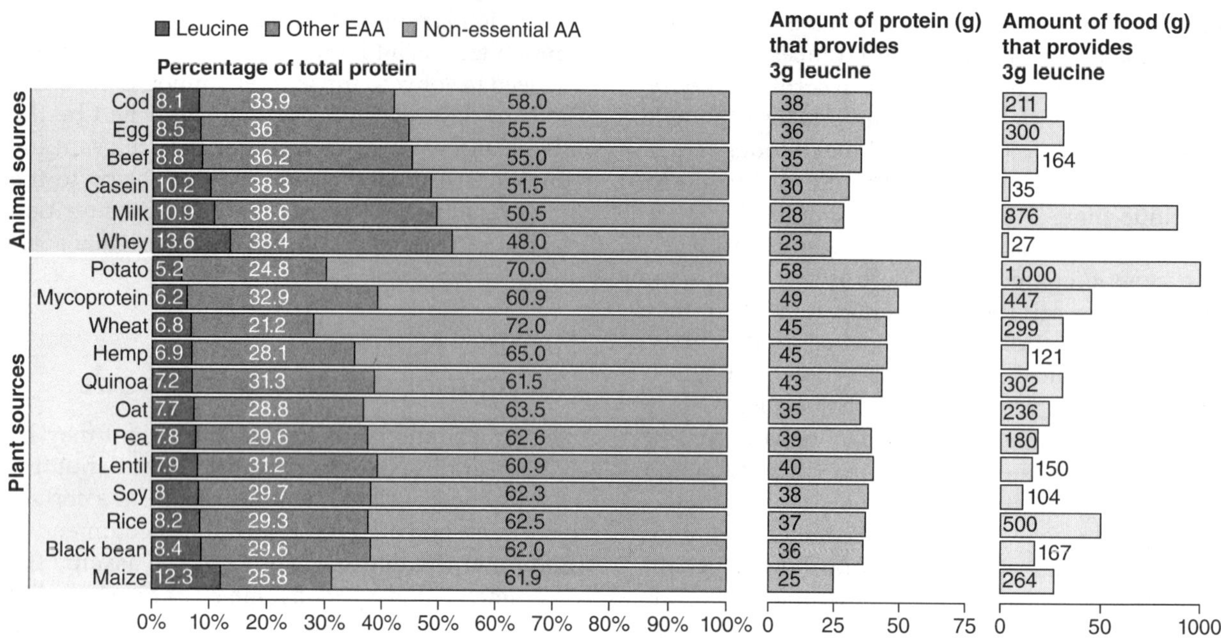

Figure 17.1 The leucine and amino acid contents of different protein sources, the amount of protein that provides 3 g of leucine, and the amount of food that provides 3 g of leucine. To convert from grams to ounces divide the amount in grams by 28.

Based on data from van Vliet, Burd, and van Loon (2015).

TABLE 17.2 Leucine and BCAA Contents of Various Protein Sources

Protein source	Leucine, g/100 g protein	BCAA, g/100 g protein
Whey protein isolate	14	26
Milk protein	10	21
Egg protein	8.5	20
Muscle (meat) protein	8	18
Soy protein isolate	8	18
Wheat protein	7	15

USDA Food Composition Databases. Available: www.https://ndb.nal.usda.gov/ndb/

that can deliver 3 g of leucine, and table 17.2 gives the leucine and BCAA contents of different protein sources.

Many studies have been done with single ingredients so clear conclusions can be drawn about that ingredient; if foods with many ingredients were used, it would be impossible to draw conclusions about the relative importance of individual ingredients. For example, protein recommendations are mostly based on studies in which a particular protein (e.g., whey) is provided to an athlete and protein synthesis rates are measured over the subsequent 4- to 5-hour period. Conclusions are then drawn about the protein, and these are used to draw up some guidelines. In reality, however, athletes don't always ingest whey protein; they ingest protein with other ingredients (e.g., whey protein plus carbohydrate), or they eat foods that contain protein, carbohydrate, fat, and perhaps fiber. It is highly unlikely that the responses to these foods are similar to the responses to isolated proteins. All these ingredients can affect absorption rates and the delivery of amino acids to the muscle. This must be kept in mind. Researchers in the future should focus on studying foods in addition to isolated ingredients to help with the translation of study findings to practical recommendations.

Sports dietitians are trained to turn the theoretical recommendations of macro- and micronutrient intakes into foods, and these are often provided in grams per kilogram of body weight per day or in grams per minute. For example, in chapter 6, we indicate that the recommended carbohydrate intake during exercise is 30 to 90 g/hour depending on the duration and intensity of the activity. Figure 17.2 shows what an athlete needs to ingest to hit that target.

In previous chapters, we mostly discuss macro- and micronutrients separately so each can be examined in detail. When advising an athlete, however, knowledge of each of these components must be translated to meaningful advice. For example, in chapter 6, we learned that carbohydrate intake may be important for performance and carbohydrate intake recommendations increase with increasing duration of exercise. In chapter 9, we learned that fluid balance can play an important role in prolonged exercise performance, especially in hot conditions. To deliver fluids effectively, it was suggested that adding carbohydrate to a drink could be beneficial; however, if too much carbohydrate is ingested, gastric emptying (and therefore fluid absorption in the gut) will be delayed. Thus, it seems there is a conflict in the advice: High carbohydrate intake may be beneficial to hydration, but it can also slow down fluid delivery, which is unwanted in situations where sweat losses are expected to be high. A partial solution to this problem would be to ingest a carbohydrate-electrolyte beverage containing less than 6 g of carbohydrate per 100 ml with most of the carbohydrate as maltodextrin so that the drink will be hypotonic compared with blood plasma. This will not completely solve the problem, however, because carbohydrate concentration appears to be more important than osmolality for gastric emptying (see chapter 5 for more information on regulation of gastric emptying).

Studies Versus Real-Life Competition

Many studies are performed in laboratory situations that do not always translate well to real-life situations. For example, sometimes experiments are conducted in heat chambers. The environmental temperature and humidity are carefully controlled, and the subject pedals a stationary cycle ergometer with a small fan to provide some cooling. The fan's cooling, however, is not comparable to the cooling a cyclist would experience on the road. When riding at high speeds, the cooling due to wind velocity is far greater than the cooling obtained from the fans used in most laboratories. In addition, most environmental chambers do not simulate radiation heat, which could play a major role in real-life situations. When we extrapolate the results from laboratory studies, we need to keep these things in mind so we don't under- or overestimate the real effects.

Carbohydrate sources	Carbohydrate content	Amount that will provide 30 g
Sports drink	6-8 g/100 mL	400-500 mL (15-18 fl oz)
Banana	24-30 g	1-1.5
Gel packet	24-30 g	1-1.5
Energy bar	20-40 g	0.7-1.5
Chews	80 g/100 g	40 g (8 chews)
Jelly beans	94 g/100 g	35 g (15 beans)

Figure 17.2 Common food products that contain 30 g of carbohydrate.

Many studies are also conducted when the participants are in a fasted state because eating before an exercise test can add complexity and cause more variability in the results. Participants are carefully instructed not to eat after 10 p.m. the night before, and they receive no breakfast before their exercise trials. Of course, this is unlikely to reflect a competition situation in which an athlete would be advised to have a good breakfast.

Nutrition to Support the Athlete's Goals

Nutrition should support the training goals, so when giving advice to an athlete, it is important to understand his or her goals. If, for example, the main goal of an endurance athlete is to enhance the oxidative capacity of the muscle, the advice could be to train in a fasted state (i.e., without breakfast) and limit carbohydrate intake during training. If, however, the goal is to perform well in a long race, the advice could be to take on sufficient carbohydrate before and during exercise.

Each training session will have specific goals that need to be supported with nutrition. In some phases of a sport season, an athlete may need to focus on body composition, and in other phases the athlete may need to focus more on performance and recovery. For example, if a soccer player is in the preparation phase of the season, in which the goal is to develop aerobic capacity, the use of high-dose antioxidant supplementation would be discouraged. However, during the competition phase of the season, antioxidant supplementation could reduce soreness and perhaps improve performance.

Periodized nutrition is the planned, purposeful, and strategic use of specific nutrition interventions to enhance the adaptations targeted by each exercise session or to obtain other nonacute effects or benefits that will enhance performance in the long term. **Nutritional training** methods that might be used in a periodized nutrition plan (Jeukendrup 2017a,b) are shown in the sidebar.

For elite athletes, a comprehensive, long-term approach to nutrition and training interactions needs to be carefully planned and monitored by the coach, athlete, and nutrition expert. Although we have very little concrete data on the effects and benefits of periodized nutrition, future developments in sport nutrition support of athletes should seek to integrate practical nutrition and training recommendations into a periodized and personalized approach for each athlete. Integration of nutrition and training methods, such as low-glycogen or fasted training, will place more emphasis on the intelligent periodization of training and nutrition interactions, which is specific to the training bout and the desired physiological adaptation (see chapter 12).

Not all the methods listed in the sidebar are appropriate for all athletes in all sports. For example, training the gut has no value for a sprinter, and training low may be detrimental during a competitive season in team sport athletes.

Consider a professional cyclist who has targeted one of the spring classics as his most important race (often referred to as the A race). This race takes place in April and covers 240 km (150 miles). Fueling during this race will be key to success. In preparation (December-January), the cyclist may include some forms of training low in his or her regular schedule. Because these training sessions are usually a little harder to complete, more recovery time must be allowed. Careful planning of training loads and training techniques should allow optimal adaptation without causing symptoms of overreaching and without compromising the immune system. Typically, riders can tolerate 1 to 2 train-low days per week during their preparation. If they **train low** more than this, they will struggle to recover or the training quality will suffer. A little closer to the start of the season (March), training intensity will increase, and although training low may still play a role, it becomes less important (maybe once per week). Training the gut may be used in the weeks leading up to the A race, and the nutrition plan for the race may be practiced in other races or in training sessions. This is done once or twice per week. As shown in this example, certain methods are selected to achieve certain goals during specific periods of the year. These nutritional training methods are incorporated into the weekly schedule that supports maximal adaptation and minimizes the risk of illness or overtraining. A streamlined integration of nutrition intake and timing of intake, on the one hand, and exercise training, on the other hand, are critical to success.

Specific Populations

Personalization is based on many factors. In the previous sections, age and sex were not mentioned, because when nutrition recommendations are based on goals, exercise intensity, and the other factors related to the event, person, and environment, age and sex are generally less important factors. Most of the differences in responses to particular nutritional strategies that are due to age or sex are relatively small from a practical point of view and are certainly small relative to some

NUTRITIONAL TRAINING METHODS IN A PERIODIZED NUTRITION PLAN 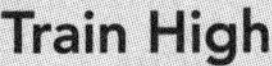

Train High

Training with high muscle and liver glycogen. Carbohydrate intake is high before training, when glycogen is important. There is also a focus on glycogen replenishment postexercise.

Training with a high-carbohydrate diet. Carbohydrate intake is high on a daily basis independent of training, but it may be especially high during and after training sessions.

Train Low

Training twice per day. The first training session will lower muscle glycogen so the second session is performed in a glycogen-depleted state. There is limited or no carbohydrate intake between the two sessions. This may increase the expression of genes relevant to training adaptation.

Training fasted. Training is performed after an overnight fast. Muscle glycogen may be normal or even high, but liver glycogen is low. Training in the fasted state may induce more profound adaptations than training in the fed state (e.g., with a high carbohydrate breakfast).

Training with low exogenous carbohydrate. During prolonged exercise, no carbohydrate or very little carbohydrate is ingested. This may exaggerate the stress response.

Low carbohydrate availability during recovery. No carbohydrate or very little carbohydrate is ingested postexercise. This may prolong the stress response.

Sleep low. Training takes place late in the day, and there is restricted carbohydrate intake before bedtime. Two studies have shown adaptation (fat oxidation) and performance improvements with this practice (for a review on this topic see Jeukendrup 2017a).

Low-carbohydrate, high-fat or ketogenic diets. Training while on a low-carbohydrate diet will result in chronically low glycogen stores.

Training the Gut

Training stomach comfort. This involves ingesting large volumes of fluid (e.g., a carbohydrate-electrolyte beverage) in the resting state in order to accustom the athlete to having a large volume of fluid in his or her stomach so that the perception of fullness decreases over time.

Training gastric emptying. Meals and fluids (usually with high carbohydrate content) are ingested to increase or improve gastric emptying of fluids and nutrients (mainly carbohydrate) and reduce stomach discomfort.

Training absorption. Daily carbohydrate intake or carbohydrate intake during exercise is increased to improve absorptive capacity of the gut and reduce intestinal discomfort.

Training competition nutrition. The competition day nutrition plan is practiced during training sessions in the weeks leading up to competition. This can include practicing all aspects of nutrition strategy as if it were the day of competition to mimic anything an athlete might encounter (e.g., having to drink from a cup, ingest a carbohydrate gel or other ergogenic aid).

Training Dehydrated

Training in a dehydrated state. Training is performed with no fluid or limited fluid intake to allow dehydration to develop to familiarize the athlete with the feelings associated with hypohydration.

Training With Supplements

Using supplements to enhance training. Supplements may allow more training to be performed (e.g., caffeine, creatine, ß-alanine, bicarbonate).

Using supplements to increase muscle mass. Supplements may initiate or increase protein synthesis or increase myofibrillar protein synthesis (e.g., whey protein isolate, essential amino acid mixture, leucine, HMB).

Using supplements to increase oxidative capacity. Supplements may increase mitochondrial biogenesis (e.g., resveratrol, quercetin, conjugated linoleic acid).

See Jeukendrup (2017a,b) for further details.

of the other factors. In the scientific literature on sport nutrition the vast majority of studies have been conducted on men aged 18 to 30 years. In this section, we discuss how some of the specific nutrition requirements may differ for young athletes, older athletes, and female athletes.

Young Athletes

Young athletes (here defined as those aged 8-17 years) have different nutritional needs because they are in a phase of growth, and they have different physiologies and metabolisms than adults. Growth of prepubertal children between the ages of 2 and 10 years occurs at an average rate of 6 cm (2 in.) per year. The median heights and weights for boys and girls are similar and average 87 cm (34 in.) and 12 kg (26 lb) at age 2 and 137 cm (54 in.) and 32 kg (71 lb) by the age of 10. The age for the onset of puberty varies among individuals. It usually occurs in boys between the ages of 12 and 16 and in girls between the ages of 11 and 14. In some African-American girls, puberty begins at about age 9. During puberty, there are large interindividual differences in development.

Children and adolescents need adequate energy intake to ensure proper growth, development, and maturation. For athletic or highly physically active children or adolescents, DRVs will need to be adjusted for the level of physical activity. The onset of the adolescent growth spurt, which requires increased energy intake, is unpredictable, and it is very difficult to estimate energy requirements. It is well known that prolonged inadequate energy intake will result in short stature, delayed puberty, poor bone health, increased risk of injuries, and menstrual irregularities or absence (Bass and Inge 2006).

Children are less metabolically efficient during motor activities, and this results in higher energy requirements per kilogram of body mass compared to adults during most forms of exercise. For example, it has been reported that children require 30% more energy during running (Krahenbuhl and Williams 1992). Therefore, estimations of energy expenditure for children cannot be based on adult data. There are several explanations for the higher energy expenditures of children during running, such as that children have a higher weight-specific resting metabolic rates and have disadvantageous stride rates and lengths (due to shorter limbs) compared with adults, meaning that children have to contract their leg muscles more frequently to cover a given distance than do adults. If the relative exercise intensity is calculated by adjusting treadmill speed to match stride frequency, the differences between adults' and children's energy expenditures and exercise economies disappear (Maliszewski and Freedson 1996).

It is important to educate children to eat healthy and balanced diets and to encourage good eating habits. Aspiring young athletes should also receive specific sport nutrition guidance that includes performance goals and health goals. This can reinforce lifelong eating habits that contribute to overall well-being and may enhance sport performance. Any bad habits developed in childhood and adolescence may be difficult to eradicate later in an athlete's sporting career and should therefore be avoided. Parents, coaches, and support staff must encourage appropriate eating behaviors, but they should avoid paying too much attention to body shape and body weight.

Exercise Metabolism

In adults, the density of mitochondria in skeletal muscle is one of the main determinants of carbohydrate and fat metabolism. In general, the greater the number and size of mitochondria, the higher fat oxidation rates are during exercise. There also seems to be an association between muscle fiber type and substrate metabolism; higher percentage type I fibers favor fat metabolism. Very few studies have investigated muscle fiber composition or mitochondrial density in children. One study reported a similar mitochondrial to myofibrillar volume ratio in children and adults (Bell et al. 1980), which indicates that with growth and maturation, the large increases in muscle mass are paralleled by increases in mitochondria within these fibers.

There appear to be some differences in substrate use between adults and children. Children have lower glycolytic capacities, higher oxidative capacities, and higher rates of fat oxidation (see Riddell 2008 for further details). During heavy exercise, muscle and blood lactate levels are lower in children than in adults, and there is a greater reliance on fat as fuel. Furthermore, prepubertal adolescents have relatively high rates of exogenous glucose oxidation, which may be because they have smaller endogenous carbohydrate reserves. These differences, however, seem to diminish throughout adolescence, especially in boys (Riddell 2008), which suggests that the hormones associated with puberty (i.e., growth hormone, IGF, testosterone, and catecholamines) play a role in regulating energy metabolism in children (Boisseau and Delamarche 2000).

Protein

In order to support their growth and development, children and adolescents have relatively high protein requirements compared to adults. The RDAs for protein in the United States and Canada are between 0.80 and 1.05 g per kilogram of body weight depending on age; the highest recommendations are for 1- to 3-year-olds and the lowest are for 18-year-olds. The protein requirements for young elite athletes are likely to be even higher. In a study of 14-year-old soccer players who played 10 to 12 h/week, nitrogen balance measurements revealed that the estimated daily protein needed to maintain nitrogen balance was 1.04 g per kilogram of body weight per day (Boisseau et al. 2007). It was suggested by the authors of the study that the recommended daily protein intake should be 1.40 g per kilogram of body weight per day (or 75 g/day for these soccer players), which would be well above the RDA of 0.8 g/kg b.m./day (52 g/day) for 14-year-olds in the general population. As is the case in adult athletes (see chapter 8), this requirement is quite easily met due to the higher daily energy intakes of highly active young people. The study was performed in France, and the suggested RDA is still well below the average protein intake of French children in this age group (2.07 g per kilogram of body weight per day). In the United States and Australia, protein intakes in children and adolescents are generally two to three times the RDA. Even in sports in which young athletes reportedly restricted their energy intakes, protein intakes were still between 1.5 and 2 g per kilogram of body weight per day. On the whole, protein requirements do not seem to be of particular concern for young athletes, but be aware that some young people have protein intakes well below the recommended amounts perhaps due to intentional energy restriction for weight loss or vegetarian diets.

Carbohydrate

It is well known that carbohydrate ingestion in adults before and during exercise can delay fatigue and improve endurance performance. Recommendations for carbohydrate intake are highly dependent on the intensity, duration, and type of exercise that is performed by young athletes. Carbohydrate loading to increase muscle glycogen levels is not advised for children (Meyer, O'Connor, and Shirreffs 2007). A relatively high carbohydrate diet is advised, but there is no need to follow a dedicated glycogen-loading regimen.

Numerous studies indicate that children benefit from carbohydrate intake during exercise, but, as in adults, this effect may only be obvious during prolonged exercise of high enough intensity. Many children will be physically active or engage in regular training but may not reach the level of physical activity that would warrant the use of carbohydrate beverages. However, young athletes who train hard and long enough (e.g., at an average intensity of over 60% of their aerobic capacity for 90 minutes or more per day) will probably benefit. Although children younger than 5 years have less efficient carbohydrate absorption, at this age their exercise will not be long enough or have a high enough intensity to require carbohydrate intake during exercise.

To date, there have been no studies investigating the performance effects of carbohydrate or the rate of carbohydrate oxidation in highly trained, elite, young athletes. Due to this dearth of information, we relied on studies undertaken on healthy, physically active boys and girls to inform this section.

Fat

Very few studies have investigated fat intake or fat requirements in physically active children. Although certain fats are important for growth and development, their link to performance is less clear. The usual general recommendation for both adults and children is that 25% to 30% of energy should come from dietary fat, but absolute fat intakes in grams per day are highly dependent on energy expenditure. As in adults, the main priorities are adequate protein and carbohydrate intakes; fat can make up the remaining energy needs. Restricting fat intake in nonobese children has been suggested to impair growth and development, although it is not clear whether this is a direct effect of low fat intake or low energy intake (Butte 2000). If weight loss is required in children who are involved in relatively hard physical training, it seems sensible to reduce fat rather than protein or carbohydrate intakes (see also the section on weight management).

Thermoregulation and Fluid Requirements

One of the main ways people lose heat is through the evaporation of sweat and the associated convection of body heat away from the surface of the skin. Because children have a higher ratio of body surface area to body mass (at the age of 8 years old it is approximately 50% higher than that of an adult) (Rowland 2008), it has been suggested that exercising children should be able to dissipate heat quicker than adults. This should give children an advantage in terms of their thermal homeostasis up to the point at which ambient temperature exceeds skin temperature, after which this advantage is supposedly reversed. In practice, however, adults and active children seem to experience similar core temperatures even when exercising at high ambient temperatures (Inbar et al. 2004). Whether the same finding would occur in young athletes compared to these active (but not competitive) children is yet to be determined.

High sweat rates in hot conditions can result in large fluid and electrolyte losses. In adults, the dehydration caused by this fluid loss has been shown to impair motor control and physical performance (Armstrong, Costill, and Fink 1985), so adults are advised to balance any fluids lost from sweating with fluid intake or to limit losses to no more than 2% of body mass.

There are large differences in sweat rates between children and adults; 9-year-old boys exposed to hot and humid conditions (45 °C [113 °F] and 97% relative humidity had an average sweat rate that was only half of that of men. This muted response (which was also observed in young girls and adult women) is probably due to the underdevelopment of the peripheral sweating mechanism in young children. Once male sex hormone production starts to increase during puberty, the sweat rate increases rapidly.

It seems tempting to speculate that a young athlete's risk of becoming dehydrated during exercise in the heat will also be reduced. Because sweating is the main way of dissipating heat during exercise, it is possible that children's thermoregulation is actually less effective and their core body temperatures could increase more rapidly than adults'. However, studies indicate that the reduced sweat rate does not impair children's ability to lose heat during exercise (Inbar et al. 2004). Instead, it seems that children use different, but equally effective, thermoregulatory mechanisms (Inbar et al. 2004; Falk and Dotan 2008), which are discussed in more detail by Falk and Dotan (2011). Because the extent of dehydration and the risk of developing a heat-related illness seem to be similar between adults and younger athletes, the recommendations regarding fluid replacement are likely to be similar, too.

Young athletes reportedly underestimate the amount of fluid they need to consume during prolonged exercise to stay hydrated, especially in hot and humid conditions and particularly when the only fluid available to them is water. Because thirst is often a poor indicator of fluid needs, it is important to encourage drinking before, during, and after exercise to prevent dehydration. Involuntary hypohydration can reach up to 1% to 2% of body mass loss in boys who are unacclimated and untrained or acclimatized and trained. Although education for parents, coaches, teachers, and young athletes can improve fluid intake, studies have also shown that there are other ways to promote thirst and therefore stimulate drinking. One of these is adding small amounts of sodium chloride to water, because this sensitizes the thirst mechanism through the maintenance of plasma osmolality and reduces the diuretic effect of ingested water while also replacing lost electrolytes (Bar-Or 2001; Rivera-Brown et al. 1999; Manore 2000). Another way is adding carbohydrate to the drink, because this increases the palatability of the beverage. The addition of flavor is another option; in one study, the addition of flavor to a carbohydrate–electrolyte drink helped reduce voluntary dehydration by 32% in heat-acclimatized, trained boys, which was enough to maintain euhydration over a 3-hour period of moderate-intensity intermittent cycling exercise in hot (30°C [86 °F]) and humid (53%-62% relative humidity) conditions (Rivera-Brown et al. 1999).

Current recommendations for fluid replacement in children are scant. The 2007 ACSM position statement titled *Exercise and Fluid Replacement* referred only to the fact that prepubescent children have a lower sweat rate than adults (Sawka et al. 2007). The 2009 and 2016 ACSM position statements titled *Nutrition and Athletic Performance* do not comment on children's or adolescents' needs at all. In contrast, the policy statement reissued by the American Academy of Pediatrics (2000) regarding the fluid replacement guidelines for children during exercise in the heat state that a child who weighs 40 kg (88 lb) should drink 150 ml (5 fl oz) of cold water or flavored, salted beverage every 20 minutes, and an adolescent who weighs 60 kg (132 lb) should drink 250 ml (8 fl oz) every 20 minutes, even if the child does not feel thirsty. In contrast to the guidelines for adults, these are far too general, because they do not consider important factors such as environmental conditions, exercise intensity, acclimatization, and individual differences. Given the current lack of studies investigating the effects of dehydration on children's performance, it is very difficult to give balanced and objective guidelines. At an elite level, it seems sensible to develop an individualized strategy that aims to reduce fluid losses in excess of 2% to 3% of body mass. This can be done by measuring body weight before and after training and correcting for fluid intake to obtain some estimate of sweat rates under different ambient conditions. This would eventually allow the coach or support staff to predict the sweat rates of young athletes in their care in similar conditions and provide a sound basis for fluid intake prescription.

Nutrition Supplements

Supplement use among young athletes is common. In a study of 32 track and field junior athletes selected for Team Great Britain at the World Junior Championships, it was found that 62% were currently using supplements (Nieper 2005). A higher percentage of girls (75%) than boys (55%) were using supplements, although this difference was not statistically significant. This trend may be attributed to a greater awareness among girls, greater genuine need for supplementation (e.g., because of menstrual loss), or possibly advertising campaigns that had a greater influence on girls (Nieper 2005). The most commonly used supplements were those related to health, such as multivitamins, vitamin C, and iron, rather than those related to performance enhancement (Nieper 2005). In a review, McDowall (2007) concluded that the prevalence of supplement use was between 22% and 71% in young athletes (aged 13-19 years). The most frequently cited reasons for using supplements were health benefits, illness prevention, enhancing performance, taste, rectifying a perceived poor diet, and increasing energy, which are similar to reasons reported by adult athletes.

In a study of 403 elite, young, UK athletes (mean age 18 years) that examined the prevalence of supplement (including sports drinks) use, single supplement use was reported by 48.1% (Petroczi et al. 2008). The most popular supplements were sports drinks, which were consumed by 41.7% of all athletes and 86.6% of the supplement users. Other popular supplements included vitamin C (22.8%), multivitamins (22.8%), whey protein (21.3%), creatine (13.4%), echinacea (7.7%), caffeine (5.7%), and iron (4.7%). A few athletes also reported taking ginseng (1.7%) or melatonin (1.0%). Among the desired outcomes resulting from supplement use, maintaining strength was the most frequently cited reason among all athletes in the sample (34.7%) and among supplement users (72.2%) followed by avoiding illness (56.1% of users) and improved endurance (55.2% of users). One-third of the supplement users listed the ability to train longer (30.4%) and recover quickly (32.5%) among the reasons, whereas 23.2% took supplements to remedy an imbalanced diet. Younger elite athletes seemed to be less health conscious and more performance focused than their adult counterparts.

The source of the advice on taking supplements varied and was different for different supplements. It appears that many young athletes decided which nutritional supplements to take without advice. There was, however, considerable overlap between self-managed supplementation and medical advice. A coach's role in advising athletes on supplements, especially in energy drinks and protein, was also apparent. Among health professionals, athletes indicated that advice was sought from nutritionists or physiotherapists. The only exception was iron supplementation, which was taken following a general practitioner's advice.

It is clear that young elite athletes perceive a need for nutritional supplementation. There must be reservations, however, about long-term use, combinations, and appropriate dosages in these athletes. These reservations concern the potential for increased health risks to an otherwise healthy population and the possibility of positive doping tests caused by supplements that contain banned substances. To minimize these potential risks of inappropriate supplement use, increased involvement of nutritionists and health professionals is desirable.

One supplement that has received substantial attention recently is caffeine. Caffeine is one of the most widely used drugs, and energy drinks that contain caffeine are now marketed specifically to young adults and children. Therefore, it is important to understand the effects of caffeine in this population. Energy drinks that contain high concentrations of sugars and caffeine represent the fastest growing segment of the beverage industry. Very few studies have examined the physiological and cognitive effects of caffeine in children; therefore, it is difficult to give sound advice on caffeine use for young athletes. There is evidence, however, that children and adolescents may be particularly vulnerable to the negative effects of caffeine (although they receive similar benefits to adults). Therefore, caffeine should be used with caution. In general, due to health concerns and lack of evidence of efficacy, supplements for younger athletes are not recommended (Meyer, O'Connor, and Shirreffs 2007).

Weight Management and Associated Dangers

Perhaps one of the greatest potential threats to child health is inappropriate weight control in young athletes that could lead to the development of an eating disorder (see chapter 16) or to impaired growth and development. If a reduction in body mass is desired, this should be accomplished gradually and limited to no more than 1.5% of body mass per week and with the supervision of a health care professional. A more rapid rate of weight loss will likely result in muscle protein breakdown, and this may interfere with growth and development. To lose about 0.5 kg (1 lb) of fat in 1 week, one must expend 14,700 kJ (3,513 kcal) more than what is consumed. It is often suggested that the preferred way to do this is to consume 7,350 kJ (1,757 kcal) fewer per week and expend 7,350 kJ (1,757 kcal) more per week by exercising, although this may not be feasible if the training load is already high. When possible, young athletes should be counseled by a registered dietician who has experience of working with young athletes and their families. A lean and light physique is often desired in certain sports, especially in endurance sports, such as distance running, and in aesthetic sports, such as gymnastics. Although in some cases there are clear links to better performance, it is important to be aware that there are also risks of energy deficiency, micronutrient deficiencies, menstrual irregularities in postpubertal girls, impaired bone development, and eating disorders.

Older Athletes

An increasing number of older adults (let's say people over 40 years of age) choose to achieve physical fitness, health, or well-being by participating in recreational or competitive sports. In this subgroup of athletes, performance is often a goal as well. Because of the link between nutrition and health and performance goals, older athletes are often very interested in the topic of nutrition. However, there are very few studies and very few nutrition guidelines for older athletes who are looking to improve their performance.

Changes in Metabolism With Age

One of the main changes with aging is the loss of muscle mass. Sarcopenia, which is characterized by losses in muscle mass, strength, and endurance, affects performance and contributes to other functional consequences of aging. With aging, changes are observed in muscle fibers, protein synthesis, and mitochondrial function. Even in healthy people, muscle strength and power begin to decline around age 25, particularly in the lower extremities, but this decline can be prevented by exercise training. At the age of about 65, the average person will have lost 25% of his or her peak youth strength. By age 80, up to 50% of peak skeletal muscle mass can be lost, which is likely related more to loss of muscle fibers than to fiber atrophy. Training can significantly delay this process, and nutrition may have a role to play as well.

Performance in strength sports declines at an earlier age (probably around 25 years), but peak performance in endurance sports may be seen around the age of 40. In triathlon, for example, performance is maintained until the age of 40; this is followed by modest declines until the age of 50. After age 50, performance times progressively decline at a steeper rate (Bernard et al. 2010; Lepers, Knechtle, and Stapley 2013). It has also been reported that after the age of 55, this decline in endurance performance is more pronounced in women compared to men (Ransdell, Vener, and Huberty 2009).

Energy, Carbohydrate, and Fluids

Energy expenditure is mostly determined by resting metabolic rate and energy expended during exercise. Because muscle is the most metabolically active tissue, a loss of muscle mass will also result in a decrease in energy expenditure. This means that daily energy intake will have to be reduced to avoid weight gain. The loss of muscle mass is a slow and gradual process, so these changes will not happen overnight, but unless a high level of physical activity is maintained or there is a reduction in energy intake, weight gain will be the logical consequence. There are plenty of examples of athletes that struggle with this, but there are also many examples of very lean older athletes.

There are no reasons for the carbohydrate or fluid intake guidelines to be different for older adults if they exercise at similar intensities to younger adults. Carbohydrate requirements are determined primarily by the goals, intensity, and duration of exercise. Older athletes may perform at lower absolute intensities, which will reduce the carbohydrate requirements, but this needs to be established on an individual basis. In many mass participation marathon events many older runners are actually much faster than the average runner, who is younger. A faster running pace means a higher exercise intensity and so the carbohydrate requirements of the older runner are higher than those of the average runner in this situation. There is no evidence that carbohydrate absorption is different in older athletes, so recommendations for daily carbohydrate intake and competition intake in endurance sports are similar to the general recommendations discussed in this book.

It is a similar story for fluids. Fluid losses are a result of metabolic rate (intensity); therefore, the same advice as provided elsewhere in this book (chapter 9) is appropriate. We recommend measuring weight loss during training or competition and drinking to prevent significant dehydration. Keep weight loss to within 2% of body mass (see chapter 9).

Protein

Aging athletes may have increased protein requirements. A common observation is that many older people seem to lose muscle mass and do not respond as well to resistance training. Different responses to resistance exercise may be because older athletes generally lift lower volumes of weight than younger athletes. It has also been suggested that a reduced anabolic responsiveness to hypertrophic exercise may be a key factor in mediating muscle adaptive remodeling in older athletes. If the same amount of protein (e.g., 20 g) is ingested by an elderly (over 60 years of age) person and a young adult, the protein synthesis rates are stimulated a little less in the older person, and this will occur with all meals throughout the day. This can explain why muscle mass decreases over time (see figure 17.3) despite the fact that the rate of protein breakdown does not seem to be different between younger and older adults.

It has been demonstrated (especially by the age of 70 and older) that protein synthesis is lower and there is some **anabolic resistance**. This is especially true at low protein intakes (see figure 17.4). At an intake of 10 g/min, young adults respond with significantly increased protein synthesis, but the elderly do not respond as well. When the protein intake (including leucine) is increased, the difference becomes smaller, and at very high intakes, the difference may be negligible. This means that protein intake recommendations for older athletes should be higher than those for young athletes. There are, however, some unanswered questions. For example, at what age do these increased requirements start? Most studies have been performed in nonathletes older than 70 who are often frail, meaning that they have low levels of physical activity. Decreases in muscle mass can be observed much earlier in life.

Female Athletes

Many publications on female athletes seem to focus on eating disorders. These are serious and important conditions with major consequences, but most female athletes do not have eating disorders. The question remains whether the nutrition recommendations we currently have can be extrapolated to women, because they are mostly based on research with men. Many differences in the physiologies and metabolisms of men and women have been consistently reported. For example, the majority of studies have found there is a relatively greater

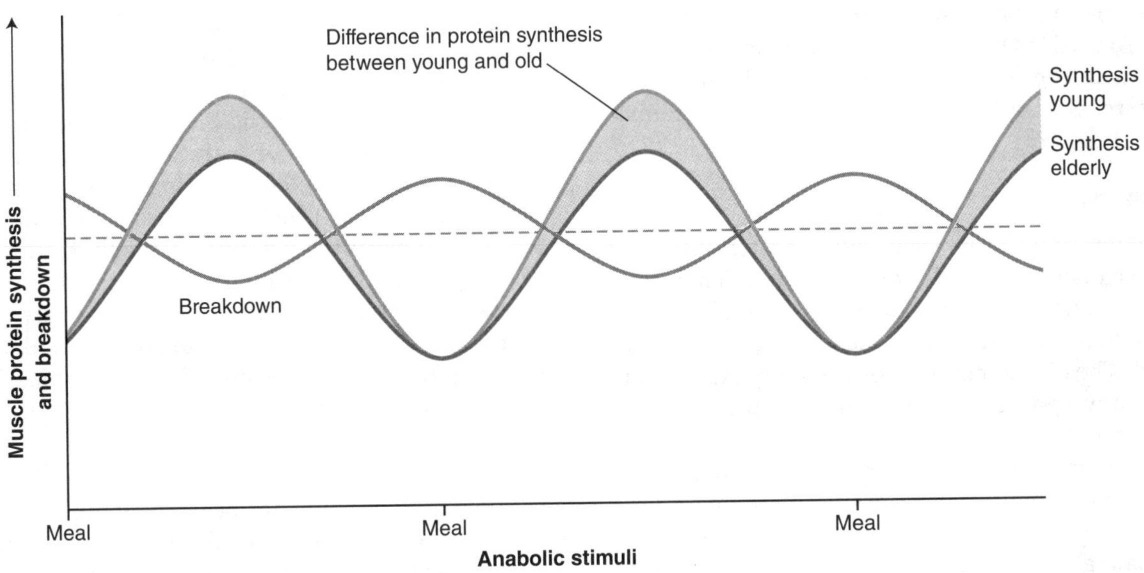

Figure 17.3 Anabolic resistance in the elderly.

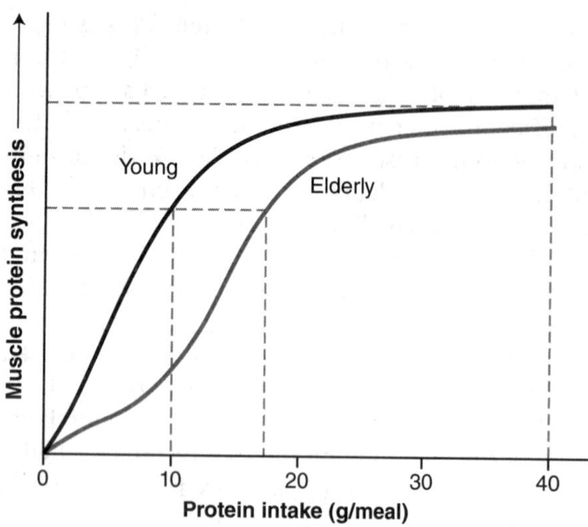

Figure 17.4 Schematic depiction of the concept of anabolic resistance in older people. At low protein intakes, muscle protein synthesis is stimulated less in the elderly. To obtain similar effects of protein synthesis, larger amounts of protein need to be ingested. At very high protein intakes per meal (40 g), differences between young and old are negligible.

fiber area of type I and type II fibers in women compared to men (Simoneau and Bouchard 1989; Staron et al. 2000). Women also have higher circulating levels of 17-ß-estradiol, which can influence fat, carbohydrate, and protein metabolism.

It has been suggested that women have a greater capacity to oxidize fat, that glycogen synthesis may be impaired in women, and that women have different hydration needs. There may also be different micronutrient needs for women. This section will evaluate the evidence to identify whether these differences warrant separate guidelines for female athletes.

Energy

Female athletes are generally smaller and have lower energy expenditures than men. Therefore, their resting metabolic rates are generally lower, and their daily energy intakes should be lower as well. The biggest contributor to energy expenditure in many sport situations is the thermic effect of exercise; therefore, this is the primary component that determines actual energy expenditure. Many male and female athletes are trying to lower their body fat to improve power-to-weight ratios. For female athletes, this often means challenging the boundaries of biological predisposition. When body fat in women is reduced to below 10%, various body functions may be impaired and menstruation may cease. If this is sustained for a long time, it will result in other health complications, including osteoporosis (see chapter 16). From a practical point of view, it is very difficult to determine energy expenditure accurately to calculate energy intake. In cycling, this may be easier because power meters can be used, and in running fairly accurate estimations can be made, but in most other sports, these estimations are relatively inaccurate. Nevertheless, it is worth trying to estimate energy availability as accurately as possible by calculating energy intake minus energy expenditure during exercise. The remaining energy is what is available for basic body functions. The target intake for a healthy female athlete should be about 188 kJ (45 kcal) per kilogram of FFM. For example, for a 60 kg (132 lb) female athlete with 20% body fat and a FFM of 48 kg (106 lb), the energy availability should be greater than $188 \times 48 = 9{,}024$ kJ (2,156 kcal). Any energy spent during training should be added to this number to get the daily energy intake.

Fat and Carbohydrate

Although some studies show that female athletes oxidize more fat during exercise than their male counterparts, these conclusions are rather academic. In most studies, conclusions are based on data expressed per kilogram of FFM to determine whether muscle is different in terms of its ability to oxidize fat in men and women. Expressed in this way, very small differences can be found in some studies but not in others. For example, in a very large sample of 300 subjects (half male and half female), we observed that fat oxidation was higher in women when expressed per kilogram of FFM. This difference, however, was small (see figure 17.5) and probably negligible related to dietary advice. When a group of male and female cyclists was carefully matched for training status, the male cyclists had higher power outputs and thus higher energy expenditures. As a logical result, the men's carbohydrate and fat oxidation rates were higher at the same relative intensity of exercise. Therefore, men oxidize more fat even though the oxidative capacity of the muscle may favor fat oxidation slightly more in women.

Carbohydrate Loading

Carbohydrate loading has been shown to result in high muscle glycogen concentrations and to help performance in some situations. Most studies examining the response of muscle glycogen to an increase in the consumption of dietary carbohy-

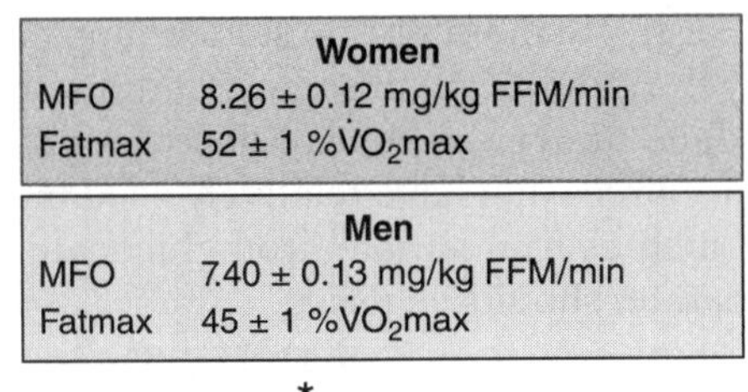

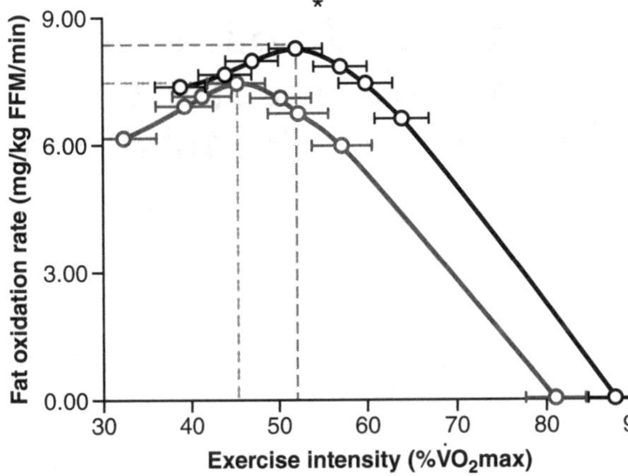

Figure 17.5 Fat oxidation in men and women as a function of exercise intensity. Fat oxidation is expressed in milligrams per kilogram of FFM. When expressed in this way, women tend to have higher maximal fat oxidation (MFO) rates at higher exercise intensities (Fatmax). Asterisk in figure indicates significantly higher maximal fat oxidation rates in women compared with men (P<0.01).

drates, however, have been conducted with predominantly male subjects. Given the attenuation in glycogen use during exercise seen in rodents with 17-ß-estradiol administration and the attenuation observed during exercise with the muscle biopsy method, it had been suggested that women would not be able to supercompensate as well as men.

In one study, muscle glycogen concentration was measured in response to a modified carbohydrate-loading protocol whereby exercise intensity was tapered for 4 days and dietary carbohydrate intake was either 57% or 75% of total energy intake (Tarnopolsky et al. 1995). After the higher carbohydrate intake, male subjects demonstrated a 41% increase in muscle glycogen and a 45% improvement in performance time in an exhaustive exercise bout following 1 hour of cycling at 75% of $\dot{V}O_2$max, whereas the women showed no increase in muscle glycogen and no effect on performance. It was hypothesized that the inability of women to carbohydrate load may have been due to a difference in the enzymatic and transport capacities for glycogen resynthesis and glucose uptake, respectively. The explanation for the difference, however, is likely much more straightforward: The men received a larger amount of carbohydrate than the women. Carbohydrate intake was 4.8 g and 6.4 g per kilogram of body weight per day for women and 6.6 g and 8.2 g per kilogram of body weight per day for men on the low- and high-carbohydrate diets, respectively. In most of the previous studies of carbohydrate loading in men, the dietary carbohydrate intake was greater than 8 g per kilogram of body weight per day. When another study was performed and men and women were given equal carbohydrate amounts per kilogram of body weight per day, there was no difference in glycogen synthesis between men and women. Therefore, there is no physiological difference, but there may be a practical difference as illustrated in the following example.

Consider a 50 kg (110 lb) female athlete who consumes 8,400 kJ/day (2,007 kcal/day). This athlete may consume about 250 grams of carbohydrate per day (or 5 g per kilogram of body weight per day), but she would have to increase her intake by around 60% to bring it up to 8 g per kilogram of body weight per day. Carbohydrate would then account for 6,700 kJ (1,601 kcal) of her total daily energy intake, which leaves only 1,700 kJ (406 kcal) for protein and fat. Although it is not impossible, this is not a practical scenario. In reality, the female athlete will probably increase her carbohydrate intake slightly, but not to 8 g per kilogram of body weight per day (as in the studies in men), and therefore glycogen synthesis may not be quite optimal.

Carbohydrate Intake During Exercise

The effects of carbohydrate intake during exercise have been studied mainly in men. There are a couple of studies, however, that specifically compared female and male athletes and observed no differences. In one study, eight moderately endurance-trained men and eight carefully matched women performed 2 hours of cycling at 67% of $\dot{V}O_2$max and ingested carbohydrate at regular intervals (Wallis et al. 2006). The total amount of carbohydrate in the men and women was the same (and was as high as 90 g/h). Ingested carbohydrate was oxidized at similar rates in men and women during exercise (see figure 17.6). As discussed in chapter 6, the main limiting factor for exogenous carbohydrate oxidation is absorption, and there is no reason to expect that women who eat a similar diet to men would have different absorptive capacities of the gut. Thus, recommendations for

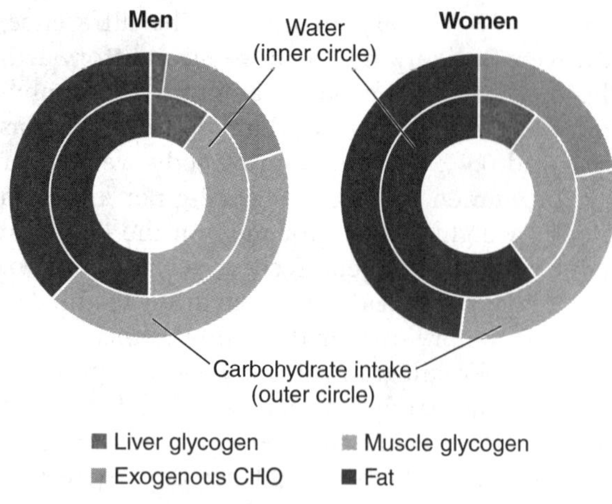

Figure 17.6 The contribution (in percentage of total energy expenditure) of different substrates to energy expenditure in men and women with ingestion of water or carbohydrate during exercise. Overall, there are no major differences in substrate use between men and women.

carbohydrate intake during exercise are not different for women.

Protein

Few studies have looked at protein requirements for female athletes, and protein intake guidelines usually don't specifically mention female athletes. Generally, it is assumed that these requirements are similar to those for men. One study measured nitrogen turnover in female endurance athletes and concluded that an intake of 1.63 g of protein per kilogram of body weight per day was required to maintain nitrogen balance (Houltham and Rowlands, 2014). This is 25% to 30% higher than previously thought (Tarnopolsky 2004), but it is similar to what would be expected for male athletes who perform similar training. Although there is a lot more research to be done, these data suggest that protein intake requirements may increase with exercise training in a similar manner to the requirements in men.

Iron

Iron recommendations for the general population are significantly higher for premenopausal women than for men (18 mg/day versus 8 mg/day) mainly due to regular losses of iron through menstrual bleeding. Female athletes may also struggle with adequate iron intake if their energy intakes are low or if they are vegetarians (see chapter 10). Therefore, it is important to pay extra attention to iron intake and to monitor iron status. Supplementation may be appropriate in some cases, but this should be done under the supervision of a professional. Iron sources that have relatively good bioavailability, such as iron sulfate, iron gluconate, and iron fumarate, should be used.

Nutrition Application in Different Sport Situations and Populations

Nutrition recommendations are usually highly specific to a sport, but they are also influenced by other factors (e.g., environmental conditions, age, sex, body size, playing position in team sports) and by goals (e.g., training adaptation, competition performance, recovery from exercise, weight loss, muscle mass gain, rehabilitation from injury). In addition, some recommendations are dictated by the rules of a sport. For example, in some sports (e.g., basketball), there is constant access to drinks, but in other sports (e.g., soccer), access to drinks is mostly limited to before the start of the game and at halftime; this affects intake patterns and specific intake advice. As another example, carbohydrate loading is used in marathon runners who have time to prepare well for a marathon race, but in team sports that have busy competition schedules, there simply isn't enough time to employ such techniques. In the next sections, we will discuss specific nutrition strategies that can be used in certain situations (e.g., preparation for competition, during competition) or by certain populations (e.g., the injured player, the player with **type 1 diabetes**) in some sports. Of course, we can't discuss all sports, and we do not address all aspects of nutrition in the sports we do discuss. We provide a few examples from popular sports and discuss some of the main nutrition issues and practicalities in these sports. We do not include citations in this part of the chapter because the information has been distilled from hundreds of articles. Instead, we a list of recommended articles for those who want to learn more about these issues.

Match Day Nutrition in Soccer

An elite soccer player typically covers at least 10 km (6 mi) in a 90-minute match, and about 600 m (0.4 mi) of this is covered at full sprint speed. Heart rate is maintained at about 85% of maximum, the mean relative exercise intensity is about 70% $\dot{V}O_2$max over the duration of the match, and the total amount of energy expended by players who complete 90 minutes is about 6,700 kJ (1,601 kcal). Performance is determined not only by running ability but also by the amount of ball possession; in-play actions, such as jumping, tackling, passing, shooting, and dribbling; and cognitive functioning (timing, reaction time, and decision making). All of these are affected by fatigue. Minimizing fatigue relative to the opposing team is an important strategy, because most goals are conceded in the last few minutes of each half and are attributed to fatigue. Generally, teams with the higher percentages of ball possessions run less distance and expend less energy. Appropriate nutrition on match days can address two of the major contributors to the development of fatigue: carbohydrate depletion and dehydration. However, practical issues and Fédération Internationale de Football Association (FIFA) rules limit opportunities for hydration and carbohydrate intake within a match, so opportunities before the match and during halftime are more important than in many other team sports.

Prematch Nutrition

Preparation for a soccer match often starts with recovery from a previous match or training session; however, extreme forms of carbohydrate loading in the days prior to a match are impractical. On match day, it is generally recommended that players consume a carbohydrate-rich meal 3 to 4 hours before warm-up so play can begin with adequate glycogen stores in the liver and muscles. As an example of the benefits of this approach, increased dribbling speed was observed when soccer players consumed a larger breakfast (2,092 vs. 1,046 kJ [500 vs. 250 kcal], 60% carbohydrate) 135 minutes before a match.

Data from many studies suggest that higher carbohydrate intakes before and during matches can delay fatigue and enhance the capacity for intermittent high-intensity exercise. Carbohydrate ingestion also seems to improve passing, dribbling speed, and shooting performance, but the effects on sprinting, jumping, and cognitive function are less consistent. Players should also aim to start the match well hydrated. This can usually be achieved by drinking 0.5 to 1 L of water 1.5 to 2 hours before kick-off. Some clubs encourage players to ingest a prematch ergogenic supplement; one strategy is to drink one concentrated beetroot juice shot (70 ml [2 fl oz] contains about 6 mmol nitrate) 2.5 hours before kick-off and a second shot that contains added caffeine (at a dose of 3 mg per kilogram of body weight) 1 hour before kickoff. Both nitrate and caffeine are known to improve endurance by different mechanisms, so combining the two could have additive effects. Caffeine may also improve cognitive function.

In-Play Nutrition

Studies using protocols that simulate soccer matches have reported performance benefits when carbohydrate is consumed during exercise at rates of about 30 to 60 g/h; furthermore, effects may be greater with higher carbohydrate intakes (>75 g/h). It seems that players are consuming amounts that are at the low end of this scale; for example, players in the English Premier League reportedly ingest 32 g/h just before and during a match. This may be attributed to the match rules, which limit intake to warm-up and halftime (a 15-minute break in the dressing room after 45 minutes of match play), and the fear or actual experience of GI problems during high-intensity exercise.

Carbohydrate consumed during exercise affects receptors in the oral cavity that detect carbohydrate ingestion and favorably alters the perception of effort. Implications for soccer are still unclear, but practical solutions that enable the use of carbohydrate mouth rinses during match play (e.g., mouth guards that serve as carbohydrate-delivery systems) could potentially enhance performance in situations where carbohydrate consumption is limited by the rules of the game and GI concerns.

Dehydration is commonly reported after a soccer match because sweat losses (governed by the intensity and duration of play and environmental conditions) exceed fluid intake (governed by hydration opportunities and individual hydration practices). In cool conditions, net fluid losses are quite small, typically 1% to 2% of body mass, which has inconsequential effects on endurance and cognitive performance. As long as dehydration is limited to moderate levels (no more than 2.5% body mass loss), it seems that current drinking practices (i.e., ensuring players start a match in a well-hydrated state and consume some fluid during the halftime interval) are not a major concern for performance in temperate conditions.

In hot conditions, greater fluid losses (e.g., match sweat rates of 2-3 L/h [0.5-0.8 gal/h]) could negatively affect players' performances. For example, in an elite soccer match played in a hot environment, players exhibited reduced performance of repeated sprint and jump activities and had a marked drop in high-intensity running toward the end of the match; this was mostly attributed to hyperthermia and dehydration. It is possible that drinking more and more frequently could prevent some of the larger effects on performance in hot environments. There are interindividual differences in fluid losses, so hydration requires an individualized approach to prevent excessive dehydration in heavy sweaters.

Halftime Nutrition

Players can rehydrate according to thirst or anticipated body mass loss at halftime. A 4% to 8% w/v carbohydrate–electrolyte beverage is probably the most appropriate choice. Taking a caffeine supplement at halftime can also be considered, particularly if caffeine was not ingested before the match. Chewing gum containing 100 mg caffeine is readily available and is a suitable choice because it allows for rapid absorption of caffeine compared with tablets or drinks.

Hydration and carbohydrate intake may require special attention in matches in which extra time (30 minutes) is played. All match nutrition strategies, including the use of supplements, should be practiced in training and during minor matches to allow individualized protocols to be developed. In training sessions, individual player sweat rates can be determined under different environmental conditions (i.e., cool, temperate, and warm weather) so fluid replacement needs during match play can be predicted with a reasonable degree of accuracy. Weighing players during matches or halftime is unrealistic.

Postmatch Nutrition

In addition to energy expended and fluid loss through sweat, players will use around 60% to 80% of their muscle glycogen stores during a match. The energy, fluid, and carbohydrate lost can be easily replaced in postmatch meals. These losses are not a major issue because the next training session or match will likely take place at least 2 to 3 days later.

Players often suffer from soreness due to eccentric exercise-induced muscle damage and soft tissue injuries from collisions and tackles during match practice or match play. Structural muscle damage is difficult to prevent altogether, but muscle soreness and the magnitude of strength and power decrements might be reduced by nutritional strategies during the postexercise period. These strategies include the intake of protein and foods rich in anti-inflammatory and antioxidant phytochemicals. Although postexercise protein intake is known to increase the muscle protein synthesis rate and decrease protein breakdown with a small degree of net protein accretion, this is a relatively slow process, and there is little evidence that this results in reduced loss of muscle function. Some studies have reported reductions in muscle soreness with intake of protein, BCAAs, or milk following damaging exercise, such as downhill running or shuttle running, but the overall effects are rather small. Inhibiting exercise-induced muscle inflammation and quenching free-radical activity, which is thought to be involved in secondary damage following muscle injury, can be achieved to some degree with large doses of individual antioxidant vitamins, but there are concerns that this may interfere with adaptive processes in muscle. There are alternatives, such as antioxidant compounds found in natural foods and beverages such as berries, cherries, cherry juice, dark chocolate, and green tea, that can reduce muscle damage and soreness. These food items are high in phytochemicals, many of which are polyphenols, such as flavonoids, flavanols, anthocyanins, catechins, and stilbenes. Several of these are more potent antioxidants than vitamins C and E. Some can be obtained in isolated form, such as quercetin, but until there is greater evidence to guide postexercise practices, it seems prudent to choose natural food sources that contain mixtures of polyphenols and use these occasionally when the priority is to reduce soreness and hasten recovery before an upcoming match. In other situations, such as during preseason training in which adaptation is the primary goal, high antioxidant intake should be avoided.

During periods when matches take place 2 to 3 times per week or long-distance travel is required, the appropriate timing, quality, and quantity of postmatch meals play critical roles in recovery. To optimize protein synthesis for repair and recovery, meals and snacks should be scheduled to target intakes of 20 to 25 g of high-quality protein in 3- to 4-hour intervals. Furthermore, consuming a high-protein meal that contains 30 to 60 g of protein prior to sleep can enhance overnight protein synthesis. There is also a need to restore liver and muscle glycogen with carbohydrate intake and to begin this at an early stage of recovery, because muscle glycogen synthesis is impaired in the presence of muscle damage, which slow postmatch recovery. To rapidly replenish glycogen stores, postmatch meals should target a carbohydrate intake of about 1 g per kilogram of body weight per hour for 4 hours. In addition, when the goal is to optimize muscle glycogen stores, daily carbohydrate intake should be increased from 5 g per kilogram of body weight per day (typical intake of a soccer player) to about 7 g per kilogram of body weight per day. The need for fluid replacement to replace sweat losses should also be addressed in first hours of postmatch recovery.

Nutrition in Marathon Running

Most marathon runners know what "hitting the wall" means; it is a well-known phenomenon during marathons. For most runners who experience this, it happens around the 32 km (20 mile) mark. The sudden lack of power and overwhelming fatigue may be the result of a combination of factors, but it is likely that carbohydrate depletion and dehydration play a role. In a marathon, nutrition can mean the difference between winning a race and not finishing a race.

Avoiding the Wall

There are a few simple strategies that can delay or completely prevent runners from hitting the wall. Runners should start the race with optimal muscle glycogen stores and liver glycogen stores and should fuel during the race (using drinks, gels, or solid foods).

To start a race with optimal glycogen stores, runners should eat carbohydrate-rich foods in the day or days before the race (usually while reducing training, which uses glycogen stores). Consuming a little more carbohydrate than normal at the expense of some protein and fat will ensure that a runner fills up the muscle glycogen stores without gaining weight. (Carbohydrate loading is sometimes confused with overeating.) Good sources of carbohydrate include pasta, rice, potatoes, and bread. Extreme muscle glycogen supercompensation diets, such as those used in the 1970s (see chapter 6), are also not necessary.

The next opportunity to make sure glycogen stores are full is during breakfast on the day of the race. As discussed in chapter 6, a good prerace breakfast includes 100 to 200 g of carbohydrate in the 3 to 4 hours before the start of the race. Many athletes, however, find it difficult to eat before a race, and race day anxiety often removes any hunger feelings. It is still important to ingest at least 100 g of carbohydrate; if eating is not an option, carbohydrate can be in liquid form. Athletes who frequently experience stomach problems should avoid breakfasts that are high in fiber, fat, and protein and may want to avoid milk products (or use lactose-free products). Good carbohydrate sources for race day include refined grains (e.g., white rice), cooked cereals, corn- and rice-based cereals, white bread, bagels (without seeds), pancakes, cooked vegetables (without seeds), cooked potatoes, ripe bananas, cooked fruits, applesauce or fruit blends, lean meat, rice cakes, honey, syrup, and pulp-free juice. Runners should plan the race day breakfast in advance to be sure necessary foods will be available (e.g., at a hotel). If the race takes place more than 4 hours after breakfast, the last meal before the race should be light and should not contain a lot of fiber (which would leave remnants and water in the intestines).

The Race

Marathon nutrition requires a bit of planning. Runners should study what is available on the course and develop a plan. The nutrition plan for a marathon should be tested several times in training. Runners should also look at the weather conditions on race day and have an idea of their sweat rates under those conditions. Based on their predicted times, runners can calculate targets for carbohydrate and fluid intake.

Runners should plan for required carbohydrate and fluid intake 10 to 15 minutes before the start of the race. The food and drink will pass through the stomach, and absorption takes minutes. Most of the carbohydrate ingested at this time will become available to the muscle during the first part of the run. What foods are best is a matter of personal preference, but gels and chews are very commonly used. The target can be achieved with many different combinations of water, sports drinks, gels, chews, bars, and regular foods.

Recommendations for carbohydrate intake during a marathon are between 30 and 90 g/h and depend on a number of factors such as pace, personal preferences, tolerance, carbohydrate content in the habitual diet, number of times the race nutrition plan has been successfully practiced, and so on. Generally, a higher carbohydrate intake (that does not cause GI discomfort) is better.

Meeting Carbohydrate Recommendations

Studies have shown little difference in carbohydrate oxidation from drinks, gels, or bars, which led researchers to conclude that runners can mix and match. The exact combination of solid foods, chews, gels, or drinks used to deliver carbohydrate depends on personal preferences. Solid foods usually provide more carbohydrates per unit of weight and are very effective energy sources to carry; however, they require chewing, and not every runner can do this during a marathon. Bars typically deliver 30 to 60 g of carbohydrate and come in many different flavors. Runners should select energy bars that are low in fat, fiber, and protein, because these ingredients slow down gastric emptying and may contribute to stomach problems. Chews are also solid, but they are generally easier to chew and do not contain much besides carbohydrate. If chewing is a challenge, gels may be the solution. Gels are a compact form of energy that contain a small volume of fluid and a relatively large amount (20-25 g) of carbohydrate. Gels come in many different flavors and sometimes also contain caffeine.

If solids and gels don't work, runners can rely on carbohydrate drinks, but when carbohydrate targets are higher (near 60 g/h), it may be difficult to reach these targets with drinks alone. Another disadvantage of drinks is that they are difficult to carry during a marathon. Although some people run with bottles or small flasks, they still have to rely on fluids provided in the race. Carbohydrate drinks typically contain 60 to 70 g of carbohydrates per liter of fluid. A 600 ml (20 fl oz) sports bottle will therefore deliver roughly 35 g of carbohydrate.

Dehydration

As discussed in chapter 9, a small amount of dehydration is unlikely to be a problem, but once you start to lose 3% of your body weight or more, performance may be affected, especially in hot conditions. To prevent significant dehydration, runners should start a race hydrated and maintain proper hydration throughout the race. About 2 hours before the race, runners should drink at least 500 ml (17 fl oz); excess fluid will be eliminated through urine. Athletes can ensure that their urine color is pale, which indicates adequate hydration. During the race, the target for fluid intake should be such that the runner loses no more than 3% body weight. This means always consuming fluid at a rate that is below the sweat rate (the longer the race, the closer the fluid consumption rate will need to be to the sweat rate). Drinking according to thirst works fine for most slower athletes, but faster athletes should develop a plan. Knowing the sweat rate can give good guidance on how much to drink during the marathon. Although a well-thought-out plan is recommended, it is still important to adapt if required. For example, when certain GI symptoms present themselves, it is best not to ignore them (e.g., drink less or, if possible, reduce the pace a little to allow better gastric emptying and absorption).

Training

One of the most important aspects of preparation is training with race nutrition. Nutritional preparation should start at least 6 to 10 weeks before the race, and runners should use the same products throughout training. Race day is not the time to experiment with new products.

Training will always involve a mix of hard and easy sessions; the same is true for nutrition. On easy days when the quality of training is not so important and the runner may want to train the body to use fat as a fuel, he or she will consume little or no carbohydrate (i.e., train low). On hard days when quality is important and the runner wants to train the body to perform just like it will in a race, the runner should follow his or her race plan.

Nutrition in Competitive Tennis

Tennis play involves repetitive short bouts of high-intensity exercise. Maintaining performance for the full duration of matches is important to success and will depend to a large degree on the ability of muscles to recover from the last sprint effort. In tennis, players perform numerous, very short sprints interspersed with variable periods of lower intensity exercise (e.g., moving side to side, forward, or backward to reach the ball; jogging; walking) or rest. The cycles of activity and rest are largely unpredictable because they are imposed by the pattern of play and will vary greatly from player to player and from one match to another.

Most tennis matches (minimum of two sets) last at least 60 minutes, and it is not uncommon for men's matches to last more than 3 hours (though 30-second breaks are taken at change of ends after every odd-numbered game).In singles matches, for every hour of tennis play completed, each player covers about 1 mi (1.5 km) while performing numerous discrete bouts of action that incorporate frequent changes of pace and direction and executing game skills such as serving, returning serve, volleying, and driving.

Energy expenditure is typically about 44 kJ/min (10 kcal/min) and players exercise at an average relative intensity close to 50% of $\dot{V}O_2$max. Thus, for a typical singles match that lasts 2 hours, the average player will expend about 5,000 kJ (1,195 kcal). In doubles matches, energy expenditure is typically about two-thirds of that recorded for singles play.

At high standards of competitive play, players suffer from noticeable fatigue during the final set, and this is reflected as a drop in work rate (less distance covered and fewer sprints) and an increase in the incidence of unforced errors. It is common to see more missed shots and mistakes in the later stages of games as players become tired. The development of fatigue during the game is likely related to depletion of the muscle glycogen stores and the development of dehydration and increased core body temperature, especially in warm environmental conditions. Players who start matches with low glycogen stores in their leg muscles will likely be close to complete glycogen depletion by the end of the second set, and this has important implications for the training and nutritional preparation of players. Blood glucose concentration remains relatively stable in the first 2 hours of tennis play but may start to fall if the match duration exceeds 3 hours. Hence, when long matches are anticipated, carbohydrate-containing drinks should be consumed at regular intervals during breaks in play (e.g., at change of ends). Ensuring good hydration status before a match is important, and attention to fluid needs during a match is essential for optimal performance and to reduce the risk of cramping, especially in hot playing conditions. The volume, frequency, and composition of fluid ingested are all important factors that need to be considered.

Fluid Intake

Besides replacing lost fluids, drinks can provide a means of supplying additional fuel (usually carbohydrate) that can be used by the working muscles and the brain. The ingestion of water and of carbohydrate have independent and additive effects on endurance performance. As a general recommendation, drinking a few mouthfuls (about 100 ml [3 fl oz]) of a sports drink at each change of ends in a tennis match will help prevent dehydration and provide an additional source of energy. These factors might be crucial if victory is to be claimed in the last set or rubber of the match.

Exactly how much players should drink during a match will depend on individual sweat rates and the playing conditions. Sweat rates vary according to fitness and acclimatization levels, intensity of exercise, and environmental conditions. Some players may lose up to 3 L (0.8 gal) of sweat per hour during strenuous play in a warm environment (e.g., 30°C [85°F]), and even at low ambient temperatures of about 12°C (54°F), sweat loss can exceed 1 L/h (0.3 gal/h). It is advisable to drink 500 ml (17 fl oz) of water about 2 hours before the start of a match. This gives plenty of time for the water to be absorbed and for any excess to be eliminated through urination. Players should go to the bathroom about 10 minutes before starting a match to empty the bladder and then drink another 250 ml (8 fl oz) of water or a sports drink just before walking on court. During a match, players should drink according to a plan rather than thirst, because several liters of fluid can be lost before thirst kicks in. A plan can be created based on known individual sweat losses (which can be measured as discussed previously).

The ideal drink for fluid replacement during tennis is one that tastes good to the player, does not cause GI discomfort when consumed in large volumes (this rules out all fizzy carbonated drinks), promotes rapid gastric emptying and fluid absorption to help maintain extracellular fluid volume, and provides some energy in the form of carbohydrate for the working muscles. Replacing the electrolytes lost in sweat can normally wait until the postmatch recovery period.

One point that is often neglected is the importance of drinking during tennis practice or friendly matches so the player is accustomed to the feeling of exercising with fluid in the stomach. This also gives the player the opportunity to experiment with different drinks and volumes to determine which formulations work best and how much fluid intake can be tolerated.

Food Intake

Carbohydrate boosts performance in tennis and other forms of prolonged exercise. Intake of fat or protein during prolonged exercise does not improve endurance. Players should aim for a carbohydrate intake of about 60 to 70 g/h for optimal carbohydrate delivery. This is the amount of carbohydrate in about 1 L of a sports drink, but a player could probably not comfortably drink this much during each hour of play. A more practical strategy would be to consume 600 ml (20 fl oz) of a sports drink and eat 1.5 bananas every hour. Ripe bananas are preferred because more of the carbohydrate is in an easily digestible form (unripe bananas contain the same amount of carbohydrate but more in the form of indigestible starch). Alternatives to bananas include grapes, mango (ripe, sliced or diced, and in a container to keep it fresh), energy bars, gels, or soft candies such as jelly beans. Keep in mind, however, that the risk of GI discomfort is greater with solid foods because they empty more slowly from the stomach than liquids.

Nutritional Strategies to Reduce Muscle Loss in Injured American Football Players

The game of American football is primarily comprised of repeated, short, maximum-intensity bouts of exercise. Each playing position on the field has specific responsibilities that may alter the physical demands of each player. For example, blocking linemen usually have more contact than skill position players (i.e., wide receivers and running backs), who often attempt to avoid contact. When the skill position players do make contact, however, the potential impact may be much greater than for linemen, because it is likely to occur at a higher velocity of movement. All players are expected to provide 100% of their effort on each play regardless of their position. The duration of each play can vary from 2 to 13 seconds, with the average play lasting 5 seconds in NCAA and National Football League (NFL) games. The average rest interval between plays in the NFL ranges from 27 to 37 seconds.

Injuries are an unavoidable aspect of participation in sport and are more common in sports such as American football and rugby, in which frequent physical contact, blocks, tackles, falls, and collisions are common in training and competitive matches. Injury risk is increased when players become fatigued, training or competition loads are increased, and the time for recovery between matches is reduced. The overall injury rate in NCAA football is 8.1 per 1,000 athlete exposures (games and practices combined), and football players are nearly seven times more likely to be injured during a game than in practice.

Many injuries result in prolonged periods of limb immobilization to reduce further potential damage and allow repair of bone or skeletal muscle and connective tissue. Immobilization results in muscle disuse and loss of muscle mass due to increased periods of negative muscle protein balance due to decreased basal muscle protein synthesis and the development of anabolic resistance to dietary protein ingestion. Muscle loss is most profound in the first 1 to 2 weeks of limb immobilization. The extent of muscle loss during injury strongly influences the level and duration of rehabilitation required.

Nutritional strategies can limit the muscle loss and decline in functional capacity that occur in injured football players. During rehabilitation and recovery, nutritional needs are much like those for any athlete seeking muscle hypertrophy to increase strength and power. Nutrient and energy deficiencies should be avoided. Daily protein intakes of 1.6 to 2.5 g per kilogram of body mass are recommended to support maintenance of muscle mass during disuse. This should be achieved through the regular consumption of meals (4-6 times/day every 3-4 h) that contain 20 to 35 g of rapidly digested protein with a high leucine content (2.5-3 g). Any other protein consumed during the day should be mostly lean, high-quality protein that contains all the essential amino acids in approximately equal proportions (e.g., beef, ham, lamb, poultry, fish). Given that the injured athlete has greatly reduced physical activity levels, maintaining muscle mass while avoiding gains in fat mass can be challenging, so selecting protein sources with relatively low fat content, avoiding other fatty foods, and reducing carbohydrate intake compared with normal training are other important considerations.

There is also a theoretical rationale for vitamin D_3 (1,000-4,000 IU/day) and omega-3 fatty acid (1-2 g/day) supplementation to help reduce muscle atrophy. Other supplements, including leucine, creatine, and HMB may also support the maintenance of muscle protein synthesis rates during recovery.

Neuromuscular electrical stimulation may be applied to evoke involuntary muscle contractions and support muscle mass maintenance in injured athletes. Resistance exercise of muscles not close to the injury site should also be employed to sustain an anabolic stimulus. During subsequent rehabilitation and recovery from immobilization, increased activity, particularly resistance exercise, will increase muscle protein synthesis and restore sensitivity to anabolic stimuli.

Nutrition for Building Muscle Mass in Game Players

Many athletes and game players may decide that they want to increase their muscle strength and power, and this can only be achieved by increasing the muscle mass of the limbs used for the sport. For soccer players, this would mean targeting the thighs and calves; for basketball players, it might mean targeting the upper arm or forearm muscles; and for American football players and rugby players, it might mean increasing muscle mass in the arms, legs, and torso. Often it will be a coach who perceives that a player may benefit from increased muscle, so young players and those with naturally slimmer builds are often the targets. Although there are training strategies to build muscle, here we will focus on nutritional strategies that maximize strength training adaptation.

Nutritional Strategies to Maximize Strength Training Adaptation

Muscle hypertrophy is mostly achieved through the generation of more myofibrils, which are composed of protein. Positive muscle protein balance (i.e., net tissue protein gain) is only achieved when the rate of new muscle protein synthesis exceeds the rate of existing muscle protein breakdown. Therefore, muscle mass increases can only be achieved through the synergistic effect of appropriate resistance training and adequate protein intake. As discussed in detail in chapter 8, the timing, amount, and composition of protein ingested can be manipulated to optimize resistance training adaptation. Timing of protein intake is an important variable to consider in optimizing skeletal muscle recovery and hypertrophy. It appears optimal to ingest protein in the immediate postexercise period in amounts of about 0.4 g per kilogram of body weight (typically 20-25 g). This is a sufficient dose to promote a marked rise in muscle protein synthesis. The protein of choice is one that is readily digestible and has a high leucine content, because this essential amino acid is key to increasing protein synthesis. Whey protein is considered ideal, but skim milk or eggs are suitable substitutes. Tables 8.4 and 8.5 list some suitable food choices that can be combined to achieve the desired amounts of protein and leucine.

If the athlete is performing the resistance exercise session in the morning, he or she should eat up to three other meals throughout the day (each with a protein dose of 0.4 g per kilogram of body weight) with the aim of achieving a total dietary protein intake of about 1.6 g per kilogram of body weight per day. Eating fewer meals with more protein is not as good as eating this optimal dose. Eating much more than 1.6 g per kilogram of body weight per day is unnecessary because it will not produce greater daily gains in muscle mass. If the athlete is performing the resistance exercise session in the late afternoon or evening, he or she should ingest some protein immediately before bedtime to maximize the anabolic response during overnight sleep. Ingesting a larger dose of protein (0.6 g per kilogram of body weight) before bedtime appears to augment acute overnight muscle protein synthesis and chronic skeletal muscle adaptations. Adequate energy is also needed to support these processes, so players should aim to maintain daily energy balance. Other protein consumed during the day should be mostly lean, high-quality protein that contains all the essential amino acids in approximately equal proportions. Protein from animal sources (e.g., beef, ham, lamb, poultry, fish) can be supplemented with soy, beans, cheese, nuts, and bread. If high leucine sources of protein are unavailable, the athlete can add a 3 g leucine supplement to the postexercise meal. The addition of any other individual amino acid is ineffective in promoting resistance exercise–induced anabolism. Creatine supplements can also be considered.

Lack of sleep in athletes contributes to a negative protein balance by reducing mechanisms that promote muscle protein synthesis and stimulating those causing muscle protein breakdown. Therefore, it is important to ensure adequate sleep (minimum of 7 hours) at night.

Nutrition in Athletes With Type 1 Diabetes

Diabetes mellitus is a metabolic syndrome that has two types, 1 and 2, that are characterized by absolute or relative insulin deficiency or insulin resistance, respectively. About 90% of people with diabetes have type 2 diabetes. Type 1 diabetes results from a highly specific immune-mediated destruction of pancreatic islet ß cells, which results in chronic elevated blood glucose concentration (known as hyperglycemia) due to absence of insulin production. The condition usually occurs in early childhood, and it is a chronic disease that can lead to many serious complications if it is not properly managed. The patient and physician must work together to optimize glucose control through insulin administration and caloric intake.

Several studies have confirmed the beneficial role of physical activity in favorably altering the prognosis of diabetes. Compared to healthy peers, athletes with diabetes experience nearly all the same health-related benefits from exercise. People with diabetes take part in physical activity for health promotion and disease management and can also participate in recreational or competitive sports. Competition at the highest level is possible; examples of outstanding athletes with diabetes include Gary Hall Jr. and Sir Steven Redgrave. Hall was an American competition swimmer who represented the United States at the 1996, 2000, and 2004 Olympics and won 10 Olympic medals. He is a former world record holder in two relay events. Redgrave is a retired British rower who won gold medals at five consecutive Olympic Games from 1984 to 2000. He has also won three Commonwealth Games gold medals and nine World Rowing Championships golds. He is the most successful male rower in Olympic history and the only man to have won gold medals at five Olympic Games in an endurance sport.

Metabolic Challenges with Exercise

For people with type 1 diabetes, injecting too much insulin, skipping meals, eating less than normal, or exercising more than usual can lead to low blood glucose (hypoglycemia). Exercise uses up energy, and there is a rapid and large increase in the uptake of glucose by the working muscle that is independent of insulin action. You may recall from chapter 3 that during endurance exercise, insulin secretion falls for healthy (nondiabetic) people, but muscle glucose uptake increases because exercise itself (via calcium-mediated mechanisms) stimulates the translocation of GLUT4 receptors to the cell surface. Therefore, if the diabetic did not eat correctly beforehand, exercise can quickly cause the blood glucose concentration to drop. For diabetics, the main risk with prolonged exercise is that it may cause a fall in the blood glucose concentration below its normal range of 4 to 6 mM. If the fall is too drastic (below 3 mM) and sustained, it can lead to fatigue, pale skin, and inability to concentrate or think clearly followed by fainting, loss of consciousness, seizure, and coma. If not corrected, it can be fatal. The early symptoms of hypoglycemia are shakiness, dizziness, sweating, hunger, irritability or moodiness, anxiety or nervousness, and headache.

With short periods of very high-intensity exercise such as sprinting, high-intensity interval training, and intense resistance exercise, people with type 1 diabetes may develop hyperglycemia. The hormonal response to predominantly anaerobic exercise is pretty much the same as in nondiabetic people; elevated catecholamines promote glucose release from the liver, which in the presence of low insulin results in mild hyperglycemia during exercise. However, insulin levels do not rise in a person with diabetes as they would after exercise in nondiabetic people, meaning that there is then the problem of sustained postexercise hyperglycemia.

A problem that is common to short-term intense exercise and more prolonged endurance exercise is the development of late hypoglycemia, which can occur 6 to 15 hours postexercise. This may be due to the recruitment of GLUT4 glucose transporters to the cell surface, which facilitate glucose uptake into muscle for glycogen resynthesis. Although this is important for the replenishment of depleted glycogen reserves and the performance of subsequent exercise, in a person with diabetes it causes hypoglycemia, and it can occur during sleep (particularly if the exercise was performed in the afternoon) when it is much less likely to be recognized.

Nutritional Strategies to Prevent Hypoglycemia

To minimize the risk of hypoglycemia during prolonged exercise, a low-fat, high-carbohydrate (at least 1 g/kg) meal should be eaten 1 to 3 hours prior to exercise, and the usual postmeal insulin dose should be reduced by 30% to 50%. Food chosen should have a low glycemic index. The athlete should check the blood glucose level about an hour before exercise to be sure it is within the usual target range before engaging in exercise. If it is too low, a small meal or snack that contains 15 to 20 g of carbohydrates should be consumed before starting exercise. Suitable snacks include granola bars, fresh or dried fruit, fruit juice, pretzels, and cookies; alternately, a 15 to 20 g glucose tablet can be ingested. If the exercise will last for an hour or longer, additional carbohydrates should be ingested during the workout at a rate of 30 to 60 g/hour (or more if the insulin dose was not reduced after the last meal before exercise). Exercise gels, sports drinks, granola bars, and candy bars can provide the body with a rapidly available source of glucose during exercise.

After prolonged exercise, it is important to restore the liver and muscle glycogen stores to reduce the risk for subsequent hypoglycemia. Carbohydrates should always be available during training sessions and in the recovery period afterward. The usual sport nutrition guidelines for postexercise recovery can be followed. The postexercise meal should be followed with appropriate insulin administration for glycemic management. The athlete should consider reducing the insulin bolus by about 50% to reduce the risk of delayed nocturnal hypoglycemia. Moderate- or high-intensity exercise can cause blood glucose to drop for up to 24 hours after exercise; therefore, the blood glucose concentration should be checked immediately after exercise and every 2 to 3 hours afterward until bedtime. If blood glucose is low, a carbohydrate snack should be ingested. It is recommended that intense exercise intense be avoided immediately before bed. In addition, reducing the evening insulin dose by about 20% or consuming a bedtime snack without insulin may help prevent nocturnal hypoglycemia after exercise.

Athletes with diabetes need to be advised on an appropriate diet that will maximize performance and reduce fatigue. Energy and macronutrient needs, especially carbohydrate and protein, must be met to allow hard training, promote adaptation, and maintain health. Current guidelines recommend 5 to 10 g of carbohydrate and 1.5 to 1.7 g of protein per kilogram of body weight per day.

Key Points

- Personalized nutrition plans provide advice on diet and supplements that is tailored to meet specific nutritional needs based on phenotype, genotype, sex, age, and particular goals.
- When giving advice to an athlete, it is always important to understand his or her goals. Nutrition should support the training goals.
- Periodized nutrition is the planned, purposeful, and strategic use of specific nutrition interventions to enhance the adaptations targeted by each exercise session or to obtain other nonacute effects or benefits that will enhance performance in the long term.
- Young athletes may have different nutritional needs because they are in a phase of growth, and they have different physiologies and metabolisms than adults. Children are less metabolically efficient during motor activities, and this results in higher energy requirements per kilogram of body mass during most forms of exercise. Children have lower glycolytic capacities, higher oxidative capacities, and higher rates of fat oxidation compared to adults.
- One of the greatest potential health threats to young athletes is inappropriate weight control that could lead to the development of eating disorders or impaired growth and development. Nutrition supplements are probably not necessary and are not recommended for young athletes.
- One of the main changes with aging is the loss of muscle mass. Sarcopenia, which is characterized by losses in muscle mass, strength, and endurance, affects performance and contributes to other functional consequences of aging.
- In older people (especially age 70 and older), protein synthesis is lower and there appears to be some anabolic resistance. Protein intake recommendations for older athletes should be higher than those for young athletes.
- When body fat in female athletes is reduced to levels below 10%, various body functions may be impaired and menstruation may cease. If this is sustained for a long time, it will result in other health complications, including osteoporosis.
- Female athletes may struggle with adequate iron intake, especially if their energy intakes are low or if they are vegetarians. Female athletes should pay extra attention to iron intake and monitor iron status. In some cases, supplementation may be appropriate.
- Nutrition recommendations are usually highly specific to a sport, but they are also influenced by other factors (e.g., environmental conditions, age, sex, body size, playing position in team sports) and by goals (e.g., training adaptation, competition performance, recovery from exercise, weight loss, muscle mass gain, rehabilitation from injury).

Recommended Readings

Anderson, L., P. Orme, R.J. Naughton, et al. 2017. Energy intake and expenditure of professional soccer players of the English premier league: Evidence of carbohydrate periodization. *Int J Sport Nutr Exerc Metab* 27 (3):228-338.

Baar, K., and L.E. Heaton. 2015. In-season recovery nutrition for American football. *Sports Sci Exch* 28 (144):1-6.

Bangsbo, J., M. Mohr, and P. Krustrup. 2006. Physical and metabolic demands of training and match-play in the elite football player. J *Sports Sci* 24 (7):665-674.

Bell, P.G., E. Stevenson, G.W. Davison, and G. Howatson. 2016. The effects of montmorency tart cherry concentrate supplementation on recovery following prolonged, intermittent exercise. *Nutrients* 8 (7):E441.

Bhogal, G., and N. Peirce. 2014. The diabetic athlete. In *Nutrition in sport*, edited by R.J.Maughan, 490-502. Oxford: Blackwell Science

Briggs, M.A., L.D. Harper, G. McNamee, E. Cockburn, P.L.S. Rumbold, E.J. Stevenson, and M. Russell. 2017. The effects of an increased calorie breakfast consumed prior to simulated match-play in Academy soccer players. *Eur J Sport Sci* 17 (7):858-866.

Brink-Elfegoun, T., S. Ratel, P.M. Leprêtre, L. Metz, G. Ennequin, E. Doré, V. Martin, D. Bishop, N. Aubineau, J.F. Lescuyer, M. Duclos, P. Sirvent, and S.L. Peltier. 2014. Effects of sports drinks on the maintenance of physical performance during 3 tennis matches: a randomized controlled study. *J Int Soc Sports Nutr* 11:46.

Burke, L.M., J.A. Hawley, S.H. Wong, and A.E. Jeukendrup. 2011. Carbohydrates for training and competition. *J Sports Sci* 29 Suppl 1:S17-27.

Burke, L.M., L.J.C. van Loon, and J.A. Hawley. 2017. Postexercise muscle glycogen resynthesis in humans. *J Appl Physiol* 122 (5):1055-1067.

Cockburn, E., E. Stevenson, P.R. Hayes, P. Robson-Ansley, and G. Howatson. 2010. Effect of milk-based carbohydrate-protein supplement timing on the attenuation of exercise-induced muscle damage. *Appl Physiol Nutr Metab* 35 (3):270-277.

Currell, K., S. Conway, and A.E. Jeukendrup. 2009. Carbohydrate ingestion improves performance of a new reliable test of soccer performance. *Int J Sport Nutr Exerc Metab* 19 (1):34-46.

Damas, F., S. Phillips, F.C. Vechin, and C. Ugrinowitsch. 2015. A review of resistance training-induced changes in skeletal muscle protein synthesis and their contribution to hypertrophy. *Sports Med* 45: 801–807.

Dirks, M.L., B.T. Wall, and L.J.C. van Loon. 2017. Interventional strategies to combat muscle disuse atrophy in humans: focus on neuromuscular electrical stimulation and dietary protein. *J Appl Physiol* doi: 10.1152/japplphysiol.00985.2016. [Epub ahead of print].

Doyle, J.A., W.M. Sherman, and R.L. Strauss. 1993. Effects of eccentric and concentric exercise on muscle glycogen replenishment. *J Appl Physiol* 74 (4):1848-1855.

Fahey, P.J., E.T. Stallkamp, and S. Kwatra. 1996. The athlete with type I diabetes: managing insulin, diet and exercise. *Am Fam Physician* 53 (5):1611-1624.

Gallen, I.W., C. Hume, and A. Lumb. 2011. Fuelling the athlete with type 1 diabetes. *Diabetes Obes Metab* 13 (2):130-136.

Gomes, R.V., A. Moreira, A.J. Coutts, C.D. Capitani, and M.S. Aoki. 2014. Effect of carbohydrate supplementation on the physiological and perceptual responses to prolonged tennis match play. J Strength *Cond Res* 28 (3):735-741.

Hoffman, J.R. 2015. Physiological demands of American football. *Sports Sci Exch* 28 (143):1-6.

Holway, F.E., and L.L. Spriet. 2011. Sport-specific nutrition: practical strategies for team sports. *J Sports Sci* 29 Suppl 1:S115-125.

Horton, W.B., and J.S. Subauste. 2016. Care of the athlete with type 1 diabetes mellitus: A clinical review. *Int J Endocrinol Metab* 14 (2):e36091. eCollection.

Jackman, S.R., O.C. Witard, A.E. Jeukendrup, et al. 2010. Branched-chain amino acid ingestion can ameliorate soreness from eccentric exercise. *Med Sci Sports Exerc* 42 (5):962-970.

Jensen, J. 2004. Nutritional concerns in the diabetic athlete. *Curr Sports Med Rep* 3 (4):192-197.

Jeukendrup, A.E. 2011. Nutrition for endurance sports: marathon, triathlon, and road cycling. *J Sports Sci* 29 Suppl 1:S91-99.

Jeukendrup, A. 2014. A step towards personalized sports nutrition: carbohydrate intake during exercise. *Sports Med* 44 Suppl 1:S25-33.

Jeukendrup, A.E. 2017a. Periodized nutrition for athletes. *Sports Med* 47 (Suppl 1):51-63.

Lumb, A.N., and I.W. Gallen. 2009. Diabetes management for intense exercise. *Curr Opin Endocrinol Diabetes Obes* 16: 150-155.

Magne, H., I. Savary-Auzeloux, D. Rémond, and D. Dardevet. 2013. Nutritional strategies to counteract muscle atrophy caused by disuse and to improve recovery. *Nutr Res Rev* 26 (2): 149-165.

Mohr, M., I. Mujika, J. Santisteban, M.B. Randers, R. Bischoff, R. Solano, A. Hewitt, A. Zubillaga, E. Peltola, and P. Krustrup. 2010. Examination of fatigue development in elite soccer in a hot environment: a multi-experimental approach. *Scand J Med Sci Sports* 20 Suppl 3:125-132.

Morton, R.W., C. McGlory, and S.M. Phillips. 2015. Nutritional interventions to augment resistance training-induced skeletal muscle hypertrophy. *Front Physiol* 6 (245): 1- 9.

NCAA injury surveillance program at www.datalyscenter.org

Olson, D., R.S. Sikka, A. Labounty, and T. Christensen. 2013. Injuries in professional football: current concepts. *Curr Sports Med Rep* 12 (6): 381-390.

Pasiakos, S.M., H.R. Lieberman, and T.M. McLellan. 2014. Effects of protein supplements on muscle damage, soreness and recovery of muscle function and physical performance: a systematic review. *Sports Med* 44 (5): 655-670.

Phillips, S.M. 2013. Protein consumption and resistance exercise: Maximizing anabolic potential. *Sport Sci Exch* 26 (107): 1-5.

Phillips, S.M. 2016. The impact of protein quality on the promotion of resistance exercise-induced changes in muscle mass. *Nutr Metab* 13:64.

Phillips, S.M., J. Sproule, and A.P. Turner. 2011. Carbohydrate ingestion during team games exercise: current knowledge and areas for future investigation. *Sports Med* 41 (7): 559-585.

Pluim, B.M. 2014. The evolution and impact of science in tennis: eight advances for performance and health. *Br J Sports Med* 48 Suppl 1:i3-5.

Ranchordas, K., J.T. Dawson, and M. Russell. 2017. Practical nutritional recovery strategies for elite soccer players when limited time separates repeated matches. *J Int Soc Sports Nutr* 14:35.

Riddell, M.C., I.W. Gallen, C.E. Smart, C.E. Taplin, P. Adolfsson, A.N. Lumb, A. Kowalski, R. Rabasa-Lhoret, R.J. McCrimmon, C. Hume, F. Annan, P.A. Fournier, C. Graham, B. Bode, P. Galassetti, T.W. Jones, I.S. Millán, T. Heise, A.L. Peters, A. Petz, and L.M. Laffel. 2017. Exercise management in type 1 diabetes: a consensus statement. *Lancet Diabetes Endocrinol* 5 (5): 377-390.

Rothenberg, P., L. Grau, L. Kaplan, and M.G. Baraga. 2016. Knee injuries in American football: An epidemiological review. *Am J Orthop* 45 (6): 368-373.

Russell, M., and M. Kingsley. 2014. The efficacy of acute nutritional interventions on soccer skill performance. *Sports Med* 44 (7): 957-970.

Shirreffs, S.M. 2010. Hydration: special issues for playing football in warm and hot environments. *Scand J Med Sci Sports* 20 Suppl 3: 90-94.

Tipton, K.D. 2013. Dietary strategies to attenuate muscle loss during recovery from injury. *Nestle Nutr Inst Workshop Ser* 75: 51-61.

Tipton, K.D., and A.A. Ferrando. 2008. Improving muscle mass: response of muscle metabolism to exercise, nutrition and anabolic agents. *Essays Biochem* 44: 85-98.

Tipton, K.D., and O.C. Witard. 2007. Protein requirements and recommendations for athletes: relevance of ivory tower arguments for practical recommendations. *Clinics Sports Med* 26: 17-36.

Trommelen, J., and L.J. van Loon. 2016. Pre-sleep protein ingestion to improve the skeletal muscle adaptive response to exercise training. *Nutrients* 8 (12): E763.

van Loon, L.J. 2013. Role of dietary protein in post-exercise muscle reconditioning. *Nestle Nutr Inst Workshop Ser* 75: 73-83.

Wall, B.T., J.P. Morton, and L.J. van Loon. 2015. Strategies to maintain skeletal muscle mass in the injured athlete: nutritional considerations and exercise mimetics. *Eur J Sport Sci* 15 (1): 53-62.

Appendix A

Key Concepts in Biological Chemistry Relevant to Sport Nutrition

The study of sport nutrition requires an understanding of some simple biochemistry and physiology. The major components that make up the body and the diet—carbohydrates, lipids, proteins, and nucleic acids—are themselves composed of smaller building blocks. This appendix contains a short review of important chemical concepts, interactions, and processes involving biomolecules and a brief summary of membrane transport mechanisms, enzyme action, the structure and function of the various cellular organelles, and the characteristics of the four major tissue types found in the human body. This appendix can be used as a reference, but an understanding of what is covered is essential to most of the principles and mechanisms discussed elsewhere in this book. This appendix may be particularly useful for those who have little background in biology and chemistry. We begin with the smallest unit that any substance can be broken down to: the atom.

Matter, Energy, Atoms, and Molecules

The human body consists only of matter and energy in their various forms. Indeed, the same can be said of the entire universe. Matter occupies space and has a mass that represents the quantity of matter that is present. We often equate mass with weight, which is the force that gravity exerts on the mass, but technically the two are different. The quantity or mass of an object does not change, regardless of its location, but its weight will vary according to the pull of gravity. For example, a rock weighing 6 kg (13 lb) on Earth weighs only about 1 kg (2 lb) on the surface of the Moon because the gravitational force of the Moon is only about one-sixth of that of Earth. Of course, matter itself remains matter whether on Earth or on the Moon.

Many thousands of types of matter exist, and all can be reduced into smaller units. The smallest units into which a substance can be broken down chemically are the elements, each of which has different and unique properties. Ninety-two elements are presently known to exist, but only about 12 are common in living organisms. The most abundant elements are oxygen, carbon, hydrogen, and nitrogen (in that order). These four elements compose 96% of the mass of a human.

Energy is the capacity of any system, including the living body, to do work (i.e., to produce a change of some sort in matter). Energy can exist in several forms, including light, heat, electrical, mechanical, and chemical energy. Energy can be transformed from one form to another. In the body, the potential chemical energy stored in foodstuffs is transformed to do various forms of work, such as movement or the synthesis of large molecules from small molecules. Matter and energy are interrelated by Einstein's famous equation:

$$E = mc^2$$

where E is energy, m is mass, and c is the speed of light (about 299,744 km/s [186,252 mi/s]). Nothing is capable of moving faster than light. Einstein's equation can, in principle, go in either direction. Thus, energy can be transformed into matter, and matter can be transformed into energy.

Atoms are the smallest unit of an element that retains all the properties of the element. The atoms of all elements can be broken down physically into the same subatomic particles: protons, neutrons, and electrons. Hence, the atoms of the various elements differ only in the numbers of protons, neutrons, and electrons they contain. Protons, which possess a positive charge, and neutrons, which are electrically neutral, are held together to form the nucleus of an atom. Electrons, which have negligible mass (only about 1/8,000 of that of a proton or a neutron) and possess a negative charge, spin around the atomic nucleus in discrete orbitals that may be spherical or dumbbell shaped. Some electrons move in orbitals close to the nucleus; others move in orbitals farther away. Electrons that are farther from the nucleus have more energy than those close to the nucleus; thus, the orbitals can be thought of as energy levels. Electrons normally stay at their particular energy level, but by gaining or losing energy, they jump from one energy level to another. Although electron orbitals can vary in shape, electrons at each energy level are usually depicted diagrammatically as moving in concentric and circular orbits, or shells, around the nucleus.

A maximum of two electrons can be held in the innermost shell. The second and third shells can each hold up to eight electrons. The fourth shell can hold up to 18 electrons.

The number of electrons is equal to the number of protons in the nucleus, resulting in an electrically neutral atom. The smallest atom is that of hydrogen, which is composed of one proton and one electron (see figure A.1*a*). The carbon atom consists of six protons, six neutrons, and six electrons, whereas an oxygen atom is made up of eight protons, eight neutrons, and eight electrons. Both oxygen and carbon have two electrons in their inner shells, but they differ in the number of electrons in the second shell. Oxygen has six electrons in the second shell and carbon has four (see figure A.1, *b* and *c*).

The chemical properties of an element and the way it reacts with other elements depend on the number of electrons in its outer shell. If this shell is full, the element does not react with others and is said to be inert. Helium, with two electrons in its outer shell, and neon, with 18 electrons in its outer shell, are examples of inert elements. Atoms whose outer shells are not full tend to move toward a more stable configuration by losing or gaining electrons or sharing electrons with other atoms. The atoms are bound together by attractive forces called chemical bonds. These bonds are a source of potential chemical energy. Breaking chemical bonds releases some energy that can be used to do work.

Nearly all the mass of an atom is in its protons and neutrons, so the combined number of these particles is the atomic mass of the element. The mass of an element is indicated by a superscript in front of the element (e.g., ^{1}H, ^{12}C, ^{16}O). The number of protons in an atom is its atomic number, which is indicated as a subscript in front of the symbol for the atom (e.g., $^{1}_{1}H$, $^{12}_{6}C$, $^{16}_{8}O$).

All atoms of a given element contain the same number of protons and electrons (which determine the chemical properties of the element), but in some elements the number of neutrons in the nucleus and, hence, the atomic mass (but not the atomic number) vary. Atoms of an element that have a different number of neutrons are called isotopes. Some isotopes are unstable and emit radiation in the form of gamma rays, electrons, or a helium nucleus (two protons and two neutrons). This radiation can be measured, and some unstable isotopes have proved useful as tracers. For example, normal carbon has an atomic mass of 12, but the radioactive isotope of carbon has a mass of 14. Glucose, a simple sugar, can be prepared using $^{14}_{6}C$, and its metabolism in the body can be followed by identifying the presence of $^{14}_{6}C$ in intermediate compounds and in expired carbon dioxide. Nowadays, the presence and quantity of stable isotopes (those that do not decay by the emission of radiation) such as $^{13}_{6}C$ can be detected, and these isotopes are increasingly used in place of the more dangerous radioactive isotopes in human metabolic studies.

Most elements in the body are not present as free atoms but are combined with other atoms to form molecules. For example, a molecule of water contains one atom of oxygen bound to two atoms of hydrogen, which is symbolized as H_2O (see figure A.2). Even the oxygen in the air that we breathe is made of molecular oxygen that consists of two atoms of oxygen bound together, which is symbolized as O_2. A molecule of a simple hexose sugar, glucose, contains 24 atoms: 6 of carbon, 12 of hydrogen, and 6 of oxygen. This formula can be expressed as $C_6H_{12}O_6$, which is known as the empirical chemical formula of glucose. The molecular mass is obtained by adding up the atomic masses present in the molecule. Thus, for glucose, we have:

$$6 \times {}^{12}C + 12 \times {}^{1}H + 6 \times {}^{16}O$$
$$= 72 + 12 + 96 = 180$$

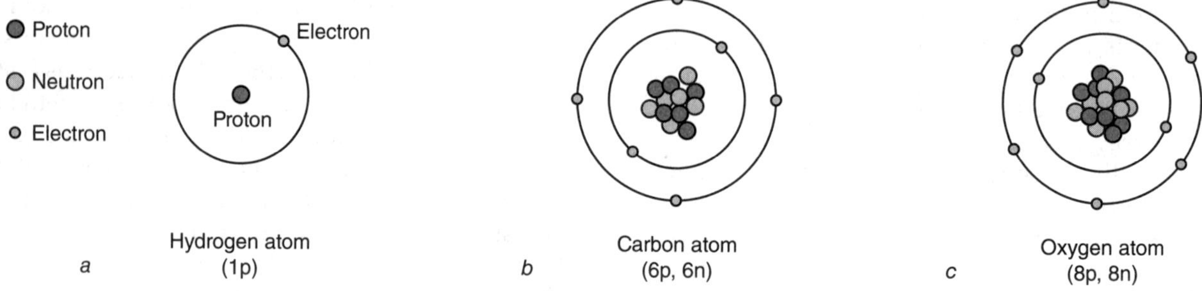

Figure A.1 Atoms of (*a*) hydrogen, (*b*) carbon, and (*c*) oxygen.

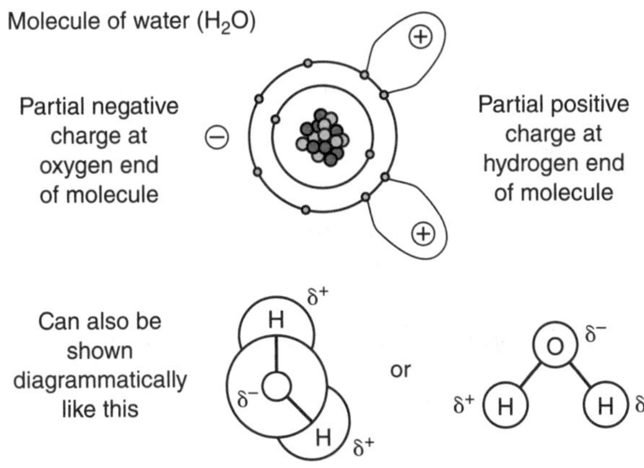

Figure A.2 A molecule of water indicating the distribution of partial charges.

TABLE A.1 Single, Double, and Triple Covalent Bonds

Bond number	Example	Energy/mol
Single	H H—C—H H	330 kJ (79 kcal)
Double	H H H—C=C—H H H	630 kJ (150 kcal)
Triple	H—C≡C—H	840 kJ (200 kcal)

The molecular mass of a substance in grams is equal to 1 mole (mol) of that substance, and the number of molecules in a mole of any substance is the same and is known as Avogadro's number, which is 6.022×10^{23}.

One mole of a substance dissolved in enough water to make 1 L is known as a 1 molar (M) solution. Biochemists usually deal with smaller concentrations, such as millimoles per liter (1 mM = 1×10^{-3} M), because many substances that are dissolved in the body fluids are found in this concentration range. For example, the concentration of glucose in blood is about 5 mM.

Chemical Bonds, Free Energy, and ATP

This section provides a brief review of chemical bonds and emphasizes bonds between the six major elements found in the living body: hydrogen (H), carbon (C), nitrogen (N), oxygen (O), phosphorus (P), and sulfur (S).

- Covalent bonds hold together two or more atoms by the interaction of their outer electrons. Covalent bonds are the strongest chemical bonds. The energy of a typical covalent bond is approximately 330 kJ/mol (79 kcal/mol), but this energy can vary from 210 kJ/mol to 460 kJ/mol (50-110 kcal/mol) depending on the elements involved. Once formed, covalent bonds rarely break spontaneously because the thermal energy of a molecule at room temperature (20 °C or 293 °K [68 °F]) is only about 2.5 kJ/mol (0.6 kcal/mol), which is much lower than the energy required to break a covalent bond. Covalent bonds are either single, double, or triple bonds (see table A.1).

- Carbon-carbon bonds are particularly strong and stable covalent bonds. The major organic elements have standard bonding capabilities: C, N, and P can form up to four covalent bonds with other atoms; O and S can form two covalent bonds; and H can form only one covalent bond. In solution, O and S can lose a proton (or hydrogen ion, H^+), thereby leaving the O or S with a negative charge (see figure A.3). Covalent bonds have partial charges when the atoms involved have different electronegativities. Water is one example of a molecule with partial charges. The symbols δ^+ and δ^- are used to indicate partial charges (see figure A.2). Oxygen, because of its high electronegativity, attracts the electrons away from the hydrogen atoms, resulting in a partial negative charge on the oxygen and a partial positive charge on each of the hydrogens. The possibility of hydrogen bonds is a consequence of these partial charges.

- Hydrogen bonds (H-bonds) are weak intramolecular or intermolecular attractions between a hydrogen atom and an electronegative atom possessing a lone pair of electrons (e.g., oxygen or nitrogen atoms). Hydrogen bonds are formed when a hydrogen atom is shared between two molecules (see figure A.4). Hydrogen bonds have polarity. A hydrogen atom covalently attached to a very electronegative atom (N, O, or P) shares its partial positive charge with a second electronegative atom (N, O, or P). Hydrogen bonds have a strength of 21 kJ/mol (5 kcal/mol). These bonds are

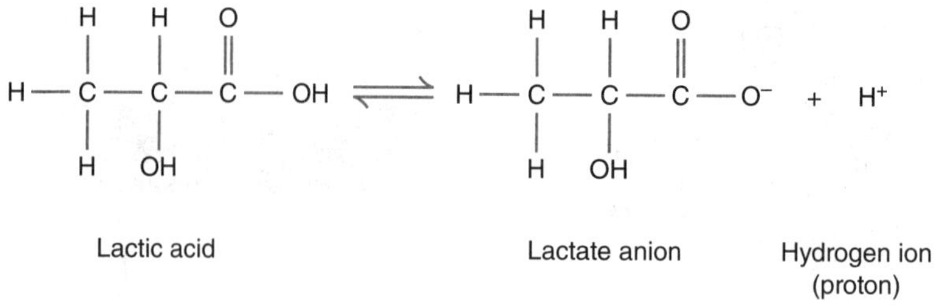

Lactic acid

Lactate anion

Hydrogen ion (proton)

Figure A.3 Dissociation of a proton (H^+) from lactic acid, leaving an oxygen (O) with a negative charge.

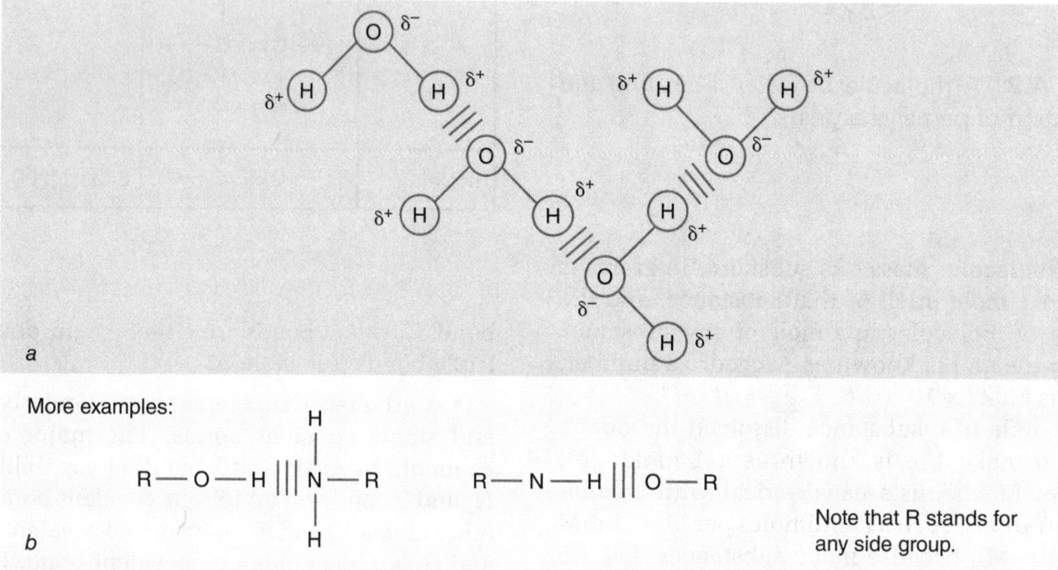

Figure A.4 (*a*) Hydrogen bonding between water molecules. A hydrogen atom covalently attached to a very electronegative atom (N, O, or P) shares its partial positive charge with a second electronegative atom (N, O, or P). (*b*) More examples of hydrogen bonding.

frequently found in proteins and nucleic acids, and by reinforcing each other, they keep the protein (or nucleic acid) structure secure. Because the hydrogen atoms in the protein can also H-bond to the surrounding water, the relative strength of protein–protein H-bonds versus protein–H_2O bonds is smaller than 21 kJ/mol.

- Ionic bonds are formed when a complete transfer of electrons from one atom to another occurs. The valence (outer shell) electrons are either lost or gained, which results in two ions: one positively charged and one negatively charged. The oppositely charged ions are held together by electrostatic forces. For example, when a sodium atom (Na) donates the one electron in its outer valence shell to a chlorine atom (Cl), which needs one electron to fill its outer valence shell, NaCl (salt) results. The symbol for sodium chloride is Na^+Cl^-. Ionic bonds have a strength of 17 to 30 kJ/mol (4-7 kcal/mol).

- Nonpolar molecules cannot form H-bonds with water and are therefore poorly soluble in water. These molecules are called hydrophobic (water-hating) molecules. Hydrophilic (water-loving) molecules can form H-bonds with water. Hydrophobic molecules tend to aggregate together in avoidance of water molecules, such as when a drop of oil is placed on water. The oil forms a thin layer over the surface of the water. If mixed together vigorously, the oil forms small globules but does not dissolve in the water. To understand the energetics driving this interaction, visualize the water molecules surrounding a single "dissolved" molecule attempting to form the greatest number of H-bonds with each other. The best energetic solution involves forcing all the nonpolar molecules together, thus reducing the total surface area that breaks up the H-bond matrix of the water.

During biochemical reactions that involve the breaking of chemical bonds, energy is released, some of which is available to do work. Some energy is also released as heat, which cannot be used to do work in the body because body temperature is regulated within a narrow range. The free energy released during the breaking of bonds, usually signified by the symbol G, can be used to do work because some of it is stored in the compound adenosine triphosphate (ATP). The free energy released when an inorganic phosphate (Pi) group is broken off ATP to form adenosine diphosphate (ADP) is used to drive several energy-requiring processes in the body, including the synthesis of macromolecules from smaller molecules (e.g., synthesis of proteins from free amino acids), membrane transport work (e.g., the movement of sodium ions out of a cell against the prevailing concentration gradient), and mechanical work (e.g., muscle contraction). Reactions that involve breaking phosphate bonds and the liberation of Pi are catalyzed by enzymes called kinases. In the case of ATP breakdown, these kinases are commonly abbreviated as ATPases.

ATP is the only form of chemical energy that is convertible into other forms of energy used by living cells. Essentially, ATP is the energy currency of the cell. Fats and carbohydrates are the main storage forms of energy in the body, and when they are broken down by oxidation reactions to carbon dioxide and water, the energy released is used to resynthesize ATP from ADP and Pi.

All biochemical reactions are inefficient, which means that not all the energy released can be conserved or used to do work. Some energy is always lost as heat. This release of heat helps maintain body temperature at about 37 °C (98.6 °F). During exercise, when the rate of catabolic reactions is markedly increased in the active muscles to provide energy for contraction, the rate of heat production also increases substantially and muscle temperature rises by 1 °C to 5 °C (1.8 °F to 9 °F).

Although ATP is considered the energy currency of the cell, it cannot be accumulated in large amounts, and the intramuscular ATP concentration is only about 5 mmol/kg of muscle tissue. During maximal exercise, ATP is sufficient to fuel about 2 seconds of muscle force generation. Experiments have shown that the muscle ATP store never becomes completely depleted, because it is efficiently resynthesized from ADP and Pi at the same rate at which it is degraded. During submaximal steady-state exercise, ATP resynthesis is achieved by mitochondrial oxidation of carbohydrates and lipids. This process is commonly referred to as aerobic metabolism because it requires oxygen. At the onset of exercise and in high-intensity exercise, however, ATP resynthesis is principally anaerobic (without the use of oxygen). Further details of the metabolic pathways involved can be found in chapter 3.

Chemical Reactions in the Body

A variety of chemical reactions take place in the body. These reactions are defined here and are accompanied by a few illustrative examples.

- Oxidation is a reaction that involves the loss of electrons from an atom. It is always accompanied by a reduction (a reaction in which a molecule gains electrons). For example, pyruvate is reduced using hydrogen donated from the reduced form of the coenzyme nicotinamide adenine dinucleotide (NADH) to form lactate. In the reverse reaction, lactate is oxidized by NAD^+ (the oxidized form of the coenzyme) when pyruvate is reformed. This reaction is also known as dehydrogenation because it is a form of oxidation that involves the loss of hydrogen atoms:

$$\text{pyruvate } CH_3\text{-CO-COOH} + NADH + H^+ \leftrightarrow \text{lactate } CH_3\text{-CHOH-COOH} + NAD^+$$

- Hydrolysis is a reaction in which an organic compound is split by interaction with water into simpler compounds. An example is the hydrolysis of phosphocreatine (PCr) to creatine (Cr) and phosphate, which is coupled to the resynthesis of ATP from ADP using the phosphate group liberated from phosphocreatine:

$$PCr + H_2O \rightarrow Cr + P$$

$$P + ADP + H^+ \rightarrow ATP + H_2O$$

- Phosphorylation is the addition of a phosphate (PO_3^{2-}) group to a molecule. Many enzymes are activated by the covalent bonding of a phosphate group. The phosphorylation of ADP forms ATP:

$$ADP + P_i \rightarrow ATP + H_2O$$

- Condensation is the union of two or more molecules with the elimination of a simpler group such as H_2O. An example is the joining of two amino acid molecules to form a dipeptide.

- Hydroxylation is the addition of a hydroxyl (OH) group to a molecule.
- Carboxylation is the addition of carbon dioxide catalyzed by an enzyme using biotin as its prosthetic group.
- Deamination is the loss of an amino (NH_2) group which liberates free ammonia (NH_3). This is important in the metabolism of amino acids such as alanine:

$$\text{alanine} \rightarrow \text{pyruvate} + NH_3$$

- Transamination is the transfer of an amino (NH_2) group from an amino acid to a keto acid. An example is the transfer of an amino group from the amino acid glutamate to the keto acid pyruvate, forming a new amino acid alanine and another keto acid α-ketoglutarate:

$$\text{glutamate} + \text{pyruvate} \rightarrow \text{alanine} + \alpha\text{-ketoglutarate}$$

- Denaturation is the alteration of the physical properties and three-dimensional structure of a protein by a chemical or physical treatment that does not disrupt the primary structure but generally results in the inactivation of the protein (e.g., the inactivation of an enzyme by the addition of a strong acid or excessive heat).

Hydrogen Ion Concentrations and Buffers

Free hydrogen ions are produced in many chemical reactions in the body. Problems such as decreased activity or even complete inactivation of enzymes and inhibition of several biological processes, including muscle contraction, can arise when free hydrogen ions accumulate inside cells. Hence, the body has several mechanisms that help to limit changes in the free hydrogen ion concentration in the fluids inside and outside cells.

An acid is a compound able to donate a hydrogen ion (H^+); examples include hydrochloric acid (HCl), carbonic acid (H_2CO_3), and lactic acid (CH_3-CHOH-COOH). A base is a compound able to accept a hydrogen ion; examples are hydroxyl ions (OH^-) and bicarbonate ions (HCO_3^-). The pH is a measure of the concentration of hydrogen ions. These values are derived, for example, from the dissociation of an acid, such as hydrochloric acid, when it is dissolved in water ($HCl \rightarrow H^+ + Cl^-$). The pH value is defined as the negative decimal logarithm of the free H^+ concentration or $[H^+]$; that is, $pH = -\log_{10}[H^+]$, where $[H^+]$ is expressed in moles per liter (mol/L or M) (the square brackets around H^+ signify a concentration; this nomenclature is commonly used in chemistry), so the concentration of free H^+ increases 10-fold for each decrease of 1 pH unit. The $[H^+]$ in pure water is 10^{-7} mol/L. Therefore, the pH of pure water is

$$pH = -\log_{10}(10^{-7}) = -(-7) = 7$$

A pH of 7 is often referred to as neutral pH. Everything below pH 7 has a higher concentration of H^+ and is considered acidic. Everything above pH 7 has a lower concentration of H^+ and is considered basic (you can also think of this as a higher concentration of OH^-). Most body fluids are close to neutral pH. For example, blood plasma has a pH of 7.4, and resting muscle intracellular fluid (sarcoplasm) has a pH of 7.0. The pH of the body fluids is tightly regulated, and even in the most severe metabolic disturbances, such as high-intensity exercise, the pH of blood does not change by more than about 0.3. Even in the exercising muscle where the additional hydrogen ions are first appearing because of the increased lactic acid production, the pH does not fall below 6.5. As previously mentioned, this stability is important because if the pH falls too low, the activity of enzymes can be inhibited, which can have fatal consequences for the cell.

Buffers act as a reservoir for hydrogen ions and thus limit, or buffer, changes in free H^+ concentration. Buffering is passive and virtually instantaneous. A buffer consists of a weak acid and its conjugate base. In solution, some (but not all) molecules of the weak acid dissociate into the conjugate base and hydrogen ions:

$$BH \leftrightarrow B^- + H^+$$

where BH is the weak acid and B^- is its conjugate base. The relationship between the concentrations of weak acid, base, and hydrogen ions can be expressed as an equation:

$$K_a \cdot [BH] = [H^+] \times [B^-]$$

where K_a is the dissociation constant of the acid, that is, the concentration of H^+ at which the concentrations of the base and acid are equal. The equation can be rearranged to give the Henderson equation:

$$[H^+] = K_a \times [BH] / [B^-]$$

Alternately, by taking the negative logarithm of each side of the equation, it becomes the Henderson-Hasselbalch equation:

$$-\log_{10}[H^+] = -\log_{10}K_a + \log_{10}[B^-] / [BH]$$

which is the same as

$$pH = pK_a + \log_{10}[B^-] / [BH]$$

which tells us that optimal buffering (minimum change in pH when H^+ ions are added) occurs at pH = pK_a and that this effect occurs when the concentrations of weak acid (BH) and base (B^-) are equal.

Carbonic acid/bicarbonate (H_2CO_3/HCO_3^-) is the most important extracellular buffer, and it has a pK_a of 6.1. Hemoglobin and other proteins and peptides containing the amino acid histidine (pK_a usually 6.0 to 8.0) and phosphates ($HPO_4^{2-}/H_2PO_4^-$), for which pK_a is 6.8, are important intracellular buffers. Because the pH of most body fluids is about 7.4, buffers with a pK_a of between 6 and 8 are the most effective.

In exercising muscle, large amounts of hydrogen ions are produced from the dissociation of lactic acid to H^+ and the lactate anion (see figure A.3). The resting intracellular pH of muscle is 7.0. A large fall in pH is undesirable because it would denature enzymes and is prevented by the presence of intracellular buffers, including carnosine (a dipeptide consisting of alanine and histidine), phosphocreatine, phosphates, and histidine-containing proteins. As the hydrogen ions diffuse out of the muscle into the blood, they are buffered by bicarbonate (in plasma) and hemoglobin (in the red blood cells). An increase in the blood lactic acid concentration of 10 mmol/L changes the blood pH by only about 0.1; this concentration of lactic acid dissolved in water alone causes the pH to drop from 7.0 to 2.0. Clearly, the body's buffer systems are very effective.

Enzymes

Enzymes act as controllable catalysts. These proteins speed up the rate of specific chemical reactions and allow them to be regulated in ways that permit the body to control the interactions between the different metabolic pathways. The direction in which the reactions proceed and the equilibrium point that is reached in a nonbiological system are governed by the laws of thermodynamics. The characteristics of enzymes that allow them to act as catalysts are briefly described.

Mechanisms of Enzyme Action and Enzyme Kinetics

The laws of thermodynamics tell us that chemical reactions proceed spontaneously only in the direction that results in the products of the reaction having a lower energy status than the substrates (see figure A.5). Enzymes act as reusable catalysts, which involves the formation of an enzyme substrate complex as an intermediate step in the reaction. The formation of this substrate lowers the energy of activation. Because less energy is now needed, the reaction is more likely to proceed. Although the enzyme participates in the reaction, it is not consumed and is therefore required only in small amounts.

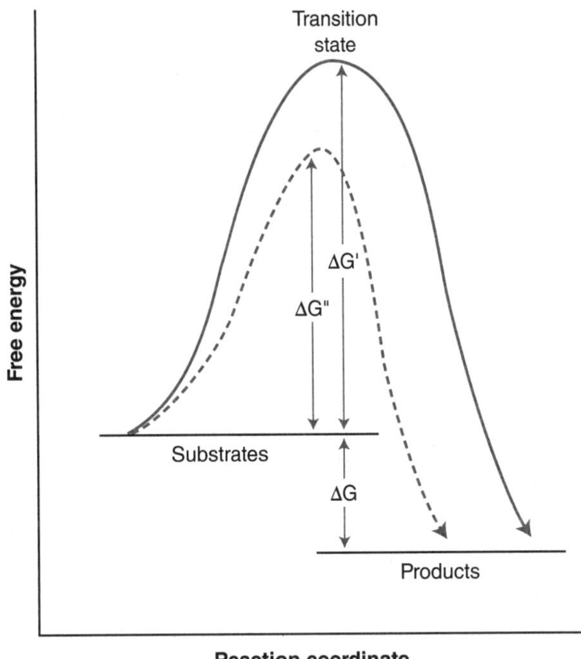

Figure A.5 Energy status of substrates and products.

The energetics of formation of the enzyme substrate complex are not well understood, but clearly some kind of weak bond forms between the substrate and the enzyme. This bond involves one or more active sites on the enzyme, and these sites have a particular shape and charge distribution that allows them to interact with the substrate. These characteristics allow enzymes to promote the rates of specific reaction in a number of ways. Where two or more substrates are involved, attachment to binding sites on the enzyme allows the substrates to be brought into close proximity in the correct orientation, thus increasing the chances that a reaction will take place. Alternatively, binding to the enzyme can cause changes in the shape of the substrate molecule that increase its susceptibility to reaction.

Enzyme Kinetics

Enzyme kinetics is the measurement of the change in substrate or product concentration as a function of time. The first stage in an enzyme-catalyzed reaction is the binding of the substrate (S) to the active site of the enzyme (E) to form an enzyme-substrate complex (ES). The substrate then reacts to form the product (P), which is released. Release of the product restores the enzyme to its original free form:

$$E + S \leftrightarrow ES \rightarrow E + P$$

The assumption is that the first stage of the process is reversible but the second is not. In almost all reactions, the substrate concentration far exceeds the enzyme concentration. This difference means that formation of the ES complex does not result in an appreciable change in the substrate concentration but does reduce the concentration of the free enzyme.

The progress curve for the reaction is initially linear, decreasing in slope as the reaction proceeds and substrate is used up, as shown in figure A.6. The initial velocity during the linear part of the curve is called V_0. The relationship between V_0 and the substrate concentration ([S]) is described by the Michaelis-Menten equation:

$$V_0 = V_{max} [S] / K_m + [S]$$

where V_{max} is the maximum velocity of the reaction at infinite [S] and K_m is the Michaelis constant equivalent to the substrate concentration in which the initial reaction velocity (V_0) is equal to one-half the maximal velocity (i.e., K_m = [S] where $V_0 = V_{max}/2$). This relationship is depicted graphically in figure A.7 and clearly shows that at low concentrations of substrate, the initial reaction rate increases linearly in response to increasing substrate concentration, but the rate approaches a limit above which it is constant and independent of substrate concentration. At this point, all the enzyme molecules are effectively saturated with substrate. The V_{max} is, therefore, a function of the amount of enzyme present.

When the substrate concentration is equal to K_m, the reaction rate is equal to half of the V_{max}. The K_m value is, therefore, equal to the substrate concentration that will result in the reaction proceeding at one-half of the maximum rate. A high K_m value is, therefore, an indication of low affinity of the enzyme for its substrate. A high substrate concentration is necessary to achieve a reaction rate equal to one-half the maximum rate. High reaction rates are only achieved when the substrate concentration is relatively high. If [S] is equal to 10 times the K_m, substituting these values into the Michaelis-Menten equation tells us that the reaction rate is 91% of V_{max}, and 99% of the maximum rate will be achieved only when the substrate concentration is 100 times the K_m.

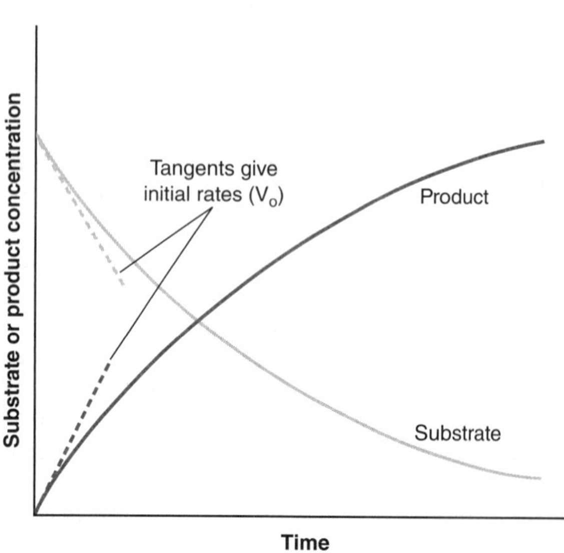

Figure A.6 Progress of an enzyme-catalyzed reaction.

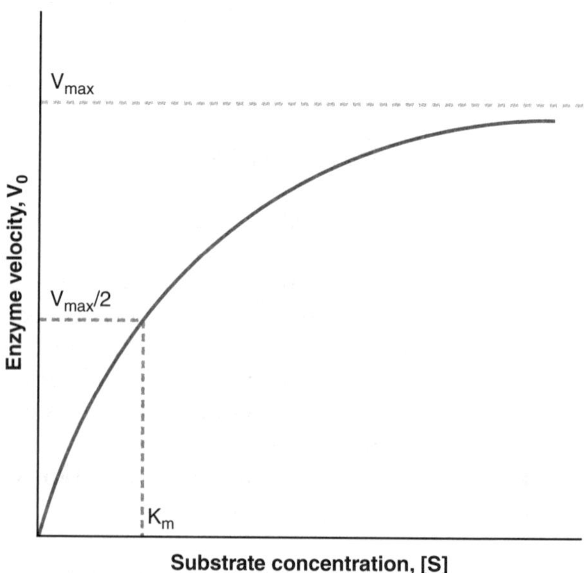

Figure A.7 Relationship between the initial reaction velocity and substrate concentration for an enzyme-catalyzed reaction.

Factors Influencing Enzyme Activity

The activity of enzymes can be assessed by the rate of substrate use or product formation under standardized conditions. The most common unit of measurement is the International Unit (IU). This measure is the amount of enzyme that converts 1 μmol of substrate to product in 1 minute under the conditions specified for that reaction. Although this measure is generally used among physiologists, the appropriate SI unit should be used. This unit is the katal (kat), which is the amount of enzyme that converts 1 mol of substrate to product in 1 second under optimum conditions. At least part of the reason for the persistence of the IU is the difficulty in defining optimum conditions for the activity of individual enzymes.

Effects of Temperature and pH

Enzyme activity is particularly sensitive to temperature and increases as the temperature increases. Any expression of enzyme activities must therefore specify the temperature at which measurements are made. Temperatures of 25 °C and 37 °C (77 °F and 98.6 °F) are normally used as standards. At high temperatures, however, enzyme activity falls sharply and irreversibly because of structural changes caused by denaturation of the protein, as shown in figure A.8. Although body core temperature is usually about 37 °C (98.6 °F), the temperature of muscle tissue may be as low as 30 °C (86 °F) in a resting person on a cold day and can rise to 42 °C (108 °F) during high-intensity

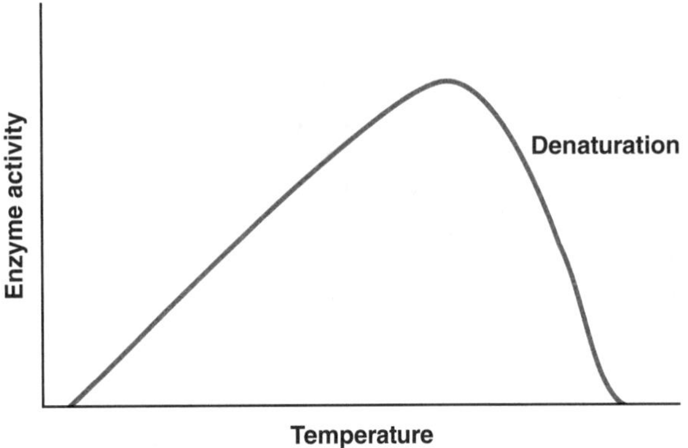

Figure A.8 Effect of temperature on enzyme activity.

exercise. Hence, warming up before an event has important implications for maximizing reaction rates and optimizing muscle performance. Except in extreme cases of heat illness, body core temperature seldom exceeds 41 °C (106 °F), but this temperature is close to the level at which some enzymes and other proteins are affected.

Changes in the ionization state of an enzyme caused by a change in the pH of the cell affect its affinity for its substrate because of changes in structure or charge distribution at the active site, as illustrated in figure A.9. The local pH may also affect the ionization state of the substrate. All enzymes have an optimum pH (where enzyme activity is at its highest, as shown in figure A.10), but optimum pH differs among different enzymes and may also be influenced by the presence of

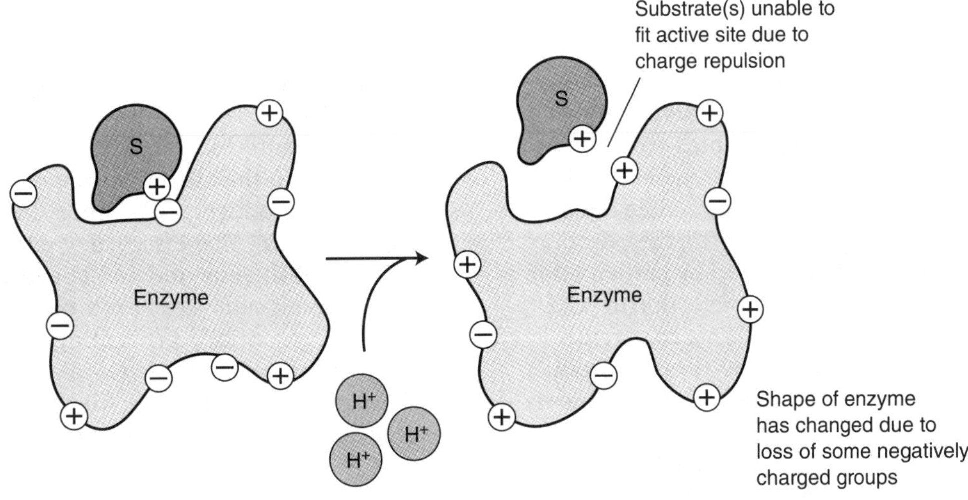

Figure A.9 Change in charge distribution of enzyme molecules caused by change in pH.

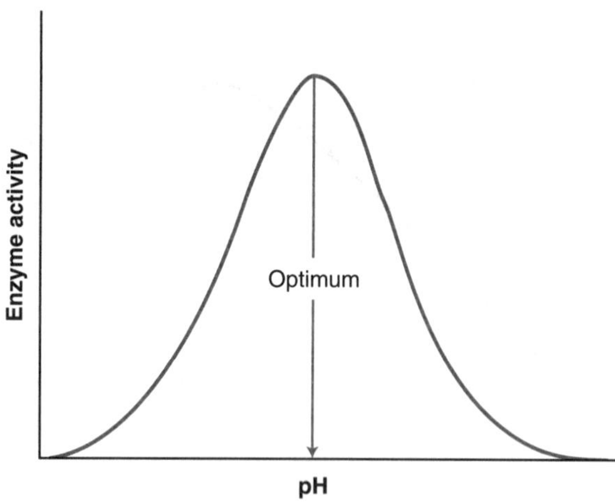

Figure A.10 Effect of pH on enzyme activity.

other activators and inhibitors. Variations in pH are generally small in most tissues, and skeletal muscle shows the largest changes in response to very high-intensity exercise; pH may fall from the resting value of about 7.0 to 6.5 or even less. Many enzymes normally function in an environment that is close to their pH optimum. For example, pepsin, which has a pH optimum of about 2.0, seems well adapted for the acid conditions of the stomach, where it hydrolyzes proteins into smaller fragments (peptides) and amino acids that can be absorbed in the small intestine. Some enzymes, however, have a pH optimum, at least in their isolated and purified form, that is far from their normal environment. Glycerol kinase has maximum activity at a pH of 9.8, a condition that is never reached in the cell.

Coenzymes, Prosthetic Groups, Cofactors, and Activators

Many enzymes require the presence of one or more coenzymes if the reaction is to proceed. For example, the conversion of lactate to pyruvate involves the removal of two hydrogen atoms from lactate and is catalyzed by lactate dehydrogenase, which requires that the coenzyme nicotinamide adenine dinucleotide (NAD^+) participate in the reaction. Coenzymes are chemically altered by participation in the reaction, in this case by conversion of NAD^+ to its reduced form, NADH. The coenzyme is, therefore, essentially a substrate for or a product of the reaction, but a characteristic of coenzymes is that they are readily regenerated by other reactions within the cell. Some coenzymes, such as NAD^+, are loosely bound to the enzyme, but others, such as biotin, are tightly bound and are referred to as prosthetic groups.

Many enzymes have low activities in the absence of cofactors, and the presence of one or another metal ion, especially the divalent metals calcium, magnesium, manganese, and zinc, is essential for activation of many enzymes. Binding to these ions alters the charge distribution and shape of the active site of the enzyme. For example, the release of calcium into the cytoplasm in response to the nerve impulse is important in the activation of phosphorylase, which allows acceleration of the glycolytic pathway.

Competitive and Noncompetitive Inhibition

Substances with a chemical structure similar to that of the normal substrate may also bind to the active site on the enzyme and thus interfere with enzyme function by reducing the number of active sites available to the proper substrate. These substances compete with the substrate for access to the active site and are therefore known as competitive inhibitors. The effect of competitive inhibition is to increase K_m. Increasing the concentration of substrate to a sufficient level will, however, swamp the effects of the inhibitor, and V_{max} is not affected by competitive inhibition.

Noncompetitive inhibitors bind to the enzyme at other sites, leaving the active site of the enzyme available to the substrate, but they have the effect of altering the conformation of the protein and thus reducing the catalytic activity of the active site. The V_{max} is reduced, but the same substrate concentration still produces one-half of the new maximum activity (i.e., K_m remains unchanged).

Allosteric and Covalent Modulation

Allosteric modulation of enzyme activity is the reversible binding of small molecules to the enzyme at sites other than the active site, producing a conformational change in the structure of the enzyme molecule. This change in shape and charge distribution results in a change (either an increase or a decrease) in the affinity of the enzyme for its substrates or products and, hence, in its activity (see figure A.11*a*). The effect may either increase the activity of the enzyme and speed up the rate of the reaction it catalyzes or inhibit the activity of the enzyme, essentially preventing the reaction it catalyzes from taking place. Covalent modulation involves phosphorylation or dephosphorylation (i.e., the addition or removal of a phosphate group, respectively) of an enzyme, which usually affects the hydroxyl (-OH) group of a serine residue in the polypeptide chain (see figure A.11*b*). As with allosteric effects, covalent modulation may either

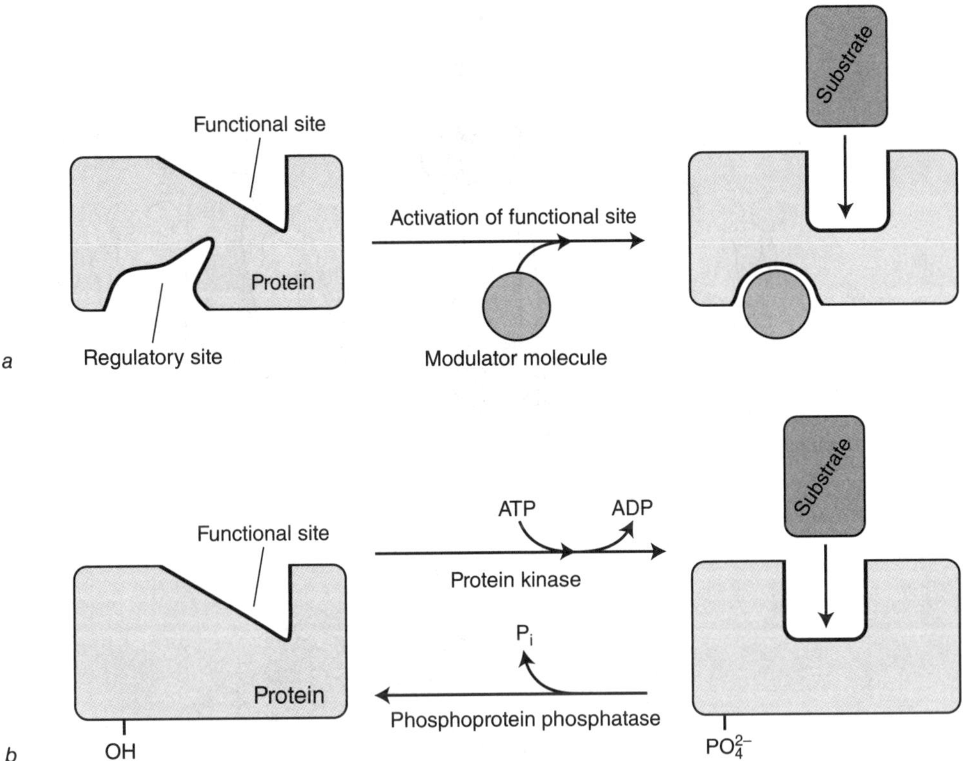

Figure A.11 (*a*) Allosteric modulation of enzyme activity and (*b*) covalent modulation of enzyme activity.

activate or inhibit enzyme activity. A good example is the activity of glycogen phosphorylase, which catalyzes the breakdown of muscle glycogen. This enzyme needs to be activated at the onset of exercise to allow the muscle glycogen store to be used as an energy source, and this increase in enzyme activity is achieved by the covalent attachment of a phosphate group by a protein kinase that was itself activated by a rise in the intracellular calcium ion concentration (for further details, see chapter 3).

Enzyme Isoforms

Some enzymes exist in more than one form. These isoforms catalyze the same reaction but are generally found in different tissues and may have different specificities or catalytic capabilities. Lactate dehydrogenase exists in two forms that are each made up of four subunits. The subunits exist in one of two forms: the H form, which is predominantly in cardiac muscle, and the M form, which is predominantly in skeletal muscle. Five different combinations of these subunits are possible. In muscle, the H form is associated with tissues that have a high capacity for oxidative metabolism and that, therefore, have a high capacity for lactate oxidation, whereas the M form is associated with tissues that have a high anaerobic capacity relative to their oxidative capability. The M form favors the conversion of pyruvate to lactate, whereas the H form favors the conversion of lactate to pyruvate. Many other enzymes exist in a variety of isoforms, but their functional significance is not well understood.

Membrane Structure and Transport

Membranes set the limits of cell boundaries. To enter a cell from the extracellular fluid, a substance must pass through the cell membrane. For example, the simple sugars that are formed from the breakdown of complex carbohydrates in the gastrointestinal tract can get into the bloodstream only by passing through the cells that line the gut. The properties of cell membranes and the components within them determine which substances can and cannot enter or leave a cell.

Cell membranes are composed of a lipid bilayer that contains mostly phospholipids and some cholesterol. Within these lipids are proteins, some of which are restricted to one side of the bilayer and some of which are embedded within the

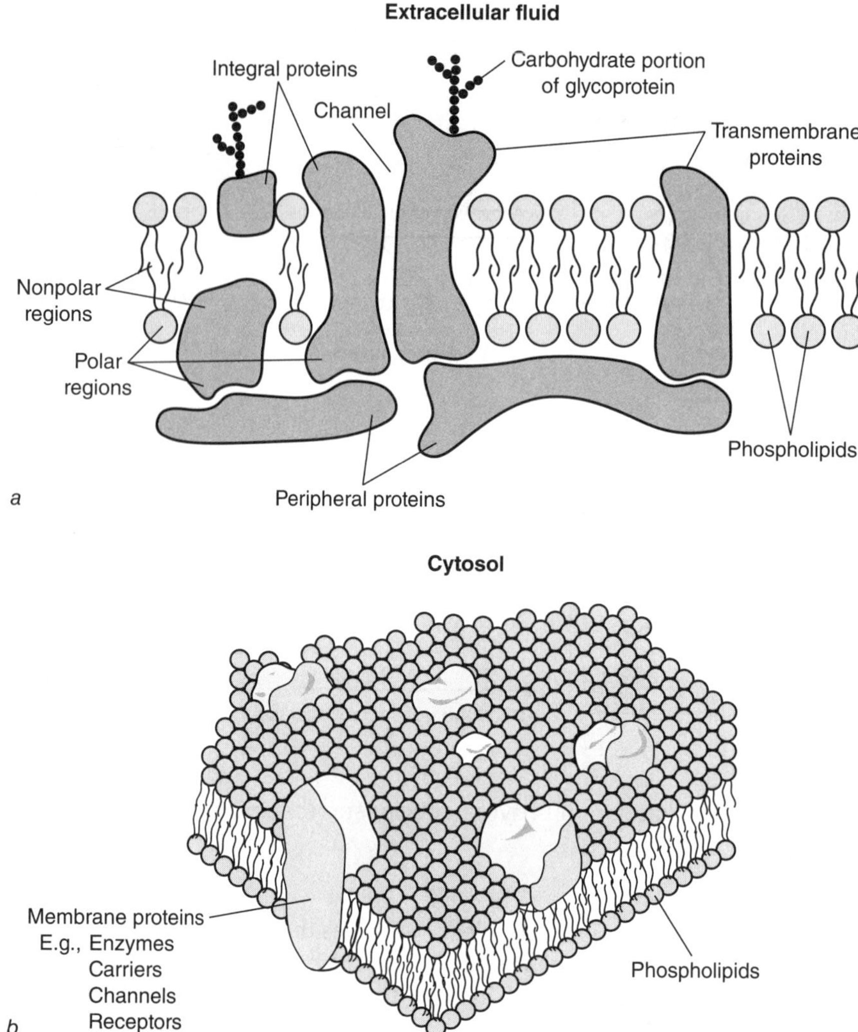

Figure A.12 Cell membranes. (*a*) A two-dimensional cross-section and (*b*) a three-dimensional view.

membrane from one side to the other (see figure A.12). These proteins have important structural roles as receptors, channels, or transporters.

Dissolved substances (solutes) move across these semipermeable membranes by simple diffusion, facilitated diffusion, or active transport. Osmosis is the movement of water across membranes.

Simple Diffusion

Solutes move from high to low concentration only by diffusion. Simple diffusion involves the movement of the solute across the lipid bilayer; therefore, to a large degree this is influenced by the solubility of the substance in lipid. Most water-soluble substances (e.g., glucose) and charged particles (e.g., sodium ions) are poorly soluble in lipid. Large molecules, such as proteins, cannot pass across membranes. Very small molecules (e.g., O_2, CO_2, H_2O, NH_3) diffuse easily across cell membranes. Rates of diffusion are affected by temperature and the concentration difference on either side of the membrane.

Facilitated Diffusion

In facilitated diffusion, solutes move only from high to low concentration by diffusion but use a specific protein carrier molecule to pass through the membrane. The protein may be a mobile carrier or a gated channel, as illustrated in figure A.13. As shown in the example of glucose membrane transport in figure A.14, the rate of transport across the membrane is far greater in facilitated diffusion compared with simple diffusion, but at high glucose concentrations, facilitated transport

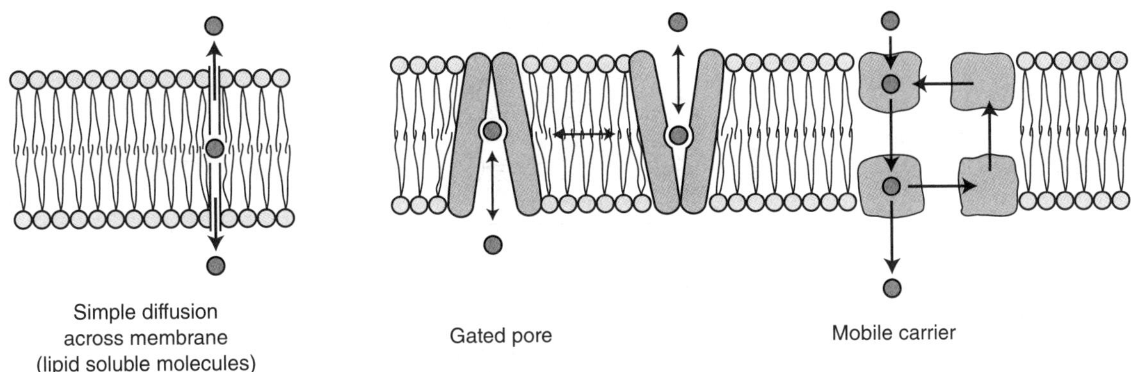

Figure A.13 Diffusion and facilitated diffusion of substances across cell membranes. In both cases, net movement of the solute molecules occurs from a high concentration of solute to a low concentration of solute.

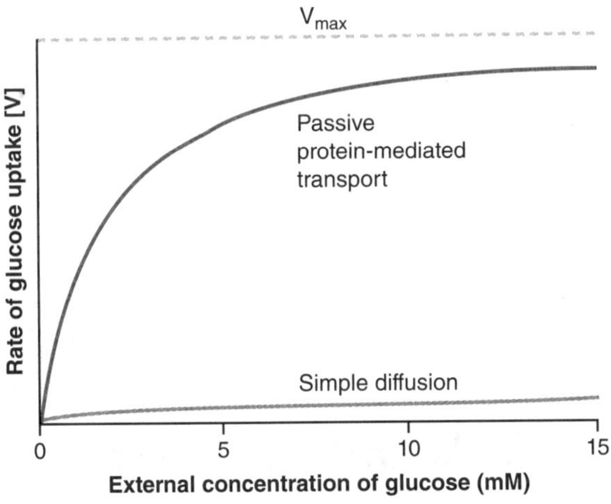

Figure A.14 Relative rates of glucose uptake into cells by simple diffusion and facilitated diffusion using a protein transporter in relation to the glucose concentration of the extracellular fluid.

exhibits saturation kinetics. The maximum speed of facilitated transport (V_{max}), indicated by the dashed line, is limited by the number of protein transporters available in the membrane. When all the transporters are full, additional movement can occur only by simple diffusion. In muscle, glucose is transported into the fibers by a protein carrier called GLUT4. The number of GLUT4 transporters in the muscle fiber membrane is influenced by exercise and the hormone insulin.

Active Transport

In active transport, substances are moved against their concentration gradient by a specific protein carrier and energy supplied directly by ATP or indirectly by ion electrochemical gradients. The sodium-potassium pump, or Na^+-K^+-ATPase pump, is a good example of an active cellular transport mechanism and is illustrated in figure A.15. Energy released from the hydrolysis of ATP moves sodium and potassium ions across the cell membrane against the prevailing concentration gradients. For each molecule of ATP hydrolyzed to ADP, three sodium ions (Na^+) are transported out of the cell and two potassium ions (K^+) are transported into the cell. Because more positively charged ions are moved out of the cell than are transported in, an electrochemical gradient is established. Inside the cell becomes negative relative to outside, with a difference in electrical potential of about 70 millivolts. Inside the cell, the Na^+ concentration is maintained at about 12 mM, whereas outside it is about 145 mM. The K^+ concentration inside the cell is about 155 mM, whereas outside it is only 4 mM. The presence of separate sodium and potassium ion channels in the membrane is also shown in figure A.15. When these channels are open, the ions move by diffusion from high to low concentration. The selective opening of sodium channels (allowing a rapid influx of positively charged Na^+ ions) causes a temporary change in the resting membrane potential called depolarization. Depolarization is important in the generation and propagation of action potentials in excitable cells such as nerve and muscle.

Cotransport (or symport) mechanisms use the electrochemical gradient set up by the Na^+-K^+-ATPase pump to transport a substance against its concentration gradient. For example, the inward transport of dietary glucose from the gut lumen

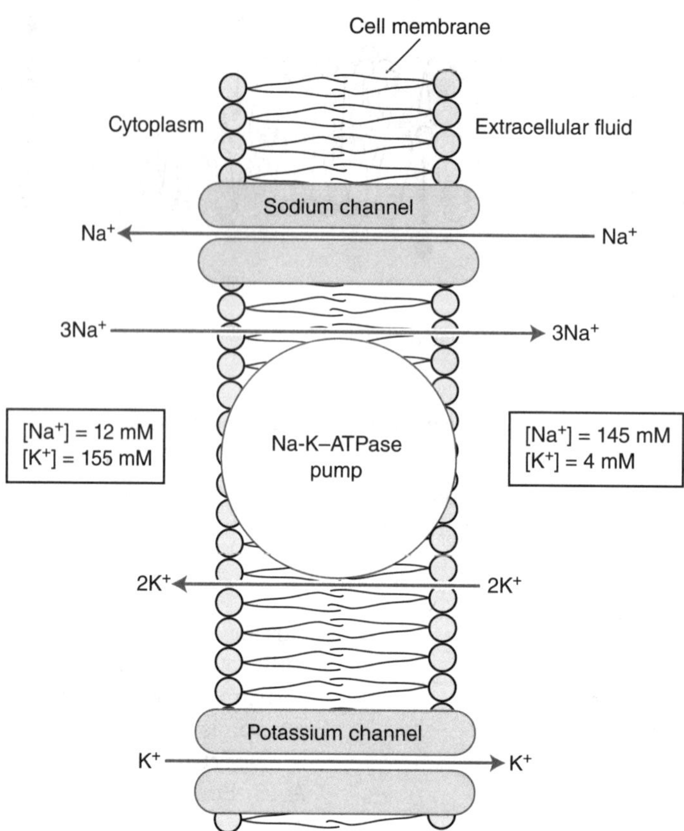

Figure A.15 The Na^+–K^+–ATPase pump. Energy released from the hydrolysis of ATP is used to move sodium and potassium ions across the cell membrane against the prevailing concentration gradients.

into intestinal epithelial cells is coupled to that of Na^+, as depicted in figure A.16. The Na^+-K^+-ATPase pump generates a large concentration difference for sodium across the membrane. The glucose–sodium symport protein uses that sodium gradient to transport glucose into the cell followed by separate transport of glucose across the basal membrane into the blood by the action of a glucose transporter (GLUT2).

Osmosis

Water can readily diffuse across membranes through the lipid bilayer and through protein pores or channels in the membrane. Osmosis is the net movement of water as a consequence of a total-solute particle concentration difference across a membrane. Water moves across a semipermeable membrane from a region of low total-solute particle concentration (osmolarity) to a region of high total-solute particle concentration until the total-solute particle concentration is equal on each side of the membrane (see figure A.17) or its movement is counteracted by the buildup of hydrostatic pressure.

Cells and Organelles

All tissues in the body are made of cells. Each cell contains several internal structures called organelles. These organelles include the nucleus, the mitochondrion, and other structures that are briefly described in this section. Not all cells contain all structures, because some cells are specialized for particular functions. For example, mature red blood cells are specialized for the transport of the respiratory pigment hemoglobin and oxygen and do not contain a nucleus or any mitochondria.

A typical cell is shown in figure A.18. The average diameter of a cell in the human body is about 10 μm (1/100th of a millimeter), although a wide variety of cell shapes and sizes exists. The cell is compartmentalized, and the organelles are distinct subcellular structures. In total, the adult human body contains about 10^{14} cells. Most cells (apart from those in adipose tissue) are 70% to 80% water.

The nucleus is the largest organelle. It is usually round or oval and surrounded by a nuclear envelope composed of two phospholipid membranes. This envelope contains pores through which messenger molecules pass to the cytoplasm. The

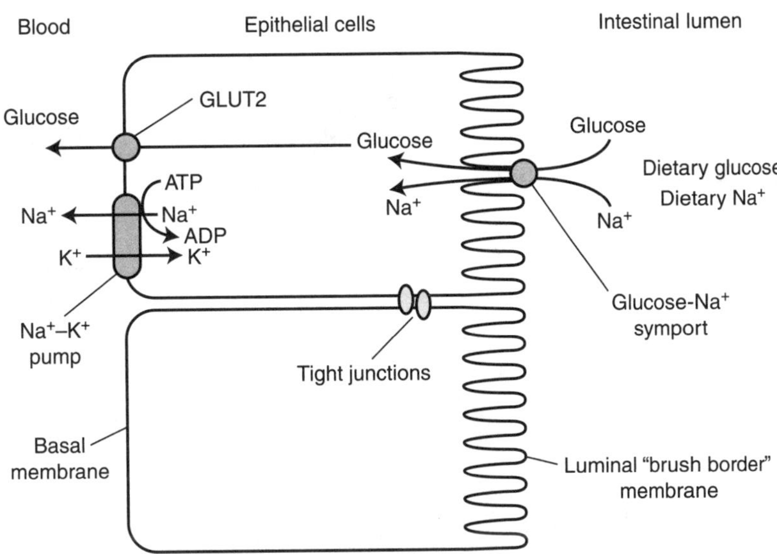

Figure A.16 Cotransport (symport) of glucose and sodium from the gut lumen into epithelial cells of the small intestine followed by separate transport across the basal membrane into the blood by the action of a glucose transporter (GLUT2) and the Na^+–K^+–ATPase pump.

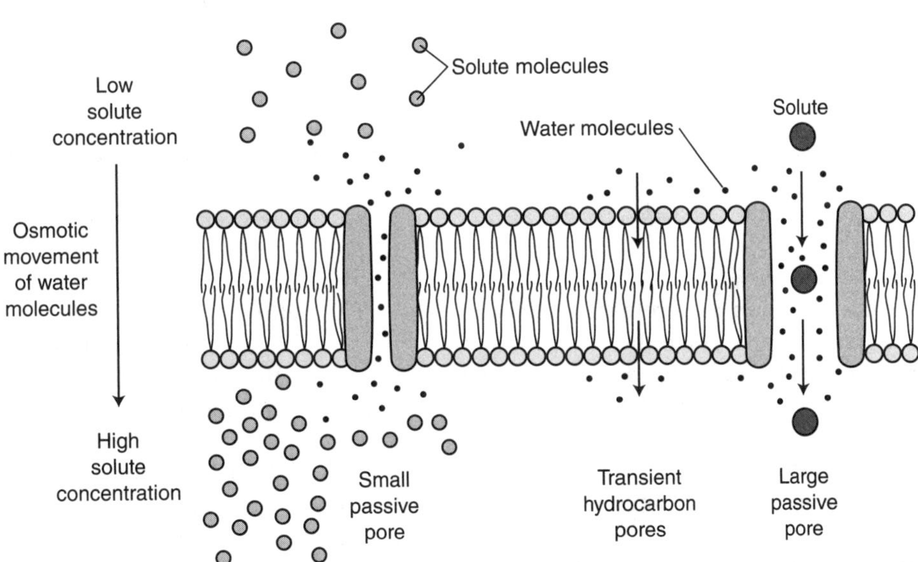

Figure A.17 Possible mechanisms for permeation of cell membranes by water. Water is a small molecule and thus permeates through the spaces between hydrophobic lipid molecules, specific water pores, or other pores (e.g., ion channels). Water molecules always move in the direction of a higher solute (dissolved particle) concentration.

nucleus stores genetic information in the form of deoxyribonucleic acid (DNA). That genetic information passes from the nucleus to the cytoplasm, where amino acids are assembled into proteins. The nucleolus is a densely staining region of the nucleus that expresses information required by ribosomal proteins.

The rough granular endoplasmic reticulum is an extensive network of folded, sheet-like membranes that has ribosomes attached to its surface. Proteins are synthesized on the ribosomes. The smooth (agranular) endoplasmic reticulum is a highly branched tubular network that does not have attached ribosomes. It contains enzymes for fatty

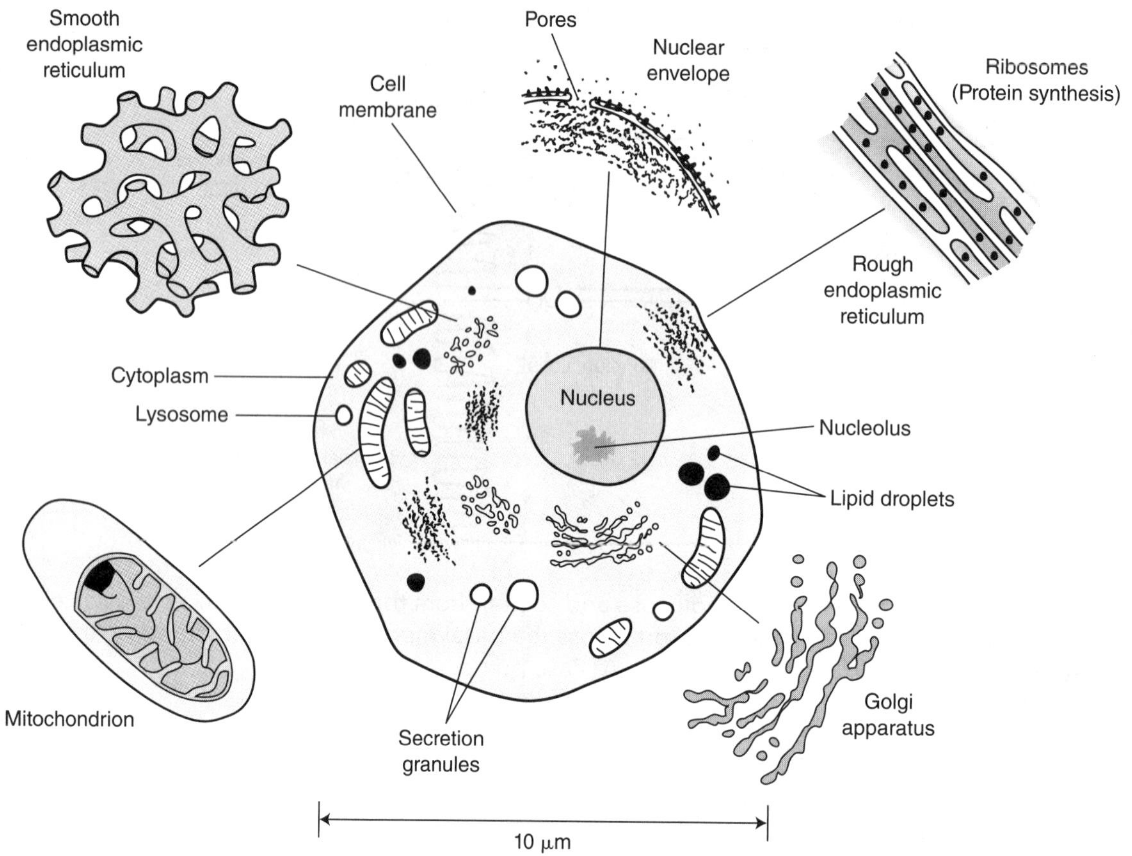

Figure A.18 A typical cell in cross-section. The structures of several organelles are shown.

acid synthesis and stores and releases calcium, which is an important process in the regulation of contraction. The specialized smooth endoplasmic reticulum in muscle is called the sarcoplasmic reticulum.

The Golgi apparatus is a series of cup-shaped flattened membranous sacs associated with numerous vesicles. It concentrates, modifies, and sorts newly synthesized proteins before their distribution, by way of vesicles, to other organelles, to the plasma membrane, or to secretions from the cell.

The mitochondrion is an oval-shaped body surrounded by two membranes. The inner membrane folds into the matrix of the mitochondrion to form cristae. This is the major site of ATP production, oxygen utilization, and carbon dioxide production. It contains the enzymes of fatty acid oxidation, the tricarboxylic acid (Krebs) cycle, and the electron-transport chain.

Lysosomes are small membranous vesicles that contain digestive enzymes. After injury, these enzymes may be activated and cause necrosis (death) of the cell.

The cytoplasm, or cytosol, is the fluid portion of the cell surrounding all the organelles. It stores energy in the form of glycogen granules and lipid droplets and contains the enzymes of anaerobic glycolysis.

Although the cell shape and size as depicted in figure A.18 are typical of many cells, other cells are distinctly specialized for the functions they perform. For example, skeletal muscle cells are long, cylindrical striated fibers (see figure A.19). The cytoplasm of muscle fibers is the sarcoplasm, and the plasma membrane is the sarcolemma. Myofibrils are the contractile elements composed of chains of sarcomeres that contain thin (actin) and thick (myosin) filaments arranged in a regular array. Surrounding the myofibrils is the sarcoplasmic reticulum, which is an elaborate, baglike membranous structure. Its interconnecting tubules lie in the narrow spaces between the myofibrils and surround and run parallel to them. It plays an important role in contraction by storing calcium ions, which when released into the sarcoplasm initiate muscle contraction. Numerous mitochon-

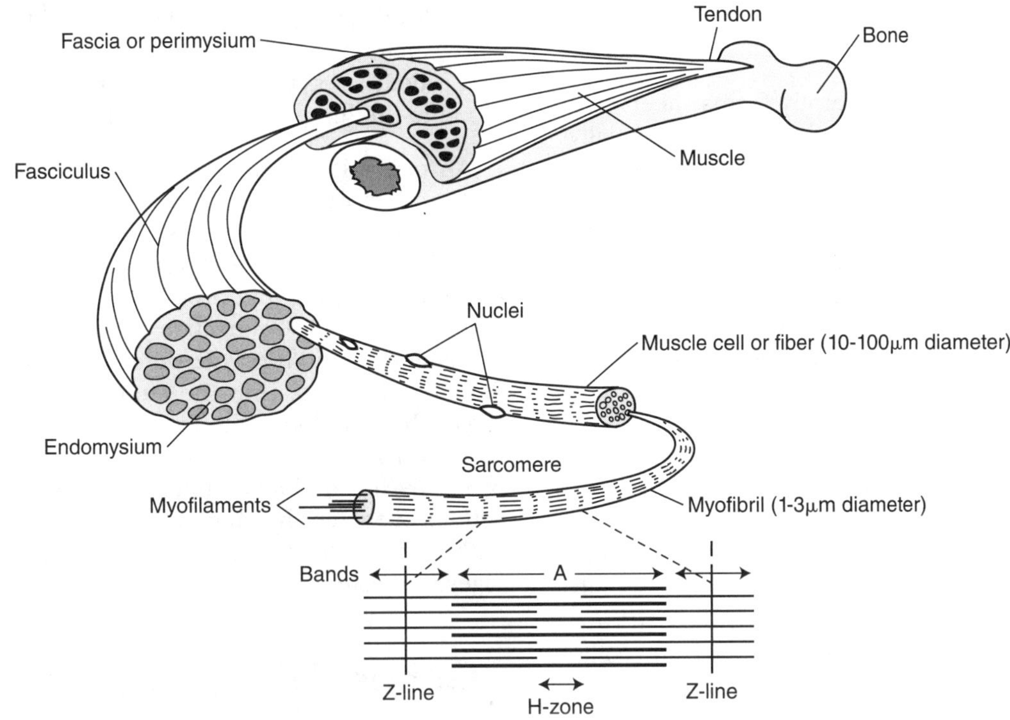

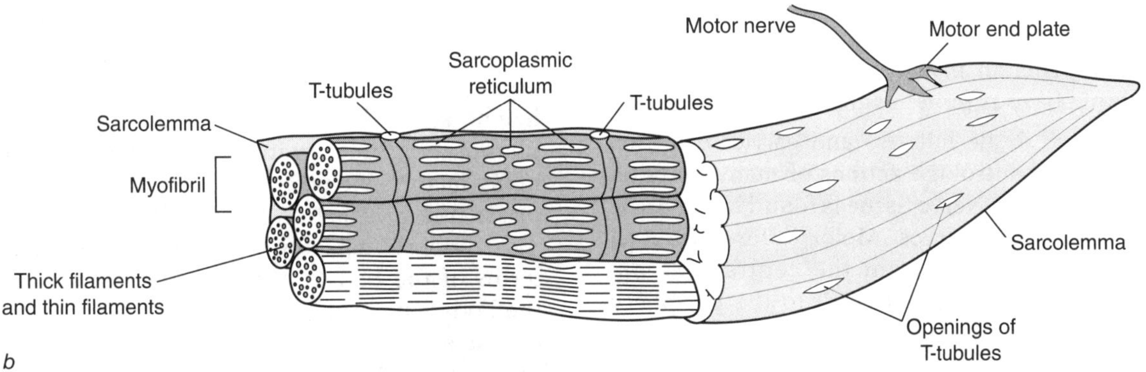

Figure A.19 (*a*) The structure of skeletal muscle and (*b*) the ultrastructure of a skeletal muscle fiber showing the location of the myofibrils (contractile proteins) and the sarcoplasmic reticulum.

dria are located near the plasma membrane mostly around the outer circumference of the muscle fiber close to the oxygen supply from the blood capillaries. Muscles contain a mixture of fiber types that are classified according to their contractile speed and metabolic characteristics. Further details can be found in chapter 3.

Tissues, Organs, and Systems

The cells of the body form larger structures called tissues (e.g., muscle) and organs (e.g., heart, lungs, and liver). A tissue is a group of similar cells specialized to carry out particular functions. An organ is a distinct body part formed from the combination of all four major tissue groups and designed to carry out a more general function than the tissues within it.

Although all somatic cells of the body except the germ cells (sperm in males, oocytes in females) contain the same genetic information, not all of this information in the DNA is expressed in the form of protein. Cellular specialization is possible because of the selective expression of genes by different cells. This specialization is what makes, for example, a skeletal muscle cell different from a nerve cell or a white blood cell. Cells can generally be classified as belonging to one of four groups of tissues: epithelial, connective, nerve, and muscle.

- Epithelial tissue generally forms sheets that protect against abrasion and the entry of potentially harmful substances or microorganisms. Epithelial tissue comprises the skin surface, the internal linings of the gastrointestinal tract, the blood and lymph vessels, the respiratory tract, the kidney tubules, the ureters, and the bladder. Parts of many glands are also formed from epithelial tissue. Some epithelial tissues synthesize and release secretions, and others absorb nutrients.
- Connective tissue connects various body parts and forms supportive or protective structures within and around tissues and organs. Connective tissue forms cartilage and bone, holds bones together, and attaches skeletal muscles to bones and skin. Most connective tissue consists of cells surrounded by an organic, semifluid, fibrous matrix. The latter is formed mostly from collagen, which is a fibrous protein that is synthesized and secreted by specialized epithelial cells called fibroblasts. Blood is a form of connective tissue. Normally the blood cells circulate within a fluid plasma, but after injury to a blood vessel, the plasma forms an insoluble clot by activating an insoluble fibrous protein called fibrinogen.
- Nerve tissue initiates and carries electrical signals that control the actions of many body tissues and organs. Nerve tissue is found in the brain, spinal cord, and nerves. Motor (efferent) nerves convey information from the central nervous system (brain and spinal cord) to the periphery. Information about changes in pressure, chemical composition, and temperature is conveyed from sensory organs in the periphery to the central nervous system by sensory (afferent) nerves.
- Muscle tissue is specialized to exert force by contracting (shortening in length). The three different types of muscle are skeletal muscle, smooth muscle, and cardiac muscle. Skeletal muscle produces body movement through its link to the bones of the skeleton and is under voluntary control. Skeletal muscle cells are long, striated, multinucleated fibers. Smooth muscle is found in internal organs, such as the walls of arteries and veins, the esophagus, the stomach, the intestines, the bladder, and the airways, and is not under voluntary control. Smooth muscle cells are spindle-shaped and smaller than skeletal muscle cells. Cardiac muscle is found in the heart and in the large blood vessels near the heart. It is involuntary like smooth muscle and striated like skeletal muscle. Cardiac muscle has branching fibers and specialized cell junctions called intercalated disks. These characteristics give it the ability to contract in a repetitive, synchronized manner that pumps blood to the lungs and other organs of the body.

An organ is a self-contained group of tissues that can perform one or more specialized functions in the body. For example, the stomach performs digestion. It contains epithelial tissue that forms a protective lining and produces digestive juices, acid, and mucus. Connective tissue supports the stomach wall and forms an outer protective layer. Smooth muscle within the stomach wall exerts forces that mix food with the digestive secretions and propel the food toward the small intestine. Nerve tissue conducts signals that coordinate the actions of the epithelial glands and muscle tissue within the stomach and with other parts of the digestive system.

Genes, DNA, and Protein Synthesis

A person's actual genetic makeup is called his or her genotype. The physical expression of the genotype as particular characteristics or traits (e.g., height, strength, hair color) is called the person's phenotype. Success in sport is determined by many factors, including motivation, effort, appropriate training, tactics, and nutrition. Perhaps the most important factor, however, is raw talent in terms of the body's phenotype—in other words, the body's physical, physiological, and metabolic characteristics. These characteristics, which in terms of athletic capability might be taken to include muscle fiber type composition, the size of the heart and lungs, and body height and mass, are all largely determined by the genotype (or genetic endowment) of the person. Certain physical characteristics are essential for success in many sports at the elite level (e.g., in the past 30 years, no male tennis player under 1.75 m [5 ft] in height has won a Grand Slam event, and NFL linebackers who weigh less than 90 kg [198 lb] are a rarity).

A person's physical characteristics are determined to a large degree by the genetic information the person carries. Only monozygotic twins, who develop from the same fertilized ovum (known as the zygote) as a result of the cell mass splitting at a very early stage of embryonic development, carry exactly the same genetic information. Nonidentical (dizygotic) twins result from the fertilization of two different ova and hence have different genotypes.

The Nature of Genetic Information

All the genetic information of every species is contained in its DNA structure, which determines the type and amount of protein synthesized in each cell of the organism. These proteins are in turn responsible for the synthesis of all other cellular components; the genetic material codes only for proteins and does this by defining their component amino acids. Proteins provide the structural basis of all tissues and organs, and it is largely the protein content of these tissues that gives them their recognizable shape. What is more important, perhaps, is that the proteins present in the various tissues confer on each tissue its metabolic capabilities. The presence or absence of a particular enzyme determines whether a tissue can carry out a particular function, and the activity (which depends on the amount of enzyme or an isoform) determines how fast that process can proceed. Proteins and amino acids also constitute, or act as precursors for, many of the body's hormones, regulatory peptides, and neurotransmitters as well as act as the receptors for these signaling systems and fulfill a variety of other functions.

Although all somatic cells of the body (i.e., all cells except the germ cells, sperm and ova) contain the same genetic material in their nuclei, not all genes are expressed (i.e., available to be translated into protein). Thus, the structural and functional characteristics of different cell types are determined by selective gene expression. Although all cells in the human body express certain genes (e.g., those that code for the enzymes of glycolysis), only some cells express genes for other specific proteins (e.g., myosin, troponin, hormone receptors, or enzymes of a metabolic pathway specific to a particular tissue type) and other genes will be repressed. This property is what makes a liver cell different from a muscle cell or a nerve cell. Alteration of gene expression is one of the means by which the body develops and adapts. Certain hormones (particularly steroid hormones such as cortisol and testosterone) are known to be important in the regulation of gene expression.

Nucleic Acids and Protein Synthesis

The development of the cell is determined by the chromosomes that are present in its nucleus, which contain the genetic information that defines the characteristics of the mature cell by regulating the synthesis of the many thousands of different proteins that give the cell its structural and functional characteristics. Chromosomes are a compact form of DNA complexed with protein called chromatin and only appear just before cell division. At other times in the cell cycle, DNA in the nucleus is in an uncoiled form, and when it is freed from contact with chromatin, it can be used as a template for ribonucleic acid (RNA) and then protein synthesis. The parts of the DNA that code for specific proteins are called genes.

All human somatic cells contain 23 pairs of chromosomes, and each cell contains thousands of different proteins. Thus, there are many genes on each chromosome. The chromosomes consist primarily of DNA; the functional unit of DNA, a deoxyribonucleotide, consists of a pentose (five-carbon) sugar molecule called deoxyribose, a phosphate group, and an organic nucleotide base that is either a purine or a pyrimidine. The four bases that are present in DNA are adenine (A), thymine (T), guanine (G), and cytosine (C). Adenine and thymine are purines, whereas guanine and cytosine are pyrimidines. The backbone of the molecule consists of two antiparallel chains of alternating deoxyribose and phosphate groups, and the DNA molecule is typically tens of millions of these units long. The chemistry of the bases in DNA allows bonding to occur between pairs of bases. Strong bonds are formed only between adenine and thymine and between guanine and cytosine, and this accounts for the two parallel strands that effectively run in opposite directions and form a double helix as illustrated in figure A.20. The hydrogen bonds that are formed are extremely stable, which accounts for the stability of the genetic information that these molecules contain, but they can be broken during the process of transcription (see the next section). The order of the nucleotide bases in DNA determines the order of the amino acids in the protein that will be synthesized, and the process is switched on and off by control sequences.

Transcription

Transcription is the process by which a complementary strand of nucleic acids (in the form of an RNA molecule) based on the DNA template is formed in the nucleus of the cell. This is needed to transfer the information that the DNA sequence contains to the protein synthetic apparatus, which is located in the cytoplasm of the cell. During the process of transcription, the hydrogen bonds joining the bases are broken, and the enzyme RNA polymerase forms a sequence of ribonucleotides

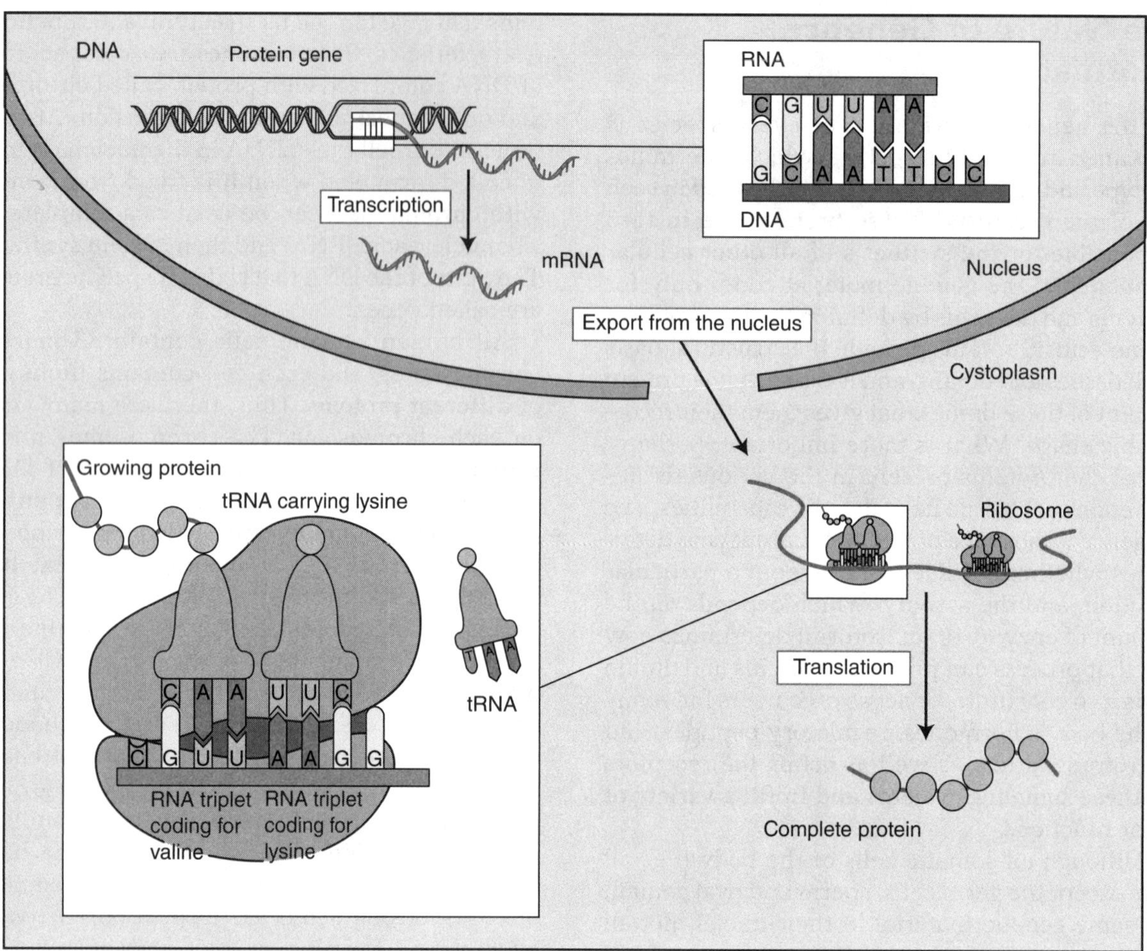

Figure A.20 The structure of DNA and the processes of transcription and translation in the synthesis of protein.

following the same base-pairing arrangement (except adenine binds with uracil [U] instead of thymine in RNA). The sequence of nucleotide bases in the original DNA molecule (or at least in one strand of it—the other strand is not used) thus determines the order of bases on the molecule of RNA, known as messenger RNA (mRNA), as shown in figure A.20. In other words, the DNA serves as a template from which a complementary RNA molecule is transcribed. The mRNA is translocated from the nucleus of the cell, where it was formed, to the cytoplasm, which is where the ribosomes, the structures on which proteins are synthesized, are located. Although a molecule of mRNA can be quite large, it can pass through the pores in the nuclear membrane.

Translation

The process of translation allows the information contained in the sequence of bases on the mRNA molecule to be used to determine the sequence of amino acids in the polypeptide chain that is synthesized. Each amino acid is denoted by a specific sequence of three base pairs, called the genetic code, and each of these sequences is known as a codon. Because there are four different nucleotide bases in RNA (adenine, guanine, cytosine, and uracil), combinations of three bases (triplets) can represent or code for up to 64 (4^3) amino acids. In fact, only 20 different amino acids are used in the synthesis of proteins, so the genetic code is said to be degenerate, which means that there is more than one codon for each amino acid. For example, the amino acid valine is coded for by the triplets GUU, GUC, GUA, and GUG; lysine is coded for by AAA and AAG; and methionine is coded for by AUG. Certain codons (UAA, UGA, and UAG) act as a code for chain termination, signaling the end of translation of the mRNA information into a polypeptide chain.

Transfer RNA molecules (tRNA) are found in the cytoplasm and contain one specific binding site (an anticodon) that recognizes and binds to the codon and another that binds to the appropriate amino acid. Ribosomes contain binding sites for two tRNA molecules and a site just below these along which the mRNA strand can progress. The amino acids are thus brought into proximity and form peptide bonds in the appropriate sequence, as illustrated in the lower part of figure A.20. The process is initiated when the first tRNA molecule together with its bound amino acid is positioned on the mRNA; this first amino acid is always methionine, and the rate at which this initiation step occurs is probably crucial in the overall control of the rate of protein synthesis. Elongation of the peptide chain is terminated when a sequence of codons that do not correspond to any of the amino acids is encountered. In this way, the sequence of bases in the mRNA determines the sequence of amino acids in the protein, which in turn determines how the protein will fold (i.e., its three-dimensional or tertiary structure). The three-dimensional structure of a protein directly determines its function.

Selective Gene Expression

Each cell in the human body contains all the genetic information necessary to make all the other cells, but this information remains repressed, and this partial expression of the genetic information is what distinguishes a muscle cell from a liver cell. This implies that a unique, tissue-specific DNA sequence is in or around certain genes expressed in a specific tissue, such as skeletal muscle. The switching on or off of the expression of certain specific genes can be influenced by hormones, nutrients, and exercise-associated signaling molecules. This is, in part, how adaptations to training (and how they are modified by nutrition) occur. For example, heavy resistance training results in a parallel increase of most proteins of skeletal muscle, which is similar to the parallel upregulation of muscle-specific proteins that occurs as myoblasts develop into myotubes during embryonic development. Another example of differential gene expression during exercise training is the increase in mitochondrial density without a change in muscle size that occurs because of endurance training. In this situation, the "exercise signal" does not interact with the same DNA regulatory sequence that controls contractile protein gene transcription. Rather, the endurance exercise factor interacts with one or more consensus DNA sequences found uniquely in the regulatory region of the mitochondrial genes. Thus, adaptations that occur in muscle with training reflect a change in the expression of the genetic material.

The control of protein synthesis and the expression of the genetic material can be achieved in a number of ways. Transcriptional control alters the concentration of mRNA, and this control is achieved by regulation of the activity of the mRNA polymerase. Repressor proteins, which are activated or inhibited depending on the availability of specific substrates, allow this control to be exerted. Several hormones exert their effects in this way. The hormone (or a hormone-receptor complex) may bind to a region of DNA on a sensor gene, which causes the transcription of an adjacent integrator gene and results in the production of an activator strand of RNA. The activator RNA then binds to a receptor gene, which permits the expression of one or more structural genes that are transcribed into mRNA molecules that leave the nucleus and are translated into proteins on the ribosomes in the cytoplasm. This process is commonly referred to as upregulation of gene expression. The opposite, downregulation of gene expression, can also occur where there is a need to reduce expression of a gene or set of genes.

The regulation of the translation process occurs at the point of assembly of the amino acids under the control of mRNA without any change in the amount of mRNA. Translational regulation controls the amounts of protein synthesized from its mRNA. The control mechanisms are primarily targeted on the control of ribosome recruitment on the initiation codon (e.g., by the phosphorylation of the eukaryotic translation initiation factor 2) but can also involve modulation of the elongation or termination of protein synthesis. In most cases, translational regulation involves specific RNA secondary structures on the mRNA and can be influenced by regulatory short sequences of RNA called microRNAs. These are small noncoding RNA molecules (that each contain about 22 nucleotides) that function in RNA silencing and post-transcriptional regulation of gene expression. MicroRNAs are produced in the nucleus and move into the cytoplasm of the cell, but some microRNAs are also found in various biological fluids, including blood plasma. MicroRNAs function via base-pairing with complementary sequences within mRNA molecules, which results in the silencing of the mRNA molecules by cleavage or destabilization of the mRNA or reduces the efficiency of the mRNA translation into proteins by ribosomes.

Appendix B

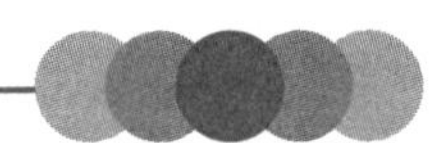

Unit Conversion Tables

A standardized system known as the System Internationale (SI) was established to measure energy, volume, weight, and length. The SI units are based on the metric system. In many countries, however, the English system of measurement is used, and in the field of nutrition, both systems are used. The following tables define the SI units and provide equivalents that allow the reader to convert between the English system and the SI system.

TABLE B.1 SI Units

Physical quantity	Name of unit	Symbol	Definition of unit
Length	Meter	m	
Mass	Kilogram	kg	
Time	Second	s	
Temperature	Degrees Kelvin Degrees Celsius	°K °C	 °C = °K - 273.15
Amount of substance	Mole	mol	
Angle	Radian	rad	
Electric current	Ampere	A	
Potential difference	Volt	V	$kg{\cdot}m^2/s^3/A = J/A/s$
Electric charge	Coulomb	C	A/s
Resistance	Ohm	Ω	$kg{\cdot}m^2/s^3/A^2 = V/A$
Energy	Joule	J	$kg{\cdot}m^2/s^2$
Force	Newton	N	$kg{\cdot}m/s^2 = J/m$
Power	Watt	W	$kg{\cdot}m^2/s^3 = J/s$
Pressure	Pascal	Pa	N/m^2
Frequency	Hertz	Hz	Cycles/s
Density	Kilogram per cubic meter or gram per cubic centimeter		kg/m^3 or g/cm^3

TABLE B.2 SI Fractions and Multiples

	Prefix	Symbol	Examples
FRACTION			
10^{-1}	Deci	d	Deciliter, dl
10^{-2}	Centi	c	Centimeter, cm
10^{-3}	Milli	m	Millisecond, ms
10^{-6}	Micro	μ	Micromole, μmol
10^{-9}	Nano	n	Nanometer, nm
10^{-12}	Pico	p	Picogram, pg
10^{-15}	Femto	f	Femtoliter, fl
MULTIPLE			
10^{3}	Kilo	k	Kilogram, kg
10^{6}	Mega	M	Megajoule, MJ
10^{9}	Giga	G	Gigaohm, GΩ

TABLE B.3 Derived SI Units and Non-SI Units Used in Biochemistry, Physiology, and Nutrition

Physical quantity	Name of unit	Symbol	Definition of unit
Length	Degree Angstrom Inch Foot	°A in ft	10^{-10} m = 10^{-1} nm 0.0254 m 0.3048 m
Mass	Pound Ounce	lb oz	454 g 28.4 g
Temperature	Degree Fahrenheit	°F	1.8 (°C) + 32
Energy	Erg Calorie Horsepower	erg cal h.p.	10^{-7} J 4.184 J 745.7 W
Force	Dyne	dyn	10^{-5} N
Velocity		V	m/s and km/h
Acceleration			m/s^2
Pressure	Bar Atmosphere Torricelli	bar atm torr	105 N/m^2 101.325 kN/m^2 133.322 N/m^2
Volume	Liter Pint Gallon Fluid ounce	L pint gal fl oz	10^{-3} m^3 0.473 × 10^{-3} m^3 3.75 L or 8 pints 29.57 × 10^{-6} m^3
Density			g/cm^3 = g/ml
Enzyme activity	International unit	IU or U	μmol/min
Concentration	Molar Weight/volume%	M %w/v	mol/L g/dl or g/100 ml
Viscosity	Poise	P	10^{-1} kg/s = 10^{-1} Pa/s
Radioactivity	Curie Roentgen	Ci R	37 × 10^{9} counts/s 22.58 × 10^{-4} counts/kg

TABLE B.4 Useful Conversion Factors (Equivalents) for Units of Length, Mass (Weight), Temperature, Energy, and Volume

Physical quantity	Name of unit	Symbol	Approximate equivalent
Length	Inch Foot Centimeter Meter	in ft cm m	2.54 cm 0.3048 m 0.394 in 3.28 ft
Mass	Ounce Pound Gram Kilogram	oz lb g kg	28.4 g 454 g 0.035 oz 2.2 lb
Temperature	Degree Fahrenheit Degree Celsius	°F °C	1.8 (°C) + 32 0.555 (°F) - 32
Energy	Calorie Joule	cal J	4.184 J 0.239 cal
Volume	Fluid ounce Pint Gallon Milliliter Liter Teaspoon Tablespoon Cup	fl oz pint gal ml L	29.57 ml 473 ml 3.75 L or 8 pints 0.034 fl oz 33.8 fl oz or 2.112 pints 5 ml or 0.17 fl oz 15 ml or 0.51 fl oz 240 ml or 8 fl oz

Appendix C

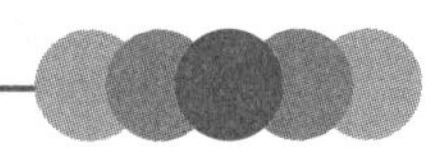

Recommended Daily Allowances for North America

TABLE C.1 Food Components and Daily Values Based on a 2,000-Calorie Diet

Food component	Daily value
Total fat	65 g
Saturated fat	20 g
Cholesterol	300 mg
Sodium	2,400 mg
Potassium	3,500 mg
Total carbohydrate	300 g
Dietary fiber	25 g
Protein	50 g
Vitamin A	5,000 IU
Vitamin C	60 mg
Calcium	1,000 mg
Iron	18 mg
Vitamin D	400 IU (10 µg)
Vitamin E	30 IU (20 mg)
Vitamin K	80 µg
Thiamin	1.5 mg
Riboflavin	1.7 mg

Food component	Daily value
Niacin	20 mg
Vitamin B_6	2 mg
Folate	400 µg
Vitamin B_{12}	6 µg
Biotin	300 µg
Pantothenic acid	10 mg
Phosphorus	1,000 mg
Iodine	150 µg
Magnesium	400 mg
Zinc	15 mg
Selenium	70 µg
Copper	2 mg
Manganese	2 mg
Chromium	120 µg
Molybdenum	75 µg
Chloride	3,400 mg

Data from U.S. Food & Drug Administration, *Food Guidance & Regulation* (2011).

TABLE C.2 Recommended Intakes for Minerals

Age (years)	9-13	14-18	19-30	31-50	51-70	≥70	9-13	14-18	19-30	31-50	51-70	≥70
	MEN						WOMEN					
Calcium (mg/day)	1,300	1,300	1,000	1,000	1,000	1,200	1,300	1,300	1,000	1,000	1,200	1,200
Chloride (g/day)*	2.3	2.3	2.3	2.3	2.0	1.8	2.3	2.3	2.3	2.3	2.0	1.8
Chromium (μg/day)*	25	35	35	35	30	30	21	24	25	25	20	20
Copper (μg/day)	700	890	900	900	900	900	700	890	900	900	900	900
Fluoride (mg/day)*	2	3	4	4	4	4	2	3	3	3	3	3
Iodine (μg/day)	120	150	150	150	150	150	120	150	150	150	150	150
Iron (mg/day)	8	11	8	8	8	8	8	15	18	18	8	8
Magnesium (mg/day)	240	410	400	420	420	420	240	360	310	320	320	320
Manganese (mg/day)*	1.9	2.2	2.3	2.3	2.3	2.3	1.6	1.6	1.8	1.8	1.8	1.8
Molybdenum (μg/day)	34	43	45	45	45	45	34	43	45	45	45	45
Phosphorus (mg/day)	1,250	1,250	700	700	700	700	1,250	1,250	700	700	700	700
Potassium (g/day)*	4.5	4.7	4.7	4.7	4.7	4.5	4.7	4.7	4.7	4.7	4.7	4.7
Selenium (μg/day)	40	55	55	55	55	55	40	55	55	55	55	55
Sodium (g/day)*	1.5	1.5	1.5	1.5	1.3	1.2	1.5	1.5	1.5	1.5	1.3	1.2
Zinc (mg/day)	8	11	11	11	11	11	8	9	8	8	8	8

Values are RDAs or AIs (the latter are denoted with asterisks).

Data from The National Academies of Science Engineering and Medicine, Health and Medicine Division, *Dietary Reference Intakes Tables and Application,* (Washington, DC: National Academies of Science, 2011).

TABLE C.3 Recommended Intakes for Vitamins

Age (years)	9-13	14-18	19-30	31-50	51-70	≥70	9-13	14-18	19-30	31-50	51-70	≥70
	MEN						WOMEN					
Biotin (μg/day)*	20	25	30	30	30	30	20	25	30	30	30	30
Choline (mg/day)*	375	550	550	550	550	550	375	400	425	425	425	425
Folate (μg/day)	300	400	400	400	400	400	300	400	400	400	400	400
Niacin (mg/day)	12	16	16	16	16	16	12	14	14	14	14	14
Pantothenic Acid (mg/day)*	4	5	5	5	5	5	4	5	5	5	5	5
Riboflavin (mg/day)	0.9	1.3	1.3	1.3	1.3	1.3	0.9	1.0	1.1	1.1	1.1	1.1
Thiamin (mg/day)	0.9	1.2	1.2	1.2	1.2	1.2	0.9	1.0	1.1	1.1	1.1	1.1
Vitamin A (μg/day)	600	900	900	900	900	900	600	700	700	700	700	700
Vitamin B_6 (mg/day)	1.0	1.3	1.3	1.3	1.7	1.7	1.0	1.2	1.3	1.3	1.5	1.5
Vitamin B_{12} (μg/day)	1.8	2.4	2.4	2.4	2.4	2.4	1.8	2.4	2.4	2.4	2.4	2.4
Vitamin C (mg/day)	45	75	90	90	90	90	45	65	75	75	75	75
Vitamin D (μg/day)	15	15	15	15	15	20	15	15	15	15	15	20
Vitamin E (mg/day)	11	15	15	15	15	15	11	15	15	15	15	15
Vitamin K (μg/day)*	60	75	120	120	120	120	60	75	90	90	90	90

Values are RDAs or AIs (the latter are denoted with asterisks).

Data from The National Academies of Science Engineering and Medicine, Health and Medicine Division, *Dietary Reference Intakes Tables and Application*, (Washington, DC: National Academies of Science, 2011).

TABLE C.4 Dietary Reference Intakes for Macronutrients and Total Water

	MALES (AGES)					
	9–13 y	14–18 y	19–30 y	31–50 y	51–70 y	≥70 y
Carbohydrate (g/day)	130	130	130	130	130	130
Fiber (g/day)*	31	38	38	38	30	30
α-Linolenic acid *(g/day)	1.2	1.6	1.6	1.6	1.6	1.6
Linoleic acid (g/day)	12	16	17	17	14	14
Protein (g/day)*	34	52	56	56	56	56
Water (L/day)**	2.4	3.3	3.7	3.7	3.7	3.7
	FEMALES (AGES)					
	9–13 y	14–18 y	19–30 y	31–50 y	51–70 y	≥70 y
Carbohydrate (g/day)	130	130	130	130	130	130
Fiber (g/day)*	26	26	25	25	21	21
α-Linolenic acid *(g/day)	1.0	1.1	1.1	1.1	1.1	1.1
Linoleic acid (g/day)	10	11	12	12	11	11
Protein (g/day)*	34	46	46	46	46	46
Water (L/day)**	2.1	2.3	2.7	2.7	2.7	2.7

Protein values calculated using the reference body weight of 0.8 g/kg. Values are RDAs or AIs (the latter are denoted with single asterisks). No values for fat are currently available. **Total daily water intake for all food and beverages.

Data from The National Academies of Science Engineering and Medicine, Health and Medicine Division, *Dietary Reference Intakes Tables and Application,* (Washington, DC: National Academies of Science, 2011).

TABLE C.5 Ranges and Recommendations for Macronutrient Distribution

	4-18 y	≥19 y (adults)
	RANGE IN NUTRITIONALLY ADEQUATE DIET (PERCENTAGE OF TOTAL ENERGY)	
Carbohydrate	45-65	45-65
Cholesterol	As low as possible	
Fat	25-35	20-35
α-Linolenic acid	0.6-1.2	0.6-1.2
Linoleic acid	5-10	5-10
Trans fatty acids	As low as possible	
Saturated fatty acids	As low as possible	
Protein	10-30	10-35
Sugar	<25	<25

Data from The National Academies of Science Engineering and Medicine, *Dietary Reference Intakes for Energy, Carbohydrate. Fiber, Fat, Fatty Acids, Cholesterol, Protein, and Amino Acids* (2002/2005). (Washington, DC: National Academies of Science, 2005).

TABLE C.6 Dietary Reference Intakes and Estimated Energy Requirements (EERs)

Height	Physical activity level	EER FOR MEN/DAY 18.5 BMI	EER FOR MEN/DAY 24.99 BMI	EER FOR WOMEN/DAY 18.5 BMI	EER FOR WOMEN/DAY 24.99 BMI
1.5 m (4.9 ft)		41.6 kg (91.7 lb)	56.2 kg (123.9 lb)	41.6 kg (91.7 lb)	56.2 kg (123.9 lb)
	Sedentary	7,732 kJ (1,848 kcal)	8,703 kJ (2,080 kcal)	6,799 kJ (1,625 kcal)	7,372 kJ (1,762 kcal)
	Low active	8,406 kJ (2,009 kcal)	9,485 kJ (2,267 kcal)	7,544 kJ (1,803 kcal)	8,184 kJ (1,956 kcal)
	Active	9,268 kJ (2,215 kcal)	10,485 kJ (2,506 kcal)	8,472 kJ (2,025 kcal)	9,196 kJ (2,198 kcal)
	Very active	10,686 kJ (2,554 kcal)	12,125 kJ (2,898 kcal)	9,586 kJ (2,291 kcal)	10,414 kJ (2,489 kcal)
1.65 m (5.41 ft)		50.4 kg (111.1 lb)	68.0 kg (149.9 lb)	50.4 kg (111.1 lb)	68.0 kg (149.9 lb)
	Sedentary	8,653 kJ (2,068 kcal)	9,828 kJ (2,349 kcal)	7,598 kJ (1,816 kcal)	8,293 kJ (1,982 kcal)
	Low active	9,431 kJ (2,254 kcal)	10,736 kJ (2,566 kcal)	8,435 kJ (2,016 kcal)	9,213 kJ (2,202 kcal)
	Active	10,837 kJ (2,490 kcal)	11,891 kJ (2,842 kcal)	9,485 kJ (2,267 kcal)	10,364 kJ (2,477 kcal)
	Very active	12,050 kJ (2,880 kcal)	13,790 kJ (3,296 kcal)	10,740 kJ (2,567 kcal)	11,744 kJ (2,807 kcal)
1.8 m (5.9 ft)		59.5 kg (131.2 lb)	81.0 kg (178.6 lb)	59.5 kg (131.2 lb)	81.0 kg (178.6 lb)
	Sedentary	9,627 kJ (2,301 kcal)	11,025 kJ (2,635 kcal)	8,431 kJ (2,015 kcal)	9,251 kJ (2,211 kcal)
	Low active	10,514 kJ (2,513 kcal)	12,067 kJ (2,884 kcal)	9,368 kJ (2,239 kcal)	10,288 kJ (2,459 kcal)
	Active	11,640 kJ (2,782 kcal)	13,389 kJ (3,200 kcal)	10,540 kJ (2,519 kcal)	11,586 kJ (2,769 kcal)
	Very active	13,493 kJ (3,225 kcal)	15,564 kJ (3,720 kcal)	12,071 kJ (2,855 kcal)	13,142 kJ (3,141 kcal)

Note: For each year below 30, add 29 kJ/day (7 kcal/day) for women and 42 kJ/day (10 kcal/day) for men. For each year above 30, subtract that amount.

Data from The National Academies of Science Engineering and Medicine, *Dietary Reference Intakes for Energy, Carbohydrate, Fiber, Fat, Fatty Acids, Cholesterol, Protein, and Amino Acids,* (Washington, DC: National Academies of Science, 2005).

TABLE C.7 Upper Intake Levels for Minerals

Age	9-13 y	14-18 y	19-70 y	≥70 y
	MEN AND WOMEN			
Calcium (mg/day)	3,000	3,000	2,500	2,000
Chloride (g/day)	3.4	3.6	3.6	3.6
Copper (µg/day)	5,000	8,000	10,000	10,000
Fluoride (mg/day)	10	10	10	10
Iodine (µg/day)	600	900	1,100	1,100
Iron (mg/day)	40	45	45	45
Magnesium (mg/day)	350	350	350	350
Manganese (mg/day)	1.9	2.2	2.3	2.3
Molybdenum (µg/day)	34	43	45	45
Phosphorus (mg/day)	4,000	4,000	4,000	3,000
Selenium (µg/day)	280	400	400	400
Sodium (g/day)	2.2	2.3	2.3	2.3
Zinc (mg/day)	23	34	40	40

Note: The upper intake level (UL) is the maximum level of nutrients (from food and supplements together) that is considered to pose no risk of adverse effects. Where data are not available for a particular mineral's UL, caution should be used in consuming more than the recommended daily intake.

Data from The National Academies of Science Engineering and Medicine, Health and Medicine Division, *Dietary Reference Intakes Tables and Application,* (Washington, DC: National Academies of Science, 2017)

TABLE C.8 Upper Intake Levels for Vitamins

Age	9-13 y	14-18 y	19-70 y	≥70 y
	MEN AND WOMEN			
Choline (mg/day)	2,000	3,000	3,500	3,500
Folate (μg/day)	600	800	1,000	1,000
Niacin (mg/day)	20	30	35	35
Vitamin A (μg/day)	1,700	2,800	3,000	3,000
Vitamin B_6 (mg/day)	60	80	100	100
Vitamin C (mg/day)	1,200	1,800	2,000	2,000
Vitamin D (μg/day)	100	100	100	100
Vitamin E (mg/day)	600	800	1,000	1,000

Note: The upper intake level (UL) is the maximum level of nutrients (from food and supplements together) that is considered to pose no risk of adverse effects. Where data are not available for a particular vitamin's UL, caution should be used in consuming more than the recommended daily intake.

Data from The National Academies of Science Engineering and Medicine, Health and Medicine Division, *Dietary Reference Intakes Tables and Application,* (Washington, DC: National Academies of Science, 2017).

Appendix D

Reference Nutrient Intakes for the United Kingdom

TABLE D.1 Reference Nutrient Intake for Protein

Age	Reference nutrient intake (g/day)
0-3 mo	12.5
4-6 mo	12.7
7-9 mo	13.7
10-12 mo	14.9
1-3 y	14.5
4-6 y	19.7
7-10 y	28.3
Males	
11-14 y	42.1
15-18 y	55.2
19-50 y	55.5
≥50 y	53.3
Females	
11-14 y	41.2
15-18 y	55.2
19-50 y	55.5
≥50 y	53.3
Pregnancy	61
During lactation	
0-4 mo	66
≥4 mo	63

Note: These figures assume complete digestibility.

From *Dietary Reference Values for Food Energy and Nutrients in the United Kingdom: Report of the Panel on Dietary Reference Values of the Committee on Medical Aspects of Food Policy* (London: Her Majesty's Stationery Office, 1991).

TABLE D.2 Reference Nutrient Intake for Vitamins

Age	Thiamin (mg/day)	Riboflavin (mg/day)	Niacin (mg/day)	Vitamin B6 (mg/day)	Vitamin B12 (μg/day)	Folate (μg/day)	Vitamin C (mg/day)	Vitamin A (mg/day)	Vitamin D (μg/day)
0-3 mo	0.2	0.4	3	0.2	0.3	50	25	350	8.5-10
4-6 mo	0.2	0.4	3	0.2	0.3	50	25	350	8.5-10
7-9 mo	0.2	0.4	4	0.3	0.4	50	25	350	8.5-10
10-12 mo	0.3	0.4	5	0.4	0.4	50	25	350	8.5-10
1-3 y	0.5	0.6	8	0.7	0.5	70	30	400	10
4-6 y	0.7	0.8	11	0.9	0.8	100	30	400	10
7-10 y	0.7	1.0	12	1.0	1	150	30	500	10
Males									
11-14 y	0.9	1.2	15	1.2	1.2	200	35	600	10
15-18 y	1.1	1.3	18	1.5	1.5	200	40	700	10
19-50 y	1.0	1.3	17	1.4	1.5	200	40	700	10
≥50 y	0.9	1.3	16	1.4	1.5	200	40	700	10
Females									
11-14 y	0.7	1.1	12	1.0	1.2	200	35	600	10
15-18 y	0.8	1.1	14	1.2	1.5	200	40	600	10
19-50 y	0.8	1.1	13	1.2	1.5	200	40	600	10
≥50 y	0.8	1.1	12	1.2	1.5	200	40	600	10
Pregnancy	0.9	1.4	13	1.2	1.5	300	50	700	10
During lactation									
0-6 mo	1.0	1.6	15	1.2	2.0	260	70	950	10
≥6 mo	1.0	1.6	15	1.2	2.0	260	70	950	10

From *Dietary Reference Values for Food Energy and Nutrients in the United Kingdom: Report of the Panel on Dietary Reference Values of the Committee on Medical Aspects of Food Policy* (London: Her Majesty's Stationery Office, 1991).

TABLE D.3 Reference Nutrient Intake for Minerals

Age	Calcium (mg/day)	Phosphorus (mg/day)	Magnesium (mg/day)	Sodium (mg/day)	Potassium (mg/day)	Chloride (mg/day)	Iron (mg/day)	Zinc (mg/day)	Copper (mg/day)	Selenium (μg/day)	Iodine (μg/day)
0-3 mo	525	400	55	210	800	320	1.7	4.0	0.2	10	50
4-6 mo	525	400	60	280	850	400	4.3	4.0	0.3	13	60
7-9 mo	525	400	75	320	700	500	7.8	5.0	0.3	10	60
10-12 mo	525	400	80	350	700	500	7.8	5.0	0.3	10	60
1-3 y	350	270	85	500	800	800	6.9	5.0	0.4	15	70
4-6 y	450	350	120	700	1,100	1,100	6.1	6.5	0.6	20	100
7-10 y	550	450	200	1,200	2,000	1,800	8.7	7.0	0.7	30	110
Males											
11-14 y	1,000	775	280	1,600	3,100	2,500	11.3	9.0	0.8	45	130
15-18 y	1,000	775	300	1,600	3,500	2,500	11.3	9.5	1.0	70	140
19-50 y	700	550	300	1,600	3,500	2,500	8.7	9.5	1.2	75	140
≥50 y	700	550	300	1,600	3,500	2,500	8.7	9.5	1.2	75	140
Females											
11-14 y	800	625	280	1,600	3,100	2,500	14.8	9.0	0.8	45	130
15-18 y	800	625	300	1,600	3,500	2,500	14.8	7.0	1.0	60	140
19-50 y	700	550	270	1,600	3,500	2,500	14.8	7.0	1.2	60	140
≥50 y	700	550	270	1,600	3,500	2,500	8.7	7.0	1.2	60	140
Pregnancy	700	550	270	1,600	3,500	2,500	14.8	7.0	1.2	60	140
During lactation											
0-4 mo	1,250	1,000	320	1,600	3,500	2,500	14.8	13.0	1.5	1.5	140
≥4 mo	1,250	1,000	320	1,600	3,500	2,500	14.8	9.5	1.5	75	140

From *Dietary Reference Values for Food Energy and Nutrients in the United Kingdom: Report of the Panel on Dietary Reference Values of the Committee on Medical Aspects of Food Policy* (London: Her Majesty's Stationery Office, 1991).

Appendix E

Recommended Dietary Intakes for Australia and New Zealand

TABLE E.1 Recommended Dietary Intakes of Vitamins, Minerals, and Protein for Adults Expressed as Mean Daily Intake

	MEN		WOMEN			
	19-70 y	**≥70 y**	**19-70 y**	**≥70 y**	**Pregnant**	**Lactating**
Vitamin A (μg retinol equivalents)	900	900	700	700	800	1,100
Thiamin (mg)	1.2	1.2	1.1	1.1	1.4	1.4
Riboflavin (mg)	1.3	1.6	1.1	1.1	1.4	1.6
Niacin (mg niacin equivalents)	16	16	14	14	18	17
Vitamin B_6 (mg)	1.3	1.7	1.3	1.5	1.9	2.0
Total folate (μg)	400	400	400	400	600	500
Vitamin B_{12} (μg)	2.4	2.4	2.4	2.4	2.6	2.8
Vitamin C (mg)	45	45	45	45	65	85
Vitamin E* (mg α-tocopherol equivalents)	10	10	7	7	7	11
Zinc (mg)	14	14	8	8	11	12
Iron (mg)	8	8	18	8	27	9
Iodine (μg)	150	150	150	150	220	270
Magnesium (mg)	420	420	320	320	350	320
Calcium (mg)	1,000	1,300	1,000	1,300	1,000	1,000
Phosphorus (mg)	1,000	1,000	1,000	1,000	1,000	1,000
Selenium (μg)	70	70	60	60	65	75
Sodium (mmol)* (mg)	20–40 460–920	20–40 460–920	20–40 460–920	20–40 460–920	20–40 460–920	20–40 460–920
Potassium (mmol)* (mg)	100 3,800	100 3,800	70 2,800	70 2,800	70 2,800	80 3,200
Protein (g)	64	81	46	57	60	67

Note: Values are RDAs or AIs (the latter are denoted with asterisks).

National Health and Medical Research Council, Australia 2014 (www.nrv.gov.au/resources/nrv-summary-tables)

Glossary

1,3-DPG (1,3-diphosphoglycerate)—An intermediate compound in glycolysis.

2,3-DPG (2,3-diphosphoglycerate)—A highly anionic organic phosphate that is present in human red blood cells at about the same molar ratio as hemoglobin. It binds to deoxyhemoglobin but not the oxygenated form, which diminishes the oxygen affinity of hemoglobin. It is essential in enabling hemoglobin to unload oxygen in tissue capillaries.

3-methylhistidine—A metabolite of the amino acid histidine. Its urinary excretion is used as an index of contractile protein breakdown.

5′ adenosine monophosphate-activated protein kinase (AMPK)—An enzyme that plays a role in cellular energy homeostasis.

5-HT (5-hydroxytryptamine)—A brain neurotransmitter. Also known as serotonin.

absorption—The transport of nutrients from the intestine into the blood or lymph system.

accelerometer—A small piece of equipment that can be attached to the body to register all accelerations the body makes. The number and the degree of the accelerations indicate the person's activity level.

acceptable macronutrient distribution range (AMDR)—The range of intake for a particular energy source (i.e., carbohydrate, fat, or protein) that is associated with reduced risk of chronic disease and that provides adequate intake of essential nutrients.

acclimatization—The adaptation of the body to an environmental extreme (e.g., heat, cold, altitude).

acetyl CoA—The major fuel for the oxidative processes in the body. It is derived from the breakdown of glycogen, glucose, and fatty acids.

acid—A substance that tends to lose a proton (e.g., a hydrogen ion).

acid–base balance—The relative balance of acid and base products in the body.

acidosis—A disturbance of the normal acid–base balance in which excess acids accumulate and cause a drop in pH (e.g., when lactic acid accumulates in muscle and blood during high-intensity exercise).

actin—One of the major contractile proteins in muscle. It is found in the thin filaments.

active transport—The movement or transport across cell membranes by membrane carriers. An expenditure of energy (adenosine triphosphate) is required.

acute-phase proteins—Several proteins released from the liver (e.g., C-reactive protein) and leukocytes that aid the body's response to injury or infection.

acyl carrier protein (ACP)—Protein that transports a fatty acyl-carnitine complex (a fatty acid linked to carnitine) across the inner mitochondrial membrane. Also known as the fatty acyl-carnitine translocase.

acyl group—The long hydrocarbon chain of a fatty acid.

adaptogens—Substances that help the body adapt to stress situations.

adenine (A)—A purine nucleotide found in DNA and several coenzymes.

adenosine monophosphate (AMP)—A product of the breakdown of adenosine diphosphate.

adequate intake (AI)—A recommended dietary intake comparable to the RDA but based on less scientific evidence.

adenosine diphosphate (ADP)—A breakdown product of adenosine triphosphate.

adenosine triphosphatase (ATPase)—An enzyme that breaks down adenosine triphosphate to adenosine diphosphate and inorganic phosphate and releases energy that can be used to fuel biological work.

adenosine triphosphate (ATP)—A high-energy compound that is the immediate source for muscular contraction and other energy-requiring processes in the cell.

adipocyte—An adipose tissue cell whose main function is to store triacylglycerol (fat).

adipose tissue—White fatty tissue that stores triacylglycerol.

adrenaline—A hormone secreted by the adrenal gland. It is a stimulant that prepares the body for fight or flight and is an important activator of fat and carbohydrate breakdown during exercise. Also known as epinephrine.

adrenocorticotrophic hormone (ACTH)—A hormone secreted from the anterior pituitary gland that stimulates release of cortisol from the adrenal glands.

aerobic—Occurring in the presence of free oxygen.

Akt—A protein kinase B enzyme that plays a key role in multiple cellular processes such as glucose metabolism, apoptosis, cell proliferation, transcription, and cell migration. Akt directly stimulates the activity of translation initiation factors and upregulates ribosome biogenesis to increase protein synthesis.

Akt-mTOR pathway—An important signaling cascade that plays a key role in increasing muscle protein synthesis and hypertrophy.

alanine—A nonessential amino acid.

alcohol—A colorless liquid that has depressant and intoxicating effects. Ethyl alcohol or ethanol (C_2H_5OH) is the alcohol found in wines, spirits, and beer.

aldosterone—A steroid hormone secreted by the adrenal cortex. It is primarily involved in fluid and electrolyte balance by controlling sodium and potassium excretion by the kidneys.

alimentary tract—See gastrointestinal tract.

alkalinizer—A group of substances with a buffering function (e.g., sodium bicarbonate, sodium citrate).

allergy—An adverse reaction of the immune system to a substance not recognized as harmful by most people's immune systems.

α-amylase or **amylase**—A digestive enzyme found in saliva that begins the digestion of starches in the mouth (also called ptyalin). It catalyzes the hydrolysis of starch by cleaving the α-1-4-glycosidic linkages between the component glucose molecules. Amylase is also present in pancreatic juice.

α-tocopherol—The most biologically active alcohol in vitamin E.

amenorrhea—The absence of at least three successive menstrual cycles in women.

amino acid—The chief structural molecule of protein that consists of an amino group (NH_2) and a carboxylic acid group (CO_2H) plus an R-group that determines the properties of the amino acid. Twenty different amino acids can be used to make proteins.

ammonia (NH_3)—A metabolic by-product of the oxidation of amino acids. It may be transformed into urea for excretion from the body.

amylopectin—A branched-chain starch (polymer of glucose).

amylose—A straight-chain starch that is more resistant to digestion compared with amylopectin.

anabolic resistance—The impaired rate of cellular anabolism (usually referring to muscle protein synthesis) in response to anabolic stimuli such as protein ingestion and resistance exercise.

anabolism—Constructive metabolism, the process whereby simple body compounds are formed into more complex ones.

anaerobic—Occurring in the absence of free oxygen.

androstenedione—An androgenic steroid produced in the body that is converted to testosterone. It is marketed as a dietary supplement.

anemia—A condition defined by an abnormally low blood hemoglobin content that results in lowered oxygen-carrying capacity.

angiogenesis— The physiological process through which new blood vessels are formed from preexisting vessels to improve blood supply to a tissue.

anion—A negatively charged ion or electrolyte (e.g., chloride, Cl^-; phosphate, HPO^{2-}_4).

anorexia athletica—A form of anorexia nervosa observed in athletes who show significant symptoms of eating disorders but do not meet the criteria of the *Diagnostic and Statistical Manual of Mental Disorders* (American Psychiatric Association) for anorexia or bulimia nervosa.

anorexia nervosa—An eating disorder characterized by abnormally small food intake and refusal to maintain a normal body weight (according to what is expected for gender, age, and height), a distorted view of body image, an intense fear of being fat or overweight and gaining weight or "feeling fat" when clearly the person is below normal weight, and the absence of at least three successive menstrual cycles in women (amenorrhea).

anthropometry—Use of body girths and diameters to evaluate body composition.

antibody—Soluble protein produced by B lymphocytes with antimicrobial effects. Also known as immunoglobulin.

antidiuretic hormone (ADH)—A hormone secreted by the posterior pituitary gland that influences water reabsorption by the kidneys.

antioxidant—Molecules that can prevent or limit the actions of free radicals, usually by removing their unpaired electron and thus converting them into something far less reactive.

appendix—A nonfunctional part of the small intestine that is short, thin, and outpouching from the cecum.

appetite—A desire for food for the purpose of enjoyment that is developed through previous experience. It is believed to be controlled in humans by an appetite center in the hypothalamus.

arginine—An essential amino acid.

arteriosclerosis—Hardening of the arteries. See also atherosclerosis.

arteriovenous (AV)—Refers to comparison of arterial and venous blood composition.

ascorbic acid—Vitamin C. Its major role is as a water-soluble antioxidant.

aspartame—An artificial sweetener made from amino acids.

atherosclerosis—A specific form of arteriosclerosis characterized by the formation of fatty plaques on the luminal walls of arteries.

atom—The smallest unit of an element that retains all the properties of the element. The atoms of all elements can be broken down physically into the same subatomic particles: protons, neutrons, and electrons. Hence, the atoms of the various elements differ only in the numbers of protons, neutrons, and electrons that they contain.

atrophy—A wasting away; a diminution in the size of a cell, tissue, organ, or part.

Atwater factors—The average net energy values for carbohydrate, fat, and protein named after Wilbur Olin Atwater: 16 kJ/g (4 kcal/g) for carbohydrate, 36 kJ/g (9 kcal/g) for fat, and 16 kJ/g (4 kcal/g) for protein.

AV differences—A difference between arterial and venous concentration of a substance that indicates net uptake or release of that substance.

average daily metabolic rate (ADMR)—The average energy expenditure over 24 hours.

basal metabolic rate (BMR)—Energy expenditure under basal, postabsorptive conditions representing the energy needed to maintain life under these basal conditions.

base—A substance that tends to donate an electron pair or coordinate an electron.

ß-alanine—A nonprotein amino acid that is synthesized from uracil in the liver and converted in muscle to the dipeptide carnosine or ß-alanyl-L-histidine that increases intracellular buffering capacity. It can be taken as an oral supplement to raise carnosine levels in muscle to improve high-intensity exercise performance.

ß-carotene—A precursor for vitamin A found in plants. Also called provitamin A.

ß-hydroxy ß-methylbutyrate (HMB)—A metabolite of the essential amino acid leucine. It is marketed as a muscle growth promotor.

ß-oxidation—Oxygen-requiring process in the mitochondria whereby two-carbon units are sequentially removed from the hydrocarbon chain of a fatty acid in the form of acetyl-CoA, which can then enter the TCA cycle.

bigorexia—A mental disorder in which a person becomes obsessed with the idea that they are not sufficiently muscular.

bile—Fluid produced by the liver and stored in the gall bladder that contains bile salts, bile pigments, cholesterol, and other molecules. The bile is secreted into the small intestine.

bile salts—Salts or derivatives of cholesterol in bile that are polar on one end and nonpolar on the other end of the molecule. Bile salts act to emulsify fat in the lumen of the small intestine.

bioavailability—In relation to nutrients in food, the amount that may be absorbed into the body.

bioelectrical impedance analysis (BIA)—A method to calculate percentage of body fat by measuring electrical resistance due to the water content of the body.

biopsy—A small sample of tissue taken for analysis.

body mass index (BMI)—Body mass in kilograms divided by height in meters squared (kg/m^2). It is used as a measure of obesity.

bomb calorimeter—An instrument to measure the energy content in which food is oxidized and the resulting heat production is measured.

branched-chain amino acid (BCAA)—Three essential amino acids that can be oxidized by muscle, including leucine, isoleucine, and valine.

breath-by-breath system—An automated system to analyze gas exchange to estimate energy expenditure and substrate use. These systems can measure carbon dioxide production and oxygen consumption from every breath.

brush border—Where the absorption of nutrients takes place in the intestine. The surface of the epithelial cells that line the intestinal wall is covered with microvilli that form the brush border.

buffer—A substance that, in solution, prevents rapid changes in hydrogen ion concentration (pH).

bulimia nervosa—An eating disorder characterized by repeated episodes of binge eating (consumption of large amounts of usually energy-dense foods) followed by purging of the stomach contents, which allows insufficient time for most of the nutrients from the heavy meal to be absorbed.

caffeine—A stimulant drug found in many food products such as coffee, tea, and cola drinks. It stimulates the central nervous system and is used as an ergogenic aid.

calorie (cal)—Traditional unit of energy. One calorie expresses the quantity of energy (heat) needed to raise the temperature of 1 g (1 ml) of water 1 °C (e.g., from 14.5 °C to 15.5 °C). A Calorie with a capital C is sometimes use to denote 1,000 calories or one kilocalorie (kcal).

calorimeter—An insulated chamber to estimate energy expenditure by measuring heat dissipation from the body. This method is called direct calorimetry.

capillary—The smallest vessel in the cardiovascular system. Capillary walls are only one cell thick. All exchanges of molecules between the blood and tissue fluid occur across the capillary walls.

carbohydrate—A compound composed of carbon, hydrogen, and oxygen in a ratio of 1:2:1 (e.g., CH_2O). Sugars, starches, and dietary fibers are sources of carbohydrate.

carboloading—Eating large quantities of carbohydrate to optimize body glycogen stores. This is a common practice of endurance athletes.

carbon dioxide (CO_2)—Gas produced during oxidation of carbohydrates and fats.

carboxylation—A reaction involving the addition of carbon dioxide that is catalyzed by an enzyme using biotin as its prosthetic group.

carboxyl group (COOH or CO_2H)—Acidic group of amino acids and components of the tricarboxylic acid cycle.

carcinogen—A cancer-inducing substance.

carnitine—A compound used to assist the transport of fatty acyl-CoA molecules from the muscle sarcoplasm across the mitochondrial inner membrane into the mitochondria for subsequent oxidation.

carnitine palmitoyl transferase (CPT)—Enzyme that links the fatty acid palmitate to carnitine so that it can be transported across the inner mitochondrial membrane for subsequent oxidation. Also known as carnitine acyl transferase (CAT).

catabolism—Destructive metabolism whereby complex chemical compounds in the body are degraded to simpler ones (e.g., glycogen to glucose, proteins to amino acids).

catalyst—A substance that accelerates a chemical reaction, usually by temporarily combining with the substrates and lowering the activation energy, and is recovered unchanged at the end of the reaction (e.g., an enzyme).

cation—A positively charged ion or electrolyte (e.g., sodium, Na^+; calcium, Ca^{2+}).

cecum—A blind pouch, open only at one end, at the beginning of the large intestine.

cell—The smallest discrete living unit of the body.

cellulose—A major component of plant cell walls and the most abundant nonstarch polysaccharide. It cannot be digested by human digestive enzymes.

cerebrospinal fluid (CSF)—The fluid found in the brain and spinal cord.

ceruloplasmin—A glycoprotein that binds copper and is thought to exert a protective effect against cellular damage caused by free radicals.

cholecystokinin—A hormone secreted by the duodenum that acts to stimulate the secretion of enzymes in pancreatic juice.

cholesterol—A lipid transported in the blood in high- and low-density lipoproteins (HDL and LDL, respectively). High HDL levels are somewhat protective against coronary heart disease.

choline—Can be found in phospholipids (phosphatidylcholine and sphingomyelin) and is a precursor for the neurotransmitter acetylcholine.

chromium—A trace element that plays a role in glucose metabolism.

chylomicrons—A class of lipoproteins that transport exogenous (dietary) cholesterol and triglycerides from the small intestine to tissues after meals.

chyme—A homogenous, souplike liquid formed from food in the gastrointestinal tract mixed with various secretions of the gastrointestinal tract.

cirrhosis—A degenerative disease of the liver. The most common cause is excessive consumption of alcohol.

cis—A prefix indicating the geometrical isomer in which the two like groups are on the same side of a double bond with restricted rotation (e.g., in unsaturated fatty acids in which the hydrogen ions are on the same side of the double bond).

closed-circuit spirometry—A method to measure resting energy expenditure in which the subject breathes through a mouthpiece into a closed system (spirometer) prefilled with 100% oxygen.

clusters of differentiation (CD)—Proteins expressed on the cell surface of leukocytes (white blood cells) that can be used to identify different types of leukocyte or subsets of lymphocytes. Also called cluster designators.

CoA-SH—Free form of coenzyme A.

coefficient of digestibility—The percentage energy of food ingested that is digested, absorbed, and available for metabolic processes in the body.

coenzyme—Small molecules that are essential in stoichiometric amounts for the activity of some enzymes. Examples include nicotinamide adenine dinucleotide (NAD), flavin adenine dinucleotide (FAD), pyridoxal phosphate (PLP), thiamin pyrophosphate (TPP), and biotin.

coenzyme A (CoA)—A molecule that acts as a carrier for acyl or acetyl groups (A stands for acetylation).

coenzyme Q10 (CoQ10)—An electron carrier that mediates transfer of electrons from flavoprotein to cytochrome c in the electron-transport chain that is located in the inner mitochondrial membrane. Also called ubiquinone.

colon—The large intestine. This part of the intestine is mainly responsible for forming, storing, and expelling feces.

colony-stimulating factor (CSF)—A cytokine that stimulates increased production and release of leukocytes (white blood cells) from the bone marrow.

complement—Soluble proteins found in body fluids and produced by the liver. Once activated, they exert several antimicrobial effects.

complex carbohydrate—A food that contains starch and other polysaccharides, such as bread, pasta, cereals, fruits, and vegetables (in contrast to simple carbohydrate foods such as glucose, milk sugar, and table sugar).

computed tomography (CT)—A method that uses ionizing radiation by an X-ray beam to create images of body segments. The CT scan produces qualitative and quantitative information about the total area of the tissue investigated and the thickness and volume of tissues within an organ.

concentration gradient—The difference in the concentration of a substance on either side of a membrane.

conduction—In relation to body temperature, the transfer of heat from one substance to another by direct contact.

conformation—The shape of molecules determined by rotation about single bonds, especially in polypeptide chains about carbon–carbon links.

convection—Heat exchange that occurs between a solid medium (e.g., the human body) and one that moves (e.g., air or water).

coronary heart disease (CHD)—Narrowing of the arteries supplying the heart muscle that can cause heart attacks.

cortisol—A steroid hormone secreted from the adrenal glands.

covalent bond—A chemical bond in which two or more atoms are held together by the interaction of their outer electrons.

covalent regulation—Control of enzyme activity by covalent bonding of phosphate groups to sites other than the active site of the enzyme.

creatine—Compound synthesized from amino acids that is the precursor of phosphocreatine, an important anaerobic energy source for high-intensity exercise.

creatine kinase (CK)—An enzyme that catalyzes the transfer of phosphate from phosphocreatine to ADP to form ATP. Also known as creatine phosphokinase.

creatinine—A product of creatine breakdown that is found in the urine. It can be measured to assess overall kidney function. An abnormally elevated blood creatinine level is seen in people with kidney insufficiency and kidney failure.

cross-bridges—Linkages formed between myosin heads of the thick filaments and actin molecules of the thin filaments during muscle contraction.

cutaneous—In the skin.

cyclic adenosine monophosphate (cAMP)—An important intracellular messenger in the action of hormones.

cytochrome—An iron-containing heme protein of the mitochondrial electron-transport chain that can be alternately oxidized and reduced.

cytokine—Protein released from cells that acts as a chemical messenger by binding to receptors on other cells. Cytokines include interleukins (IL), tumor necrosis factors (TNF), colony-stimulating factors (CSF), and interferons (IFN).

cytosine (C)—A pyrimidine nucleotide found in DNA.

cytosolic fatty acid–binding protein (FABPc)—A protein found in liver and muscle that binds fatty acids in the cytosol of the cell. It is involved in transport from the plasma membrane to mitochondria.

cytotoxic—Ability to kill other cells (e.g., those infected with a virus).

daily reference value (DRV)—Recommended daily intakes for the macronutrients (carbohydrate, fat, and protein) and for cholesterol, sodium, and potassium. On a food label, the DRV is based on an 8.4 MJ (2,000 kcal) diet.

daily value (DV)— Recommended intake values that appear on food labels. They are based on the reference daily intakes and the daily reference values that are recommended for healthy people in the United States. DVs are based on a daily energy intake of 8.4 MJ (2,000 kcal).

deamination—Reaction involving the loss of an amino (NH_2) group.

decarboxylation—Reaction involving the loss of a carbon dioxide group.

dehydration—Reaction involving the loss of a water molecule or loss of body water (e.g., with sweating).

dehydroepiandrosterone (DHEA)—A steroid hormone produced endogenously by the adrenal gland. It may be marketed as a nutritional sport ergogenic as derived from herbal precursors. It is often referred to as the youth hormone.

delta efficiency (DE)—The change in energy expended per minute relative to the change in actual work accomplished per minute.

denaturation—Alteration of the physical properties and three-dimensional structure of a protein by a chemical or physical treatment that does not disrupt the primary structure but generally results in the inactivation of the protein (e.g., the inactivation of enzyme activity by the addition of a strong acid).

dental caries—Erosion or decay of the tooth caused by the effects of bacteria in the mouth.

densitometry—Method used to estimate the density (mass per unit volume) of the tissues or the whole body.

diabetes mellitus—A disorder of carbohydrate metabolism caused by disturbances in production or use of insulin. It causes high blood glucose levels and loss of sugar in the urine.

diacylglycerol—Glycerol backbone with two fatty acids. It is formed by the removal of one fatty acid from triacylglycerol. Also known as diglyceride.

diarrhea—Frequent passage of a watery fecal discharge because of a gastrointestinal disturbance or infection.

diastolic—The time between ventricular contractions (systole) in which ventricular filling occurs.

dietary reference intake (DRI)—The latest nutrient recommendations by the Food and Nutrition Board of the National Academy of Sciences.

diet-induced thermogenesis (DIT)—The energy needed for the digestion, assimilation, and metabolism of food that is consumed. Also called the thermic effect of food (TEF).

diffusion—The movement of molecules from a region of high concentration to one of low concentration, which is brought about by their kinetic energy.

digestion—The process of breaking down food to its smallest components so that it can be absorbed in the intestine.

dihydroxyacetone (DHA)—When linked to phosphate is a metabolite in glycolysis. In combination with pyruvate, it is marketed as an ergogenic aid.

dihydroxyphenylalanine (DOPA)—A neurotransmitter in the brain.

direct calorimetry—A method of determining energy expenditure by measuring heat dissipation from the body, usually using an insulated chamber or suit.

disaccharide—A sugar that yields two monosaccharides on hydrolysis. Sucrose, the most common disaccharide, is composed of glucose and fructose.

diuretics—Drugs that act on the kidney to promote urine formation.

DNA (deoxyribonucleic acid)—The compound that forms genes (i.e., the genetic material).

dopamine—A catecholamine neurotransmitter and hormone formed by decarboxylation of dihydroxyphenylalanine (DOPA). It is a precursor of epinephrine (adrenaline) and norepinephrine (noradrenaline).

Douglas bag—A plastic bag (named after British scientist Claude Douglas) used to collect expired gases for a certain period of time and to measure the volume, the oxygen concentration, and the carbon dioxide concentration of this gas. From the measurements of inhaled and exhaled air, energy expenditure and substrate use can be calculated.

dry matter, dry material, or **dry mass (d.m.)**—Usually refers to tissue weight after removal of water.

dry weight (d.w.)—Usually refers to tissue weight after removal of water.

dual-energy X-ray absorptiometry (DXA or DEXA)— A high-tech technique that has become the clinical standard to measure bone density. The principle is based on absorption of low-energy X-rays.

duodenum—The first 20 to 30 cm (8-12 in.) of the small intestine.

eating disorder—A psychological disorder centering on the avoidance or purging of food, such as anorexia nervosa and bulimia nervosa.

eating disorders not otherwise specified (EDNOS)—An eating disorder that does not meet the criteria for anorexia nervosa or bulimia nervosa.

eccentric exercise—Types of exercise that involve lengthening of the muscle during activation, which can cause damage to some of the myofibers. Types of exercise that have a significant eccentric component include downhill running, bench stepping, and lowering of weights.

economy—Oxygen uptake needed to exercise at a certain work load or speed.

efficiency—The actual work performed after muscle contraction expressed as a percentage of the total work or energy expended.

eicosanoids—Derivatives of fatty acids in the body that act as cell-to-cell signaling molecules. They include prostaglandins, thromboxanes, and leukotrienes.

electrolyte—A substance that conducts an electric current when dissolved in water. Electrolytes, which include acids, bases, and salts, usually dissociate into ions carrying either a positive charge (cation) or a negative charge (anion).

electron-transport chain (ETC)—Proteins located on the inner mitochondrial membrane that transfer electrons from the reduced forms of the coenzymes nicotinamide adenine dinucleotide (NADH) and flavin adenine dinucleotide ($FADH_2$) to oxygen and allow protons to be pumped into the space between the inner and outer mitochondrial membranes. The flow of hydrogen ions (protons) back into the inner mitochondrial matrix through the adenosine triphosphate (ATP) synthase complex is used to drive ATP synthesis.

element—The smallest units into which a substance can be broken down chemically. Each element has different and unique properties. At least 94 elements are known to exist, but only about 12 are common in living organisms. The most abundant are oxygen, carbon, hydrogen, and nitrogen (in that order). Those four elements constitute 96% of the mass of a human.

emetics—Drugs that promote vomiting.

endocrine—Ductless glands that secrete hormones into the blood.

endogenous—From within the body.

energy—The ability to perform work. Energy exists in various forms, including mechanical, heat, and chemical energy.

energy availability—The amount of energy obtained through dietary intake minus the energy expended during exercise.

energy balance—The balance between energy intake and energy expenditure.

energy density—The amount of energy (or calories) per gram of food. Lower energy density foods provide fewer calories per gram of food.

energy expenditure (EE)—The energy expended per unit of time to produce power.

energy expenditure for activity (EEA)—The energy cost associated with physical activity (exercise).

enzyme—A protein with specific catalytic activity. They are designated by the suffix *-ase,* which is frequently attached to the type of reaction catalyzed. Virtually all metabolic reactions in the body are dependent on and controlled by enzymes.

ephedrine—An α-adrenergic and ß-adrenergic agonist that may also enhance release of norepinephrine. It has been used in the treatment of several disorders, including asthma, heart failure, rhinitis, and urinary incontinence and for its central nervous system stimulatory effects in the treatment of narcolepsy and depression. Ephedrine is on the International Olympic Committee list of banned substances.

epigallocatechin gallate (EGCG)—A polyphenol found in tea and purported to have ergogenic properties.

epimerization—A type of asymmetric transformation in organic molecules.

epinephrine—A hormone secreted by the adrenal gland. It is a stimulant, prepares the body for fight or flight, and is an important activator of fat and carbohydrate breakdown during exercise. Also known as adrenaline.

ergogenic—Performance-enhancing.

ergogenic aids—Substances that improve exercise performance and are used in attempts to increase athletic or physical performance capacity.

ergolytic—Performance-impairing.

erythrocyte—Red blood cell that contains hemoglobin and transports oxygen.

esophageal sphincter—A ringlike band of smooth muscle fibers that act as a valve between the esophagus and the stomach.

esophagus—Part of the intestinal tract located between the mouth and the stomach.

essential amino acids—Amino acids that must be obtained in the diet and cannot be synthesized in the body. Also known as indispensable amino acids.

essential fatty acids—Unsaturated fatty acids that cannot be synthesized in the body and must be obtained in the diet (e.g., linoleic acid and linolenic acid).

estimated average requirement (EAR)—The nutrient intake value that is estimated to meet the requirements of an average individual in a certain age and gender group.

estradiol—A hormone synthesized mainly in the ovary but also in the placenta, testis, and possibly adrenal cortex.

euhydration—Normal state of body hydration (water content).

evaporation—The loss of water that occurs when water on a surface changes from a liquid to a gas.

excretion—The removal of metabolic wastes.

exogenous—From outside the body.

exogenous carbohydrate oxidation—Oxidation of carbohydrates that have been ingested or infused but are not from body stores.

extracellular fluid—Body fluid that is located outside the cells including the blood plasma, interstitial fluid, cerebrospinal fluid, synovial fluid, and ocular fluid.

fasting—Starvation; abstinence from eating that may be partial or complete.

fat—Fat molecules contain the same structural elements as carbohydrates, but they have little oxygen relative to carbon and hydrogen and are poorly soluble in water. Also known as lipids.

fat-free mass (FFM)—Lean mass of a tissue or the whole body.

FAT/CD36—Fatty acid translocator involved in the transport of fatty acids across the plasma membrane

fatty acid (FA)—A type of fat having a carboxylic acid group (COOH) at one end of the molecule and a methyl (CH_3) group at the other end separated by a hydrocarbon chain that can vary in length. A typical structure of a fatty acid is $CH_3(CH_2)_{14}COOH$ (palmitic acid or palmitate).

fatty acid–binding protein (FABP)—A protein found in liver and muscle that binds fatty acids to maintain a low intracellular free fatty acid concentration.

feces—The excrement discharged from the intestines that consists of bacteria, cells from the intestines, secretions, and a small amount of food residue.

female athlete triad syndrome—A syndrome characterized by the three conditions prevalent in female athletes: amenorrhea, disordered eating, and osteoporosis.

ferritin—A protein that is used to store iron. It is mostly found in the liver, spleen, and bone marrow. Soluble ferritin is released from cells into the blood plasma in direct proportion to cellular ferritin content. Hence, the serum ferritin concentration can be used to indicate the status of the body's iron stores.

fiber—Indigestible carbohydrate.

fish oil—Oils high in unsaturated fats extracted from the bodies of fish or fish parts, especially the livers. The oils are used as dietary supplements.

flavin adenine dinucleotide, oxidized form (FAD)—A coenzyme important in energy metabolism.

flavin adenine dinucleotide, reduced form ($FADH_2$)—Reduced form of the coenzyme FAD.

flavin mononucleotide, oxidized form (FMN)—A coenzyme important in energy metabolism.

flavin mononucleotide, reduced form ($FMNH_2$)—Reduced form of the coenzyme FMN.

flux—The rate of flow through a metabolic pathway.

folic acid or **folate**—A water-soluble vitamin required in the synthesis of nucleic acids. It appears to be essential in preventing certain types of anemia.

food diary—A written record of sequential food intake over a period of time. Details associated with the food intake are often recorded as well.

food groups—A collection of foods that share similar nutritional properties or biological classifications. Nutrition guides typically divide foods into food groups and recommend daily servings of each group for a healthy diet. Common examples of food groups include dairy, meat, fruit, vegetables, grains, and beans.

food intolerance—A condition in which symptoms of abdominal discomfort with flatulence and bloating or diarrhea occur every time a particular food is consumed. The usual cause is when the body fails to produce a sufficient amount of a particular enzyme needed to digest a food component before it can be absorbed.

free fatty acid (FFA)—A fatty acid that is not esterified to glycerol or any other molecule.

free radical—An atom or molecule that possess at least one unpaired electron in its outer orbit. Important free radicals include the superoxide ($\cdot O_2^-$), hydroxyl ($\cdot OH$), and nitric oxide ($\cdot NO$) radicals. They are highly reactive and may cause damage to lipid membranes, causing membrane instability and increased permeability. Free radicals can also cause oxidative damage to proteins, including enzymes, and damage to DNA.

free tryptophan (fTRP)—Tryptophan that is not bound to protein.

fructose-1,6-diphosphate (FDP)—A metabolic intermediate in glycolysis.

fructose-1,6-diphosphatase (FDPase)—An enzyme that catalyzes the conversion of fructose-1,6-diphosphate to fructose-6-phosphate, a reaction involved in gluconeogenesis.

fructose-6-phosphate (F-6-P)—A metabolic intermediate in glycolysis.

gallbladder—A digestive organ that stores bile (produced in the liver), which is used in the digestion and absorption of fats in the duodenum.

gamma-amino butyric acid (GABA)—A neurotransmitter in the brain.

gastric emptying—The rate at which substances (food and fluids) leave the stomach into the small intestine. A high gastric emptying rate is desirable for sports drinks.

gastric juice—The secretions by the gastric mucosa. Gastric juice contains water, hydrochloric acid, and pepsinogen as major components.

gastrin—A hormone secreted by the stomach that stimulates gastric secretion of hydrochloric acid and pepsin.

gastrointestinal tract—The main site in the body used for digestion and absorption of nutrients. It consists of the mouth, esophagus, stomach, small intestine, large intestine, rectum, and anus. Also called the alimentary tract.

gene—A specific sequence in DNA that codes for a particular protein. Genes are located on the chromosomes. Each gene is found in a definite position (locus).

gene transcription—The process by which RNA polymerase produces single-stranded RNA complementary to one strand of the DNA. This is the first step in the process of synthesizing protein based on the information encoded in the genes.

genotype—The genetic composition or assortment of genes that together with environmental influences determines the appearance or phenotype of a person.

geometrical isomerism—A form of stereoisomerism in which the difference in chemical properties arises because of hindered rotation about a double bond. An unsaturated fatty acid containing one carbon double bond has two isomers depending on whether the hydrogen atoms are on the same (*cis*) side or the opposite (*trans*) side of the molecule.

ginseng—A root that has been a popular nutritional supplement and medication in Asia for centuries.

glandulars—Extracts from animal glands (such as the adrenals, thymus, pituitary, and testes) that are claimed to enhance the function of the equivalent gland in the human body. Glandular extracts are degraded during the digestive process, however, so they cannot exert a pharmacological effect.

glomerular filtration rate—A measure of the ability of the kidneys to filter and remove waste products.

gluconeogenesis—The synthesis of glucose from noncarbohydrate precursors such as glycerol, keto acids, or amino acids.

glucose-1-phosphate (G1P)—A compound formed from the breakdown of glycogen.

glucose-6-phosphate (G6P)—A compound formed by the addition of a phosphate group to a glucose molecule by the action of hexokinase. It can also be formed from G1P by glucose phosphate isomerase. G6P is the starting substrate for glycolysis.

GLUT—A glucose (or other monosaccharide) transporter found in cell membranes including those of the muscle and liver.

GLUT2—An isoform of the glucose transporter found in the liver and epithelial cell membranes of the gut.

GLUT4—An isoform of the glucose transporter found in the sarcolemma of muscle fibers.

GLUT5—An isoform of the glucose transporter found in the epithelial cell membranes of the gut. This one is specifically for fructose.

glutamate—An amino acid that acts as a neurotransmitter and a precursor of other neurotransmitters.

glutamine—One of the 20 amino acids commonly found in proteins.

glycemic index (GI)—A ranking or number that reflects the effects of ingested carbohydrates in a particular type of food on a person's blood glucose (also called blood sugar) concentration. The glycemic index of a food is expressed against a reference food (usually glucose).

glycemic load (GL)— A number that estimates how much food will raise a person's blood glucose level after eating it. Glycemic load is based on the glycemic index (GI), and is calculated by multiplying the grams of available carbohydrate in the food (for a typical serving size) by the food's GI and then dividing by 100.

glycerokinase—An enzyme involved in phosphorylation of glycerol to glycerol-3-phosphate.

glycerol—A three-carbon molecule that is the backbone structure of triglycerides.

glycogen—A polymer of glucose that is used to store carbohydrate in the liver and muscles.

glycogenolysis—The breakdown of glycogen into glucose-1-phosphate by the action of phosphorylase.

glycolysis—The sequence of reactions that converts glucose (or glycogen) to pyruvate.

glycoprotein—A protein that is attached to one or more sugar molecules.

glycosidic bond—A chemical bond in which the oxygen atom is the common link between a carbon of one sugar molecule and a carbon of another. Glycogen, the glucose polymer, is a branched-chain polysaccharide that consists of glucose molecules linked by glycosidic bonds.

gonadotrophic hormones—Hormones released from the anterior pituitary gland that promote sex steroid hormone synthesis by the ovaries in women and the testes in men.

gross efficiency (GE)—The ratio of the total work accomplished to the energy expended. Humans are approximately 20% efficient.

gross energy value—The amount of energy in food when measured in a bomb calorimeter. This energy is more than the energy that would be available to the human body if the food were eaten.

guanine (G)—A purine nucleotide base found in DNA.

guanosine diphosphate (GDP)—A compound formed from the breakdown of guanosine triphosphate.

guanosine triphosphate (GTP)—A high-energy phosphate compound similar to adenosine triphosphate.

gum—A form of water-soluble dietary fiber found in plants.

H^+—A hydrogen ion or proton.

half-life—The time in which half the quantity or concentration of a substance is eliminated or removed from the body.

HCO_3^-—Bicarbonate ion, which is the principal extracellular buffer.

heartburn—Indigestion and a burning pain as a result of acidic gastric juices entering the esophagus.

heatstroke—An elevated body temperature of 105.8 °F (41 °C) or higher caused by exposure to excessive heat or high levels of heat production and diminished heat loss. It may result in tissue damage and is potentially fatal.

heat syncope—Fainting caused by excessive heat exposure.

helix—A spiral that has a uniform diameter and periodic spacing between the coils. It is a common secondary structure of proteins and DNA.

hematocrit—The proportion of the blood volume that is occupied by the cellular elements (red cells, white cells, and platelets). Also known as the packed cell volume.

hematuria—The presence of red blood cells or hemoglobin in the urine.

heme—The molecular ring structure that is incorporated in the hemoglobin molecule and enables this protein to carry oxygen.

hemicellulose—A form of dietary fiber found in plants. It differs from cellulose in that it can be hydrolyzed by acid outside of the body.

hemochromatosis—The presence of excessive iron in the body that results in an enlarged liver and liver damage in susceptible people.

hemodilution—A thinning of the blood caused by an expansion of the plasma volume without an equivalent rise in red blood cells.

hemoglobin—The red, iron-containing respiratory pigment found in red blood cells. It is important in the transport of respiratory gases and in the regulation of blood pH.

hemolysis—The destruction of red blood cells within the circulation.

hemorrhage—Damage to blood vessel walls that results in bleeding.

hepatic glucose output—The glucose released from the liver as a result of glycogenolysis or gluconeogenesis.

hexokinase—An enzyme that catalyzes the phosphorylation of glucose to form glucose-6-phosphate.

high-density lipoprotein (HDL)—A protein–lipid complex in the blood plasma that facilitates the transport of triacylglycerols, cholesterol, and phospholipids.

high-density lipoprotein cholesterol (HDL-C)—One way in which lipids are transported in the blood.

homeostasis—The tendency to maintain uniformity or stability of the internal environment of the cell or of the body.

hormone—An organic chemical produced in cells of one part of the body (usually an endocrine gland) that diffuses or is transported by the blood circulation to cells in other parts of the body where it regulates and coordinates their activities.

hormone-sensitive lipase (HSL)—An enzyme that splits triacylglycerols into fatty acids and glycerol. It is regulated by hormones (mainly by epinephrine and insulin).

humoral—Fluid-borne.

hydration—A reaction involving the incorporation of a molecule of water into a compound or a term relating to the state of the body water content.

hydrochloric acid (HCl)—Part of the gastric digestive juices.

hydrogen bond—A weak intermolecular or intramolecular attraction resulting from the interaction of a hydrogen atom and an electronegative atom that has a lone pair of electrons (e.g., oxygen or nitrogen). Hydrogen bonding is important in DNA and RNA and is responsible for much of the tertiary structure of proteins.

hydrolysis—A reaction in which an organic compound is split by interaction with water into simpler compounds.

hydroxylation—A reaction involving the addition of a hydroxyl (OH) group to a molecule.

hyperhydration—Body-water content that is above the normal level.

hyperthermia—Elevated body temperature (>37 °C [98.6 °F]).

hypertonic—Having a higher concentration of dissolved particles (osmolality) than that of another solution with which it is being compared (usually blood plasma, which has an osmolality of 290 mOsm/kg).

hyperventilation—A state in which an increased amount of air enters the pulmonary alveoli (increased alveolar ventilation), which results in reduction of carbon dioxide tension and eventually alkalosis.

hypohydration—A state of dehydration that occurs when the body loses more fluid than is ingested. Common causes of dehydration include vigorous exercise (especially in the heat), diarrhea, vomiting, fever, or excessive sweating.

hyponatremia—Below-normal serum sodium concentration (<140 mmol/L).

hypothalamus—The region at base of brain responsible for integration of sensory input and effector responses in the regulation of body temperature. It also contains the centers that control hunger, appetite, and thirst.

hypothermia—Lower than normal body temperature.

hypotonic—Having a lower concentration of dissolved particles (osmolality) than that of another solution with which it is being compared (usually blood plasma, which has an osmolality of 290 mOsm/kg).

hypovolemia—Reduced blood volume.

immune system—Cells and soluble molecules involved in tissue repair after injury and in the protection of the body against infection.

immunodepression—The lowered functional activity of the immune system.

immunoglobulin (Ig)—A soluble protein with antimicrobial effects that is produced by B-lymphocytes. Also known as an antibody.

incisors—Anterior teeth that are used for cutting food.

indirect calorimetry—A method to measure energy expenditure and substrate utilization on the basis of gas exchange measurements. The term *indirect* refers to the measurement of oxygen uptake and carbon dioxide production rather than the direct measurement of heat transfer.

inflammation—The body's response to injury, which includes redness (increased blood flow) and swelling (edema) caused by increased capillary permeability.

insoluble fiber—Fiber that does not dissolve in water.

insomnia—Difficulty in falling asleep or staying asleep.

insulin—A hormone secreted by the pancreas that is involved in carbohydrate metabolism and particularly in the control of the blood glucose concentration.

insulin-like growth factor (IGF)—A peptide, formerly called somatomedin, that functions primarily to stimulate growth but that also possesses some ability to decrease blood glucose levels.

interferon (IFN)—A type of cytokine. Some interferons inhibit viral replication in infected cells.

interleukin—A type of cytokine produced by leukocytes and some other tissues. It acts as a chemical messenger, like a hormone, but usually with localized effects.

interstitial—Fluid-filled spaces that lie between cells.

intramuscular triacylglycerol (IMTG)—A storage form of fat found in muscle fibers.

in vitro—Outside the living body in an artificial environment.

in vivo—Within the living body.

ion—Any atom or molecule that has an electrical charge due to loss or gain of valency (outer shell) electrons. Ions may carry a positive charge (cation) or a negative charge (anion).

ionic bond—A bond in which valence electrons are either lost or gained and atoms that are oppositely charged are held together by electrostatic forces.

ischemia—Reduced blood supply to a tissue or organ.

isoforms—Chemically distinct forms of an enzyme with identical activities that are usually coded by different genes. Also called isoenzymes.

isomer—One of two or more substances that have identical molecular compositions and relative molecular mass but different structures because of a different arrangement of atoms within the molecule.

isotonicity—Having the same concentration of dissolved particles (osmolality) as that of another solution with which it is being compared (usually blood plasma, which has an osmolality of 290 mOsm/kg).

isotope—One of a set of chemically identical species of an atom. Items within the set of the species have the same atomic number but different mass numbers (e.g., 12-isotopes, 13-isotopes, and 14-isotopes of carbon whose atomic number is 12). Isotopes contain equal numbers of protons but different numbers of neutrons in their nuclei; hence, they differ in relative atomic mass but not in chemical properties.

jejunum—The middle and longest part of the small intestine where a lot of the absorption of nutrients takes place. The jejunum is approximately 1 to 2 m (3 to 6 ft) long.

joule (J)—The SI unit of energy. One joule is the amount of energy needed to move a mass of 1 g at a velocity of 1 m/s.

Ka—Rate constant of a reaction (e.g., for the dissociation of a weak acid into its conjugate base).

Kerckring folds—Folds in the intestinal mucosa of the gastrointestinal tract.

keto acid—An acid that contains a ketone group (-C=O in addition to the acid group(s).

ketogenesis—The synthesis of ketones such as acetoacetate, 3-hydroxybutyrate, and acetone.

ketone bodies—Acidic organic compounds that are produced during the incomplete oxidation of fatty acids in the liver. They contain a carboxyl group (-COOH) and a ketone group (-C=O). Examples include acetoacetate and 3-hydroxybutyrate.

ketone esters—Synthetically made compounds that link an alcohol to a ketone body that is metabolized in the liver to a ketone. Ketone esters are used primarily in research (at the moment) for testing their efficacy in elevating ketone body levels.

ketone salts—Naturally derived compounds that simply mix sodium (and/or potassium or calcium) with 3-hydroxybutyrate to improve absorption.

kinase—An enzyme that regulates a phosphorylation-dephosphorylation reaction (i.e., the addition or removal of a phosphate group). This process is one important way in which enzyme activity can be regulated.

kilojoule (kJ)—Unit of energy (kJ = 10^3 J).

lactase—The enzyme responsible for splitting lactose into galactose and glucose.

lactate dehydrogenase (LDH)—The enzyme that catalyzes the reversible reduction of pyruvate to lactate.

lacteal—The lymphatic vessel that drains the villi in the gut wall.

lactic acid—The metabolic end product of anaerobic glycolysis.

lactose—Milk sugar, a disaccharide that links a molecule of glucose and a molecule of galactose.

lacto vegetarian—A vegetarian who consumes milk products but not eggs.

laxatives—Drugs that act on the gut to promote defecation.

lean body mass (LBM)—All parts of the body excluding fat.

lecithin—The common name for phosphatidylcholine, which is the most abundant phospholipid found in cell membranes. It occurs naturally in a variety of food items (e.g., beans, eggs, wheat germ).

legume—The high-protein seed or pod of vegetables (e.g., beans, peas, lentils).

leptin—A regulatory hormone produced by fat cells. When released into the circulation, it influences the hypothalamus to control appetite.

leucine—An essential amino acid and the only one that has a direct stimulatory effect on muscle protein synthesis.

leukocytes—White blood cells that are important in inflammation and immune defense.

leukocytosis—An increased number of leukocytes in the circulation.

lingual lipase—A fat-splitting enzyme secreted by cells at the base of the tongue.

linoleic acid—An essential fatty acid.

linolenic acid—An essential fatty acid.

lipase—An enzyme that catalyzes the hydrolysis of triacylglycerols into fatty acids and glycerol.

lipid—A compound composed of carbon, hydrogen, oxygen, and sometimes other elements. Lipids dissolve in organic solvents but not in water and include triacylglycerol, cholesterol, and phospholipids. Lipid is a general name for oils, fats, waxes, and related compounds. Oil is liquid at room temperature, whereas fat is solid.

lipid peroxidation—Oxidation of fatty acids in lipid structures (e.g., membranes) caused by the actions of free radicals.

lipolysis—The breakdown of triacylglycerols into fatty acids and glycerol.

lipoprotein lipase (LPL)—An enzyme that catalyzes the breakdown of triacylglycerols in plasma lipoproteins.

long-chain fatty acid (LCFA)—The most abundant type of fatty acid. LCFAs have hydrocarbon chains of 12 or more carbon atoms. LCFAs are part of triacylglycerols. Palmitic acid and oleic acid are the most abundant LCFAs in humans.

long-chain triacylglycerols—Triacylglycerols that consist of glycerol and three long-chain fatty acids.

low-density lipoprotein (LDL)—A protein-lipid complex in the blood plasma that facilitates the transport of triacylglycerols, cholesterol, and phospholipids.

low-density lipoprotein cholesterol (LCL-C)—One way in which cholesterol is transported in the blood. High blood levels are associated with increased incidence of coronary heart disease.

lymphocyte—A type of white blood cell that is important in the acquired immune response. It includes both T cells and B cells, and the latter produce antibodies.

lysosome—A membranous vesicle found in the cell cytoplasm. Lysosomes contain digestive enzymes capable of autodigesting the cell.

lysozymes—Enzymes that break down proteins and attack bacteria.

macrominerals—Dietary elements essential to life processes that each constitute at least 0.01% of total body mass. The seven macrominerals are potassium, sodium, chloride, calcium, magnesium, phosphorus, and sulfur.

macronutrients—Nutrients that are ingested in relatively large amounts: carbohydrate, fat, protein.

macrophage —A type of leukocyte found in tissues that can ingest and destroy foreign material and initiate the acquired immune response. Tissue macrophages are derived from the monocytes in the blood.

magnetic resonance imaging (MRI)—An imaging technique that generates pictures of body tissues and compartments. The results are somewhat similar to those obtained by a CT scan, but an MRI uses electromagnetic radiation rather than ionizing radiation.

making weight—The practice of rapid weight loss based on the belief that training at a heavier body weight, then dropping weight shortly before competition, gives an athlete an advantage.

maltodextrin—A glucose polymer (that commonly contains 6-12 glucose molecules) that exerts lesser osmotic effects compared with glucose and is used in a variety of sports drinks as the main source of carbohydrate.

maltose—A disaccharide that yields two molecules of glucose upon hydrolysis.

mammalian target of rapamycin (mTor)—A protein kinase that regulates cell growth, cell proliferation, cell motility, cell survival, protein synthesis, and transcription. Signaling through mTOR is activated by amino acids, insulin, and growth factors and is impaired by nutrient or energy deficiency. mTOR regulates numerous components involved in protein synthesis, including initiation and elongation factors, and the biogenesis of ribosomes.

masticating—Chewing food.

mechanical digestion—Breaking down food by chewing.

medium-chain fatty acid (MCFA)—A fatty acid with 8 or 10 carbon atoms.

medium-chain triacylglycerol (MCT)—A triacylglycerol (triglyceride) that contains fatty acids with hydrocarbon chain lengths of 6 to 12 carbons.

megadose—An excessive amount of a substance in comparison to a normal dose (such as the RDA). It is usually used to refer to vitamin supplements.

menarche—The onset of menstruation in adolescent girls.

menstruation—Monthly bleeding and discharge of the outer uterine wall in healthy women.

metabolic acidosis—A metabolic derangement of acid-base balance where the blood pH is abnormally low.

metabolic equivalents (METS)—A measurement of energy expenditure expressed as multiples of the resting metabolic rate. One MET equals an oxygen uptake rate of approximately 3.5 ml of oxygen per kilogram of body weight per minute.

metabolite—A product of a metabolic reaction.

metalloenzyme—An enzyme that needs a mineral component (e.g., copper, iron, magnesium, zinc) to function effectively.

Michaelis constant (Km)—The concentration of substrate that permits half the maximal rate of an enzyme-catalyzed reaction.

microbiota—The microorganisms that are found in a particular environment or location such as those that occupy the gut or the skin.

microminerals—Dietary elements essential to life processes that each make up less than 0.01% of total body mass and are needed in quantities of less than 100 mg a day. Among the 14 microminerals are iron, zinc, copper, chromium, and selenium. Also called trace elements.

micronutrients—Organic vitamins and inorganic minerals that must be consumed in relatively small amounts in the diet to maintain health.

microvilli—Very small (1 mm) fingerlike projections of a cell membrane. They occur on the luminal surface of the cells in the small intestine.

mineral—An inorganic element found in nature; the term is usually reserved for those elements that are solid. In nutrition, the term *mineral* is usually used to classify dietary elements that are essential to life processes such as calcium and iron.

mitochondria—Oval or spherical organelles that contain the enzymes of the tricarboxylic acid cycle and electron transport chain. They are sites of oxidative phosphorylation (resynthesis of adenosine triphosphate involving the use of oxygen).

mitochondrial biogenesis—The process by which cells increase their numbers of mitochondria to increase the capacity for aerobic adenosine triphosphate production.

mitochondrial matrix—The substance that occupies the space enclosed by the inner membrane of a mitochondrion. It contains enzymes, filaments of DNA, ribosomes, granules, and inclusions of protein crystals, glycogen, and lipids.

mitogen—A chemical that can stimulate lymphocytes to proliferate (undergo rapid cell divisions).

molar (mol)—Unit of concentration.

mole—The amount of a chemical compound whose mass in grams is equivalent to its molecular weight, which is the sum of the atomic weights of its constituent atoms.

molecule—An aggregation of at least two atoms of the same or different elements held together by special forces (covalent bonds) and having a precise chemical formula (e.g., O_2, $C_6H_{12}O_6$).

monoacylglycerol—A glycerol backbone with one fatty acid. Also known as monoglyceride.

monocyte—A type of leukocyte found in the blood that can ingest and destroy foreign material and initiate the acquired immune response. When monocytes infiltrate tissues they become macrophages.

monosaccharide—A simple sugar that cannot be hydrolyzed to smaller units (e.g., glucose, fructose, galactose).

motility—The movement of food through the gastrointestinal tract by coordinated muscular contractions of the intestine.

motor unit—All the muscle fibers supplied by a single motor neuron.

mucosa—Layers of cells that line the mouth, nasal passages, airways, and gut that present a barrier to pathogen entry into the body.

muscle hypertrophy—The growth and increase of the size of muscle cells. The most common type of muscular hypertrophy occurs as a result of resistance exercise such as weightlifting.

myofibril—Threadlike (1- to 3-mm thick) structures that contain the contractile proteins and are continuous from end to end in the muscle fiber.

myoglobin—A protein that functions as an intracellular respiratory pigment that is capable of binding oxygen and releasing it only at very low partial pressures.

myosin—One of the major contractile proteins in muscle found in the thick filaments.

MyPlate—The current nutrition guide published by the USDA Center for Nutrition Policy and Promotion. It is a chart that depicts a place setting with a plate and glass divided into the five food groups.

MyPyramid—The American food guide pyramid produced by the USDA Center for Nutrition Policy and Promotion that was used from 2005 to 2011. It was replaced by MyPlate.

nandrolone—A steroid with androgenic and anabolic properties.

natural killer (NK) cell—A type of lymphocyte that is important in eliminating viral infections and preventing cancer.

natural killer cytotoxic activity (NKCA)—The ability of natural killer cells to destroy virally infected cells and tumor cells.

net efficiency (NE)—The work accomplished divided by the energy expended minus resting energy expenditure.

neurotransmitters—Endogenous signaling molecules that transfer information from one nerve ending to the next.

neutrophil—A type of white blood cell that can ingest and destroy foreign material. It is important as a first line of defense against bacteria.

NH_2—Amino group.

NH^+_4—Ammonium ion.

nicotinamide adenine dinucleotide, oxidized form (NAD^+)—A coenzyme that is important in energy metabolism.

nicotinamide adenine dinucleotide, reduced form (NADH)—A reduced form of the coenzyme NAD.

nicotinamide adenine dinucleotide phosphate, oxidized form ($NADP^+$)—A coenzyme that is important in anabolic reactions, such as lipid and nucleic acid synthesis, which require NADPH as a reducing agent.

nicotinamide adenine dinucleotide phosphate, reduced form (NADPH)—A reduced form of the coenzyme NADP.

nitrogen balance—A dietary state in which the input and output of nitrogen are balanced so the body neither gains nor loses tissue protein.

NO—Nitric oxide.

NO·—Nitric oxide radical.

NO^-_2—Nitrite ion.

NO^-_3—Nitrate ion. This ergogenic aid reduces the oxygen cost of exercise. It is naturally abundant in beetroot and rhubarb.

nonessential amino acids—Amino acids that can be synthesized in the body.

nonesterified fatty acid (NEFA)—A free fatty acid (FFA) or fatty acid (FA).

norepinephrine—Catecholamine neurohormone, the neurotransmitter of most of the sympathetic nervous system (of adrenergic neurons). Also known as noradrenaline.

nutraceutical—A nutrient that may function as a pharmaceutical (drug) when taken in certain quantities.

nutrient—A substance found in food that provides energy or promotes growth and repair of tissues.

nutrient density—Amount of essential nutrients expressed per unit of energy in the food.

nutrigenomics—The study of interactions between genes and nutrients that is mainly concerned with the effects of foods and food constituents on gene expression.

nutrition—The result of the processes of ingestion, digestion, absorption, and metabolism of food and the subsequent assimilation of nutrient materials into the tissues.

nutritional training—See periodized nutrition.

O_2—Oxygen molecule.

$\cdot O^-_2$ (superoxide radical)—A highly reactive free radical.

obesity—An excessive accumulation of body fat. This term is usually reserved for people who are 20% or more above the average weight for their size.

OH—Hydroxyl group.

OH^- (hydroxyl radical)—A highly reactive free radical.

oligosaccharide—A saccharide polymer containing a small number (typically three to nine) of monosaccharides (simple sugars).

omega-3 fatty acid—A polyunsaturated fatty acid. Examples include eicosapentaenoic acid (EPA), docosahexaenoic acid (DHA), and α-linolenic acid (ALA).

orthorexia nervosa—An eating disorder characterized by an excessive preoccupation with eating healthy food.

osmolality—A measure of the total dissolved particle concentration. Units are mOsm/kg.

osmolarity—A measure of the total concentration of a solution; the number of moles of solute per liter of solvent typically expressed in mOsm/L.

osmoreceptors—Sensory cells in the hypothalamus capable of detecting changes in osmolarity of the blood.

osmosis—The diffusion of water molecules from the lesser to the greater concentration of solute (dissolved substance) when two solutions are separated by a membrane that selectively prevents the passage of solute molecules but is permeable to water molecules.

osteoblasts—Cells responsible for mineralization of bone.

osteoclasts—Cells responsible for breakdown (demineralization) of bone.

osteoporosis—A weakening of the bone structure that occurs when the rate of demineralization exceeds the rate of bone formation.

overhydration—Body-water content that is above the normal level. This is usually caused by drinking too much water, which can result in potentially harmful water intoxication.

ovo-lacto vegetarian—A vegetarian who consumes eggs and milk products.

ovulation—The monthly release of an ovum (egg) from the ovaries in women.

oxidation—A reaction involving the loss of electrons from an atom. It is always accompanied by a reduction. For example, pyruvate is reduced by the reduced form of the coenzyme nicotinamide adenine dinucleotide (NADH) in the rection catalyzed by lactate dehydrogenase to form lactate. In the reverse reaction, lactate is oxidized by nicotinamide adenine dinucleotide (NAD^+) when pyruvate is reformed.

oxidative phosphorylation—Resynthesis of adenosine triphosphate involving the use of oxygen.

pancreas—An organ located below and behind the stomach. It secretes insulin and glucagon, which are involved in plasma glucose regulation, and pancreatic enzymes, which are involved in the digestion of fats and protein in the small intestine.

pancreatic duct—The connecting tube between the pancreas and the duodenum through which pancreatic juice is transported into the duodenum.

pancreatic juice—The secretions of the pancreas that are transported by the pancreatic duct to the duodenum. Pancreatic juice contains bicarbonate and the digestive enzymes amylase, lipase, and trypsin.

parathyroid hormone (PTH)—A hormone secreted from the parathyroid glands that is involved in regulation of the blood plasma calcium ion concentration.

pathogen—A microorganism that can cause symptoms of disease.

pectin—A form of soluble dietary fiber found in some fruits.

pepsin—A group of proteases (enzymes that digest proteins) involved in food digestion that are secreted in pancreatic juice.

pepsinogen—The inactive form (storage form) of pepsin. Pepsinogen is stored in the cells of the stomach wall.

peptide—A small compound formed by the bonding of two to nine amino acids.

peptide bond—The bond formed by the condensation of the amino group and the carboxyl group of a pair of amino acids. Peptides are constructed from a linear array of amino acids joined together by a series of peptide bonds.

periodized nutrition—The strategic use of nutrition or exercise training combined with nutrition to obtain adaptations that improve exercise performance in the long term. Also known as nutritional training.

peristalsis—Waves of contraction in the smooth muscle of the digestive tract. It involves circular and longitudinal muscle fibers at successive locations along the tract and serves to propel the contents of the tract in one direction.

peroxisome proliferator-activated receptor γ coactivators (PGCs)—A family of transcription coactivators that are important in driving mitochondrial biogenesis. A transcription coactivator is a protein or protein complex that increases the probability of a gene being transcribed by interacting with transcription factors but does not itself bind to DNA in a sequence-specific manner.

personalized nutrition—A tailored diet and supplement plan that provides effective nutrition for a person depending on his or her phenotype, genotype, sex, age, and goals.

pH—A measure of acidity or alkalinity; $pH = -\log_{10}[H^+]$.

phagocyte—A leukocyte that is capable of ingesting and digesting microorganisms.

phenotype—The appearance or physiological characteristic of an individual that results from the interaction of the genotype and the environment.

phosphagens—The high-energy phosphate compounds adenosine triphosphate and phosphocreatine.

phosphocreatine (PCr)—An important energy source in very high-intensity exercise. Also called creatine phosphate.

phosphofructokinase (PFK)—The rate-limiting enzyme in glycolysis.

phospholipids—Fats that contain a phosphate group that yield fatty acids, glycerol, and a nitrogenous compound on hydrolysis (e.g., lecithin). Phospholipids are important components of membranes.

phosphorylase—An enzyme that breaks down the glucose polymer glycogen into molecules of glucose-1-phosphate. This breakdown of stored carbohydrate takes place in the liver and muscles.

phosphorylation—A reaction that involves the addition of a phosphate (PO^{2-}_3) group to a molecule. Many enzymes are activated by the covalent bonding of a phosphate group. The oxidative phosphorylation of adenosine diphosphate forms adenosine triphosphate.

photosynthesis—The process by which green plants and algae absorb light energy and use it to synthesize organic compounds including glucose.

phytonutrients—Certain organic components of plants that are thought to promote human health. They differ from vitamins because they are not considered essential nutrients, which means that people will not develop nutritional deficiencies without them. Examples include carotenoids, flavonoids, and coumarins.

Pi—Inorganic phosphate (HPO^{2-}_4).

plaque—The material that accumulates on the inner layer of the arteries and contributes to atherosclerosis. It contains cholesterol, lipids, platelets, and other debris. Plaque on the inner layers of the arterial wall can cause coronary heart disease.

plasma—The liquid portion of the blood in which the blood cells are suspended. It typically accounts for 55% to 60% of the total blood volume. It differs from serum in that it contains fibrinogen, which is the clot-forming protein.

plasma membrane fatty acid–binding protein (FABPpm)—A protein found in liver and muscle that is involved in transport of fatty acids across the plasma membrane.

polypeptide—A peptide that, upon hydrolysis, yields more than 10 amino acids.

polyphenols—A large class of naturally occurring compounds that includes the flavonoids, flavonols, flavanones, and anthocyanidins. These compounds contain a number of phenolic hydroxyl (-OH) groups attached to ring structures, which confers them with powerful antioxidant activity.

polysaccharide—A polymer of more than about 10 monosaccharide residues linked glycosidically in branched or unbranched chains. Examples include starch and glycogen.

polyunsaturated fatty acid (PUFA)—A fatty acid that contains more than one carbon–carbon double bond.

postabsorptive state—The period after a meal has been absorbed from the gastrointestinal tract.

power—Work performed per unit of time.

prebiotic—A nondigestible food ingredient that promotes the growth of beneficial microorganisms in the intestines.

precursor—A substance from which another substance, which is usually more active or mature, is formed.

probiotic—A supplement that is usually derived from dairy foods or a dietary supplement that contains live bacteria that replace or add to the beneficial bacteria normally present in the gut.

prohormone—A protein hormone that is in an inactive state until it undegoes processing to remove parts of its polypeptide sequence to make it biologically active. It is also a term used to describe a chemical precursor to a steroid hormone such as testosterone.

prosthetic group—A coenzyme that is tightly bound to an enzyme.

protease—An enzyme that catalyzes the digestion or cleavage of proteins.

proteins—Biological macromolecules that are composed of a chain of covalently linked amino acids. Proteins may have structural or functional roles.

protein balance—A state in which the rates of protein synthesis and degradation are equal such that the body neither gains nor loses tissue protein.

protein degradation—The process in which the individual amino acids from a protein are disconnected.

protein energy malnutrition (PEM)—The inadequate intake of dietary protein and energy.

protein synthesis—The process in which individual amino acids, whether of exogenous or endogenous origin, are connected to each other in peptide linkage in a specific order dictated by the sequence of nucleotides in DNA.

ptyalin—A digestive enzyme found in saliva that begins the digestion of starches in the mouth. Also called α-amylase.

pyloric sphincter—A circular muscle that controls the entry of stomach contents into the duodenum. The pyloric sphincter serves as a gate, closing the opening from the stomach to the intestine.

pylorus—The opening from the stomach into the duodenum.

pyrogen—A substance that causes body temperature to be elevated and be regulated at a higher set point.

pyruvate—A three-carbon molecule that is the end product of glycolysis.

pyruvate dehydrogenase (PDH)—The enzyme that catalyzes the conversion of pyruvate to acetyl-CoA.

quercetin—A flavonoid polyphenol compound.

R-group—The side chain of an amino acid.

radiation—The transfer of energy waves that are emitted by one object and absorbed by another (e.g., solar energy from sunlight).

radiolabeled isotopes—An isotope is of a set of chemically identical species of an atom. Items within the set of the species have the same atomic number but different mass numbers because they contain equal numbers of protons but different numbers of neutrons in their nuclei. Radiolabeled isotopes (e.g., carbon-14, ^{14}C) transmit radiation and are used as tracers in studies of metabolism.

rate-limiting enzyme—An enzyme in a metabolic pathway that regulates the slowest step in the pathway and limits the rate of flux through the pathway.

rating of perceived exertion (RPE)—A subjective numerical rating that is used to express the perceived difficulty of a given exercise task.

reactive hypoglycemia— A decrease in blood glucose concentration to hypoglycemic levels (<3.5 mmol/L) in response to carbohydrate feeding before exercise. Also called rebound hypoglycemia.

reactive oxygen species (ROS)—Collective name for free radicals and other highly reactive molecules derived from molecular oxygen. ROS include superoxide radical ($O_2^{-}\cdot$), hydroxyl radical ($OH^{-}\cdot$), hydrogen peroxide (H_2O_2), and perchlorous acid (HOCl).

recommended dietary allowance (RDA)—The recommended intake of a particular nutrient that meets the needs of nearly all (97%) healthy individuals of similar age and gender. The RDAs are established by the Food and Nutrition Boards of the National Academy of Sciences.

rectum—Last portion of the colon connected to the anus.

reduction—A reaction in which a molecule gains electrons.

reesterification—A process during which fatty acids are not released into the circulation but are used to form new triacylglycerols within the adipose tissue.

reference daily intake (RDI)—Nutrient intake standards set by the FDA based on the 1968 RDA for various vitamins and minerals. RDIs have been set for infants, toddlers, people older than 4 years of age, and pregnant and lactating women.

reference nutrient intake (RNI)—The level of intake required to meet the known nutritional needs of more than 97.5% of healthy persons. In the United Kingdom, the RNI is similar to the original recommended dietary allowance.

refined sugar—Sweet, crystalline carbohydrate typically found as sucrose. It is extracted from processed sugar cane or sugar beets and used as a food and beverage sweetener.

relative humidity—The percentage of moisture in the air compared with the amount of moisture needed to cause saturation.

reperfusion—Restoration of the blood supply to a tissue or organ.

respiration chamber—A chamber in which the exchange of carbon dioxide and oxygen is measured to estimate energy expenditure and substrate use.

respiratory exchange ratio (RER)—The ratio of carbon dioxide produced divided by oxygen consumed, which represents a measure of substrate use at the whole-body level.

respiratory quotient (RQ)—The ratio of the rate of carbon dioxide production divided by the rate of oxygen consumption, which can be used to establish the approximate pattern of substrate use by an organ or tissue (e.g., muscle).

resting metabolic rate (RMR)—Energy expenditure under resting conditions.

resveratrol—A polyphenol compound found in certain plants and in red wine that has antioxidant and potentially ergogenic properties. It has been reported to increase exercise performance in rodents.

ribonucleic acid (RNA)—A nucleic acid that is essential for protein synthesis. Different forms of RNA include mRNA: messenger RNA; miRNA: micro RNA; rRNA: ribosomal RNA; and tRNA: transfer RNA.

ribosome—An extremely small organelle composed of protein and ribonucleic acid that is either free in the cytoplasm or attached to the membranes of the endoplasmic reticulum of a cell. It is the site of protein synthesis.

saccharine—An artificial sweetener made from coal tar.

salt—Sodium chloride; a white crystalline substance that gives seawater its characteristic taste and is used for seasoning or preserving food. In chemistry, a salt is any chemical compound formed from the reaction of an acid with a base with all or part of the hydrogen of the acid replaced by a metal or other cation.

sarcolemma—The cell membrane of a muscle fiber.

sarcomere—The smallest contractile unit or segment of a muscle fiber. It is defined as the region between two Z lines.

sarcoplasm—The cytoplasm or intracellular fluid within a muscle fiber.

sarcoplasmic reticulum—An elaborate, baglike, membranous structure found within a muscle cell. Its interconnecting membranous tubules lie in the narrow spaces between the myofibrils and surround and run parallel to them.

serotonin—A brain neurotransmitter. Also known as 5-hydroxytryptamine (5-HT).

serum—The fluid that is left after blood has clotted.

short-chain fatty acid (SCFA)—A fatty acid that contains six or fewer carbon atoms.

signal transduction pathways—A series of chemical reactions in a cell that occur when a molecule, such as a hormone, attaches to a receptor on the cell membrane. The pathway is actually a cascade of biochemical reactions inside the cell that eventually reach the target molecule to influence enzyme activity or gene expression.

smooth muscle—A specialized type of nonstriated muscle tissue that is composed of single nucleated fibers. It contracts in an involuntary rhythmic fashion in the walls of visceral organs. It is also found in the walls of blood vessels.

sodium glucose transporter (SGLT)—A carrier protein that cotransports sodium and glucose across a cell membrane.

sodium pump—The common name for the sodium-potassium adenosine triphosphatase that helps establish the resting membrane potential of a cell.

soluble fiber—Fiber that dissolves well in water.

solute—A substance dissolved in a solvent liquid such as water.

solvent—A liquid medium in which particles can dissolve.

specific heat—The amount of energy or heat needed to raise the temperature of a unit of mass (e.g., 1 g of body tissue) by 1 °C. Units are J/g/°C.

sphingomyelin—A type of lipid found in the membranes of Schwann cells that provide an insulating sheath around nerve axons.

spirometry—A method to measure breathing.

stable isotope—An isotope that is not radioactive (e.g., carbon-13, ^{13}C). Stable isotopes are used as tracers in studies of metabolism.

standard deviation (SD)—A measure of variability about the mean; 68% of the population is within one standard deviation above and below the mean (average) value, and about 95% of the population is within two standard deviations of the mean (average) value.

starch—A carbohydrate made of multiple units of glucose attached together by bonds that can be broken down by human digestion processes. Also known as complex carbohydrate.

steroid—A complex molecule derived from the lipid cholesterol that contains four interlocking carbon rings.

STPD—Abbreviation indicating that a gas volume has been expressed as if it were at standard temperature (0°C), standard pressure (760 mm Hg absolute), and dry; under these conditions a mole of gas occupies 22.4 L.

substrate—The reactant molecule in a reaction catalyzed by an enzyme.

substrate-level phosphorylation—Synthesis of high-energy phosphate bonds through reaction of inorganic phosphate with an activated and usually organic substrate.

succinate dehydrogenase (SDH)—An enzyme of the tricarboxylic acid cycle.

sucrose—Table sugar; a disaccharide that consists of a combination of glucose and fructose.

sugar—Any of the class of soluble, crystalline, typically sweet-tasting carbohydrates found in plant and animal tissues and exemplified by glucose and sucrose.

supercompensation of muscle glycogen—Higher than normal muscle glycogen concentrations that can be achieved with a combination of exercise and diet.

superoxide dismutase (SOD)—An enzyme in body cells that helps neutralize free radicals.

Système Internationale (SI)—The International System of Units; a worldwide uniform system of units.

systolic—Indicating the maximum arterial pressure during contraction of the left ventricle of the heart.

testosterone—The male sex hormone responsible for male secondary sex characteristics at puberty. It has anabolic and androgenic effects and is responsible for aggressive behavior.

thermic effect of exercise (TEE)—The energy required for exercise. Increased muscle contraction increases heat production.

thermogenesis—The production of heat. Metabolic processes in the body constantly generate heat.

thermoreceptors—Sensory cells that are capable of detecting changes in temperature.

thermoregulation—The maintenance of a stable and safe body core temperature, usually around 37°C (98°F).

thymine (T)—A pyrimidine nucleotide found in DNA.

tissue—An organized association of similar cells that perform a common function (e.g., muscle tissue).

tracer—An element or compound that contains atoms that can be distinguished from their normal counterparts by physical means (e.g., radioactivity assay or mass spectrometry) and can thus be used to follow (trace) the metabolism of the normal substances.

train high—A general term to describe training with high carbohydrate. Muscle and liver glycogen levels are high at the start of exercise or carbohydrates are ingested during exercise.

train low—A general term to describe training with low carbohydrate availability. This low carbohydrate availability could be low muscle glycogen, low liver glycogen, low carbohydrate intake during or after exercise, or combinations thereof.

trans—A prefix indicating the geometrical isomer in which the two like groups are on opposite sides of a double bond with restricted rotation (e.g., in unsaturated fatty acids in which the hydrogen ions are on the opposite side of the double bond).

transamination—A reaction that involves the transfer of an amino (NH_2) group from an amino acid to a keto acid.

***trans* fatty acids**—Unsaturated fatty acids that contain at least one double bond in the *trans* configuration.

transfer ribonucleic acid (tRNA)—This transports amino acids to ribosomes where protein synthesis takes place.

transit time—The time that food stays in the gastrointestinal tract.

translation—The process by which ribosomes and transfer ribonucleic acid decipher the genetic code in messenger RNA to synthesize a specific polypeptide or protein.

triacylglycerol—The storage form of fat (lipid) composed of three fatty acid molecules linked to a three-carbon glycerol molecule. Also known as triglyceride.

tricarboxylic acid (TCA)—A compound that contains three carboxyl (-COOH) groups (e.g., citric acid).

tricarboxylic acid cycle (TCA cycle)—A series of reactions that are important in energy metabolism and take place in the mitochondrion. Also known as the Krebs cycle (after Hans Krebs, who first described the reactions involved) or the citric acid cycle (because citrate is one of the key intermediates in the process).

triplet code—The sequences of three nucleotides that compose the codons, which are the units of genetic information in DNA or RNA that specify the order of amino acids in a peptide or protein.

tryptophan (TRP)—An essential amino acid and a precursor of the neurotransmitter serotonin in the brain.

tumor necrosis factor (TNF)—A cytokine that promotes inflammation.

type 1 diabetes mellitus—A chronic condition in which the pancreas makes little or no insulin because the beta cells have been destroyed and the body is not able to use glucose (blood sugar) for energy. Also called insulin-dependent diabetes mellitus.

type 2 diabetes mellitus—A long-term metabolic disorder that is characterized by high blood sugar, insulin resistance, and relative lack of insulin. It develops when a person is overweight or obese. Also called non-insulin-dependent diabetes mellitus (NIDDM).

type I fibers—Small-diameter muscle cells that contain relatively slow-acting myosin adenosine triphosphatases and hence contract slowly. Their red color is caused by the presence of myoglobin. These fibers possess a high capacity for oxidative metabolism, are extremely fatigue resistant, and are specialized for the performance of repeated contractions over prolonged periods.

type II fibers—Muscle cells that are much paler than type I fibers because they contain little myoglobin. They possess rapidly acting myosin adenosine triphosphatases, so their contraction (and relaxation) times are relatively fast. A high activity of glycogen phosphorylase and glycolytic enzymes endows type II fibers with a high capacity for rapid (but relatively short-lived) adenosine triphosphate production.

unsaturated fatty acid (UFA)—A fatty acid that contains at least one double bond within its hydrocarbon chain.

upper limit (UL)—The maximum level of daily nutrient intake that is unlikely to pose health risks to the greatest number of individuals in the group for whom it is designed.

uracil (U)—A pyrimidine nucleotide found in RNA.

urea—The end product of protein metabolism. The chemical formula is $CO(NH_2)_2$.

uric acid—A breakdown product of nucleic acids present in small quantities in the urine of people and most mammals.

uridine diphosphate (UDP)—A coenzyme involved in glycogen synthesis.

urine—Waste fluid produced in the kidneys and excreted from the body that contains urea, ammonia, and other metabolic wastes.

vanadium—A trace element that has a role in glucose metabolism.

vegan—A person who does not eat animal products.

vegetarian—A person who does not eat meat and whose diet is plant based.

very low-density lipoprotein (VLDL)—A protein–lipid complex in the blood plasma that transports triacylglycerols, cholesterol, and phospholipids.

villi—Small (1 mm), fingerlike folds of the mucosa of the small intestine.

vitamin—An organic substance that is necessary in small amounts for the normal metabolic functioning of the body. Vitamins must be present in the diet because the body cannot synthesize them (or cannot synthesize adequate amounts).

vitamin B_1—Thiamin.

vitamin B_2—Riboflavin.

vitamin B_6—Pyridoxine.

vitamin B_{12}—Cyanocobalamin.

vitamin C—Ascorbic acid.

vitamin D—Cholecalciferol, the product of irradiation of 7-dehydrocholesterol found in the skin.

vitamin E—α-tocopherol.

vitamin K—Menoquinone.

V_{max}—Maximal velocity of an enzymatic reaction when substrate concentration is not limiting.

$\dot{V}O_2$—Rate of oxygen uptake.

$\dot{V}O_2$max—Maximal oxygen uptake; the highest rate of oxygen consumption by the body that can be determined in an incremental exercise test to exhaustion.

water—The universal solvent of life (H_2O). The body is composed of 60% water.

watt (W)—Unit of power or work rate (J/s).

weight cycling—A cycle in which the considerable effort applied to achieve weight loss is exceeded by the effort required to maintain the new lower body weight. After the weight is lost, it is regained in a relatively short period. Also referred to as the yo-yo effect.

wet-bulb globe thermometer index (WBGT index)—A heat-stress index based on four factors measured by the wet-bulb globe thermometer.

whey protein—A rapidly digested protein with a high leucine content that is derived from milk.

white blood cells (WBC)—Important cells of the immune system that defend the body against invading microorganisms. Also called leukocytes.

work efficiency (WE)—The work accomplished divided by the energy expended minus the energy cost in the unloaded condition.

w.w.—Wet weight.

yohimbine—An alkaloid substance derived from yohimbine bark, which functions as an α_2-adrenoreceptor blocker (monamine oxidase inhibitor).

yo-yo effect—See weight cycling.

References

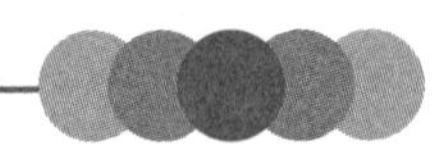

Aarsland, A., D. Chinkes, and R.R. Wolfe. 1997. Hepatic and whole-body fat synthesis in humans during carbohydrate overfeeding. *Am J Clin Nutr* 65 (6): 1774-1782.

Abbasi, A., E. Fehrenbach, M. Hauth, M. Walter, J. Hudemann, V. Wank, A.M. Niess, and H. Northoff. 2013. Changes in spontaneous and LPS-induced ex vivo cytokine production and mRNA expression in male and female athletes following prolonged exhaustive exercise. *Exerc Immunol Rev* 19:8-28.

Abbasi, A., M. Hauth, M. Walter, J. Hudemann, V. Wank, A.M. Niess, and H. Northoff. 2014. Exhaustive exercise modifies different gene expression profiles and pathways in LPS-stimulated and un-stimulated whole blood cultures. *Brain Behav Immun* 39:130-141.

Abbott, W.G., B.V. Howard, L. Christin, et al. 1988. Short-term energy balance: Relationship with protein, carbohydrate, and fat balances. *Am J Physiol* 255 (3 Pt 1): E332-E337.

Achten, J., M. Gleeson, and A.E. Jeukendrup. 2002. Determination of the exercise intensity that elicits maximal fat oxidation. *Med Sci Sports Exerc* 34 (1): 92-97.

Achten, J., S.L. Halson, L. Moseley, M.P. Rayson, A. Casey, and A.E. Jeukendrup. 2004. Higher dietary carbohydrate content during intensified running training results in better maintenance of performance and mood state. *J Appl Physiol* 96 (4): 1331-1340.

Achten, J., and A.E. Jeukendrup. 2003. The effect of pre-exercise carbohydrate feedings on the intensity that elicits maximal fat oxidation. *J Sports Sci* 21:1017-1024.

Achten, J., M.C. Venables, and A.E. Jeukendrup. 2003. Fat oxidation rates are higher during running compared to cycling over a wide range of intensities. *Metabolism* 52 (6): 747-752.

Acker, S.A.B.E., M.N.J.L. Tromp, G.R.M.M. Haenen, J.F. Wim, V. Vijgh, and A. Bast. 1995. Flavonoids as scavengers of nitric oxide radical. *Bio Chem Res Rev* 3:755-757.

Ackland, T.R., T.G. Lohman, J. Sundgot-Borgen, R.J. Maughan, N.L. Meyer, A.D. Stewart, and W. Müller. 2012. Current status of body composition assessment in sport: Review and position statement on behalf of the ad hoc research working group on body composition health and performance, under the auspices of the I.O.C. Medical Commission. *Sports Med* 42 (3): 227-249.

Afshar, M., S. Richards, D. Mann, A. Cross, G.B. Smith, G. Netzer, E. Kovacs, and J. Hasday. 2015. Acute immunomodulatory effects of binge alcohol consumption. *Alcohol* 49 (1): 57-64.

Akerstrom, T.C., J.B. Birk, D.K. Klein, C. Erikstrup, P. Plomgaard, B.K. Pedersen, and J. Wojtaszewski. 2006. Oral glucose ingestion attenuates exercise-induced activation of 5′-AMP-activated protein kinase in human skeletal muscle. *Biochem Biophys Res Commun* 342:949-955.

Akerstrom, T.C.A., C.P. Fischer, P. Plomgaard, C. Thomsen, G. van Hall, and B. Klarlund Pedersen. 2009. Glucose ingestion during endurance training does not alter adaptation. *J Appl Physiol* 106:1771-1779.

Al-Jaderi, Z., and A.A. Maghazachi. 2013. Effects of vitamin D3, calcipotriol and FTY720 on the expression of surface molecules and cytolytic activities of human natural killer cells and dendritic cells. *Toxins* 5 (11): 1932-1947.

Allen, J.D., J. McLung, A.G. Nelson, and M. Welsch. 1998. Ginseng supplementation does not enhance healthy young adults' peak aerobic exercise performance. *J Am Coll Nutr* 17 (5): 462-466.

Allgrove, J.E., E. Farrell, M. Gleeson, G. Williamson, and K. Cooper. 2011. Regular dark chocolate consumption's reduction of oxidative stress and increase of free-fatty-acid mobilization in response to prolonged cycling. *Int J Sport Nutr Exerc Metab* 21 (2): 113-123.

Alonso, J.M., P. Edouard, G. Fischetto, B. Adams, F. Depiesse, and M. Mountjoy. 2012. Determination of future prevention strategies in elite track and field: Analysis of Daegu 2011 IAAF Championships injuries and illnesses surveillance. *Br J Sports Med* 46:505-514.

Ameri, P., A. Giusti, M. Boschetti, G. Murialdo, F. Minuto, and D. Ferone. 2013. Interactions between vitamin D and IGF-1: From physiology to clinical practice. *Clin Endocrinol* 79:457-463.

American Academy of Pediatrics. 2000. Climatic heat stress and the exercising child and adolescent. *Pediatrics* 106:158-159.

American College of Sports Medicine. 2007. Exercise and fluid replacement. *Med Sci Sports Exerc* 39:377-390.

American College of Sports Medicine. 2015. Protein Intake for Optimal Muscle Maintenance. www.acsm.org/docs/default-source/brochures/protein-intake-for-optimal-muscle-maintenance.pdf.

American Dietetic Association. 1997. Health implications of dietary fiber. *Am Diet Assoc* 97:1157-1160.

American Psychiatric Association. 1994. *Diagnostic and statistical manual of mental disorders.* 4th ed. Washington, DC: American Psychiatric Association.

American Psychiatric Association. 2013. *Diagnostic and statistical manual of mental disorders.* 5th ed. Washington, DC: American Psychiatric Association.

Andersen, A.E. 1990. Diagnosis and treatment of males with eating disorders. In *Males with eating disorders,* ed. A.E. Andersen, 133-162. New York: Brunner/Mazel.

Andersen, A.E. 1995. Eating disorders in males. In *Eating disorders and obesity: A comprehensive handbook,* ed. K.D. Brownell and C.G. Fairburn, 177-192. London: Guildford Press.

Anderson, M.J., J.D. Cotter, A.P. Garnham, D.J. Casley, and M.A. Febbraio. 2001. Effect of glycerol-induced hyperhydration on thermoregulation and metabolism during exercise in the heat. *Int J Sport Nutr Exerc Metab* 11 (3): 315-333.

Anderson, R.A., and A.S. Kozlovsky. 1985. Chromium intake, absorption and excretion of subjects consuming self-selected diets. *Am J Clin Nutr* 41 (6): 1177-1183.

Andrews, S., L.A. Balart, M.C. Bethea, et al. 1998. *Sugarbusters.* London: Vermillion.

Angeline, M.E., A.O. Gee, M. Shindle, R.F. Warren, and S.A. Rodeo. 2013. The effects of vitamin D deficiency in athletes. *Am J Sports Med* 41:461-464.

Angus, D.J., M. Hargreaves, J. Dancey, and M.A. Febbraio. 2000. Effect of carbohydrate or carbohydrate plus medium-chain triglyceride ingestion on cycling time trial performance. *J Appl Physiol* 88 (1): 113-119.

Anthony, J.C., T.G. Anthony, and D.K. Layman. 1999. Leucine supplementation enhances skeletal muscle recovery in rats following exercise. *J Nutr* 129 (6): 1102-1106.

Anton, S.D., A. Hida, K. Heekin, K. Sowalsky, C. Karabetian, H. Mutchie, C. Leeuwenburgh, T.M. Manini, and T.E. Barnett. 2017. Effects of popular diets without specific calorie targets on weight loss outcomes: Systematic review of findings from clinical trials. *Nutrients* 9 (8): E822.

Applegate, E. 1999. Effective nutritional ergogenic aids. *Int J Sport Nutr* 9 (2): 229-239.

Applegate, E.A., and L.E. Grivetti. 1997. Search for the competitive edge: A history of dietary fads and supplements. *J Nutr* 127 (5 Suppl): S869-S873.

Aranow, C. 2011. Vitamin D and the immune system. *J Invest Med* 59:881-886.

Ardawi, M.S.M., and E.A. Newsholme. 1994. *Glutamine metabolism in lymphoid tissues,* edited by D. Haussinger and H. Sies, 235-246. Berlin: Springer-Verlag.

Areta, J.L., L.M. Burke, M.L. Ross, D.M. Camera, D.W.D. West, E.M. Broad, N.A. Jeacocke, D.R. Moore, T. Stellingwerff, S.M. Phillips, J.A. Hawley, and V.G. Coffey. 2013. Timing and distribution of protein ingestion during prolonged recovery from resistance exercise alters myofibrillar protein synthesis. *J Physiol* 591:2319-2331.

Arkinstall, M.J., C.R. Bruce, V. Nikolopoulos, et al. 2001. Effect of carbohydrate ingestion on metabolism during running and cycling. *J Appl Physiol* 91 (5): 2125-2134.

Armstrong, L.E. 2002. Caffeine, body fluid-electrolyte balance, and exercise performance. *Int J Sport Nutr Exerc Metab* 12 (2): 189-206.

Armstrong, L.E., D.L. Costill, and W.J. Fink. 1985. Influence of diuretic-induced dehydration on competitive running performance. *Med Sci Sports Exerc* 17:456-461.

Armstrong, L., A. Pumerantz, M. Roti, D. Judelson, G. Watson, J. Dias, B. Sokmen, D. Casa, C. Maresh, H. Lieberman, and M. Kellogg. 2005. Fluid, electrolyte, and renal indices of hydration during 11 days of controlled caffeine consumption. *Int J Sport Nutr Exerc Metab* 15 (3): 252-265.

Artioli, G.G., B. Gualano, A. Smith, J. Stout, and A.H. Lancha Jr. 2010. Role of beta-alanine supplementation on muscle carnosine and exercise performance. *Med Sci Sports Exerc* 42 (6): 1162-1173.

Atherton, P.J., J. Babraj, K. Smith, J. Singh, M.J. Rennie, and H. Wackerhage. 2005. Selective activation of AMPK-PGC-1alpha or PKB-TSC2-mTOR signaling can explain specific adaptive responses to endurance or resistance training-like electrical muscle stimulation. *FASEB J* 19:786-788.

Atherton, P.J., T. Etheridge, P.W. Watt, D. Wilkinson, A. Selby, D. Rankin, K. Smith, and M.J. Rennie. 2010. Muscle full effect after oral protein: Time-dependent concordance and discordance between human muscle protein synthesis and mTORC1 signaling. *Am J Clin Nutr* 92:1080-1088.

Atkins, R.C. 1992. *Doctor Atkins' new diet revolution.* New York: Avon Books.

Atkinson, F.S., K. Foster-Powell, and J.C. Brand-Miller. 2008. International table of glycolic index and glycolic load values: 2008. *Diab Care* 31 (12): 2281-2283.

Aulin, K.P. 2000. Minerals: Calcium. In *Nutrition in sport,* edited by R.J. Maughan, 318-325. Oxford: Blackwell Science.

Aune, D., E. Giovannucci, P. Boffetta, L.T. Fadnes, N. Keum, T. Norat, D.C. Greenwood, E. Riboli, L.J. Vatten, and S. Tonstad. 2017. Fruit and vegetable intake and the risk of cardiovascular disease, total cancer and all-cause mortality: A systematic review and dose-response meta-analysis of prospective studies. *Int J Epidemiol* (February 22). https://doi.org/10.1093/ije/dyw319.

Australian Dietary Guidelines. 2015. www.eatforhealth.gov.au/guidelines/about-australian-dietary-guidelines.

Baar, K., and L.E. Heaton. 2015. In-season recovery nutrition for American football. *Sport Sci Exch* 28 (144): 1-6.

Baar, K., A.R. Wende, T.E. Jones, M. Marison, L.A. Nolte, M. Chen, D.P. Kelly, and J.O. Holloszy. 2002. Adaptations of skeletal muscle to exercise: Rapid increase in the transcriptional coactivator PGC-1. *FASEB J* 16:1879-1886.

Bach, A.C., and V.K. Babayan. 1982. Medium-chain triglycerides: An update. *Am J Clin Nutr* 36:950-962.

Bagby, G.J., H.J. Green, S. Katsuta, and P.D. Gollnick. 1978. Glycogen depletion in exercising rats infused with glucose, lactate or pyruvate. *J Appl Physiol* 45 (3): 425-429.

Bailey, S.J., J. Fulford, A. Vanhatalo, P.G. Winyard, J.R. Blackwell, F.J. DiMenna, D.P. Wilkerson, N. Benjamin, and A.M. Jones. 2010. Dietary nitrate supplementation enhances muscle contractile efficiency during knee-extensor exercise in humans. *J Appl Physiol* 109 (1): 135-148.

Bailey, S.J., P. Winyard, A. Vanhatalo, J.R. Blackwell, F.J. Dimenna, D.P. Wilkerson, J. Tarr, N. Benjamin, and A.M. Jones. 2009. Dietary nitrate supplementation reduces the O_2 cost of low-intensity exercise and enhances tolerance to high-intensity exercise in humans. *J Appl Physiol* 107 (4): 1144-1155.

Baker, L.B., R.P. Nuccio, and A.E. Jeukendrup. 2014. Acute effects of dietary constituents on motor skill and cognitive performance in athletes. *Nutr Rev* 72 (12): 790-802.

Ballantyne, C.S., S.M. Phillips, J.R. MacDonald, M.A. Tarnopolsky, and J.D. MacDougall. 2000. The acute effects of androstenedione supplementation in healthy young males. *Can J Appl Physiol* 25 (1): 68-78.

Ballor, D.L., and R.E. Keesey. 1991. A meta-analysis of the factors affecting exercise-induced changes in body mass, fat mass and fat-free mass in males and females. *Int J Obes* 15 (11): 717-726.

Balsom, P.D., B. Ekblom, K. Soderlund, B. Sjodin, and E. Hultman. 1993. Creatine supplementation and dynamic high-intensity intermittent exercise. *Scand J Med Sci Sports* 3:143-149.

Balsom, P.D., S.D.R. Harridge, K. Soderlund, B. Sjodin, and B. Ekblom. 1993. Creatine supplementation per se does not enhance endurance exercise performance. *Acta Physiol Scand* 149:521-523.

Balsom, P.D., K. Wood, P. Olsson, and B. Ekblom. 1999. Carbohydrate intake and multiple sprint sports: With special reference to football (soccer). *Int J Sports Med* 20 (1): 48-52.

Banderet, L.E., and H.R. Lieberman. 1989. Treatment with tyrosine, a neurotransmitter precursor, reduces environmental stress in humans. *Brain Res Bull* 22 (4): 759-762.

Barnett, C., D.L. Costill, M.D. Vukovich, K.J. Cole, B.H. Goodpaster, S.W. Trappe, and W.J. Fink. 1994. Effect of L-carnitine supplementation on muscle and blood carnitine content and lactate accumulation during high-intensity sprint cycling. *Int J Sports Nutr* 4 (3): 280-288.

Barnosky, A.R., K.K. Hoddy, T.G. Unterman, and K.A. Varady. 2014. Intermittent fasting vs daily calorie restriction for type 2 diabetes prevention: A review of human findings. *Transl Res* 164 (4): 302-311.

Bar-Or, O. 2001. Nutritional considerations for the child athlete. *Can J Appl Physiol* 26 (Suppl): S186-S191.

Barrett, B. 2003. Medicinal properties of Echinacea: Critical review. *Phytomedicine* 10:66-86.

Barrett, B.P., R.L. Brown, K. Locken, R. Maberry, J.A. Bobula, and D. D'Alessio. 2002. Treatment of the common cold with unrefined Echinacea: A randomized, double-blind, placebo-controlled trial. *Ann Intern Med* 137:939-946.

Barron, J.L., T.D. Noakes, W. Levy, C. Smith, and R.P. Millar. 1985. Hypothalamic dysfunction in overtrained athletes. *J Clin Endocrinol Metab* 60 (4): 803-806.

Barry, A., T. Cantwell, F. Doherty, J.C. Folan, M. Ingoldsby, J.P. Kevany, J.D. O'Broin, H. O'Connor, B. O'Shea, B.A. Ryan, and J. Vaughan. 1981. A nutritional study of Irish athletes. *Br J Sports Med* 5:99.

Bass, S., and K. Inge. 2006. Nutrition for special populations: Children and young athletes. In *Clinical Sports Nutrition*, edited by L.M. Burke and V. Deakin, 589-632. Sydney: McGraw Hill.

Bassit, R.A., L.A. Sawada, R.F.P. Bacurau, F. Navarro, E. Martins, R.V.T. Santos, E.C. Caperuto, P. Rogeri, and L.F.B.P. Costa-Rosa. 2002. Branched-chain amino acid supplementation and the immune response of long-distance athletes. *Nutrition* 18:376-379.

Baumgartner, R.N., W.C. Chumlea, and A.F. Roche. 1990. Bioelectric impedance for body composition. *Exerc Sport Sci Rev* 18:193-224.

Beaumont, R., P. Cordery, M. Funnell, S. Mears, L. James, and P. Watson. 2017. Chronic ingestion of a low dose of caffeine induces tolerance to the performance benefits of caffeine. *J Sports Sci* 35 (19): 1920-1927.

Beckers, E.J., A.E. Jeukendrup, F. Brouns, A.J.M. Wagenmakers, and W.H.M. Saris. 1992. Gastric emptying of carbohydrate-medium chain triglyceride suspensions at rest. *Int J Sports Med* 13 (8): 581-584.

Beelen, M., J. Berghuis, B. Bonaparte, S.B. Ballak, A.E. Jeukendrup, and L.J. van Loon. 2009. Carbohydrate mouth rinsing in the fed state: Lack of enhancement of time-trial performance. *Int J Sport Nutr Exerc Metab* 19 (4): 400-409.

Beidleman, B.A., J.L. Puhl, and M.J. De Souza. 1995. Energy balance in female distance runners. *Am J Clin Nutr* 61 (2): 303-311.

Bell, P.G., M.P. McHugh, E. Stenenson, and G. Howatson. 2014. The role of cherries in exercise and health. *Scand J Med Sci Sports* 24 (3): 477-490.

Bell, R.D., J.D. Macdougall, R. Billeter, and H. Howald. 1980. Muscle-fiber types and morphometric analysis of skeletal-muscle in 6-year-old children. *Med Sci Sports Exerc* 12:28-31.

Below, P., R. Mora-Rodriguez, J. Gonzalez-Alonso, and E.F. Coyle. 1995. Fluid and carbohydrate ingestion independently improve performance during 1 h of intense cycling. *Med Sci Sports Exerc* 27:200-210.

Bendik I., A. Friedel, F.F. Roos, P. Weber, and M. Eggersdorfer. 2014. Vitamin D: A critical and essential micronutrient for human health. *Front Physiol* 5:248.

Bennell, K., G. Matheson, and W. Heevwisse. 1999. Risk factors for stress fractures. *Sports Med* 28:91-122.

Bennet, W.M., A.A. Connacher, C.M. Scrimgeour, and M.J. Rennie. 1990. The effect of amino acid infusion on leg protein turnover assessed by L-[15N]phenylalanine and L-[1-13C]leucine exchange. *Eur J Clin Invest* 20 (1): 41-50.

Bennet, W.M., and M.J. Rennie. 1991. Protein anabolic actions of insulin in the human body. *Diabetic Med* 8:199-207.

Bentley, J. 2017. US trends in food availability and a dietary assessment of loss adjusted food availability 1970-2014. Economic Information Bulletin Number 166, US Department of Agriculture. https://www.ers.usda.gov/webdocs/publications/82220/eib-166.pdf?v=42762.

Berg, A., H. Northoff, and D. Konig. 1998. Influence of Echinacin (E31) treatment on the exercise-induced immune response in athletes. *J Clin Res* 1:367-380.

Bergstrom, J., and E. Hultman. 1966. Muscle glycogen synthesis after exercise: An enhancing factor localized in muscle cells in man. *Nature* 210:309-310.

Bergstrom, J., and E. Hultman. 1967a. A study of glycogen metabolism during exercise in man. *Scand J Clin Invest* 19:218-228.

Bergstrom, J., and E. Hultman. 1967b. Synthesis of muscle glycogen in man after glucose and fructose infusion. *Acta Med Scand* 182 (1): 93-107.

Bermon, S. 2007. Airway inflammation and upper respiratory tract infection in athletes: Is there a link? *Exerc Immunol Rev* 13:6-14.

Bermon, S., L.M. Castell, P.C. Calder, N.C. Bishop, E. Blomstrand, F.C. Mooren, K. Krüger, A.N. Kavazis, J.C. Quindry, D.S. Senchina, D.C. Nieman, M. Gleeson, D.B. Pyne, C.M. Kitic, G.L. Close, D.E. Larson-Meyer, A. Marcos, S.N. Meydani, D. Wu, N.P. Walsh, and R. Nagatomi. 2017. Consensus statement: Immunonutrition and exercise. *Exerc Immunol Rev* 23:8-50.

Bernard, T., F. Sultana, R. Lepers, C. Hausswirth, and J. Brisswalter. 2010. Age-related decline in olympic triathlon performance: Effect of locomotion mode. *Exp Aging Res* 36:64-78.

Beumont, P.J.V. 1995. The clinical presentation of anorexia and bulimia nervosa. In *Eating disorders and obesity: A comprehensive handbook*, edited by K.D. Brownell and C.G. Fairburn, 151-158. London: Guildford Press.

Beumont, P.J.V., B. Arthur, J.D. Russell, and S.W. Touyz. 1994. Excessive physical activity in dieting disorder patients: Proposals for a supervised exercise program. *Int J Eating Disorders* 15:21-36.

Bibbò, S., G. Ianiro, V. Giorgio, F. Scaldaferri, L. Masucci, A. Gasbarrini, and G. Cammarota. 2016. The role of diet on gut microbiota composition. *Eur Rev Med Pharmacol Sci* 20 (22): 4742-4749.

Bierkamper, G.G., and A.M. Goldberg. 1980. Release of acetylcholine from the vascular perfused rat phrenic nerve-hemidiaphragm. *Brain Res* 202 (1): 234-237.

Biolo, G., K. Tipton, S. Klein, and R. Wolfe. 1997. An abundant supply of amino acids enhances the metabolic effect of exercise on muscle protein. *Am J Physiol* 273 (1 Pt 1): E122-E129.

Biolo, G., B.D. Williams, R.Y. Fleming, and R.R. Wolfe. 1999. Insulin action on muscle protein kinetics and amino acid transport during recovery after resistance exercise. *Diabetes* 48 (5): 949-957.

Birch, R., D. Noble, and P.L. Greenhaff. 1994. The influence of dietary creatine supplementation on work output and metabolism during repeated bouts of maximal isokenetic cycling in man. *Eur J Appl Physiol* 69 (3): 268-276.

Bischoff-Ferrari, H.A., E.J. Orav, W.C. Willett, and B. Dawson-Hughes. 2014. The effect of vitamin D supplementation on skeletal, vascular, or cancer outcomes. *Lancet Diabetes Endocrinol* 2 (5): 363-364.

Bishop, N.C., A.K. Blannin, and M. Gleeson. 2000. Effect of carbohydrate and fluid intake during prolonged exercise on saliva flow and IgA secretion. *Med Sci Sports Exerc* 32:2046-2051.

Bishop, N.C., A.K. Blannin, L. Rand, R. Johnson, and M. Gleeson. 1999. Effects of carbohydrate and fluid intake on the blood leucocyte response to prolonged exercise. *J Sports Sci* 17:26-27.

Bishop, N.C., A.K. Blannin, P.J. Robson, N.P., Walsh, and M. Gleeson. 1999. The effects of carbohydrate supplementation on neutrophil degranulation responses to a soccer-specific exercise protocol. *J Sports Sci* 17:787-779.

Bishop, N.C., A.K. Blannin, N.P. Walsh, and M. Gleeson. 2001. Effect of dietary carbohydrate status on bacterial lipopolysaccharide-stimulated neutrophil degranulation response following cycling to fatigue. *Int J Sports Med* 22:226-231.

Bishop, N.C., C. Fitzgerald, P.J. Porter, G.A. Scanlon, and A.C. Smith. 2005. Effect of caffeine ingestion on lymphocyte counts and subset activation in vivo following strenuous cycling. *Eur J Appl Physiol* 93 (5-6): 606-613.

Bishop, N.C., G.J. Walker, L.A. Bowley, et al. 2005. Lymphocyte responses to influenza and tetanus toxoid in vitro following intensive exercise and carbohydrate ingestion on consecutive days. *J Appl Physiol* 99 (4): 1327-1335.

Blaak, E. 2001. Gender differences in fat metabolism. *Curr Opin Clin Nutr Metab Care* 4 (6): 499-502.

Blannin, A.K., L.J. Chatwin, R. Cave, and M. Gleeson. 1996. Effects of submaximal cycling and long-term endurance training on neutrophil phagocytic activity in middle aged men. *Br J Sports Med* 30:125-129.

Blom, P.C.S., A.T. Høstmark, O. Vaage, K.R. Kardel, and S. Maehlum. 1987. Effect of different post-exercise sugar diets on the rate of muscle glycogen resynthesis. *Med Sci Sports Exerc* 19:491-496.

Blomstrand, E., S. Andersson, P. Hassmen, B. Ekblom, and E.A. Newsholme. 1995. Effect of branched-chain amino acid and carbohydrate supplementation on the exercise-induced change in plasma and muscle concentration of amino acids in human subjects. *Acta Physiol Scand* 153 (2): 87-96.

Blomstrand, E., P. Hassmen, S. Ek, B. Ekblom, and E.A. Newsholme. 1997. Influence of ingesting a solution of branched-chain amino acids on perceived exertion during exercise. *Acta Physiol Scand* 159 (1): 41-49.

Blomstrand, E., P. Hassmen, B. Ekblom, and E.A. Newsholme. 1991. Administration of branched-chain amino acids during sustained exercise—effects on performance and on plasma concentration of some amino acids. *Eur J Appl Physiol* 63 (2): 83-88.

Bloomfield, S.A. 2001. Optimizing bone health: Impact of nutrition, exercise and hormones. *Sports Science Exchange 82* 14(3). www.gssiweb.com/en/sports-science-exchange/Article/sse-82-optimizing-bone-health-impact-of-nutrition-exercise-and-hormones.

Blot, W. 1997. Vitamin/mineral supplementation and cancer risk: International chemoprevention trials. *Proc Soc Exp Biol Med* 261:291-296.

Blundell, J.E., C. Gibbons, P. Caudwell, G. Finlayson, and M. Hopkins. 2015. Appetite control and energy balance: Impact of exercise. *Obes Rev Suppl* 1:67-76.

Blundell, J.E., R.J. Stubbs, D.A. Hughes, S. Whybrow, and N.A. King. 2003. Cross talk between physical activity and appetite control: Does physical activity stimulate appetite? *Proc Nutr Soc* 62 (3): 651-661.

Boden, G., X. Chen, J. Ruiz, G.D. van Rossum, and S. Turco. 1996. Effects of vanadyl sulfate on carbohydrate and lipid metabolism in patients with non-insulin-dependent diabetes mellitus. *Metabolism* 45 (9): 1130-1135.

Bohe, J., A. Low, R.R. Wolfe, and M.J. Rennie. 2003. Human muscle protein synthesis is modulated by extracellular, not intramuscular amino acid availability: A dose-response study. *J Physiol* 552 (Pt 1): 315-324.

Boirie, Y., M. Dangin, P. Gachon, M.-P. Vasson, J.-L. Maubois, and B. Beaufrere. 1997. Slow and fast dietary proteins differently modulate postprandial protein accretion. *Proc Natl Acad Sci USA* 94 (26): 14930-14935.

Boisseau, N., and P. Delamarche. 2000. Metabolic and hormonal responses to exercise in children and adolescents. *Sports Med* 30:405-422.

Boisseau, N., M. Vermorel, M. Rance, P. Duche, and P. Patureau-Mirand. 2007. Protein requirements in male adolescent soccer players. *Eur J Appl Physiol* 100:27-33.

Bolster, D.R., M.A. Pikosky, P.C. Gaine, W. Martin, R.R. Wolfe, K.D. Tipton, D. Maclean, C.M. Maresh, and N.R. Rodriguez. 2005. Dietary protein intake impacts human skeletal muscle protein fractional synthetic rates after endurance exercise. *Am J Physiol Endocrinol Metab* 289:E678-E683.

Bond, H., L. Morton, and A.J. Braakhuis. 2012. Dietary nitrate supplementation improves rowing performance in well-trained rowers. *Int J Sport Nutr Exerc Metab* 22 (4): 251-256.

Bonen, A., D.J. Dyck, A. Ibrahimi, and N.A. Abumrad. 1999. Muscle contractile activity increases fatty acid metabolism and transport and FAT/CD36. *Am J Physiol* 276 (4 Pt 1): E642-E649.

Boorsma, R.K., J. Whitfield, and L.L. Spriet. 2014. Beetroot juice supplementation does not improve performance of elite 1500-m runners. *Med Sci Sports Exerc* 46 (12): 2326-2334.

Booth, A.O., C.E. Huggins, N. Wattanapenpaiboon, and C.A. Nowson. 2015. Effect of increasing dietary calcium through supplements and dairy food on body weight and body composition: A meta-analysis of randomised controlled trials. *Br J Nutr* 114 (7): 1013-1025.

Borchers, A.T., C. Selmi, F.J. Meyers, C.L. Keen, and M.E. Gershwin. 2009. Probiotics and immunity. *J Gastroenterol* 44 (1): 26-46.

Borsheim, E., and R. Bahr. 2003. Effect of exercise intensity, duration and mode on post-exercise oxygen consumption. *Sports Med* 33 (14): 1037-1060.

Borsheim, E., K. Tipton, S. Wolf, and R. Wolfe. 2002. Essential amino acids and muscle protein recovery from resistance exercise. *Am J Physiol Endocrinol Metab* 283 (4): E648-E657.

Bouchard, C. 1994. Genetics of obesity: Overview and research directions. In *The genetics of obesity,* edited by C. Bouchard, 223-233. Boca Raton, FL: CRC Press.

Bouchard, C., A. Tremblay, J.P. Despres, A. Nadeau, P.J. Lupien, G. Theriault, J. Dullault, S. Moorjani, S. Pinault, and G. Fournier. 1990. The response to long-term overfeeding in identical twins. *N Engl J Med* 322 (21): 1477-1482.

Boudou, P., E. Sobngwi, F. Mauvais-Jarvis, P. Vexiau, and J.-F. Gautier. 2003. Absence of exercise-induced variations in adiponectin levels despite decreased abdominal adiposity and improved insulin sensitivity in type 2 diabetic men. *Eur J Endocrinol* 149 (5): 421-424.

Boutcher, S.H. 2011. High-intensity intermittent exercise and fat loss. *J Obesity* (November 24). http://doi.org/10.1155/2011/868305.

Bowtell, J.L., K. Gelly, M.L. Jackman, A. Patel, M. Simeoni, and M.J. Rennie. 1999. Effect of oral glutamine on whole body carbohydrate storage during recovery from exhaustive exercise. *J Appl Physiol* 86:1770-1777.

Bradbury, K.E., P.N. Appleby, and T.J. Key. 2014. Fruit, vegetable, and fiber intake in relation to cancer risk: Findings from the European Prospective Investigation into Cancer and Nutrition (EPIC). *Am J Clin Nutr* 100 (Suppl 1):394S-398S.

Bredle, D.L., J.M. Stager, W.F. Brechue, and M.O. Farber. 1988. Phosphate supplementation, cardiovascular function, and exercise performance in humans. *J Appl Physiol* 65 (4): 1821-1826.

Bremer, J. 1983. Carnitine-metabolism and functions. *Phys Rev* 63 (4): 1420-1479.

Brewerton, T.D., E.J. Stellefson, N. Hibbs, E.L. Hodges, and C.E. Cochrane. 1995. Comparison of eating disorder patients with and without compulsive exercising. *Int J Eating Disorders* 17:413-416.

Brilla, L.R., and T.E. Landerholm. 1990. Effect of fish oil supplementation on serum lipids and aerobic fitness. *J Sports Med Phys Fitness* 30:173-180.

Broeder, C.E., K.A. Burrhus, L.S. Svanevik, et al. 1997. Assessing body composition before and after resistance or endurance training. *Med Sci Sports Exerc* 29 (5): 705-712.

Brooks, G.A. 1986. The lactate shuttle during exercise and recovery. *Med Sci Sports Exerc* 18 (3): 360-368.

Brouns, F., and E. Beckers. 1993. Is the gut an athletic organ? Digestion, absorption and exercise. *Sports Med* 15 (4): 242-257.

Brouns, F., W.H. Saris, E. Beckers, H. Adlercreutz, G.J. van der Vusse, H.A. Keizer, H. Kuipers, P. Menheere, A.J. Wagenmakers, and F. ten Hoor. 1989. Metabolic changes induced by sustained exhaustive cycling and diet manipulation. *Int J Sports Med* 10 (Suppl 1): S49-S62.

Brouns, F., W.H.M. Saris, J. Stroecken, E. Beckers, R. Thijssen, N.J. Rehrer, and F. ten Hoor. 1989a. Eating, drinking, and cycling. A controlled Tour de France simulation study, part I. *Int J Sports Med* 10 (Suppl 1): S32-S40.

Brouns, F., W.H.M. Saris, J. Stroecken, E. Beckers, R. Thijssen, N.J. Rehrer, and F. ten Hoor. 1989b. Eating, drinking, and cycling. A controlled Tour de France simulation study, part II: Effect of diet manipulation. *Int J Sports Med* 10 (Suppl 1): S41-S48.

Brouns, F., J. Senden, E.J. Beckers, and W.H.M. Saris. 1995. Osmolarity does not affect the gastric emptying rate of oral rehydration solutions. *JPEN* 19:403-406.

Brouwer, I.A., A.J. Wanders, and M.B. Katan. 2010. Effect of animal and industrial trans fatty acids on HDL and LDL cholesterol levels in humans: A quantitative review. *PLoS One* 5 (3): e9434.

Brown, G.D. and S. Gordon. 2003. Fungal beta-glucans and mammalian immunity. *Immunity* 19:311-315.

Brown, G., M. Vukovich, and D.S. King. 2006. Testosterone prohormone supplements. *Med Sci Sports Exerc* 38 (8): 1451-1461.

Brownell, K.D., S.N. Steen, and J.H. Wilmore. 1987. Weight regulation practices in athletes: Analysis of metabolic and health effects. *Med Sci Sports Exerc* 6:546-560.

Brownlie, T., V. Utermohlen, P.S. Hinton, C. Giordano, and J.D. Haas. 2002. Marginal iron deficiency without anemia impairs aerobic adaptation among previously untrained women. *Am J Clin Nutr* 75:734-742.

Brune, M., B. Magnusson, H. Persson, and L. Hallberg. 1986. Iron losses in sweat. *Am J Clin Nutr* 43:438-443.

Brutsaert, T.D., S. Hernandez-Cordero, J. Rivera, T. Viola, G. Hughes, and J.D. Haas. 2003. Iron supplementation improves progressive fatigue resistance during dynamic knee extensor exercise in iron-depleted, nonanemic women. *Am J Clin Nutr* 77:441-448.

Bucci, L.R., J.F. Hickson, Jr., I. Wolinsky, and J.M. Pivarnik. 1992. Ornithine supplementation and insulin release in bodybuilders. *Int J Sport Nutr* 2 (3): 287-291.

Burckes-Miller, M.E., and D.R. Black. 1988. Male and female college athletes: Prevalence of anorexia nervosa and bulimia nervosa. *Athletic Training* 2:137-140.

Burd, N.A., Tang, J.E., Moore, D.R., and Phillips, S.M. 2009. Exercise training and protein metabolism: Influences of contraction, protein intake, and sex-based differences. *J Appl Physiol* 106:1692-1701.

Burd, N.A., D.W. West, D.R. Moore, P.J. Atherton, A.W. Staples, T. Prior, J.E. Tang, M.J. Rennie, S.K. Baker, and S.M. Phillips. (2011). Enhanced amino acid sensitivity of myofibrillar protein synthesis persists for up to 24h after resistance exercise in young men. *J Nutr* 141:568-573.

Burdon, C.A., I. Spronk, H.L. Cheng, and H.T. O'Connor. 2016. Effect of glycemic index of a pre-exercise meal on endurance exercise performance: A systematic review and meta-analysis. *Sports Med* 47 (6): 1087-1101.

Burgomaster, K.A., K.R. Howarth, S.M. Phillips, M. Rakobowchuk, M.J. Macdonald, S.L. McGee, and M.J. Gibala. 2008. Similar metabolic adaptations during exercise after low volume sprint interval and traditional endurance training in humans. *J Physiol* 586 (1): 151-160.

Burke, L.M., Ross, M.L., Garvican-Lewis, L.A., Welvaert, M., Heikura, I.A., Forbes, S.G., Mirtschin, J.G., Cato, L.E., Strobel, N., Sharma, A.P., and Hawley, J.A. 2017. Low carbohydrate, high fat diet impairs exercise economy and negates the performance benefit from intensified training in elite race walkers. *J Physiol.* 595 (9): 2785-2807.

Burke, L.M. 2001. Nutritional practices of male and female endurance cyclists. *Sports Med* 31 (7): 521-532.

Burke, L.M. 2010. Fueling strategies to optimize performance: Training high or training low? *Scand J Med Sci Sports* 20 (Suppl. 2): 48-58.

Burke, L.M., D.J. Angus, G.R. Cox, K.M. Gawthorn, J.A. Hawley, M.A. Febbraio, and M. Hargreaves. 1999. Fat adaptation with carbohydrate recovery promotes metabolic adaptation during prolonged cycling. *Med Sci Sports Exerc* 31 (5): 297.

Burke, L.M., A. Claassen, J.A. Hawley, and T.D. Noakes. 1998. Carbohydrate intake during prolonged cycling minimizes effect of glycemic index of preexercise meal. *J Appl Physiol* 85:2220-2226.

Burke, L.M., G.R. Collier, and M. Hargreaves. 1993. Muscle glycogen storage after prolonged exercise: Effect of glycemic index of carbohydrate feedings. *J Appl Physiol* 75 (2): 1019-1023.

Burke, L.M., and V. Deakin. 2000. *Clinical sports nutrition.* 2nd ed. New York: McGraw-Hill.

Burke, L.M., J.A. Hawley, M.L Ross, D.R. Moore, S.M. Phillips, G.R. Slater, T. Stellingwerff, K.D. Tipton, A.P. Garnham, and V.G. Coffey. 2012. Preexercise aminoacidemia and muscle protein synthesis after resistance exercise. *Med Sci Sports Exerc* 44:1968-1977.

Burke, L.M., J.A. Hawley, S.H. Wong, and A.E. Jeukendrup. 2011. Carbohydrates for training and competition. *J Sports Sci* 29 (Suppl 1): S17-S27.

Burke, L.M., B. Kiens, and J.L. Ivy. 2004. Carbohydrates and fat for training and recovery. *J Sports Sci* 22:15-30.

Burke, L.M., D.B. Pyne, and R.D. Telford. 1996. Effect of oral creatine supplementation on single-effort sprint performance in elite swimmers. *Int J Sport Nutr* 6 (3): 222-233.

Burke, L.M., M.L. Ross, L.A. Garvican-Lewis, M. Welvaert, I.A. Heikura, S.G. Forbes, J.G. Mirtschin, L.E. Cato, N. Strobel, A.P. Sharma, and J.A. Hawley. 2017. Low carbohydrate, high fat diet impairs exercise economy and negates the performance benefit from intensified training in elite race walkers. *J Physiol* 595 (9): 2785-2807.

Burke, L.M., L.J. van Loon, and J.A. Hawley. 2017. Postexercise muscle glycogen resynthesis in humans. *J Appl Physiol* 122 (5): 1055-1067.

Burke, L.M., J.A. Winter, D. Cameron-Smith, M. Enslen, M. Farnfield, and J. Decombaz. 2012. Effect of intake of different dietary protein sources on plasma amino acid profiles at rest and after exercise. *Int J Sport Nutr Exerc Metab* 22:452-462.

Burns, J.M., D.L. Costill, W.J. Fink, J.B. Mitchell, and J.A. Hol. 1988. Effects of choline on endurance performance. *Med Sci Sports Exerc* 20 (2): S25.

Buscemi, N., B. Vandermeer, N. Hooton, R. Pandya, L. Tjosvold, L. Hartling, G. Baker, T.P. Klassen, and S. Vohra. 2005. The efficacy and safety of exogenous melatonin for primary sleep disorders: A meta-analysis. *J Gen Intern Med* 20 (12): 1151-1158.

Bussau, V.A., T.J. Fairchild, A. Rao, P. Steele, and P.A. Fournier. 2002. Carbohydrate loading in human muscle: An improved 1 day protocol. *Eur J Appl Physiol* 87 (3): 290-295.

Busschaert, C., I. De Bourdeaudhuij, V. Van Holle, S.F. Chastin, G. Cardon, and K. De Cocker. 2015. Reliability and validity of three questionnaires measuring context-specific sedentary behaviour and associated correlates in adolescents, adults and older adults. *Int J Behav Nutr Phys Act* 12:117.

Butte, N.F. 2000. Fat intake of children in relation to energy requirements. *Am J Clin Nutr* 72 (5 Suppl): 1246S-1252S.

Butterfield, G.E., and D.H. Calloway. 1984. Physical activity improves protein utilization in young men. *Br J Nutr* 51 (2): 171-184.

Byrne, A., and D.G. Byrne. 1993. The effect of exercise on depression, anxiety, and other mood states: A review. *J Psychosomatic Res* 37:565-574.

Byrne, S., and N. McLean. 2002. Elite athletes: Effects of pressure to be thin. *J Sci Med Sport* 5:80-94.

Cade, R., M. Conte, C. Zauner, D. Mars, J. Peterson, D. Lunne, N. Hommen, and D. Packer. 1984. Effects of phosphate loading on 2,3-diphosphoglycerate and maximal oxygen uptake. *Med Sci Sports Exerc* 16 (3): 263-268.

Calder, P.C. 2006. N-3 polyunsaturated fatty acids, inflammation, and inflammatory diseases. *Am J Clin Nutr* 83:1505S-1519S.

Calle, E.E., M.J. Thun, J.M. Petrelli, et al. 1999. Body-mass index and mortality in a prospective cohort of U.S. adults. *N Engl J Med* 341 (15): 1097-1105.

Cannon, J.G., S.F. Orencole, R.A. Fielding, M. Meydani, S.N. Meydani, M.A. Fiatarone, et al. 1990. Acute phase response in exercise: Interaction of age and vitamin E on neutrophils and muscle enzyme release. *Am J Physiol* 259:R1214-R1219.

Caris, A.V., F.S. Lira, M.T. de Mello, L.M. Oyama, and R.V.T. dos Santos. 2014. Carbohydrate and glutamine supplementation modulates the Th1/Th2 balance after exercise performed at a simulated altitude of 4500 m. *Nutrition* 30:1331-1336.

Carter, J.M., A.E. Jeukendrup, and D.A. Jones. 2004. The effect of carbohydrate mouth rinse on 1-h cycle time trial performance. *Med Sci Sports Exerc* 36 (12): 2107-2111.

Casey, A., D. Constantin-Teodosiu, S. Howell, E. Hultman, and P.L. Greenhaff. 1996. Creatine ingestion favorably affects performance and muscle metabolism during maximal exercise in humans. *Am J Physiol* 271 (1 Pt 1): E31-E37.

Casey, A., and P.L. Greenhaff. 2000. Does dietary creatine supplementation play a role in skeletal muscle metabolism and performance? *Am J Clin Nutr* 72 (2 Suppl): 607S-617S.

Casey, A., R. Mann, K. Banister, J. Fox, P.G. Morris, I.A. Macdonald, and P.L. Greenhaff. 2000. Effect of carbohydrate ingestion on glycogen resynthesis in human liver and skeletal muscle, measured by (13)C MRS. *Am J Physiol Endocrinol Metab* 278 (1): E65-E75.

Castell, L.M., and E.A. Newsholme. 1996. Does glutamine have a role in reducing infections in athletes? *Eur J Appl Physiol* 73:488-490.

Castell, L.M., J.R. Poortmans, R. Leclercq, M. Brasseur, J. Duchateau, and E.A. Newsholme. 1997. Some aspects of the acute phase response after a marathon race, and effect of glutamine supplementation. *Eur J Appl Physiol* 75:47-53.

Castell, L.M., J.R. Poortmans, and E.A. Newsholme. 1996. Does glutamine have a role in reducing infections in athletes? *Eur J Appl Physiol* 73:488-490.

Centers for Disease Control and Prevention. 2013. Alcohol-Related Disease Impact (ARDI) application 2013. Available at www.cdc.gov/ARDI

Centers for Disease Control and Prevention. 1998. Hyperthermia and dehydration-related deaths associated with intentional rapid weight loss in three collegiate wrestlers—North Carolina, Wisconsin, and Michigan, November–December 1997. *MMWR Morb Mortal Wkly Rep* 47 (6): 105-108.

Chambers, E.S., M.W. Bridge, and D.A. Jones. 2009. Carbohydrate sensing in the human mouth: Effects on exercise performance and brain activity. *J Physiol* 15:1779-94.

Chan, J.L., and C.S. Mantzoros. 2005. Role of leptin in energy-deprivation states: Normal human physiology and clinical implications for hypothalamic amenorrhea and anorexia nervosa. *Lancet* 366 (9479): 74-85.

Chandler, J., and J. Hawkins. 1984. The effect of bee pollen on physiological performance. *Int J Biosci Res* 6:107.

Chaouloff, F., G.A. Kennett, B. Serrurrier, D. Merino, and G. Curzon. 1986. Amino acid analysis demonstrates that increased plasma free tryptophan causes the increase of brain tryptophan during exercise in the rat. *J Neurochem* 46 (5): 1647-1650.

Chasiotis, D. 1983. The regulation of glycogen phosphorylase and glycogen breakdown in human skeletal muscle. *Acta Physiol Scand Suppl* 518:1-68.

Cheung, S.S., G.W. McGarr, M.M. Mallette, P.J. Wallace, C.L. Watson, I.M. Kim, and M.J. Greenway. 2015. Separate and combined effects of dehydration and thirst sensation on exercise performance in the heat. *Scand J Med Sci Sports* 25 (Suppl 1): 104-111.

Chia, J.S., L.A. Barrett, J.Y. Chow, and S.F. Burns. 2017. Effects of caffeine supplementation on performance in ball games. *Sports Med* (July 24). http://doi.org/10.1007/s40279-017-0763-6.

Chilibeck, P.D., C. Magnus, and M. Anderson. 2007. Effect of in-season creatine supplementation on body composition and performance in rugby union football players. *Appl Physiol Nutr Metab* 32 (6): 1052-1057.

Christensen, E.H. 1932. Der Stoffwechsel und die Respiratorischen Funktionen bei schwerer körperlicher Arbeit. *Skand Arch Physiol* 81:160-171.

Christensen, E.H., and O. Hansen. 1939. Arbeitsfähigkeit und Ernährung. *Skand Arch Physiol* 81:160-171.

Christensen. P.M., M. Nyberg, and J. Bangsbo. 2013. Influence of nitrate supplementation on VO_2kinetics and endurance of elite cyclists. *Scand J Med Sci Sports* 23 (1): e21-e31.

Churchward-Venne, T.A., L. Breen, D.M. DiDonato, A.J. Hector, C.J. Mitchell, D.R. Moore, T. Stellingwerff, D. Breuille, E.A. Offord, S.K. Baker, and S.M. Phillips. 2014. Leucine supplementation of a low-protein mixed macronutrient beverage enhances myofibrillar protein synthesis in young men: A double-blind, randomized trial. *Am J Clin Nutr* 99:276-286.

Civitarese, A.E., M.K. Hesselink, A.P. Russell, E. Ravussin, and P. Schrauwen. 2005. Glucose ingestion during exercise blunts exercise-induced gene expression of skeletal muscle fat oxidative genes. *Am J Physiol Endocrinol Metab* 289:E1023-E1029.

Clairmont, A., D. Tessman, A. Stock, S. Nicolai, W. Stahl, and H. Sies. 1996. Induction of gap junctional intercellular communication by vitamin D in human skin fibroblasts is dependent on the nuclear vitamin D receptor. *Carcinogenesis* 17 (6): 1389-1391.

Clancy, S.P., P.M. Clarkson, M.E. DeCheke, K. Nosaka, P.S. Freedson, J.J. Cunningham, and B. Valentine. 1994. Effects of chromium picolinate supplementation on body composition, strength, and urinary chromium loss in football players. *Int J Sport Nutr* 4 (2): 142-153.

Clancy, R.L., M. Gleeson, A. Cox, et al. 2006. Reversal in fatigued athletes of a defect in interferon γ secretion after administration of Lactobacillus acidophilus. *Br J Sports Med* 40:351-354.

Clemes, S.A., S. O'Connell, L.M. Rogan, and P.L. Griffiths. 2010. Evaluation of a commercially available pedometer used to promote physical activity as part of a national programme. *Br J Sports Med* 44:1178-83.

Close, G.L., J. Russell, J.N. Cobley, D.J. Owens, G. Wilson, W. Gregson, W.D. Fraser, and J.P. Morton. 2013. Assessment of vitamin D concentration in non-supplemented professional athletes and healthy adults during the winter months in the UK: Implications for skeletal muscle function. *J Sports Sci* 31 (4): 344-353.

Close, G.L., T. Ashton, T. Cable, D. Doran, C. Holloway, F. McArdle, and D.P. MacLaren. 2006. Ascorbic acid supplementation does not attenuate post-exercise muscle soreness following muscle-damaging exercise but may delay the recovery process, *Brit J Nutr* 95:976-981.

Cluberton, L.J., S.L. McGee, R.M. Murphy, and M. Hargreaves. 2005. Effect of carbohydrate ingestion on exercise-induced alterations in metabolic gene expression. *J Appl Physiol* 99:1359-1363.

Cockburn, E., P. Robson-Ansley, P.R. Hayes, and E. Stevenson. 2012. Effect of volume of milk consumed on the attenuation of exercise-induced muscle damage. *Eur J Appl Physiol* 112 (9): 3187-3194.

Coffey, V.G., Z. Zhong, A. Shield, B.J. Canny, A.V. Chibalin, J.R. Zierath, J.A. Hawley. 2006. Early signaling responses to divergent exercise stimuli in skeletal muscle from well-trained humans. *FASEB J* 20:190-192.

Cohen, N., M. Halberstam, P. Shlimovich, C.J. Chang, H. Shamoon, and L. Rossetti. 1995. Oral vanadyl sulfate improves hepatic and peripheral insulin sensitivity in patients with non-insulin-dependent diabetes mellitus. *J Clin Invest* 95:2501-2509.

Collins, M.A., M.L. Millard-Stafford, P.B. Sparling, et al. 1999. Evaluation of the BOD POD for assessing body fat in collegiate football players. *Med Sci Sports Exerc* 31 (9): 1350-1356.

Collomp, K., S. Ahmaidi, M. Audran, et al. 1991. Effects of caffeine ingestion on performance and anaerobic metabolism during the Wingate test. *Int J Sports Med* 12 (5): 439-443.

Conlay, L.A., R.J. Wurtman, K. Blusztajn, I.L. Coviella, T.J. Maher, and G.E. Evoniuk. 1986. Decreased plasma choline concentrations in marathon runners. *N Engl J Med* 315 (14): 892.

Conger, S.A., G.L. Warren, M.A. Hardy, and M.L. Millard-Stafford. 2011. Does caffeine added to carbohydrate provide additional ergogenic benefit for endurance? *Int J Sport Nutr Exerc Metab* 21 (1): 71-84.

Conlee, R.K., R.L. Hammer, W.W. Winder, M.L. Bracken, A.G. Nelson, and D.W. Barnett. 1990. Glycogen repletion and exercise endurance in rats adapted to a high fat diet. *Metabolism* 39 (3): 289-294.

Constantin-Teodosiu, D., J.I. Carlin, G. Cederblad, R.C. Harris, and E. Hultman. 1991. Acetyl group accumulation and pyruvate dehydrogenase activity in human muscle during incremental exercise. *Acta Physiol Scand* 143 (4): 367-372.

Coris, E.E., A.M. Ramirez, and D.J. Van Durme. 2004. Heat illness in athletes: The dangerous combination of heat, humidity and exercise. *Sports Medicine* 34 (1): 9-16.

Costa, C., A. Tsatsakis, C. Mamoulakis, M. Teodoro, G. Briguglio, E. Caruso, D. Tsoukalas, D. Margina, E. Dardiotis, D. Kouretas, and C. Fenga. 2017. Current evidence on the effect of dietary polyphenols intake on chronic diseases. *Food Chem Toxicol* 110:286-299.

Costill, D.L., A. Bennett, G. Branam, and D. Eddy. 1973. Glucose ingestion at rest and during prolonged exercise. *J Appl Physiol* 34 (6): 764-769.

Costill, D.L., R. Bowers, G. Branam, and K. Sparks. 1971. Muscle glycogen utilization during prolonged exercise on successive days. *J Appl Physiol* 31:834-838.

Costill, D.L., E. Coyle, G. Dalsky, W. Evans, W. Fink, and D. Hoopes. 1977. Effects of elevated plasma FFA and insulin on muscle glycogen usage during exercise. *J Appl Physiol* 43 (4): 695-699.

Costill, D.L., G.P. Dalsky, and W.J. Fink. 1978. Effects of caffeine ingestion on metabolism and exercise performance. *Med Sci Sports Exerc* 10 (3): 155-158.

Costill, D.L., and W.J. Fink. 1974. Plasma volume changes following exercise and thermal dehydration. *J Appl Physiol* 37:521-525.

Costill, D.L., M.G. Flynn, J.P. Kirwan, J.A. Houmard, J.B. Mitchell, R. Thomas, and S.H. Park. 1988. Effects of repeated days of intensified training on muscle glycogen and swimming performance. *Med Sci Sports Exerc* 20:249-254.

Costill, D.L., and J.M. Miller. 1980. Nutrition for endurance sport: Carbohydrate and fluid balance. *Int J Sports Med* 1:2-14.

Costill, D.L., and B. Saltin. 1974. Factors limiting gastric emptying during rest and exercise. *J Appl Physiol* 37 (5): 679-683.

Costill, D.L., W.M. Sherman, W.J. Fink, C. Maresh, M. Witten, and J.M. Miller. 1981. The role of dietary carbohydrates in muscle glycogen resynthesis after strenuous running. *Am J Clin Nutr* 34:1831-1836.

Cox, A.J., D.B. Pyne, P.U. Saunders, and P.A. Fricker. 2010. Oral administration of the probiotic Lactobacillus fermentum VRI-003 and mucosal immunity in endurance athletes. *Br J Sports Med* 44 (4): 222-226.

Cox, G.R., B. Desbrow, P.G. Montgomery, M.E. Anderson, C.R. Bruce, T.A. Macrides, D.T. Martin, A. Moquin, A. Roberts, J.A. Hawley, and L.M. Burke. 2002. Effect of different protocols of caffeine intake on metabolism and endurance performance. *J Appl Physiol* 93 (3): 990-999.

Cox, P.J., T. Kirk, T. Ashmore, K. Willerton, R. Evans, A. Smith, A.J. Murray, B. Stubbs, J. West, S.W. McLure, M.T. King, M.S. Dodd, C. Holloway, S. Neubauer, S. Drawer, R.L. Veech, J.L. Griffin, and K. Clarke. 2016. Nutritional ketosis alters fuel preference and thereby endurance performance in athletes. *Cell Metab* 24 (2): 256-268.

Coyle, E.F., and A.R. Coggan. 1984. Effectiveness of carbohydrate feeding in delaying fatigue during prolonged exercise. *Sports Med* 1:446-458.

Coyle, E.F., A.R. Coggan, M.K. Hemmert, and J.L. Ivy. 1986. Muscle glycogen utilization during prolonged strenuous exercise when fed carbohydrate. *J Appl Physiol* 61 (1): 165-172.

Coyle, E.F., A.E. Jeukendrup, M.C. Oseto, B.J. Hodgkinson, and T.W. Zderic. 2001. Low-fat diet alters intramuscular substrates and reduces lipolysis and fat oxidation during exercise. *Am J Physiol Endocrinol Metab* 280 (3): E391-E398.

Coyle, E.F., A.E. Jeukendrup, A.J.M. Wagenmakers, and W.H.M. Saris. 1997. Fatty acid oxidation is directly regulated by carbohydrate metabolism during exercise. *Am J Physiol* 273:E268-E275.

Craig, E.N., and E.G. Cummings. 1966. Dehydration and muscular work. *J Appl Physiol* 21:670-674.

Crook, T.H., J. Tinklenberg, J. Yesavage, W. Petrie, M.G. Nunzi, and D.C. Massari. 1991. Effects of phosphatidylserine in age-associated memory impairment. *Neurology* 41 (5): 644-649.

Crooks, C., M.L. Cross, C. Wall, and A. Ali. 2010. Effect of bovine colostrum supplementation on respiratory tract mucosal defenses in swimmers. *Int J Sport Nutr Exerc Metab* 20:224-235.

Crooks, C.V., C.R. Wall, M.L. Cross, et al. 2006. The effect of bovine colstrum supplementation on salivary IgA in distance runners. *Int J Sport Nutr Exerc Metabol* 16:47-64.

Cumming, D. 1996. Exercise-associated amenorrhoea, low bone density and oestradiol replacement therapy. *Arch Intern Med* 156:2193-2195.

Curatolo, P.W., and D. Robertson. 1983. The health consequences of caffeine. *Ann Intern Med* 98 (5 Pt 1): 641-653.

Currell, K., and A.E. Jeukendrup. 2008a. Superior endurance performance with ingestion of multiple transportable carbohydrates. *Med Sci Sports Exerc* 40 (2): 275-281.

Currell, K., and A.E. Jeukendrup. 2008b. Validity, reliability and sensitivity of measures of sporting performance. *Sports Med* 38 (4): 297-316.

DaCosta, M., and K.A. Halmi. 1992. Classification of anorexia nervosa: Question of subtypes. *Int J Eating Disorders* 11:305-314.

Davies, K.J.A., A.T. Quintanilha, G.A. Brooks, and L. Packer. 1982. Free radicals and tissue damage produced by exercise. *Biochem Physiol Res Communications* 107:1198-1205.

Davis, C. 1992. Body image, dieting behaviours and personality factors: A study of high performance female athletes. *Int J Sport Psychol* 23:179-192.

Davis, C., S.H. Kennedy, E. Ralevski, and M. Dionne. 1994. The role of physical activity in the development and maintenance of eating disorders. *Psycholog Med* 24:957-967.

Davis, J.M., C.J. Carlstedt, S. Chen, M.D. Carmichael, and E.A. Murphy. 2010. The dietary flavonoid quercetin increases VO_2max and endurance capacity. *Int J Sport Nutr* 20 (1): 56-62.

Davis, J.M., E.A. Murphy, A.S. Brown, M.D. Carmichael, A. Ghaffar, and E.P. Mayer. 2004. Effects of oat beta-glucan on innate immunity and infection after exercise stress. *Med Sci Sports Exerc* 36:1321-1327.

Davis, J.M., E.A. Murphy, J.L. McClellan, M.D. Carmichael, and J.D. Gangemi. 2008. Quercetin reduces susceptibility to influenza infection following stressful exercise. *Am J Physiol* 295 (2): R505-R509.

Davis, S.E., G.B. Dwyer, K. Reed, et al. 2002. Preliminary investigation: The impact of the NCAA Wrestling Weight Certification Program on weight cutting. *J Strength Cond Res* 16 (2): 305-307.

Davison, G., and B.C. Diment. 2010. Bovine colostrum supplementation attenuates the decrease of salivary lysozyme and enhances the recovery of neutrophil function after prolonged exercise. *Br J Nutr* 103 (10): 1425-1432.

Davison, G., M. Gleeson, and S. Phillips. 2007. Antioxidant supplementation and immunoendocrine responses to prolonged exercise. *Med Sci Sports Exerc* 39 (4): 645-652.

Davison, G., C. Kehaya, B.C. Diment, and N.P. Walsh. 2016. Carbohydrate supplementation does not blunt the prolonged exercise-induced reduction of in vivo immunity. *Eur J Nutr* 55 (4): 1583-1593.

Deakin, V. 2000. Iron depletion in athletes. In *Clinical sports nutrition,* edited by V. Deakin, 273-311. New York: McGraw-Hill.

Dean, S. 2017. Medical nutrition therapy for thyroid, adrenal, and other endocrine disorders. In *Krause's food and the nutrition care process*, edited by L.K.Mahn and J.L.Raymond, 619-630, 14th ed. Saint Louis, MO: Elsevier.

De Bock, K., W. Derave, B.O. Eijnde, M.K. Hesselink, E. Koninckx, A.J. Rose, P. Schrauwen, A. Bonen, E.A. Richter, and P. Hespel. 2008. Effect of training in the fasted state on metabolic responses during exercise with carbohydrate intake. *J Appl Physiol* 104 (4): 1045-1055.

de Castro, J.M. 1987. Macronutrient relationships with meal patterns and mood in the spontaneous feeding behavior of humans. *Physiol Behav* 39 (5): 561-569.

de Castro, J.M., and D.K. Elmore. 1988. Subjective hunger relationships with meal patterns in the spontaneous feeding behavior of humans: Evidence for a causal connection. *Physiol Behav* 43 (2): 159-165.

Decombaz, J., R. Jentjens, M. Ith, E. Scheurer, T. Buehler, A. Jeukendrup, and C. Boesch. 2011. Fructose and galactose enhance postexercise human liver glycogen synthesis. *Med Sci Sports Exerc* 43 (10): 1964-1971.

de Koning, L., V.S. Malik, M.D. Kellogg, E.B. Rim, W.C. Willett, and F.B. Hu. 2012. Sweetened beverage consumption, incident coronary heart disease and biomarkers of risk in men. *Circulation* 125:1735-1741.

De Luca, L., and S. Ross. 1996. Beta-carotene increases lung cancer incidence in cigarette smokers. *Nutr Rev* 54:178-180.

Depaola, D.P., M.P. Faine, and C.A. Pamer. 1999. Nutrition in relation to dental medicine. In *Modern nutrition in health and disease,* edited by M.E. Shils, J.A. Olson, M. Shike, and A.C. Ross, 1099-1124. Baltimore: Williams & Wilkins.

Derave, W., Everaert, I., Beeckman, S., and Baguet, A. 2010. Muscle carnosine metabolism and beta-alanine supplementation in relation to exercise and training. *Sports Med* 40 (3): 247-263.

Derave, W., M.S. Ozdemir, R. Harris, A. Pottier, H. Reyngoudt, K. Koppo, J.A. Wise, and E. Achten. 2007. Beta-alanine supplementation augments muscle carnosine content and attenuates fatigue during repeated isokinetic contraction bouts in trained sprinters. *J Appl Physiol* 103 (5): 1736-1743.

Derman, W., M. Schwellnus, E. Jordaan, C.A. Blauwet, C. Emery, P. Pit-Grosheide, N.A. Marques, O. Martinez-Ferrer, J. Stomphorst, P. Van de Vliet, N. Webborn, and S.E. Willick. 2013. Illness and injury in athletes during the competition period at the London 2012 Paralympic Games: Development and implementation of a web-based surveillance system (WEB-IISS) for team medical staff. *Br J Sports Med* 47:420–425.

de Ruyter, J. C., M.R. Olthof, J.C. Seidell, and M.B. Katan. 2012. A trial of sugar-free or sugar-sweetened beverages and body weight in children. *New Eng J Med* 367 (15): 1397-1406.

DeSilva, P., and S.B.G. Eysenck. 1987. Personality and addictiveness in anorexic and bulimic patients. *Pers Indiv Differ* 8:749-751.

Devries, M.C., S.A. Lowther, A.W. Glover, M.J. Hamadeh, and M.A. Tarnopolsky. 2007. IMCL area density, but not IMCL utilization, is higher in women during moderate-intensity endurance exercise, compared with men. *Am J Physiol Regul Integr Comp Physiol* 293 (6): R2336-R2342.

Diaz, K.M., D.J. Krupka, M.J. Chang, J. Peacock, Y. Ma, J. Goldsmith, J.E. Schwartz, and K.W. Davidson. 2015. Fitbit®: An accurate and reliable device for wireless physical activity tracking. *Int J Cardiol* 185:138-140.

Dill, D.B., H.T. Edwards, and J.H. Talbott. 1932. Factors limiting the capacity for work. *J Physiol* 1932:49-62.

Diogenes GI Database. 2010. www.diogenes-eu.org/GI-Database/Default.htm.

Dodd, S.L., E. Brooks, S.K. Powers, and R. Tulley. 1991. The effects of caffeine on graded exercise performance in caffeine naive versus habituated subjects. *Eur J Appl Physiol* 62:424-429.

Doherty, M., and P.M. Smith. 2004. Effects of caffeine ingestion on exercise testing: A meta-analysis. *Int J Sport Nutr Exerc Metab* 14 (6): 626-646.

Doherty, M., and P.M. Smith. 2005. Effects of caffeine ingestion on rating of perceived exertion during and after exercise: A meta-analysis. *Scand J Med Sci Sports* 15 (2): 69-78.

Dohm, G.L., R.T. Beeker, R.G. Israel, and E.B. Tapscott. 1986. Metabolic responses after fasting. *J Appl Physiol* 61 (4): 1363-1368.

Dohm, G.L., E.B. Tapscott, H.A. Barakat, and G.J. Kasperek. 1983. Influence of fasting on glycogen depletion in rats during exercise. *J Appl Physiol* 55 (3): 830-833.

Donini, L.M., D. Marsili, M.P. Graziani, et al. 2004. Orthorexia nervosa: A preliminary study with a proposal for diagnosis and an attempt to measure the dimension of the phenomenon. *Eat Weight Disord* 9 (2): 151-157.

Douglas, R.M., H. Hemila, E. Chalker, and B. Treacy. 2007. Vitamin C for preventing and treating the common cold. *Cochrane Database Syst Rev 18(*3): CD000980.

Drinkwater, B.L., K. Nilson, C.H. Chesnut 3rd, et al. 1984. Bone mineral content of amenorrheic and eumenorrheic athletes. *N Engl J Med* 311 (5): 277-281.

Duchman, S.M., A.J. Ryan, H.P. Schedl, R.W. Summers, T.L. Bleiler, and C.V. Gisolfi. 1997. Upper limit for intestinal absorption of a dilute glucose solution in men at rest. *Med Sci Sports Exerc* 29 (4): 482-488.

Duffy, D.J., and R.K. Conlee. 1986. Effects of phosphate loading on leg power and high intensity treadmill exercise. *Med Sci Sports Exerc* 18 (6): 674-677.

Dulloo, A.G., and J. Jacquet. 1998. Adaptive reduction in basal metabolic rate in response to food deprivation in humans: A role for feedback signals from fat stores. *Am J Clin Nutr* 68 (3): 599-606.

Dummer, G.M., L.W. Rosen, and W.W. Heusner. 1987. Pathogenic weight-control behaviors of young competitive swimmers. *Physician Sports Med* 5:75-86.

Dunn, T.M., and S. Bratman. 2016. On orthorexia nervosa: A review of the literature and proposed diagnostic criteria. *Eat Behav* 21:11-17.

Dupre, J., J.D. Curtis, R.W. Waddell, and J.C. Beck. 1968. Alimentary factors in the endocrine response to administration of arginine in man. *Lancet* 2 (7558): 28-29.

Durnin, J.V., and J. Womersley. 1974. Body fat assessed from total body density and its estimation from skin fold thickness: Measurements on 481 men and women aged from 16 to 72 years. *Br J Nutr* 32 (1): 77-97.

Duthie, G.G. 1999. Determination of activity of antioxidants in human subjects. *Pro Nutr Soc* 58:1015-1024.

Dyck, D.J., S.A. Peters, P.S. Wendling, A. Chesley, E. Hultman, and L.L. Spriet. 1996. Regulation of muscle glycogen phosphorylase activity during intense aerobic cycling with elevated FFA. *Am J Physiol* 265:E116-E125.

Dyck, D.J., C.T. Putman, G.J.F. Heigenhauser, E. Hultman, and L.L. Spriet. 1993. Regulation of fat-carbohydrate interaction in skeletal muscle during intense aerobic cycling. *Am J Physiol* 265:E852-859.

Eden, B., and P. Abernethy. 1994. Nutritional intake during an ultraendurance running race. *Int J Sports Nutr* 4:166–174.

Edwards, H.T., R. Margaria, and D.B. Dill. 1934. Metabolic rate, blood sugar and the utilization of carbohydrate. *Am J Physiol* 108:203-209.

Egan, B., and J.R. Zierath. Exercise metabolism and the molecular regulation of skeletal muscle adaptation. *Cell Metabolism* 17 (2): 162-184.

Eichner, E.R. 2000. Minerals: Iron. In *Nutrition in sport,* edited by R.J. Maughan, 326-338. Oxford: Blackwell Science.

Elango, R., R.O. Ball, and P.B. Pencharz. 2012. Recent advances in determining protein and amino acid requirements in humans. *Br J Nutr* 108 (Suppl 2):S22–S30.

el-Khoury, A.E., A. Forslund, R. Olsson, S. Branth, A. Sjödin, A. Andersson, A. Atkinson, A. Selvaraj, L. Hambraeus, and V.R. Young. 1997. Moderate exercise at energy balance does not affect 24-h leucine oxidation or nitrogen retention in healthy men. *Am J Physiol* 273(2 Pt 1):E394-E407.

Elliot, T.A., M.G. Cree, A.P. Sanford, R.R. Wolfe, and K.D. Tipton. 2006. Milk ingestion stimulates net muscle protein synthesis following resistance exercise. *Med Sci Sports Exerc* 38 (4): 667-674.

Elowsson, P., A.H. Forslund, H. Mallmin, et al. 1998. An evaluation of dual-energy X-ray absorptiometry and underwater weighing to estimate body composition by means of carcass analysis in piglets. *J Nutr* 128 (9): 1543-1549.

Engels, H.J., and J.C. Wirth. 1997. No ergogenic effects of ginseng (Panax ginseng C.A. Meyer) during graded maximal aerobic exercise. *J Am Diet Assoc* 97 (10): 1110-1115.

Epling, W.F., and W.D. Pierce. 1988. Activity-based anorexia: A biobehavioral perspective. *Int J Eating Disorders* 7:475-485.

Eshak, E.S., H. Iso, Y. Kokubo, I. Saito, K. Yamagishi, M. Inoue, and S. Tsugane. 2012. Soft drink intake in relation to incident ischemic heart disease, stroke, and stroke subtypes in Japanese men and women: The Japan Public Health Centre–based study cohort I. *Am J Clin Nutr* 96:1390-1397.

Essig, D., D.L. Costill, and P.J. Van Handel. 1980. Effects of caffeine ingestion on utilization of muscle glycogen and lipid during leg ergometer cycling. *Int J Sports Med* 1:86-90.

Evain-Brion, D., M. Donnadieu, M. Roger, and J.C. Job. 1982. Simultaneous study of somatotrophic and corticotrophic pituitary secretions during ornithine infusion test. *Clin Endocrinol* 17 (2): 119-122.

Evans, G.W. 1989. The effect of chromium picolinate on insulin controlled parameters in humans. *Int J Biosoc Med Res* 11:163-180.

Evenson, K.R., M.M. Goto, and R.D. Furberg. 2015. Systematic review of the validity and reliability of consumer-wearable activity trackers. *Int J Behav Nutr Phys Act* 12:159.

Fahey, T.D., J.D. Larsen, G.A. Brooks, W. Colvin, S. Henderson, and D. Lary. 1991. The effects of ingesting polylactate or glucose polymer drinks during prolonged exercise. *Int J Sport Nutr* 1 (3): 249-256.

Fairchild, T.J., S. Fletcher, P. Steele, C. Goodman, B. Dawson, and P. Fournier. 2002. Rapid carbohydrate loading after a short bout of near maximal-intensity exercise. *Med Sci Sports Exerc* 34 (6): 980-986.

Falk, B., R. Burstein, I. Ashkenazi, et al. 1989. The effect of caffeine ingestion on physical performance after prolonged exercise. *Eur J Appl Physiol* 59:168-173.

Falk, B., and R. Dotan. 2008. Children's thermoregulation during exercise in the heat: A revisit. *Appl Physiol Nutr Metab* 33:420-427.

Falk, B., and R. Dotan. 2011. Temperature regulation and elite young athletes. *Med Sport Sci* 56:126-149.

Fallowfield, J.L., C. Williams, J. Booth, B.H. Choo, and S. Growns. 1996. Effect of water ingestion on endurance capacity during prolonged running. *J Sports Sci* 14:497-502.

Fares, E.J., and B. Kayser. 2011. Carbohydrate mouth rinse effects on exercise capacity in pre- and postprandial states. *Journal of Nutrition and Metabolism*, vol. 2011, Article ID 385962, 6 pages. doi:10.1155/2011/385962.

Ferguson, T., A.V. Rowlands, T. Olds, and C. Maher. 2015. The validity of consumer-level, activity monitors in healthy adults worn in free-living conditions: A cross-sectional study. *Int J Behav Nutr Phys Act* 12:42.

Fernandez-San-Martin, M.I., R. Masa-Font, L. Palacios-Soler, P. Sancho-Gómez, C. Calbó-Caldentey, and G. Flores-Mateo. 2010. Effectiveness of valerian on insomnia: A meta-analysis of randomized placebo-controlled trials. *Sleep Med* 11 (6): 505-511.

Ferreira, L.F., and B.J. Behnke. 2011. A toast to health and performance! Beetroot juice lowers blood pressure and the O_2 cost of exercise. *J Appl Physiol* 110 (3): 585-586.

Fery, F., and E.O. Balasse. 1983. Ketone body turnover during and after exercise in overnight-fasted and starved humans. *Am J Physiol* 245:E18-E25.

Field, A.E., T. Byers, D.J. Hunter, et al. 1999. Weight cycling, weight gain, and risk of hypertension in women. *Am J Epidemiol* 150 (6): 573-579.

Fielding, R.A., T.J. Manfredi, W. Ding, M.A. Fiatarone, W.J. Evans, and J.G. Cannon. 1993. Acute phase response in exercise. III. Neutrophil and IL-1b accumulation in skeletal muscle. *Am J Physiol* 265:R166-R172.

Fischer, C.P., N.J. Hiscock, M. Penkowa, et al. 2004. Supplementation with vitamins C and E inhibits the release of interleukin-6 from contracting human skeletal muscle. *J Physiol* 558:633-645.

Flatt, J.-P. 1995. Use and storage of carbohydrate and fat. *Am J Clin Nutr* 61:952S-959S.

Fogelholm, G.M., R. Koskinen, and J. Laasko. 1993. Gradual and rapid weight loss: Effects on nutrition and performance in male athletes. *Med Sci Sports Exerc* 25:371-377.

Fogelholm, G.M., H.K. Naveri, K.T. Kiilavuori, and M.H. Harkonen. 1993. Low dose amino acid supplementation: No effects on serum growth hormone and insulin in male weightlifters. *Int J Sports Nutr* 3:290-297.

Fogelholm, M. 1994a. Vitamins, minerals and supplementation in soccer. *J Sports Sci* 12:S23-S27.

Fogelholm, M. 1994b. Effects of body weight reduction on sports performance. *Sports Med* 4:249-267.

Fontani, G., F. Corradeschi, A. Felici, F. Alfatti, S. Migliorini, and L. Lodi. 2005. Cognitive and physiological effects of Omega-3 polyunsaturated fatty acid supplementation in healthy subjects. *Eur J Clin Invest* 35:691-699.

Food and Nutrition Board. 2005. *Dietary reference intakes for energy, carbohydrate, fiber, fat, fatty acids, cholesterol, protein, and amino acids (macronutrients)*. Washington, DC: National Academies Press.

Foster, C., D.L. Costill, and W.J. Fink. 1979. Effects of preexercise feedings on endurance performance. *Med Sci Sports* 11 (1): 1-5.

Fowler, P.M., R. Duffield, and D. Lu. 2016. Effects of long-haul transmeridian travel on subjective jet-lag and self-reported sleep and upper respiratory symptoms in professional Rugby League players. *Int J Sports Physiol Perform* 11 (7): 876-884.

Frexes-Steed, M., D.B. Lacy, J. Collins, and N.N. Abumrad. 1992. Role of leucine and other amino acids in regulating protein metabolism in vivo. *Am J Physiol* 262 (6 Pt 1): E925-E935.

Fujii, N., T. Hayashi, M.F. Hirshman, J.T. Smith, S.A. Habinowski, L. Kaijser, J. Mu, O. Ljungqvist, M.J. Birnbaum, L.A. Witters, A. Thorell, and L.J. Goodyear. 2000. Exercise induces isoform-specific increase in 5′AMP-activated protein kinase activity in human skeletal muscle. *Biochem Biophys Res Commun* 273:1150-1155.

Fuchs, C.J., J.T. Gonzalez, M. Beelen, N.M. Cermak, F.E. Smith, P.E. Thelwall, R. Taylor, T.I. Trenell, E. Stevenson, and L.J. van Loon. 2016. Sucrose ingestion after exhaustive exercise accelerates liver, but not muscle glycogen repletion compared with glucose ingestion in trained athletes. *J Appl Physiol* 120 (11): 1328-1334.

Fujita, S., H.C. Dreyer, M.J. Drummond, E.L. Glynn, E. Volpi, and B.B. Rasmussen. 2009. Essential amino acid and carbohydrate ingestion before resistance exercise does not enhance postexercise muscle protein synthesis. *J Appl Physiol* 106:1730-1739.

Fung, T., V. Malik, K. Rexrode, J.E. Manson, W.C. Willett, and F.B. Hu. 2009. Sweetened beverage consumption and risk of coronary heart disease in women. *Am J Clin Nutr* 89 (4): 1037-1042.

Gadpalle, W.J., C.F. Sandborn, and W.W. Wagner. 1987. Athletic amenorhea, major affective disorders and eating disorders. *Am J Psychiatry* 144:939-943.

Galbo, H. 1983. *Hormonal and metabolic adaptation to exercise.* New York: Verlag.

Galloway, S.D., M.S. Tremblay, J.R. Sexsmith, and C.J. Roberts. 1996. The effects of acute phosphate supplementation in subjects of different aerobic fitness levels. *Eur J Appl Physiol* 72 (3): 224-230.

Galloway, S.D.R., and R.J. Maughan. 2000. The effects of fluid and substrate provision on thermoregulatory and metabolic responses to prolonged exercise in a hot environment. *J Sports Sci* 18:339-351.

Gam, S., K.J. Guelfi, and P.A. Fournier. 2013. Opposition of carbohydrate in a mouth-rinse solution to the detrimental effect of mouth rinsing during cycling time trials. *Int J Sport Nutr Exerc Metab*. 23:48-56.

Gant, N., A. Ali, and A. Foskett. 2010. The influence of caffeine and carbohydrate coingestion on simulated soccer performance. *Int J Sport Nutr Exerc Metab* 20 (3): 191-197.

Gardiner, J.E., and M.C. Gwee. 1974. The distribution in the rabbit of choline administered by injection or infusion. *J Physiol (Lond)* 239 (3): 459-476.

Garner, M.D., P.E. Garfinkel, W. Rockert, and M.P. Olmsted. 1987. A prospective study of eating disturbances in the ballet. *Psychother Psychosomat* 48:170-175.

Garvican, L.A., L. Lobigs, R. Telford, K. Fallon, and C.J. Gore. 2011. Haemoglobin mass in an anaemic female endurance runner before and after iron supplementation. *Int J Sports Physiol Perform* 6:137-40.

Geleijnse, J.M., L.J. Launer, D.A. Van der Kuip, A. Hofman, and J.C. Witteman. 2002. Inverse association of tea and flavonoid intakes with incident myocardial infarction: The Rotterdam Study. *Am J Clin Nutr* 75 (5): 880-886.

Geng, T., L. Qi, and T. Huang. 2018. Effects of dairy products consumption on body weight and body composition among adults: An updated meta-analysis of 37 randomized control trials. *Mol Nutr Food Res* 62(1). doi: 10.1002/mnfr.201700410.

Gibala, M.J., and S.L. McGee. 2008. Metabolic adaptations to short-term high-intensity interval training: A little pain for a lot of gain? *Exerc Sport Sci Rev* 36 (2): 58-63.

Gibson, S.A. 1996. Are high-fat, high-sugar foods and diets conducive to obesity? *Int J Food Sci Nutr* 47 (5): 405-415.

Girandola, R.N., R.A. Wiswell, and R. Bulbulian. 1980. Effects of pangamic acid (B-15) ingestion on metabolic response to exercise. *Biochem Med* 24 (2): 218-222.

Girgis, C.M., R.J. Clifton-Bligh, N. Turner, S.L. Lau, and J.E. Gunton. 2014. Effects of vitamin D in skeletal muscle: Falls, strength, athletic performance and insulin sensitivity. *Clin Endocrinol* 80:169-181.

Glazer, J.L. 2008. Eating disorders among male athletes. *Curr Sports Med Rep* 7 (6): 332-337.

Gleeson, M. 1998. Temperature regulation during exercise. *Int J Sports Med* 19 (Suppl 2): S96-S99.

Gleeson, M. 2000. Minerals and exercise immunology. In *Nutrition and exercise immunology,* edited by D.C. Nieman and B.K. Pedersen, 137-154. Boca Raton, FL: CRC Press.

Gleeson, M. 2006. Immune system adaptation in elite athletes. *Curr Opin Clin Nutr Metab Care* 9 (6): 659-665.

Gleeson, M. 2008. Dosing and efficacy of glutamine supplementation in human exercise and sport training. *J Nutr* 138 (10): 2045S-2049S.

Gleeson, M. 2013. Exercise, nutrition and immunity. In *Diet, immunity and inflammation,* edited by P.C. Calder and P. Yaqoob, 652-685. Cambridge: Woodhead Publishing.

Gleeson, M. 2014. Biochemistry of exercise. In *Sports nutrition*, edited by R.J. Maughan, 36-58. Chichester, UK: Blackwell.

Gleeson, M. 2016. Immunological aspects of sport nutrition. *Immunol Cell Biol* 94:117-123.

Gleeson, M., and N.C. Bishop. 2000a. Elite athlete immunology: Importance of nutrition. *Int J Sports Med* 21 (Suppl 1): S44-S50.

Gleeson, M., and N.C. Bishop. 2000b. Modification of immune responses to exercise by carbohydrate, glutamine and antioxidant supplements. *Immunol Cell Biol* 78:554-561.

Gleeson, M., and N.C. Bishop. 2013. URI in athletes: Are mucosal immunity and cytokine responses key risk factors? *Exerc Sport Sci Rev* 41:148-153.

Gleeson, M., N.C.Bishop, D.J. Stensel, M.R. Lindley, S.S. Mastana, and M.A. Nimmo. 2011. The anti-inflammatory effects of exercise: Mechanisms and implications for the prevention and treatment of disease. *Nat Rev Immunol* 11:607-615.

Gleeson, M., N.C. Bishop, and N.P. Walsh, eds. 2013. *Exercise immunology*. Abingdon: Routledge.

Gleeson, M., A.K. Blannin, N.P. Walsh, N.C. Bishop, and A.M. Clark. 1998. Effect of low and high carbohydrate diets on the plasma glutamine and circulating leukocyte responses to exercise. *Int J Sport Nutr* 8:49-59.

Gleeson, M., R.J. Maughan, and P.L. Greenhaff. 1986. Comparison of the effects of pre-exercise feeding of glucose, glycerol and placebo on endurance and fuel homeostasis in man. *Eur J Appl Physiol* 55 (6): 645-653.

Gleeson, M., J. Siegler, L.M. Burke, S. Stear, and L.M. Castell. 2012. A to Z of nutritional supplements: Dietary supplements, sports nutrition foods and ergogenic aids for health and performance—Part 31. (Probiotics). *Br J Sports Med* 46:377-378.

Global News Wire. 2017. Dietary supplements market will reach USD 220.3 billion in 2022: Zion Market Research. https://globenewswire.com/news-release/2017/01/11/905073/0/en/Global-Dietary-Supplements-Market-will-reach-USD-220-3-Billion-in-2022-Zion-Market-Research.html.

Gniadecki, R., B. Gajkowska, and M. Hansen. 1997. 1,25-dihydroxyvitamin D3 stimulates the assembly of adherens junctions in keratinocytes: Involvement of protein kinase C. *Endocrinology* 138(6): 2241-2248.

Godek, S.F., A.R. Bartolozzi, and J.J. Godek. 2005. Sweat rate and fluid turnover in American football players compared with runners in a hot and humid environment. *Br J Sports Med* 39:205-211.

Goedecke, J.H., R. Elmer-English, S.C. Dennis, I. Schloss, T.D. Noakes, and E.V. Lambert. 1999. Effects of medium-chain triacylglycerol ingested with carbohydrate on metabolism and exercise performance. *Int J Sports Nutr* 9 (1): 35-47.

Going, S.B., M.P. Massett, M.C. Hall, et al. 1993. Detection of small changes in body composition by dual-energy x-ray absorptiometry. *Am J Clin Nutr* 57 (6): 845-850.

Goldberg, A.L., and T.W. Chang. 1978. Regulation and significance of amino acid metabolism in skeletal muscle. *Fed Proc* 37:2301-2307.

Golden, N.H. 2002. A review of the female athlete triad (amenorrhea, osteoporosis and disordered eating). *Int J Adolesc Med Health* 14:9-17.

Gomez-Cabrera, M.C., C. Borras, F.V. Pallardo, J. Sastre, L.L. Ji, and J. Vina. 2005. Decreasing xanthine oxidase-mediated oxidative stress prevents useful cellular adaptations to exercise in rats. *J Physiol* 567:113-120.

Gomez-Cabrera, M.C., E. Domenech, M. Romagnoli, A. Arduini, C. Borras, F.V. Pallardo, J. Sastre, and J. Vina. 2008. Oral administration of vitamin C decreases muscle mitochondrial biogenesis and hampers training-induced adaptations in endurance performance. *Am J Clin Nutr* 87 (1): 142-149.

Gonçalves, L.S., V.S. Painelli, G. Yamaguchi, L.F. Oliveira, B. Saunders, R.P. da Silva, E. Maciel, G.G. Artioli, H. Roschel, and B. Gualano. 2017. Dispelling the myth that habitual caffeine consumption influences the performance response to acute caffeine supplementation. *J Appl Physiol* 123 (1): 213-220.

Gontzea, I., R. Sutzeescu, and S. Dumitrache. 1975. The influence of adaptation to physical effort on nitrogen balance in man. *Nutr Rep Internat* 11 (3): 231-236.

Gonzalez, J.T., C.J. Fuchs, J.A. Betts, and L.J. van Loon. 2016. Liver glycogen metabolism during and after prolonged endurance-type exercise. *Am J Physiol Endocrinol Metab* 311 (3): E543-E553.

González-Alonso, J., C. Teller, S.L. Andersen, F.B. Jensen, T. Hyldig, and B. Nielsen. 1999. Influence of body temperature on the development of fatigue during prolonged exercise in the heat. *J Appl Physiol* 86 (3): 1032-1039.

Goulet, E.D. 2011. Effect of exercise-induced dehydration on time-trial exercise performance: A meta-analysis. *Br J Sports Med* 45 (14): 1149-1156.

Graham, T.E., E. Hibbert, and P. Sathasivam. 1998. Metabolic and exercise endurance effects of coffee and caffeine ingestion. *J Appl Physiol* 85 (3): 883-889.

Graham, T.E., and L.L. Spriet. 1991. Performance and metabolic responses to a high caffeine dose during prolonged exercise. *J Appl Physiol* 71 (6): 2292-2298.

Graham, T.E., and L.L. Spriet. 1995. Metabolic, catecholamine, and exercise performance responses to various doses of caffeine. *J Appl Physiol* 78 (3): 867-874.

Graham, T.E., J.W. Rush, and M.H. van Soeren. 1994. Caffeine and exercise: Metabolism and performance. *Can J Appl Physiol* 19 (2): 111-138.

Granados, J., T.L. Gillum, K.M. Christmas, and M.R. Kuennen. 2014. Prohormone supplement 3ß-hydroxy-5α-androst-1-en-17-one enhances resistance training gains but impairs user health. *J Appl Physiol* 116 (5): 560-569.

Graudal, N.A., A.M. Galloe, and P. Garred. 1998. Effects of sodium restriction on blood pressure, renin, aldosterone, catecholamines, cholesterols, and triglyceride: A meta-analysis. *JAMA* 279 (17): 1383-1391.

Gray, M.E., and L.W. Titlow. 1982. The effect of pangamic acid on maximal treadmill performance. *Med Sci Sports Exerc* 14 (6): 424-427.

Green, A.L., D.A. Sewell, L. Simpson, E. Hultman, and P.L. Greenhaff. 1995. Carbohydrate ingestion stimulates creatine uptake in human skeletal muscle. *J Physiol* 489:27P.

Green, A.L., E.J. Simpson, J.J. Littlewood, I.A. MacDonald, and P.L. Greenhaff. 1996. Carbohydrate ingestion augments creatine retention during creatine feeding in humans. *Acta Physiol Scand* 158:195-202.

Green, H.J. 1995. Metabolic determinants of activity induced muscular fatigue. In *Exercise metabolism,* edited by M. Hargreaves, 211-256. Champaign, IL: Human Kinetics.

Green, N.R., and A.A. Ferrando. 1994. Plasma boron and the effects of boron supplementation in males. *Environ Health Perspect* 102 (Suppl 7): 73-77.

Greenhaff, P.L. 1998. The nutritional biochemistry of creatine. *Nutr Biochem* 11:1610-1618.

Greenhaff, P.L., K. Bodin, R.C. Harris, D.A. Jones, D.B. McIntyre, K. Soderlund, and D.L. Turner. 1993. The influence of oral creatine supplementation on muscle phosphocreatine resynthesis following intense contraction in man. *J Physiol* 467:75P.

Greenhaff, P.L., K. Bodin, K. Soderlund, and E. Hultman. 1994. Effect of oral creatine supplementation on skeletal muscle phosphocreatine resynthesis. *Am J Physiol* 266:E725-E730.

Greenhaff, P.L., A. Casey, A.H. Short, R. Harris, K. Soderlund, and E. Hultman. 1993. Influence of oral creatine supplementation of muscle torque during repeated bouts of maximal voluntary exercise in man. *Clin Sci* 84:565-571.

Greenhaff, P.L., and J.A. Timmons. 1998a. Pyruvate dehydrogenase complex activation status and acetyl group availability as a site of interchange between anaerobic and oxidative metabolism during intense exercise. *Adv Exp Med Biol* 441:287-298.

Greenhaff, P.L., and J.A. Timmons. 1998b. Interaction between aerobic and anaerobic metabolism during intense muscle contraction. *Exerc Sport Sci Rev* 26:1-30.

Greenleaf, J.E. 1979. Hyperthermia in exercise. In *International review of physiology: Environmental physiology III,* Vol. 20, edited by D. Robertshaw, 1-50. Baltimore: University Park Press.

Greer, F., C. McLean, and T.E. Graham. 1998. Caffeine, performance, and metabolism during repeated Wingate exercise tests. *J Appl Physiol* 85 (4): 1502-1508.

Guezennec, C.Y., J.F. Nadaud, P. Satabin, F. Léger, and P. Lafargue. 1989. Influence of polyunsaturated fatty acid diet on the hemorrheological response to physical exercise in hypoxia. *Int J Sports Med* 10 (4): 286-291.

Halberstam, M., N. Cohen, P. Shlimovich, L. Rossetti, and H. Shamoon. 1996. Oral vanadyl sulfate improves insulin sensitivity in NIDDM but not in obese nondiabetic subjects. *Diabetes* 45:659-666.

Hall, J.N., S. Moore, S.B. Harper, and J.W. Lynch. 2009. Global variability in fruit and vegetable consumption. *Am J Prev Med* 36 (5): 402-409, e405.

Hall, K.D., T. Bemis, R. Brychta, K.Y. Chen, A. Courville, E.J. Crayner, S. Goodwin, J. Guo, L. Howard, N.D. Knuth, B.V. Miller 3rd, C.M. Prado, M. Siervo, M.C. Skarulis, M. Walter, P.J. Walter, and L. Yannai. 2015. Calorie for calorie, dietary fat restriction results in more body fat loss than carbohydrate restriction in people with obesity. *Cell Metab* 22 (3): 427-436.

Hall, K.D., K.Y. Chen, J. Guo, Y.Y. Lam, R.L. Leibel, L.E. Mayer, M.L. Reitman, M. Rosenbaum, S.R. Smith, B.T. Walsh, and E. Ravussin. 2016. Energy expenditure and body composition changes after an isocaloric ketogenic diet in overweight and obese men. *Am J Clin Nutr* 104 (2): 324-333.

Hall, K.D., and J. Guo. 2017. Obesity energetics: Body weight regulation and the effects of diet composition. *Gastroenterology* 152 (7): 1718-1727.

Hallmark, M.A., T.H. Reynolds, C.A. DeSouza, C.O. Dotson, R.A. Anderson, and M.A. Rogers. 1996. Effects of chromium and resistive training on muscle strength and body composition. *Med Sci Sports Exerc* 28 (1): 139-144.

Halson, S. 2013. Nutritional interventions to enhance sleep. *Sports Sci Exch* 26 (116): 1-5.

Halson, S.L. 2014. Sleep in elite athletes and nutritional interventions to enhance sleep. *Sports Med* 44 (Suppl 1): S13-S23.

Halson, S.L., G.I. Lancaster, J. Achten, M. Gleeson, and A.E. Jeukendrup. 2004. Effects of carbohydrate supplementation on performance and carbohydrate oxidation after intensified cycling training. *J Appl Physiol* 97 (4): 1245-1253.

Hamilton, B. 2010. Vitamin D and human skeletal muscle. *Scand J Med Sci Sports* 20:182-190.

Handzlik, M., and M. Gleeson. 2013. Likely additive ergogenic effects of combined pre-exercise dietary nitrate and caffeine ingestion in trained cyclists. *ISRN Nutr* (December 14). http://doi.org/10.5402/2013/396581.

Hansen, A.K., C.P. Fischer, P. Plomgaard, J.L. Andersen, B. Saltin, B.K. Pedersen. 2005. Skeletal muscle adaptation: Training twice every second day vs. training once daily. *J Appl Physiol* 98:93-99.

Hao, Q., Z. Lu, B.R. Dong, C.Q. Huang, and T. Wu. 2011. Probiotics for preventing acute upper respiratory tract infections. *Cochrane Database Syst Rev* (September 7): CD006895.

Hargreaves, M. 1995. *Exercise metabolism*. Champaign, IL: Human Kinetics.

Hargreaves, K.M., J.A. Hawley, and A.E. Jeukendrup. 2004. Pre-exercise carbohydrate and fat ingestion: Effects on metabolism and performance. *J Sports Sci* 22:31-38.

Hargreaves, K.M., and W.M. Pardridge. 1988. Neutral amino acid transport at the human blood-brain barrier. *J Biol Chem* 263 (36): 19392-19397.

Harper, A.E. 1999. Nutritional essentiality: Evolution of the concept. *Nutr Today* 36:216-222.

Harris, R.C., K. Soderlund, and E. Hultman. 1992. Elevation of creatine in resting and exercised muscle of normal subjects by creatine supplementation. *Clin Sci* 83:367-374.

Harris, R.C., M.J. Tallon, M. Dunnett, L. Boobis, J. Coakley, H.J. Kim, J.L. Fallowfield, C.A. Hill, C. Sale, and J.A. Wise. 2006. The absorption of orally supplied beta-alanine and its effect on muscle carnosine synthesis in human vastus lateralis. *Amino Acids* 30 (3): 279-289.

Hartman, J.W., J.E. Tang, S.B. Wilkinson, M.A. Tarnopolsky, R.L. Lawrence, A.V. Fullerton, and S.M. Phillips. 2007. Consumption of fat-free fluid milk after resistance exercise promotes greater lean mass accretion than does consumption of soy or carbohydrate in young, novice, male weightlifters. *Am J Clin Nutr* 86 (2): 373-381.

Haskell, W.L., I.M. Lee, R.R. Pate, et al. 2007. Physical activity and public health: Updated recommendation for adults from the American College of Sports Medicine and the American Heart Association. *Med Sci Sports Exerc* 39:1423-1434.

Hasten, D.L., E.P. Rome, B.D. Franks, and M. Hegsted. 1992. Effects of chromium picolinate on beginning weight training students. *Int J Sport Nutr* 2 (4): 343-350.

Haubrich, D.R., P.F. Wang, D.E. Clody, and P.W. Wedeking. 1975. Increase in rat brain acetylcholine induced by choline or deanol. *Life Sci* 17 (6): 975-980.

Hausswirth, C., J. Louis, A. Aubry, G. Bonnet, R. Duffield, and Y. Le Meur. 2014. Evidence of disturbed sleep and increased illness in overreached endurance athletes. *Med Sci Sports Exerc* 46 (5): 1036-1045.

Havel, R.J., B. Pernow, and N.L. Jones. 1967. Uptake and release of free fatty acids and other metabolites in the legs of exercising men. *J Appl Physiol* 23 (1): 90-99.

Hawley, J.A., A.N. Bosch, S.M. Weltan, S.C. Dennis, and T.D. Noakes. 1994. Glucose kinetics during prolonged exercise in euglycemic and hyperglycemic subjects. *Pflügers Arch* 426:378-386.

Hawley, J.A., Burke, L.M., Phillips, S.M., and Spriet, L.L. 2011. Nutritional modulation of training-induced skeletal muscle adaptations. *J Appl Physiol* 110:834-845.

Hawley, J.A., E.J. Schabort., T.D. Noakes, and S.C. Dennis. 1997. Carbohydrate loading and exercise performance. *Sports Med* 24 (1): 1-10.

Haywood, B.A., K.E. Black, D. Baker, J. McGarvey, P. Healey, and R.C. Brown. 2014. Probiotic supplementation reduces the duration and incidence of infections but not severity in elite rugby union players. *J Sci Med Sport* 17:356-360.

He, C.-S., X.H. Aw Yong, N.P. Walsh, and M. Gleeson. 2016. Is there an optimal vitamin D status for immunity in athletes and military personnel? *Exerc Immunol Rev* 22:42-64.

He, C.-S., M. Handzlik, W.D. Fraser, A. Muhamad, H. Preston, A. Richardson, and Gleeson, M. 2013. Influence of vitamin D status on respiratory infection incidence and immune function during 4 months of winter training in endurance sport athletes. *Exerc Immunol Rev* 19:86-101.

Heaton, L.E., J.K. Davis, E.S. Rawson, R.P. Nuccio, O.C. Witard, W. Stein, K. Baar, J.M. Carter, and L.B. Baker. 2017. Selected in-season nutritional strategies to enhance recovery for team sport athletes: A practical overview. *Sports Med* 47 (11): 2201-2218.

Heikkinen, A., A. Alaranta, I. Helenius, and T. Vasankari. 2011. Dietary supplementation habits and perceptions of supplement use among elite Finnish athletes. *Int J Sport Nutr Exerc Metab* 21 (4): 271-279.

Heinonen, O.J. 1996. Carnitine and physical exercise. *Sports Med* 22 (2): 109-132.

Helge, J.W., B. Wulff, and B. Kiens. 1998. Impact of a fat-rich diet on endurance in man: Role of the dietary period. *Med Sci Sports Exerc* 30:456-461.

Hemila, H. 2011. Zinc lozenges may shorten the duration of colds: A systematic review. *Open Resp Med J* 5:51-58.

Henry, C.J.K., H.J. Lightowler, C.M. Stirk, H. Renton, and S. Hails. 2005. Glycaemic index and glycaemic load values of commercially available products in the UK. *Br J Nutr* 94:922-930.

Henson, D.A., D.C. Nieman, J.C.D. Parker, M.K. Rainwater, D.E. Butterworth, B.J. Warren, A. Utter, J.M. Davis, O.R. Fagoaga, and S.L. Nehlsen-Cannarella. 1998. Carbohydrate supplementation and the lymphocyte proliferative response to long endurance running. *Int J Sports Med* 19:574-580.

Herbert, V. 1979. Pangamic acid ("vitamin B_{15}"). *Am J Clin Nutr* 32 (7): 1534-1540.

Hertog, M.C.L., E.M. Feskens, P.C.H. Hollman, and M.B. Katan. 1993. Dietary antioxidant flavonoids and risk of coronary heart disease: The Zutphen elderly study. *Lancet* 342:1007-1011.

Hespel, P., Maughan, R.J., and Greenhaff, P.L. 2006. Dietary supplements for football. *J Sports Sci* 24:749-761.

Heymsfield, S.B., R. Smith, M. Aulet, et al. 1990. Appendicular skeletal muscle mass: Measurement by dual-photon absorptiometry. *Am J Clin Nutr* 52 (2): 214-218.

Hickson, M. 2015. Nutritional interventions in sarcopenia: A critical review. *Proc Nutr Soc* 74 (4): 378-386.

Hill, C.A., R.C. Harris, H.J. Kim, B.D. Harris, C. Sale, L.H. Boobis, C.K. Kim, and J.A. Wise. 2007. Influence of beta-alanine supplementation on skeletal muscle carnosine concentrations and high intensity cycling capacity. *Amino Acids* 32 (2): 225-233.

Hinton, P.S., C. Giordano, T. Brownlie, and J.D. Haas. 2000. Iron supplementation improves endurance after training in iron-depleted, nonanemic women. *J Appl Physiol* 88:1103-1111.

Hiscock, N., and B.K. Pedersen. 2002. Exercise-induced immunosuppression—plasma glutamine is not the link. *J Appl Physiol* 93:813-822.

Hobson, R.M., B. Saunders, G.Ball, R.C. Harris, and C. Sale. 2012. Effects of beta-alanine supplementation on exercise performance: A review by meta-analysis. *Amino Acids* 43:25-37.

Hodgson, A.B., R.K. Randell, and A.E. Jeukendrup. 2013. The effect of green tea extract on fat oxidation at rest and during exercise: Evidence of efficacy and proposed mechanisms. *Adv Nutr* 4 (2): 129-140.

Hogervorst, E., S. Bandelow, J. Schmitt, R. Jentjens, M. Oliveira, J. Allgrove, T. Carter, and M. Gleeson. 2008. Caffeine improves physical and cognitive performance during exhaustive exercise. *Med Sci Sports Exerc* 40 (10): 1841-1851.

Hogervorst, E., W.J. Riedel, E. Kovacs, F. Brouns, and J. Jolles. 1999. Caffeine improves cognitive performance after strenuous physical exercise. *Int J Sports Med* 20 (6): 354-361.

Holloszy, J.O., and W. Booth. 1976. Biochemical adaptations to endurance exercise in muscle. *Ann Rev Physiol* 38:273-291.

Holloszy, J.O., and E.F. Coyle. 1984. Adaptations of skeletal muscle to endurance exercise and their metabolic consequences. *J Appl Physiol* 56 (4): 831-838.

Hooper, L., N. Martin, A. Abdelhamid, and G. Davey Smith. 2015. Reduction in saturated fat intake for cardiovascular disease. *Cochrane Database Syst Rev* (June 10): CD011737.

Hopkins, W.G. 2000. Measures of reliability in sports medicine and science. *Sports Med* 30 (1): 1-15.

Hoppeler, H., and M. Fluck. 2003. Plasticity of skeletal muscle mitochondria: Structure and function. *Med Sci Sports Exerc* 35:95-104.

Horowitz, J.F., R. Mora-Rodriguez, L.O. Byerley, and E.F. Coyle. 2000. Preexercise medium-chain triglyceride ingestion does not alter muscle glycogen use during exercise. *J Appl Physiol* 88 (1): 219-225.

Horowitz, J.F., R. Mora-Rodriguez, L.O. Byerley, and E.F. Coyle. 1997. Lipolytic suppression following carbohydrate ingestion limits fat oxidation during exercise. *Am J Physiol* 273:E768-E775.

Horswill, C.A. 1995. Effects of bicarbonate, citrate, and phosphate loading on performance. *Int J Sports Nutr* 5:S111-S119.

Houltham, S.D., and D.S. Rowlands 2014. A snapshot of nitrogen balance in endurance-trained women. *Appl Physiol Nutr Metab* 39 (2): 219-225.

Houmard, J.A., D.L. Costill, J.A. Davis, J.B. Mitchell, D.D. Pascoe, and R.A. Robergs. 1990. The influence of exercise intensity on heat acclimation in trained subjects. *Med Sci Sports Exerc* 22 (5): 615-620.

Howarth, K.R., N.A. Moreau, S.M. Phillips, and M.J. Gibala. 2009. Coingestion of protein with carbohydrate during recovery from endurance exercise stimulates skeletal muscle protein synthesis in humans. *J Appl Physiol* 106 (4): 1394-1402.

Howatson, G., P.G. Bell, J. Tallent, B. Middleton, M.P. McHugh, and J. Ellis. 2012. Effect of tart cherry juice (Prunus cerasus) on melatonin levels and enhanced sleep quality. *Eur J Nutr* 51 (8): 909-916.

Howell, S., and R. Kones. 2017. "Calories in, calories out" and macronutrient intake: The hope, hype, and science of calories. *Am J Physiol Endocrinol Metab.* 313(5):E608-E612.

Hoy, M.K., and J.D. Goldman. 2014. Fiber intake of the U.S. population: What we eat in America, NHANES 2009-2010. Food Surveys Research Group Dietary Data Brief No. 12. September.

Hu, D., J. Huang, Y. Wang, D. Zhang, and Y. Qu. 2014. Fruits and vegetables consumption and risk of stroke: A meta-analysis of prospective cohort studies. *Stroke* 45 (6): 1613-1619.

Hubert, P., N.A. King, and J.E. Blundell. 1998. Uncoupling the effects of energy expenditure and energy intake: Appetite response to short-term energy deficit induced by meal omission and physical activity. *Appetite* 31:9-19.

Hulston, C.J., and A.E. Jeukendrup. 2008. Substrate metabolism and exercise performance with caffeine and carbohydrate intake. *Med Sci Sports Exerc* 40 (12): 2096-2104.

Hultman, E. 1967. Physiological role of muscle glycogen in man, with special reference to exercise. *Circ Res* 10:I99-I114.

Hultman, E., and L.H. Nilsson. 1971. Liver glycogen in man: Effects of different diets and muscular exercise. In *Muscle metabolism during exercise, II,* edited by B. Pernow and B. Saltin, 143-151. New York: Plenum.

Hultman, E., K. Soderlund, J.A. Timmons, G. Cederblad, and P.L. Greenhaff. 1996. Muscle creatine loading in men. *J Appl Physiol* 81 (1): 232-237.

Hultman, E., P.L. Greenhaff, J.M. Ren, and K. Soderlund. 1991. Energy metabolism and fatigue during intense muscle contraction. *Biochem Soc Trans* 19 (2): 347-353.

Hunt, C., N.K. Chakaravorty, G. Annan, N. Habibzadeh, and C.J. Schorah. 1994. The clinical effects of vitamin C supplementation in elderly hospitalized with acute respiratory infections. *Int J Vit Nutr Res* 64:202-207.

Hunt, J.N., and I. Donald. 1954. The influence of volume on gastric emptying. *J Physiol* 126:459-474.

Inbar, O., N. Morris, Y. Epstein, and G. Gass. 2004. Comparison of thermoregulatory responses to exercise in dry heat among prepubertal boys, young adults and older males. *Exp Physiol* 89:691-700.

Inder, W.J., M.P. Swanney, R.A. Donald, T.C.R. Prickett, and J. Hellemans. 1998. The effect of glycerol and desmopressin on exercise performance and hydration in triathletes. *Med Sci Sports Exerc* 30:1263-1269.

Irwin, C., B. Desbrow, A. Ellis, B. O'Keeffe, G. Grant, and M. Leveritt. 2011. Caffeine withdrawal and high-intensity endurance cycling performance. *J Sports Sci* 29:509-515.

Issekutz, B., H.I. Miller, P. Paul, and K. Rodahl. 1964. Source of fat in exercising dogs. *Am J Physiol* 207 (3): 583-589.

Isselbacher, K.J. 1968. Mechanisms of absorption of long and medium chain triglycerides. In *Medium chain triglycerides,* edited by J.R. Senior, 21-37. Philadelphia: University of Pensylvania Press.

Ivy, J.L. 1998. Glycogen resynthesis after exercise: Effect of carbohydrate intake. *Int J Sports Med* 19:S142-S145.

Ivy, J.L., A.L. Katz, C.L. Cutler, W.M. Sherman, and E.F. Coyle. 1988. Muscle glycogen synthesis after exercise: Effect of time of carbohydrate ingestion. *J Appl Physiol* 64:1480-1485.

Ivy, J.L., and C.-H. Kuo. 1998. Regulation of GLUT4 protein and glycogen synthase during musle glycogen synthesis after exercise. *Acta Physiol Scand* 162:295-304.

Ivy, J.L., D.L. Costill, W.J. Fink, and R.W. Lower. 1979. Influence of caffeine and carbohydrate feedings on endurance performance. *Med Sci Sports* 11:6-11.

Ivy, J.L., M.C. Lee, J.T. Brozinick, and M.J. Reed. 1988. Muscle glycogen storage after different amounts of carbohydrate ingestion. *J Appl Physiol* 65:2018-2023.

Ivy, J.L., P.T. Res, R.C. Sprague, and M.O. Widzer. 2003. Effect of a carbohydrate-protein supplement on endurance performance during exercise of varying intensity. *Int J Sport Nutr Exerc Metab* 13 (3): 382-395.

Jackman, M., P. Wendling, D. Friars, and T.E. Graham. 1996. Metabolic catecholamine, and endurance responses to caffeine during intense exercise. *J Appl Physiol* 81 (4): 1658-1663.

Jackson, A.S., and M.L. Pollock. 1978. Generalized equations for predicting body density of men. *Br J Nutr* 40 (3): 497-504.

Jackson, M.J. 2000. Exercise and oxygen radical production by muscle. In *Handbook of oxidants and antioxidants in exercise,* edited by C.K. Sen, L. Packer, and O.P. Hanninnen Osmo, 297-321. Amsterdam: Elsevier.

Jagetia, G.C., and B.B. Aggarwal. 2007. "Spicing up" of the immune system by curcumin. *J Clin Immunol* 27 (1): 19-35.

Jakubowicz, D., N. Beer, and R. Rengifo. 1995. Effect of dehydroepiandrosterone on cyclic-guanosine monophosphate in men of advancing age. *Ann N Y Acad Sci* 774:312-315.

James, L.J., J. Moss, J Henry, C. Papadopoulou, and S.A. Mears. 2017. Hypohydration impairs endurance performance: A blinded study. *Physiol Rep* 5 (12). pii: e13315.

James, R.M., S. Ritchie, I. Rollo, and L.J. James. 2016. No dose response effect of carbohydrate mouth rinse on cycling time-trial performance. *Int J Sport Nutr Exerc Metab* 27:25-31.

Jansson, E., and L. Kaijser. 1982. Effect of diet on the utilization of blood-borne and intramuscular substrates during exercise in man. *Acta Physiol Scand* 115:19-30.

Jeffery, R.W., W.L. Hellerstedt, S.A. French, et al. 1995. A randomized trial of counseling for fat restriction versus calorie restriction in the treatment of obesity. *Int J Obes Relat Metab Disord* 19 (2): 132-137.

Jentjens, R.L., and A.E. Jeukendrup. 2002. Effect of acute and short-term administration of vanadyl sulphate on insulin sensitivity in healthy active humans. *Int J Sport Nutr Exerc Metab* 12 (4): 470-479.

Jentjens, R.L., and A.E. Jeukendrup. 2003. Effects of pre-exercise ingestion of trehalose, galactose and glucose on subsequent metabolism and cycling performance. *Eur J Appl Physiol* 88 (4-5): 459-465.

Jentjens, R.L., and A.E. Jeukendrup. 2005. High rates of exogenous carbohydrate oxidation from a mixture of glucose and fructose ingested during prolonged cycling exercise. *Br J Nutr* 93 (4): 485-492.

Jentjens, R.L., L. Moseley, R.H. Waring, L.K. Harding, and A.E. Jeukendrup. 2004. Oxidation of combined ingestion of glucose and fructose during exercise. *J Appl Physiol* 96 (4): 1277-1284.

Jentjens, R.L., C. Shaw, T. Birtles, R.H. Waring, L.K. Harding, and A.E. Jeukendrup. 2005. Oxidation of combined ingestion of glucose and sucrose during exercise. *Metabolism* 54 (5): 610-618.

Jentjens, R.L., K. Underwood, J. Achten, K. Currell, C.H. Mann, and A.E. Jeukendrup. 2006. Exogenous carbohydrate oxidation rates are elevated after combined ingestion of glucose and fructose during exercise in the heat. *J Appl Physiol* 100 (3): 807-816.

Jentjens, R.L., L.J. van Loon, C.H. Mann, A.J. Wagenmakers, and A.E. Jeukendrup. 2001. Addition of protein and amino acids to carbohydrates does not enhance postexercise muscle glycogen synthesis. *J Appl Physiol* 91 (2): 839-846.

Jentjens, R.L., M.C. Venables, and A.E. Jeukendrup. 2004. Oxidation of exogenous glucose, sucrose, and maltose during prolonged cycling exercise. *J Appl Physiol* 96 (4): 1285-1291.

Jeppesen, J. and B. Kiens. 2012. Regulation and limitations to fatty acid oxidation during exercise. *J Physiol* 590 (5): 1059-1068.

Jeukendrup, A.E. 2002. Regulation of skeletal muscle fat metabolism. *Ann N Y Acad Sci* 967:217-35.

Jeukendrup, A.E. 2004. Carbohydrate intake during exercise and performance. *Nutrition* 20 (7-8): 669-677.

Jeukendrup, A.E. 2008. Carbohydrate feeding during exercise. *Eur J Sport Sci* 8 (2): 77-86.

Jeukendrup, A.E. 2011. Nutrition for endurance sports: Marathon, triathlon, and road cycling. *J Sports Sci* 29 (Suppl 1): S91-S99.

Jeukendrup, A.E. 2013a. Oral carbohydrate rinse: Placebo or beneficial? *Curr Sports Med Rep* 12 (4): 222-227.

Jeukendrup, A. 2013b. The new carbohydrate intake recommendations. *Nestle Nutr Inst Workshop Ser* 75:63-71.

Jeukendrup, A.E. 2014. A step towards personalized sports nutrition: carbohydrate intake during exercise. *Sports Med.* 44 Suppl 1:S25-33.

Jeukendrup, A.E. 2017a. Periodized nutrition for athletes. *Sports Med* 47 (Suppl 1): 51-63.

Jeukendrup, A.E. 2017b. Training the gut for athletes. *Sports Med* 47 (Suppl 1): 101-110.

Jeukendrup, A.E., F. Brouns, A.J.M. Wagenmakers, and W.H.M. Saris. 1997. Carbohydrate-electrolyte feedings improve 1 h time trial cycling performance. *Int J Sports Med* 18 (2): 125-129.

Jeukendrup, A.E., N.P. Craig, and J.A. Hawley. 2000. The bioenergetics of world class cycling. *J Sci Med Sport* 3 (4): 414-433.

Jeukendrup, A.E., M.K.C. Hesselink, A.C. Snyder, H. Kuipers, and H.A. Keizer. 1992. Physiological changes in male competitive cyclists after two weeks of intensified training. *Int J Sports Med* 13:534-541.

Jeukendrup, A.E., and R.L. Jentjens. 2000. Oxidation of carbohydrate feedings during prolonged exercise: Current thoughts, guidelines and directions for future research. *Sports Med* 29 (6): 407-424.

Jeukendrup, A.E., and S.C. Killer. 2010. The myths surrounding pre-exercise carbohydrate feeding. *Ann Nutr Metab* 57 (Suppl 2): 18-25.

Jeukendrup, A.E., L. Moseley, G.I. Mainwaring, S. Samuels, S. Perry, and C.H. Mann. 2006. Exogenous carbohydrate oxidation during ultraendurance exercise. *J Appl Physiol* 100 (4): 1134-1141.

Jeukendrup, A.E., W.H.M. Saris, F. Brouns, and A.D.M. Kester. 1996. A new validated endurance performance test. *Med Sci Sport Exerc* 28 (2): 266-270.

Jeukendrup, A.E., W.H.M. Saris, P. Schrauwen, F. Brouns, and A.J.M. Wagenmakers. 1995. Metabolic availability of medium chain triglycerides co-ingested with carbohydrates during prolonged exercise. *J Appl Physiol* 79 (3): 756-762.

Jeukendrup, A.E., J.J.H.C. Thielen, A.J.M. Wagenmakers, F. Brouns, and W.H.M. Saris. 1998. Effect of MCT and carbohydrate ingestion on substrate utilization and cycling performance. *Am J Clin Nutr* 67:397-404.

Jeukendrup, A.E., K. Vet-Joop, A. Sturk, J.H. Stegen, J. Senden, W.H. Saris, and A.J. Wagenmakers. 2000. Relationship between gastro-intestinal complaints and endotoxaemia, cytokine release and the acute-phase reaction during and after a long-distance triathlon in highly trained men. *Clin Sci (Colch)* 98 (1): 47-55.

Jeukendrup, A.E., A.J. Wagenmakers, J.H. Stegen, A.P. Gijsen, F. Brouns, and W.H. Saris. 1999. Carbohydrate ingestion can completely suppress endogenous glucose production during exercise. *Am J Physiol* 276 (4 Pt 1): E672-E683.

Jeukendrup, A.E., A.J.M. Wagenmakers, L.M.L.A. Van Etten, R.L.P. Jentjens, G.J. Oomen, J.H.C.H. Stegen, P.F. Schoffelen, and W.H.M. Saris. 2000. Negative fat balance in weight stable physically active humans on a low-fat diet. *J Physiol* 523:223P.

Jeukendrup, A.E., and G.A. Wallis. 2005. Measurement of substrate oxidation during exercise by means of gas exchange measurements. *Int J Sports Med* 26 (Suppl 1): S28-S37.

Ji, L.L. 2007. Antioxidant signaling in skeletal muscle: A brief review. *Experimental Gerontology* 42 (7): 582-593.

Johannes, C.B., R.K. Stellato, H.A. Feldman, C. Longcope, and J.B. McKinlay. 1999. Relation of dehydroepiandrosterone and dehydroepiandrosterone sulfate with cardiovascular disease risk factors in women: Longitudinal results from the Massachusetts Women's Health Study. *J Clin Epidemiol* 52 (2): 95-103.

Johansson, L., K. Solvoll, G.E. Bjorneboe, and C.A. Drevon. 1998. Under- and overreporting of energy intake related to weight status and lifestyle in a nationwide sample. *Am J Clin Nutr* 68 (2): 266-274.

Johnstone, A.M. 2007. Fasting—The ultimate diet? *Obesity Rev* 8:211-222.

Jones, A.W., S.J. Cameron, R. Thatcher, M.S. Beecroft, L.A. Mur, and G. Davison. 2014. Effects of bovine colostrum supplementation on upper respiratory illness in active males. *Brain Behav Immun* 39:194-203.

Jones, G. 2008. Caffeine and other sympathomimetic stimulants: Modes of action and effects on sports performance. *Essays Biochem* 44:109-123.

Jongkees, B.J., B. Hommel, S. Kühn, and L.S. Colzato. 2015. Effect of tyrosine supplementation on clinical and healthy populations under stress or cognitive demands—A review. *J Psychiatr Res* 70:50-57.

Jordy, A.B. and B. Kiens. 2014. Regulation of exercise-induced lipid metabolism in skeletal muscle. *Exp Physiol* 99 (12): 1586-1592.

Jouris, K. B., J. L. McDaniel, and E. P. Weiss. 2011. The effect of omega-3 fatty acid supplementation on the inflammatory response to eccentric strength exercise. *J Sports Sci Med* 10:432-438.

Jówko, E., B. Długołecka, B. Makaruk, and I. Cieśliński. 2015. The effect of green tea extract supplementation on exercise-induced oxidative stress parameters in male sprinters. *Eur J Nutr* 54 (5): 783-791.

Jówko, E., P. Ostaszewski, M. Jank, J. Sacharuk, A. Zieniewicz, J. Wilczak, and S. Nissen. 2001. Creatine and beta-hydroxy-beta-methylbutyrate (HMB) additively increase lean body mass and muscle strength during a weight-training program. *Nutrition* 17 (7-8): 558-566.

Jozsi, A.C., T.A. Trappe, R.D. Starling, B. Goodpaster, S.W. Trappe, W.J. Fink, D.L. Costill. 1996. The influence of starch structure on glycogen resynthesis and subsequent cycling performance. *Int J Sports Med* 17 (5): 373-378.

Judelson, D.A., C.M. Maresh, J.M. Anderson, et al. 2007. Hydration and muscular performance: Does fluid balance affect strength, power and high-intensity endurance? *Sports Medicine* 37 (10): 907-921.

Kagan, A., B.R. Harris, W. Winkelstein, Jr., K.G. Johnson, H. Kato, S.L. Syme, G.G. Rhoads, M.L. Gay, M.Z. Nichaman, H.B. Hamilton, and J. Tillotson. 1974. Epidemiologic studies of coronary heart disease and stroke in Japanese men living in Japan, Hawaii and California: Demographic, physical, dietary and biochemical characteristics. *J Chronic Dis* 27 (7-8): 345-364.

Kaiser, K.A., J.M. Shikany, K.D. Keating, and D.B. Allison. 2013. Will reducing sugar-sweetened beverage consumption reduce obesity? Evidence supporting conjecture is strong, but evidence when testing effect is weak. *Obes Rev* 14:620-633.

Kamada, T., S. Tokuda, S.-I. Aozaki, and S. Otsuji. 1993. Higher levels of erethrocyte membrane fluidity in sprinters and long-distance runners. *J Appl Physiol* 74 (1): 354-358.

Kaminski, M., and R. Boal. 1992. An effect of ascorbic acid on delayed-onset muscle soreness. *Pain* 50:317-321.

Kandelman, D. 1997. Sugar, alternative sweeteners and meal frequency in relation to caries prevention: New perspectives. *Br J Nutr* 77 (Suppl 1): S121-S128.

Kantamala, D., M. Vongsakul, and J. Satayavivad. 1990. The in vivo and in vitro effects of caffeine on rat immune cell activities: B, T and NK cells. *Asian Pac J Allergy Immunol* 8:77-82

Karlsson, J., and B. Saltin. 1970. Lactate, ATP, and CP in working muscles during exhaustive exercise in man. *J Appl Physiol* 29 (5): 596-602.

Kasperek, G.J., and R.D. Snider. 1989. Total and myofibrillar protein degradation in isolated soleus muscles after exercise. *Am J Physiol* 257 (1 Pt 1): E1-E5.

Kato, H., K. Suzuki, M. Bannai, and D.R. Moore. 2016. Protein requirements are elevated in endurance athletes after exercise as determined by the indicator amino acid oxidation method. *PLoS One* 11(6):e0157406.

Kazis, K., and E. Iglesias. 2003. The female athlete triad. *Adolesc Med* 14:87-95.

Keeffe, E.B., D.K. Lowe, J.R. Goss, and R. Wayne. 1984. Gastrointestinal symptoms of marathon runners. *West J Med* 141:481-484.

Keesey, R.E., and M.D. Hirvonen. 1997. Body weight set-points: Determination and adjustment. *J Nutr* 127 (9): 1875S-1883S.

Keizer, H., H. Kuipers, and G. van Kranenburg. 1987. Influence of liquid and solid meals on muscle glycogen resynthesis, plasma fuel hormone response, and maximal physical working capacity. *Int J Sports Med* 8:99-104.

Keizer, H., H. Kuipers, G. van Kranenburg, and P. Geurten. 1987. Influence of liquid and solid meals on glycogen resynthesis, plasma fuel hormone response, and maximal physical working capacity. *Int J Sports Med* 8 (2): 99-104.

Kekkonen, R.A., T.J. Vasankari, T. Vuorimaa, et al. 2007. The effects of probiotics on respiratory infections and gastrointestinal symptoms during training in marathon runners. *Int J Sport Nutr Exerc Metabol* 17:352-363.

Kelly, J.M., B.A. Gorney, and K.K. Kalm. 1978. The effects of a collegiate wrestling season on body composition, cardiovascular fitness and muscular strength and endurance. *Med Sci Sports* 10 (2): 119-124.

Keys, A., A. Menotti, M.J. Karvonen, C. Aravanis, H. Blackburn, R. Buzina, B.S. DjordjevicS, A.S. Dontas, F. Fidanza, and M.H. Keys. 1986. The diet and 15-year death rate in the seven countries study. *Am J Epidemiol* 124 (6): 903-915.

Khatta, M., B.S. Alexander, C.M. Krichten, M.L. Fisher, R. Freudenberger, S.W. Robinson, and S.S. Gottlieb. 2000. The effect of coenzyme Q10 in patients with congestive heart failure. *Ann Intern Med* 132 (8): 636-640.

Killer, S.C., I.S. Svendsen, A.E. Jeukendrup, and M. Gleeson. 2015. Evidence of disturbed sleep and mood state in well-trained athletes during short-term intensified training with and without a high carbohydrate nutritional intervention. *J Sports Sci* (September 25): 1-9.

Kim, Y.S., T.J. Sayers, N.H. Colburn, J.A. Milner, and H.A. Young. 2015. Impact of dietary components on NK and Treg cell function for cancer prevention. *Mol Carcinog* 54:669-678.

King, N.A., V.J. Burley, and J.E. Blundell. 1994. Exercise-induced suppression of appetite: Effects on food intake and implications for energy balance. *Eur J Clin Nutr* 48 (10): 715-724.

King, D.S., R.L. Sharp, M.D. Vukovich, G.A. Brown, T.A. Reifenrath, N.L. Uhl, and K.A. Parsons. 1999. Effect of oral androstenedione on serum testosterone and adaptations to resistance training in young men: A randomized controlled trial. *JAMA* 281 (21): 2020-2028.

Kit, B.K., T.H. Fakhouri, S. Park, S.J. Nielsen, and C.L. Ogden. 2013. Trends in sugar-sweetened beverage consumption among youth and adults in the United States: 1999-2010. *Am J Clin Nutr* 98 (1): 180-188.

Klein, S., E.F. Coyle, and R.R. Wolfe. 1994. Fat metabolism during low-intensity exercise in endurance trained and untrained men. *Am J Physiol* 267:E934-E940.

Klein, S., J.-M. Weber, E.F. Coyle, and R.R. Wolfe. 1996. Effect of endurance training on glycerol kinetics during strenuous exercise in humans. *Metabolism* 45 (3): 357-361.

Knapik, J., C. Meredith, B. Jones, R. Fielding, V. Young, and W. Evans. 1991. Leucine metabolism during fasting and exercise. *J Appl Physiol* 70 (1): 43-47.

Knapik, J.J., C.N. Meredith, B.H. Jones, L. Suek, V.R. Young, and W.J. Evans. 1988. Influence of fasting on carbohydrate and fat metabolism during rest and exercise in men. *J Appl Physiol* 64 (5): 1923-1929.

Knapik, J.J., R.A Steelman, S.S. Hoedebecke, K.G. Austin, E.K. Farina, and H.R. Lieberman. 2016. Prevalence of dietary supplement use by athletes: Systematic review and meta-analysis. *Sports Med* 46 (1): 103-123.

Knopf, R.F., J.W. Conn, J.C. Floyd, Jr., S.S. Fajans, J.A. Rull, E.M. Guntsche, and C.A. Thiffault. 1966. The normal endocrine response to ingestion of protein and infusions of amino acids: Sequential secretion of insulin and growth hormone. *Trans Assoc Am Physicians* 79:312-321.

Koenigsberg, P.S., K.K. Martin, H.R. Hlava, and M.L. Riedesel. 1995. Sustained hyperhydration with glycerol ingestion. *Life Sci* 57 (7): 645-653.

Kohrt, W.M. 1995. Body composition by DXA: Tried and true? *Med Sci Sports Exerc* 27 (10): 1349-1353.

Kongsbak M., T.B. Levring, C. Geisler, and M.R. von Essen. 2013. The vitamin d receptor and T cell function. *Front Immunol* 4:148.

Konig, D., A. Berg, C. Weinstock, J. Keul, and H. Northoff. 1997. Essential fatty acids, immune function and exercise. *Exerc Immunol Rev* 3:1-31.

Koopman, R., M. Beelen, T. Stellingwerff, B. Pennings, W.H.M. Saris, A.K. Kies, H. Kuipers, and L.J. van Loon. 2007. Coingestion of carbohydrate with protein does not further augment postexercise muscle protein synthesis. *Am J Physiol Endocrinol Metab* 293:E833-E842.

Koopman, R., D.L. Pannemans, A.E. Jeukendrup, A. Gijsen, J.M.G. Senden, D. Halliday, W.H.M. Saris, L.J.C. van Loon, and A.J.M. Wagenmakers. 2004. Combined ingestion of protein and carbohydrate improves protein balance during ultra-endurance exercise. *Am J Physiol Endocrinol Metab* 287 (4): E712-E720.

Koopman, R., A.J.M. Wagenmakers, R.J.F. Manders, A.H.G. Zorenc, J.M.G. Senden, M. Gorselink, H.A. Keizer, and L.J.C. van Loon. 2005. Combined ingestion of protein and free leucine with carbohydrate increases postexercise muscle protein synthesis in vivo in male subjects. *Am J Physiol Endocrinol Metab* 288 (4): E645-653.

Kopp-Hoolihan, L. 2001. Prophylactic and therapeutic uses of probiotics: A review. *J Am Diet Assoc* 101:229-238.

Koubi, H.E., D. Desplanches, C. Gabrielle, J.M. Cottet-Emard, B. Sempore, and R.J. Favier. 1991. Exercise endurance and fuel utilization: A reevaluation of the effects of fasting. *J Appl Physiol* 70 (3): 1337-1343.

Koulmann, N., C. Jimenez, D. Regal, et al. 2000. Use of bioelectrical impedance analysis to estimate body fluid compartments after acute variations of the body hydration level. *Med Sci Sports Exerc* 32 (4): 857-864.

Kovacs, E.M.R., J.H.C.H. Stegen, and F. Brouns. 1998. Effect of caffeinated drinks on substrate metabolism, caffeine excretion, and performance. *J Appl Physiol* 85:709-715.

Kraemer, W.J., J.F. Patton, S.E. Gordon, et al. 1995. Compatibility of high-intensity strength and endurance training on hormonal and skeletal muscle adaptations. *J Appl Physiol* 78 (3): 976-989.

Krahenbuhl, G.S., and T.J. Williams. 1992. Running economy: Changes with age during childhood and adolescence. *Med Sci Sports Exerc* 24:462-466.

Krajcovicova-Kudlackova M, Buckova K, Klimes I, and E. Seboková. 2003. Iodine deficiency in vegetarians and vegans. *Ann Nutr Metab* 47 (5): 183-185.

Kreider, R.B., M. Ferreira, M. Wilson, P. Grindstaff, S. Plisk, J. Reinardy, E. Cantler, and A.L. Almada. 1998. Effects of creatine supplementation on body composition, strength, and sprint performance. *Med Sci Sports Exerc* 30 (1): 73-82.

Kreider, R.B., G.W. Miller, D. Schenck, C.W. Cortes, V. Miriel, C.T. Somma, P. Rowland, C. Turner, and D. Hill. 1992. Effects of phosphate loading on metabolic and myocardial responses to maximal and endurance exercise. *Int J Sport Nutr* 2 (1): 20-47.

Kreider, R.B., G.W. Miller, M.H. Williams, C.T. Somma, and T.A. Nasser. 1990. Effects of phosphate loading on oxygen uptake, ventilatory anaerobic threshold, and run performance. *Med Sci Sports Exerc* 22 (2): 250-256.

Krentz, E.M., and P. Warschburger. 2011. Sports-related correlates of disordered eating in athletic sports. *Psych Sport Exerc* 12:375-382.

Krogh, A., and J. Lindhard. 1920. The relative value of fat and carbohydrate as sources of muscular energy. *Biochem J* 14:290-363.

Kron, L., J.L. Katz, G. Gorzynski, and H. Weiner. 1978. Hyperactivity in anorexia nervosa: A fundamental clinical feature. *Comp Psych* 19:433-440.

Kuipers, H., W.H.M. Saris, F. Brouns, H.A. Keizer, and C. ten Bosch. 1989. Glycogen synthesis during exercise and rest with carbohydrate feeding in males and females. *Int J Sports Med* 10 (Suppl 1): S63-S67.

Kumanyika, S.K., and J.A. Cutler. 1997. Dietary sodium reduction: Is there cause for concern? *J Am Coll Nutr* 16 (3): 192-203.

Laaksi, I. 2012. Vitamin D and respiratory infection in adults. *Proc Nutr Soc* 71:90-97.

Laaksi, I., J.P. Ruohola, V. Mattila, A. Auvinen, T. Ylikomi, and H. Pihlajamaki. 2010. Vitamin D supplementation for the prevention of acute respiratory tract infection: A randomized, double-blinded trial among young Finnish men. *J Infect Dis* 202:809-814.

Lambert, C.P., D. Ball, J.B. Leiper, and R.J. Maughan. 1999. The use of a deuterium tracer technique to follow the fate of fluids ingested by human subjects: Effects of drink volume and tracer concentration and content. *Exp Physiol* 84 (2): 391-399.

Lambert, M.I., J.A. Hefer, R.P. Millar, and P.W. Macfarlane. 1993. Failure of commercial oral amino acid supplements to increase serum growth hormone concentrations in male body-builders. *Int J Sport Nutr* 3 (3): 298-305.

Lamont, L.S., A.J. McCullough, and S.C. Kalhan. 1999. Comparison of leucine kinetics in endurance-trained and sedentary humans. *J Appl Physiol* 86 (1): 320-325.

Lamprecht, M., ed. 2015. *Antioxidants in sport nutrition*. Boca Raton, FL: CRC Press/Taylor & Francis.

Lancaster, G.I., Q. Khan, P.T. Drysdale, et al. 2005. Effect of prolonged exercise and carbohydrate ingestion on type 1 and type 2 lymphocyte distribution and intracellular cytokine production in humans. *J Appl Physiol* 98:565-571.

Lancha Jr, A.H., S. Painelli Vde, B. Saunders, and G.G. Artioli. 2015. Nutritional strategies to modulate intracellular and extracellular buffering capacity during high-intensity exercise. *Sports Med* 45 (Suppl 1): S71-S81.

Lane, S.C., S.R. Bird, L.M. Burke, and J.A. Hawley. 2013. Effect of a carbohydrate mouth rinse on simulated cycling time-trial performance commenced in a fed or fasted state. *Appl Physiol Nutr Metab* 38:134-9.

Lane, S.C., J.A. Hawley, B. Desbrow, A.M. Jones, J.R. Blackwell, M.L. Ross, A.J. Zemski, and L.M. Burke. 2014. Single and combined effects of beetroot juice and caffeine supplementation on cycling time trial performance. *Appl Physiol Nutr Metab* 39 (9): 1050-1057.

Lang, F., G.L. Busch, M. Ritter, H. Volkl, S. Waldegger, E. Gulbins, and D. Haussinger. 1998. Functional significance of cell volume regulatory mechanisms. *Physiol Rev* 78 (1): 247-306.

Lanou, A.J., and N.D. Barnard. 2008. Dairy and weight loss hypothesis: An evaluation of the clinical trials. *Nutr Rev* 66 (5): 272-279.

Lansley, K.E., P.G. Winyard, S.J. Bailey, A. Vanhatalo, D.P. Wilkerson, J.R. Blackwell, M. Gilchrist, N. Benjamin, and A.M. Jones 2011. Acute dietary nitrate supplementation improves cycling time trial performance. *Med Sci Sports Exerc* 43 (6): 1125-1131.

Lansley, K.E., Winyard, P.G., Fulford, J., Vanhatalo, A., Bailey, S.J., Blackwell, J.R., DiMenna, F.J., Gilchrist, M., Benjamin, N., and Jones, A.M. 2011. Dietary nitrate supplementation reduces the O_2 cost of walking and running: A placebo-controlled study. *J Appl Physiol* 110 (3): 591-600.

Larsen, F.J., Schiffer, T.A., Borniquel, S., Sahlin, K., Ekblom, B., Lundberg, J.O., and Weitzberg, E. 2011. Dietary inorganic nitrate improves mitochondrial efficiency in humans. *Cell Metab* 13 (2): 149-159.

Larsen, F.J., Weitzberg, E., Lundberg, J.O., and Ekblom, B. 2007. Effects of dietary nitrate on oxygen cost during exercise. *Acta Physiol (Oxf)* 191 (1): 59-66.

Latzka, W.A., M.N. Sawka, S.J. Montain, G.S. Skrinar, R.A. Fielding, R.P. Matott, and K.B. Pandolf. 1997. Hyperhydration: Thermoregulatory effects during compensable exercise-heat stress. *J Appl Physiol* 83 (3): 860-866.

Latzka, W.A., M.N. Sawka, S.J. Montain, G.S. Skrinar, R.A. Fielding, R.P. Matott, and K.B. Pandolf. 1998. Hyperhydration: Tolerance and cardiovascular effects during uncompensable exercise-heat stress. *J Appl Physiol* 84:1858-1864.

Layman, D., and D. Walker. 2006. Potential importance of leucine in treatment of obesity and the metabolic syndrome. *J Nutr* 136 (1 Suppl): 319S-323S.

Lebenstedt, M., P. Platte, and K.M. Pirke. 1999. Reduced resting metabolic rate in athletes with menstrual disorders. *Med Sci Sports Exerc* 31 (9): 1250-1256.

Ledikwe, J.H., H.M. Blanck, L. Kettel Khan, M.K. Serdula, J.D. Seymour, B.C. Tohill, and B.J. Rolls. 2006. Dietary energy density is associated with energy intake and weight status in US adults. *American Journal of Clinical Nutrition* 83 (6): 1362-1368.

Leenders, N.M., D.R. Lamb, and T.E. Nelson. 1999. Creatine supplementation and swimming performance. *Int J Sport Nutr* 9 (3): 251-262.

Lee-Young, R.S., M.J. Palmer, K.C. Linden, K. LePlastrier, B.J. Canny, M. Hargreaves, G.D. Wadley, B.E. Kemp, and G.K. McConell. 2006. Carbohydrate ingestion does not alter skeletal muscle AMPK signaling during exercise in humans. *Am J Physiol Endocrinol Metab* 291:E566-E573.

Leibel, R.L., M. Rosenbaum, and J. Hirsch. 1995. Changes in energy expenditure resulting from altered body weight. *N Engl J Med* 332 (10): 621-628.

Leiper, J.B., N.P. Broad, and R.J. Maughan. 2001. Effect of intermittent high-intensity exercise on gastric emptying in man. *Med Sci Sports Exerc* 33 (8): 1270-1278.

Leiper, J.B., A.S. Prentice, C. Wrightson, and R.J. Maughan. 2001. Gastric emptying of a carbohydrate-electrolyte drink during a soccer match. *Med Sci Sports Exerc* 33 (11): 1932-1938.

Lemos, T., and D. Gallagher. 2017. Current body composition measurement techniques. *Curr Opin Endocrinol Diabetes Obes* 24 (5): 310-314.

Lepers, R., B. Knechtle, and P.J. Stapley. 2013. Trends in triathlon performance: Effects of sex and age. *Sports Med* 43:851-863.

Levine, S.A., B. Gordon, and C.L. Derick. 1924. Some changes in chemical constituents of blood following a marathon race. *JAMA* 82:1778-1779.

Lichtenstein, A.H. 2014. Dietary trans fatty acids and cardiovascular disease risk: Past and present. *Curr Atheroscler Rep* 16 (8): 433.

Lichtenstein, A.H., L.M. Ausman, S.M. Jalbert, and E.J. Schaefer. 1999. Effects of different forms of dietary hydrogenated fats on serum lipoprotein cholesterol levels. *N Engl J Med* 340 (25): 1933-1940.

Lieberman, H.R. 2003. Nutrition, brain function and cognitive performance. *Appetite* 40 (3): 245-254.

Lin, J., K.M. Rexrode, F. Hu, C.M. Albert, C.U. Chae, E.B. Rimm, M.J. Stampfer, and J.E. Manson. 2007. Dietary intakes of flavonols and flavones and coronary heart disease in US women. *Am J Epidemiol* 165 (11): 1305-1313.

Linde, K., B. Barrett, K. Wolkart, R. Bauer, and D. Melcahrt. 2006. Echinacea for preventing and treating the common cold. *Cochrane Database Syst Rev* (February 20): CD000530.

Linderman, J.K., and K.L. Gosselink. 1994. The effects of sodium bicarbonate ingestion on exercise performance. *Sports Med* 18 (2): 75-80.

Liu, X.M., Y.J. Liu, Y. Huang, H.J. Yu, S. Yuan, B.W. Tang, P.G. Wang, and Q.Q. He. 2017. Dietary total flavonoids intake and risk of mortality from all causes and cardiovascular disease in the general population: A systematic review and meta-analysis of cohort studies. *Mol Nutr Food Res* (January 5). http://doi.org/10.1002/mnfr.201601003.

Lohman, T.G., and S.B. Going. 1993. Multicomponent models in body composition research: Opportunities and pitfalls. *Basic Life Sci* 60:53-58.

Loucks, A. 2006. The evolution of the female athlete triad. In *Clinical sports nutrition,* 3rd ed., edited by L. Burke and V. Deakin, 227-235. New York: McGraw-Hill.

Loucks, A.B. 2004. Energy balance and body composition in sports and exercise. *J Sports Sci* 22 (1): 1-14.

Loucks, A.B., B. Kiens, and H.H. Wright. 2011. Energy availability in athletes. *J Sports Sci* 29 (Suppl 1): S7-S15.

Loucks, A.B., and J.R. Thuma. 2003. Luteinizing hormone pulsatility is disrupted at a threshold of energy availability in regularly menstruating women. *J Clin Endocr Metab* 88:297-311.

Loy, S.F., R.K. Conlee, W.W. Winder, A.G. Nelson, D.A. Arnall, and A.G. Fisher. 1986. Effect of 24-hour fast on cycling endurance time at two different intensities. *J Appl Physiol* 61 (2): 654-659.

Lukaski, H.C., W.W. Bolonchuk, W.A. Siders, and D.B. Milne. 1996. Chromium supplementation and resistance training: Effects on body composition, strength, and trace element status of men. *Am J Clin Nutr* 63 (6): 954-965.

Lyons, T.P., M.L. Riedesel, L.E. Meuli, and T.W. Chick. 1990. Effects of glycerol-induced hyperhydration prior to exercise in the heat on sweating and core temperature. *Med Sci Sports Exerc* 22 (4): 477-483.

Mackinnon, L.T. 1999. *Advances in exercise and immunology.* Champaign, IL: Human Kinetics.

Macknin, M.L. 1999. Zinc lozenges for the common cold. *Cleveland Clin J Med* 66:27-32.

MacLaren, D., and Morton, J. 2011. *Biochemistry for sport and exercise metabolism.* London: Wiley.

MacLean, D.A., T.E. Graham, and B. Saltin. 1994. Branched-chain amino acids augment ammonia metabolism while attenuating protein breakdown during exercise. *Am J Physiol* 267 (6 Pt 1): E1010-E1022.

Macnaughton, L.S., S.L. Wardle, O.C. Witard, C. McGlory, D.L Hamilton, S. Jeromson, C.E. Lawrence, G.A. Wallis, and K.D. Tipton. 2016. The response of muscle protein synthesis following whole-body resistance exercise is greater following 40 g than 20 g of ingested whey protein. *Physiol Rep* 4 (15): e12893.

MacRae, H., and K.M. Mefferd. 2006. Dietary antioxidant supplementation combined with quercetin improves cycling time trial performance. *Int J Sport Nutr Exerc Metab* 16 (4): 405-419.

Madsen, K., D.A. MacLean, B. Kiens, and D. Christensen. 1996. Effects of glucose, glucose plus branched-chain amino acids, or placebo on bike performance over 100 km. *J Appl Physiol* 81 (6): 2644-2650.

Malik, V.S., A. Pan, W.C. Willett, and F.B. Hu. 2013. Sugar-sweetened beverages and weight gain in children and adults: A systematic review and meta-analysis. *Am J Clin Nutr* 98:1084-1102.

Malik, V.S., M.B. Schulze, and F.B. Hu. 2006. Intake of sugar-sweetened beverages and weight gain: A systematic review. *Am J Clin Nutr* 84:274-288.

Maliszewski, A.F., and P.S. Freedson. 1996. Is running economy different between children and adults? *Ped Exerc Sci* 8:351-360.

Malm, C., M. Svensson, B. Ekblom, and B. Sjodin. 1997. Effects of ubiquinone-10 supplementation and high intensity training on physical performance in humans. *Acta Physiol Scand* 161 (3): 379-384.

Mannix, E.T., J.M. Stager, A. Harris, and M.O. Farber. 1990. Oxygen delivery and cardiac output during exercise following oral phosphate-glucose. *Med Sci Sports Exerc* 22 (3): 341-347.

Manore, M.M. 2000. Effect of physical activity on thiamine, riboflavin, and vitamin B-6 requirements. *Am J Clin Nutr* 72:598S-606S.

Manore, M.M. 2002. Dietary recommendations and athletic menstrual dysfunction. *Sports Med* 32:887-901.

Marchbank, T., G. Davison, J.R. Oakes, M.A. Ghatei, M. Patterson, M.P. Moyer, and R.J. Playford. 2011. The neutraceutical bovine colostrum truncates the increase in gut permeability caused by heavy exercise in athletes. *Am J Gastrointest Liver Physiol* 300:G477-G484.

Marmy-Conus, N., S. Fabris, J. Proietto, and M. Hargreaves. 1996. Preexercise glucose ingestion and glucose kinetics during exercise. *J Appl Physiol* 81 (2): 853-857.

Marshall, I. 2000. Zinc for the common cold. *Cochrane Database Syst Rev 2:*CD001364.

Martin, B., S. Robinson, and D. Robertshaw. 1978. Influence of diet on leg uptake of glucose during heavy exercise. *Am J Clin Nutr* 31:62-67.

Martin, C.K., L.K. Heilbronn, L. de Jonge, J.P. DeLany, J. Volaufova, S.D. Anton, L.M. Redman, S.R. Smith, and E. Ravussin. 2007. Effect of calorie restriction on resting metabolic rate and spontaneous physical activity. *Obesity (Silver Spring)* 15 (12): 2964-2973.

Martinsen, M., S. Bratland-Sanda, A.K. Eriksson, et al. 2010. Dieting to win or to be thin? A study of dieting and disordered eating among adolescent elite athletes and nonathlete controls. *Br J Sports Med* 44 (1): 70-76.

Matsakas, A., and Patel, K. 2009. Intracellular signalling pathways regulating the adaptation of skeletal muscle to exercise and nutritional changes. *Histol Histopathol* 24:209-222.

Matson, L.G., and Z. Vu Tran. 1993. Effects of sodium bicarbonate ingestion on anaerobic performance: A meta-analytic review. *Int J Sport Nutrition* 3:2-28.

Matsuzaki, T. 1998. Immunomodulation by treatment with Lactobacillus casei strain Shirota. *Int J Food Microbiol* 41 (2): 133-140.

Matthews, C.E., I.S. Ockene, P.S. Freedson, M.C. Rosal, P.A. Merriam, and J.R. Hebert. 2002. Moderate to vigorous physical activity and the risk of upper-respiratory tract infection. *Med Sci Sports Exerc* 34:1242-1248.

Matthews, D.E. 1999. Proteins and amino acids. In *Modern nutrition in health and disease,* edited by M.E. Shils, J.A. Olson, M. Shike, and A.C. Ross, 11-30. Baltimore: Williams & Wilkins.

Maughan, R.J. 1985. Thermoregulation and fluid balance in marathon competition at low ambient temperature. *Int J Sports Med* 6:15-19.

Maughan, R.J. 1991. Fluid and electrolyte loss and replacement in exercise. *J Sports Sci* 9:117-142.

Maughan, R.J., L.M. Burke, J. Dvorak, D.E. Larson-Meyer, P. Peeling, S.M. Phillips, E.S. Rawson, N.P. Walsh, I. Garthe, H. Geyer, R. Meeusen, L.J.C. van Loon, S.M. Shirreffs, L.L. Spriet, M. Stuart, A. Vernec, K. Currell, V.M. Ali, R.G. Budgett, A. Ljungqvist, M. Mountjoy, Y.P. Pitsiladis, T. Soligard, U. Erdener, and L. Engebretsen. 2018. IOC consensus statement: Dietary supplements and the high-performance athlete. *Br J Sports Med* 52 (7): 439-455.

Maughan, R.J., A.E. Donnelly, M. Gleeson, P.H. Whiting, K.A. Walker, and P.J. Clough. 1989. Delayed-onset muscle damage and lipid peroxidation in man after a downhill run. *Muscle Nerve* 12:332-336.

Maughan, R.J., C.E. Fenn, M. Gleeson, and J.B. Leiper. 1987. Metabolic and circulatory responses to the ingestion of glucose polymer and glucose/electrolyte solutions during exercise in man. *Eur J Appl Physiol* 56:356-362.

Maughan, R.J., and M. Gleeson. 1988. Influence of a 36 h fast followed by refeeding with glucose, glycerol or placebo on metabolism and performance during prolonged exercise in man. *Eur J Appl Physiol* 57 (5): 570-576.

Maughan, R.J., and M. Gleeson. 2004. *The biochemical basis of sports performance.* Oxford: Oxford University Press.

Maughan, R.J., and M. Gleeson. 2010. *The biochemical basis of sports performance.* 2nd ed. Oxford: Oxford University Press.

Maughan, R.J., M. Gleeson, P.L. Greenhaff. 1997. *Biochemistry of exercise and training.* Oxford: Oxford University Press.

Maughan, R.J., P.L. Greenhaff, J.B. Leiper, D. Ball, C.P. Lambert, and M. Gleeson. 1997. Diet composition and the performance of high-intensity exercise. *J Sports Sci* 15 (3): 265-275.

Maughan, R.J., J.B. Leiper, and S.M. Shirreffs. 1996. Restoration of fluid balance after exercise-induced dehydration: Effects of food and fluid intake. *Eur J Appl Physiol* 73:317-325.

Maughan, R.J., and R. Murray, eds. 2000. *Sports drinks: Basic science and practical aspects.* Boca Raton, FL: CRC Press.

Maughan, R.J., and D.J. Sadler. 1983. The effects of oral administration of salts of aspartic acid on the metabolic response to prolonged exhausting exercise in man. *Int J Sports Med* 4 (2): 119-123.

Maughan, R.J., and S.M. Shirreffs. 2011. IOC consensus conference on nutrition in sport, 25-27 October 2010, International Olympic Committee, Lausanne, Switzerland. *J Sports Sci* 29 (Suppl 1): S1.

Maughan, R.J., C. Williams, D.M. Campbell, and D. Hepburn. 1978. Fat and carbohydrate metabolism during low intensity exercise: Effects of the availability of muscle glycogen. *Eur J Appl Physiol* 39:7-16.

McCarty, M.F. 1996. Chromium (III) picolinate (letter). *FASEB J* 10 (2): 365-369.

McDowall, J.A. 2007. Supplement use by young athletes. *J Sports Sci Med* 6:337-342.

McElroy, B.H., and S.P. Miller. 2002. Effectiveness of zinc gluconate glycine lozenges (Cold-Eeze) against the common cold in school-aged subjects: A retrospective chart review. *Am J Ther* 9:472-475.

McFarlin, B.K., K.C. Carpenter, T. Davidson, and M.A. McFarlin. 2013. Baker's yeast beta glucan supplementation increases salivary IgA and decreases cold/flu symptomatic days after intense exercise. *J Diet Suppl* 10(3): 171-183.

McGee, S.L., K.F. Howlett, R.L. Starkie, D. Cameron-Smith, B.E. Kemp, and M. Hargreaves. 2003. Exercise increases nuclear AMPK alpha2 in human skeletal muscle. *Diabetes* 52:926-928.

McLay, R.T., C.D. Thomson, S.M. Williams, and N.J. Rehrer. 2007. Carbohydrate loading and female endurance athletes: Effect of menstrual-cycle phase. *Int J Sport Nutr Exerc Metab* 17 (2): 189-205.

McLellan, T.M., and D.G. Bell. 2004. The impact of prior coffee consumption on the subsequent ergogenic effect of anhydrous caffeine. *Int J Sport Nutr Exerc Metab* 14 (6): 698-708.

McLellan, T.M., S.M. Pasakios, and H.R. Lieberman. 2014. Effects of protein in combination with carbohydrate supplements on acute or repeat endurance exercise performance: A systematic review. *Sports Med* 44 (4): 535-550.

McMurray, R.G., V. Ben-Ezra, W.A. Forsythe, et al. 1985. Responses of endurance-trained subjects to caloric deficits induced by diet or exercise. *Med Sci Sports Exerc* 17 (5): 574-579.

McNaughton, L.R. 1990. Sodium citrate and anaerobic performance: Implications of dosage. *Eur J Appl Physiol* 61 (5-6): 392-397.

McNaughton, L., and R. Cedaro. 1992. Sodium citrate ingestion and its effects on maximal anaerobic exercise of different durations. *Eur J Appl Physiol* 64 (1): 36-41.

McNaughton, L., B. Dalton, and G. Palmer. 1999. Sodium bicarbonate can be used as an ergogenic aid in high-intensity, competitive cycle ergometry of 1 h duration. *Eur J Appl Physiol* 80 (1): 64-69.

McNaughton, L., B. Dalton, and J. Tarr. 1999. Inosine supplementation has no effect on aerobic or anaerobic cycling performance. *Int J Sport Nutr* 9:333-344.

Meeusen, R., M. Duclos, C. Foster, A. Fry, M. Gleeson, D. Nieman, J. Raglin, G. Rietjens, J. Steinacker, and A. Urhausen. 2013. Prevention, diagnosis, and treatment of the overtraining syndrome: Joint consensus statement of the European College of Sport Science and the American College of Sports Medicine. *Med Sci Sports Exerc* 45 (1): 186-205.

Mendenhall, L.A., Swanson, S.C., Hasbash, D.L., and Coggan, A.R. 1994. Ten days of exercise training reduces glucose production and utilization during moderate-intensity exercise. *Am J Physiol* 266 (1 Pt 1): E136-E143.

Meneton, P., X. Jeunemaitre, H.E. de Wardener, and G.A. MacGregor. 2005. Links between dietary salt intake, renal salt handling, blood pressure, and cardiovascular diseases. *Physiol Rev* 85:679-715.

Mengheri, E. 2008. Health, probiotics and inflammation. *J Clin Gastroenterol* 42 (2): S177-S178.

Mensink, R.P., and M.B. Katan. 1990. Effect of dietary trans fatty acids on high-density and low-density lipoprotein cholesterol levels in healthy subjects. *N Engl J Med* 323 (7): 439-445.

Meydani, M., W.J. Evans, A. Handleman, R.A. Biddle, R.A. Fielding, S.N. Meydani, et al. 1993. Protective effect of vitamin E on exercise-induced oxidative damage in young and older adults. *Am J Physiol* 264:R992-R998.

Meyer, F., H. O'Connor, and S.M. Shirreffs. 2007. Nutrition for the young athlete. *J Sports Sci* 25 (Suppl 1): S73-S82.

Michalska, A., N. Szejko, A. Jakubczyk, and M. Wojnar. 2016. Nonspecific eating disorders: A subjective review. *Psychiatr Pol* 50 (3): 497-507.

Mickleborough, T.D., S.K. Head, and M.R. Lindley. 2011. Exercise-induced asthma: Nutritional management. *Curr Sports Med Rep* 10 (4): 197-202.

Mikkelsen, P.B., S. Toubro, and A. Astrup. 2000. Effect of fat-reduced diets on 24-h energy expenditure: Comparisons between animal protein, vegetable protein, and carbohydrate. *Am J Clin Nutr* 72 (5): 1135-1141.

Miller, S.L., K.D. Tipton, D.L. Chinkes, S.E. Wolf, and R.R. Wolfe. 2003. Independent and combined effects of amino acids and glucose after resistance exercise. *Med Sci Sports Exerc* 35 (3): 449-455.

Miller, W.C., R. Bryce, and R.K. Conlee. 1984. Adaptations to a high-fat diet that increase exercise endurance in male rats. *J Appl Physiol* 56 (1): 78-83.

Minocha, A. 2009. Probiotics for preventive health. *Nutr Clin Prac* 24 (2): 227-241.

Mishell, D.R. 1993. Non-contraceptive benefits of oral contraceptives. *J Reprod Med* 38:1021-1029.

Mitchell, C.J., T.A. Churchward-Venne, D.D. West, N.A. Burd, L. Breen, S.K. Baker, and S.M. Phillips. 2012. Resistance exercise load does not determine training-mediated hypertrophic gains in young men. *J Appl Physiol* 113:71-77.

Mitchell, J.B., F.X. Pizza, A. Paquet, J.B. Davis, M.B. Forrest, and W.A. Braun. 1998. Influence of carbohydrate status on immune responses before and after endurance exercise. *J Appl Physiol* 84:1917-1925.

Modlesky, C.M., K.J. Cureton, R.D. Lewis, et al. 1996. Density of the fat-free mass and estimates of body composition in male weight trainers. *J Appl Physiol* 80 (6): 2085-2096.

Molfino, A., G. Gioia, F. Rossi Fanelli, and M. Muscaritoli. 2013.Beta-hydroxy-beta-methylbutyrate supplementation in health and disease: A systematic review of randomized trials. *Amino Acids* 45 (6): 1273-1292.

Montagnani, G.F., B. Arena, and N. Maffulli. 1992. Oestradiol and progesterone during exercise in healthy untrained women. *Med Sci Sports Exerc* 24:764-768.

Montain, S.J., M.K. Hopper, A.R. Coggan, and E.F. Coyle. 1991. Exercise metabolism at different time intervals after a meal. *J Appl Physiol* 70 (2): 882-888.

Monteleone, P., L. Beinat, C. Tanzillo, M. Maj, and D. Kemali. 1990. Effects of phosphatidylserine on the neuroendocrine response to physical stress in humans. *Neuroendocrinology* 52 (3): 243-248.

Monteleone, P., M. Maj, L. Beinat, M. Natale, and D. Kemali. 1992. Blunting by chronic phosphatidylserine administration of the stress-induced activation of the hypothalamo-pituitary-adrenal axis in healthy men. *Eur J Clin Pharmacol* 42 (4): 385-388.

Moore, D.R., T.A. Churchward-Venne, O. Witard, L. Breen, N.A. Burd, K.D. Tipton, and S.M. Phillips. 2015. Protein ingestion to stimulate myofibrillar protein synthesis requires greater relative protein intakes in healthy older versus younger men. *J Gerontol Ser A Biol Sci Med Sci* 70:57-62.

Moore, D.R., N.C. Del Bel, K.I. Nizi, J.W. Hartman, J.E. Tang, D. Armstrong, and SM. Phillips. 2007. Resistance training reduces fasted- and fed-state leucine turnover and increases dietary nitrogen retention in previously untrained young men. *J Nutr* 137 (4) :985-991.

Moore, D.R., M.J. Robinson, J.L. Fry, J.E. Tang, E.I. Glover, S.B. Wilkinson, T. Prior, M.A. Tarnopolsky, and S.M. Phillips. 2009. Ingested protein dose response of muscle and albumin protein synthesis after resistance exercise in young men. *Am J Clin Nutr* 89 (1): 161-168.

Mooren, F.C. 2015. Nutritional supplements in sport, exercise and health. In *An A-Z guide,* edited by L.M. Castell, S.J. Stear, and L.M. Burke, 178-179. London: Routledge.

Moran, D.S., J.P. McClung, T. Kohen, and H.R. Lieberman. 2013. Vitamin D and physical performance. *Sports Med* 43:601-611.

Morrison, M.A., L.L. Spriet, and D.J. Dyck. 2000. Pyruvate ingestion for 7 days does not improve aerobic performance in well-trained individuals. *J Appl Physiol* 89:549-556.

Mortola, J.F., and S.S. Yen. 1990. The effects of oral dehydroepiandrosterone on endocrine-metabolic parameters in postmenopausal women. *J Clin Endocrinol Metab* 71 (3): 696-704.

Morton, J.F., and J.F. Guthrie. 1998. Changes in children's total fat intakes and their group sources of fat, 1989-91 versus 1994-95: Implications for diet quality. *Fam Econ Nutr Rev* 11:44-57.

Morton, J.P., Z. Iqbal, B. Drust, D. Burgess, G.L. Close, and P.D. Brukner. 2012. Seasonal variation in vitamin D status in professional soccer players of the English Premier League. *Appl Physiol Nutr Metab* 37(4): 798-802.

Morton, R.W., C. McGlory, and S.M. Phillips. 2015. Nutritional interventions to augment resistance training-induced skeletal muscle hypertrophy. *Front Physiol* 6: 245.

Moseley, L., G.I. Lancaster, and A.E. Jeukendrup. 2003. Effects of timing of pre-exercise ingestion of carbohydrate on subsequent metabolism and cycling performance. *Eur J Appl Physiol* 88 (4-5): 453-458.

Mosley, M., and Spencer, M. 2014. *The fast diet: Lose weight, stay healthy, live longer*. New York: Atria Books.

Mosley P.E. 2009. Bigorexia: Bodybuilding and muscle dysmorphia. *Eur Eat Disord Rev* 17 (3): 191-198.

Mountjoy, M., J. Sundgot-Borgen, L. Burke, S. Carter, N. Constantini, C. Lebrun, N. Meyer, R. Sherman, K. Steffen, R. Budgett, and A. Ljungqvist. 2014. The IOC consensus statement: Beyond the Female Athlete Triad—Relative Energy Deficiency in Sport (RED-S). *Br J Sports Med* 48 (7): 491-497.

Mourier, A., A.X. Bigard, E. de Kerviler, B. Roger, H. Legrand, and C.Y. Guezennec. 1997. Combined effects of caloric restriction and branched-chain amino acid supplementation on body composition and exercise performance in elite wrestlers. *Int J Sports Med* 18 (1): 47-55.

Mujika, I., J.C. Chatard, L. Lacoste, F. Barale, and A. Geyssant. 1996. Creatine supplementation does not improve sprint performance in competitive swimmers. *Med Sci Sports Exerc* 28 (11): 1435-1441.

Murray, K.O., H.L. Paris, A.D. Fly, R.F. Chapman, T.D. Mickleborough. Carbohydrate mouth rinse improves cycling time-trial performance without altering plasma insulin concentration. *J Sports Sci Med.* 17:145-152.

Murray, R., D.E. Eddy, G.L. Paul, J.G. Seifert, and G.A. Halaby. 1991. Physiological responses to glycerol ingestion during exercise. *J Appl Physiol* 71 (1): 144-149.

Murray, A.J., N.S. Knight, M.A. Cole, L.E. Cochlin, E. Carter, K. Tchabanenko, T. Pichulik, M.K. Gulston, H.J. Atherton, M.A. Schroeder, R.M. Deacon, Y. Kashiwaya, M.T. King, R. Pawlosky, J.N. Rawlins, D.J. Tyler, J.L. Griffin, J. Robertson, R.L. Veech, and K. Clarke. 2016. Novel ketone diet enhances physical and cognitive performance. *FASEB J* 30 (12): 4021-4032.

Mursu, J., S. Voutilainen, T. Nurmi, T.P. Tuomainen, S. Kurl, and J.T. Salonen. 2008. Flavonoid intake and the risk of ischaemic stroke and CVD mortality in middle-aged Finnish men: The Kuopio Ischaemic Heart Disease Risk Factor Study. *Br J Nutr* 100 (4): 890-895.

Myburgh, K.H. 2014. Polyphenol supplementation: Benefits for exercise performance or oxidative stress? *Sports Med* (Suppl 1): S57-S70.

Myburgh, K.H., L.K. Bachrach, and B. Lewis. 1993. Low bone mineral density at axial and appendicular sites in amenorrhoeic athletes. *Med Sci Sports Exerc* 25:1197-1202.

Myerson, M., B. Gutin, M.P. Warren, et al. 1991. Resting metabolic rate and energy balance in amenorrheic and eumenorrheic runners. *Med Sci Sports Exerc* 23 (1): 15-22.

Nachtigall, D., P. Nielsen, R. Fischer, R. Engelgardt, and E.E. Gabbe. 1996. Iron deficiency in distance runners: A reinvestigation using 59Fe-labelling and non-invasive liver iron quantification. *Int J Sports Med* 17:473-479.

Naclerio, F., E. Larumbe-Zabala, R. Cooper, A. Jimenez, and M. Goss-Sampson. 2014. Effect of a carbohydrate-protein multi-ingredient supplement on intermittent sprint performance and muscle damage in recreational athletes. *Appl Physiol Nutr Metab* 39 (10): 1151-1158.

Nadel, E.R., E. Cafarelli, M.F. Roberts, and C.B. Wenger. 1979. Circulatory regulation during exercise in different ambient temperatures. *J Appl Physiol* 46:430-437.

Nadel, E.R., S.M. Fortney, and C.B. Wenger. 1980. Effect of hydration state on circulatory and thermal regulations. *J Appl Physiol* 49:715-721.

Nagao, F., M. Nakayama, T. Muto, and K. Okumura. 2000. Effects of a fermented milk drink containing Lactobacillus casei strain Shirota on the immune system in healthy human subjects. *Biosci Biotechnol Biochem* 64 (12): 2706-2708.

Nair, K.S., D.E. Matthews, S.L. Welle, and T. Braiman. 1992. Effect of leucine on amino acid and glucose metabolism in humans. *Metabolism* 41 (6): 643-648.

Narkar, V.A., M. Downes, R.T. Yu, E. Embler, Y.X. Wang, E. Banayo, M.M. Mihaylova, M.C. Nelson, Y. Zou, H. Juguilon, H. Kang, R.J. Shaw, and R.M. Evans. 2008. AMPK and PPARdelta agonists are exercise mimetics. *Cell* 134:405-415.

Nattiv, A., A.B. Loucks, M.M. Manore, C.F. Sanborn, J. Sundgot-Borgen, M.P.Warren, and American College of Sports Medicine. 2007. American College of Sports Medicine position stand. The female athlete triad. *Med Sci Sports Exerc* 39 (10): 1867-1882.

Nehlsen-Cannarella, S.L., O.R. Fagoaga, D.C. Nieman, D.A. Henson, D.E. Butterworth, R.L. Schmitt, E.M. Bailey, B.J. Warren, A. Utter, and J.M. Davis. 1997. Carbohydrate and the cytokine response to 2.5 h of running. *J Appl Physiol* 82:1662-1667.

Nelson, J.L., and R.A. Rogbergs. 2007. Exploring the potential ergogenic effects of glycerol hyperhydration. *Sports Medicine* 37 (11): 981-1000.

Nestler, J.E., C.O. Barlascini, J.N. Clore, and W.G. Blackard. 1988. Dehydroepiandrosterone reduces serum low density lipoprotein levels and body fat but does not alter insulin sensitivity in normal men. *J Clin Endocrinol Metab* 66 (1): 57-61.

Neufer, P.D., A.J. Young, and M.N. Sawka. 1989. Gastric emptying during exercise: Effects of heat stress and hypohydration. *Eur J Appl Physiol* 58:433-439.

Neville, V., M. Gleeson, and J.P. Folland. 2008. Salivary IgA as a risk factor for upper respiratory infections in elite professional athletes. *Med Sci Sports Exerc* 40:1228-1236.

Newsholme, E.A., I.N. Acworth, and E. Blomstrand. 1987. Amino acids, brain neurotransmitters and a functional link between muscle and brain that is important in sustained exercise. In *Advances in myochemistry,* edited by G. Benzi, 127-147. London: John Libby Eurotext.

Newsholme, E.A., E. Blomstrand, and B. Ekblom. 1992. Physical and mental fatigue: Metabolic mechanisms and importance of plasma amino acids. *Brit Med Bull* 48 (3): 477-495.

Newsholme, E.A., M. Parry-Billings, N. McAndrew, and R. Budgett. 1991. A biochemical mechanism to explain some mechanisms of overtraining. In *Advances in nutrition and top sport*, Vol. 32, edited by F. Brouns, 79-93. Basel: Karger.

Nielsen, F.H. 1996. Other trace elements. In *Present knowledge of nutrition,* edited by E.E. Ziegler and L.J. Filer, 355-358. Washington, DC: ILSI Press.

Nielsen, F.H., C.D. Hunt, L.M. Mullen, and J.R. Hunt. 1987. Effect of dietary boron on mineral, estrogen, and testosterone metabolism in postmenopausal women. *FASEB J* 1 (5): 394-397.

Nieman, D.C. 1994. Exercise, infection, and immunity. *Int J Sports Med* 15 (Suppl 3): S131-S141.

Nieman, D.C., D.A. Henson, M.D. Austin, and W. Sha. 2011. Upper respiratory tract infection is reduced in physically fit and active adults. *Br J Sports Med* 45:987-992.

Nieman, D.C., D.A. Henson, O.R. Fagoaga, et al. 2002. Change in salivary IgA following a competitive marathon race. *Int J Sports Med* 23:69-75.

Nieman, D.C., D.A. Henson, S.J. Gross, et al. 2007. Quercetin reduces illness but not immune perturbations after intensive exercise. *Med Sci Sports Exerc* 39:1561-1569.

Nieman, D.C., D.A. Henson, S.R. McAnulty, et al. 2002. Influence of vitamin C supplementation on oxidative and immune changes after an ultramarathon. *J Appl Physiol* 92:1970-1977.

Nieman, D.C., D.A. Henson, S.R. McAnulty, F. Jin, and K.R. Maxwell. 2009. n-3 polyunsaturated fatty acids do not alter immune and inflammation measures in endurance athletes. *Int J Sport Nutr Exerc Metab* 19 (5): 536-546.

Nieman, D.C., D.A. Henson, M. McMahon, J.L. Wrieden, J.M. Davis, E.A. Murphy, S.J. Gross, L.S. McAnulty, and C.L. Dumke. 2008. Beta-glucan, immune function, and upper respiratory tract infections in athletes. *Med Sci Sports Exerc* 40 (8): 1463-1471.

Nieman, D.C., D.A. Henson, K.R. Maxwell, A.S. Williams, S.R. McAnulty, F. Jin, R.A. Shanely, and T.C. Lines. 2009. Effects of quercetin and EGCG on mitochondrial biogenesis and immunity. *Med Sci Sports Exerc* 41 (7): 1467-1475.

Nieman, D.C., L.M. Johansen, J.W. Lee, and K. Arabatzis. 1990. Infectious episodes in runners before and after the Los Angeles Marathon. *J Sports Med Phys Fitness* 30:316-328.

Nieman, D.C., A.R. Miller, D.A. Henson, B.J. Warren, G. Gusewitch, R.L. Johnson, J.M. Davis, D.E. Butterworth, and S.L. Nehlsen-Cannarella. 1993. Effects of high- versus moderate-intensity exercise on natural killer activity. *Med Sci Sports Exerc* 25:1126-1134.

Nieman, D.C., S.L. Nehlsen-Cannarella, O.R. Fagoaga, et al. 1998a. Effects of mode and carbohydrate on the granulocyte and monocyte response to intensive, prolonged exercise. *J Appl Physiol* 84 (4): 1252-1259.

Nieman, D.C., S.L. Nehlsen-Cannarella, O.R. Fagoaga, et al. 1998b. Influence of mode and carbohydrate on the cytokine response to heavy exertion. *Med Sci Sports Exerc* 30 (5): 671-678.

Nieman, D.C., S.L. Nehlsen-Cannarella, O.R. Fagoaga, D.A. Henson, M. Shannon, J.M. Davis, M.D. Austin, C.L. Hisey, J.C. Holbeck, J.M. Hjertman, M.R. Bolton, and B.K. Schilling. 1999. Immune response to two hours of rowing in elite female rowers. *Int J Sports Med* 20:476-481.

Nieman, D.C., and B.K. Pedersen, eds. 2000. *Nutrition and exercise immunology.* Boca Raton, FL: CRC Press.

Nieman, D.C., A.S. Williams, R.A. Shanely, F. Jin, S.R. McAnulty, N.T. Triplett, M.D. Austin, and D.A. Henson. 2010. Quercetin's influence on exercise performance and muscle mitochondrial biogenesis. *Med Sci Sports Exerc* 42 (2): 338-345.

Nieper, A. 2005. Nutritional supplement practices in UK junior national track and field athletes. *Br J Sports Med* 39:645-649.

Nilsson, L.H., and E Hultman. 1973. Liver glycogen in man: The effects of total starvation or a carbohydrate-poor diet followed by carbohydrate refeeding. *Scand J Clin Lab Invest* 32:325-330.

Nissen, S.L., and R.L. Sharp. 2003. Effect of dietary supplements on lean mass and strength gains with resistance exercise: A meta-analysis. *J Appl Physiol* 94 (2): 651-659.

Nissen, S.L., R.L. Sharp, L. Panton, M. Vukovich, S. Trappe, and J.C. Fuller Jr. 2000. Beta-hydroxy-beta-methylbutyrate (HMB) supplementation in humans is safe and may decrease cardiovascular risk factors. *J Nutr* 130 (8): 1937-1945.

Nissen, S.L., R. Sharp, M. Ray, J.A. Rathmacher, D. Rice, J.C. Fuller, Jr., A.S. Connelly, and N. Abumrad. 1996. Effect of leucine metabolite beta-hydroxy-beta-methylbutyrate on muscle metabolism during resistance-exercise training. *J Appl Physiol* 81 (5): 2095-2104.

Nitzke, S., J. Freeland-Graves, and American Dietetic Association. 2007. Position of the American Dietetic Association: Total diet approach to communicating food and nutrition information. *J Am Dietetic Assoc* 107 (7): 1224-32.

Noakes, T.D. 1986. *Lore of running.* Cape Town: Oxford University Press.

Noakes, T.D. 2007. The limits of human endurance: What is the greatest endurance performance of all time? Which factors regulate performance at extreme altitude? *Adv Exp Med Biol* 618:255-276.

Noakes, T.D., N. Goodwin, B.L. Rayner, T. Branken, and R.K.N. Taylor. 1985. Water intoxication: A possible complication during endurance exercise. *Med Sci Sports Exerc* 17:370-375.

Noakes, T.D., and J. Windt. 2017. Evidence that supports the prescription of low-carbohydrate high-fat diets: A narrative review. *Br J Sports Med* 51 (2): 133-139.

Nose, H., G.W. Mack, X. Shi, and E.R. Nadel. 1988. Role of osmolality and plasma volume during rehydration in humans. *J Appl Physiol* 65:325-331.

Notivol, R., I. Carrio, L. Cano, M. Estorch, and F. Vilardell. 1984. Gastric emptying of solid and liquid meals in healthy young subjects. *Scand J Gastroenterol* 19 (8): 1107-1113.

Nybo, L., P. Rasmussen, and M.N. Sawka. 2014. Performance in the heat-physiological factors of importance for hyperthermia-induced fatigue. *Compr Physiol* 4 (2): 657-689.

O'Connell, E.J., J.E. Allgrove, L.V. Pollard, M. Xiang, and L.S. Harbige. 2009. A pilot study investigating the effects of Yakult fermented milk drink (L. casei Shirota) on salivary IFN-γ, sIgA, IgA1 and IgA2 in healthy volunteers. In *Proceedings of the Yakult International Symposium.* June 18-19: Amsterdam (The Netherlands).

Odland, L.M., G.J.F. Heigenhauser, G.D. Lopaschuk, and L.L. Spriet. 1996. Human skeletal muscle malonyl-COA at rest and during prolonged submaximal exercise. *Am J Physiol* 270:E541-E44.

Odland, L.M., R.A. Howlett, G.J. Heigenhauser, E. Hultman, and L.L. Spriet. 1998. Skeletal muscle malonyl-COA content at the onset of exercise at varying power outputs in humans. *Am J Physiol* 274 (6 Pt 1): E1080-E1085.

Okudan, N., M. Belviranli, H Pepe, and H Gokbel. 2015. The effects of beta alanine plus creatine administration on performance during repeated bouts of supramaximal exercise in sedentary men. *J Sports Med Phys Fitness* 55 (11): 1322-1328.

Olsen, N.J., and B.L. Heitmann. 2009. Intake of calorically sweetened beverages and obesity. *Obes Rev* 10:68-75.

Olveira, G., and I. González-Molero. 2016. An update on probiotics, prebiotics and symbiotics in clinical nutrition. *Endocrinol Nutr* 63 (9): 482-494.

Oostenbrug, G.S., R.P. Mensink, T. De Vries, M.R. Hardeman, F. Brouns, and G. Hornstra. 1997. Exercise performance, red blood cell characteristics and lipid peroxidation: Effect of fish oil and vitamin E. *J Appl Physiol* 83 (3): 746-752.

Oppliger, R.A., H.S. Case, C.A. Horswill, et al. 1996. American College of Sports Medicine position stand: Weight loss in wrestlers. *Med Sci Sports Exerc* 28 (6): ix-xii.

Oppliger, R.A., D.H. Nielsen, C.G. Vance. 1991. Wrestlers' minimal weight: Anthropometry, bioimpedance, and hydrostatic weighing compared. *Med Sci Sports Exerc* 23 (2): 247-253.

Oscai, L.B., D.A. Essig, and W.K. Palmer. 1990. Lipase regulation of muscle triglyceride hydrolysis. *J Appl Physiol* 69 (5): 1571-1577.

Outram, S., and B. Stewart. 2015. Doping through supplement use: A review of the available empirical data. *Int J Sport Nutr Exerc Metab* 25 (1) :54-59.

Owens, D.J., W.D. Fraser, and G.L. Close. 2015. Vitamin D and the athlete: Emerging insights. *Eur J Sport Sci* 15:73-84.

Packer, L. 1997. Oxidants, antioxidant nutrients and the athlete. *J Sports Sci* 15:353-363.

Paddon-Jones, D., A. Keech, and D. Jenkins. 2001. Short-term beta-hydroxy-beta-methylbutyrate supplementation does not reduce symptoms of eccentric muscle damage. *Int J Sport Nutr Exerc Metab* 11 (4): 442-450.

Paddon-Jones, D., E. Westman, R.D. Mattes, R.R. Wolfe, A. Astrup, and M. Westerterp-Plantenga. 2008. Protein, weight management, and satiety. *Am J Clin Nutr* 87 (5): 1558S-1561S.

Pagala, M.K., T. Namba, and D. Grob. 1984. Failure of neuromuscular transmission and contractility during muscle fatigue. *Muscle Nerve* 7 (6): 454-464.

Pálmer, H.G., J.M. González-Sancho, J. Espada, M.T. Berciano, I. Puig, J. Baulida, M. Quintanilla, A. Cano, A.G. de Herreros, M. Lafarga, and A. Muñoz. 2001. Vitamin D(3) promotes the differentiation of colon carcinoma cells by the induction of E-cadherin and the inhibition of beta-catenin signaling. *J Cell Biol* 154(2): 369-387.

Pan, D.A., S. Lillioja, A.D. Kriketos, M.R. Milner, L.A. Baur, C. Bogardus, A.B. Jenkins, and L.H. Storlien. 1997. Skeletal muscle triglyceride levels are inversely related to insulin action. *Diabetes* 46:983-988.

Pannemans, D.L.E., A.J.M. Wagenmakers, K.R. Westerterp, G. Schaafsma, and D. Halliday. 1998. Effect of protein source and quantity on protein metabolism in elderly women. *Am J Clin Nutr* 68 (6): 1228-1235.

Panton, L.B., J.A. Rathmacher, S. Baier, and S. Nissen. 2000. Nutritional supplementation of the leucine metabolite beta-hydroxy-beta-methylbutyrate (Hmb) during resistance training. *Nutrition* 16 (9): 734-739.

Papacosta, E., G. Nassis, and M. Gleeson. 2015. Effects of acute post-exercise chocolate milk consumption during intensive judo training on the recovery of salivary hormones, salivary IgA, mood state, muscle soreness and judo-related performance. *Appl Physiol Nutr Metab* 40:1-7.

Papet, I., P. Ostaszewski, F. Glomot, C. Obled, M. Faure, G. Bayle, S. Nissen, M. Arnal, and J. Grizard. 1997. The effect of a high dose of 3-hydroxy-3-methylbutyrate on protein metabolism in growing lambs. *Br J Nutr* 77 (6): 885-896.

Parry-Billings, M., R. Budgett, Y. Koutedakis, E. Blomstrand, S. Brooks, C. Williams, P.C. Calder, S. Pilling, R. Baigrie, and E.A. Newsholme. 1992. Plasma amino acid concentrations in the overtraining syndrome: Possible effects on the immune system. *Med Sci Sports Exerc* 24 (12): 1353-1358.

Pasakios, S.M., H.R. Lieberman, and T.M. McLellan. 2014. Effects of protein supplements on muscle damage, soreness and recovery of muscle function and physical performance: A systematic review. *Sports Med* 44 (5): 655-670.

Pasman, W.J., M.A. van Baak, A.E. Jeukendrup, and A. deHaan. 1995. The effect of varied dosages of caffeine on endurance performance time. *Int J Sports Med* 16 (4): 225-230.

Patton, G.C., R. Selzer, C. Coffey, J.B. Carlin, and R.Wolfe. 1999. Onset of adolescent eating disorders: Population based cohort study over 3 years. *Br Med J* 318 (7186): 765-768.

Peake, J.M., O. Neubauer, P.A. Della Gatta, and K. Nosaka. 2017. Muscle damage and inflammation during recovery from exercise. *J Appl Physiol* 122 (3): 559-570.

Pedersen, B.K., and H. Bruunsgaard. 1995. How physical exercise influences the establishment of infections. *Sports Med* 19:393-400.

Pedersen, B.K., and Febbraio, M. A. 2008. Muscle as an endocrine organ: Focus on muscle-derived interleukin-6. *Physiol Rev* 88:1379-1406.

Pedersen, B.K., J. Helge, E. Richter, T. Rhode, K. Ostrowski, and B. Kiens. 2000. Training and natural immunity: Effects of diets rich in fat or carbohydrate. *Eur J Appl Physiol* 82:98-102.

Pedersen, D.J., S.J. Lessard, V.G. Coffey, E.G. Churchley, A.M. Wootton, T. Ng, M.J. Watt, and J.A. Hawley. 2008. High rates of muscle glycogen resynthesis after exhaustive exercise when carbohydrate is coingested with caffeine. *J Appl Physiol* 105 (1): 7-13.

Peeling, P., M.J. Binnie, P.S.R. Goods, M. Sim, and L.M. Burke. 2018. Evidence-based supplements for the enhancement of athletic performance. *Int J Sport Nutr Exerc Metab* 28 (2): 178-187.

Peeling, P., and C. Goodman. 2015. Iron. In *Nutritional supplements in sport, exercise and health*, edited by L.M. Castell, S.J. Stear, and L.M. Burke, 158-161. London: Routledge.

Pendergast, D.R., P.J. Horvath, J.J. Leddy, and J.T. Venkatraman. 1996. The role of dietary fat on performance, metabolism and health. *Am J Sports Med* 24 (6): S53-S58.

Pennings, B., Y. Boirie Y, J.M. Senden, A.P. Gijsen, H. Kuipers H, and L.J. van Loon. 2011. Whey protein stimulates postprandial muscle protein accretion more effectively than do casein and casein hydrolysate in older men. *Am J Clin Nutr* 93 (5): 997-1005.

Perry, B., and Y. Wang. 2012. Appetite regulation and weight control: The role of gut hormones. *Nutr Diabetes* 2 (1): e26.

Perry, C.G., G.J. Heigenhauser, A. Bonen, and L.L. Spriet. 2008. High-intensity aerobic interval training increases fat and carbohydrate metabolic capacities in human skeletal muscle. *Appl Physiol Nutr Metab* 33 (6): 1112-1123.

Perusse, L., and C. Bouchard. 2000. Gene-diet interactions in obesity. *Am J Clin Nutr* 72 (5 Suppl): 1285S-1290S.

Peternelj, T.T., and J.S. Coombes. 2011. Antioxidant supplementation during exercise training: Beneficial or detrimental? *Sports Med* 41 (12): 1043-1069.

Peters, E.M., and E.D. Bateman. 1983. Ultramarathon running and URTI: An epidemiological survey. *S Afr Med J* 64:582-584.

Peters, E.M., and J.M. Goetzsche. 1997. Dietary practices of South African ultradistance athletes. *Int J Sport Nutr* 7:80-103.

Peters, E.M., J.M. Goetzsche, B. Grobbelaar, and T.D. Noakes. 1993. Vitamin C supplementation reduces the incidence of post-race symptoms of upper respiratory tract in ultramarathon runners. *Am J Clin Nutr* 57:170-174.

Peters, E.M., J.M. Goetzsche, L.E. Joseph, and T.D. Noakes. 1996. Vitamin C as effective as combinations of anti-oxidant nutrients in reducing symptoms of upper respiratory tract infections in ultramarathon runners. *S Afr J Sports Med* 11:23-27.

Petroczi, A., D.P. Naughton, G. Pearce, R. Bailey, A. Bloodworth, and M. McNamee. 2008. Nutritional supplement use by elite young UK athletes: Fallacies of advice regarding efficacy. *J Int Soc Sports Nutr* 5:22.

Pew. 2013. Tracking for Health. Pew Research Center's Internet & American Life Project. www.pewinternet.org/Reports/2013/Tracking-for-Health.aspx.

Peyrebrune, M.C., M.E. Nevill, F.J. Donaldson, and D.J. Cosford. 1998. The effects of oral creatine supplementation on performance in single and repeated sprint swimming. *J Sports Sci* 16 (3): 271-279.

Phillips, G.C. 2007. Glutamine: the nonessential amino acid for performance enhancement. *Curr Sports Med Rep* 6 (4): 265-268.

Phillips, S.M. 2011. The science of muscle hypertrophy: Making dietary protein count. *Proc Nutr Soc* 70:100-103.

Phillips, S.M. 2012. Dietary protein requirements and adaptive advantages in athletes. *Brit J Nutr* 108 (Suppl 2): S158-S167.

Phillips, S.M. 2013. Protein consumption and resistance exercise: Maximizing anabolic potential. *Sport Science Exchange* 26 (107): 1-5.

Phillips, S.M. 2015. Nutritional supplements in support of resistance exercise to counter age-related sarcopenia. *Adv Nutr* 6 (4): 452-460.

Phillips, S.M. 2016. The impact of protein quality on the promotion of resistance exercise-induced changes in muscle mass. *Nutr Metab* 13:64.

Phillips, S.M., A.A. Aragon, P.J. Arciero, S.M. Arent, et al. 2017. Changes in body composition and performance with supplemental HMB-FA + ATP. *J Strength Cond Res* (March 13). http://doi.org/10.1519/JSC.0000000000001760.

Phillips, S.M., K.D. Tipton, A. Aarsland, S.E. Wolf, and R.R. Wolfe. 1997. Mixed muscle protein synthesis and breakdown after resistance exercise in humans. *Am J Physiol* 273 (1 Pt 1): E99-E107.

Phillips, S.M., K.D. Tipton, A.A. Ferrando, and R.R. Wolfe. 1999. Resistance training reduces the acute exercise-induced increase in muscle protein turnover. *Am J Physiol* 276 (1 Pt 1): E118-E124.

Phinney, S.D., B.R. Bistrian, W.J. Evans, E. Gervino, and G.L. Blackburn. 1983. The human metabolic response to chronic ketosis without caloric restriction: Preservation of submaximal exercise capability with reduced carbohydrate oxidation. *Metabolism* 32 (9): 769-776.

Phinney, S.D., B.R. Bistrian, R.R. Wolfe, and G.L. Blackburn. 1983. The human metabolic response to chronic ketosis without caloric restriction: Physical and biochemical adaptation. *Metabolism* 32 (8): 757-768.

Phinney, S.D., E.S. Horton, E.A.H. Sims, J.S. Hanson, E. Danforth, and B.M. LaGrange. 1980. Capacity for moderate exercise in obese subjects after adaptation to a hypocaloric, ketogenic diet. *J Clin Invest* 66:1152-1161.

Phoenix, J., R.H. Edwards, and M.J. Jackson. 1991. The effect of vitamin E analogues and long hydrocarbon chain compounds on calcium-induced muscle damage: A novel role for alpha-tocopherol? *Biochim Biophys Acta* 1097:212-218.

Pilegaard, H., C. Keller, A. Steensberg, J.W. Helge, B.K. Pedersen, B. Saltin, and P.D. Neufer. 2002. Influence of pre-exercise muscle glycogen content on exercise-induced transcriptional regulation of metabolic genes. *J Physiol* 541:261-271.

Pilegaard, H., Domino, K., Noland, T., Juel, C., Hellsten, Y., Halestrap, A.P., and Bangsbo, J. 1999. Effect of high-intensity exercise training on lactate/H+ transport capacity in human skeletal muscle. *Am J Physiol* 276 (2 Pt 1): E255-E261.

Pilegaard, H., B. Saltin, and P.D. Neufer. 2003. Exercise induces transient transcriptional activation of the PGC-1alpha gene in human skeletal muscle. *J Physiol* 546:851-858.

Pinchan, G., R.K. Gauttam, O.S. Tomar, and A.C. Babaj. 1988. Effects of primary hypohydration on physical work capacity. *Int J Biometeorol* 32:176-180.

Pinckaers, P.J., T.A. Churchward-Venne, D. Bailey, and L.J. van Loon. 2017. Ketone bodies and exercise performance: The next magic bullet or merely hype? *Sports Med* 47 (3): 383-391.

Pirnay, F., J.M. Crielaard, N. Pallikarakis, M. Lacroix, F. Mosora, G. Krzentowski, A.S. Luyckx, and P.J. Lefebvre. 1982. Fate of exogenous glucose during exercise of different intensities in humans. *J Appl Physiol* 53:1620-1624.

Pirnay, F., A.J. Scheen, J.F. Gautier, M. Lacroix, and P.J. Lefèbvre. 1995. Exogenous glucose oxidation during exercise in relation to the power output. *Int J Sports Med* 16 (7): 456-460.

Pizza, F.X., J.M. Peterson, J.H. Baas, and T.J. Koh. 2005. Neutrophils contribute to muscle injury and impair its resolution after lengthening contractions in mice. *J Physiol* 562 (3): 899-913.

Polivy, J., and C.P. Herman. 1995. Dieting and its relation to eating disorders. In *Eating disorders and obesity: A comprehensive handbook,* edited by K.D. Brownell and C.G. Fairburn, 83-86. London: Guildford Press.

Pomeroy, C., and S.F. Mitchell. 1992. Medical issues in the eating disorders. In *Eating, body weight and performance in athletes: Disorders of modern society,* edited by K.D. Brownell, J. Rodin, and J.H. Wilmore, 202-221. Philadelphia: Lea & Febiger.

Pope Jr, H.G., K.A. Phillips, and R. Olivardia. 2000. *The Adonis complex: The secret crisis of male body obsession.* New York: Free Press.

Poppitt, S.D., and A.M. Prentice. 1996. Energy density and its role in the control of food intake: Evidence from metabolic and community studies. *Appetite* 26 (2), 153-174.

Potteiger, J.A., G.L. Nickel, M.J. Webster, M.D. Haub, and R.J. Palmer. 1996. Sodium citrate ingestion enhances 30 km cycling performance. *Int J Sports Med* 17 (1): 7-11.

Pottier, A., J. Bouckaert, W. Gilis, T. Roels, and W. Derave. 2010. Mouth rinse but not ingestion of a carbohydrate solution improves 1-h cycle time trial performance. *Scand J Med Sci Sports* 20 (1): 105-111.

Powers, S.K., and M.J. Jackson. 2008. Exercise-induced oxidative stress: Cellular mechanisms and impact on muscle force production. *Physiol Rev* 88:1243-1276.

Powers, S.K., A.N. Kavazis, and J.M. McClung. 2007. Oxidative stress and disuse muscle atrophy. *J Appl Physiol* 102:2389-2397.

Powers, S., W.B. Nelson, and E. Larson-Meyer. 2011. Antioxidant and vitamin D supplements for athletes: Sense or nonsense? *J Sports Sci* 29:S47-S55.

Prado de Oliveira, E., R.C Burin, and A.E.Jeukendrup. 2014. Gastrointestinal complaints during exercise: Prevalence, etiology, and nutritional recommendations. *Sports Med* 44 (Suppl 1):S79–S85.

Prietl, B., G. Treiber, T.R.Pieber, and K. Amrein. 2013. Vitamin D and immune function. *Nutrients* 5(7): 2502-2521.

Pujol, P., J. Huguet, F. Drobnic, et al. 2000. The effect of fermented milk containing Lactobacillus casei on the immune response to exercise. *Sports Med Train Rehab* 9:209-223.

Pyne, D.B., N.P. West, A.J. Cox, and A.W. Cripps. 2015. Probiotics supplementation for athletes—Clinical and physiological effects. *Eur J Sport Sci* 15:63-72.

Quadrilatero, J., and L. Hoffman-Goetz. 2004. N-acetyl-L-cysteine prevents exercise-induced intestinal lymphocyte apoptosis by maintaining intracellular glutathione levels and reducing mitochondrial membrane depolarization. *Biochem Biophys Res Comm* 319:894-901.

QuickStats. 2017. Percentage of total daily kilocalories consumed from sugar-sweetened beverages among children and adults, by sex and income level: National Health and Nutrition Examination Survey, United States, 2011-2014. *MMWR Morb Mortal Wkly Rep* 66 (6): 181.

Racinais, S., J.M. Alonso, A.J. Coutts, A.D. Flouris, O. Girard, J. González-Alonso, C. Hausswirth, O. Jay, J.K. Lee, N. Mitchell, G.P. Nassis, L. Nybo, B.M. Pluim, B. Roelands, M.N. Sawka, J.E. Wingo, and J.D. Périard. 2015. Consensus recommendations on training and competing in the heat. *Scand J Med Sci Sports* 25 (Suppl 1):6-19.

Randle, P.J., P.B. Garland, C.N. Hales, and E.A. Newsholme. 1963. The glucose fatty acid cycle: Its role in insulin sensitivity and the metabolic disturbances of diabetes mellitus. *Lancet* 1:786-789.

Rankin, P., E. Stevenson, and E. Cockburn. 2015. The effect of milk on the attenuation of exercise-induced muscle damage in males and females. *Eur J Appl Physiol* 115 (6): 1245-1261.

Rankinen, T., L. Perusse, S.J. Weisnagel, et al. 2002. The human obesity gene map: The 2001 update. *Obes Res* 10 (3): 196-243.

Ransdell, L., J. Vener, and J. Huberty. 2009. Master athletes: An analysis of running, swimming and cycling performance by age and gender. *J Exerc Sci Fitness* 7 (Suppl): S61-S73.

Rasmussen, B.B., K.D. Tipton, S.L. Miller, S.E. Wolf, and R.R. Wolfe. 2000. An oral essential amino acid-carbohydrate supplement enhances muscle protein anabolism after resistance exercise. *J Appl Physiol* 88 (2): 386-392.

Rasmussen, B.B., E. Volpi, D.C. Gore, and R.R. Wolfe. 2000. Androstenedione does not stimulate muscle protein anabolism in young healthy men. *J Clin Endocrinol Metab* 85 (1): 55-59.

Reale, R., G. Slater, I.C. Dunican, G.R. Cox, and L.M. Burke. 2017. The effect of water loading on acute weight loss following fluid restriction in combat sports athletes. *Int J Sport Nutr Exerc Metab* 28:1-22.

Rector, R.S., R. Rogers, M. Ruebel, et al. 2008. Participation in road cycling vs running is associated with lower bone mineral density in men. *Metabolism* 57 (2): 226-232.

Rehrer, N.J., E.J. Beckers, F. Brouns, F. ten Hoor, and W.H. Saris. 1990. Effects of dehydration on gastric emptying and gastrointestinal distress while running. *Med Sci Sports Exerc* 22 (6): 790-795.

Rehrer, N.J., M. van Kemenade, W. Meester, F. Brouns, and W.H.M. Saris. 1992. Gastrointestinal complaints in relation to dietary intake in triathletes. *Int J Sport Nutr* 2:48-59.

Rehrer, N.J., A.J.M. Wagenmakers, E.J. Beckers, D. Halliday, J.B. Leiper, F. Brouns, R.J. Maugham, K. Westerterp, and W.H.M. Saris. 1992. Gastric emptying, absorption and carbohydrate oxidation during prolonged exercise. *J Appl Physiol* 72 (2): 468-475.

Reid, M.B. 2008. Free radicals and muscle fatigue: Of ROS, canaries, and the IOC. *Free Rad Biol Med* 44:169-179.

Reidy, P.T., D.K. Walker, J.M. Dickinson, D.M. Gundermann, M.J. Drummond, K.L. Timmerman, C.S. Fry, M.S. Borack, M.B. Cope, R. Mukherjea, K. Jennings, E. Volpi, and B.B. Rasmussen. 2013. Protein blend ingestion following resistance exercise promotes human muscle protein synthesis. *J Nutr* 143:410-416.

Reitelseder, S., J. Agergaard, S. Doessing, I.C. Helmark, P. Lund, N.B. Kristensen, J. Frystyk, A. Flyvbjerg, P. Schjerling, G. van Hall, M. Kjaer, and L. Holm.et al. 2011. Whey and casein labeled with L-[1-13C]leucine and muscle protein synthesis: Effect of resistance exercise and protein ingestion. *Am J Physiol Endocrinol Metab* 300:E231-E242.

Remely, M., I. Tesar, B. Hippe, S. Gnauer, P. Rust, and A.G. Haslberger. 2015. Gut microbiota composition correlates with changes in body fat content due to weight loss. *Benef Microbes* 6 (4): 431-439.

Ren, J.M., C.F. Semenkovich, E.A. Gulve, J. Gao, and J.O. Holloszy. 1994. Exercise induces rapid increases in GLUT4 expression, glucose transport capacity, and insulin-stimulated glycogen storage in muscle. *J Biol Chem* 269 (20): 14396-14401.

Rennie, M.J. 2005. Body maintenance and repair: How food and exercise keep the musculoskeletal system in good shape. *Exp Physiol* 90:427-436.

Rennie, M.J., P.A. MacLellan, H.S. Hundal, B. Weryl, K. Smith, P.M. Taylor, C. Egan, and P.W. Watt. 1989. Skeletal muscle glutamine concentration and muscle protein turnover. *Clin Exp* 38:47-51.

Rennie, M.J., and K.D. Tipton. 2000. Protein and amino acid metabolism during and after exercise and the effects of nutrition. *Annu Rev Nutr* 20:457-483.

Res, P.T., B. Groen, B. Pennings, M. Beelen, G.A. Wallis, A.P. Gijsen, J.M. Senden, and L.J. van Loon. 2012. Protein ingestion before sleep improves postexercise overnight recovery. *Med Sci Sports Exerc* 44:1560-1569.

Riddell, M.C. 2008. The endocrine response and substrate utilization during exercise in children and adolescents. *J Appl Physiol* 105:725-733.

Riddoch, C., and T. Trinick. 1988. Gastrointestinal disturbances in marathon runners. *Br J Sports Med* 22 (2): 71-4.

Riley, M.L., R.G. Israel, D. Holbert, E.B. Tapscott, and G.L. Dohm. 1988. Effect of carbohydrate ingestion on exercise endurance and metabolism after 1-day fast. *Int J Sports Med* 9:320-324.

Rimm, E.B., M.B. Katan, A. Ascherio, M.J. Stampfer, and W.C. Willett. 1996. Relation between intake of flavonoids and risk for coronary heart disease in male health professionals. *Ann Intern Med* 125 (5): 384-389.

Rippe, J.M., and T.J. Angelopoulos. 2016. Sugars, obesity, and cardiovascular disease: Results from recent randomized control trials. *Eur J Nutr* 55 (Suppl 2): 45-53.

Ristow, M., K. Zarse, A. Oberbach, N. Klöting, M. Birringer, M. Kiehntopf, M. Stumvoll, C.R. Kahn, and M. Blüher. 2009. Antioxidants prevent health-promoting effects of physical exercise in humans. *Proc Natl Acad Sci* 106 (21): 8665-8670.

Rivera-Brown, A.M., R. Gutierrez, J.C. Gutierrez, W.R. Frontera, and O. Bar-Or. 1999. Drink composition, voluntary drinking, and fluid balance in exercising, trained, heat-acclimatized boys. *J Appl Physiol* 86:78-84.

Roberts, J.D., M.G. Roberts, M.D. Tarpey, J.C. Weekes, and C.H. Thomas. 2015. The effect of a decaffeinated green tea extract formula on fat oxidation, body composition and exercise performance. *J Int Soc Sports Nutr* 12 (1): 1.

Robertson, T.L., H. Kato, G.G. Rhoads, A. Kagan, M. Marmot, S.L. Syme, T. Gordon, R.M. Worth, J.L. Belsky, D.S. Dock, M. Miyanishi, and S. Kawamoto. 1977. Epidemiologic studies of coronary heart disease and stroke in Japanese men living in Japan, Hawaii and California: Incidence of myocardial infarction and death from coronary heart disease. *Am J Cardiol* 39 (2): 239-243.

Rohde, T., S. Asp, D. Maclean, and B.K. Pedersen. 1998. Competitive sustained exercise in humans, and lymphokine activated killer cell activity—An intervention study. *Eur J Appl Physiol* 78:448-453.

Rollo, I., M. Cole, R. Miller, and C. Williams. 2010. Influence of mouth rinsing a carbohydrate solution on 1-h running performance. *Med Sci Sports Exerc* 42:798-804.

Rollo, I., C. Williams, N. Gant, and M. Nute. 2008. The influence of carbohydrate mouth rinse on self-selected speeds during a 30-min treadmill run. *Int J Sport Nutr Exerc Metab* 18:585-600.

Rollo, I., C. Williams, and M. Nevill. 2011. Influence of ingesting versus mouth rinsing a carbohydrate solution during a 1-h run. *Med Sci Sports Exerc* 43:468-75.

Romeo, J., J. Warnberg J, E. Nova, et al. 2007. Moderate alcohol consumption and the immune system. A review. *Br J Nut* 98 (1): S111-S116.

Romer, L.M., J.P. Barrington, and A.E. Jeukendrup. 2001. Effects of oral creatine supplementation on high intensity, intermittent exercise performance in competitive squash players. *Int J Sports Med* 22 (8): 546-552.

Romijn, J.A., E.F. Coyle, L.S. Sidossis, A. Gastaldelli, J.F. Horowitz, E. Endert, and R.R. Wolfe. 1993. Regulation of endogenous fat and carbohydrate metabolism in relation to exercise intensity. *Am J Physiol* 265:E380-E391.

Romijn, J.A., E.F. Coyle, L.S. Sidossis, X.-J. Zhang, and R.R. Wolfe. 1995. Relationship between fatty acid delivery and fatty acid oxidation during strenuous exercise. *J Appl Physiol* 79 (6): 1939-1945.

Rontoyannis, G.P., T. Skoulis, and K.N. Pavlou. 1989. Energy balance in ultramarathon running. *Am J Clin Nutr 49* (5 Suppl):976-9.

Rosen, L.W., and D.O. Hough. 1988. Pathogenic weight control behaviors of female college gymnasts. *Physician Sports Med* 9:141-144.

Rosenberger, M., M. Buman, W. Haskell, M. McConnell, and L. Carstensen. 2016. Twenty-four hours of sleep, sedentary behavior, and physical activity with nine wearable devices. *Med Sci Sports Exerc* 48 (3): 457-465.

Rosenthal, L.A., D.D. Taub, M.A. Moors, and K.J. Blank. 1992. Methylxanthine-induced inhibition of the antigen- and superantigen-specific activation of T and B lymphocytes. *Immunopharmacol* 24:302-217

Ross, A.C., J.E. Manson, S.A. Abrams, J.F. Aloia, P.M. Brannon, S.K. Clinton, R.A. Durazo-Arvizu, J.C. Gallagher, R.L. Gallo, G. Jones, C.S. Kovacs, S.T. Mayne, C.J. Rosen, and S.A. Shapses. 2011. The 2011 report on dietary reference intakes for calcium and vitamin D from the Institute of Medicine: What clinicians need to know. *J Clin Endocrinol Metab* 96:53-58.

Ross, S. 2000. Functional foods: The Food and Drug Administration perspective. *Am J Clin Nutr* 71 (6 Suppl): 1735S-1738S.

Rossiter, H.B., E.R. Cannell, and P.M. Jakeman. 1996. The effect of oral creatine supplementation on the 1000-m performance of competitive rowers. *J Sports Sci* 14 (2): 175-179.

Roth, A., and G. Fonagy. 1998. *What works for whom?* New York: Guildford Press.

Rowland, T. 2008. Thermoregulation during exercise in the heat in children: Old concepts revisited. *J Appl Physiol* 105 (2): 718-724.

Roxas, M., and J. Jurenka. 2007. Colds and influenza: A review of diagnosis and conventional, botanical, and nutritional considerations. *Alt Med Rev* 12 (1): 25-48.

Rucinski, A. 1989. Relationship of body image and dietary intake of competitive ice skaters. *J Am Dietetic Assoc* 89:98-100.

Rueda, R. 2007. The role of dietary gangliosides on immunity and the prevention of infection. *Br J Nutr* 98:S68-S73.

Rugg-Gunn, A. 2013. Dental caries: Strategies to control this preventable disease. *Acta Med Acad* 42 (2): 117-130.

Rustad, P.I., M. Sailer, K.T. Cumming, P.B. Jeppesen, K.J. Kolnes, O. Sollie, J. Franch, J.L. Ivy, H. Daniel, and J. Jensen. 2016. Intake of protein plus carbohydrate during the first two hours after exhaustive cycling improves performance the following day. *PLoS One*11(4):e0153229.

Sabatini, S. 2001. The female athlete triad. *Am J Med Sci* 322:193-195.

Sale, C., and R.C. Harris. 2014. Buffering agents. In *Sports nutrition,* edited by R.J. Maughan, 324-335. Chichester, UK: Blackwell.

Sale, C., C.A. Hill, J. Ponte, and R.C. Harris. 2012. Beta-alanine supplementation improves isometric endurance of the knee extensor muscles. *J Int Soc Sports Nutr* 9:26.

Sale, C., Saunders, B., and Harris, R.C. 2010. Effect of beta-alanine supplementation on muscle carnosine concentrations and exercise performance. *Amino Acids* 39 (2): 321-333.

Saltin, B. 1973. Metabolic fundamentals in exercise. *Med Sci Sports Exerc* 5:137-146.

Saltin, B., A.P. Gagge, and J.A.J. Stolwijk. 1968. Muscle temperature during submaximal exercise in man. *J Appl Physiol* 25:679-688.

Sandage, B.W., R.N. Sabounjian, R. White, and R.J. Wurtman. 1992. Choline citrate may enhance athletic performance. *Physiologist* 35:236A.

Saris, W.H.M., B.H. Goodpaster, A.E. Jeukendrup, F. Brouns, D. Halliday, and A.J.M. Wagenmakers. 1993. Exogenous carbohydrate oxidation from different carbohydrate sources during exercise. *J Appl Physiol* 755:2168-2172.

Sarna, S., and J. Kaprio. 1994. Life expectancy of former elite athletes. *Sports Med* 17 (3): 49-51.

Sasaki, J.E., A. Hickey, M. Mavilia, J. Tedesco, D. John, S. Kozey, S. Keadle, and P.S. Freedson. 2014. Validation of the Fitbit wireless activity tracker for prediction of energy expenditure. *J Phys Act Health* 12:149-154.

Sasaki, H., J. Maeda, S. Usui, and T. Ishiko. 1987. Effect of sucrose and caffeine ingestion on performance of prolonged strenuous running. *Int J Sports Med* 8:261-265.

Saunders, B., K. Elliott-Sale, G.G. Artioli, P.A. Swinton, E. Dolan, H. Roschel, C. Sale, and B. Gualano. 2017. ß-alanine supplementation to improve exercise capacity and performance: A systematic review and meta-analysis. *Br J Sports Med* 51 (8): 658-669.

Saunders, M.J. 2011. Carbohydrate-protein intake and recovery from endurance exercise: Is chocolate milk the answer? *Curr Sports Med Rep* 10 (4): 203-210.

Saunders, M.J., J.E. Blevins, and C.E. Broeder. 1998. Effects of hydration changes on bioelectrical impedance in endurance trained individuals. *Med Sci Sports Exerc* 30 (6): 885-892.

Saunders, M.J., M.D. Kane, and M.K. Todd. 2004. Effects of a carbohydrate-protein beverage on cycling endurance and muscle damage. *Med Sci Sports Exerc* 36 (7): 1233-1238.

Saunders, M.J., N.D. Luden, and J.E. Herrick. 2007. Consumption of an oral carbohydrate-protein gel improves cycling endurance and prevents postexercise muscle damage. *J Strength Cond Res* 21 (3): 678-684.

Saunders, M.J., R.W. Moore, A.K. Kies, N.D. Luden, and C.A. Pratt. 2009. Carbohydrate and protein hydrolysate coingestions improvement of late-exercise time-trial performance. *Int J Sport Nutr Exerc Metab* 19 (2): 135-149.

Savoie, F.A., R.W. Kenefick, B.R. Ely, S.N. Cheuvront, and E.D. Goulet. 2015. Effect of hypohydration on muscle endurance, strength, anaerobic power and capacity and vertical jumping ability: A meta-analysis. *Sports Med* 45 (8): 1207-1227.

Sawka, M.N., L.M. Burke, E.R. Eichner, R.J. Maughan, S.J. Montain, and N.S. Stachenfeld. 2007. American College of Sports Medicine position stand: Exercise and fluid replacement. *Med Sci Sports Exerc* 39:377-390.

Sawka, M.N., S.N. Cheuvront, and R.W. Kenefick. 2015. Hypohydration and human performance: Impact of environment and physiological mechanisms. *Sports Med* 45 (Suppl 1): S51-S60.

Sawka, M.N., and S.J. Montain. 2000. Fluid and electrolyte supplementation for exercise heat stress. *Am J Clin Nutr* 72 (2): 564S-572S.

Sawka, M.N., and K.B. Pandolf. 1990. Effects of body water loss on physiological function and exercise performance. In *Perspectives in exercise science and sports medicine,* Vol. 3, edited by C.V. Gisolfi and D.R. Lamb, 1-38. Carmel, IN: Benchmark Press.

Sawka, M.N., and C.B. Wenger. 1988. Physiological responses to acute-exercise heat stress. In *Human performance physiology and environmental medicine at terrestrial extremes,* edited by K. Pandolf, 1-38. Indianapolis, IN: Benchmark Press.

Sawka, M.N., A.J. Young, B.S. Cadarette, L. Levine, and K.B. Pandolf. 1985. Influence of heat stress and acclimation on maximal aerobic power. *Eur J Appl Physiol* 53:294-298.

Sawka, M.N., A.J. Young, R.P. Francesconi, S.R. Muza, and K.B. Pandolf. 1985. Thermoregulatory and blood responses during exercise at graded hypohydration levels. *J Appl Physiol* 59:1394-1401.

Sawka, M.N., A.J. Young, W.A. Latzka, P.D. Neufer, M.D. Quigley, and K.B. Pandolf. 1992. Human tolerance to heat strain during exercise: Influence of hydration. *J Appl Physiol* 73:368-375.

Scherr, J., D.C. Nieman, T. Schuster, J. Habermann, M. Rank, S. Braun, A. Pressler, B. Wolfarth, and M. Halle. 2012. Nonalcoholic beer reduces inflammation and incidence of respiratory tract illness. *Med Sci Sports Exerc* 44 (1): 18-26.

Schlundt, D.G., J.O. Hill, J. Pope-Cordle, et al. 1993. Randomized evaluation of a low fat ad libitum carbohydrate diet for weight reduction. *Int J Obes Relat Metab Disord* 17 (11): 623-629.

Schoenfeld, B.J., A.A. Aragon, and J.W. Krieger. 2013. The effect of protein timing on muscle strength and hypertrophy: A meta-analysis. *J Int Soc Sports Nutr* 10:53.

Schwellnus, M.P., W.E. Derman, E. Jordaan, et al. 2012. Elite athletes travelling to international destinations >5 time zone differences from their home country have a 2-3-fold increased risk of illness. *Br J Sports Med* 46:816-821.

Schwellnus, M., T. Soligard, J.M. Alonso, R. Bahr, B. Clarsen, P. Dijkstra, T.J. Gabbett, M. Gleeson, M. Hägglund, M.R. Hutchinson, C.J. Van Rensburg, K. Khan, R. Meeusen, J.W. Orchard, B.M. Pluim, M. Raftery, U. Erdener, R. Budgett, and L. Engebretsen. 2016. How much is too much? (Part 2) International Olympic Committee consensus statement on load in sport and risk of illness. *Br J Sports Med* 50 (17): 1043-1052.

Scott, J.W., F.A. Ross, J.K. Liu, and D.G. Hardie. 2007. Regulation of AMP-activated protein kinase by a pseudosubstrate sequence on the gamma subunit. *EMBO J* 26:806-815.

Sears, B. 1995. *The zone: A dietary road map*. New York: Harper Collins.

Segura, R., and J.L. Ventura. 1988. Effect of L-tryptophan supplementation on exercise performance. *Int J Sports Med* 9:301-305.

Segura-García, C., M.C. Papaianni, F. Caglioti et al. 2012. Orthorexia nervosa: A frequent eating disordered behavior in athletes. *Eat Weight Disord* 17 (4): e226-e233.

Senate Select Committee on Nutrition and Human Needs. 1977. *Dietary goals for the United States.* Washington, DC: U.S. Government Printing Office.

Sheppard, L., A.R. Kristal, and L.H. Kushi. 1991. Weight loss in women participating in a randomized trial of low-fat diets. *Am J Clin Nutr* 54 (5): 821-828.

Sherman, W.M., and D.L. Costill. 1984. The marathon: Dietary manipulation to optimize performance. *Am J Sports Med* 12 (1): 44-51.

Sherman, W.M., D.L. Costill, W.J. Fink, and J.M. Miller. 1981. The effect of exercise and diet manipulation on muscle glycogen and its subsequent utilization during performance. *Int J Sports Med* 2:114-118.

Sherman, W.M., J.A. Doyle, D.R. Lamb, and R.H. Strauss. 1993. Dietary carbohydrate, muscle glycogen, and exercise performance during 7 d of training. *Am J Clin Nutr* 57:27-31.

Shi, X., R.W. Summers, H.P. Schedl, S.W. Flanagan, R. Chang, and C.V. Gisolfi. 1995. Effects of carbohydrate type and concentration and solution osmolality on water absorption. *Med Sci Sports Exerc* 27 (12): 1607-1615.

Shils, M.E., J.A. Olson, M. Shike, and A.C. Ross. 1999. *Modern nutrition in health and disease.* 9th ed. Baltimore: Williams & Wilkins.

Shing, C.M., J.M. Peake, K. Suzuki, D.G. Jenkins, and J.S. Coombes. 2013. A pilot study: Bovine colostrum supplementation and hormonal and autonomic responses to competitive cycling. *J Sports Med Phys Fitness* 53:490-501.

Shing, C.M., J.M. Peake, K. Suzuki, M. Okutsu, R. Pereira, L. Stevenson, D.G. Jenkins, and J.S. Coombes. 2007. Effects of bovine colostrum supplementation on immune variables in highly trained cyclists. *J Appl Physiol* 102:1113-1122.

Shirreffs, S.M., and R.J. Maughan. 1997. Restoration of fluid balance after exercise-induced dehydration: Effects of alcohol consumption. *J Appl Physiol* 83:1152-1157.

Shirreffs, S.M., and R.J. Maughan. 1998. Volume repletion following exercise-induced volume depletion in man: Replacement of water and sodium losses. *Am J Physiol* 274:F868-F875.

Shirreffs, S.M., and R.J. Maughan. 2000. Rehydration and recovery of fluid balance after exercise. *Exer Sports Sci Rev* 28:27-32.

Shirreffs, S.M., A.J. Taylor, J.B. Leiper, and R.J. Maughan. 1996. Post-exercise rehydration in man: Effects of volume consumed and drink sodium content. *Med Sci Sports Exerc* 28:1260-1271.

Shuler, F.D., M.K. Wingate, G.H. Moore, and C. Giangarra. 2012. Sports health benefits of vitamin D. *Sports Health* 4(6): 496-501.

Sidossis, L.S., A. Gastaldelli, S. Klein, and R.R. Wolfe. 1997. Regulation of plasma fatty acid oxidation during low- and high-intensity exercise. *Am J Physiol* 272:E1065-E1070.

Silber, B.Y., and J.A. Schmitt. 2010. Effects of tryptophan loading on human cognition, mood, and sleep. *Neurosci Biobehav Rev* 34 (3): 387-407.

Silva, A.C., M.S. Santos-Neto, A.M. Soares, M.C. Fonteles, R.L. Guerrant, and A.A. Lima. 1998. Efficacy of a glutamine-based oral rehydration solution on the electrolyte and water absorption in a rabbit model of secretory diarrhea induced by cholera toxin. *J Pediatr Gastroenterol Nutr* 26 (5): 513-519.

Simi, B., B. Sempore, M.-H. Mayet, and R.J. Favier. 1991. Additive effects of training and high-fat diet on energy metabolism during exercise. *J Appl Physiol* 71 (1): 197-203.

Simoneau, J.A., and C. Bouchard. 1989. Human variation in skeletal muscle fiber-type proportion and enzyme activities. *Am J Physiol* 257:E567-E572.

Simonsen, J.C., W.M. Sherman, D.R. Lamb, A.R. Dernbach, J.A. Doyle, and R. Strauss. 1991. Dietary carbohydrate, muscle glycogen, and power output during rowing training. *J Appl Physiol* 70:1500-1505.

Singh, A., M.L. Failla, and, P.A. Deuster. 1994. Exercise-induced changes in immune function: Effects of zinc supplementation. *J Appl Physiol* 76:2298-2301.

Siri, W.E. 1956. The gross composition of the body. *Adv Biol Med Physiol* 4:239-280.

Sirrs, S.M., and R.A. Bebb. 1999. DHEA: Panacea or snake oil? *Can Fam Physician* 45:1723-1728.

Sjodin, A.M., A.B. Andersson, J.M. Hogberg, and K.R. Westerterp. 1994. Energy balance in cross-country skiers: A study using doubly labeled water. *Med Sci Sports Exerc* 26 (6): 720-724.

Skeaff, C.M., and J. Miller. 2009. Dietary fat and coronary heart disease: Summary of evidence from prospective cohort and randomised controlled trials. *Ann Nutr Metab* 55 (1-3): 173-201.

Slater, G., D. Jenkins, P. Logan, H. Lee, M. Vukovich, J.A. Rathmacher, and A.G. Hahn. 2001. Beta-hydroxy-beta-methylbutyrate (hmb) supplementation does not affect changes in strength or body composition during resistance training in trained men. *Int J Sport Nutr Exerc Metab* 11 (3): 384-396.

Slattery K., D. Bentley, and A.J. Coutts. 2015. The role of oxidative, inflammatory and neuroendocrinological systems during exercise stress in athletes: Implications of antioxidant supplementation on physiological adaptation during intensified physical training. *Sports Med* 45 (4): 453-471.

Sly, L.M., M. Lopez, W.M. Nauseef, and N.E. Reiner. 2001. 1-alpha, 5-Dihydroxyvitamin D3-induced monocyte antimycobacterial activity is regulated by phosphatidylinositol 3-kinase and mediated by the NADPH-dependent phagocyte oxidase. *J Biol Chem* 276(38): 35482-35493.

Slyper, A.H. 2013. The influence of carbohydrate quality on cardiovascular disease, the metabolic syndrome, type 2 diabetes, and obesity: An overview. *J Pediatr Endocrinol Metab* 26 (7-8): 617-629.

Smathers, A.M., M.G. Bemben, and D.A. Bemben. 2009. Bone density comparisons in male competitive road cyclists and untrained controls. *Med Sci Sports Exerc* 41 (2): 290-296.

Smith, G.I., P. Atherton, D.N. Reeds, B.S. Mohammed, D. Rankin, M.J. Rennie, and B. Mittendorfer. 2011a. Dietary Omega-3 fatty acid supplementation increases the rate of muscle protein synthesis in older adults: A randomized controlled trial. *Am J Clin Nutr* 93:402-412.

Smith, G.I., P. Atherton, D.N. Reeds, B.S. Mohammed, D. Rankin, M.J. Rennie, and B. Mittendorfer. 2011b. Omega-3 polyunsaturated fatty acids augment the muscle protein anabolic response to hyperinsulinaemia-hyperaminoacidaemia in healthy young and middle-aged men and women. *Clin Sci* 121:267-278.

Smith, J.W., D.D. Pascoe, D.H. Passe, B.C. Ruby, L.K. Stewart, L.B. Baker, and J.J. Zachwieja. 2013. Curvilinear dose-response relationship of carbohydrate (0-120 g·h(-1)) and performance. *Med Sci Sports Exerc* 45 (2): 336-341.

Smyth, P.P., and L.H. Duntas. 2005. Iodine uptake and loss-can frequent strenuous exercise induce iodine deficiency? *Horm Metab Res* 37 (9): 555-558.

Snijders, T., P.T. Res, J.S.J. Smeets, S. Vliet, J. VanKranenburg, K. VanMaase, A.K. Kies, L.B. Verdijk, and L.J. van Loon.et al. 2015. Protein ingestion before sleep increases muscle mass and strength gains during prolonged resistance-type exercise training in healthy young men. *J Nutr* 145:1178-1784.

Snow-Harter, C.M. 1994. Bone health and prevention of osteoporosis in active and athletic women. *Clin Sport Med* 13:389-404.

Snyder, A.C., K.P. O'Hagan, P.S. Clifford, et al. 1993. Exercise responses to in-line skating: Comparisons to running and cycling. *Int J Sports Med* 14 (1): 38-42.

Sole, C.C., and T.D. Noakes. 1989. Faster gastric emptying for glucose-polymer and fructose solutions than for glucose in humans. *Eur J Appl Physiol* 58:605-612.

Somerville, V.S., A.J. Braakhuis, and W.G. Hopkins. 2016. Effect of flavonoids on upper respiratory tract infections and immune function: A systematic review and meta-analysis. *Adv Nutr* 7:488-497.

Somerville, V., C. Bringans, and A. Braakhuis. 2017. Polyphenols and performance: A systematic review and meta-analysis. *Sports Med* 47 (8): 1589-1599.

Song, Q.-H., R.M. Xu, Q.-H. Zhang, G.-Q. Shen, M. Ma, X.P. Zhao, Y.-H. Guo, and Y. Wang. 2015. Glutamine supplementation and immune function during heavy load training. *Int J Clin Pharmacol Ther* 53:372-376.

Spector, S.A., M.R. Jackman, L.A. Sabounjian, C. Sakkas, D.M. Landers, and W.T. Willis. 1995. Effect of choline supplementation on fatigue in trained cyclists. *Med Sci Sports Exerc* 27 (5): 668-673.

Spriet, L.L. 1991. Phosphofructokinase activity and acidosis during short-term tetanic contractions. *Can J Physiol Pharmacol* 69:298-304.

Spriet, L.L. 1995a. Anaerobic metabolism during high-intensity exercise. In *Exercise metabolism,* edited by M. Hargreaves, 1-39. Champaign, IL: Human Kinetics.

Spriet, L.L. 1995b. Caffeine and performance. *Int J Sports Nutr* 5:S84-S99.

Spriet, L.L., D.A. MacLean, D.J. Dyck, E. Hultman, G. Cederblad, and T.E. Graham. 1992. Caffeine ingestion and muscle metabolism during prolonged exercise in humans. *Am J Physiol* 262:E891-E898.

Spurr, G.B., A.M. Prentice, P.R. Murgatroyd, G.R. Goldberg, J.C. Reina, and N.T. Christman. 1988. Energy expenditure from minute-by-minute heart-rate recording: Comparison with indirect calorimetry. *Am J Clin Nutr* 48:552-559.

Stackhouse, S.K., D.S. Reisman, and S.A. Binder-Macleod. 2001. Challenging the role of pH in skeletal muscle fatigue. *Physical Therapy* 81:1897–1903.

Stackpool, C.M., J.P. Porcari, R.P. Mikat, C. Gillette, and C. Foster. 2014. The accuracy of various activity trackers in estimating steps taken and energy expenditure. *Journal of Fitness Research* 3:32-48.

Stanko, R.T., R.J. Robertson, R.W. Galbreath, J.J. Reilly, K.D. Greenawalt, and F.L. Goss. 1990. Enhanced leg exercise endurance with a high-carbohydrate diet and dihydroxyacetone and pyruvate. *J Appl Physiol* 69 (5): 1651-1656.

Stanko, R.T., R.J. Robertson, R.J. Spina, J.J. Reilly, Jr., K.D. Greenawalt, and F.L. Goss. 1990. Enhancement of arm exercise endurance capacity with dihydroxyacetone and pyruvate. *J Appl Physiol* 68 (1): 119-124.

Starling, R.D., T.A. Trappe, K.R. Short, M. Sheffield-Moore, A.C. Jozsi, W.J. Fink, and D.L. Costill. 1996. Effect of inosine supplementation on aerobic and anaerobic cycling performance. *Med Sci Sports Exerc* 28 (9): 1193-1198.

Staron, R.S., F.C. Hagerman, R.S. Hikida, T.F. Murray, D.P. Hostler, M.T. Crill, K.E. Ragg, and K. Toma. 2000. Fiber type composition of the vastus lateralis muscle of young men and women. *J Histochem Cytochem* 48:623-629.

Starritt, E.C., R.A. Howlett, G.J. Heigenhauser, and L.L. Spriet. 2000. Sensitivity of CPT I tomalonyl-COA in trained and untrained human skeletal muscle. *Am J Physiol Endocrinol Metab* 278 (3): E462-E468.

Stearns, D.M., J.J. Belbruno, and K.E. Wetterhahn. 1995. A prediction of chromium (III) accumulation in humans from chromium dietary supplements. *FASEB J* 9 (15): 1650-1657.

Stearns, D.M., Sr., J.P. Wise, S.R. Patierno, and K.E. Wetterhahn. 1995. Chromium (III) picolinate produces chromosome damage in Chinese hamster ovary cells. *FASEB J* 9 (15): 1643-1648.

Steensberg, A., C. Keller, T. Hillig, C. Fresig, J.F. Wojtaszewski, B.K. Pedersen, H. Pilegaard, and M. Sander. 2007. Nitric oxide production is a proximal signalling event controlling exercise-induced mRNA expression in human skeletal muscle. *FASEB J* 21 (11): 2683-2694.

Stellingwerff T., and G.R. Cox. 2014. Systematic review: Carbohydrate supplementation on exercise performance or capacity of varying durations. *Appl Physiol Nutr Metab* 39 (9): 998-1011.

Stellingwerff, T., L.L. Spriet, M.J. Watt, N.E. Kimber, M. Hargreaves, J.A. Hawley, and L.M. Burke. 2006. Decreased PDH activation and glycogenolysis during exercise following fat adaptation with carbohydrate restoration. *Am J Physiol Endocrinol Metab* 290 (2): E380-388.

Stensrud, T., F. Ingjer, H. Holm, and S.B. Strømme. 1992. L-tryptophan supplementation does not improve running performance. *Int J Sports Med* 13 (6): 481-485.

Stephens, F.B., D. Constantin-Teodosiu, D. Laithwaite, E.J. Simpson, and P.L. Greenhaff. 2006. Insulin stimulates L-carnitine accumulation in human skeletal muscle. *FASEB J* 20 (2): 377-379.

Stephens, F.B., C.E. Evans, D. Constantin-Teodosiu, and P.L. Greenhaff. 2007. Carbohydrate ingestion augments L-carnitine retention in humans. *J Appl Physiol* 102 (3): 1065-1070.

Stephens, F.B., and Greenhaff, P.L. 2014. Creatine. In *Sports nutrition*, edited by R.J. Maughan, 301-312. Oxford: Wiley, Blackwell.

Stephens, F.B., B.T. Wall, K. Marimuthu, C.E. Shannon, D. Constantin-Teodosiu, I.A. Macdonald, and P.L. Greenhaff. 2013. Skeletal muscle carnitine loading increases energy expenditure modulates fuel metabolism gene networks and prevents body fat accumulation in humans. *J Physiol* 591 (Pt 18): 4655-4666.

Stewart, I., L. McNaughton, P. Davies, and S. Tristram. 1990. Phosphate loading and the effects on $\dot{V}O_2$max in trained cyclists. *Res Q Exerc Sport* 61 (1): 80-84.

Stoecker, B.J. 1996. Chromium. In *Present knowledge in nutrition*, edited by E.E. Ziegler and L.J. Filer, 344-353. Washington, DC: ILSI Press.

Stolarczyk, L.M., V.H. Heyward, M.D. Van Loan, et al. 1997. The fatness-specific bioelectrical impedance analysis equations of Segal et al.: Are they generalizable and practical? *Am J Clin Nutr* 66 (1): 8-17.

Storm, F., B.W. Heller, and C. Mazzà. 2015. Step detection and activity recognition accuracy of seven physical activity monitors. *PLoS One* 10 (3): e0118723.

Stout, J.R., J.T. Cramer, M. Mielke, J. O'Kroy, D.J. Torok, and R.F.Zoeller. 2006. Effects of twenty-eight days of beta-alanine and creatine monohydrate supplementation on the physical working capacity at neuromuscular fatigue threshold. *J Strength Cond Res* 20 (4): 928-931.

St-Pierre, J., J.A. Buckingham, S.J. Roebuck, and M.D. Brand. 2002. Topology of superoxide production from different sites in the mitochondrial electron transport chain. *J Biol Chem* 277:44784-44790.

Stubbs, R.J., C.J. Habron, P.R. Murcatroyd, and A.M. Prentice. 1995. Covert manipulation of dietary fat and energy density: Effect on substrate flux and food intake in men eating ad libitum. *Am J Clin Nutr* 62:316-329.

Stubbs, R.J., C.J. Harbron, and A.M. Prentice. 1996. Covert manipulation of the dietary fat to carbohydrate ratio of isoenergetically dense diets: Effect on food intake in feeding men ad libitum. *Int J Obes Relat Metab Disord* 20 (7): 651-660.

Stubbs, R.J., P. Ritz, W.A. Coward, and A.M. Prentice. 1995. Covert manipulation of the ratio of dietary fat to carbohydrate and energy density: Effect on food intake and energy balance in free-living men eating ad libitum. *Am J Clin Nutr* 62 (2): 330-337.

Sundgot-Borgen, J. 1994a. Eating disorders in female athletes. *Sports Med* 3:176-188.

Sundgot-Borgen, J. 1994b. Risk and trigger factors for the development of eating disorders in female elite athletes. *Med Sci Sports Exerc* 4:414-419.

Sundgot-Borgen, J. 2000. Eating disorders in athletes. In *Nutrition in sport*, edited by R.J. Maughan, 510-522. Oxford: Blackwell Science.

Sundgot-Borgen, J., and S. Larsen. 1993. Pathogenic weight-control methods and self-reported eating disorders in female elite athletes and controls. *Scand J Med Sci Sports* 3:150-155.

Sutton, J.R., and O. Bar-Or. 1980. Thermal illness in fun running. *Am Heart J* 100:778-781.

Svendsen, I.S., I.M Taylor, E. Tonnesen, et al. 2016. Training- and competition-related risk factors for respiratory tract and gastrointestinal infections in elite cross-country skiers. *Br J Sports Med* 50:809-815.

Svensson, M., C. Malm, M. Tonkonogi, B. Ekblom, B. Sjodin, and K. Sahlin. 1999. Effect of Q10 supplementation on tissue Q10 levels and adenine nucleotide catabolism during high-intensity exercise. *Int J Sport Nutr* 9 (2): 166-180.

Swensen, T., G. Crater, D.R. Bassett, Jr., and E.T. Howley. 1994. Adding polylactate to a glucose polymer solution does not improve endurance. *Int J Sports Med* 15 (7): 430-434.

Symons, T.B., M. Sheffield-Moore, R.R. Wolfe, and D. Paddon-Jones. 2009. A moderate serving of high-quality protein maximally stimulates skeletal muscle protein synthesis in young and elderly subjects. *J Am Diet Assoc* 109:1582-1586.

Tang, J.E., J.W. Hartman, and S.M. Phillips. 2006. Increased muscle oxidative potential following resistance training induced fibre hypertrophy in young men. *Appl Physiol Nutr Metab* 31 (5): 495-501.

Tang, J.E., D.R. Moore, G.W. Kujbida, M.A. Tarnopolsky, and S.M. Phillips. 2009. Ingestion of whey hydrolysate, casein, or soy protein isolate: effects on mixed muscle protein synthesis at rest and following resistance exercise in young men. *J Appl Physiol* 107:987-992.

Tappy, L. 1996. Thermic effect of food and sympathetic nervous system activity in humans. *Reprod Nutr Dev* 36 (4): 391-397.

Tappy, L., and K.A. Lê. 2010. Metabolic effects of fructose and the worldwide increase in obesity. *Physiol Rev* 90 (1): 23-46.

Tappy, L., and K.A. Lê. 2015. Health effects of fructose and fructose-containing caloric sweeteners: Where do we stand 10 years after the initial whistle blowings? *Curr Diab Rep* 15 (8): 54.

Tarnopolsky, M.A. 2004. Protein requirements for endurance athletes. *Nutrition* 20:662-668.

Tarnopolsky, M.A., S.A. Atkinson, S.M. Phillips, and J.D. MacDougall. 1995. Carbohydrate loading and metabolism during exercise in men and women. *J Appl Physiol* 78 (4): 1360-1368.

Tarnopolsky, M.A., M. Bosman, J.R. MacDonald, D. Vandeputte, J. Martin, and B.D. Roy. 1997. Post-exercise protein-carbohydrate and carbohydrate supplements increase muscle glycogen in men and women. *J Appl Physiol* 83 (6): 1877-1883.

Tartibian, B., B. H. Maleki, and A. Abbasi 2009. The effects of ingestion of omega-3 fatty acids on perceived pain and external symptoms of delayed onset muscle soreness in untrained men. *Clin J Sport Med* 19:115-119.

Te Morenga, L., S. Mallard, and J. Mann. 2013. Dietary sugars and body weight: Systematic review and meta-analysis of randomized controlled trials and cohort studies. *BMJ* 346:e7492.

Temple, J.L., C. Bernard, S.E. Lipshultz, J.D. Czachor, J.A. Westphal, and M.A. Mestre. 2017. The safety of ingested caffeine: A comprehensive review. *Front Psychiatry* (May 26): 80.

Terjung, R.L., P. Clarkson, E.R. Eichner, P.L. Greenhaff, P.J. Hespel, R.G. Israel, W.J. Kraemer, R.A. Meyer, L.L. Spriet, M.A. Tarnopolsky, A.J. Wagenmakers, and M.H. Williams. 2000. American College of Sports Medicine roundtable: The physiological and health effects of oral creatine supplementation. *Med Sci Sports Exerc* 32 (3): 706-717.

Tenforde, A.S., M.T. Barrack, A. Nattiv, and M. Fredericson. 2016. Parallels with the female athlete triad in male athletes. *Sports Med* 46 (2): 171-182.

Thein-Nissenbaum, J.M., M.J. Rauh, K.E. Carr, et al. 2011. Associations between disordered eating, menstrual dysfunction, and musculoskeletal injury among high school athletes. *J Orthop Sports Phys Ther* 41 (2): 60-69.

Thomas D.T., K.A. Erdman, and L.M. Burke. 2016. American College of Sports Medicine Joint Position Statement: Nutrition and athletic performance. *Med Sci Sports Exerc* 48 (3): 543-568.

Thompson, R.A., and R.T. Sherman. 2010. *Eating disorders in sport*. New York: Routledge, Taylor and Francis Group.

Thompson, R.A., and R. Trattner-Sherman. 1993. *Helping athletes with eating disorders.* Champaign, IL: Human Kinetics.

Thorning, T.K., A. Raben, T. Tholstrup, S.S. Soedamah-Muthu, I. Givens, and A. Astrup. 2016. Milk and dairy products: Good or bad for human health? An assessment of the totality of scientific evidence. *Food Nutr Res* 60:32527.

Thorogood, M. 1996. Nutrition. In *Prevention of cardiovascular disease: An evidence-based approach*, edited by M. Lawrence, A. Neil, D. Mant, and G. Fowler, 54-66. Kings Lynn: Oxford University Press.

Threapleton, D.E., D.C. Greenwood, C.E. Evans, C.L. Cleghorn, C. Nykjaer, C. Woodhead, J.E. Cade, C.P. Gale, and V.J. Burley. 2013. Dietary fibre intake and risk of cardiovascular disease: Systematic review and meta-analysis. *BMJ* 347:f6879.

Tiidus, P.M., Tupling, A.R., and Houston, M.E. 2012. *Biochemistry primer for exercise science.* 4th ed. Champaign, IL: Human Kinetics.

Timmons, J.A., S.M. Poucher, D. Constantin-Teodosiu, V. Worrall, I.A. Macdonald, and P.L. Greenhaff. 1996. Increased acetyl group availability enhances contractile function of canine skeletal muscle during ischemia. *J Clin Invest* 97:879-883.

Tiollier, E., C.D.T.M. Chennaoui, D. Gomez-Merino, et al. 2007. Effect of a probiotics supplementation on respiratory infections and immune and hormonal parameters during intense military training. *Military Med* 172:1006-1011.

Tippett, K.S., and L.E. Cleveland., eds. 1999. How current diets stack up: Comparison with dietary guidelines. *Agriculture Information Bulletin* 750:51-70.

Tipton, K.D. 2013. Dietary strategies to attenuate muscle loss during recovery from injury. *Nestle Nutr Inst Workshop Ser* 75:51-61.

Tipton, C.M., and R.A. Oppliger. 1993. Nutritional and fitness considerations for competitive wrestlers. *World Rev Nutr Diet* 71:84-96.

Tipton, K.D., T.A. Elliott, M.G. Cree, A.A. Aarsland, A.P. Sanford, and R.R. Wolfe. 2007. Stimulation of net muscle protein synthesis by whey protein ingestion before and after exercise. *Am J Physiol Endocrinol Metab* 292 (1): E71-E76.

Tipton, K.D., A.A. Ferrando, S.M. Phillips, D. Doyle, Jr., and R.R. Wolfe. 1999. Postexercise net protein synthesis in human muscle from orally administered amino acids. *Am J Physiol* 276 (4 Pt 1): E628-E634.

Tipton, K.D., B.B. Rasmussen, S.L. Miller, S.E. Wolf, S.K. Owens-Stovall, B.E. Petrini, and R.R. Wolfe. 2001. Timing of amino acid-carbohydrate ingestion alters anabolic response of muscle to resistance exercise. *Am J Physiol Endocrinol Metab* 281 (2): E197-E206.

Todd, J.J., L.K. Pourshahidi, E.M. McSorley, S.M. Madigan, and P.J. Magee. 2015. Vitamin D: Recent advances and implications for athletes. *Sports Med* 45:213-229.

Tomás-Barberán, F.A., M.V. Selma, and J.C. Espín. 2016. Interactions of gut microbiota with dietary polyphenols and consequences to human health. *Curr Opin Clin Nutr Metab Care* 19 (6): 471-476.

Tonevitsky, A.G., D.V. Maltseva, A. Abbasi, T.R. Samatov, D.A. Sakharov, M.U. Shkurnikov, A.E. Lebedev, V.V. Galatenko, A.I. Grigoriev, and H. Northoff. 2013. Dynamically regulated miRNA-mRNA networks revealed by exercise. *BMC Physiol* 13:9.

Torstveit, M.K., and J. Sundgot-Borgen. 2014. Eating disorders in male and female athletes. In *Sports nutrition*, edited by R. J. Maughan, 513-525. Oxford: Blackwell Science.

Touyz, S.W., P.J.V. Beumont, and S. Hook. 1987. Exercise anorexia: A new dimension in anorexia nervosa? In *Handbook of Eating Disorders: Part 1,* edited by P.J.V. Beumont, G.D. Burrows, and R.C. Casper, 143-157. Amsterdam: Elsevier.

Trapp, E.G., D.J. Chisholm, J. Freund, and S.H. Boutcher. 2008. The effects of high-intensity intermittent exercise training on fat loss and fasting insulin levels of young women. *Int J Obesity* 32 (4): 684-691.

Trappe, T.A., F. White, C.P. Lambert, D. Cesar, M. Hellerstein, and W.J. Evans. 2002. Effect of ibuprofen and acetaminophen on postexercise muscle protein synthesis. *Am J Physiol Endocrinol Metab* 282:E551-556.

Tremblay, M.S., S.D. Galloway, and J.R. Sexsmith. 1994. Ergogenic effects of phosphate loading: Physiological fact or methodological fiction? *Can J Appl Physiol* 19 (1): 1-11.

Trexler, E.T., A.E. Smith-Ryan, J.R. Stout, J.R., Hoffman, C.D. Wilborn, C. Sale, R.B. Kreider, R. Jäger, C.P. Earnest, L. Bannock, B. Campbell, D. Kalman, T.N. Ziegenfuss, and J. Antonio. 2015. International Society of Sports Nutrition position stand: Beta-alanine. *J Int Soc Sports Nutr* (July 15). http://doi.org/10.1186/s12970-015-0090-y.

Tsintzas, K., and C. Williams. 1998. Human muscle glycogen metabolism during exercise: Effect of carbohydrate supplementation. *Sports Med* 25 (1): 7-23.

Tsintzas, O.K., C. Williams, L. Boobis, and P. Greenhaff. 1995. Carbohydrate ingestion and glycogen utilisation in different muscle fibre types in man. *J Physiol* 489 (1): 243-250.

Turcotte, L.P., E.A. Richter, and B. Kiens. 1995. Lipid metabolism during exercise. In *Exercise metabolism,* edited by M. Hargreaves, 99-130. Champaign, IL: Human Kinetics.

U.K. National Diet and Nutrition Survey Rolling Programme for 2008/2009 to 2011/2012. 2014. www.gov.uk/government/collections/national-diet-and-nutrition-survey.

U.K. National Diet and Nutrition Survey Rolling Programme for 2012/2013 to 2013/2014. 2016. www.gov.uk/government/uploads/system/uploads/attachment_data/file/551352/NDNS_Y5_6_UK_Main_Text.pdf.

USADA. n.d. Supplement 441: Realize, Recognize, Reduce. www.usada.org/substances/supplement-411/reduce-risk-testing-positive-experiencing-adverse-health-effects.

U.S. Department of Agriculture. 2005. *Dietary guidelines for Americans, 2005.* www.health.gov/dietaryguidelines.

U.S. Department of Agriculture. 2015. *2015-2020 dietary guidelines for Americans.* https://health.gov/dietaryguidelines/2015/guidelines.

U.S. Department of Agriculture. 2003. *USDA national nutrient database for standard reference.* www.nal.usda.gov/fnic/foodcomp/Data/index.html.

Vandenberghe, K., M. Goris, P. Van Hecke, M. Van Leemputte, L. Vangerven, and P. Hespel. 1997. Long-term creatine intake is beneficial to muscle performance during resistance training. *J Appl Physiol* 83 (6): 2055-2063.

Vandenbogaerde, T.J., and W.G. Hopkins. 2011. Effects of acute carbohydrate supplementation on endurance performance: A meta-analysis. *Sports Med* 41 (9): 773-792.

van der Meulen, J.H., A. McArdle, M.J. Jackson, and J.A. Faulkner. 1997. Contraction-induced injury to the extensor digitorum longus muscles of rats: The role of vitamin E. *J Appl Physiol* 83:817-823.

van Erp-Baart, A.M.J., W.H.M. Saris, R.A. Binkhorst, J.A. Vos, and J.W.H. Elvers. 1989a. Nationwide survey on nutritional habits in elite athletes. Part I: Energy carbohydrate, protein. *Int J Sports Med* 10 (Suppl 1): S3-S10.

van Erp-Baart, A.M.J., W.H.M. Saris, R.A. Binkhorst, J.A. Vos, and J.W.H. Elvers. 1989b. Nationwide survey on nutritional habits in elite athletes. Part II: Mineral and vitamin intake. *Int J Sports Med* 10 (1): S11-S16.

van Essen, M.J., and M.J. Gibala. 2006. Failure of protein to improve time trial performance when added to a sports drink. *Med Sci Sports Exerc* 38 (8): 1476-1483.

Van Etten, L.M., F.T. Verstappen, and K.R. Westerterp. 1994. Effect of body build on weight-training-induced adaptations in body composition and muscular strength. *Med Sci Sports Exerc* 26 (4): 515-521.

van Hall, G. 2015. The physiological regulation of skeletal muscle fatty acid supply and oxidation during moderate-intensity exercise. *Sports Med* 45 (Suppl 1): S23-S32.

van Hall, G., J.S.H. Raaymakers, W.H.M. Saris, and A.J.M. Wagenmakers. 1995. Ingestion of branched-chain amino acids and tryptophan during sustained exercise in man: Failure to affect performance. *J Physiol* 486 (3): 789-794.

Van Loan, M.D., N.L. Keim, K. Berg, et al. 1995. Evaluation of body composition by dual energy X-ray absorptiometry and two different software packages. *Med Sci Sports Exerc* 27 (4): 587-591.

van Loon, L.J., P. Greenhaff, D. Constantin-Teodosiu, W.H. Saris, and A.J. Wagenmakers. 2001. The effects of increasing exercise intensity on muscle fuel utilisation in humans. *J Physio* 536 (Pt 1): 295-304.

van Loon, L.J., W.H. Saris, M. Kruijshoop, and A.J. Wagenmakers. 2000. Maximizing postexercise muscle glycogen synthesis: Carbohydrate supplementation and the application of amino acid or protein hydrolysate mixtures. *Am J Clin Nutr* 72 (1): 106-111.

Van Nieuwenhoven, M.A., R.-J.M. Brummer, and F. Brouns. 2000. Gastrointestinal function during exercise: Comparison of water, sports drink, and sports drink with caffeine. *J Appl Physiol* 89 (3): 1079-1085.

van Oort, M.M., J.M. van Doorn, A. Bonen, J.F.C. Glatz, D.J. van der Horst, K.W. Rodenburg, and J.J.F.P. Luiken. 2008. Insulin-induced translocation of CD36 to the plasma membrane is reversible and shows similarity to that of GLUT4. *Biochim Biophys Acta* 1781 (1-2): 61-71.

Van Soeren, M.H., and T.E. Graham. 1998. Effect of caffeine on metabolism, exercise endurance, and catecholamine responses after withdrawal. *J Appl Physiol* 85 (4): 1493-1501.

Van Soeren, M.H., P. Sathasivam, L.L. Spriet, and T.E. Graham. 1993. Caffeine metabolism and epinephrine responses during exercise in users and nonusers. *J Appl Physiol* 75 (2): 805-812.

Van Thienen, R., K. Van Proeyen, B. Vanden Eynde, J. Puype, T. Lefere, and P. Hespel. 2009. Beta-alanine improves sprint performance in endurance cycling. *Med Sci Sports Exerc* 41 (4): 898-903.

Van Tonder, A., M. Schwellnus, S. Swanevelder, E. Jordaan, W. Derman, and D.C. Janse van Rensburg. 2016. A prospective cohort study of 7031 distance runners shows that 1 in 13 report systemic symptoms of an acute illness in the 7-day period before a race, increasing their risk of not finishing the race 1.9 times for those runners who started the race: SAFER study IV. *Br J Sport Med* 50:939-945.

van Vliet, S., N.A. Burd, and L.J. van Loon. 2015. The skeletal muscle anabolic response to plant- versus animal-based protein consumption. *J Nutr* 145 (9): 1981-1991.

Van Zeyl, C.G., E.V. Lambert, J.A. Hawley, T.D. Noakes, and S.C. Dennis. 1996. Effects of medium-chain triglyceride ingestion on carbohydrate metabolism and cycling performance. *J Appl Physiol* 80:2217-2225.

Varnier, M., P. Sarto, D. Martines, L. Lora, F. Carmignoto, G.P. Leese, and R. Naccarato. 1994. Effect of infusing branched-chain amino acid during incremental exercise with reduced muscle glycogen content. *Eur J Appl Physiol* 69 (1): 26-31.

Venables, M.C., L. Shaw, A.E. Jeukendrup, A. Roedig-Penman, M. Finke, R.G. Newcombe, J. Parry, and A.J. Smith. 2005. Erosive effect of a new sports drink on dental enamel during exercise. *Med Sci Sports Exerc* 37 (1): 39-44.

Vergauwen, L., F. Brouns, and P. Hespel. 1998. Carbohydrate supplementation improves stroke performance in tennis. *Med Sci Sports Exerc* 30 (8): 1289-1295.

Verma, S., M.C. Cam, and J.H. McNeill. 1998. Nutritional factors that can favorably influence the glucose/insulin system: Vanadium. *J Am Coll Nutr* 17:11-18.

Veverka, D.V., C. Wilson, M.A. Martinez, R. Wenger, and A. Tamosuinas. 2009. Use of zinc supplements to reduce upper respiratory infections in United States Air Force Academy cadets. *Complement Ther Clin Pract* 15(2): 91-95.

Vist, G.E., and R.J. Maughan. 1994. Gastric emptying of ingested solutions in man: Effect of beverage glucose concentration. *Med Sci Sports Exerc* 26 (10): 1269-1273.

Vist, G.E., and R.J. Maughan. 1995. The effect of osmolality and carbohydrate content on the rate of gastric emptying of liquids in man. *J Physiol* 486 (Pt 2): 523-531.

Vitetta, L., D. Briskey, H. Alford, S. Hall, and S. Coulson. 2014. Probiotics, prebiotics and the gastrointestinal tract in health and disease. *Inflammopharmacology* 22 (3): 135-154.

Volek, J.S., D.J. Freidenreich, C. Saenz, L.J. Kunces, B.C. Creighton, J.M. Bartley, P.M. Davitt, C.X. Munoz, J.M. Anderson, C.M. Maresh, E.C. Lee, M.D. Schuenke, G. Aerni, W.J. Kraemer, and S.D. Phinney. 2016. Metabolic characteristics of keto-adapted ultra-endurance runners. *Metabolism* 65 (3): 100-110.

Volek, J.S., W.J. Kraemer, J.A. Bush, M. Boetes, T. Incledon, K.L. Clark, and J.M. Lynch. 1997. Creatine supplementation enhances muscular performance during high-intensity resistance exercise. *J Am Diet Assoc* 97 (7): 765-770.

Volek, J.S., R. Silvestre, J.P. Kirwan, M.J. Sharman, D.A. Judelson, B.A. Spiering, J.L. Vingren, C.M. Maresh, J.L. Vanheest, and W.J. Kraemer. 2006. Effects of chromium supplementation on glycogen synthesis after high-intensity exercise. *Med Sci Sports Exerc* 38 (12): 2102-2109.

Volman, J.J., J.D. Ramakers, and J. Plat. 2008. Dietary modulation of immune function by b-glucans. *Physiol Behav* 94 (2): 276-284.

Volpe, S.L., L.J. Taper, and S. Meacham. 1993. The relationship between boron and magnesium status and bone mineral density in the human: A review. *Magnes Res* 6 (3): 291-296.

von Allworden, H.N., S. Horn, J. Kahl, and W. Feldheim. 1993. The influence of lecithin on plasma choline concentrations in triathletes and adolescent runners during exercise. *Eur J Appl Physiol* 67 (1): 87-91.

von Essen, M.R., M. Kongsbak, P. Schjerling, K. Olgaard, N. Odum, and C. Geisler. 2010. Vitamin D controls T cell antigen receptor signaling and activation of human T cells. *Nat Immunol* 11(4): 344-349.

Vukovich, M.D., D.L. Costill, and W.J. Fink. 1994. Carnitine supplementation: Effect on muscle carnitine and glycogen content during exercise. *J Appl Physiol* 26 (9): 1122-1129.

Vukovich, M.D., D.L. Costill, M.S. Hickey, S.W. Trappe, K.J. Cole, and W.J. Fink. 1993. Effect of fat emulsion infusion and fat feeding on muscle glycogen utilization during cycle exercise. *J Appl Physiol* 75 (4): 1513-1518.

Wachter, S., M. Vogt, R. Kreis, C. Boesch, P. Bigler, H. Hoppeler, and S. Krahenbuhl. 2002. Long-term administration of L-carnitine to humans: Effect on skeletal muscle carnitine content and physical performance. *Clin Chim Acta* 318 (1-2): 51-61.

Wagenmakers, A.J.M. 1991. L-carnitine supplementation and performance in man. In *Advances in nutrition and top sport,* Vol. 32, edited by F. Brouns, 110-127. Basel: Karger.

Wagenmakers, A.J. 1999a. Amino acid supplements to improve athletic performance. *Curr Opin Clin Nutr Metab Care* 2 (6): 539-544.

Wagenmakers, A.J.M. 1999b. Nutritional supplements: Effects on exercise performance and metabolism. In *The metabolic basis of performance in exercise and sport,* edited by D.R. Lamb and R. Murray, 209-220. Carmel, IN: Cooper.

Wagenmakers, A.J.M., J.H. Brookes, J.H. Coakley, T. Reilly, and R.H.T. Edwards. 1989. Exercise-induced activation of branched-chain 2-oxo acid dehydrogenase in human muscle. *Eur J Appl Physiol* 59:159-167.

Wagner, D.R., V.H. Heyward, and A.L. Gibson. 2000. Validation of air displacement plethysmography for assessing body composition. *Med Sci Sports Exerc* 32 (7): 1339-1344.

Wahrenberg, H., J. Bolinder, and P. Arner. 1991. Adrenergic regulation of lipolysis in human fat cells during exercise. *Eur J Clin Invest* 21:534-541.

Walberg, J.L., M.K. Leidy, D.J. Sturgill, D.E. Hinkle, S.J. Ritchey, and D.R. Sebolt. 1988. Macronutrient content of a hypoenergy diet affects nitrogen retention and muscle function in weight lifters. *Int J Sports Med* 9 (4): 261-266.

Walker, G.J., P. Caudwell, N. Dixon, and N.C. Bishop. 2006. The effect of caffeine ingestion on neutrophil oxidative burst responses following prolonged exercise. *Int J Sport Nutr Exerc Metab* 16 (1): 24-35.

Wall, B.T., J.P. Morton, and L.J.C. van Loon. 2015. Strategies to maintain skeletal muscle mass in the injured athlete: Nutritional considerations and exercise mimetics. *Eur J Sport Sci* 15 (1): 53-62.

Wall, B.T., F.B. Stephens, D. Constantin-Teodosiu, K. Marimuthu, I.A. Macdonald, and P.L. Greenhaff. 2011. Chronic oral ingestion of L-carnitine and carbohydrate increases muscle carnitine content and alters muscle fuel metabolism during exercise in humans. *J Physiol* 589 (Pt 4): 963-973.

Wallace, M.B., J. Lim, A. Cutler, and L. Bucci. 1999. Effects of dehydroepiandrosterone vs androstenedione supplementation in men. *Med Sci Sports Exerc* 31 (12): 1788-1792.

Waller, M.F., and E.M. Haymes. 1996. The effects of heat and exercise on sweat iron loss. *Med Sci Sports Exer* 28:197-203.

Wallis, G.A., R. Dawson, J. Achten, J. Webber, and A.E. Jeukendrup. 2006. Metabolic response to carbohydrate ingestion during exercise in males and females. *Am J Physiol Endocrinol Metab* 290 (4): E708-E715.

Wallis, G.A., D.S. Rowlands, C. Shaw, R.L.P.G. Jentjens, and A.E. Jeukendrup. 2005. Oxidation of combined ingestion of maltodextrins and fructose during exercise. *Med Sci Sports Exerc* 37 (3): 426-432.

Walsh, N.P., A.K. Blannin, N.C. Bishop, P.J. Robson, and M.Gleeson. 2000. Oral glutamine supplementation does not attenuate the fall in human neutrophil lipopolysaccharide-stimulated degranulation following prolonged exercise. *Int J Sport Nutr* 10:39-50.

Walsh, N.P., A.K. Blannin, P.J. Robson, and M. Gleeson. 1998. Glutamine, exercise and immune function: Links and possible mechanisms. *Sports Med* 26:177-191.

Walsh, N.P., M. Gleeson, D.B. Pyne, D.C. Nieman, F.S. Dhabhar, R.J. Shephard, S.J. Oliver, S. Bermon, and A. Kajėnienė. 2011. Position statement part two: Maintaining immune health. *Exerc Immunol Rev* 17:64-103.

Walsh, N.P., M. Gleeson, R.J. Shephard, M. Gleeson, J.A. Woods, N.C. Bishop, M. Fleshner, C. Green, B.K. Pedersen, L. Hoffman-Goetz, C.J. Rogers, H. Northoff, A. Abbasi, and P. Simon. 2011. Position statement part one: Immune function and exercise. *Exerc Immunol Rev* 17:6-63.

Walters T.J., K.L. Ryan, L.M. Tate, and P.A. Mason. 2000. Exercise in the heat is limited by a critical internal temperature. *J Appl Physiol* 89 (2): 799-806.

Wannamethee, S.G., A.G. Shaper, and M. Walker. 2002. Weight change, weight fluctuation, and mortality. *Arch Intern Med* 162 (22): 2575-2580.

Wapnir, R.A., M.C. Sia, and S.E. Fisher. 1996. Enhancement of intestinal water absorption and sodium transport by glycerol in rats. *J Appl Physiol* 81 (6): 2523-2527.

Warren, B.J., A.L. Stanton, and D.L. Blessing. 1990. Disordered eating patterns in competitive female athletes. *Int J Eating Disorders* 5:565-569.

Warren, J.A., R.R. Jenkins, L. Packer, E.H. Witt, and R.B. Armstrong. 1992. Elevated muscle vitamin E does not attenuate eccentric exercise-induced muscle injury. *J Appl Physiol* 72:2168-2175.

Weaver, C., and S. Rajaram. 1992. Exercise and iron status. *J Nutrition* 122:782-787.

Weck, M., S.R. Bornstein, and M. Blüher. 2012. Strategies for successful weight reduction: Focus on energy balance. *Dtsch Med Wochenschr* 137:2223-2228.

Wee, S.L., C. Williams, S. Gray, and J. Horabin. 1999. Influence of high and low glycemic index meals on endurance running capacity. *Med Sci Sports Exerc* 31 (3): 393-399.

Weigle, D.S., P.A. Breen, C.C. Matthys, H.S. Callahan, K.E. Meeuws, V.R. Burden, and J.Q. Purnell. 2005. A high-protein diet induces sustained reductions in appetite, ad libitum caloric intake, and body weight despite compensatory changes in diurnal plasma leptin and ghrelin concentrations. *Am J Clin Nutr* 82 (1): 41-48.

Welle, S., R. Jozefowicz, and M. Statt. 1990. Failure of dehydroepiandrosterone to influence energy and protein metabolism in humans. *J Clin Endocrinol Metab* 71 (5): 1259-1264.

Wemple, R.D., D.R. Lamb, and K.H. McKeever. 1997. Caffeine vs caffeine-free sports drinks: Effects on urine production at rest and during prolonged exercise. *Int J Sports Med* 18 (1): 40-46.

West, N.P., D.B. Pyne, J.M. Peake, and A.W. Cripps. 2009. Probiotics, immunity and exercise: A review. *Exerc Immunol Rev* 15:107-126.

West, N.P., D.B. Pyne, A.W. Cripps, W.G. Hopkins, D.C. Eskesen, A. Jairath, C.T. Christophersen, M.A. Conlon, and P.A. Fricker. 2011. Lactobaccillus fermentum (PCC®) supplementation and gastrointestinal and respiratory tract illness symptoms: A randomised control trial in athletes. *Nutr J* 10:30.

West, N.P., P.L. Horn, D.B. Pyne, V.J. Gebski, S.J. Lahtinen, P.A. Fricker, and A.W. Cripps. 2014. Probiotic supplementation for respiratory and gastrointestinal illness symptoms in healthy physically active individuals. *Clin Nutr* 2014 33:581-587.

Westerblad, H., D.G. Allen, and J. Lannergren. 2002. Muscle fatigue: Lactic acid or inorganic phosphate the major cause? *News Physiol Sci* 17 (1): 17-21.

Westerterp, K.R. 1993. Food quotient, respiratory quotient, and energy balance. *Am J Clin Nutr* 57 (5 Suppl): 759S-764S.

Westerterp, K.R. 2013. Metabolic adaptations to over-and-underfeeding: Still a matter of debate? *Eur J Clin Nutr* 67:443-445.

Westerterp, K.R., J.H. Donkers, E.W. Fredrix, and P. Boekhoudt. 1995. Energy intake, physical activity and body weight: A simulation model. *Br J Nutr* 73:337-347.

Weyers, A.M., S.A. Mazzetti, D.M. Love, et al. 2002. Comparison of methods for assessing body composition changes during weight loss. *Med Sci Sports Exerc* 34 (3): 497-502.

Whitham, M., and J. McKinney. 2007. Effect of a carbohydrate mouthwash on running time-trial performance. *J Sports Sci* 25:1385-92.

WHO. 1996. *Trace elements in human nutrition and health.* Geneva: WHO Press.

WHO. 2015a. *Guideline: Sugars intake for adults and children.* Geneva: WHO Press.

WHO. 2015b. Healthy Diet Factsheet. www.who.int/mediacentre/factsheets/fs394/en.

Wiles, J.D., S.R. Bird, J. Hopkins, and M. Riley. 1992. Effect of caffeinated coffee on running speed, respiratory factors, blood lactate and perceived exertion during 1500-m treadmill running. *Br J Sports Med* 26 (2): 116-191.

Wilkes, D., Gledhill, N., and Smyth, R. 1983. Effect of acute induced metabolic alkalosis on 800-m racing time. *Med Sci Sports Exerc* 15:277-280.

Wilkinson, S.B., P.L. Kim, D. Armstrong, and S.M. Phillips. 2006. Addition of glutamine to essential amino acids and carbohydrate does not enhance anabolism in young human males following exercise. *Appl Physiol Nutr Metab* 31 (5): 518-529.

Wilkinson, S.B., S.M. Phillips, P.J. Atherton, R. Patel, K.E. Yarasheski, M.A. Tarnopolsky, M.J. Rennie. 2008. Differential effects of resistance and endurance exercise in the fed state on signaling molecule phosphorylation and protein synthesis in human muscle. *J Physiol* 586:3701-3717.

Wilkinson, S.B., M.A. Tarnopolsky, M.J. MacDonald, J.R. Macdonald, D. Armstrong, and S. M. Phillips. 2007. Consumption of fluid skim milk promotes greater muscle protein accretion following resistance exercise than an isonitrogenous and isoenergetic soy protein beverage. *Am J Clin Nutr* 85:1031-1040.

Willett, W.C. 2000. Diet and cancer. *Oncologist* 5:393-404.

Williams, C., and J.T. Devlin. 1992. *Foods, Nutrition, and Sports Performance*. London: E & F Spon.

Williams, J.H., J.F. Signorile, W.F. Barnes, and T.W. Henrich. 1988. Caffeine, maximal power output and fatigue. *Br J Sports Med* 22 (4): 132-134.

Williams, M.H. 1993. Nutritional supplements for strength trained athletes. *Sports Sci Exch* 6 (6): 1-4.

Williams, M.H., R.B. Kreider, and J.D. Branch. 1999. *Creatine: The power supplement.* Champaign, IL: Human Kinetics.

Williams, M.H., R.B. Kreider, D.W. Hunter, et al. 1990. Effect of inosine supplementation on 3-mile treadmill run performance and $\dot{V}O_2$ peak. *Med Sci Sports Exerc* 22 (4): 517-522.

Wilmore, J.H., K.C. Wambsgans, M. Brenner, et al. 1992. Is there energy conservation in amenorrheic compared with eumenorrheic distance runners? *J Appl Physiol* 72 (1): 15-22.

Wilson, J.G., J.M. Wilson, and A.H. Manninen. 2008. Effects of beta-hydroxy-beta-methylbutyrate (HMB) on exercise performance and body composition across varying levels of age, sex, and training experience: A review. *Nutr Metab (Lond)* 5:1.

Winder, W.W., and D.G. Hardie. 1996. Inactivation of acetyl-CoA carboxylase and activation of AMP-activated protein kinase in muscle during exercise. *Am J Physiol* 270:E299-304.

Witard, O.C., S.R. Jackman, L. Breen, K. Smith, A. Selby, and K.D. Tipton. 2014. Myofibrillar muscle protein synthesis rates subsequent to a meal in response to increasing doses of whey protein at rest and after resistance exercise. *Am J Clin Nutr* 99:86-95.

Witard, O.C., J.E. Turner, S.R. Jackman, A.K. Kies, A.E. Jeukendrup, J.A. Bosch, and K.D. Tipton. 2013. High dietary protein restores overreaching induced impairments in leukocyte trafficking and reduces the incidence of upper respiratory tract infection in elite cyclists. *Brain Behav Immun* 39:211-219.

Wojtaszewski, J.F., C. MacDonald, J.N. Nielsen, Y. Hellsten, D.G. Hardie, B.E. Kemp, B. Kiens, and E.A. Richter. 2003. Regulation of 5′AMP-activated protein kinase activity and substrate utilization in exercising human skeletal muscle. *Am J Physiol Endocrinol Metab* 284:E813-E822.

Wolfe, R.R. 1992. *Radioactive and stable isotope tracers in biomedicine.* New York: Wiley-Liss.

Wolfe, R.R., S. Klein, F. Carraro, and J.-M. Weber. 1990. Role of triglyceride-fatty acid cycle in controlling fat metabolism in humans during and after exercise. *Am J Physiol* 258:E382-E389.

Wright, D.C., D.H. Han, P.M. Garcia-Roves, P.C. Geiger, T.E. Jones, J.O. Holloszy. 2007. Exercise-induced mitochondrial biogenesis begins before the increase in muscle PGC-1alpha expression. *J Biol Chem* 282:194-199.

Wurtman, R.J., and M.C. Lewis. 1991. Exercise, plasma composition and neurotransmission. *Med Sport Sci* 32:94-109.

Wylie, L.J., J. Kelly, S.J. Bailey, J.R. Blackwell, P.F. Skiba, P.G. Winyard, A.E. Jeukendrup, A. Vanhatalo, and A.M. Jones. 2013. Beetroot juice and exercise: Pharmacodynamic and dose-response relationships. *J Appl Physiol* 115 (3): 325-336.

Wylie, L.J., M. Mohr, P. Krustrup, S.R. Jackman, G. Ermιdis, J. Kelly, M.I. Black, S.J. Bailey, A. Vanhatalo, and A.M. Jones. 2013. Dietary nitrate supplementation improves team sport-specific intense intermittent exercise performance. *Eur J Appl Physiol* 113 (7): 1673-1684.

Wynne, K., S. Stanley, B. McGowann, and S. Bloom. 2005. Appetite control. *J Endocrinol* 184:291-318.

Wyss, M., and R. Kaddurah-Daouk. 2000. Creatine and creatinine metabolism. *Physiol Rev* 80 (3): 1107-1213.

Yang, Y., A. Creer, B. Jemiolo, and S. Trappe. 2005. Time course of myogenic and metabolic gene expression in response to acute exercise in human skeletal muscle. *J Appl Physiol* 98:1745-1752.

Yaspelkis, B.B., J.G. Patterson, P.A. Anderla, Z. Ding, and J.L. Ivy. 1993. Carbohydrate supplementation spares muscle glycogen during variable-intensity exercise. *J Appl Physiol* 75 (4): 1477-1485.

Yeo, S.E., R.L.P.G. Jentjens, G.A. Wallis, and A.E. Jeukendrup. 2005. Caffeine increases exogenous carbohydrate oxidation during exercise. *J Appl Physiol* 99:844-850.

Yeo, W.K., C.D. Paton, A.P. Garnham, L.M. Burke, A.L. Carey, and J.A. Hawley. 2008. Skeletal muscle adaptation and performance responses to once a day versus twice every second day endurance training regimens. *J Appl Physiol* 105:1462-1470.

Yfanti, C., Akerström, T., Nielsen, S., Nielsen, A.R., Mounier, R., Mortensen, O.H., Lykkesfeldt, J, Rose, A.J., Fischer, C.P., and Pedersen, B.K. 2010. Antioxidant supplementation does not alter endurance training adaptation. *Med Sci Sports Exerc* 42 (7): 1388-1395.

Zawadzki, K.M., B.B. Yaspelkis III, and J.L. Ivy. 1992. Carbohydrate-protein complex increases the rate of muscle glycogen storage after exercise. *J Appl Physiol* 72 (5): 1854-1859.

Zeisel, S.H. 1998. *Choline and phosphatidylcholine.* Washington, DC: ILSI Press.

Zeisel, S.H., K.A. Da Costa, P.D. Franklin, E.A. Alexander, J.T. Lamont, N.F. Sheard, and A. Beiser. 1991. Choline, an essential nutrient for humans [see comments]. *FASEB J* 5 (7): 2093-2098.

Zemel, M.B. 2004. Role of calcium and dairy products in energy partitioning and weight management. *Am J Clin Nutr* 79 (5): 907S-912S.

Zemel, M.B., J. Richards, S. Mathis, A. Milstead, L. Gebhardt, and E. Silva. 2005. Dairy augmentation of total and central fat loss in obese subjects. *Int J Obes (Lond)* 29 (4): 391-397.

Zemel, M.B., H. Shi, B. Greer, D. Dirienzo, and P.C. Zemel. 2000. Regulation of adiposity by dietary calcium. *FASEB J* 14 (9): 1132-1138.

Zenith International. 2013. Soft Drinks. www.zenithinternational.com/reports_data/market_reports/soft_drinks.

Zerba, E., T.E. Komorowski, and J.A. Faulkner. 1990. Free radical injury to skeletal muscles of young, adult, and old mice. *Am J Physiol* 258:C429-C435.

Ziegenfuss, T.N., J.M. Berardi, and L.M. Lowery. 2002. Effects of prohormone supplementation in humans: A review. *Can J Appl Physiol* 27 (6): 628-646.

Zinker, B.A., K. Britz, and G.A. Brooks. 1990. Effects of a 36-hour fast on human endurance and substrate utilization. *J Appl Physiol* 69 (5): 1849-1855.

Zoeller, R.F., J.R. Stout, J.A. O'Kroy, D.J. Torok, and M. Mielke. 2007. Effects of twenty-eight days of beta-alanine and creatine monohydrate supplementation on aerobic power, ventilatory and lactate thresholds, and time to exhaustion. *Amino Acids* 33 (3): 505-510.

Index

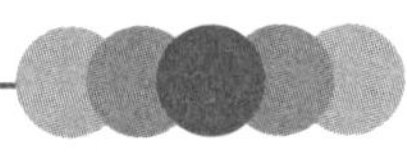

Note: The italicized *f* and *t* following page numbers refer to figures and tables, respectively.

F

W

Y

Z

About the Authors

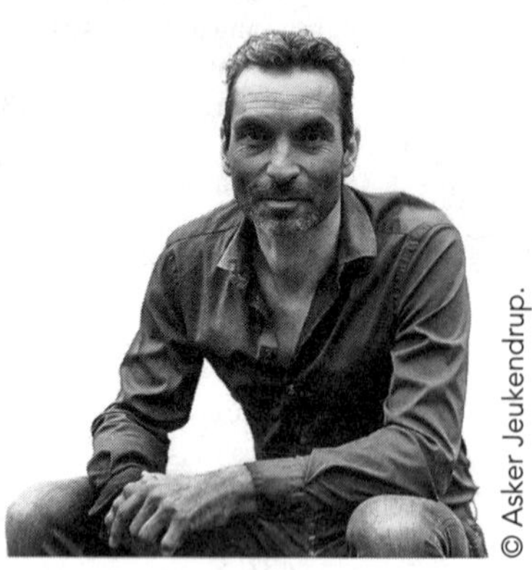
© Asker Jeukendrup.

Asker Jeukendrup, PhD, is a professor at Loughborough University in the UK, the director of mysportscience Ltd performance consulting, and cofounder and co-CEO of CORE Nutrition Planning. After obtaining his degrees at Maastricht University in the Netherlands, he spent a year at the University of Texas at Austin before accepting a position at the University of Birmingham UK. In Birmingham, he served for 12 years as the director of the Human Performance Laboratory, heading up the Exercise Metabolism Research Group. His research focused on the metabolic responses to exercise, the regulation of carbohydrate and fat metabolism during exercise, adaptations to training, and the influence of nutrition on metabolism and exercise nutrition. He is considered a leading expert in the general areas of sports nutrition, training and overtraining, and recovery.

Jeukendrup received several awards for his achievements including the Danone Chair at the University of Brussels in 2005. In 2011 he accepted a position as Global Senior Director of Exercise Physiology where he headed the Gatorade Sports Science Institute, defining strategies for research, education, and sport science services for the largest sports nutrition company in the world. He is a registered sport and exercise nutritionist, having worked with many elite athletes and clubs, including the Rabobank, Lotto-Soudal and Lotto Jumbo professional cycling teams, Chelsea Football Club, FC Barcelona, Red Bull Salzburg, UK Athletics, the British Olympic Association, African runners, and several Olympic and world champions. Currently Asker is Performance Manager Nutrition for the Dutch Olympic Committee and Head of Performance Nutrition for the Lotto Jumbo pro cycling team.

Jeukendrup has published extensively in sport nutrition. He is a fellow of the American College of Sports Medicine and the European College of Sport Sciences. In his leisure time, he enjoys running, cycling, and competing in triathlons. To date, he has completed 21 Ironman-distance races, including the Ironman Hawaii six times.

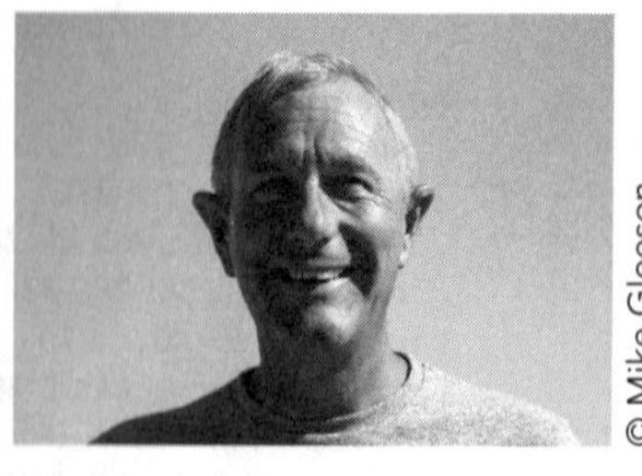
© Mike Gleeson.

Michael Gleeson, PhD, is a professor of exercise biochemistry in the School of Sport, Exercise and Health Sciences at Loughborough University in Loughborough, Leicestershire, UK. Gleeson is considered a world authority on exercise biochemistry, immunology, and nutrition, and has worked with numerous world-class athletes and professional football clubs. He has taught sport nutrition at the university level and has published several books and over 250 scientific articles in scientific and medical journals. He has a particular interest and expertise in the effects of exercise, training, and nutrition on immune function and has been both vice president and president of the International Society of Exercise and Immunology.

Gleeson is also a fellow of the European College of Sport Sciences and a member of the American College of Sports Medicine, the Physiological Society, and the British Association of Sport and Exercise Sciences. He enjoys playing tennis, hill walking, and watching football and films.